Varcarolis' FOUNDATIONS of PSYCHIATRIC-MENTAL HEALTH NURSING

A Clinical Approach

8 EDITION

MARGARET (PEGGY) JORDAN HALTER, PhD, APRN

Clinical Nurse Specialist
Cleveland Clinic Akron General
Akron, Ohio;
Adjunct Faculty
Ohio State University
Columbus, Ohio

ELSEVIER

ELSEVIER

3251 Riverport Lane
St. Louis, Missouri 63043

VARCAROLIS' FOUNDATIONS OF PSYCHIATRIC-MENTAL HEALTH NURSING: A CLINICAL APPROACH, EIGHTH EDITION ISBN: 978-0-323-38967-9

Notices

Knowledge and best practice in this field are constantly changing. As new research and experience broaden our understanding, changes in research methods, professional practices, or medical treatment may become necessary.

Practitioners and researchers must always rely on their own experience and knowledge in evaluating and using any information, methods, compounds, or experiments described herein. In using such information or methods, they should be mindful of their own safety and the safety of others, including parties for whom they have a professional responsibility.

With respect to any drug or pharmaceutical products identified, readers are advised to check the most current information provided (i) on procedures featured or (ii) by the manufacturer of each product to be administered, to verify the recommended dose or formula, the method and duration of administration, and contraindications. It is the responsibility of practitioners, relying on their own experience and knowledge of their patients, to make diagnoses, to determine dosages and the best treatment for each individual patient, and to take all appropriate safety precautions.

To the fullest extent of the law, neither the Publisher nor the authors, contributors, or editors assume any liability for any injury and/or damage to persons or property as a matter of products' liability, negligence or otherwise, or from any use or operation of any methods, products, instructions, or ideas contained in the material herein.

Library of Congress Cataloging-in-Publication Data

Names: Halter, Margaret J. (Margaret Jordan), editor.
Title: Varcarolis' foundations of psychiatric mental health nursing : a clinical approach / [edited by] Margaret Jordan Halter.
Other titles: Foundations of psychiatric mental health nursing
Description: Eighth edition. | St. Louis, Missouri : Elsevier, [2018] | Preceded by Varcarolis' foundations of psychiatric mental health nursing. 7th ed. / [edited by] Margaret Jordan Halter. c2014. | Includes bibliographical references and index.
Identifiers: LCCN 2017015075 | ISBN 9780323389679 (pbk. : alk. paper)
Subjects: | MESH: Mental Disorders--nursing | Psychiatric Nursing
Classification: LCC RC440 | NLM WY 160 | DDC 616.89/0231--dc23 LC record available at https://lccn.loc.gov/2017015075

Senior Content Strategist: Yvonne Alexopoulos
Content Development Manager: Lisa P. Newton
Publishing Services Manager: Jeff Patterson
Senior Project Manager: Tracey Schriefer
Design Direction: Paula Catalano

Printed in Canada

Last digit is the print number: 9 8 7 6 5 4 3 2 1

This book is dedicated to people who are living with and recovering from mental illness and to the future registered nurses who will focus on supporting their recovery.

My dream is that scientific understanding and advances will not only provide even better treatments, but will also prevent, and even cure, psychiatric disorders.

Dedicated to my husband, Paul.
Your kindness and love of life shine
through your daughters and granddaughters.

I miss you every day.

ACKNOWLEDGMENTS

My ancestors were storytellers. Boxes of diaries, articles, and books fill an unused closet and detail many of their moves and thoughts. The family tree includes a newspaper editor, a historian, a poet, and a nonfiction writer. One great aunt, Ella Chalfant, published a book titled *A Goodly Heritage* in 1955. Her book centered on inheritance laws in the 1800s and featured copies of wills demonstrating the disenfranchisement of women (e.g., a husband needed to will a wife her own clothing on his death). She was likely an early feminist.

As a registered nurse, I did have the opportunity to write some non-fiction in the form of nurses notes. As a tenure-track faculty member, I was required to write some stories in the form of presentations, research, and publications.

A 2004 phone call finally put me on the path to join my ancestors in their vocation. A pleasant voice with a slight New York accent says, "Peggy? Hi, this is Betsy Varcarolis." I knew the name at once—my undergraduates used her book. She went on, "The reason I'm calling is that I very much enjoyed your article, 'Stigma and help seeking related to depression: A study of nursing students.' I would like to feature it as an Evidence-Based Practice box in the fifth edition of my book." I was thrilled—what an honor!

This was the beginning. After that call, my work progressed from chapter reviewer to chapter writer to textbook editor. I spent several years as an apprentice of Elizabeth Varcarolis, the creative power who conceived of *Foundations of Psychiatric Mental Health Nursing* in 1990. She went on to make this textbook a leader in the specialty of psychiatric nursing. Betsy has the rare gift of making the complex understandable and of making impersonal learning a joint process in which the experts talk with the students rather than just providing information.

In this 8th edition of the book, Elizabeth Varcarolis continues to be honored for her work with her name in the title. Sincere thanks and gratitude go out to Betsy for enriching my life. The profession of psychiatric nursing, countless students, and recipients of psychiatric-mental health care have benefited from her wisdom. I wish for Betsy all the best as she enjoys her retirement hand-in-hand with her husband, Paul.

My heartfelt appreciation also goes out to the talented group of writers who contributed to the 8th edition. We have a talented pool of veteran writers, and their knowledge and passion continue to influence psychiatric nursing. A few new writers whose expertise was both recognized and sought after agreed to join us in this edition. It has truly been a joy working with each of you. Thanks for the countless hours you spent researching, writing, and rewriting!

A huge debt of gratitude goes to the many educators and clinicians who reviewed the manuscript and offered valuable suggestions, ideas, opinions, and criticisms. All comments were appreciated and helped refine and strengthen the individual chapters.

Throughout this project, a number of people at Elsevier provided superb support. I am grateful for Tracey Schriefer, our Senior Project Manager, who nudged me to meet deadlines, and Paula Catalano, a talented and creative designer. Yvonne Alexopoulos, Senior Content Strategist, kept me on a straight path and helped me work through some thorny issues. Lisa Newton, Content Development Manager, was my ever-optimistic colleague who celebrated each milestone with a smiley emoji and an exclamation mark! My sincere thanks go out to my whole Elsevier family.

Peggy Halter

CONTRIBUTOR LIST

Lois Angelo, APRN
Case Manager
Newton-Wellesley Hospital
Newton, Massachusetts

Natalie K. Boysen, BSN, RN
Genesis East Medical Center
Emergency Services
Davenport, Iowa

Leslie A. Briscoe, MSN, RN, PMHCNP
Psychiatric Nurse Practitioner
Louis Stokes Cleveland VA Medical Center
Geriatric Psychiatry: Outpatient and Consultation/Liaison Service
Cleveland, Ohio
Nursing Editorial Advisory Panel
Wolters Kluwer Publishing
Clinical Drug Information / Nursing division
Hudson, Ohio

Alison M. Colbert, PhD, APRN, BC
Assistant Professor
Duquesne University School of Nursing
Pittsburgh, Pennsylvania

Carissa Enright, MSN, RN, PMHNP BC
Associate Clinical Professor
Texas Woman's University
Dallas, Texas

Jill Espelin, DNP, PMHNP-BC, CNE, APRN
Assistant Professor
Central Connecticut State University
New Britain, Connecticut

Jodie A. Flynn, MSN, RN, SANE-A, SANE-P, D-ABMDI
Instructor
Capital University
Columbus, Ohio

Christina Fratena, MSN, PMHCNS-BC
Clinical Instructor of Nursing
Malone University
Canton, Ohio

Faye J. Grund, PhD, APRN, PMHNP-BC
Dean
Dwight Schar College of Nursing and Health Sciences
Ashland University
Mansfield, Ohio

Mary A. Gutierrez, PharmD, BCPP
Professor of Pharmacy Practice (Psychiatry)
Chapman University School of Pharmacy
Irvine, California

Monica J. Halter, APRN, PMHNP-BC
Psychiatric Nurse Practitioner
Psychological and Behavioral Consultants
Cleveland, Ohio

Edward A. Herzog, APRN-CNS
Senior Lecturer, College of Nursing
Kent State University
Kent, Ohio

Jerika T. Lam, PharmD, AAHIVP, FCSHP
Assistant Professor of Pharmacy Practice
Chapman University School of Pharmacy
Irvine, California

Laura G. Leahy, DrNP, APN, PMH-CNS/FNP, BC
Family Psychiatric Advanced Practice Nurse
APN Solutions, LLC
Sewell, New Jersey

Lorann Murphy, MSN, PsychBC
Clinical Nurse Specialist
Lutheran Hospital
Cleveland, Ohio

Cindy Parsons, DNP, PMHNP-BC, FAANP
Associate Professor of Nursing
University of Tampa
Tampa, Florida

Donna Rolin, PhD, APRN, PM-HCNS-BC, PMHNP-BC
Assistant Professor
Director of Family Psychiatric Mental Health Nurse Practitioner Graduate Program
University of Texas at Austin, School of Nursing
Austin, Texas

L. Kathleen Sekula, PhD, PMHCNS, FAAN
Professor
Coordinator: Forensic Graduate Programs
Duquesne University School of Nursing
Pittsburgh, Pennsylvania

Jane Stein-Parbury, RN, BSN, MEd, PhD, FRCNA
Adjunct Professor
University of Technology Sydney
Sydney, Australia

Christine Tackett, MSN RN
Associate Professor
Herzing University
Akron, Ohio

Christine Tebaldi, RN, MS, PMHNP-BC
Director, Clinical Business Development
McLean Hospital
Belmont, Massachusetts

Elizabeth M. Varcarolis, RN, MA
Professor Emeritus
Formerly Deputy Chairperson and Psychiatric Nursing Coordinator Department of Nursing
Borough of Manhattan Community College, Associate Fellow
Albert Ellis Institute for Rational Emotional Behavioral Therapy (REBT)
Former Major, Army Nurse Corps Reserve
New York, New York

Kathleen Wheeler, PhD, PMHNP-BC, APRN, FAAN
Professor
Fairfield University Egan School of Nursing
Fairfield, Connecticut

Kimberly M. Wolf, PhD, MS, PM-HCNS-BC
Hennepin County Medical Center Inpatient Provider
Minneapolis, Minnesota
Associated Clinic of Psychology Outpatient Provider
Minneapolis, Minnesota
University of North Dakota PMHNP Program Director
Grand Forks, North Dakota
Duquesne University Adjunct Faculty
Pittsburgh, Pennsylvania

Sandy Snelson Yaklin, MSN, APRN, PMHNP-BC, CNE, CHPN
Bluebonnet Trails Community Service
Round Rock, Texas

Rick Zoucha, PhD, PMHCNS-BC, CTN-A, FAAN
Joseph A. Lauritis, C.S.Sp. Endowed Chair for Teaching and Technology
Professor and Chair of Advanced Role and PhD Programs
Duquesne University
Pittsburgh, Pennsylvania

ANCILLARY WRITERS

Teresa S. Burckhalter, MSN, RN, BC
Adjunct Faculty
University of South Carolina Beaufort
Beaufort, South Carolina
Test Bank

BJ Garrett, MSN, NE, RN
Associate Professor
Austin Community College
Austin, Texas
Chapter Review Questions

Linda Turchin, RN, MSN, CNE
Associate Professor of Nursing
Fairmont State University
Fairmont, West Virginia
Case Studies and Nursing Care Plans
Chapter Review Questions
Pre/Posttests
Student Review Questions

Linda Wendling, MS, MFA
Learning Theory Consultant
University of Missouri–St. Louis
St. Louis, Missouri
TEACH for Nurses and PowerPoints

REVIEWERS

Nancy Bryan, RN, MSN
Nurse Educator
Roseman University of Health Sciences
College of Nursing
Henderson, Nevada

Lori J. Cline, RN, MNSc
Lecturer, Clinical Instructor, and Group Therapist
College of Nursing – University of Central Arkansas and University of Arkansas at Little Rock
Group Therapy – Little Rock Community Mental Health Center
Little Rock, Arkansas

Leslie A. Folds, EdD, PMHCNS-BC, CNE
Associate Professor of Nursing
Belmont University
Nursing Department
Nashville, Tennessee

Susan Justice, MSN, RN, CNS
Assistant Clinical Professor, Lead Faculty
UT Arlington College of Nursing
Arlington, Texas

Chris Paxos, PharmD, BCPP, BCPS, CGP
Associate Professor, Pharmacy Practice
Assistant Professor, Psychiatry
Northeast Ohio Medical University
Pharmacotherapy Specialist, Psychiatry
Cleveland Clinic Akron General
Rootstown, Ohio

Victoria Plagenz, RN, BSN, MS, PhD
Assistant Professor
University of Great Falls
Nursing
Great Falls, Montana

Jeffrey A. Robbins, RN, BSN, MBA
Clinical Nursing Instructor, Psychiatric Nursing
UTA College of Nursing
Arlington, Texas

TO THE INSTRUCTOR

We are living in an age of fast-paced discoveries in neurobiology, genetics, and psychopharmacology. Researchers continue to seek the most effective evidence-based approaches for patients and their families. Legal issues and ethical dilemmas faced by the health care system are magnified accordingly. Given these challenges, keeping up and knowing how best to teach our students and serve our patients can seem overwhelming. With contributions from many knowledgeable and experienced nurse educators, our goal is to bring to you the most current and comprehensive trends and evidence-based practices in psychiatric-mental health nursing.

CONTENT NEW TO THIS EDITION

The following changes reflect contemporary nursing practice and psychiatric-mental health care and are considered in detail in this 8th edition:

- Full *Diagnostic and Statistical Manual of Mental Disorders,* 5th edition *(DSM-5)* diagnostic criteria are provided for major disorders within the clinical chapters.
- Genetic underpinnings of psychiatric disorders and genetic implications for testing and treatment choices are emphasized.
- Chapter 30 reintroduces completely updated dying, death, and grieving concepts and nursing care.
- The five chapter review questions included in previous editions of *Foundations* have been doubled to ten.
- The latest U.S. Food and Drug Administration approved medications are featured in all clinical chapters.
- Screenings and severity rating scales are introduced in Chapter 1 and included throughout most clinical chapters that provide quantifiable data to supplement categorical criteria.
- The *Manual of Psychiatric Nursing Care Planning* has been updated and realigned to more closely match this edition of *Foundations.* These revisions increase continuity between academic learning and clinical support.

Refer to the *To the Student* section of this introduction on page xii for examples of thoroughly updated **familiar features with a fresh perspective,** including Evidence-Based Practice boxes, Considering Culture boxes, Health Policy boxes, Key Points to Remember, Assessment Guidelines, Vignettes, and other features.

ORGANIZATION OF THE TEXT

Chapters are grouped in units to emphasize the clinical perspective and facilitate location of information. The order of the clinical chapters approximates those found in the *DSM-5.* All clinical chapters are organized in a clear, logical, and consistent format with the nursing process as the strong, visible framework. The basic outline for clinical chapters is:

- **Introduction:** Provides a brief overview of the disorder and identifies disorders that fall under the umbrella of the general chapter name.
- **Epidemiology:** Helps the student understand the extent of the problem and characteristics of those who may be more likely to be affected. This section includes information such as 12-month prevalence, lifetime prevalence, age of onset, and gender differences.
- **Comorbidity:** Describes the most common conditions that are associated with the psychiatric disorder. Knowing that comorbid disorders are often part of the clinical picture of specific disorders helps students as well as clinicians understand how to better assess and care for their patients.
- **Risk Factors:** Provides current views of causation. This section is being updated to increasingly focus on genetic and neurobiological factors in the etiology of psychiatric diagnoses.
- **Clinical Picture:** This section presents an overview of the disorder(s), *DSM-5* criteria for many of the disorders, and strong source material.
- **Assessment:**
  - **General Assessment:** Identifies assessment for specific disorders, including assessment tools and rating scales. The rating scales included help to highlight important areas in the assessment of a variety of behaviors or mental conditions.
  - **Self-Assessment:** Discusses the nurse's thoughts and feelings that should be addressed to enhance self-growth and provide the best possible and most appropriate care to the patient.
  - **Assessment Guidelines:** Provides a summary of specific areas to assess by disorder.
- **Diagnosis:** NANDA-I–approved nursing diagnoses are used in all nursing process sections. Some critical issues in psychiatric-mental health nursing are best addressed by essential non-NANDA-I diagnoses such as *disturbed thought processes* and *nonadherence.*
- **Outcomes Identification:** *Nursing Outcomes Classification (NOC)* provides a link to the NANDA-I diagnoses. They are introduced in Chapter 1 and used throughout the text when appropriate.
- **Planning:** Students are encouraged to develop patient-centered priorities in conjunction with patients, families, and others.
- **Implementation:** Interventions follow the standards set forth in the *Psychiatric-Mental Health Nursing: Scope and Standards of Practice* (2014). This publication was developed collaboratively by the American Nurses Association, the American Psychiatric Nurses Association, and the International Society of Psychiatric-Mental Health Nurses. These standards are incorporated throughout the chapters.

Nursing Intervention Classifications (NIC) (2013) also provides direction for interventions.

- **Evaluation:** Evaluation of nursing care is addressed as essential in order to support current planning and intervening. Evaluation also provides direction in modifying the plan of care and updating priorities.

TEACHING AND LEARNING RESOURCES

For Instructors

Instructor Resources on Evolve, available at http://evolve.elsevier.com/Varcarolis, provide a wealth of material to help you make your psychiatric nursing instruction a success. In addition to all of the Student Resources, the following are provided for faculty:

- **TEACH for Nurses Lesson Plans**, based on textbook chapter Learning Objectives, serve as ready-made, modifiable lesson plans and a complete roadmap to link all parts of the educational package. These concise and straightforward lesson plans can be modified or combined to meet your particular scheduling and teaching needs.
- **PowerPoint Presentations** are organized by chapter with approximately 750 slides for in-class lectures. These are detailed and include customizable text and image lecture slides to enhance learning in the classroom or in web-based course modules. If you share them with students, they can use the note feature to help them with your lectures.
- **Audience Response Questions for i> clicker and other systems** are provided with two to five multiple-answer questions per chapter to stimulate class discussion and assess student understanding of key concepts.
- The **Test Bank** has more than 1800 test items, complete with the correct answer, rationale, cognitive level of each question, corresponding step of the nursing process, appropriate NCLEX Client Needs label, and text page reference(s).
- A ***DSM-5* Webinar** explaining the changes in structure and disorders from the DSM-IV-TR is available for reference.

For Students

Student Resources on Evolve, available at http://evolve.elsevier.com/Varcarolis, provide a variety of valuable learning resources. The Evolve Resources page near the front of the book gives login instructions and a description of each resource.

- **Animations** of the neurobiology of select psychiatric disorders and medications make complex concepts come to life with multidimensional views. You can find these illustrations in the textbook with the icon next to them.
- The **Answer Keys to Critical Thinking Guidelines** provide possible outcomes for the Critical Thinking questions at the end of each chapter.
- **Case Studies and Nursing Care Plans** provide detailed case studies and care plans for specific psychiatric disorders to supplement those found in the textbook.
- **Glossary** provides an alphabetical list of nursing terms with accompanying definitions.
- **NCLEX® Review Questions,** provided for each chapter, will help you prepare for course examinations and for your RN licensure examination.
- **Pretests and Posttests** provide interactive self-assessments for each chapter of the textbook, including instant scoring and feedback at the click of a button.

We are grateful to educators who send suggestions and provide feedback and strive to incorporate these ideas from this huge pool of experts into reprints and revisions of *Foundations*. We hope that this 8th edition continues to help students learn and appreciate the scope and practice of psychiatric-mental health nursing.

Peggy Halter

TO THE STUDENT

Psychiatric-mental health nursing challenges us to understand the complexities of the brain and human behavior. We focus on the origin of psychiatric disorders, including biological determinants along with environmental factors. In the chapters that follow, you will learn about people who experience psychiatric disorders and how to provide them with quality nursing care in any setting. As you read, keep in mind these special features.

READING AND REVIEW TOOLS

Objectives and Key Terms and Concepts introduce the chapter topics and provide a concise overview of the material discussed.

Key Points to Remember listed at the end of each chapter reinforce essential information.

Critical Thinking activities at the end of each chapter are scenario-based critical thinking problems for practice in applying what you have learned. **Answer Guidelines** can be found on the Evolve website.

Ten multiple-choice **Chapter Review** questions at the end of each chapter help you review the chapter material and study for exams. **Answers** are conveniently provided following the questions. **Answers** along with **rationales** and textbook **page references** are located on the Evolve website.

ADDITIONAL LEARNING RESOURCES

Your **Evolve Resources** at http://evolve.elsevier.com/Varcarolis offer more helpful study aids, such as additional Case Studies and Nursing Care Plans.

CHAPTER FEATURES

Vignettes are short stories that describe the unique circumstances surrounding individual patients with psychiatric disorders.

Self-Assessment sections explore thoughts and feelings you may experience working with patients who have psychiatric disorders. These thoughts and feelings may need to be addressed to enhance self-growth and provide the best possible and most appropriate care to the patient.

Assessment Guidelines in the clinical chapters provide summary points for patient assessment.

Evidence-Based Practice boxes demonstrate how current research findings affect psychiatric-mental health nursing practice and standards of care.

Guidelines for Communication boxes provide tips for communicating therapeutically with patients and their families.

Considering Culture boxes reinforce the importance of providing culturally competent care.

FDA-Approved Drug tables present the latest information on medications used to treat psychiatric disorders.

Patient and Family Teaching boxes underscore the nurse's role in helping patients and families understand psychiatric disorders, treatments, complications, and medication side effects, among other important issues.

Case Studies and Nursing Care Plans present individualized histories of patients with specific psychiatric disorders following the steps of the nursing process. Interventions with rationales and evaluation statements are presented for each patient goal.

CONTENTS

UNIT I Foundations in Theory

UNIT II Foundations for Practice

UNIT IV Psychobiological Disorders

UNIT V Trauma Interventions

UNIT VI Interventions for Special Populations

1

Mental Health and Mental Illness

Margaret Jordan Halter

Visit the Evolve website for a pretest on the content in this chapter: http://evolve.elsevier.com/Varcarolis Pre-Test interactive review

OBJECTIVES

1. Describe the continuum of mental health and mental illness.
2. Explore the role of resilience in the prevention of and recovery from mental illness and consider resilience in response to stress.
3. Identify how culture influences the view of mental illnesses and behaviors associated with them.
4. Discuss the nature/nurture origins of psychiatric disorders.
5. Summarize the social influences of mental healthcare in the United States.
6. Explain how epidemiological studies can improve medical and nursing care.
7. Identify how the *Diagnostic and Statistical Manual, Fifth Edition (DSM-5)* is used for diagnosing psychiatric conditions.
8. Describe the specialty of psychiatric-mental health nursing.
9. Compare and contrast a *DSM-5* medical diagnosis with a nursing diagnosis.
10. Discuss future challenges and opportunities for mental healthcare in the United States.
11. Describe direct and indirect advocacy opportunities for psychiatric-mental health nurses.

OUTLINE

KEY TERMS AND CONCEPTS

basic level registered nurse
clinical epidemiology
comorbid condition
cultural competence
Diagnostic and Statistical Manual of Mental Disorders, Fifth Edition (DSM-5)
diathesis-stress model
electronic healthcare
epidemiology
incidence
mental health
mental health continuum
mental illness
Nursing Interventions Classification (NIC)
Nursing Outcomes Classification (NOC)
phenomena of concern
prevalence
psychiatric-mental health registered nurse (PMH-RN)
psychiatric-mental health advanced practice registered nurse (PMH-APRN)
psychiatric-mental health nursing
recovery
resilience
stigma

If you are a fan of vintage films, you may have witnessed a scene similar to this: A doctor, wearing a lab coat, carrying a clipboard, and displaying an expression of deep concern, enters a hospital waiting room. He approaches an obviously distraught gentleman seated there. The doctor says, "I'm afraid your wife has suffered a nervous breakdown."

From that point on in the film, the woman's condition is only vaguely hinted at. The husband dutifully drives through the asylum gates and enters the stately building. Sounds of sobbing or shrieking patients are heard. Patients are rocking on the floor or shuffling down the hall.

As he nears his wife's room, the staff regard him with sad expressions and keep a polite distance. He may find his wife lying in her bed motionless, standing by the window and staring vacantly into the distance, or sitting among other non-interacting patients in the hospital's garden. The viewer can only speculate about the true nature of the woman's illness.

MENTAL HEALTH AND MENTAL ILLNESS

We have come a long way in acknowledging and addressing mental illness since the days of nervous breakdowns. In your psychiatric-mental health nursing course, you will learn about psychiatric disorders, associated nursing care, and treatments. As a foundation for this learning, we will begin by exploring what it means to be mentally healthy.

First, overall health is not possible without good mental health. The World Health Organization (WHO, 2014) describes health as "a state of complete physical, mental, and social well-being and not merely the absence of disease or infirmity." There is a strong relationship between physical health and mental health: Poor physical health can lead to mental distress and disorders, and poor mental health can lead to physical problems.

What does it mean to be mentally healthy? The WHO, again, provides us with a useful definition. **Mental health** is a state of well-being in which each individual is able to realize his or her own potential, cope with the normal stresses of life, work productively, and make a contribution to the community. Mental health provides people with the capacity for rational thinking, communication skills, learning, emotional growth, resilience, and self-esteem. Some of the attributes of mentally healthy people are shown in Fig. 1.1.

Society's definition of mental illness evolves over time. It is a definition shaped by the prevailing culture and societal values, and it reflects changes in cultural norms, social expectations, political climates, and even reimbursement criteria by third-party payers.

In the past, the term *mental illness* was applied to behaviors considered "strange" and "different"—behaviors that occurred infrequently and deviated from an established norm. Such criteria are inadequate because they suggest that mental health is based on conformity. Applying that definition to nonconformists and independent thinkers such as Abraham Lincoln, Mahatma Gandhi, and Florence Nightingale might result in a judgment of mental illness. Although the sacrifices of a Mother Teresa or the dedication of Martin Luther King Jr. are uncommon, virtually none of us would consider these much-admired behaviors to be signs of mental illness.

Mental illness refers to all psychiatric disorders that have definable diagnoses. These disorders are manifested in significant dysfunctions that may be related to developmental, biological, or psychological disturbances in mental functioning. The ability to think may be impaired—as in Alzheimer's disease. Emotions may be affected—as in major depression. Behavioral alterations may be apparent—as in schizophrenia. Or the patient may display some combination of the three alterations.

Mental illness is such a common problem that most of us know someone with a disorder. You may even have one yourself. According to the US Department Health and Human Services (HHS), in 2014:

- One in five American adults experienced a mental health issue.
- One in ten young people experienced a period of major depression.
- One in twenty-five Americans lived with a serious mental illness such as schizophrenia, bipolar disorder, or major depression.
- Suicide was the 10th leading cause of death in the United States.

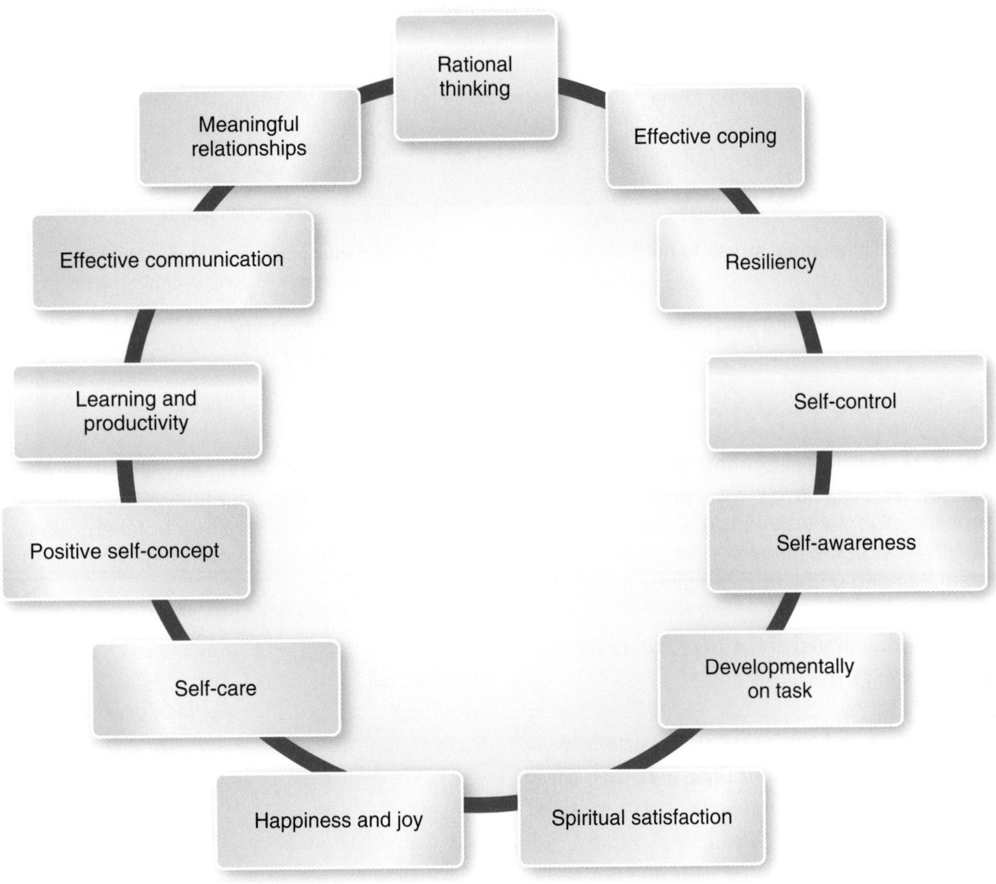

FIG. 1.1 Some attributes of mental health.

MENTAL HEALTH CONTINUUM

You may wonder if there is some middle ground between mental health and mental illness. After all, it is a rare person who does not have doubts as to his or her sanity at one time or another. The answer is that there is definitely a middle ground. In fact, mental health and mental illness can be conceptualized as points along a **mental health continuum** (Fig. 1.2).

On one end of the continuum is mental health. Well-being describes the general condition of people in this category. Well-being is characterized by adequate to high-level functioning. While individuals at this end of the continuum may experience stress and discomfort resulting from problems of everyday life, they experience no serious impairments in daily functioning.

For example, you may spend a day or two in a gray cloud of self-doubt and recrimination over a failed exam, a sleepless night filled with worry about trivial concerns, or months of genuine sadness and mourning after the death of a loved one. During those low times, you are fully or vaguely aware that you are not functioning well. However, time, exercise, a balanced diet, rest, interaction with others, and mental reframing may alleviate these problems or concerns.

At the opposite end of the continuum is mental illness. Individuals may have emotional problems or concerns and experience mild to moderate discomfort and distress. Mild impairment in functioning such as insomnia, lack of concentration, or loss of appetite may be felt. If the distress increases or persists, individuals might seek professional help. Problems in this category tend to be temporary, but individuals with mild depression, generalized anxiety disorder, and attention-deficit disorder may fit into this group.

The most severely affected individuals fall into the mental illness portion of the continuum. At this point, individuals experience altered thinking, mood, and behavior. It may include relatively common disorders such as depression and anxiety, as well as major disorders such as schizophrenia. The distinguishing factor in mental illness is typically chronic or long-term impairments that range from moderate to disabling.

All of us fall somewhere on the mental health–mental illness continuum and shift gradually or suddenly. Many people will never move into the mental illness stage. On the other hand, many people who do reach a more severe level of impairment can experience recovery that ranges from a glimmer of hope to leading a satisfying life.

People who have experienced mental illness can testify to the existence of changes in functioning. The following comments of a 40-year-old woman illustrate the continuum between illness

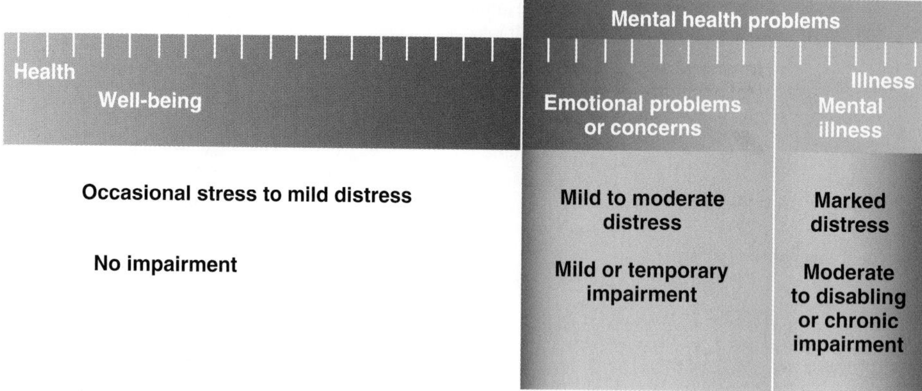

FIG. 1.2 Mental health-mental well-being continuum. (From University of Michigan, "Understanding U." [2007]. *What is mental health?* Retrieved from https://hr.umich.edu/benefits-wellness/health/mhealthy/mental-emotional-well-being/understanding-mental-emotional-health/mental-emotional-health-classes-training-events/online-tutorial-supervisors/section-1-what-you-need-know-about-mental-health-problems-substance-misuse).

and health as her condition ranged from deep depression to mania to well-being (recovery):

Depression *It was horror and hell. I was at the bottom of the deepest and darkest pit there ever was. I was worthless and unforgivable. I was as good as—no, worse than—dead.*

Mania *I was incredibly alive. I could sense and feel everything. I was sure I could do anything, accomplish any task, and create whatever I wanted if only other people wouldn't get in my way.*

Well-being (Recovery) *I am much calmer. I realize now that, when I was manic, it was a pressure-cooker feeling. When I am happy now, or loving, it is more peaceful and real. I have to admit that I sometimes miss the intensity—the sense of power and creativity—of those manic times. I never miss anything about the depressed times, but of course the power and the creativity never bore fruit. Now I do get things done, some of the time, like most people. And people treat me much better now. I guess I must seem more real to them. I certainly seem more real to me (Altrocchi, 1980).*

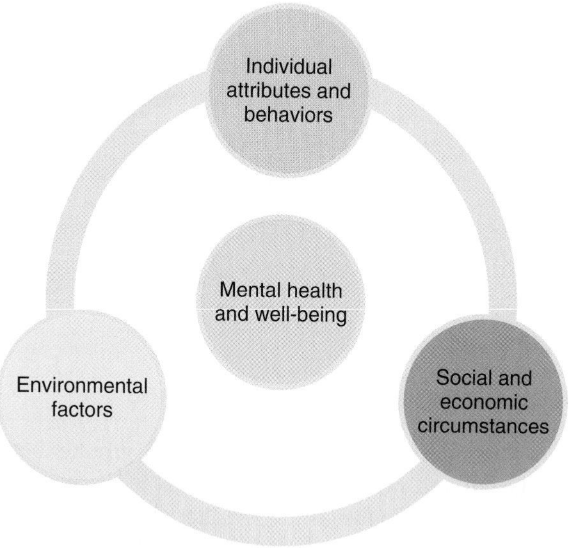

Individual attributes and behaviors

Mental health and well-being

Environmental factors

Social and economic circumstances

FIG. 1.3 Contributing factors to mental health and well-being. From World Health Organization. (2012). *Risks to mental health: An overview of vulnerabilities and risk factors.* Retrieved from http://www.who.int/mental_health/mhgap/risks_to_mental_health_EN_27_08_12.pdf

RISK AND PROTECTIVE FACTORS

Many factors can affect the severity and progression of a mental illness, as well as the mental health of a person who does not have a mental illness. Individual characteristics and attributes influence mental health and well-being (WHO, 2012). Socioeconomic circumstances and the environment also influence mental health (Fig. 1.3).

Individual Attributes and Behaviors

Individual attributes refer to characteristics that are both inborn and learned that make us who we are. We all have unique ways of managing thoughts and feelings and navigating the everyday pressures of life. The ability to respond to social cues and participate in social activities influences our view of ourselves and how others view us.

Biological and genetic factors can also influence mental health. Prenatal exposure to alcohol and oxygen deprivation at birth are two examples of biological factors. Genetic factors are huge predictors of mental health and are implicated in nearly every psychiatric disorder.

What makes some people adapt to tragedy, loss, trauma, and severe stress better than others? The answer may be the individual attribute of resilience. **Resilience** is the ability and capacity for people to secure the resources they need to support their well-being. It

BOX 1.1 The Resilience Factor Test

Use the following scale to rate each item listed below:
1 = Not true of me
2 = Sometimes true
3 = Moderately true
4 = Usually true
5 = Very true

1. Even if I plan ahead for a discussion with my spouse, my boss, or my child, I still find myself acting emotionally.
2. I am unable to harness positive emotions to help me focus on a task.
3. I can control the way I feel when adversity strikes.
4. I get carried away by my feelings.
5. I am good at identifying what I am thinking and how it affects my mood.
6. If someone does something that upsets me, I am able to wait until an appropriate time when I have calmed down to discuss it.
7. My emotions affect my ability to focus on what I need to get done at home, school, or work.
8. When I discuss a hot topic with a colleague or family member, I am able to keep my emotions in check.

Add Your Score on the Following Items:	Add Your Score on the Following Items:
3 _____	1 _____
5 _____	2 _____
6 _____	4 _____
8 _____	7 _____
Positive total = _____	Negative total = _____

Positive total minus negative total = _____

A score higher than 13 is rated as above average in emotional regulation.
A score between 6 and 13 is inconclusive.
A score lower than 6 is rated as below average in emotional regulation.

If your emotional regulation is below average, you may need to master some calming skills. Here are a few tips:

- When anxiety strikes, your breathing may become shallow and quick. You can help control the anxiety by controlling your breathing. Inhale slowly through your nose, breathing deeply from your belly, not your chest.
- Stress will make your body tight and stiff. Again, you can counter the effects of stress on the body and brain if you relax your muscles.
- Try positive imagery; create an image that is relaxing such as visualizing yourself on a secluded beach.
- Resilience is within your reach.

From Reivich, K., & Shatte, A. (2002). *The resilience factor: 7 essential skills for overcoming life's obstacles.* New York, NY: Broadway Books.

is a quality found in some children of poverty and abuse who seek out trusted adults. These adults provide them with the psychological and physical resources that allow them to excel.

Being resilient does not mean being unaffected by stressors. People who are resilient are effective at regulating their emotions and not falling victim to negative, self-defeating thoughts. You can get an idea of how good you are at regulating your emotions by taking the Resilience Factor Test in Box 1.1.

Social and Economic Circumstances

Your immediate social surroundings impact personal attributes. The earliest social group, the family, has tremendous effects on developing and vulnerable humans. The family sets the stage in promoting confidence and coping skills or for instilling anxiety and feelings of inadequacy.

The social environment extends to schools and peer groups. Again, this environment has the ability to affect mental health positively and negatively. For example, socioeconomic status dictates the sort of resources available to support mental health and reduce concerns over basic needs such as food, clothing, and shelter. Educational advancement is a tremendous supporter of mental health by providing opportunities for a satisfying career, security, and economic benefits.

Environmental Factors

The overall environment that affects mental health relates to the political climate and cultural considerations. Access and lack of access to basic needs and commodities such as healthcare, water, safety services, and a strong highway system have a profound effect on community mental health. Social and economic policies, which are formed at the global, national, state, and local government levels, also impact mental health. For example, in the United States, laws have been gradually shifting toward better reimbursement for mental health services. This shift makes it easier to access and improve mental healthcare.

Predominant cultural beliefs, attitudes, and practices influence mental health. There is no standard measure for mental health, partly because it is culturally defined. One approach to differentiating mental health from mental illness is to consider what a particular culture regards as acceptable or unacceptable. In this view, those with mental illness are those who violate social norms and thus threaten (or make anxious) those observing them. For example, traditional Japanese culture may consider suicide to be an act of honor, and Middle Eastern "suicide bombers" are considered holy warriors or martyrs. Contrast these viewpoints with Western culture where people who attempt or complete suicides are nearly always considered mentally ill.

Throughout history, people have interpreted health or sickness according to their own current views. A striking example of how cultural change influences the interpretation of mental illness is an old definition of *hysteria*. According to *Webster's Dictionary* (Porter, 1913), hysteria was:

> *A nervous affection…in women, in which the emotional and reflex excitability is exaggerated, and the will power correspondingly diminished, so that the patient loses control over the emotions, becomes the victim of imaginary sensations, and often falls into paroxysm or fits.*

Treatment for this condition, thought to be the result of sexual deprivation, often involved sexual activity. Thankfully, this diagnosis fell into disuse as women's rights improved, the family atmosphere became less restrictive, and societal tolerance of sexual practices increased.

Cultures differ not only in their views regarding mental illness but also the types of behavior categorized as mental illness. Culture-bound syndromes seem to occur in specific sociocultural contexts, and people in those cultures easily recognized them. For example, one syndrome recognized in parts of Southeast Asia is running amok, in which a person (usually a male) runs around engaging in almost indiscriminate violent behavior. In the United States, anorexia nervosa is recognized as a disorder characterized by voluntary starvation. The disorder is well known in Europe, North America, and Australia but unheard of in many other parts of the world.

Perceptions of Mental Health and Mental Illness

Mental Illness Versus Physical Illness

People often make a distinction between mental illnesses and physical illnesses. This is a peculiar distinction. *Mental* refers to the brain, the most complex part of the body, responsible for the higher thought processes that set us apart from all other creatures. Surely the workings of the brain—the synaptic connections, the areas of functioning, the spinal innervations and connections—are *physical*.

One problem with this distinction is that it implies that psychiatric disorders are "all in the head." Most damaging is the belief that these disorders are under personal control and indistinguishable from a choice to engage in bad behavior. These beliefs support the **stigma** to which people with mental illness are often subjected. Stigma, the belief that the overall person is flawed, is characterized by social shunning, disgrace, and shame.

Perhaps the difference between mental and physical illness lies in the tradition of explaining the unexplainable through superstition. Consider that the frightening convulsions of epilepsy were once explained as demon possession or a curse. Unfortunate individuals with epilepsy were subjected to horrible treatment including shunning, imprisonment, and exorcisms. Today, people recognize that seizures are part of a disorder and not under personal control. How do we know? Because we can *see* epilepsy on brain scans as areas of overactivity and excitability.

There are no specific biological tests to diagnose most psychiatric disorders—no cranium culture for depression and no magnetic resonance imaging (MRI) for obsessive-compulsive disorder (OCD). However, researchers are convinced that the root of most mental disorders lies in intercellular abnormalities. We can now see clear signs of altered brain function in several mental disorders including schizophrenia, OCD, stress disorders, and depression.

Nature Versus Nurture

For centuries, people believed that extremely unusual behaviors resulted from supernatural (usually evil) forces. In the late 1800s, the mental health pendulum swung briefly to a biological focus with the "germ theory of diseases." Germ theory explained mental illness in the same way other illnesses were being described—that is, a specific agent in the environment caused them. This theory was abandoned rather quickly because clinicians and researchers could not identify causative factors for mental illnesses. There was no "mania germ" that could be viewed under a microscope and subsequently treated.

Although biological treatments for mental illness continued to be explored, psychological theories dominated and focused on the science of the mind and behavior. These theories explained the origin of mental illness as faulty psychological processes that could be corrected by increasing personal insight and understanding. For example, a patient experiencing depression and apathy could be assisted to explore feelings from childhood when overly protective parents strictly discouraged attempts at independence.

This psychological focus was challenged in 1952 when chlorpromazine (Thorazine) was found to have a calming effect on agitated, out-of-control patients. Imagine what this discovery must have been like for clinicians. Out of desperation they had resorted to every biological treatment imaginable including wet wraps, insulin shock therapy, and psychosurgery (in which holes were drilled in the head of a patient and probes inserted into the brain) as attempts to change behavior. The scientific community began to believe that if psychiatric problems respond to medications that alter neurochemistry, then a disruption of intercellular components must already be present.

A **diathesis-stress model**—in which diathesis represents biological predisposition and stress represents environmental stress or trauma—is the most accepted explanation for mental illness. This nature-*plus*-nurture argument asserts that most psychiatric disorders result from a combination of genetic vulnerability and negative environmental stressors. One person may develop major depression largely as the result of an inherited and biological vulnerability that alters brain chemistry. Another person with little vulnerability may develop depression as a result of a stressful environment that causes changes in brain chemistry.

Social Influences on Mental Healthcare

Consumer Movement and Mental Health Recovery

Over 100 years ago, tremendous energy was directed toward improving equality in the United States. Black men were given the right to vote in 1870 as were women, finally, in 1920. Treating people fairly and challenging labels became a focus of the American culture.

With regard to treatment of people with mental illness, decades of institutionalization had created significant political and social concerns. Groups of people with mental illnesses—frequently called mental health consumers—began to advocate for their rights and fought against discrimination and forced treatment.

In 1979 people with mental illnesses and their families formed a nationwide advocacy group, the National Alliance on Mental Illness (NAMI). In the 1980s, individuals in the consumer movement organized by NAMI began to resist the traditional arrangement of mental healthcare providers dictating treatment without the input of the patient. This paternalistic relationship was demoralizing, and it also implied that patients were not competent to make their own decisions. Consumers demanded increased involvement in decisions concerning their treatment.

The consumer movement also promoted the concept of **recovery**, a new and an old idea. On one hand, it represents a concept that has been around a long time: that some people—even those with the most serious illnesses such as schizophrenia—recover. One recovery was depicted in the movie *A Beautiful Mind*. In this film, a brilliant mathematician, John Nash, seems to have emerged from a continuous cycle of devastating psychotic relapses to a state of stabilization and recovery (Howard, 2001).

A newer conceptualization of recovery evolved into a consumer-focused process. According to the Substance Abuse and Mental Health Services Administration (SAMHSA, 2012), recovery is "a process of change through which individuals improve their health and wellness, live a self-directed life, and strive to reach their full potential." The focus is on the consumer and what he or she can do. A real-life example of recovery follows:

VIGNETTE: Jeff began hearing voices when he was 19 and was diagnosed with schizophrenia the same year. He dropped out of college, lost his part-time job at a factory, and began collecting Social Security Disability Income. For 20 years, Jeff was told what medication to take, where to live, and what to do.

At the community health center where he received services, he met a fellow patient, Linda, who was involved with a recovery support group. She gave him a pamphlet with a list of the 10 guiding principles of recovery:

1. **Recovery emerges from hope:** Recovery provides the essential motivating message of a better future: That people can and do overcome the barriers and obstacles that confront them. Hope is the catalyst of the recovery process.
2. **Recovery is person driven:** Self-determination and self-direction are the foundations for recovery. Consumers lead, control, exercise choice over, and determine their own path of recovery.
3. **Recovery occurs through many pathways:** Individuals are unique with distinct needs, strengths, preferences, goals, culture, and background (including past trauma) that affect their pathways to recovery. Recovery is nonlinear and may involve setbacks. Abstinence from the use of alcohol, nonprescribed medications, and tobacco is essential. A supportive environment is essential, especially for children.
4. **Recovery is holistic:** Recovery encompasses an individual's whole life including mind, body, spirit, and community.
5. **Recovery is supported by peers and allies:** Mutual support and aid groups play an invaluable role in recovery. Peers improve social learning, provide experiential knowledge and skills, and a sense of belonging. Helping others helps one's self.
6. **Recovery is supported through relationships and social networks:** The presence and involvement of people who believe in the personal's ability to recover; who offer hope, support, and encouragement; and who suggest strategies and resources for change are important.
7. **Recovery is culturally based and influenced:** Culture and cultural background are keys in determining a person's journey and unique pathway to recovery. Services should be culturally grounded, attuned, sensitive, congruent, and competent, as well as personalized to meet unique needs.
8. **Recovery is supported by addressing trauma:** Trauma (e.g., physical or sexual abuse, domestic violence, war, disaster) is associated with substance use and mental health problems. Services and supports should be trauma-informed to foster safety and trust, as well as promote choice, empowerment, and collaboration.
9. **Recovery involves individual, family, and community strengths and responsibility:** Individuals, families, and communities have strengths and resources that serve as a foundation for recovery.
10. **Recovery is based on respect:** Community, systems, and societal acceptance and appreciation of consumers—including protecting their rights and eliminating discrimination and stigma—are crucial in achieving recovery.

Jeff's involvement in the recovery support group changed his view of himself, and he began to take the lead role in his own care. According to Jeff, "Nobody knows your body better than you do, and some, maybe some mental health providers or doctors, think, 'Hey, I am the professional, and you're the person seeing me. I know what's best for you.' But technically, it isn't true. They only provide you with the tools to get better. They can't crawl inside you and see how you are."

Jeff asked for and received newer, more effective medications. He moved into his own apartment and returned to community college and focused on information technology. Jeff now attends recovery support groups regularly and has taken up bicycling. He has his high and low days but maintains goals, hope, and a purpose for his life.

Adapted from Substance Abuse and Mental Health Administration. (2012). *SAMHSA's working definition of recovery updated.* Retrieved from http://blog.samhsa.gov/2012/03/23/defintion-of-recovery-updated/#.VpQInpMrLBI.

Decade of the Brain

In 1990 President George H.W. Bush designated the last decade of the 1900s as the Decade of the Brain. The overriding goal of this designation was to make legislators and the public aware of the advances that had been made in neuroscience and brain research. This US initiative stimulated a worldwide growth of scientific research. Advances and progress made during the Decade of the Brain include:

- Understanding the genetic basis of embryonic and fetal neural development
- Mapping genes involved in neurological illnesses including mutations associated with Parkinson's disease, Alzheimer's disease, and epilepsy
- Discovering that the brain uses a relatively small number of neurotransmitters but has a vast assortment of neurotransmitter receptors
- Uncovering the role of cytokines (proteins involved in the immune response) in such disorders as depression
- Refining neuroimaging techniques
- Bringing together computer modeling and laboratory research, which resulted in the new discipline of computational neuroscience.

Surgeon General's Report on Mental Health

The first Surgeon General's report on the topic of mental health was published in 1999 (**HHS**). This landmark document was based on an extensive review of the scientific literature in consultation with mental health providers and consumers. The two most important messages from this report were that (1) mental health is fundamental to overall health, and (2) there are effective treatments. The report is reader-friendly and a good introduction to mental health and illness. You can review the report at http://www.surgeongeneral.gov/library/mentalhealth/home.html.

Human Genome Project

The Human Genome Project was a 13-year project that lasted from 1990–2003 and was completed on the 50th anniversary of the discovery of the DNA double helix. The project has strengthened biological and genetic explanations for psychiatric conditions. The goals of the project (US Department of Energy, 2008) were to do the following:

- **Identify** the approximately 20,000 to 25,000 genes in human DNA.
- **Determine** the sequences of the 3 billion chemical base pairs that make up human DNA.
- **Store** this information in databases.
- **Improve** tools for data analysis.
- **Address** the ethical, legal, and social issues that may arise from the project.

Researchers are continuing to make progress in understanding genetic underpinnings of diseases and disorders. You will be learning about these advances in the clinical chapters that follow.

President's New Freedom Commission on Mental Health

The President's New Freedom Commission on Mental Health chaired by Michael Hogan released its recommendations for mental healthcare in America in 2003. This was the first commission since First Lady Rosalyn Carter's (wife of President Jimmy Carter) in 1978. The report stated that the system of delivering mental healthcare in America was in a shambles. It called for a streamlined system with less fragmentation in the delivery of care. The commission advocated for early diagnosis and treatment, adoption of principles of recovery, and increased assistance in helping people find housing and work. Box 1.2 describes the goals necessary for such a transformation of mental healthcare in the United States.

Institute of Medicine

The *Improving the Quality of Health Care for Mental and Substance-Use Conditions: Quality Chasm Series* was released in 2005 by the Health and Medicine Division (HMD) of the National Academies of Medicine, formerly the Institute of Medicine (IOM). It highlighted effective treatments for mental illness and addressed the huge gap between the best care and the worst. It focused on such issues as the problem of coerced (forced) treatment, a system that treats mental health issues separately from physical health problems, and lack of quality control. The report encouraged healthcare workers to focus on safe, effective, patient-centered, timely, efficient, and equitable care.

Another important and related publication issued by the Institute of Medicine in 2011 is *The Future of Nursing: Focus on Education*. This report contends that the old way of training nurses is not adequate for the 21st century's complex requirements. It calls for highly educated nurses who are prepared to care for an aging and diverse population with an increasing incidence of chronic disease. They recommended that nurses be trained in leadership, health policy, system improvement, research, and teamwork.

Quality and safety education for nurses. Recommendations from both documents were addressed by a group called Quality and Safety Education for Nurses (QSEN; pronounced *Q-sen*) and were funded by the Robert Wood Johnson Foundation. They have developed a structure to support the education of future nurses who possess the knowledge, skills, and attitudes to continuously improve the safety and quality of healthcare. Consider this tragic story:

Betsy Lehman was a health reporter for the Boston Globe who was married to a cancer researcher. When she herself was diagnosed with cancer she was prescribed an incorrect, extremely high dose of an anticancer drug. Ms. Lehman sensed something was wrong and appealed to the healthcare providers who did not respond to her concerns. The day before she died, she begged others to help because the professionals were not listening (Robert Wood Johnson Foundation, 2011).

How could her death have been prevented? Consider the key areas of care promoted by QSEN and how they could have prevented Ms. Lehman's death:

1. **Patient-centered care:** Care should be given in an atmosphere of respect and responsiveness, and the patient's values, preferences, and needs should guide care.
2. **Teamwork and collaboration:** Nurses and interprofessional teams need to maintain open communication, respect, and shared decision making.
3. **Evidence-based practice:** Optimal healthcare is the result of integrating the best current evidence while considering the patient/family values and preferences.
4. **Quality improvement:** Nurses should be involved in monitoring the outcomes of the care that they give. They should also be care designers and test changes that will result in quality improvement.
5. **Safety:** The care provided should not add further injury (e.g., nosocomial infections). Harm to patients and providers are minimized through both system effectiveness and individual performance.
6. **Informatics:** Information and technology are used to communicate, manage knowledge, mitigate error, and support decision making.

BOX 1.2 Goals for a Transformed Mental Health System in the United States

Goal 1

Americans understand that mental health is essential to overall health.

Goal 2

Mental healthcare is consumer- and family-driven.

Goal 3

Disparities in mental health services are eliminated.

Goal 4

Early mental health screening, assessment, and referral to services are common practice.

Goal 5

Excellent mental healthcare is delivered, and research is accelerated.

Goal 6

Technology is used to access mental healthcare and information.

Data from US Department of Health and Human Services, President's New Freedom Commission on Mental Health. (2003). *Achieving the promise: Transforming mental health care in America.* USDHHS Publication No. SMA-03-3832. Retrieved from http://www.mentalhealthcommission.gov/reports/finalreport/fullreport-02.htm

Brain Research through Advancing Innovative Neurotechnologies (BRAIN) Initiative

In 2013 President Barack Obama announced that $300 million in public and private funding would be devoted to the Brain Research through Advancing Innovative Neurotechnologies (BRAIN) Initiative. This money would be used to develop innovative techniques and technologies to unravel the mystery of how the brain functions. The goal is to uncover news ways to prevent, treat, and cure psychiatric disorders, epilepsy, and traumatic brain injury.

According to the National Institutes of Health (2016) more than $70 million is going to over 170 researchers working at 60 different institutions. These researchers are examining such topics as:

- Developing computer programs that may help researchers detect and diagnose autism and Alzheimer's disease from brain scans
- Building a cap that uses ultrasound waves to precisely stimulate brain cells
- Creating a "neural dust" system made of tiny electric sensors for wirelessly recording brain activity
- Improving current rehabilitation technologies for helping the lives of stroke patients
- Studying how the brain reads and speaks

Research Domain Criteria (RDoC) Initiative

In other specialty areas, symptom-based classification has been replaced by more scientific understanding of the problem. For example, physicians do not make a cardiac diagnosis depending on the type of chest pain a person is having but rather on diagnosing the specific problem such as myocarditis. Psychiatry continues to rely heavily on symptoms in the absence of objective and measurable data.

In 2013 the National Institute of Mental Health (NIMH) announced that it would no longer fund *DSM* diagnosis-based studies. Instead it would put all of its time, effort, and money into something called the Research Domain Criteria (RDoC) Initiative. This promising initiative challenges researchers to seek causes for mental disorders at the molecular level. NIMH hopes to transform the current diagnostic procedure by using genetics, imaging, and fresh information to create a new classification system.

LEGISLATION AND MENTAL HEALTH FUNDING

Mental Health Parity

Imagine insurance companies singling out a group of disorders such as digestive diseases for reduced reimbursement. Imagine people with colon cancer being assigned higher co-pays than other cancers. Imagine limiting the number of treatments for which patients could be reimbursed for Crohn's disease over a lifetime. People would be outraged by such discrimination. Yet this is exactly what has happened with psychiatric disorders. Too often, insurance companies:

- Did not cover mental healthcare at all
- Identified yearly or lifetime limits on mental health coverage
- Limited hospital days or outpatient treatment sessions
- Assigned higher co-payments or deductibles

In response to this problem, advocates fought for parity. This term means equivalence or equal treatment. The Mental Health Parity Act was passed in 1996. This legislation required insurers that provide mental health coverage to offer annual and lifetime benefits at the same level provided for medical/surgical coverage. Unfortunately, by the year 2000, the Government Accounting Office found that although 86% of health plans complied with the 1996 law, 87% of those plans actually imposed new limits on mental health coverage.

The Wellstone-Domenici Parity Act was enacted in 2008 for group health plans with more than 50 employees. The law required that any plan providing mental health coverage must do so in a manner that is functionally equivalent or on par with coverage of other health conditions. This parity pertains to deductibles, co-payments, coinsurance, and out-of-pocket expenses, as well as treatment limitations (e.g., frequency of treatment and number/frequency of visits).

Patient Protection and Affordable Care Act of 2010

Parity laws were a good first step in providing more equitable coverage for mental healthcare. However, parity laws do not *require* health plans to cover psychiatric care. Furthermore, the parity laws only applied to large insurers. The Patient Protection and Affordable Care of 2010 (ACA) improves coverage for most Americans who are uninsured through a combination of expanded Medicaid eligibility (for the very poor), creation of Health Insurance Exchanges in the states (to serve as a broker to help uninsured consumers choose among various plans), and the so-called "insurance mandate," a requirement that people without coverage obtain it. The ACA improves mental healthcare coverage in several ways (Norris, 2016):

- Eliminates medical underwriting in the individual and small group markets, so medical history no longer results in enrollment denials for preexisting conditions or higher premiums.
- Requires all individual and small group health plans to cover 10 essential health benefits with no annual or lifetime dollar limits. Mental health and addiction treatment are among the essential benefits.
- Makes health insurance with mental health benefits available for many individuals who previously had been uninsured. Significant numbers of these (mostly low-income) persons had untreated mental health problems.
- Provides for prescription coverage for all new individual and small group health plans, including medications to treat behavioral health problems.
- Requires all non-grandfathered health plans—including large group plans—to cover a range of preventive care at no cost to the patient.
- Allows young adults to remain on their parents' health plans until age 26. This is important to mental health since most psychiatric disorders emerge in adolescence or early 20s.

Although the ACA has dramatically improved mental healthcare coverage, there are still problems. Problems include finding a mental health professional for care within certain plans and limited coverage for some brand-name drugs, especially antipsychotics. Also, health insurance companies may be more than twice as likely to deny authorization for mental healthcare compared with authorization for general medical care (NAMI, 2015). Hopefully, these deficiencies will be addressed as the ACA continues to be evaluated and evolves.

EPIDEMIOLOGY OF MENTAL DISORDERS

Epidemiology, as it applies to psychiatric-mental health, is the quantitative study of the distribution of mental disorders in human populations. Understanding this distribution helps identify high-risk groups and risk factors associated with illness onset, duration, and recurrence.

According to SAMHSA (2014), nearly 44 million adults in the United States experienced a diagnosable mental illness in 2013. In fact, neuropsychiatric disorders are the leading category of disease with twice the disability as the next category, cardiovascular diseases. More than a third of this disability is caused by depression.

Individuals may have more than one mental disorder or another medical disorder. The simultaneous existence of two or more disorders is known as a **comorbid condition**. For example, schizophrenia is frequently comorbid with diabetes.

Two different but related words used in epidemiology are **incidence** and **prevalence**. *Incidence* conveys information about the risk of contracting a disease. It refers to the number of new cases of mental disorders in a healthy population within a given period of time, usually annually. An example of incidence is the number of Atlanta adolescents who were diagnosed with major depression between 2000 and 2001.

Prevalence describes the *total number of cases*, new and existing, in a given population during a specific period of time, regardless of when they became ill. An example of prevalence is the number of adolescents who screened positive for major depression in New York City schools between 2000 and 2010.

A disease with a short duration such as the common cold tends to have a high incidence (many new cases in a given year) and a low prevalence (not many people suffering from a cold at any given time). Conversely, a chronic disease such as diabetes will have a low incidence because the person will be dropped from the list of new cases after the first year (or whatever time increment is being used).

Lifetime risk data, or the risk that one will develop a disease in the course of a lifetime, will be higher than both incidence and prevalence. According to Kessler, Berglund, and colleagues (2005), 46.4% of all Americans will meet the criteria for a psychiatric disorder in their lifetimes. Table 1.1 shows the prevalence of some psychiatric disorders in the United States.

Originally, epidemiology meant the study of epidemics. **Clinical epidemiology** is a broad field that examines health and illness at the population level. Studies use traditional epidemiological methods and are conducted in groups usually defined by the illness or symptoms or by the diagnostic procedures or treatments given for the illness or symptoms. Clinical epidemiology includes the following:

- Studies of the natural history—what happens if there is no treatment and the problem is left to run its course—of an illness
- Studies of diagnostic screening tests
- Observational and experimental studies of interventions used to treat people with the illness or symptoms

Analysis of epidemiological studies can reveal the frequency with which psychological symptoms appear together with physical illness. For example, epidemiological studies demonstrate that depression is a significant risk factor for death in people

TABLE 1.1 Twelve-Month Prevalence of Psychiatric Disorders in the United States

Disorder	Prevalence Over 12 Months (%)	12 Month % Receiving Treatment	Comments
Schizophrenia	1.1	45.8	Affects men and women equally
Major depressive disorder	6.7	51.7	Leading cause of disability in United States and established economies worldwide Nearly twice as many women (6.5%) as men (3.3%) suffer from major depressive disorder every year
Bipolar disorder	2.6	48.8	Affects men and women equally
Generalized anxiety disorder	3.1	43.2	Can begin across life cycle; risk is highest between childhood and middle age
Panic disorder	2.7	59.1	Typically develops in adolescence or early adulthood About one in three people with panic disorder develop agoraphobia
Obsessive-compulsive disorder	1	No data	First symptoms begin in childhood or adolescence
Posttraumatic stress disorder (PTSD)	3.5	49.9	Can develop at any time About 30% of Vietnam veterans experienced PTSD after the war; percentage high among first responders to Sept. 11, 2001, US terrorist attacks
Social phobia	6.8	40.1	Typically begins in childhood or adolescence
Agoraphobia	0.08	45.8	Begins in young adulthood
Specific phobia	8.7	32.4	Begins in childhood
Any personality disorder	9.1	No data	Antisocial personality disorder more common in men
Alzheimer's disease	10 (65+) 50 (85 years+)		Rare, inherited forms can strike in the 30s-40s

Data from Kessler, R.C., Chiu, W.T., Demler, O., & Walters, E.E. (2005). Prevalence, severity, and comorbidity of twelve-month DSM-IV disorders in the National Comorbidity Survey Replication (NCS-R). *Archives of General Psychiatry, 62*(6), 617-27.

with cardiovascular disease and premature death in people with breast cancer.

Classification of Mental Disorders

Nursing care, as opposed to medical care, is care based on responses to illness. Registered nurses do not diagnose, prescribe, and treat major depression. They treat the problems associated with depression such as insomnia or hopelessness. Nurses provide effective care using the nursing process as a guide to holistic care. Nurses, physicians, and other healthcare providers are part of an interprofessional team. When the team is well coordinated, it can provide optimal care for the biological, psychological, social, and spiritual needs of patients.

To carry out their diverse professional responsibilities, educators, clinicians, and researchers need clear and accurate guidelines for identifying and categorizing mental illness. For clinicians in particular, such guidelines help in planning and evaluating their patients' treatment.

At present, there are two major classification systems used in the United States: the ***Diagnostic and Statistical Manual, Fifth Edition (DSM-5)*** and the *International Classification of Disease, Tenth Revision, Clinical Modification* (*ICD-10-CM*) (WHO, 2016). Both are important in terms of planning for patient care and determining reimbursement for services. However, the *DSM-5* is the dominant method of categorizing and diagnosing mental illness in the United States and is the framework for clinical disorders in this textbook.

The *DSM-5*

The *Diagnostic and Statistical Manual (DSM)* is a publication of the American Psychiatric Association (APA). First published in 1952, the latest 2013 edition describes criteria for 157 disorders. The development of the *DSM-5* was influenced by clinical field trials conducted by psychiatrists, psychiatric–mental health advanced practice registered nurses, psychologists, licensed clinical social workers, licensed counselors, and licensed marriage and family therapists.

The *DSM* identifies disorders based on specific criteria. It is used in inpatient, outpatient, partial hospitalization, consultation-liaison, clinics, private practice, primary care, and community settings. The *DSM* also serves as a tool for collecting epidemiological statistics about the diagnosis of psychiatric disorders.

The following is a list of disorder categories in the *DSM-5*. You may notice that the order of the list is similar to the way the chapters are organized in this textbook.

1. Neurodevelopmental Disorders
2. Schizophrenia Spectrum Disorders
3. Bipolar and Related Disorders
4. Depressive Disorders
5. Anxiety Disorders
6. Obsessive-Compulsive Disorders
7. Trauma and Stressor-Related Disorders
8. Dissociative Disorders
9. Somatic Symptom Disorders
10. Feeding and Eating Disorders
11. Elimination Disorders
12. Sleep-Wake Disorders
13. Sexual Dysfunctions
14. Gender Dysphoria
15. Disruptive, Impulse Control, and Conduct Disorders
16. Substance-Related and Addictive Disorders
17. Neurocognitive Disorders
18. Personality Disorders
19. Paraphilic Disorders
20. Other Disorders

A common misconception is that a classification of mental disorders classifies *people*, when the *DSM* actually classifies *disorders*. For this reason, the *DSM* and this textbook avoid the use of labels such as "a schizophrenic" or "an alcoholic." Viewing the person as a person and not an illness requires more accurate terms such as "an individual with schizophrenia" or "my patient has major depression."

The *ICD-10-CM*

In an increasingly global society, it is important to view the United States' diagnosis and treatment of mental illness as part of a bigger picture. The international standard of disease classification is the *International Classification of Diseases, Tenth Revision (ICD-10)* (WHO, 2016). The United States has adapted this resource with a "clinical modification," hence its title of *ICD-10-CM*.

PSYCHIATRIC-MENTAL HEALTH NURSING

In most clinical settings, nurses work with people going through a variety of crises. These crises may be based on physical, psychological, mental, and spiritual distress. Most of you have already come across people going through difficult times in their lives. While you may have handled these situations well, there may have been times when you wished you had additional skills and knowledge.

The psychiatric nursing rotation will greatly increase your insight into the experiences of others with mental health alterations. Exploring mental health and mental illness may even help you increase insight into yourself. You will learn essential information about psychiatric disorders and, hopefully, have the opportunity to develop new skills for dealing with a variety of behaviors associated with them. The rest of this chapter is devoted to psychiatric nursing—what psychiatric nurses do, their scope of practice, and the challenges and evolving roles for the future healthcare environment.

What Is Psychiatric-Mental Health Nursing?

Psychiatric-mental health nursing is the nursing specialty that is dedicated to promoting mental health through the assessment, diagnosis, and treatment of behavioral problems, mental disorders, and comorbid conditions across the lifespan (American Nurses Association et al., 2014). Psychiatric-mental health nurses work with people throughout their life span: children, adolescents, adults, and the elderly.

Psychiatric-mental health nurses assist people who are in crisis or who are experiencing life problems, as well as those with long-term mental illness. These nurses work with patients with dual diagnoses (e.g., a mental disorder and a comorbid substance disorder), homeless persons and families, forensic

BOX 1.3 Phenomena of Concern for Psychiatric-Mental Health Nurses

Phenomena of concern for psychiatric-mental health nurses include:

- Promotion of optimal mental and physical health and well-being
- Prevention of mental and behavioral distress and illness
- Promotion of social inclusion of mentally and behaviorally fragile individuals
- Co-occurring mental health and substance use disorders
- Co-occurring mental health and physical disorders
- Alterations in thinking, perceiving, communicating, and functioning related to psychological and physiological distress
- Psychological and physiological distress resulting from physical, interpersonal, and/or environment trauma or neglect
- Psychogenesis and individual vulnerability
- Complex clinical presentations confounded by poverty and poor, inconsistent, or toxic environmental factors
- Alterations in self-concept related to loss of physical organs and/or limbs, psychic trauma, developmental conflicts, or injury
- Individual, family, or group isolation and difficulty with interpersonal relations
- Self-harm and self-destructive behaviors including mutilation and suicide
- Violent behavior including physical abuse, sexual abuse, and bullying
- Low health literacy rates contributing to treatment nonadherence

From American Psychiatric Nurses Association, International Society of Psychiatric-Mental Health Nurses, & American Nurses Association. (2014). *Psychiatric-mental health nursing: Scope and standards of practice (2nd ed.)*. Silver Spring, MD: NursesBooks.org.

patients (i.e., people in jail), and individuals who have survived abusive situations. Psychiatric-mental health nurses work with individuals, couples, families, and groups in every nursing setting. They work with patients in hospitals, in their homes, in halfway houses, in shelters, in clinics, in storefronts, on the street—virtually everywhere.

The *Psychiatric-Mental Health Nursing: Scope and Standards of Practice* defines the specific activities of the psychiatric-mental health nurse. This publication—jointly written in 2014 by the American Nurses Association (ANA), the American Psychiatric Nurses Association (APNA), and the International Society of Psychiatric-Mental Health Nurses (ISPN)—defines the focus of **psychiatric-mental health nursing** as "promoting mental health through the assessment, diagnosis, and treatment of human responses to mental health problems and psychiatric disorders" (p. 14).

The psychiatric-mental health nurse uses the same nursing process you have already learned to assess and diagnose patients' illnesses, identify outcomes, and plan, implement, and evaluate nursing care. Box 1.3 describes **phenomena of concern**—human experiences and responses—for psychiatric-mental health nurses.

Classification of Nursing Diagnoses, Outcomes, and Interventions

To provide the most appropriate and scientifically sound care, the psychiatric-mental health nurse uses standardized classification systems developed by professional nursing groups. The book *Nursing Diagnoses: Definitions and Classification 2015–2017* of the North American Nursing Diagnosis Association International (NANDA-I; Herdman & Kamitsuru, 2014) provides standardized diagnoses, many of which are related to psychosocial/psychiatric nursing care. These diagnoses provide a common language to aid in the selection of nursing interventions and ultimately lead to outcome achievement.

DSM-5 and NANDA-I–Approved Nursing Diagnoses

Psychiatric-mental health nursing includes the diagnosis and treatment of human responses to actual or potential mental health problems. "A nursing diagnosis is a clinical judgment concerning a human response to health conditions/life processes, or vulnerability for that response by an individual, family, group, or community" (Herdman & Kamitsuru, 2014, p. 25). While the *DSM-5* is used to diagnose a psychiatric disorder, a well-defined nursing diagnosis provides the framework for identifying appropriate nursing interventions for dealing with the patient's reaction to the disorder.

Nursing Outcomes Classification (NOC)

The ***Nursing Outcomes Classification (NOC)*** is a comprehensive source for standardized outcomes and definitions of these outcomes (Moorhead et al., 2013). A five-point Likert scale is used with all outcomes and indicators. A rating of 5 is always the best possible score and a rating of 1 is always the worst possible scale. Words used in the scales include 1 = Extremely compromised to 5 = Not compromised and 1=Never demonstrated to 5 = Consistently demonstrated.

The 490 outcomes are listed in alphabetical order. Outcomes are organized into seven domains: functional health, physiological health, psychosocial health, health knowledge and behavior, perceived health, family health, and community health. The psychosocial health domain includes four classes: psychological well-being, psychosocial adaptation, self-control, and social interaction.

Nursing Interventions Classification (NIC)

The ***Nursing Interventions Classification (NIC)*** is another book used to standardize, define, and measure nursing care. The *NIC* (Bulechek et al., 2013) defines a nursing intervention as "any treatment, based upon clinical judgment and knowledge, that a nurse performs to enhance patient/client outcomes" (p. xv) including direct and indirect care through a series of nursing activities. There are seven domains: basic physiological, complex physiological, behavioral, safety, family, health system, and community. Two domains relate specifically to psychiatric nursing: behavioral, including communication, coping, and education, and safety, covering crisis and risk management.

Levels of Psychiatric-Mental Health Clinical Nursing Practice

Psychiatric-mental health nurses are registered nurses educated in nursing and licensed to practice in their individual states. Psychiatric nurses are qualified to practice at two levels, basic and advanced, depending on educational preparation. Table 1.2 describes basic and advanced psychiatric nursing interventions.

TABLE 1.2 Basic Level and Advanced Practice Psychiatric-Mental Health Nursing Interventions

Basic Level Intervention	Description
Coordination of care	Coordinates implementation of the nursing care plan and documents coordination of care
Health teaching and health maintenance	Individualized anticipatory guidance to prevent or reduce mental illness or enhance mental health (e.g., community screenings, parenting classes, stress management)
Milieu therapy	Provides, structures, and maintains a safe and therapeutic environment in collaboration with patients, families, and other healthcare clinicians
Pharmacological, biological, and integrative therapies	Applies current knowledge to assessing patient's response to medication, provides medication teaching, and communicates observations to other members of the healthcare team
Advanced Practice Intervention	**Description**
All of the Above Plus:	
Medication prescription and treatment	Prescription of psychotropic medications with appropriate use of diagnostic tests; hospital admitting privileges
Psychotherapy	Individual, couple, group, or family therapy using evidence-based therapeutic frameworks and the nurse-patient relationship
Consultation	Sharing of clinical expertise with nurses or those in other disciplines to enhance their treatment of patients or address systems issues

Data from American Psychiatric Nurses Association, International Society of Psychiatric-Mental Health Nurses, & American Nurses Association. (2014). *Psychiatric-mental health nursing: Scope and standards of practice.* Silver Spring, MD: NurseBooks.org.

Basic Level

Basic level registered nurses are professionals who have completed a nursing program, passed the state licensure examination, and are qualified to work in most any general or specialty area. The **psychiatric-mental health registered nurse (PMH-RN)** is a nursing graduate who possesses a diploma, an associate degree, or a baccalaureate degree and chooses to work in the specialty of psychiatric-mental health nursing. At the basic level, nurses work in various supervised settings and perform multiple roles such as staff nurse, case manager, home care nurse, and so on.

After 2 years of full-time work as a registered nurse, 2,000 clinical hours in a psychiatric setting, and 30 hours of continuing education in psychiatric nursing, a baccalaureate-prepared nurse may take a certification examination administered by the American Nurses Credentialing Center (the credentialing arm of the ANA) to demonstrate clinical competence in psychiatric-mental health nursing. After passing the examination, a board-certified credential is added to the RN title resulting in RN-BC. Certification gives nurses a sense of mastery and accomplishment, identifies them as competent clinicians, and satisfies a requirement for reimbursement by employers in some states.

Advanced Practice

One of the first advanced practice nursing roles in the United States was the psychiatric clinical nurse specialist in the 1950s. These expert nurses were originally trained to provide individual therapy and group therapy in state psychiatric hospitals and to provide training for other staff. Eventually they, along with psychiatric nurse practitioners who were introduced in the mid-1960s, gained diagnostic privileges, prescriptive authority, and the ability to provide psychotherapy.

Currently, the **psychiatric-mental health advanced practice registered nurse (PMH-APRN)** is a licensed registered nurse with a Master of Science in Nursing (MSN) or Doctor of Nursing Practice (DNP) in psychiatric nursing. This DNP is not to be confused with a doctoral degree in nursing (PhD), which is a research degree, whereas the DNP is a practice doctorate. The PMH-APRN may function autonomously depending on the state and is eligible for specialty privileges. Some advanced practice nurses continue their education to the PhD level.

Unlike other specialty areas, there is no significant difference between a psychiatric nurse practitioner (NP) and a clinical nurse specialist (CNS) as long as the CNS has achieved prescriptive authority. Certification is required and is obtained through the American Nurses Credentialing Center. Only one examination—the Psychiatric-Mental Health Nurse Practitioner—Board Certified (PMHNP-BC)—is currently available. Three other examinations have been discontinued:

- Adult Psychiatric-Mental Health Nurse Practitioner—Board Certified (PMHNP-BC)
- Adult Psychiatric-Mental Health Clinical Nurse Specialist—Board Certified (PMHCNS-BC)
- Child/Adolescent Psychiatric-Mental Health Clinical Nurse Specialist—Board Certified (PMHCNS-BC)

While these examinations are no longer given, you will still find many nurses who practice in these roles. Their credentials will continue to be renewed if professional development and practice hour requirements are met.

FUTURE ISSUES FOR PSYCHIATRIC-MENTAL HEALTH NURSES

Significant trends will affect the future of psychiatric nursing in the United States. These trends include educational challenges, an aging population, increasing cultural diversity, and expanding technology.

Educational Challenges

As with other specialty areas in a hospital setting, psychiatric nurses are caring for more acutely ill patients. In the 1980s, it was common for patients who were depressed and suicidal to have insurance coverage for about 2 weeks. Now patients are lucky to be covered for 3 days, if they are covered at all. This means that nurses need to be more skilled and be prepared to discharge patients for whom the benefit of their care will not always be evident.

Providing educational experiences for nursing students is challenging as a result of this level of acute care and also due to the declining inpatient populations. Clinical rotations in general medical centers are becoming more difficult to obtain. Faculty are fortunate to secure rotations in state psychiatric hospitals, veterans administration facilities, and community settings.

Community psychiatric settings also provide students with valuable experience, but the logistics of placing and supervising students in multiple sites has required creativity on the part of nursing educators. Some schools have established integrated rotations that, theoretically, allow students to work outside the psychiatric setting with patients who have mental health issues—for example, caring for a person with major depressive disorder on an orthopedic floor. Some faculty are concerned that without serious commitment, this type of specialty integration may water down a previously rich experience.

Nurse-led medical/health homes and clinics are becoming increasingly common. Community nursing centers that can secure funding serve low-income and uninsured people. In this model, psychiatric-mental health nurses work with primary care nurses to provide comprehensive care, usually funded by scarce grants from academic centers. These centers use a nontraditional approach of combining primary care and health promotion interventions. Advanced practice psychiatric nurses have also been extremely successful in setting up private practices where they provide both psychotherapy and medication management.

An Aging Population

As the number of older adults grows, the prevalence of Alzheimer's disease and other dementias requiring skilled nursing care in inpatient settings is likely to increase. Healthier older adults will need more services at home, in retirement communities, or in assisted living facilities. For more information on the needs of older adults, refer to Chapters 23, 28, and 31.

Cultural Diversity

Cultural diversity is steadily increasing in the United States. The United States Census Bureau (2015) notes that the United States will have a majority minority population by 2044. Psychiatric-mental health nurses will need to increase their **cultural competence**. Simply put, cultural competence means that nurses adjust *their* practices to meet their patients' cultural beliefs, practices, needs, and preferences.

Science, Technology, and Electronic Healthcare

Genetic mapping from the Human Genome Project has resulted in a steady stream of research discoveries concerning genetic markers implicated in a variety of psychiatric illnesses. This information could be helpful in identifying at-risk individuals and in targeting medications specific to certain genetic variants and profiles. However, the legal and ethical implications of responsibly using this technology are staggering. For example:

- Would you want to know you were at risk for a psychiatric illness such as bipolar disorder?
- Who should have access to this information—your primary care provider, insurer, future spouse, or a lawyer in a child-custody battle?
- Who will regulate genetic testing centers to protect privacy and prevent 21st-century problems such as identity theft and fraud?

Despite these concerns, the next decade holds great promise in the diagnosis and treatment of psychiatric disorders, and nurses will be central as educators and caregivers. Scientific advances through research and technology are certain to shape psychiatric-mental health nursing practice. Magnetic resonance imaging research, in addition to comparing healthy people to people diagnosed with mental illness, is now focusing on the development of preclinical profiles of children and adolescents. The hope of this type of research is to identify people at risk for developing mental illness, which allows earlier interventions to try to decrease impairment.

Electronic healthcare services provided from a distance are gaining wide acceptance. In the early days of the internet, consumers were cautioned against the questionable wisdom of seeking advice through an unregulated medium. However, the internet has transformed the way we approach healthcare needs and allows people to be their own advocates.

Telepsychiatry through audio and visual media is an effective way to reach underserved populations and those who are homebound. This allows for assessment and diagnosis, medication management, and even group therapy. Psychiatric nurses may become more active in developing websites for mental health education, screening, or support, especially to reach geographically isolated areas. Many health agencies hire nurses to staff help lines or hotlines, and as provision of these cost-effective services increases, so too will the need for bilingual resources.

ADVOCACY AND LEGISLATIVE INVOLVEMENT

Through direct care and indirect action, nurses advocate for the psychiatric patient. As a patient advocate, the nurse reports incidents of abuse or neglect to the appropriate authorities for immediate action. The nurse also upholds patient confidentiality, which has become more of a challenge as the use of electronic medical records increases. Another form of nursing advocacy is supporting the patient's right to make decisions regarding treatment.

On an indirect level, the nurse may choose to be active in consumer mental health groups (such as NAMI) and state and local mental health associations to support consumers of mental healthcare. The nurse can also be vigilant about reviewing local and national legislation affecting healthcare to identify potential detrimental effects on the mentally ill. Especially during times of fiscal crisis, lawmakers are inclined to decrease or eliminate funding for vulnerable populations who do not have a strong political voice.

The APNA devotes significant energy to monitoring legislative, regulatory, and policy matters affecting psychiatric nursing and mental health. As the 24-hours-a-day, 7-days-a-week caregivers and members of the largest group of healthcare professionals, nurses have the potential to exert tremendous influence on legislation.

However, when commissions and task forces are developed, nurses are not usually the first group to be considered to provide input and expertise for national, state, and local decision makers. In fact, nursing presence is often absent at the policymaking table. Consider the President's New Freedom Commission for Mental Health, which included psychiatrists (medical doctors), psychologists (PhDs), academics, and policymakers—but no nurses. It is difficult to understand how the largest contingent of mental healthcare providers in the United States could be excluded from a group that would determine the future of mental healthcare.

It is in the best interest of consumers of mental healthcare that all members of the collaborative healthcare team, including nurses, be involved in decisions and legislation that will affect their care. Current political issues that need monitoring and support include mental health parity, discriminatory media portrayal, standardized language and practices, and advanced practice issues, such as prescriptive authority over schedule II drugs and government and insurance reimbursement for nursing care.

KEY POINTS TO REMEMBER

- Overall health is not possible without good mental health.
- Mental illness refers to all psychiatric disorders with definable diagnoses that cause significant dysfunction in developmental, biological, or psychological disturbances.
- A mental health and mental illness continuum is a useful representation for demonstrating how functioning may change over time. Mental health and illness are not either/or propositions, but are instead endpoints on a continuum.
- Risk factors such as inborn vulnerability, a poor social environment, economic hardship, and poor health policy may increase the risk of adverse mental health outcomes.
- Protective factors such as resiliency improve a person's ability to respond to stress, trauma, and loss.
- The distinction between mental and physical illness is artificial. Mental illness is brain-based and is therefore a physical illness.
- Psychiatric disorders are generally the result of nature and nurture. A diathesis-stress model—in which diathesis represents biological predisposition and stress represents environmental stress or trauma—is the most accepted explanation for mental illness.
- The recovery movement has shifted the focus of decision making from a paternalistic system, where compliance is emphasized, to a focus on self-determination and self-direction.
- Government programs and initiatives such as the Decade of the Brain, the Human Genome Project, Brain Research through Advancing Innovative Neurotechnology, and Research Domain Criteria are expanding our knowledge of the brain and will provide the basis for future treatments.
- Until recently, funding for psychiatric care had not been equal to that of other medical care. Mental health parity refers to equality in funding.
- The study of epidemiology can help identify high-risk groups and behaviors. In turn, this can lead to a better understanding of the causes of some disorders. Prevalence rates help us identify the proportion of a population experiencing a specific mental disorder at a given time.
- The *DSM-5* provides criteria for psychiatric disorders and a basis for the development of comprehensive and appropriate interventions.
- Standardized nursing classification systems (NANDA-I, *NOC, NIC*) are used to form and communicate patient problems, outcomes, and interventions specific to nursing care.
- Psychiatric-mental health nurses function at a basic or advanced level of practice with clearly defined roles.
- As a result of social, cultural, scientific, and political factors, the future holds many challenges and possibilities for the psychiatric-mental health nurse.

CRITICAL THINKING

1. Brian, a college sophomore with a grade-point average of 3.4, is brought to the emergency department after a suicide attempt. He has been extremely depressed since the death of his girlfriend 5 months previously when the car he was driving crashed. His parents are devastated, and they believe that taking one's own life prevents a person from going to heaven.

   Brian has epilepsy and has had more seizures since the auto accident. He says he should be punished for his carelessness and does not care what happens to him. He has stopped going to classes and no longer shows up for his part-time job of tutoring young children in reading.

   a. What might be a possible *DSM-5* (medical) diagnosis?
   b. What are some factors that you should assess regarding aspects of Brian's overall health and other influences that can affect mental health?
   c. If an antidepressant medication could help Brian's depression, explain why this alone would not meet his multiple needs. What issues do you think have to be addressed if Brian is to receive a holistic approach to care?
   d. Formulate two potential nursing diagnoses for Brian.
   e. Would Brian's parents' religious beliefs factor into your plan of care? If so, how?
2. In a small group, share experiences you have had with others from unfamiliar cultural, ethnic, religious, or racial backgrounds, and identify two positive learning experiences from these encounters.
3. Would you feel comfortable referring a family member to a mental health clinician? What factors influence your feelings?
4. How could basic and advanced practice psychiatric-mental health nurses work together to provide the highest quality of care?
5. Would you consider joining a professional group or advocacy group that promotes mental health? Why or why not?

CHAPTER REVIEW

Questions

1. When providing respectful, appropriate nursing care, how should the nurse identify the patient and his or her observable characteristics?
   a. The manic patient in room 234
   b. The patient in room 234 is a manic
   c. The patient in room 234 is possibly a manic
   d. The patient in room 234 is displaying manic behavior
2. Recognizing the frequency of depression among the American population, the nurse should advocate for which mental health promotion intervention?
   a. Including discussions on depression as part of school health classes
   b. Providing regular depression screening for adolescent and teenage students
   c. Increasing the number of community-based depression hotlines available to the public
   d. Encouraging senior centers to provide information on accessing community depression resources
3. Which statement made by a patient demonstrates a healthy degree of resilience? *Select all that apply.*
   a. "I try to remember not to take other people's bad moods personally."
   b. "I know that if I get really mad I'll end up being depressed."
   c. "I really feel that sometimes bad things are meant to happen."
   d. "I've learned to calm down before trying to defend my opinions."
   e. "I know that discussing issues with my boss would help me get my point across."
4. Which statement demonstrates the nurse's understanding of the effect of environmental factors on a patient's mental health?
   a. "I'll need to assess how the patient's family views mental illness."
   b. "There is a history of depression in the patient's extended family."
   c. "I'm not familiar with the patient's Japanese's cultural view on suicide."
   d. "The patient's ability to pay for mental health services needs to be assessed."
5. When considering stigmatization, which statement made by the nurse demonstrates a need for immediate intervention by the nurse manager?
   a. "Depression seems to be a real problem among the teenage population."
   b. "My experience has been that the Irish have a problem with alcohol use."
   c. "Women are at greater risk for developing suicidal thoughts then acting on them."
   d. "We've admitted several military veterans with post-traumatic stress disorder this month."
6. A nursing student new to psychiatric-mental health nursing asks a peer what resources he can use to figure out which symptoms are present in a specific psychiatric disorder. The best answer would be:
   a. *Nursing Interventions Classification (NIC)*
   b. *Nursing Outcomes Classification (NOC)*
   c. NANDA-I nursing diagnoses
   d. *DSM-5*
7. Epidemiological studies contribute to improvements in care for individuals with mental disorders by:
   a. Providing information about effective nursing techniques.
   b. Identifying risk factors that contribute to the development of a disorder.
   c. Identifying individuals in the general population who will develop a specific disorder.
   d. Identifying which individuals will respond favorably to a specific treatment.
8. Which of the following activities would be considered nursing care and appropriate to be performed by a basic level nurse for a patient suffering from mental illness?
   a. Treating major depression
   b. Teaching coping skills for a specific family dynamic
   c. Conducting psychotherapy
   d. Prescribing antidepressant medication
9. Which statement about mental illness is true?
   a. Mental illness is a matter of individual nonconformity with societal norms.
   b. Mental illness is present when irrational and illogical behavior occurs.
   c. Mental illness changes with culture, time in history, political systems, and the groups defining it.
   d. Mental illness is evaluated solely by considering individual control over behavior and appraisal of reality.
10. The World Health Organization describes health as "a state of complete physical, mental, and social wellbeing and not merely the absence of disease or infirmity." Which statement is true in regards to overall health? *Select all that apply.*
   a. There is no relationship between physical and mental health.
   b. Poor physical health can lead to mental distress and disorders.
   c. Poor mental health does not lead to physical illness.
   d. There is a strong relationship between physical health and mental health.
   e. Mental health needs take precedence over physical health needs.

Answers

1. **d;** 2. **b;** 3. **a, d, e;** 4. **c;** 5. **b;** 6. **d;** 7. **b, d;** 8. **b;** 9. **c;** 10. **b, d**

Visit the Evolve website for a posttest on the content in this chapter: http://evolve.elsevier.com/Varcarolis

Post-Test interactive review

REFERENCES

Altrocchi, J. (1980). *Abnormal behavior*. New York, NY: Harcourt Brace Jovanovich.

American Nurses Association, American Psychiatric Nurses Association, & International Society of Psychiatric-Mental Health Nurses. (2014). *Psychiatric-mental health nursing: Scope and standards of practice*. Silver Spring, MD: NursesBooks.org.

American Psychiatric Association. (2013). *Diagnostic and statistical manual of mental disorders* (5th ed.). Washington, DC: Author.

Bulechek, G. M., Butcher, H. K., Dochterman, J. M., & Wagner, C. (2013). *Nursing interventions classification (NIC)* (6th ed.). St. Louis, MO: Mosby.

Department of Health and Human Services. (2003). *New freedom commission on mental health*. Publication number SMA-03-3831. Rockville, MD.

Herdman, T. H., & Kamitsuru, S. (2014). *NANDA international nursing diagnoses: Definitions and classification, 2015-2017* (10th ed.). Oxford, UK: Wiley-Blackwell.

Howard, R., Director. (2001). *A beautiful mind* [film]. Los Angeles: Universal Pictures.

Institute of Medicine (IOM). (2005). *Improving the quality of health care for mental and substance-use conditions: Quality chasm series*. Washington, DC: National Academies Press.

Institute of Medicine (IOM). (2011). *The future of nursing: Focus on education*. Retrieved from http://nationalacademies.org/hmd/reports/2010/the-future-of-nursing-leading-change-advancing-health/report-brief-education.aspx.

Kessler, R. C., Berglund, P., Demler, O., Jin, R., & Walters, E. E. (2005). Lifetime prevalence and age-of-onset distributions of DSM-IV disorders in the national comorbidity survey replication. *Archives of General Psychiatry, 62*, 593–602.

Moorhead, S., Johnson, M., Maas, M. L., & Swanson, E. (2013). *Nursing outcomes classification (NOC)* (5th ed.). St Louis, MO: Mosby.

National Alliance on Mental Illness. (2015). *The long road ahead*. Retrieved from https://www.nami.org/About-NAMI/Publications-Reports/Public-Policy-Reports/A-Long-Road-Ahead/2015-ALongRoadAhead.pdf.

National Institutes of Health. (2016). *NIH nearly doubles investment in BRAIN initiative research*. Retrieved from https://www.nimh.nih.gov/news/science-news/2016/nih-nearly-doubles-investment-in-brain-initiative-research.shtml.

Norris, L. (2016). *How Obamacare improved mental health coverage*. Retrieved from https://www.healthinsurance.org/blog/2016/02/16/how-obamacare-improved-mental-health-coverage/.

Porter, N. (Ed.). (1913). *Webster's revised unabridged dictionary*. Boston, MA: Merriam.

Robert Wood Johnson Foundation. (2011). *QSEN branches out*. Retrieved from http://www.rwjf.org/humancapital/product.jsp?id=72552.

Substance Abuse and Mental Health Services Administration. (2012). *SAMHSA announces a working definition of "recovery" from mental disorders and substance use disorders*. Retrieved from http://www.samhsa.gov/newsroom/advisories/1112223420.aspx.

Substance Abuse and Mental Health Services Administration. (2014). *Nearly one in five adult Americans experienced mental illness in 2013*. Retrieved from http://www.samhsa.gov/newsroom/press-announcements/201411200115.

United States Census Bureau. (2015). *Projections of the size and composition of the US population: 2014 to 2060*. Retrieved from http://www.census.gov/content/dam/Census/library/publications/2015/demo/p25-1143.pdf.

United States Department of Energy. (2008). *The human genome project information*. Retrieved from http://www.ornl.gov/sci/techresources/Human_Genome/home.shtml.

United States Department of Health and Human Services,. (1999). *Mental health: A report of the Surgeon General*. Washington, DC: US Government Printing Office.

United States Department of Health and Human Services. (2014). *Mental health myths and facts*. Retrieved from http://www.mentalhealth.gov/basics/myths-facts/.

World Health Organization. (2014). *Mental health: A state of well-being*. Retrieved from http://www.who.int/features/factfiles/mental_health/en/.

World Health Organization. (2016). *ICD-10: International statistical classification of diseases, tenth revision, clinical modification*. New York, NY: Author.

2

Theories and Therapies

Margaret Jordan Halter

ⓔ Visit the Evolve website for a pretest on the content in this chapter: http://evolve.elsevier.com/Varcarolis Pre-Test interactive review

OBJECTIVES

1. Describe the evolution of theories of psychiatric disorders.
2. Distinguish between dominant theories and associated therapies for psychiatric alterations.
3. Identify the implications of psychiatric theories and therapies for nursing care.
4. Discuss the major components of Peplau's Theory of Interpersonal Relationships.
5. Apply developmental theories to patients across the lifespan.

OUTLINE

KEY TERMS AND CONCEPTS

automatic thoughts
behavioral therapy
biofeedback
classical conditioning
cognitive-behavioral therapy (CBT)
cognitive distortions
conditioning
conscious
countertransference
defense mechanisms
ego
extinction
id
interpersonal therapy
negative reinforcement

operant conditioning
positive reinforcement
preconscious
psychodynamic therapy
punishment
reinforcement
superego
systematic desensitization
transference
unconscious

Every professional discipline, from math and science to philosophy and psychology, bases its work and beliefs on theories. Most of these theories can be best described as explanations, hypotheses, or hunches, rather than testable facts.

The word *theory* may conjure up some dry, conceptual images. You may vaguely recall the physicists' theory of relativity or the geologists' plate tectonics. Compared with most other theories, however, psychological theories are filled with familiar concepts and terms. Psychological theories have filtered their way into parts of mainstream thinking and speech. For example, advertisers use the behaviorist trick of linking a seductive woman to the utilitarian minivan. And who has not attributed language mistakes to subconscious motivation? As the fictional king greets his queen: "Good morning, my beheaded…I mean my beloved!" we comprehend the Freudian slip.

Dealing with other people is one of the most universally anxiety-provoking activities, and psychological theories provide plausible explanations for perplexing behavior. Maybe the guy at the front desk who never greets you in the morning does not really despise you. Maybe he has an inferiority complex because his mother was cold and his father was absent from the home.

This chapter will provide you with snapshots of some of the most influential psychological theories. It also gives you an overview of the treatments, or therapies, that the theories inspired. We will also address the contributions that the theories have made to the practice of psychiatric-mental health nursing.

PSYCHOANALYTIC THEORIES AND THERAPIES

Psychoanalytic Theory

Sigmund Freud (1856–1939), an Austrian neurologist, revolutionized thinking about mental health disorders. He introduced a groundbreaking theory of personality structure, levels of awareness, anxiety, the role of defense mechanisms, and the stages of psychosexual development.

Originally, he was searching for biological treatments for psychological disturbances and even experimented with using cocaine as medication. He soon abandoned this physiological approach and focused on psychological treatments. Freud came to believe that the vast majority of mental disorders resulted from unresolved issues that originated in childhood.

Levels of Awareness

Freud believed that there were three levels of psychological awareness in operation. He used the image of an iceberg to describe these levels of awareness (Fig. 2.1).

Conscious. The **conscious** part of the mind is the tip of the iceberg. It contains all the material a person is aware of at any one time including perceptions, memories, thoughts, fantasies, and feelings.

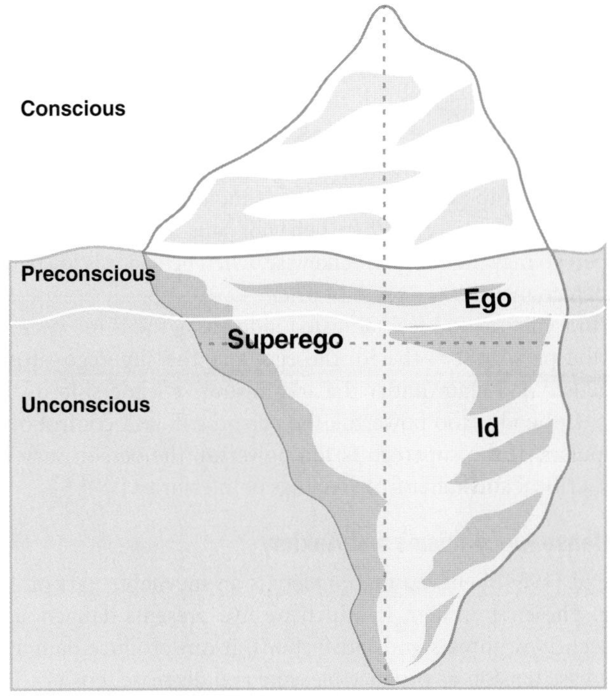

FIG. 2.1 The mind as an iceberg.

Preconscious. Just below the surface of awareness is the **preconscious**, which contains material that can be retrieved rather easily through conscious effort.

Unconscious. The **unconscious** includes all repressed memories, passions, and unacceptable urges lying deep below the surface. Memories and emotions associated with trauma may be stored in the unconscious because the individual finds it too painful to deal with them. The unconscious exerts a powerful yet unseen effect on the conscious thoughts and feelings of the individual. The individual is usually unable to retrieve unconscious material without the assistance of a trained therapist.

Personality Structure

Freud (1960) delineated three major and distinct but interactive systems of the personality: the id, the ego, and the superego.

Id. At birth we are all **id**. The id is totally unconscious and impulsive. It is the source of all drives, instincts, reflexes, and needs. The id cannot tolerate frustration and seeks to discharge tension and return to a more comfortable level of energy. The id lacks the ability to problem solve and is illogical. A hungry, screaming infant is the perfect example of id.

Ego. Within the first few years of life as the child begins to interact with others, the **ego** develops. The ego resides in the conscious, preconscious, and unconscious levels of awareness. The problem solver and reality tester, the ego attempts to navigate the outside world. It is able to differentiate subjective experiences, memory images, and objective reality.

The ego follows the reality principle, which says to the id, "You have to delay gratification for right now," then sets a course of action. For example, a hungry man feels tension arising from the id that wants to be fed. His ego allows him not only to think about his hunger but also to plan where he can eat and to seek that destination. This process is known as reality testing because the individual is factoring in reality to implement a plan to decrease tension.

Superego. The **superego**, which develops between the ages of 3 and 5, represents the moral component of personality. The superego resides in the conscious, preconscious, and unconscious levels of awareness. The superego consists of the conscience (all the "should nots" internalized from parents and society) and the ego ideal (all the "shoulds" internalized from parents and society). When behavior falls short of ideal, the superego may induce guilt. Likewise, when behavior is ideal, the superego may allow a sense of pride.

In a mature and well-adjusted individual, the three systems of the personality—the id, the ego, and the superego—work together as a team under the administrative leadership of the ego. If the id is too powerful, the person will lack control over impulses. If the superego is too powerful, the person may be self-critical and suffer from feelings of inferiority.

Defense Mechanisms and Anxiety

Freud (1969) believed that anxiety is an inevitable part of living. The environment in which we live presents dangers and insecurities, threats and satisfactions. It can produce pain and increase tension or produce pleasure and decrease tension. The ego develops defenses, or **defense mechanisms**, to ward off anxiety by preventing conscious awareness of threatening feelings.

Defense mechanisms share two common features: (1) they all (except suppression) operate on an unconscious level and (2) they deny, falsify, or distort reality to make it less threatening. Although we cannot survive without defense mechanisms, it is possible for our defense mechanisms to distort reality to such a degree that we experience difficulty with healthy adjustment and personal growth. Chapter 15 provides a full list and description of defense mechanisms.

Psychosexual Stages of Development

Freud believed that human development proceeds through five stages from infancy to adulthood. He believed that experiences during the first 5 years determined an individual's lifetime adjustment pattern and personality traits. By the time a child enters school, subsequent growth consists of elaborating on this basic structure. Freud's psychosexual stages of development are in Table 2.1.

Psychoanalytic Therapy

Classical psychoanalysis, as developed by Sigmund Freud, is seldom used today. Freud's premise that early intrapsychic conflict as the cause for all mental illness is no longer widely thought to be valid. Such therapy requires an unrealistically lengthy period of treatment (i.e., three to five times a week for many years), making it prohibitively expensive and uncovered by insurance.

The purpose of these sessions is to uncover unconscious conflicts. Free association, dream and fantasy analysis, defense mechanism recognition, and interpretation are tools used by the analyst.

Two concepts from classic psychoanalysis that are important for nurses to know are transference and countertransference (Freud, 1969). **Transference** refers to unconscious feelings that the patient has toward a healthcare worker that were originally felt in childhood for a significant other. The patient may say something like, "You remind me exactly of my sister." The transference may be positive (affectionate) or negative (hostile). Psychoanalysis actually encourages transference as a way to understand original relationships. Such exploration helps the patient to better understand certain feelings and behaviors.

Countertransference refers to unconscious feelings that the healthcare worker has toward the patient. For instance, if the patient reminds you of someone you do not like, you may unconsciously react as if the patient were that individual. Strong negative or positive feelings toward the patient could be a red flag for countertransference. Such responses underscore the importance of maintaining self-awareness and seeking supervisory guidance as therapeutic relationships progress. Chapter 8 talks more about countertransference and the nurse-patient relationship.

Psychodynamic Therapy

Psychodynamic therapy follows the psychoanalytic model by using many of the tools of psychoanalysis such as free association, dream analysis, transference, and countertransference. However, the therapist has increased involvement and interacts with the patient more freely than in traditional psychoanalysis. The therapy is oriented toward the here and now and makes less of an attempt to reconstruct the developmental origins of conflicts. Psychodynamic therapy tends to last longer than other common therapeutic modalities and may extend for more than 20 sessions, which insurance companies often reject.

The best candidates for psychodynamic therapy are relatively healthy and well-functioning individuals, sometimes referred to as the "worried well" who have a clear area of difficulty and are intelligent, psychologically minded, and well motivated for change. Patients with psychosis, severe depression, borderline personality disorders, and severe character disorders are not appropriate candidates for this type of treatment.

At the start of treatment, the patient and therapist agree on what the focus will be and concentrate their work on that focus. Sessions are held weekly, and the total number of sessions to be held is determined at the outset of therapy. There is a rapid, back-and-forth pattern between patient and therapist with both participating actively. The therapist intervenes constantly to keep the therapy on track, either by redirecting the patient's attention or by interpreting deviations from the focus to the patient.

Implications of Psychoanalytic Theory for Nursing Practice

Freud's theory offers a comprehensive explanation of complex human processes. It emphasizes the importance of childhood experiences on personality development. Nurses can be sources of support and education for both parents and children to promote a healthy emotional environment.

TABLE 2.1 **Freud's Psychosexual Stages of Development**

Stage (Age)	Source of Satisfaction	Primary Conflict	Tasks	Desired OutComes	Other Possible Personality Traits
Oral (0-1 yr)	Mouth (sucking, biting, chewing)	Weaning	Mastery of gratification of oral needs; beginning of ego development (4-5 mo)	Development of trust in the environment, with the realization that needs can be met	Fixation at the oral stage is associated with passivity, gullibility, and dependence; the use of sarcasm; may develop orally focused habits (e.g., smoking, nail-biting).
Anal (1-3 yr)	Anal region (expulsion and retention of feces)	Toilet training	Beginning of development of a sense of control over instinctual drives; ability to delay immediate gratification to gain a future goal	Control over impulses	Fixation at the anal stage is associated with anal retentiveness (stinginess, rigid thought patterns, obsessive-compulsive disorder) or anal-expulsive character (messiness, destructiveness, cruelty).
Phallic (oedipal; 3-6 yr)	Genitals (masturbation)	Oedipus and Electra	Sexual identity with parent of same sex; beginning of superego development	Identification with parent of the same sex	Fixation may result in reckless, self-assured, and narcissistic, person. Lack of resolution may result in inability to love and difficulties with sexual identity.
Latency (6-12 yr)	—	—	Growth of ego functions (social, intellectual, mechanical) and the ability to care about and relate to others outside the home (peers of the same sex)	The development of skills needed to cope with the environment	Fixations can result in difficulty identifying with others and in developing social skills, leading to a sense of inadequacy and inferiority.
Genital (12 yr and beyond)	Genitals (sexual intercourse)	—	Development of satisfying sexual and emotional relationship; emancipation from parents—planning of life goals and development of a sense of personal identity	The ability to be creative and find pleasure in love and work	Inability to negotiate this stage may derail emotional and financial independence, may impair personal identity and future goals, and disrupt ability to form satisfying intimate relationships.

Data from Gleitman, H. (1981). *Psychology*. New York, NY: W. W. Norton.

Freud's theory of the unconscious mind is particularly valuable as a baseline for considering the complexity of human behavior. By considering conscious and unconscious influences, a nurse can identify and begin to think about the root causes of patient suffering. Freud emphasized the importance of individual talk sessions characterized by attentive listening with a focus on underlying themes as an important tool of healing in psychiatric care.

INTERPERSONAL THEORIES AND THERAPIES

Interpersonal Theory

Harry Stack Sullivan (1892–1949), an American-born psychiatrist, developed a model for understanding psychiatric alterations that focused on interpersonal problems. Sullivan (1953) believed that human beings are driven by the need for interaction. Indeed, he viewed loneliness as the most painful human condition. He emphasized the early relationship with the primary parenting figure, or *significant other* (a term he coined), as crucial for personality development.

According to Sullivan, the purpose of all behavior is to get needs met through interpersonal interactions and to reduce or avoid anxiety. He defined *anxiety* as any painful feeling or emotion that arises from social insecurity or prevents biological needs from being satisfied. Sullivan coined the term *security operations* to describe measures the individual employs to reduce anxiety and enhance security. Collectively, all of the security operations an individual uses to defend against anxiety and ensure self-esteem make up the *self-system*.

Interpersonal Therapy

Interpersonal therapy is an effective short-term therapy. The assumption is that psychiatric disorders are influenced by interpersonal interactions and the social context. The goal of interpersonal therapy is to reduce or eliminate psychiatric symptoms (particularly depression) by improving interpersonal functioning and satisfaction with social relationships.

Interpersonal therapy has proven successful in the treatment of depression. Treatment is based on the notion that disturbances in important interpersonal relationships (or a deficit in one's capacity to form those relationships) can play a role in initiating or maintaining clinical depression. In interpersonal therapy, the therapist identifies the nature of the problem to be resolved and then selects strategies consistent with that problem area. Three types of problems in particular respond well to interpersonal therapy (Weissman et al., 2007):

1. **Grief and loss:** Complicated bereavement after death, divorce, or other loss
2. **Interpersonal disputes:** Conflicts with a significant other
3. **Role transition:** Problematic change in life status or social or vocational role

Implications of Interpersonal Theory to Nursing

Peplau's Theory of Interpersonal Relationships

Hildegard Peplau (1909–1999; Fig. 2.2), influenced by the work of Sullivan and learning theory, developed the first systematic theoretical framework for psychiatric nursing in her groundbreaking book *Interpersonal Relations in Nursing* (1952). Peplau not only established the foundation for the professional practice of psychiatric nursing but also continued to enrich psychiatric nursing theory and work for the advancement of nursing practice throughout her career.

Peplau was the first nurse to identify psychiatric-mental health nursing both as an essential element of general nursing and as a specialty area that embraces specific governing principles. She was also the first nurse theorist to describe the nurse-patient relationship as the foundation of nursing practice. She also shifted the focus from what nurses do *to* patients to what nurses do *with* patients.

Her theory is mainly concerned with the processes by which the nurse helps patients make positive changes in their health-care status and well-being. She believed that illness offered a unique opportunity for experiential learning, personal growth, and improved coping strategies. Psychiatric nurses play a central role in facilitating this growth.

Peplau proposed an approach in which nurses are both participants and observers in therapeutic conversations. She believed it was essential for nurses to observe the behavior not only of the patient but also of themselves. This self-awareness on the part of the nurse is essential in keeping the focus on the patient and in keeping the social and personal needs of the nurse out of the nurse-patient conversation.

Perhaps Peplau's most universal contribution to the everyday practice of psychiatric-mental health nursing is her application of Sullivan's theory of anxiety to nursing practice. She described the effects of different levels of anxiety (mild, moderate, severe, and panic) on perception and learning. She promoted interventions to lower anxiety with the aim of improving patients' abilities to think and function at more satisfactory levels. Chapter 15 presents more on the application of Peplau's theory of anxiety and interventions.

Table 2.2 lists selected nursing theorists and summarizes their major contributions and the impact of these contributions on psychiatric-mental health nursing.

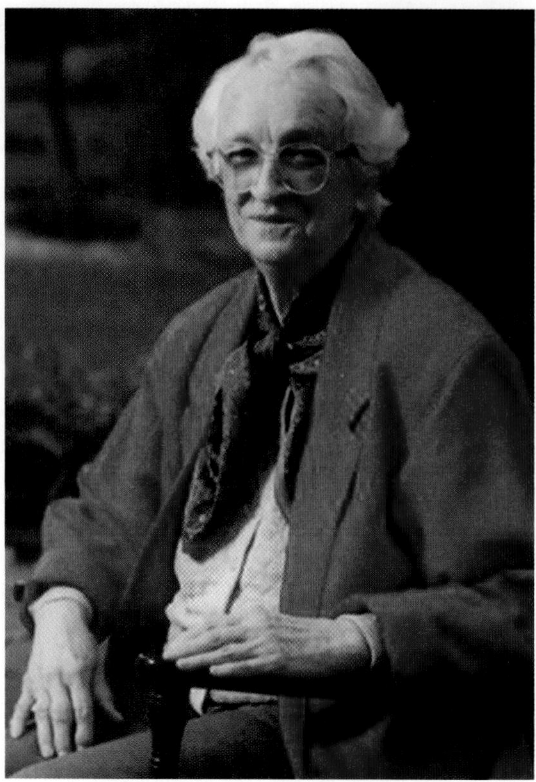

FIG. 2.2 Hildegard Peplau.

BEHAVIORAL THEORIES AND THERAPIES

Behavioral theories developed as a protest response to Freud's assumption that a person's destiny was carved in stone at a very early age. Behaviorists have no concern with inner conflicts but argue that personality simply consists of learned behaviors. Consequently, personality becomes synonymous with behavior—if behavior changes, so does the personality. Behaviorists believe that behavior can be influenced through a process referred to as conditioning. **Conditioning** involves pairing a behavior with a condition that reinforces or diminishes the behavior's occurrence.

Classical Conditioning Theory

Ivan Pavlov (1849–1936) was a Russian physiologist. He won a Nobel Prize for his outstanding contributions to the physiology of digestion, which he studied through his well-known experiments with dogs. In incidental observation of the dogs, Pavlov noticed that the dogs were able to anticipate when food would be forthcoming and would begin to salivate even before actually tasting the meat.

Pavlov formalized his observations of behaviors in dogs in a theory of **classical conditioning**. Pavlov (1928) found that when a neutral stimulus (a bell) was repeatedly paired with another stimulus (food that triggered salivation), eventually the sound of the bell alone could elicit salivation in the dogs. A human example of this response is a boy becoming ill after eating spoiled coleslaw at a picnic. Later in life, he feels nauseated whenever he smells coleslaw. It is important to recognize that classical conditioned responses are *involuntary*—not under conscious personal control—and are not spontaneous choices.

TABLE 2.2 Selected Nursing Theorists, Their Major Contributions, and Their Impact on Psychiatric-Mental Health Nursing

Nursing Theorist	Focus of Theory	Contribution to Psychiatric-Mental Health Nursing
Patricia Benner	Caring as foundation for nursing	Benner encourages nurses to provide caring and comforting interventions. She emphasizes the importance of the nurse-patient relationship and the importance of teaching and coaching the patient and bearing witness to suffering as the patient deals with illness.
Dorothea Orem	Goal of self-care as integral to the practice of nursing	Orem emphasizes the role of the nurse in promoting self-care activities of the patient; this has relevance to the seriously and persistently mentally ill patient.
Sister Callista Roy	Continual need for people to adapt physically, psychologically, and socially	Roy emphasizes the role of nursing in assisting patients to adapt so that they can cope more effectively with changes.
Betty Neuman	Impact of internal and external stressors on the equilibrium of the system	Neuman emphasizes the role of nursing in assisting patients to discover and use stress-reducing strategies.
Joyce Travelbee	Meaning in the nurse-patient relationship and the importance of communication	Travelbee emphasizes the role of nursing in affirming the suffering of the patient and in being able to alleviate that suffering through communication skills used appropriately through the stages of the nurse-patient relationship.

Data from Benner, P., & Wrubel, J. (1989). *The primacy of caring: Stress and coping in health and illness.* Menlo Park, CA: Addison-Wesley; Leddy, S., & Pepper, J. M. (1993). *Conceptual bases of professional nursing* (3rd ed., pp. 174–175). Philadelphia, PA: Lippincott; Neuman, B., & Young, R. (1972). A model for teaching total-person approach to patient problems. *Nursing Research, 21,* 264–269; Orem, D. E. (1995). *Nursing: Concepts of practice* (5th ed.). New York, NY: McGraw-Hill; Roy, C., & Andrews, H. A. (1991). *The Roy adaptation model: The definitive statement.* Norwalk, CT: Appleton & Lange; Travelbee, J. (1961). *Intervention in psychiatric nursing.* Philadelphia, PA: F. A. Davis.

Behavioral Theory

John B. Watson (1878–1958) was an American psychologist who rejected the unconscious motivation of psychoanalysis for being too subjective. He developed the school of thought referred to as *behaviorism,* which he believed was more objective or measurable. Watson (1919) contended that personality traits and responses—adaptive and maladaptive—were socially learned through classical conditioning. In a famous (but terrible) experiment, Watson stood behind Little Albert, a 9-month-old who liked animals, and made a loud noise with a hammer every time the infant reached for a white rat. After this experiment, Little Albert became terrified at the sight of white fur or hair, even in the absence of a loud noise. Watson concluded that controlling the environment could mold behavior and that anyone could be trained to be anything, from a beggar man to a merchant.

Operant Conditioning Theory

B. F. Skinner (1904–1990) represented the second wave of behavioral theorists. Skinner (1987) researched **operant conditioning,** a method of learning that occurs through rewards and punishment for *voluntary* behavior. Behavioral responses are elicited through **reinforcement,** which causes a behavior to occur *more* frequently.

Skinner conducted experiments with laboratory animals in what is now referred to as a Skinner Box. The contents of this box included a lever and an electric grid (Fig. 2.3). To cause behavior *more* frequently, Skinner used two methods. When a hungry rat pressed the lever, it would receive a food pellet. He learned to go straight to the lever for food. This is **positive reinforcement** of the behavior. Another rat was placed in the cage with an electrical charge on the grid under his feet. If he accidentally pressed the lever, the charge would turn off. He learned to go straight to the lever to eliminate the shock. This removal of an objectionable or averse stimulus is **negative reinforcement.**

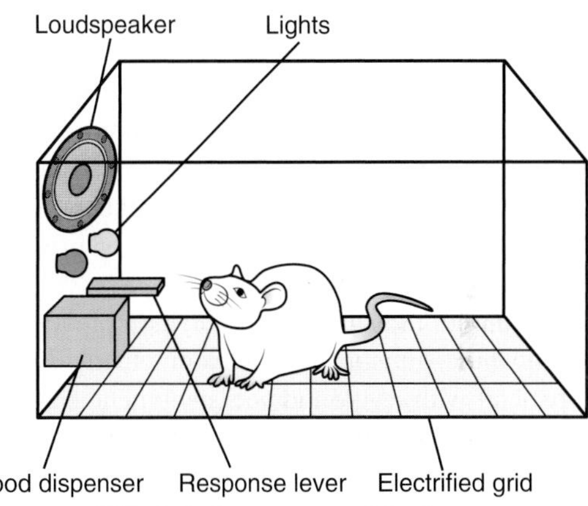

FIG. 2.3 Operant conditioning.

Other techniques can cause behaviors to occur *less* frequently. One technique is an unpleasant consequence, or **punishment.** Driving too fast may result in a speeding ticket, which—in mature and healthy individuals—decreases the chances that speeding will occur.

Absence of reinforcement, or **extinction,** also decreases behavior by withholding a reward that has become habitual. If a person tells a joke and no one laughs, for example, the person is less apt to tell jokes because his joke-telling behavior is not being reinforced. Teachers employ this strategy in the classroom when they ignore acting-out behavior that had previously been rewarded by more attention.

Behavioral Therapy

Behavioral therapy is based on the assumption that changes in maladaptive behavior can occur without insight into the underlying cause. This approach works best when it is directed at specific problems and the goals are well defined. Behavioral therapy is effective in treating people with phobias, alcoholism, schizophrenia, and many other conditions. Four types of behavioral therapy are discussed here: modeling, operant conditioning, systematic desensitization, and aversion therapy.

Modeling

In modeling, the therapist provides a role model for specific identified behaviors, and the patient learns through imitation. The therapist may do the modeling, provide another person to model the behaviors, or present a video for the purpose. Bandura, Blanchard, and Ritter (1969) were able to help people reduce their phobias about nonpoisonous snakes. They did this by having them first view closeups of filmed encounters between people and snakes that resulted in successful outcomes. Afterward they viewed live encounters between people and snakes that also had successful outcomes.

In a similar fashion, some behavior therapists use role playing in the consulting room. They demonstrate patterns of behavior that might prove more effective than those usually engaged in and then have the patients practice these new behaviors. For example, a student who does not know how to ask a professor for an extension on a term paper would watch the therapist portray a potentially effective way of making the request. The clinician would then help the student practice the new skill in a similar role-playing situation.

Operant Conditioning

Operant conditioning is the basis for behavior modification and uses positive reinforcement to increase desired behaviors. For example, when desired goals are achieved or behaviors are performed, patients might be rewarded with tokens. These tokens can be exchanged for food, small luxuries, or privileges. This reward system is known as a *token economy*.

Operant conditioning has been useful in improving the verbal behaviors of mute, autistic, and developmentally disabled children. In patients with severe and persistent mental illness, behavior modification has helped increase levels of self-care, social behavior, group participation, and more. You may find this a useful technique as you proceed through your clinical rotations.

A familiar case in point of positive reinforcement is the mother who takes her preschooler along to the grocery store, and the child starts acting out, demanding candy, nagging, crying, and yelling. Here are examples of three ways the child's behavior can be reinforced:

Action	Result
1. The mother gives the child the candy.	The child continues to use this behavior. This is positive reinforcement of negative behavior.
2. The mother scolds the child.	Acting out may continue, because the child gets what he really wants—attention. This positively rewards negative behavior.
3. The mother ignores the acting out but gives attention to the child when he is acting appropriately.	The child gets a positive reward for appropriate behavior.

Systematic Desensitization

Systematic desensitization is another form of behavior modification therapy that involves the development of behavior tasks customized to the patient's specific fears; these tasks are presented to the patient while using learned relaxation techniques. The process involves four steps:

1. The patient's fear is broken down into its components by exploring the particular stimulus cues to which the patient reacts. For example, certain situations may precipitate a phobic reaction, whereas others do not. Crowds at parties may be problematic, whereas similar numbers of people in other settings do not cause the same distress.
2. The patient is exposed to the fear little by little. For example, a patient who has a fear of flying is introduced to short periods of visual presentations of flying—first with still pictures, then with videos, and finally in a busy airport. The situations are confronted while the patient is in a relaxed state. Gradually, over a period of time, exposure is increased until anxiety about or fear of the object or situation has ceased.
3. The patient is instructed in how to design a hierarchy of fears. For fear of flying, a patient might develop a set of statements representing the stages of a flight, order the statements from the most fearful to the least fearful, and use relaxation techniques to reach a state of relaxation as they progress through the list.
4. The patient practices these techniques every day.

Aversion Therapy

Aversion therapy is used to treat behaviors such as alcoholism, paraphilic disorders, shoplifting, violent and aggressive behavior, and self-mutilation. Aversion therapy is the pairing of a negative stimulus with a specific target behavior, thereby suppressing the behavior. This treatment may be used when other less drastic measures have failed to produce the desired effects.

Simple examples of extinguishing undesirable behavior through aversion therapy include painting foul-tasting substances on the fingernails of nail biters or the thumbs of thumb suckers. Other examples of aversive stimuli are chemicals that induce nausea and vomiting, unpleasant odors, unpleasant verbal stimuli (e.g., descriptions of disturbing scenes), costs or fines in a token economy, and denial of positive reinforcement (e.g., isolation).

Before initiating any aversive protocol, the therapist, treatment team, or society *must* answer the following questions:

- Is this therapy in the best interest of the patient?
- Does its use violate the patient's rights?
- Is it in the best interest of society?

If the therapist believes aversion therapy as the most appropriate treatment, ongoing supervision, support, and evaluation of those administering it must occur.

Biofeedback

Biofeedback is also a form of behavioral therapy and is successfully used today, especially for controlling the body's physiological response to stress and anxiety. Chapter 10 discusses biofeedback in further detail.

Implications of Behavioral Theory to Nursing

Behavior and health are inextricably linked. Consider the toll that such behaviors as smoking, overeating, alcohol and substance use problems, and inactivity take on the body and mind. A behavioral model provides a concrete method for modifying or replacing undesirable behaviors. An example of a nurse teaching a behavioral technique is smoking cessation. For example, a therapist teaches patients to modify routines to reduce smoking cues such as avoiding bars.

Nurses may work in units based on behavioral principles, particularly with children and adolescents. *Token economies* represent extensions of Skinner's thoughts on learning. In a token economy, patients' positive behaviors are reinforced with tokens. These tokens may be small plastic disks, checkmarks, or coins with no real value that can be used in exchange for materials (e.g., candy, gum, books) or services (e.g., phone calls, time off the unit, recognition).

COGNITIVE THEORIES AND THERAPIES

While behaviorists focused on increasing, decreasing, or eliminating measurable behaviors, they did not focus on the thoughts, or cognitions, that were involved in these behaviors. Rather than thinking of people as passive recipients of environmental conditioning, cognitive theorists proposed that there is a dynamic interplay between individuals and the environment. These theorists believe that thoughts come before feelings and actions, and thoughts about the world and our place in it are based on our own unique perspectives, which may or may not be based on reality. This section presents two of the most influential theorists and their therapies.

Rational-Emotive Therapy

Albert Ellis (1913–2007) developed rational-emotive therapy in 1955. The aim of rational-emotive therapy is to remove core irrational beliefs by helping people recognize thoughts that are not accurate, sensible, or useful. These thoughts tend to take the form of *shoulds* (e.g., "I should always be polite."), *oughts* (e.g., "I ought to consistently win my tennis games."), and musts (e.g., "I must be thin."). Ellis described negative thinking as a simple A-B-C process. *A* stands for the activating event, *B* stands for beliefs about the event, and *C* stands for emotional consequence as a result of the event.

A Activating Event	→	**B Beliefs**	→	**C Emotional Consequence**

Perception influences all thoughts, which in turn influence our behaviors. It often boils down to the simple notion of perceiving the glass as half full or half empty. For example, imagine you have just received an invitation to a birthday party (activating event). You think, "I hate parties. Now I have to hang out with people who don't like me instead of watching my favorite television shows. They probably just invited me to get a gift" (beliefs). You will probably be miserable (emotional consequence) if you go. On the other hand, you may think, "I love parties! This will be a great chance to meet new people, and it will be fun to shop for the perfect gift" (beliefs). You could have a delightful time (emotional consequence).

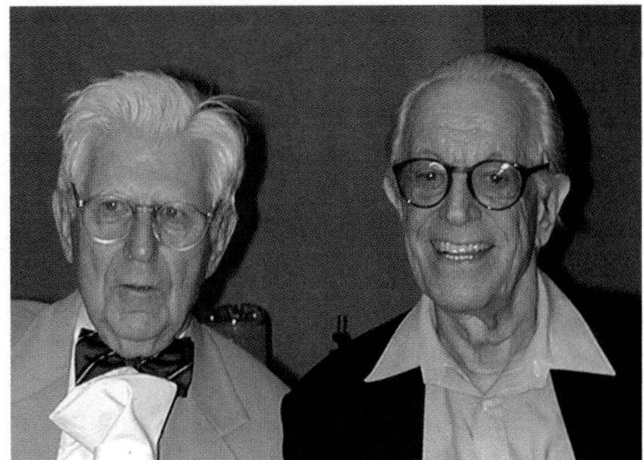

FIG. 2.4 Aaron Beck and Albert Ellis. (Courtesy of Fenichel, 2000.)

Although Ellis (Fig. 2.4) recognized the role of past experiences on current beliefs, the focus of rational-emotive therapy is on present attitudes, painful feelings, and dysfunctional behaviors. If our beliefs are negative and self-deprecating, we are more susceptible to depression and anxiety. Ellis noted that while we cannot change the past, we can change the way we are now. He was pragmatic in his approach to mental illness and colorful in his therapeutic advice. "It's too [darn] bad you panic, but you don't die from it! Get them over the panic about panic, you may find the panic disappears" (Ellis, 2000).

Cognitive-Behavioral Therapy

Aaron T. Beck (see Fig. 2.4) was originally trained in psychoanalysis. He noticed that people with depression thought differently than people who were not depressed. They had stereotypical patterns of negative and self-critical thinking that seemed to distort their ability to think and process information. To challenge these negative patterns, he developed **cognitive-behavioral therapy (CBT)**, which is based on both cognitive psychology and behavioral theory.

Beck's method (Beck et al., 1979), the basis for CBT, is an active, directive, time-limited, structured approach. This evidence-based therapy is used to treat a variety of psychiatric disorders such as depression, anxiety, phobias, and pain. It is based on the underlying theoretical principle that feelings and behaviors are largely determined by the way people think about the world and their place in it (Beck, 1967). Their cognitions (verbal or pictorial events in their streams of consciousness) are based on attitudes or assumptions developed from previous experiences. These cognitions may be fairly accurate or distorted.

According to Beck, people have *schemas*, or unique assumptions about themselves, others, and the world in general. For example, if a man has the schema, "The only person I can trust is myself," he will have expectations that everyone else has questionable motives, are dishonest, and will eventually hurt him. Other negative schemas include incompetence, abandonment, evilness, and vulnerability. People are typically not aware of such cognitive biases.

Rapid, unthinking responses based on schemas are known as **automatic thoughts**. These responses are particularly intense and frequent in psychiatric disorders such as depression and anxiety. Often automatic thoughts, or **cognitive distortions**, are irrational and lead to false assumptions and misinterpretations. For example, if a woman interprets all experiences in terms of whether she is competent and adequate, thinking may be dominated by the cognitive distortion, "Unless I do everything perfectly, I'm a failure." Consequently, the person reacts to situations in terms of adequacy, even when these situations are unrelated to whether she is personally competent. Table 2.3 describes common cognitive distortions.

Therapeutic techniques are designed to identify, reality test, and correct distorted conceptualizations and the dysfunctional beliefs underlying them. Patients are taught to challenge their own negative thinking and substitute it with positive, rational thoughts. They learn to recognize when thinking is based on distortions and misconceptions.

Homework assignments play an important role in CBT. A particularly useful technique is the use of a four-column format to record the precipitating event or situation, the resulting automatic thought, and the proceeding feeling(s) and behavior(s). Finally, a challenge to the negative thoughts based on rational evidence and thinking is listed in the last column. The following is an example of the type of analysis done by a patient receiving CBT.

A 24-year-old nurse who was recently discharged from the hospital for severe depression presented this record (Beck, 1979):

Event	Feeling	Cognitions	Other Possible Interpretations
While at a party, Cory asked me, "How is it going?" a few days after I was discharged from the hospital.	Anxious	Cory thinks I am crazy. I must really look bad for him to be concerned.	He really cares about me. He noticed that I look better than before I went into the hospital and wants to know if I feel better too.

Table 2.4 compares and contrasts psychodynamic, interpersonal, cognitive-behavioral, and behavioral therapies.

Implications of Cognitive Theories for Nursing

Recognizing the interplay between events, negative thinking, and negative responses can be beneficial from both a patient-care standpoint and a personal one. As a supportive therapeutic measure, helping the patient identify negative thought patterns is a worthwhile intervention. Workbooks are available to aid in the process of identifying cognitive distortions.

The cognitive approach can also help nurses understand their own responses to a variety of difficult situations. One example might be the anxiety that some students feel regarding the psychiatric nursing clinical rotation. Students may overgeneralize ("All psychiatric patients are dangerous.") or personalize ("My patient doesn't seem to be better. I'm probably not doing him any good.") the situation. The key to effectively using this approach in clinical situations is to challenge the negative thoughts not based on facts then replace them with more realistic appraisals.

HUMANISTIC THEORIES

In the 1950s humanistic theories arose as a protest against both the behavioral and psychoanalytic schools, which were thought to be pessimistic, deterministic, and dehumanizing. Humanistic theories focus on human potential and free will to choose life patterns supportive of personal growth. Humanistic frameworks emphasize a person's capacity for self-actualization. This approach focuses on understanding the patient's perspective as he or she subjectively experiences it. There are a number of humanistic theorists, and this text will explore Abraham Maslow and his theory of self-actualization.

Theory of Human Motivation

Abraham Maslow (1908–1970) is considered the father of humanistic psychology. He criticized other therapies for focusing too intently on humanity's frailties and not enough on its strengths. Maslow contended that the focus of psychology must go beyond experiences of hate, pain, misery, guilt, and conflict to include love, compassion, happiness, exhilaration, and well-being.

Hierarchy of Needs

Maslow believed that human beings are motivated by unmet needs. Maslow (1968) focused on human need fulfillment, which he categorized into six incremental stages, beginning with physiological survival needs and ending with self-transcendent needs (Fig. 2.5). The hierarchy of needs is conceptualized as a pyramid with the strongest, most fundamental needs placed on the lower levels. The higher levels—the more distinctly human needs—occupy the top sections of the pyramid. When lower-level needs are met, higher needs are able to emerge.

- **Physiological needs:** The most basic needs are the physiological drives—needing food, oxygen, water, sleep, sex, and a constant body temperature. If all needs were deprived, this level would take priority over the rest.
- **Safety needs:** Once physiological needs are met, safety needs emerge. They include security; protection; freedom from fear, anxiety, and chaos; and the need for law, order, and limits. Adults in a stable society usually feel safe, but they may feel threatened by debt, job insecurity, or lack of insurance. It is during times of crisis, such as war, disasters, assaults, and social breakdown, when safety needs take precedence. Children, who are more vulnerable and dependent, respond far more readily and intensely to safety threats.
- **Belonging and love needs:** People have a need for intimate relationships, love, affection, and belonging and will seek to overcome feelings of loneliness and alienation. Maslow stresses the importance of having a family and a home and being part of identifiable groups.

TABLE 2.3 **Common Cognitive Distortions**

Distortion	Definition	Example
All-or-nothing thinking	Thinking in black and white, reducing complex outcomes into absolutes	Although Lindsey earned the second highest score in the state's cheerleading competition, she consistently referred to herself as "a loser."
Overgeneralization	Using a bad outcome (or a few bad outcomes) as evidence that nothing will ever go right again	Andrew had a minor traffic accident. He is reluctant to drive and says, "I shouldn't be allowed on the road."
Labeling	A form of generalization in which a characteristic or event becomes definitive and results in an overly harsh label for self or others	"Because I failed the advanced statistics exam, I am a failure. I might as well give up. I may as well quit and look for an easier major."
Mental filter	Focusing on a negative detail or bad event and allowing it to taint everything else	Anne's boss evaluated her work as exemplary and gave her a few suggestions for improvement. She obsessed about the suggestions and ignored the rest.
Disqualifying the positive	Maintaining a negative view by rejecting information that supports a positive view as being irrelevant, inaccurate, or accidental	"I've just been offered the job I thought I always wanted. There must have been no other applicants."
Jumping to conclusions	Making a negative interpretation despite the fact that there is little or no supporting evidence	"My fiancé, Juan, didn't call me for 3 hours, which just proves he doesn't love me anymore."
a. Mind-reading	Inferring negative thoughts, responses, and motives of others	Isabel is giving a presentation and a man in the audience is sleeping. She panics, "I must be boring."
b. Fortune-telling error	Anticipating that things will turn out badly as an established fact	"I'll ask her out, but I know she won't have a good time."
Magnification or minimization	Exaggerating the importance of something (such as a personal failure or the success of others) or reducing the importance of something (such as a personal success or the failure of others)	"I'm alone on a Saturday night because no one likes me. When other people are alone, it's because they want to be."
a. Catastrophizing	Catastrophizing is an extreme form of magnification in which the very worst is assumed to be a probable outcome	"If I don't make a good impression on the boss at the company picnic, she will fire me."
Emotional reasoning	Drawing a conclusion based on an emotional state	"I'm nervous about the exam. I must not be prepared. If I were, I wouldn't be afraid."
"Should" and "must" statements	Rigid self-directives that presume an unrealistic amount of control over external events	Renee believes that a patient with diabetes has high blood sugar today because she's not a very good nurse and that her patients should always get better.
Personalization	Assuming responsibility for an external event or situation that was likely outside personal control	"I'm sorry your party wasn't more fun. It's probably because I was there."

Modified from Burns, D. D. (1989). *The feeling good handbook.* New York, NY: William Morrow.

- **Esteem needs:** People need to have a high self-regard and have it reflected to them from others. If self-esteem needs are met, they feel confident, valued, and valuable. When self-esteem is compromised, they feel inferior, worthless, and helpless.
- **Self-actualization:** Human beings are preset to strive to be everything they are capable of becoming. Maslow said, "What a man *can* be, he *must* be." What people are capable of becoming is highly individual—an artist must paint, a writer must write, and a healer must heal. The drive to satisfy this need is felt as a sort of restlessness, a sense that something is missing. It is up to each person to choose a path that will bring about inner peace and fulfillment.

Although Maslow's early work included only five levels of needs, he later took into account two additional factors: (1) cognitive needs (the desire to know and understand) and (2) aesthetic needs (Maslow, 1970). He describes the acquisition of knowledge (our first priority) and the need to understand (our second priority) as being hard-wired and essential. The aesthetic need for beauty and symmetry is universal.

You may be interested to know that Maslow (1970) developed his theory by investigating people whom he believed were self-actualized. Among these people were historical figures such as Abraham Lincoln, Thomas Jefferson, Harriet Tubman, Walt Whitman, Ludwig van Beethoven, William James, and Franklin D. Roosevelt. Other people he investigated were living at the time of his studies. They include Albert Einstein, Eleanor Roosevelt, and Albert Schweitzer. Box 2.1 identifies basic personality characteristics that distinguish self-actualizing people.

Implications of Motivation Theory for Nursing

The value of Maslow's model in nursing practice is twofold. First, an emphasis on human potential and the patient's strengths is key to successful nurse-patient relationships. Second, the model helps establish what is most important in the sequencing of nursing actions. For example, to collect any but the most essential information when a patient is struggling with drug withdrawal may be dangerous. Following Maslow's model as a way of prioritizing actions, the nurse meets the patient's physiological need for stable vital signs and pain relief before collecting general information for a nursing database.

TABLE 2.4 **Comparison of Psychoanalytic, Interpersonal, Cognitive-Behavioral, and Behavioral Therapies**

Aspects of Therapy	Psychodynamic Therapy	Interpersonal Therapy	Cognitive-Behavioral Therapy	Behavioral Therapy
Treatment focus	Unresolved past relationships and core conflicts	Current interpersonal relationships and social supports	Thoughts and cognitions	Learned maladaptive behavior
Therapist role	Significant other Transference object	Problem solver	Active, directive, challenging	Active, directive teacher
Primary disorders treated	Anxiety Depression Personality disorders	Depression	Depression Anxiety/panic Eating disorders	Posttraumatic stress disorder Obsessive-compulsive disorder Panic disorder
Length of therapy	20+ sessions	Short term (12-20 sessions)	Short term (5-20 sessions)	Varies, typically fewer than 10 sessions
Technique	Therapeutic alliance Free association Understanding transference Challenging defense mechanisms	Facilitate new patterns of communication and expectations for relationships	Evaluating thoughts and behaviors Modifying dysfunctional thoughts and behaviors	Relaxation Thought stopping Self-reassurance Seeking social support

Data from Dewan, M. J., Steenbarger, B. N., & Greenberg, R. P. (2014). Brief psychotherapies. In R. E. Hales, S. C. Yudofsky, & L.W. Roberts (Eds.), *Textbook of Psychiatry* (6th ed., pp. 1037–1064). Arlington, VA: American Psychiatric Publishing.

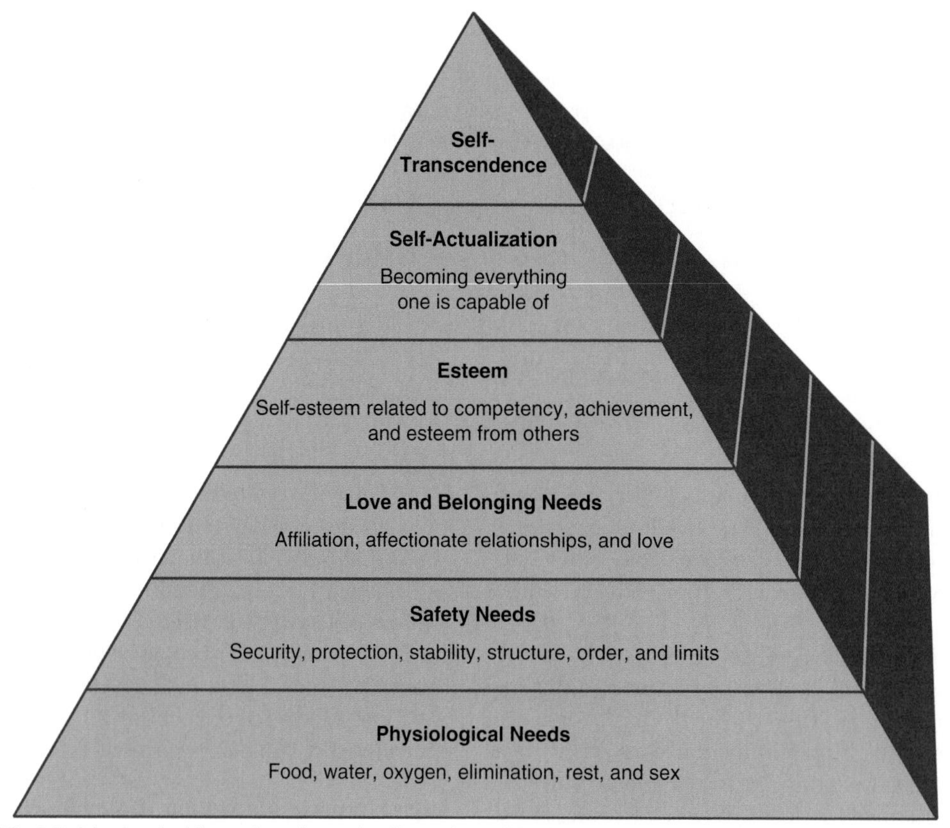

FIG. 2.5 Maslow's hierarchy of needs. (Data from Maslow, A. H. [1972]. *The farther reaches of human nature*. New York, NY: Viking.)

BIOLOGICAL THEORIES AND THERAPIES

Biological Model

A biological model, or medical model, of mental illness assumes that abnormal behavior is the result of a physical problem. It focuses on neurological, chemical, biological, and genetic issues. Adherents of this dominant model seek to understand how the body and brain interact to create emotions, memories, and perceptual experiences. The biological model locates the illness or disease in the body—usually in the limbic system of the brain and the synapse receptor sites of the central nervous system—and targets the site of the illness using physical interventions such as drugs, diet, or surgery.

BOX 2.1 Some Characteristics of Self-Actualized Persons

- Accurate perception of reality. Not defensive in their perceptions of the world.
- Acceptance of themselves, others, and nature.
- Spontaneity, simplicity, and naturalness. Self-actualized individuals do not live programmed lives.
- Problem-centered rather than self-centered orientation. Possibly the most important characteristic. Possibly the most important characteristic is a sense of a mission to which they dedicate their lives.
- Pleasure in being alone and in ability to reflect on events.
- Active social interest.
- People who are self-actualized don't take life for granted.
- Mystical or peak experiences. A peak experience is a moment of intense ecstasy, similar to a religious or mystical experience, during which the self is transcended.
- Self-actualized people may become so involved in what they are doing that they lose all sense of time and awareness of self (*flow experience*).
- Lighthearted sense of humor that indicates "we're in it together" and lacks sarcasm or hostility.
- Fairness and respect for people of different races, ethnicities, religions, and political views.
- Creativity, especially in managing their lives.
- Resistance to conformity (enculturation). Self-actualization results in autonomous, independent, and self-sufficient individuals.

Adapted from Maslow, A. H. (1970). *Motivation and personality*. New York, NY: Harper & Row.

The recognition that psychiatric illnesses are as physical in origin as diabetes and coronary heart disease serves to decrease the stigma surrounding them. Just as someone with diabetes or heart disease cannot be held responsible for being ill, patients with schizophrenia or bipolar affective disorder are no more to blame.

Biological Therapies

Psychopharmacology therapy. In 1950 a French drug firm synthesized chlorpromazine—a powerful antipsychotic medication—and psychiatry experienced a revolution. The advent of psychopharmacology—the use of medications to treat mental illness—presented a strong alternative to psychological approaches for mental illness. The dramatic experience of observing patients freed from the bondage of psychosis and mania by powerful drugs such as chlorpromazine and lithium left witnesses convinced of the critical role of the brain in psychiatric illness.

Since the discovery of chlorpromazine (later sold under the trade name Thorazine), many other medications have proven effective in controlling psychosis, mania, depression, and anxiety. These medications greatly reduce the need for hospitalization and dramatically improve the lives of people suffering from serious psychiatric difficulties. Today, psychoactive medications exert differential effects on different neurotransmitters and help restore brain function, allowing patients with mental illness to continue living productive lives with greater satisfaction and far less emotional pain.

Brain stimulation therapies. In addition to psychotherapy and psychopharmacology as treatment for mental illness are the brain stimulation therapies. The oldest of these therapies is electroconvulsive therapy (ECT). All of these methods involve focused electrical stimulation of the brain. In addition to treating psychiatric disorders, they also treat traditional neurological disorders such as Parkinson's disease, epilepsy, and pain conditions. Table 2.5 provides a summary of Food and Drug Administration–approved brain stimulation treatments and their use.

Implications of the Biological Model for Nursing

Historically, psychiatric-mental health nurses always have attended to the physical needs of psychiatric patients. Nurses administer medications. They also monitor sleep, activity, nutrition, hydration, elimination, and other functions. Nurses are responsible for preparing patients for somatic therapies such as electroconvulsive therapy. Physical needs and physical care in psychiatric nursing are provided as part of a holistic approach to healthcare. Basic nursing strategies such as focusing on the qualities of a therapeutic relationship, understanding the patient's perspective, and communicating in a way that facilitates the patient's recovery take place alongside physical care.

DEVELOPMENTAL THEORIES

Cognitive Development

Jean Piaget (1896–1980) was a Swiss psychologist and researcher. While working at a boys' school run by Alfred Binet, developer of the Binet Intelligence Test, Piaget helped to score these tests. He became fascinated by the fact that young children consistently gave wrong answers on intelligence tests, wrong answers that revealed a discernible pattern of cognitive processing that was different from that of older children and adults. He concluded that cognitive development was a dynamic progression from primitive awareness and simple reflexes to complex thought and responses. Our mental representations of the world, or schemata, depend on the cognitive stage we have reached.

- *Sensorimotor stage (birth to 2 years).* Begins with basic reflexes and culminates with purposeful movement, spatial abilities, and hand-eye coordination. Physical interaction with the environment provides the child with a basic understanding of the world. By about 9 months, object permanence is achieved, and the child can conceptualize objects that are no longer visible. This explains the delight of the game of peek-a-boo as an emerging skill, as the child begins to anticipate the face hidden behind the hands.
- *Preoperational stage (2 to 7 years).* Operations is a term used to describe thinking about objects. Children are not yet able to think abstractly or generalize qualities in the absence of specific objects, but rather think in a concrete fashion. Egocentric thinking is demonstrated through a tendency to expect others to view the world as they do. They are also unable to conserve mass, volume, or number. An example of this inability is thinking that a tall, thin glass holds more liquid than a short, wide glass.
- *Concrete operational stage (7 to 11 years).* Logical thought appears and abstract problem solving is possible. The child is able to see a situation from another's point of view and can

TABLE 2.5 Summary of Approved Brain Stimulation Treatments and Their Use

Treatment	Convulsive?	Site	Disorders
Electroconvulsive therapy (ECT)	Yes	Cortical	Depression, mania, catatonia
Transcranial magnetic stimulation-repetitive (rTMS)	No	Cortical	Depression
Vagus nerve stimulation (VNS)	No	Cervical cranial nerve	Depression
Deep brain stimulation (DBS)	No	Subcortical	Depression, obsessive-compulsive disorder

take into account a variety of solutions to a problem. Conservation is possible. For example, two small cups hold an amount of liquid equal to a tall glass. They are able to classify based on discrete characteristics, order objects in a pattern, and understand the concept of reversibility.

- *Formal operational stage (11 years to adulthood).* Conceptual reasoning commences at approximately the same time as does puberty. At this stage, the child's basic abilities to think abstractly and problem solve mirror those of an adult.

Theory of Psychosocial Development

Erik Erikson (1902–1994), an American psychoanalyst, began as a follower of Freud. Erikson (1963) came to believe that Freudian theory was restrictive and negative in its approach. He also stressed that more than the limited mother-child-father triangle influences an individual's development. He emphasized the role of culture and society on personality development. According to Erikson, personality was not set in stone at age 5, as Freud suggested, but continued to evolve throughout the life span.

Erikson described development as occurring in eight predetermined and consecutive life stages (psychosocial crises), each of which results in a positive or negative outcome. The successful or unsuccessful completion of each stage will affect the individual's progression to the next (Table 2.6). For example, Erikson's crisis of industry versus inferiority occurs from the ages of 7 to 12. During this stage, the child's task is to gain a sense of personal abilities and competence and to expand relationships beyond the immediate family to include peers. The attainment of this task (industry) brings with it the virtue of confidence. The child who fails to navigate this stage successfully is unable to master age-appropriate tasks, cannot make a connection with peers, and will feel like a failure (inferiority).

Theory of Object Relations

The theory of object relations was developed by interpersonal theorists who emphasize past relationships in influencing a person's sense of self as well as the nature and quality of relationships in the present. The term *object* refers to another person, particularly a significant person.

Margaret Mahler (1895–1985) was a Hungarian-born child psychologist who worked with emotionally disturbed children. She developed a framework for studying how an infant transitions from complete self-absorption, with an inability to separate from its mother, to a physically and psychologically differentiated toddler. Mahler (1975) believed that psychological problems were largely the result of a disruption of this separation.

During the first 3 years, the significant other (e.g., the mother) provides a secure base of support that promotes enough confidence for the child to separate. This is achieved by a balance of holding (emotionally and physically) a child enough for the child to feel safe while encouraging independence and natural exploration.

Problems may arise in this process. If a toddler leaves his or her mother on the park bench and wanders off to the sandbox, the child should be encouraged with smiles and reassurance, "Go on honey. It's safe to go away a little." Then the mother needs to be reliably present when the toddler returns, thereby rewarding his or her efforts. Mahler notes that raising healthy children does not require that parents never make mistakes and that "good enough parenting" will promote successful separation-individuation.

Theories of Moral Development

Stages of Moral Development

Lawrence Kohlberg (1927–1987) was an American psychologist whose work reflected and expanded on Piaget's by applying his theory to moral development, a development that coincided with cognitive development (Crain, 1985). While visiting Israel, Kohlberg became convinced that children living in a kibbutz had advanced moral development, and he believed that the atmosphere of trust, respect, and self-governance nurtured this development. In the United States, he created schools or "just communities" that were grounded on these concepts. Based on interviews with youths, Kohlberg developed a theory of how people progressively develop a sense of morality (Kohlberg & Turiel, 1971).

His theory provides a framework for understanding the progression from black-and-white thinking about right and wrong to a complex, variable, and context-dependent decision-making process regarding the rightness or wrongness of action.

Preconventional level

Stage 1: Obedience and punishment. The hallmarks of this stage are a focus on rules and on listening to authority. People at this stage believe that obedience is the method to avoid punishment.

Stage 2: Individualism and exchange. Individuals become aware that not everyone thinks the way that they do, and that different people see rules differently. If they or others decide to break the rules, they are risking punishment.

Conventional level

Stage 3: Good interpersonal relationships. Children begin to view rightness or wrongness as related to motivations, personality, or the goodness or badness of the person. Generally speaking, people should get along and have similar values.

TABLE 2.6 Erikson's Eight Stages of Development

Approximate Age	Developmental Task	Psychosocial Crisis	Successful Resolution of Crisis	Unsuccessful Resolution of Crisis
Infancy (0-1½ yr)	Forming attachment to mother, which lays foundations for later trust in others	Trust versus mistrust	Sound basis for relating to other people; trust in people; faith and hope about environment and future "If he's late in picking me up, there must be a good reason."	General difficulties relating to people effectively; suspicion; trust-fear conflict; fear of future "I can't trust anyone; no one has ever been there when I needed them."
Early childhood (1½-3 yr)	Gaining some basic control of self and environment (e.g., toilet training, exploration)	Autonomy versus shame and doubt	Sense of self-control and adequacy; will power "I'm sure that with the proper diet and exercise program, I can achieve my target weight."	Independence/fear conflict; severe feelings of self-doubt "I could never lose the weight they want me to, so why even try?"
Preschool (3-6 yr)	Becoming purposeful and directive	Initiative versus guilt	Ability to initiate one's own activities; sense of purpose "I like to help mommy set the table for dinner."	Aggression/fear conflict; sense of inadequacy or guilt "I wanted the candy, so I took it."
School age (6-12 yr)	Developing social, physical, and school skills	Industry versus inferiority	Competence; ability to work "I'm getting really good at swimming since I've been taking lessons."	Sense of inferiority; difficulty learning and working "I can't read as well as the others in my class; I'm just dumb."
Adolescence (12-20 yr)	Making transition from childhood to adulthood; developing sense of identity	Identity versus role confusion	Sense of personal identity; fidelity "I'm going to go to college to be an engineer; I hope to get married before I am 30."	Confusion about who one is; weak sense of self "I belong to the gang because without them, I'm nothing."
Early adulthood (20-35 yr)	Establishing intimate bonds of love and friendship	Intimacy versus isolation	Ability to love deeply and commit oneself "My husband has been my best friend for 25 years."	Emotional isolation; egocentricity "There's no one out there for me."
Middle adulthood (35-65 yr)	Fulfilling life goals that involve family, career, and society; developing concerns that embrace future generations	Generativity versus self-absorption	Ability to give and to care for others "I'm joining the political action committee to help people get the healthcare they need."	Self-absorption; inability to grow as a person "After I work all day, I just want to watch television and don't want to be around people."
Later years (65 yr to death)	Looking back over one's life and accepting its meaning	Integrity versus despair	Sense of integrity and fulfillment; willingness to face death; wisdom "I've led a happy, productive life, and I still have plenty to give."	Dissatisfaction with life; denial of or despair over prospect of death "What a waste my life has been; I'm going to die alone."

Data from Erikson, E. H. (1963). *Childhood and society.* New York, NY: W. W. Norton; Altrocchi, J. (1980). *Abnormal psychology* (p. 196). New York, NY: Harcourt Brace Jovanovich.

Stage 4: Maintaining the social order. A "rules are rules" mindset returns. However, the reasoning behind it is not simply to avoid punishment; it is because the person has begun to adopt a broader view of society. Listening to authority maintains the social order; bureaucracies and big government agencies often seem to operate with this tenet.

Postconventional level

Stage 5: Social contract and individual rights. People in stage 5 still believe that the social order is important, but the social order must be *good*. For example, if the social order is corrupt, then rules should be changed and it is a duty to protect the rights of others.

Stage 6: Universal ethical principles. Actions should create justice for everyone involved. We are obliged to break unjust laws.

Ethics of Care Theory

Carol Gilligan (born 1936) is an American psychologist, ethicist, and feminist who inspired the normative ethics of care theory. She worked with Kohlberg as he developed his theory of moral development and later criticized his work for being based on a sample of boys and men. Additionally, she believed that he used a scoring method that favored males' methods of reasoning, resulting in lower moral development scores for girls as

TABLE 2.7 Gilligan's Stages of Moral Development

Stage	Goal	Action
Preconventional	Goal is individual survival—selfishness	Caring for self
Conventional	Self-sacrifice is goodness—responsibility to others	Caring for others
Postconventional	Principle of nonviolence—do not hurt others or self	Balancing caring for self with caring for others

TABLE 2.8 Additional Theorists Whose Contributions Influence Psychiatric-Mental Health Nursing

Theorist	School of Thought	Major Contributions	Relevance to Psychiatric Mental Health Nursing
Carl Rogers	Humanism	Developed a person-centered model of psychotherapy. Emphasized the concepts of: Congruence—authenticity of the therapist in dealings with the patient. Unconditional acceptance and positive regard—climate in the therapeutic relationship that facilitates change. Empathetic understanding—therapist's ability to apprehend the feelings and experiences of the patient as if these things were happening to the therapist.	Encourages nurses to view each patient as unique. Emphasizes attitudes of unconditional positive regard, empathetic understanding, and genuineness that are essential to the nurse-patient relationship. *Example:* The nurse asks the patient, "What can I do to help you regain control over your anxiety?"
Jean Piaget	Cognitive development	Identified stages of cognitive development, including sensorimotor (0-2 yr); preoperational (2-7 yr); concrete operational (7-11 yr); and formal operational (11 yr-adulthood). These describe how cognitive development proceeds from reflex activity to application of logical solutions to all types of problems.	Provides a broad base for cognitive interventions, especially with patients with negative self-views. *Example:* The nurse shows an 8-year-old all the equipment needed to start an IV when discussing the fact that he will need one before surgery.
Lawrence Kohlberg	Moral development	Posited a six-stage theory of moral development.	Provides nurses with a framework for evaluating moral decisions.
Albert Ellis	Existentialism	Developed approach of rational emotive behavioral therapy that is active and cognitively oriented; confrontation used to force patients to assume responsibility for behavior; patients are encouraged to accept themselves as they are and are taught to take risks and try out new behaviors.	Encourages nurses to focus on "here-and-now" issues and to help the patient live fully in the present and look forward to the future. *Example:* The nurse encourages the patient to vacation with her family even though she will be wheelchair-bound until her leg fracture heals.
Albert Bandura	Social learning theory	Responsible for concepts of modeling and self-efficacy: person's belief or expectation that he or she has the capacity to affect a desired outcome through his or her own efforts.	Includes cognitive functioning with environmental factors, which provides nurses with a comprehensive view of how people learn. *Example:* The nurse helps the teenage patient identify three negative outcomes of tobacco use.
Viktor Frankl	Existentialism	Developed "logotherapy," a form of support offered to help people find their sense of self-respect. Logotherapy is a future-oriented therapy focused on one's need to find meaning and value in living as one's most important life task.	Focuses nurse beyond mere behaviors to understanding the meaning of these behaviors to the patient's sense of life meaning. *Example:* The nurse listens attentively as the patient describes what it's been like since her daughter died.

Data from Bandura, A. (1977). *Social learning theory.* Englewood Cliffs, NJ: Prentice-Hall; Bernard, M. E., & Wolfe, J. L. (Eds.). (1993). *The RET resource book for practitioners.* New York, NY: Institute for Rational-Emotive Therapy; Ellis, A. (1989). *Inside rational emotive therapy.* San Diego, CA: Academic Press; Frankl, V. (1969). *The will to meaning.* Cleveland, OH: New American Library; Kohlberg, L. (1986). A current statement on some theoretical issues. In S. Modgil & C. Modgil (Eds.), *Lawrence Kohlberg.* Philadelphia, PA: Palmer; Rogers, C. R. (1961). *On becoming a person.* Boston, MA: Houghton Mifflin.

compared with boys. Based on Gilligan's critique, Kohlberg later revised his scoring methods, which resulted in greater similarity between girls' and boys' scores.

Gilligan (1982) suggests that a morality of care should replace Kohlberg's "justice view" of morality, which maintains that we should do what is right no matter the personal cost or the cost to those we love. Gilligan's care view emphasizes the importance of forming relationships, banding together, and putting the needs of those for whom we care above the needs of strangers. Gilligan asserts that a female approach to ethics has always been in existence but has been trivialized. Like Kohlberg, Gilligan asserts that moral development progresses through three major divisions: preconventional, conventional, and postconventional. These transitions are not dictated by cognitive ability but rather through personal development and changes in a sense of self (Table 2.7).

CONCLUSION

This chapter introduced you to some of the historically significant theories and therapies widely used today and the theoretical implications for nursing care. Table 2.8 lists additional theorists whose contributions influence psychiatric-mental health nursing.

There are literally hundreds of therapies in use today. The Substance Abuse and Mental Health Services Administration (SAMHSA) maintains a National Registry of Evidence-based Practices and Programs. New therapies are entered into the database all the time. Examples of therapies that were added in 2015 include AlcoholEdu for College and Internal Family Systems Therapy. The registry can be accessed at http://www.nrepp.samhsa.gov/AllPrograms.aspx.

You will be introduced to other therapeutic approaches later in the book. Crisis intervention (Chapter 26) is an approach you will find useful not only in psychiatric-mental health nursing but also in other nursing specialties. This book will also discuss group therapy (Chapter 34) and family interventions (Chapter 35), which are appropriate for the basic level practitioner.

KEY POINTS TO REMEMBER

- Freud articulated levels of awareness (unconscious, preconscious, conscious) and demonstrated the influence of our unconscious behavior on everyday life as evidenced by the use of defense mechanisms.
- Freud identified three psychological processes of personality (id, ego, and superego) and described how they operate and develop.
- Freud articulated one of the first modern developmental theories of personality based on five psychosexual stages.
- Various psychoanalytic therapies have been used over the years. Currently, a short-term, time-limited version of psychotherapy is common.
- Harry Stack Sullivan proposed the interpersonal theory of personality development, which focuses on interpersonal processes that can be observed in a social framework.
- Interpersonal therapy seeks to improve interpersonal relationships and improve communication patterns.
- Hildegard Peplau, a nursing theorist, developed an interpersonal theoretical framework that has become the foundation of psychiatric mental health nursing practice.
- Behavioral theorists argue that changing a behavior changes a personality.
- Pavlov focused on classical conditioning (in which an involuntary reaction is caused by a stimulus), while Skinner experimented with operant conditioning (in which voluntary behavior is learned through reinforcement).
- Common behavioral treatments include modeling, operant conditioning, systematic desensitization, aversion therapy, and biofeedback.
- Cognitive theory is based on the belief that thoughts come before feelings and actions. Thoughts may not be a clear representation of reality and may be distorted.
- Cognitive-behavioral therapy is the most commonly used, accepted, and empirically validated psychotherapeutic approach. It focuses on identifying, understanding, and changing distorted thought patterns.
- Abraham Maslow, the founder of humanistic psychology, offered the theory of self-actualization and human motivation that is basic to all nursing education. He argued that humans are motivated by unmet needs. Basic needs must be met before higher level needs.
- A biological model of mental illness and treatment dominates care for psychiatric disorders. Current biological treatments include psychopharmacology therapy and brain stimulation therapy.
- Erik Erikson expanded on Freud's developmental stages to include middle age through old age. Erikson called his stages psychosocial stages and emphasized the social aspect of personality development.
- Lawrence Kohlberg provides us with a framework to understand the progression of moral development from black-and-white thinking to a complex decision-making process that coincides with intellectual development.
- Carol Gilligan expanded on Kohlberg's moral theory of development to emphasize relationships and tending to the needs of others.

CRITICAL THINKING

1. Consider how the theorists and theories discussed in this chapter have had an effect on your practice of nursing:
   a. How do Freud's concepts of the conscious, preconscious, and unconscious affect your understanding of patients' behaviors?
   b. Do you believe Erikson's psychosocial stages represent a sound basis for identifying disruptions in stages of development in your patients? Support your position with a clinical example.
   c. What are the implications of Sullivan's focus on the importance of interpersonal relationships for your interactions with patients?
   d. Peplau believed that nurses must exercise self-awareness within the nurse-patient relationship. Describe situations in your student experience in which this self-awareness played a vital role in your relationships with patients.
   e. Identify someone you believe to be self-actualized. What characteristics does this person have that support your assessment? How do you make use of Maslow's hierarchy of needs in your nursing practice?
   f. What do you think about the behaviorist point of view that to change behaviors is to change personality?
2. Which of the therapies described in this chapter do you think can be the most helpful to you in your nursing practice? What are your reasons for this choice?

CHAPTER REVIEW

Questions

1. A male patient reports to the nurse, "I'm told I have memories of childhood abuse stored in my unconscious mind. I want to work on this." Based on this statement, what information should the nurse provide the patient?
   - **a.** To seek the help of a trained therapist to help uncover and deal with the trauma associated with those memories.
   - **b.** How to use a defense mechanism such as suppression so that the memories will be less threatening.
   - **c.** Psychodynamic therapy will allow the surfacing of those unconscious memories to occur in just a few sessions.
   - **d.** Group sessions are valuable to identify underlying themes of the memories being suppressed.
2. Which question should the nurse ask when assessing for what Sullivan's Interpersonal Theory identifies as the most painful human condition?
   - **a.** "Is self-esteem important to you?"
   - **b.** "Do you think of yourself as being lonely?"
   - **c.** "What do you do to manage your anxiety?"
   - **d.** "Have you ever been diagnosed with depression?"
3. When discussing therapy options, the nurse should provide information about interpersonal therapy to which patient? *Select all that apply.*
   - **a.** The teenager who is the focus of bullying at school
   - **b.** The older woman who has just lost her life partner to cancer
   - **c.** The young adult who has begun demonstrating hoarding tendencies
   - **d.** The adolescent demonstrating aggressive verbal and physical tendencies
   - **e.** The middle-aged adult who recently discovered her partner has been unfaithful
4. When considering the suggestions of Hildegard Peplau, which activity should the nurse regularly engage in to ensure that the patient stays the focus of all therapeutic conversations?
   - **a.** Assessing the patient for unexpressed concerns and fears
   - **b.** Evaluating the possible need for additional training and education
   - **c.** Reflecting on personal behaviors and personal needs
   - **d.** Avoiding power struggles with the manipulative patient
5. Which action reflects therapeutic practices associated with operant conditioning?
   - **a.** Encouraging a parent to read to their children to foster a love for learning
   - **b.** Encouraging a patient to make daily journal entries describing their feelings
   - **c.** Suggesting to a new mother that she spend time cuddling her newborn often during the day
   - **d.** Acknowledging a patient who is often verbally aggressive for complimenting a picture another patient drew
6. A nurse is assessing a patient who graduated at the top of his class but now obsesses about being incompetent in his new job. The nurse recognizes that this patient may benefit from the following type of psychotherapy:
   - **a.** Interpersonal
   - **b.** Operant conditioning
   - **c.** Behavioral
   - **d.** Cognitive-behavioral
7. According to Maslow's hierarchy of needs, the most basic needs category for nurses to address is:
   - **a.** physiological
   - **b.** safety
   - **c.** love and belonging
   - **d.** self-actualization
8. In an outpatient psychiatric clinic, a nurse notices that a newly admitted young male patient smiles when he sees her. One day the young man tells the nurse, "You are pretty like my mother." The nurse recognizes that the male is exhibiting:
   - **a.** Transference
   - **b.** Id expression
   - **c.** Countertransference
   - **d.** A cognitive distortion
9. Linda is terrified of spiders and cannot explain why. Because she lives in a wooded area, she would like to overcome this overwhelming fear. Her nurse practitioner suggests which therapy?
   - **a.** Behavioral
   - **b.** Biofeedback
   - **c.** Aversion
   - **d.** Systematic desensitization
10. A patient is telling a tearful story. The nurse listens empathically and responds therapeutically with:
    - **a.** "The next time you find yourself in a similar situation, please call me."
    - **b.** "I am sorry this situation made you feel so badly. Would you like some tea?"
    - **c.** "Let's devise a plan on how you will react next time in a similar situation."
    - **d.** "I am sorry that your friend was so thoughtless. You should be treated better."

Answers

1. **a**; 2. **b**; 3. **a, b, e** ; 4. **c**; 5. **d**; 6. **d**; 7. **a**; 8. **a**; 9. **d**; 10. **c**

Visit the Evolve website for a posttest on the content in this chapter: http://evolve.elsevier.com/Varcarolis

Post-Test interactive review

REFERENCES

Bandura, A., Blanchard, A. B., & Ritter, B. (1969). The relative efficacy of desensitization and modeling approaches for inducing behavioral, affective, and attitudinal changes. *Journal of Personality and Social Psychology, 13*, 173–179.

Beck, A. T. (1967). *Depression: clinical, experimental and theoretical aspects*. New York, NY: Harper & Row.

Beck, A. T., Rush, A. J., Shaw, B. F., & Emery, G. (1979). *Cognitive therapy of depression*. New York, NY: Guilford Press.

Crain, W. C. (1985). *Theories of development*. New York, NY: Prentice-Hall.

Ellis, A. (2000). *On therapy: A dialogue with Aaron T. Beck and Albert Ellis*. Washington, DC: Discussion at the American Psychological Association's 108th Convention.

Erikson, E. H. (1963). *Childhood and society*. New York, NY: W. W. Norton.

Freud, S. (1960). *The ego and the id* (J. Strachey, trans.). New York, NY: W. W. Norton (Original work published in 1923).

Freud, S. (1969). *An outline of psychoanalysis* (J. Strachey, trans.). New York, NY: W. W. Norton (original work published in 1940).

Gilligan, C. (1982). *In a different voice*. Boston, MA: Harvard University Press.

Kohlberg, L., & Turiel, E. (1971). Moral development and moral education. In G. S. Lesser (Ed.), *Psychology and educational practice* (pp. 410–465). Glenview, IL: Scott, Foresman, & Company.

Mahler, M. S., Pine, F., & Bergman, A. (1975). *The psychological birth of the human infant*. New York: Basic Books.

Maslow, A. H. (1968). *Toward a psychology of being*. Princeton, NJ: Van Nostrand.

Maslow, A. H. (1970). *Motivation and personality* (2nd ed.). New York, NY: Harper & Row.

Pavlov, I. (1928). *Lectures on conditioned reflexes* (W. H. Grant, trans.). New York, NY: International Publishers.

Peplau, H. E. (1952). *Interpersonal relations in nursing: A conceptual frame of reference for psychodynamic nursing*. New York, NY: Putnam.

Skinner, B. F. (1987). Whatever happened to psychology as the science of behavior? *American Psychologist, 42*, 780–786.

Substance Abuse and Mental Health Services Administration. (2012). *National Registry of Evidence-Based Practices and Programs*. Retrieved from http://www.nrepp.samhsa.gov/ViewAll.aspx.

Sullivan, H. S. (1953). *The interpersonal theory of psychiatry*. New York, NY: W. W. Norton.

Watson, J. B. (1919). *Psychology from the standpoint of a behaviorist*. Philadelphia, PA: Lippincott.

Weissman, M. M., Markowitz, J. W., & Klerman, G. L. (2007). *Clinician's quick guide to interpersonal psychotherapy*. Oxford, United Kingdom: Oxford University Press.

3

Psychobiology and Psychopharmacology

Mary A. Gutierrez, Jerika T. Lam

ⓔ Visit the Evolve website for a pretest on the content in this chapter: http://evolve.elsevier.com/Varcarolis Pre-Test interactive review

OBJECTIVES

1. Discuss major functions of the brain and how psychotropic drugs can alter these functions.
2. Identify how specific brain functions are altered in certain mental disorders (e.g., depression, anxiety, schizophrenia).
3. Describe how a neurotransmitter functions as a chemical messenger.
4. Describe how the use of imaging techniques can be helpful for understanding mental illness.
5. Identify the main neurotransmitters that are affected by the following psychotropic drugs and their subgroups:
   Antianxiety and hypnotic drugs
   Antidepressant drugs
   Cholinesterase inhibitors
   Mood stabilizers
   Antipsychotic drugs
   Psychostimulants
6. Identify special dietary and drug restrictions in a teaching plan for a patient taking a monoamine oxidase inhibitor.
7. Identify specific cautions you might incorporate into your medication teaching plan with regard to herbal treatments.

OUTLINE

KEY TERMS AND CONCEPTS

antagonists
antianxiety (anxiolytic) drugs
cholinesterase inhibitors
circadian rhythms
first-generation antipsychotics
hypnotic
limbic system
lithium
monoamine oxidase inhibitors (MAOIs)
mood stabilizers
neurons
neurotransmitter
norepinephrine and serotonin specific antidepressant (NaSSA)
pharmacodynamics
pharmacogenetics
pharmacokinetics
psychotropic medication
receptors
reuptake
selective serotonin reuptake inhibitors (SSRIs)
second-generation antipsychotics
synapse
therapeutic index
tricyclic antidepressants (TCAs)

A number of factors, such as genetics, neurodevelopmental factors, drugs, infection, and traumatic experiences can interact and produce a psychiatric disorder. No matter the cause, physical changes in the brain can result in disturbances in the patient's behavior and mental experiences. These physiological alterations are the targets of the **psychotropic** (Greek for *psyche,* or mind, + *trepein,* to turn) **medications** used to treat mental disease.

Despite the fact that psychotropic drugs have been used for more than half a century, we do not understand how some of these drugs improve psychiatric symptoms. Early biological theories associated a single neurotransmitter with a specific disorder. Experts now view the dopamine theory of schizophrenia and the monoamine theory of depression as overly simplistic. Other neurotransmitters, hormones, and coregulators play important and complex roles. Recent discoveries have influenced the direction of research and treatment.

Before looking at specific drugs, this chapter begins with an overview of normal functions of the brain and how these functions are carried out. Theories of the psychobiological basis of various types of emotional and physiological dysfunctions are presented next. Finally, the chapter reviews the major classification of drugs used to treat mental disorders, explains how they work, and identifies both the beneficial and the problematic effects of psychiatric drugs. Additionally, detailed information regarding adverse and toxic effects, nursing implications, and teaching tools are presented in the appropriate clinical chapters (Chapters 11 to 24).

STRUCTURE AND FUNCTION OF THE BRAIN

Functions and Activities of the Brain

Regulating behavior and carrying out mental processes are important, but not the only, responsibilities of the brain. Box 3.1 summarizes some of the major functions and activities of the brain.

Maintenance of Homeostasis

The brain serves as the coordinator and director of the body's response to both internal and external changes. Appropriate responses require a constant monitoring of the environment, interpretation and integration of the incoming information, and control

BOX 3.1 Functions of the Brain

- Monitor changes in the external world.
- Monitor the composition of body fluids.
- Regulate the contractions of the skeletal muscles.
- Regulate the internal organs.
- Initiate and regulate the basic drives: hunger, thirst, sex, aggressive self-protection.
- Mediate conscious sensation.
- Store and retrieve memories.
- Regulate mood (affect) and emotions.
- Think and perform intellectual functions.
- Regulate the sleep cycle.
- Produce and interpret language.
- Process visual and auditory data.

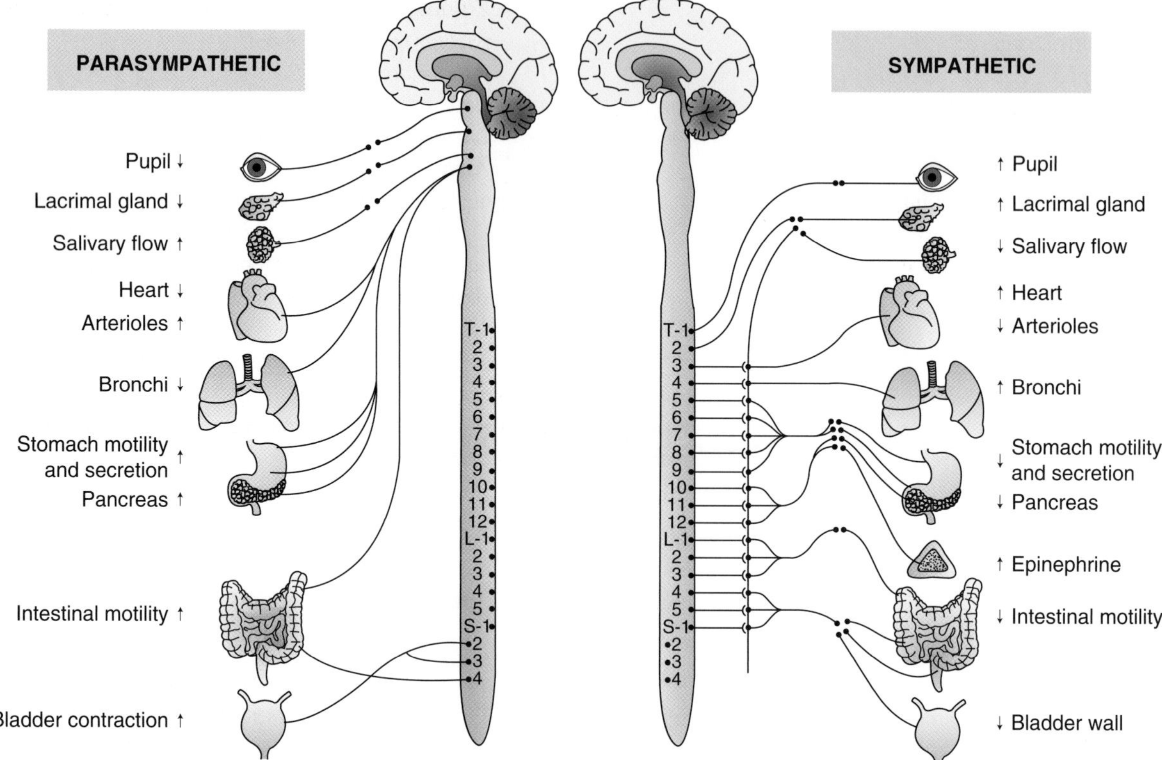

FIG. 3.1 The autonomic nervous system has two divisions: the sympathetic and parasympathetic. The sympathetic division is dominant in stress situations, such as those involving fear and anger (known as the fight-or-flight response).

over the appropriate organs of response. The goal of these responses is to maintain homeostasis and, therefore, to maintain life.

Various sense organs relay information about the external world to the brain by the peripheral nerves. Sensations such as light, sound, or touch must ultimately be interpreted as a lamp, doorbell, or a tap on the back. These sensations can be altered, particularly in psychotic disorders such as schizophrenia where an individual experiences a sensation, such as voices, that does not originate in the external world.

To respond to the external world, the brain controls skeletal muscles. This control includes the ability to initiate contraction. It also fine-tunes and coordinates contraction so that a person can, for example, guide the fingers to the correct keys on a piano. Unfortunately, both psychiatric disease and its treatment with psychotropic drugs can be associated with disturbance of movement.

It is important to remember that the skeletal muscles controlled by the brain include the diaphragm, which is essential for breathing, and the muscles of the throat, tongue, and mouth, which are essential for speech. Therefore drugs that affect brain function can stimulate or depress respiration or lead to slurred speech.

The brain not only monitors the external world but also monitors internal functions. It continuously receives information about blood pressure, body temperature, blood gases, and the chemical composition of the body fluids so that it can direct the appropriate responses required to maintain homeostasis. For example, if blood pressure drops, the brain must direct the heart to pump more blood and the smooth muscles of the arterioles to constrict. This increase in cardiac output and vasoconstriction allows the body to return blood pressure to its normal level.

Regulation of the Autonomic Nervous System and Hormones

The autonomic nervous system and the endocrine system serve as links between the brain and the cardiac muscle, smooth muscle, and glands of which the internal organs are composed (Fig. 3.1). If the brain needs to stimulate the heart, it must activate the sympathetic nerves to the sinoatrial node and the ventricular myocardium. If the brain needs to bring about vasoconstriction, it must activate the sympathetic nerves to the smooth muscles of the arterioles.

The homeostatic linkage between the brain and the internal organs explains why mental disturbances, such as anxiety, alter internal function. Anxiety can activate the sympathetic nervous system, leading to symptoms such as increased heart rate and blood pressure, shortness of breath, and sweating.

The brain also influences the internal organs by regulating hormonal secretions of the pituitary gland, which in turn regulates other glands. A specific area of the brain, the hypothalamus, secretes hormones called releasing factors. These hormones act on the pituitary gland to stimulate or inhibit the synthesis and release of pituitary hormones. Once in the general circulation they influence various internal activities. An example of this linkage is the release of gonadotropin-releasing hormone by the hypothalamus at the time of puberty. This hormone stimulates the pituitary to release two gonadotropins—follicle-stimulating

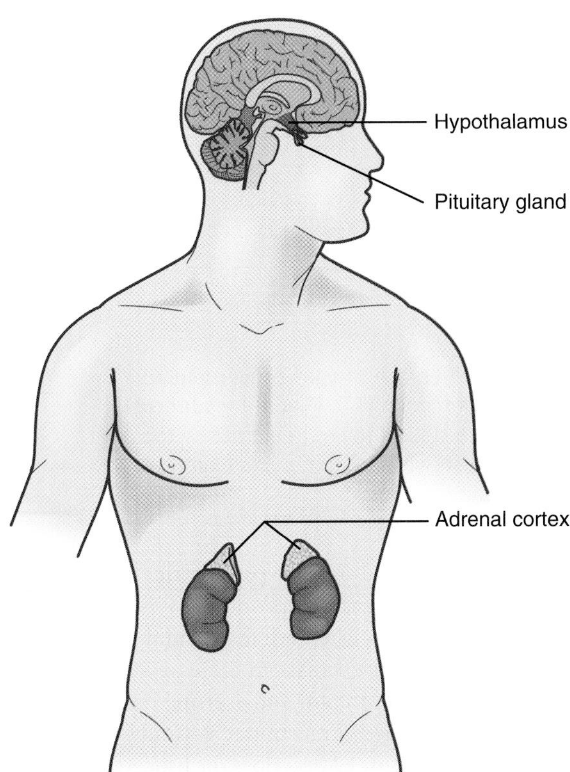

FIG. 3.2 The hypothalamic-pituitary-adrenal axis.

hormone and luteinizing hormone—which activates the ovaries or testes. This linkage may explain why anxiety or depression (e.g., premenstrual dysphoric disorder) in some women is associated with the menstrual cycle.

The relationship between the brain, the pituitary gland, and the adrenal glands is particularly important in normal and abnormal mental function. The steps in this system are:

1. The hypothalamus secretes corticotropin-releasing hormone (CRH).
2. CRH stimulates the pituitary to release adrenocorticotropic hormone.
3. Adrenocorticotropin stimulates the cortex of each adrenal gland (located on top of the kidneys) to secrete the hormone cortisol.

This system is referred to as the hypothalamic-pituitary-adrenal axis (HPTA). It is part of the normal response to a variety of mental and physical stressors (Fig. 3.2). All three hormones—CRH, corticotropin, and cortisol—influence the functions of the nerve cells of the brain. There is considerable evidence that this system influences most psychiatric disturbances. For example, elevated cortisol levels are found in people with major depressive disorder. Elevated cortisol levels suppress the immune response and make depressed individuals more vulnerable to infection.

Control of Biological Drives and Behavior

To understand the basis of psychiatric disorders, it is helpful to distinguish between the various types of brain activity. An understanding of these activities shows where to look for disturbed function and what to hope for in treatment. The brain is responsible for such basic drives as sex and hunger. Disturbances of these drives (e.g., overeating or undereating, loss of sexual interest) can be an indication of an underlying psychiatric disorder such as depression.

Cycle of sleep and wakefulness. Various regions of the brain regulate and coordinate the entire cycle of sleep and wakefulness, as well as the intensity of alertness while the person is awake. Sleep is essential for both physiological and psychological well-being. Sleep pattern disturbances occur in virtually every psychiatric disorder. An important gauge in the process of recovery from these disorders is improvement of sleep.

Drugs used to treat psychiatric problems may also interfere with the normal regulation of sleep and alertness. Drugs with a sedative-hypnotic effect can reduce alertness and can cause drowsiness. These drugs require caution while engaging in activities that require a great deal of attention, such as driving a car or operating machinery. One way of minimizing the danger is to take sedating drugs at night just before bedtime.

Circadian rhythms. **Circadian rhythms** are the fluctuation of various physiological and behavioral patterns over a 24-hour cycle. Changes in sleep, body temperature, secretion of hormones such as corticotropin and cortisol, and secretion of neurotransmitters such as norepinephrine and serotonin are influenced by these rhythms. Both norepinephrine and serotonin are thought to be involved in mood. There is evidence that the circadian rhythm of neurotransmitter secretion is altered in psychiatric disorders, particularly in those that involve mood.

Conscious Mental Activity

All aspects of conscious mental experience and sense of self originate from the activity of the brain. Conscious mental activity can be a basic, meandering stream of consciousness that flows from thoughts of future responsibilities, memories, fantasies, and so on. Conscious mental activity can also be much more complex when it is applied to problem solving and the interpretation of the external world. Unfortunately, conscious mental experiences can become distorted in psychiatric illness. A person with schizophrenia may have chaotic and incoherent speech and thought patterns (e.g., unconnected phrases and topics) and delusional interpretations of personal interactions such as beliefs about people or events not supported by data or reality.

Memory

An extremely important component of mental activity is memory, the ability to retain and recall past experiences. From both an anatomical and a physiological perspective, there is a major difference in the processing of short- and long-term memory. This can be seen dramatically in some forms of cognitive mental disorders such as Alzheimer's disease in which a person has no recall of the events of the previous few minutes but may have vivid recall of events that occurred decades earlier.

Social Skills

An important, and often neglected, aspect of brain functioning involves social skills that make interpersonal relationships possible. In almost all types of mental illness, from mild anxiety to severe schizophrenia, difficulties in interpersonal relationships are important parts of the disorder. As with sleep, improvements in these relationships are important gauges of recovery.

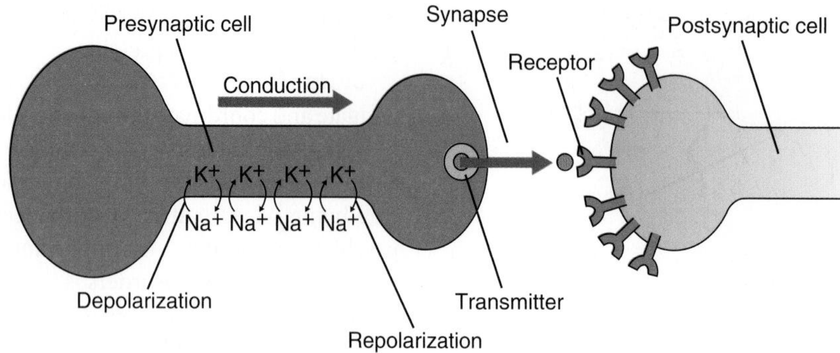

FIG. 3.3 Activities of neurons. Conduction along a neuron involves the inward movement of sodium ions (Na^+) followed by the outward movement of potassium ions (K^+). When the current reaches the end of the cell, a neurotransmitter is released. The neurotransmitter crosses the synapse and attaches to a receptor on the postsynaptic cell. The attachment of neurotransmitter to receptor either stimulates or inhibits the postsynaptic cell.

Cellular Composition of the Brain

The brain is composed of approximately 100 billion **neurons**, nerve cells that conduct electrical impulses. Most functions of the brain, from regulation of blood pressure to the conscious sense of self, result from the actions of individual neurons and the interconnections between them. Although neurons come in a great variety of shapes and sizes, all carry out the same three types of physiological actions:

1. Responding to stimuli
2. Conducting electrical impulses
3. Releasing chemicals called neurotransmitters

Neurons have the ability to communicate by conducting an electrical impulse from one end of the cell to the other. All cellular membranes are electrically charged due to ions inside and outside the cell. Communication between neurons occurs mainly through sodium (Na^+) and potassium (K^+) ions. In a resting state, there is an unequal distribution of these two on the inside of the cell membrane and the outside. There are lots of positively charged potassium ions just inside the membrane and lots of sodium ions (along with some potassium ions) on the outside. The intracellular space is more negative when compared with the extracellular space.

Stimulation of the nerve cell membrane changes this resting state within milliseconds. First, the stimulus causes the sodium gates to open. Sodium ions flow into the nerve cell and potassium ions flow out. The entry of positively charged ions into the cell actually reverses the electrical potential from a negative one to a positive one. The current at the end of the cell is conducted along the membrane until it reaches the other end (Fig. 3.3).

Once an electrical impulse reaches the end of a neuron, a neurotransmitter is released. A **neurotransmitter** is a chemical substance that functions as a neuromessenger. Neurotransmitters are released from the axon terminal at the presynaptic neuron on excitation. The neurotransmitter then crosses the space, or **synapse**, to an adjacent postsynaptic neuron where it attaches to **receptors** on the neuron's surface.

It is this interaction from one neuron to another, by way of a neurotransmitter and receptor that allows the activity of one neuron to influence the activity of other neurons. It is the interaction between neurotransmitter and receptor that is a major target of the drugs used to treat psychiatric disease. Table 3.1 lists important neurotransmitters and the types of receptors to which they attach. Also listed are the mental disorders associated with an increase or decrease in these neurotransmitters.

After attaching to a receptor and exerting its influence on the postsynaptic cell, the neurotransmitter separates from the receptor and is destroyed. Box 3.2 describes the process of neurotransmitter destruction. Neurotransmitters can be destroyed two ways. Specific enzymes destroy some neurotransmitters (e.g., acetylcholine) at the postsynaptic cell. The enzyme that destroys acetylcholine is called acetylcholinesterase (referred to as cholinesterase from here on). Most enzymes start with the name of the neurotransmitter they destroy and end with the suffix –ase.

Other neurotransmitters (e.g., norepinephrine) are taken back into the presynaptic cell from which they were originally released by a process called cellular **reuptake**. These neurotransmitters are either reused or destroyed by intracellular enzymes. In the case of the monoamine neurotransmitters (e.g., norepinephrine, dopamine, serotonin), the destructive enzyme is called monoamine oxidase (MAO).

Organization of the Brain

Brainstem

The most primitive area of the brain is the brainstem. It connects directly to the spinal cord and is central to the survival of all animals by controlling such functions as heart rate, breathing, digestion, and sleeping.

Ascending pathways in the brainstem, referred to as mesolimbic and mesocortical pathways, seem to play a strong role in modulating the emotional value of sensory material. These pathways project to areas of the cerebrum collectively known as the **limbic system**. The limbic system plays a crucial role in emotional status and psychological function using norepinephrine, serotonin, and dopamine as their neurotransmitters.

The role of these pathways in normal and abnormal mental activity is significant. For example, experts believe that the release of dopamine from the mesolimbic pathway plays a role in psychological reward and drug addiction. The neurotransmitters released by these neurons are major targets of the drugs used to treat psychiatric disorders.

TABLE 3.1 **Transmitters and Receptors**

Transmitters	Receptors	Effects/Comments	Association with Mental Health
Monoamines			
Dopamine (DA)	D_1, D_2, D_3, D_4, D_5	Involved in fine muscle movement Involved in integration of emotions and thoughts Involved in decision making Stimulates hypothalamus to release hormones (sex, thyroid, adrenal)	*Decrease:* Parkinson's disease Depression *Increase:* Schizophrenia Mania
Norepinephrine (NE) (noradrenaline)	α_1, α_2, β_1, β_2	Level in brain affects mood Attention and arousal Stimulates sympathetic branch of autonomic nervous system for "fight or flight" in response to stress	*Decrease:* Depression *Increase:* Mania Anxiety states Schizophrenia
Serotonin (5-HT)	5-HT_1, 5-HT_2, 5-HT_3, 5-HT_4, others	Plays a role in sleep regulation, hunger, mood states, and pain perception Hormonal activity Plays a role in aggression and sexual behavior	*Decrease:* Depression
Histamine	H_1, H_2	Involved in alertness Involved in inflammatory response Stimulates gastric secretion	*Decrease:* Sedation Weight gain
Amino Acids			
γ-aminobutyric acid (GABA)	$GABA_A$, $GABA_B$	Plays a role in inhibition; reduces aggression, excitation, and anxiety May play a role in pain perception Has anticonvulsant and muscle-relaxing properties May impair cognition and psychomotor functioning	*Decrease:* Anxiety disorders Schizophrenia Mania Huntington's disease *Increase:* Reduction of anxiety
Glutamate	NMDA, AMPA	Is excitatory AMPA plays a role in learning and memory	*Decrease (NMDA):* Psychosis *Increase (NMDA):* Prolonged increased state can be neurotoxic Neurodegeneration in Alzheimer's disease *Increase (AMPA):* Improvement of cognitive performance in behavioral tasks
Cholinergics			
Acetylcholine (ACh)	Nicotinic, muscarinic (M_1, M_2, M_3)	Plays a role in learning, memory Regulates mood: mania, sexual aggression Affects sexual and aggressive behavior Stimulates parasympathetic nervous system	*Decrease:* Alzheimer's disease Huntington's disease Parkinson's disease *Increase:* Depression
Peptides (Neuromodulators)			
Substance P	SP	Centrally active SP antagonist has antidepressant and anti-anxiety effects in depression Promotes and reinforces memory Enhances sensitivity to pain receptors to activate	Involved in regulation of mood and anxiety Role in pain management
Somatostatin	SRIF	Altered levels associated with cognitive disease	*Decrease:* Alzheimer's disease Decreased levels of SRIF found in spinal fluid of some depressed patients *Increase:* Huntington's disease
Neurotensin	NT	Endogenous antipsychotic-like properties	Decreased levels found in spinal fluid of patients with schizophrenia

AMPA, α-Amino-3-hydroxy-5-methyl-4-isoxazolepropionic acid; *NMDA, N*-methyl-D-aspartate.

BOX 3.2 Destruction of Neurotransmitters

A full explanation of the various ways in which psychotropic drugs alter neuronal activity requires a brief review of the manner in which neurotransmitters are destroyed after attaching to the receptors. To avoid continuous and prolonged action on the postsynaptic cell, the neurotransmitter is released shortly after attaching to the postsynaptic receptor. Once released, the neurotransmitter is destroyed in one of two ways.

One way is the immediate inactivation of the neurotransmitter at the postsynaptic membrane. An example of this method of destruction is the action of the enzyme cholinesterase on the neurotransmitter acetylcholine. Cholinesterase is present at the postsynaptic membrane and destroys acetylcholine shortly after it attaches to nicotinic or muscarinic receptors on the postsynaptic cell.

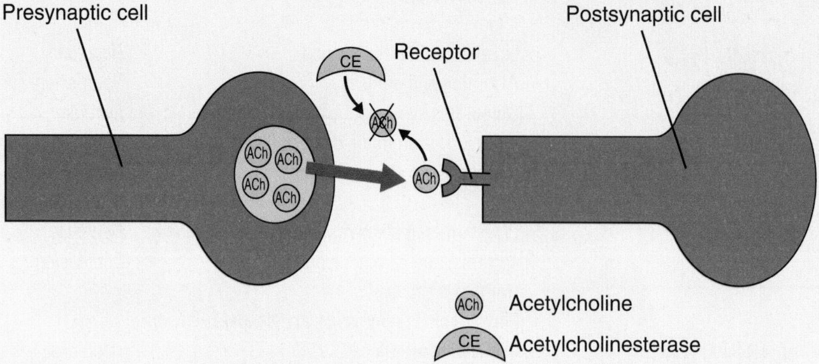

A second method of neurotransmitter inactivation is a little more complex. After interacting with the postsynaptic receptor, the neurotransmitter is released and taken back into the presynaptic cell, the cell from which it was released. This process, referred to as the reuptake of neurotransmitter, is a common target for drug action. Once inside the presynaptic cell, an enzyme within the cell recycles or inactivates the neurotransmitter. The monoamine neurotransmitters norepinephrine, dopamine, and serotonin are all inactivated in this manner by the enzyme monoamine oxidase.

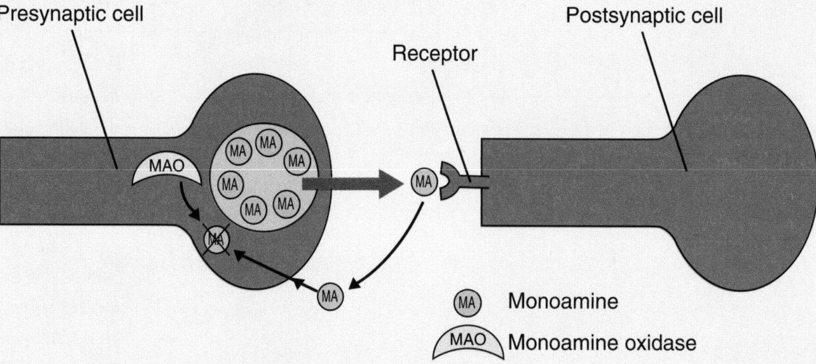

Looking at this second method, you might naturally ask what prevents the enzyme from destroying the neurotransmitter before its release. The answer is that before release the neurotransmitter is stored within a membrane and is protected. After release and reuptake, the neurotransmitter is either destroyed by the enzyme or reenters the membrane to be used again.

Hypothalamus

In a small area above the brainstem lies the hypothalamus, which plays a vital role in:

- Controlling basic drives such as hunger, thirst, and sex
- Linking higher brain activities, such as thought, emotion, and the functioning of the internal organs
- Processing sensory information that is then sent to the cerebral cortex
- Regulating the entire cycle of sleep and wakefulness and the ability of the cerebrum to carry out conscious mental activity

Cerebellum

Located behind the brainstem where the spinal cord meets the brain, the cerebellum (Fig. 3.4) receives information from the sensory systems, the spinal cord, and other parts of the brain and then regulates voluntary motor movements. It plays a crucial role in coordinating contractions so that movement is accomplished in a smooth and directed manner. It is also involved in balance and the maintenance of equilibrium.

Cerebrum

The human brainstem and cerebellum are similar in both structure and function to these same structures in other mammals. The development of a much larger and more elaborate cerebrum is what distinguishes human beings from the rest of the animal kingdom.

The cerebrum, situated on top of and surrounding the brainstem, is responsible for mental activities and a conscious sense

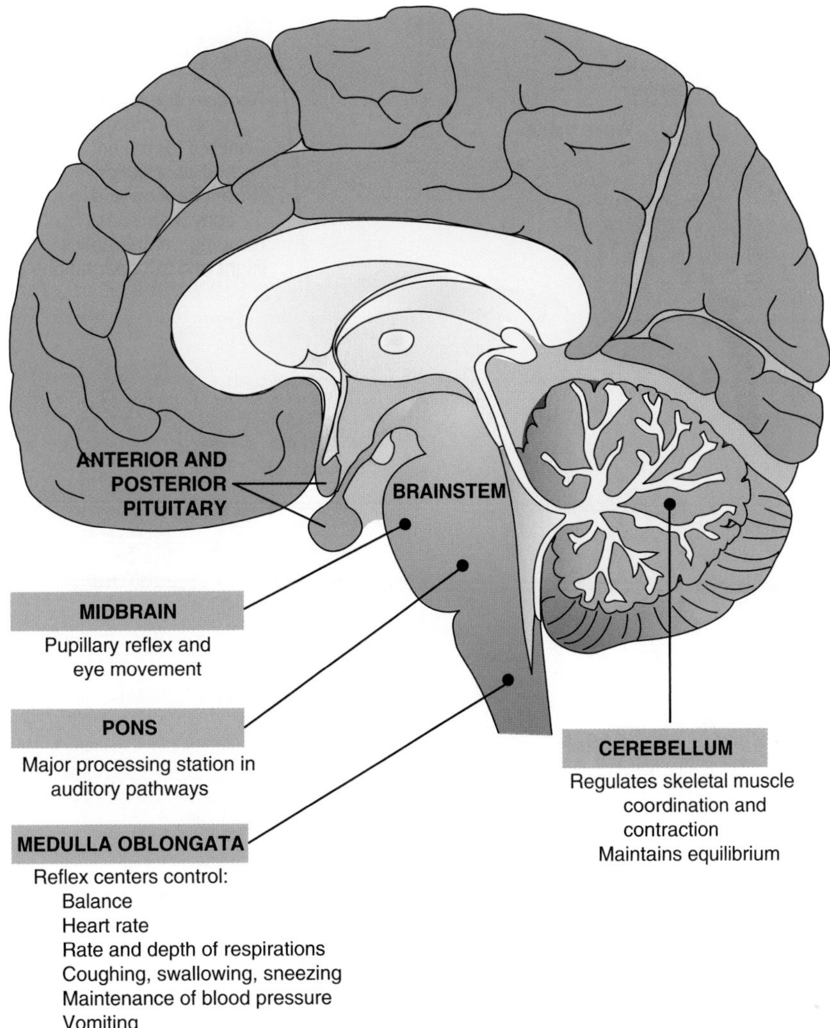

FIG. 3.4 The functions of the brainstem and cerebellum.

of being. This is responsible for our conscious perception of the external world and our own body, emotional status, memory, and control of skeletal muscles that allow willful direction of movement. The cerebrum is also responsible for language and the ability to communicate.

The surface of the cerebrum is called the cerebral cortex. There are four major lobes of the cortex, each responsible for specific functions. For example, conscious sensation and the initiation of movement reside in the frontal lobe, the sensation of touch resides in the parietal lobe, sounds are based in the temporal lobe, and vision is housed in the occipital lobe. Likewise, a specific area of the frontal cortex controls the initiation of skeletal muscle contraction. Of course, all areas of the cortex are interconnected so that you can form an appropriate picture of the world and, if necessary, link it to a proper response (Fig. 3.5).

Both sensory and motor aspects of language reside in specialized areas of the cerebral cortex. Sensory language functions include the ability to read, understand spoken language, and know the names of objects perceived by the senses. Motor functions involve the physical ability to use muscles properly for speech and writing. In both neurological and psychological dysfunction, the use of language may become compromised or distorted. The change in language ability may be a factor in determining a diagnosis.

Underneath the cerebral cortex are pockets of gray matter deep within the cerebrum. Some of these, the basal ganglia, are involved in the regulation of movement. Others, the amygdala and hippocampus in the limbic system, are involved in emotions, learning, memory, and basic drives. Anxiety disorders can be associated with abnormalities in the amygdala, which cause intense fear such as in panic disorder. Significantly, there is an overlap of these areas both anatomically and in the types of neurotransmitters involved. One important consequence is that drugs used to treat emotional disturbances may cause movement disorders, and drugs used to treat movement disorders may cause emotional changes.

Visualizing the Brain

A variety of noninvasive imaging techniques are used to visualize brain structure, functions, and metabolic activity. Table 3.2 identifies some common brain imaging techniques and preliminary findings as they relate to psychiatry. There are two types of neuroimaging techniques: structural and functional. Structural imaging techniques (e.g., computed tomography [CT] and

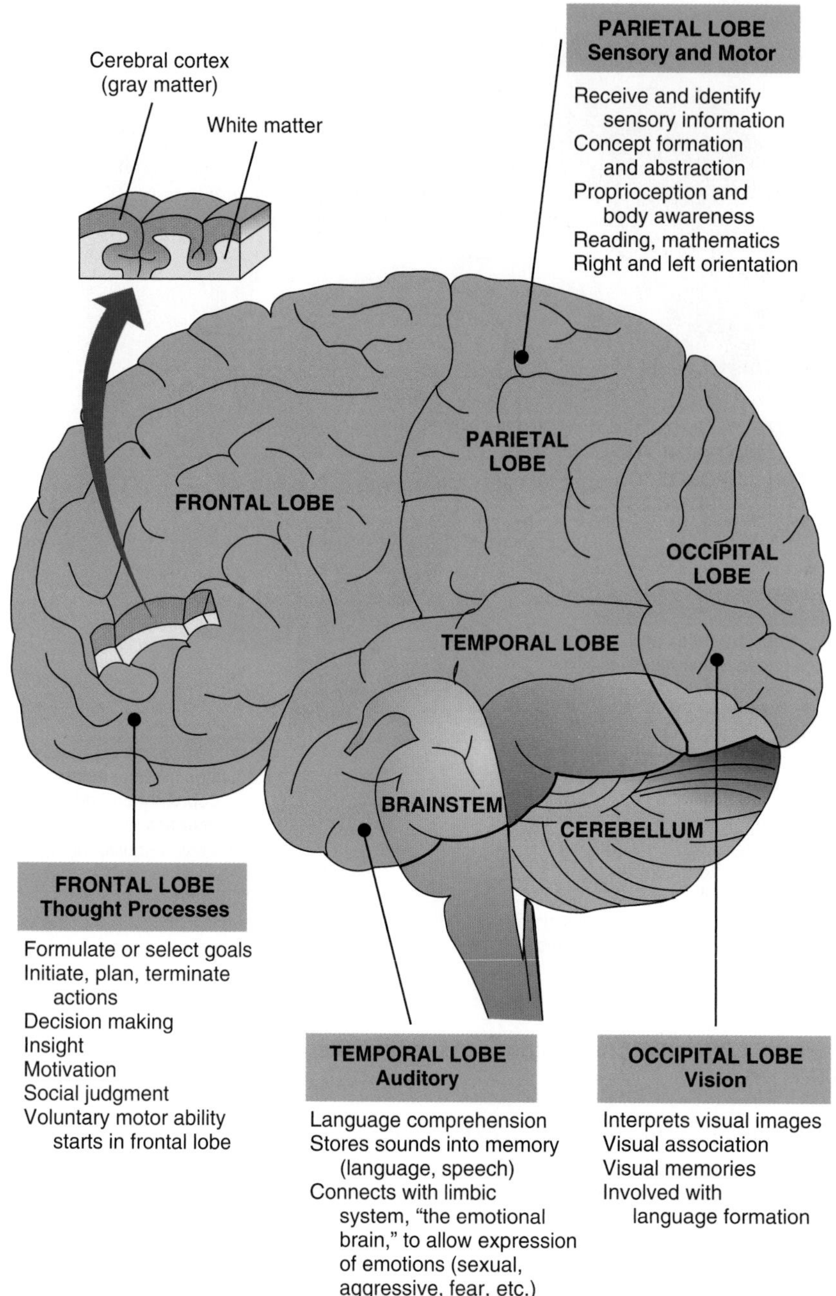

FIG. 3.5 The functions of the cerebral lobes: frontal, parietal, temporal, and occipital.

magnetic resonance imaging [MRI]) provide overall images of the brain and layers of the brain. Functional imaging techniques (e.g., positron emission tomography [PET] and single photon emission computed tomography [SPECT]) reveal physiological activity in the brain.

PET scans are particularly useful in identifying physical and chemical changes as they occur in living tissue. For scanning the brain, a radioactive atom is applied to glucose to create a radionuclide (also referred to as a tag), because the brain uses glucose for its metabolism.

In unmedicated patients with schizophrenia, PET scans may show a decreased use of glucose in the frontal lobes. Twin studies demonstrate lower brain activity in the frontal lobe of a twin diagnosed with schizophrenia compared with the twin who does not have the diagnosis. The area affected in the frontal cortex of the twin with schizophrenia is an area associated with reasoning skills, which are greatly impaired in people with schizophrenia.

PET scans of individuals with depression show decreased brain activity in the prefrontal cortex. Fig. 3.6 shows a patient with depression with reduced brain activity compared with someone who does not have depression. Fig. 3.7 shows three views of a PET scan of the brain of a patient with Alzheimer's disease.

Modern imaging techniques have become important tools in assessing molecular changes in mental disease and marking the receptor sites of drug action. From a psychiatric perspective, it is important to understand what areas of the brain are implicated in dysfunction.

TABLE 3.2 **Common Brain Imaging Techniques**

Technique	Description	Uses	Psychiatric Relevance and Preliminary Findings
Electrical: Recording Electrical Signals from the Brain			
Electroencephalograph (EEG)	A recording of electrical signals from the brain made by hooking up electrodes to the subject's scalp.	Can show the state a person is in—asleep, awake, anesthetized—because the characteristic patterns of current differ for each of these states.	Provides support from a wide range of sources that brain abnormalities exist; may lead to further testing.
Structural: Show Gross Anatomical Details of Brain Structures			
Computerized axial tomography (CT)	A series of x-ray images is taken of the brain and a computer analysis produces "slices" providing a precise 3D-like reconstruction of each segment.	Can detect: Lesions Abrasions Areas of infarct Aneurysm	Schizophrenia Cortical atrophy Third ventricle enlargement Cognitive disorders Abnormalities
Magnetic resonance imaging (MRI)	A magnetic field is applied to the brain. The nuclei of hydrogen atoms absorb and emit radio waves that are analyzed by computer, which provides 3D visualization of the brain's structure in sectional images.	Can detect: Brain edema Ischemia Infection Neoplasm Trauma	Schizophrenia Enlarged ventricles Reduction in temporal lobe and prefrontal lobe
Functional: Show Some Activity of the Brain			
Functional magnetic resonance imaging (fMRI)	Measures brain activity indirectly by changes in blood oxygen in different parts of the brain as subjects participate in various activities.	See MRI	See MRI
Positron-emission tomography (PET)	Radioactive substance (tracer) is injected, travels to the brain, and shows up as bright spots on the scan. Data collected by the detectors are relayed to a computer, which produces images of the activity and 3D visualization of the CNS.	Can detect: Oxygen utilization Glucose metabolism Blood flow Neurotransmitter-receptor interaction	Schizophrenia Increased D_2, D_3 receptors in caudate nucleus Abnormalities in limbic system Mood disorder Abnormalities in temporal lobes Adult ADHD Decreased utilization of glucose
Single photon emission computed tomography (SPECT)	Similar to PET but uses radionuclides that emit γ-radiation (photons). Measures various aspects of brain functioning and provides images of multiple layers of the CNS (as does PET).	Can detect: Circulation of cerebrospinal fluid Similar functions to PET	See PET

3D, Three-dimensional; *ADHD,* attention-deficit/hyperactivity disorder; *CNS,* central nervous system.

Can We Measure Neurotransmitters?

The answer is that there is no perfect or easy way to measure levels of neurotransmitters. In fact, much of what we know about neurotransmitters and brain disturbances comes from pharmacology of the drugs used to treat these conditions. For example, we knew that drugs that were effective in reducing the delusions and hallucinations of schizophrenia blocked the D_2 receptors for dopamine. With this knowledge, researchers concluded that delusions and hallucinations result from overactivity of dopamine at these receptors.

Diagnoses of mental illnesses are based on signs and symptoms and not quantifiable, biological evidence. Change may be on the way! In 2013 the National Institute of Mental Health began an initiative called the Research Domain Criteria (RDoC) to develop a biologically valid framework for understanding mental disorders. They hope to bring together the power of modern research approaches in genetics, neuroscience, and behavioral science to the problem of mental illness.

National Institute of Mental Health. (n.d.). *Research domain criteria.* Retrieved from https://www.nimh.nih.gov/research-priorities/rdoc/index.shtml.

Disturbances of Mental Function

Most origins of mental dysfunction are unknown. Some known causes include drugs (e.g., lysergic acid diethylamide [LSD]), long-term use of high daily doses of prednisone, excess levels of hormones (e.g., thyroxine, cortisol), infection (e.g., encephalitis, acquired immunodeficiency syndrome [AIDS]), and physical trauma. Even when the cause is known, the link between the causative factor and the mental dysfunction is difficult to understand.

Genetics

There is often a genetic predisposition for psychiatric disorders. The incidence of both thought and mood disorders are higher in relatives of people who have these diseases than in the general population. Monozygotic (identical) twins provide us with an understanding of inheritance of a disorder through a concept

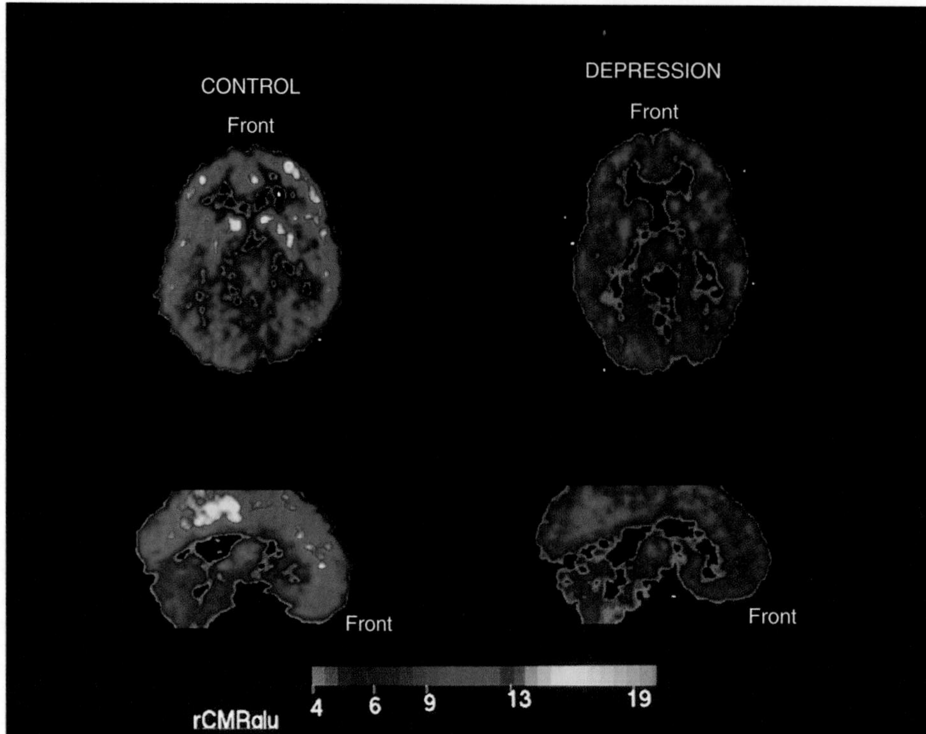

FIG. 3.6 Positron emission tomographic (PET) scans of a patient with depression *(right)* and a person without depression *(left)* reveal reduced brain activity *(darker colors)* in depression, especially in the prefrontal cortex. A form of radioactively tagged glucose was used as a tracer to visualize levels of brain activity. (From Mark George, MD, courtesy of National Institute of Mental Health, Biological Psychiatry Branch.)

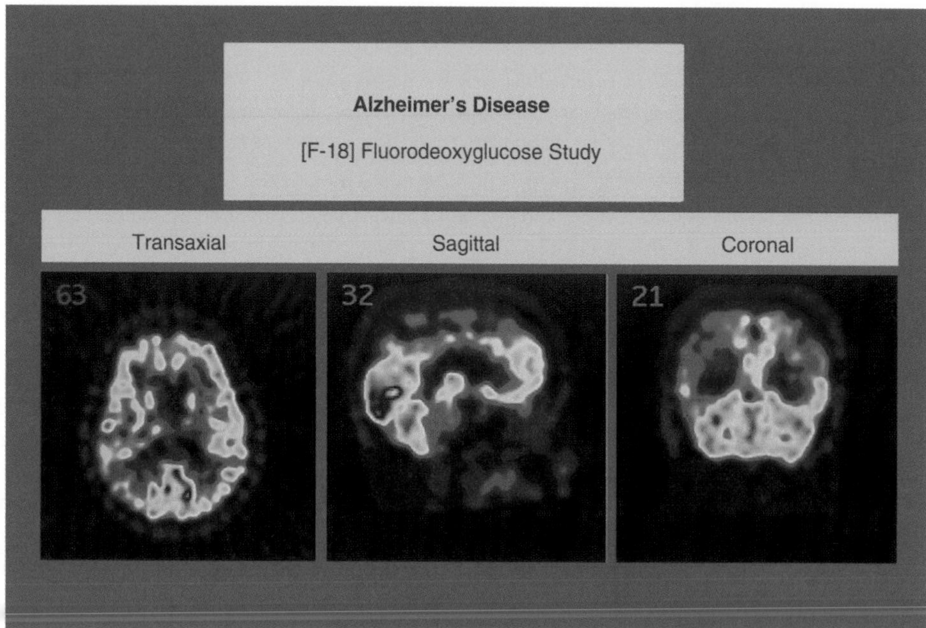

FIG. 3.7 Positron emission tomographic (PET) scan of a patient with Alzheimer's disease demonstrates a classic pattern for areas of hypometabolism in the temporal and parietal regions of the brain. Areas of reduced metabolism *(dark blue and black regions)* are very noticeable in the sagittal and coronal views. (Courtesy of PET Imaging Center, Department of Radiology, University of Iowa Hospitals and Clinics, Iowa City.)

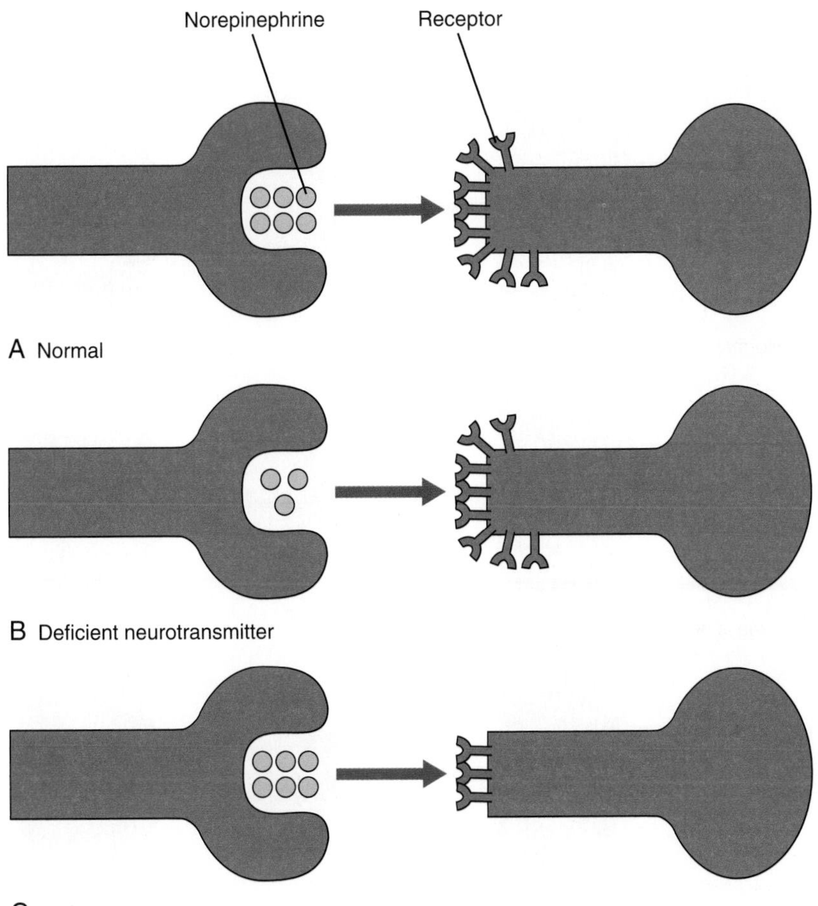

FIG. 3.8 Normal transmission of neurotransmitters (A). Deficiency in transmission may be resulting from deficient release of neurotransmitter, as shown in (B), or to a reduction in receptors, as shown in (C).

known as concordance rate. Concordance refers to how often an illness will affect both twins even when they are raised apart. A 100% concordance rate would mean that if one twin has a disorder, the other one would also have it. For schizophrenia, the concordance rate is 50%, meaning that inheritance is half of the equation and that other factors are involved.

Neurotransmitters

Major components in the brain's chemical stew are the monoamine neurotransmitters (norepinephrine, dopamine, and serotonin), the amino acid neurotransmitters (glutamate and γ-aminobutyric acid [GABA]), the neuropeptides (CRH and endorphin), and acetylcholine. Alteration of these chemicals is the basis of psychiatric illness and is the target for pharmacological treatment.

Understanding alterations in neurotransmitters will lead to better treatments and possibly prevent mental disorders. Research interest is focused on certain neurotransmitters and their receptors, particularly in the limbic system, which links the frontal cortex, basal ganglia, and upper brainstem.

Let us consider major depression. We believe that a deficiency of norepinephrine, serotonin, dopamine, or a combination of these is the biological basis of depression. How this deficiency happens is illustrated in Fig. 3.8. Fig. 3.8A shows normal transmission of neurotransmitters. In Fig. 3.8B we see a deficiency in the amount of neurotransmitter in the presynaptic cell. Fig. 3.8C shows a deficiency or loss of the ability of postsynaptic receptors to respond to the neurotransmitters.

Changes in neurotransmitter release and receptor response can be both a cause and a consequence of intracellular changes in the neurons involved. Thought disorders such as schizophrenia are associated with excess transmission of dopamine from the presynaptic neuron. As illustrated in Fig. 3.9, this may be caused by excessive release of the neurotransmitter or to an increase in receptor responsiveness.

Besides dopamine, the neurotransmitter glutamate may have a role in schizophrenia's pathology. Glutamate may have a direct influence on the activity of dopamine-releasing cells (Howes et al., 2015). First, glutamate activity increases in the hippocampus, then hippocampus metabolism is increased, and then the hippocampus begins to atrophy or shrink the brain's memory center. This process happens early in the disease and may become a primary tool for early diagnosis and a target for treatment.

The neurotransmitter GABA seems to play a role in modulating neuronal excitability and anxiety. Not surprisingly, many

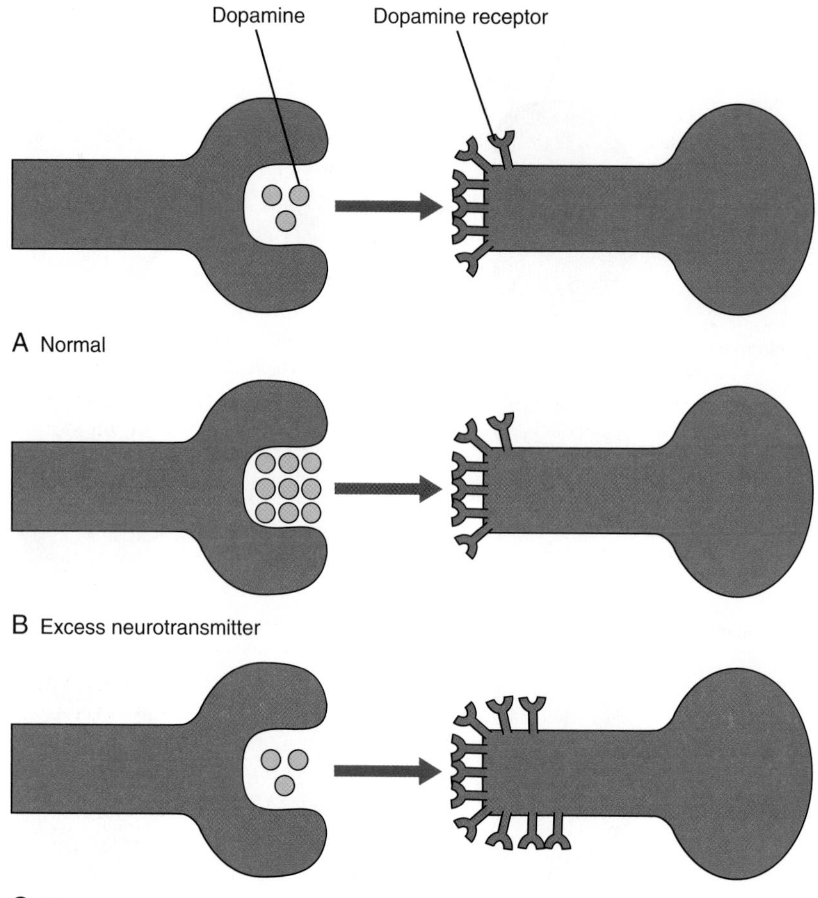

FIG. 3.9 Transmission of neurotransmitters (A). Excess transmission may be resulting from excess release of neurotransmitter, as shown in (B), or to excess responsiveness of receptors, as shown in (C).

antianxiety (anxiolytic) drugs act by increasing the effectiveness of this neurotransmitter. This is accomplished primarily by increasing receptor responsiveness.

It is important to keep in mind that a vast network of neurons interconnects the various areas of the brain. This network serves to integrate the many activities of the brain. A limited number of neurotransmitters are used in the brain and, thus, a particular neurotransmitter is often used by different neurons to carry out quite different activities.

For example, dopamine is not only involved in thought processes but also the regulation of movement. As a result, alterations in neurotransmitter activity, resulting from a mental disturbance or to the drugs used to treat the disturbance, can affect both thinking and movement. Basic body processes such as sleep patterns, body movement, and autonomic functions can be affected by alterations in mental status whether arising from disease or from medication.

ACTION OF PSYCHOTROPIC DRUGS

Two essential concepts to understand when studying drugs are pharmacodynamics and pharmacokinetics. **Pharmacodynamics** is fairly straightforward. It is the study of what drugs do to the body and how they do it. It includes drug action and drug responses. Both the action and responses are dose-related.

The term **pharmacokinetics** comes from two Greek words: *pharmakon* (drug) and *kinesis* (motion). As these words imply, pharmacokinetics is the movement of a drug through the body. Four basic processes of pharmacokinetics which determine the concentration of a drug at its sites of action are easily remembered with the acronym ADME:

Absorption—How is the drug absorbed into the blood?
Distribution—How is it distributed in the body?
Metabolism—How is the drug transformed for use and excretion?
Excretion—How does the body excrete it?

An understanding of pharmacokinetics helps maximize the drug's benefit, while minimizing harm. The benefits are derived by achieving a high enough level of the drug at the site of action, while minimizing harm by using the lowest possible dose. Pharmacokinetics helps us choose the most effective route, dosage, and schedule.

Pharmacokinetics and pharmacodynamics are impacted by genetic factors that give rise to interindividual and cross-ethnic variations in drug response. The Considering Culture box discusses how the area of pharmacogenetics influences the way healthcare providers tailor their prescriptions for patients.

 CONSIDERING CULTURE

Pharmacogenetics

Pharmacogenetics explains how genetic variation leads to differences in drug tolerability and responses in individuals and ethnic groups. One of the interesting genetically based variations is the cytochrome P450 (CYP) enzyme, which is the enzyme responsible for metabolizing most psychotropic medications.

People who metabolize drugs poorly will experience more adverse drug reactions. It is important to consider pharmacogenetics for patients who are experiencing significant adverse effects at low daily doses. On the other hand, people who hypermetabolize drugs may have less of a therapeutic response to treatment.

Poor metabolism of one of these enzymes, CYP 2D6, occurs in about 10% of Caucasians. Poor metabolism of another of these enzymes, CYP 2C19, occurs in about 20% of Asian subgroups.

Carbamazepine (Tegretol) is an anticonvulsant used for mood stabilization with bipolar disorder. Individuals of Asian and Southern Asian Indian ancestry with the HLA-B*1502 allele have a higher risk of dangerous or fatal skin reactions when taking carbamazepine. These emergency reactions are Stevens-Johnson syndrome and toxic epidermal necrolysis, which are characterized by the shedding of skin and mucous membranes. The US Food and Drug Administration (FDA) recommends screening for HLA-B*1502 in individuals who may be genetically at risk before starting this drug.

There are still challenges to achieving the goals of personalized treatments in psychiatry. With more evidence on predictable impact in clinical care, the value of pharmacogenetics will be appreciated to maximize drug therapy response and minimize adverse effects for many.

Hamilton S. P. (2015). The promise of psychiatric pharmacogenomics. *Biological Psychiatry, 77*, 29–35.

The liver metabolizes most drugs into active metabolites—chemicals that also have pharmacological actions. Researchers use this knowledge in designing new drugs that make use of the body's own mechanisms to activate a chemical for pharmacological use.

An ideal psychiatric drug would relieve the mental disturbance of the patient without inducing additional cerebral (mental) or somatic (physical) effects. Unfortunately, in psychopharmacology—as in most areas of pharmacology—there are no drugs that are both fully effective and free of undesired side effects. Researchers work toward developing medications that target the symptoms while producing fewer side effects.

Because all activities of the brain involve actions of neurons, neurotransmitters, and receptors, these are the targets of pharmacological intervention. Most psychotropic drugs act by either increasing or decreasing the activity of certain neurotransmitter-receptor systems.

Drug Agonism and Antagonism

Two important terms that you will see in connection with many of the psychotropic drugs are agonist and antagonist. The word agonist comes from the Latin word *agōnista* that means contender. **Agonist** drugs mimic the effects of neurotransmitters naturally found in the human brain by binding to and stimulating the receptor site.

The word antagonist is derived from the Latin word *antagōnista* that means adversary or opponent. Rather than binding to and stimulating the receptor site, drugs with **antagonistic** properties block the neurotransmitters, thereby obstructing the neurotransmitter's action.

Antianxiety and Hypnotic Drugs

The major inhibitory (calming) neurotransmitter in the central nervous system (CNS) is GABA. The most commonly used antianxiety agents are the benzodiazepines.

Benzodiazepines

Benzodiazepines potentiate, or promote, the activity of GABA by binding to a specific receptor on the GABA receptor complex. This binding results in an increased frequency of chloride channel opening causing membrane hyperpolarization, which reduces the cellular excitation. If cellular excitation is decreased, the result is a calming effect. Fig. 3.10 shows that benzodiazepines, such as diazepam (Valium), clonazepam (Klonopin), and alprazolam (Xanax), enhance the effects of GABA.

All benzodiazepines can cause sedation at higher therapeutic doses. There are five benzodiazepines approved by the FDA for treatment of insomnia with a predominantly **hypnotic** (sleep-inducing) effect: flurazepam (Dalmane), temazepam (Restoril), triazolam (Halcion), estazolam (ProSom), and quazepam (Doral). Other benzodiazepines, such as lorazepam (Ativan) and alprazolam (Xanax), reduce anxiety without being as sleep-producing when used at lower therapeutic doses.

The fact that the benzodiazepines inhibit neurons probably accounts for their usefulness as anticonvulsants and for their ability to reduce the neuronal overexcitement of alcohol withdrawal. When used alone, even at high dosages, these drugs rarely inhibit the brain to the degree of respiratory depression, coma, and death. However, when combined with other CNS depressants, such as alcohol, opiates, or tricyclic antidepressants, the inhibitory actions of the benzodiazepines can lead to life-threatening CNS depression.

Any drug that inhibits electrical activity in the brain can interfere with motor ability, attention, and judgment. Healthcare providers must caution a patient taking benzodiazepines about engaging in activities that could be dangerous if reflexes and attention are impaired, including specialized activities, such as working in construction, and more common activities, such as driving a car. In older adults, the use of benzodiazepines may contribute to falls and bone fractures. Ataxia is a common side effect secondary to the abundance of GABA receptors in the cerebellum.

Short-Acting Sedative-Hypnotic Sleep Agents

The Z-hypnotics include zolpidem (Ambien), zaleplon (Sonata), and eszopiclone (Lunesta). They have sedative effects without the antianxiety, anticonvulsant, or muscle relaxant effects of benzodiazepines. They are selective for $GABA_A$ receptors containing alpha-1 subunits. The drugs' affinity to alpha-1 subunits confers the potential for amnestic and ataxic side effects, and their onset of action is faster than that of most benzodiazepines. It is important to inform patients taking nonbenzodiazepine hypnotic agents about the quick onset of action and to take them when they are ready to go to sleep.

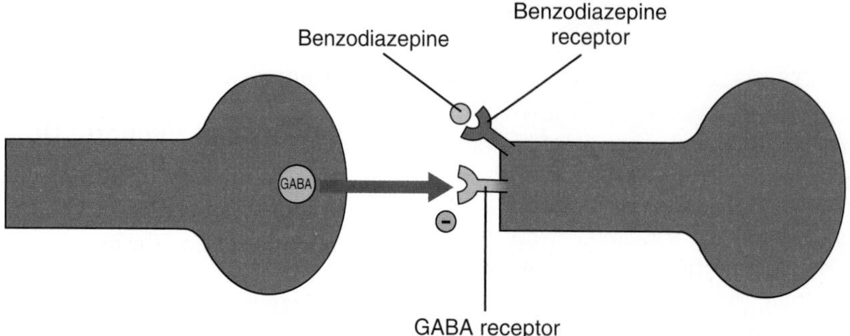

FIG. 3.10 Action of the benzodiazepines. Drugs in this group attach to receptors adjacent to the receptors for the neurotransmitter γ-aminobutyric acid (GABA). Drug attachment to these receptors results in a strengthening of the inhibitory effects of GABA. In the absence of GABA there is no inhibitory effect of benzodiazepines.

Most of these drugs have short half-lives, which determine the duration of action. Eszopiclone has the longest duration of action (an average of 7 to 8 hours of sleep per therapeutic dose) while the other two are much shorter. Eszopiclone also has a unique side effect of an unpleasant bitter taste upon awakening. Although tolerance and dependence are reportedly less than with benzodiazepines, the Z-hypnotics are categorized as schedule IV, similar to the benzodiazepines, by the US Drug Enforcement Administration (DEA). There have been reports of sleepwalking, eating, and even driving after the use of Z-hypnotics. These CNS adverse effects have been reported with other hypnotics as well. Doses for immediate-release zolpidem are now lower for women and the elderly.

Melatonin Receptor Agonists

Melatonin is a naturally occurring hormone that is only excreted at night as part of the normal circadian rhythm. Ramelteon (Rozerem) is a melatonin (MT) receptor agonist and acts much the same way as endogenous melatonin. It has a high selectivity and potency at the MT1 receptor site—which regulates sleepiness—and at the MT2 receptor site—which regulates circadian rhythms. This is one of two hypnotic medications approved for the treatment of insomnia not classified as a scheduled substance, lacking abuse potential, by the DEA. Side effects include headache and dizziness. Long-term use of ramelteon above therapeutic doses can lead to increased prolactin and associated side effects (e.g., sexual dysfunction).

Doxepin

Doxepin (Silenor) is the low-dose formulation (3-mg and 6-mg tablets) of an old tricyclic antidepressant. Doxepin is indicated for the treatment of insomnia characterized by difficulty in maintaining sleep. The mechanism of action for its sedative effect is most likely from a strong histamine-1 receptor blockade.

Patients with severe urinary retention or on MAOIs should avoid this medication. The use of other CNS depressants and sedating antihistamines should also be avoided. Doxepin was mainly studied in the geriatric population where it showed an improvement in total sleep duration with no significant decrease in time of sleep onset.

Suvorexant

The orexins are neurotransmitters produced in the hypothalamus that promote normal wakefulness. Suvorexant (Belsomra) is an orexin receptor antagonist. It selectively blocks the binding of orexin to suppress wakefulness. There are some important precautions including:

- Daytime impairment (e.g., falling asleep while driving)
- Additive CNS depression when used together with other CNS depressants
- Abnormal thinking and behavioral changes
- Worsening depression or increases in suicidal ideation
- Sleep paralysis
- Hypnagogic and hypnopompic hallucinations
- Cataplexy-like symptoms associated with the higher doses

Buspirone

Buspirone (BuSpar) is a drug that reduces anxiety without having strong sedative-hypnotic properties. Because this agent does not leave the patient sleepy or sluggish, patients tolerate it better than the benzodiazepines. It is not a CNS depressant and, therefore, does not have as great a danger of interaction with other CNS depressants such as alcohol.

Although the mechanism of action of buspirone is not clear, one possibility is illustrated in Fig. 3.11. Buspirone seems to act as a partial serotonin-1A agonist (booster). It also has a moderate affinity for D_2 receptors, and side effects include dizziness and insomnia.

Refer to Chapter 15 on anxiety disorders for a discussion of the adverse reactions, dosages, nursing implications, and patient and family teaching points for the antianxiety drugs. Refer to Chapter 19 on sleep disorders for a more detailed discussion on medications to promote sleep.

Treating Anxiety Disorders with Antidepressants

The symptoms, neurotransmitters, and circuits associated with anxiety disorders overlap extensively with those of depressive disorders (refer to Chapters 14 and 15). Many antidepressants have proven to be effective treatments for anxiety disorders. Selective

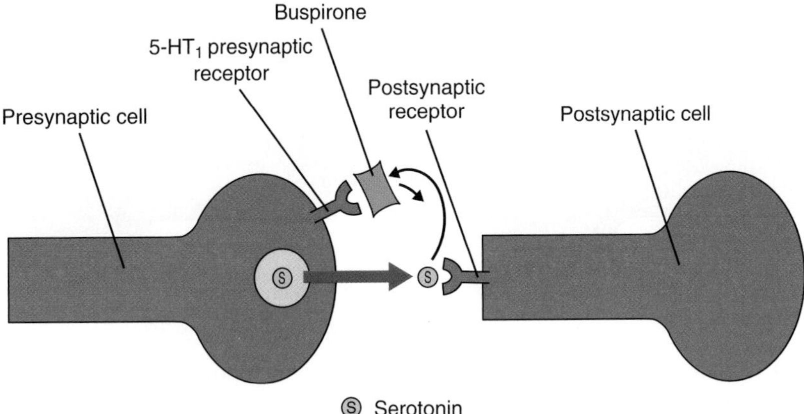

FIG. 3.11 Action of buspirone. A proposed mechanism of action of buspirone is that it blocks feedback inhibition by serotonin. This leads to increased release of serotonin by the presynaptic cell. *5-HT₁*, Serotonin.

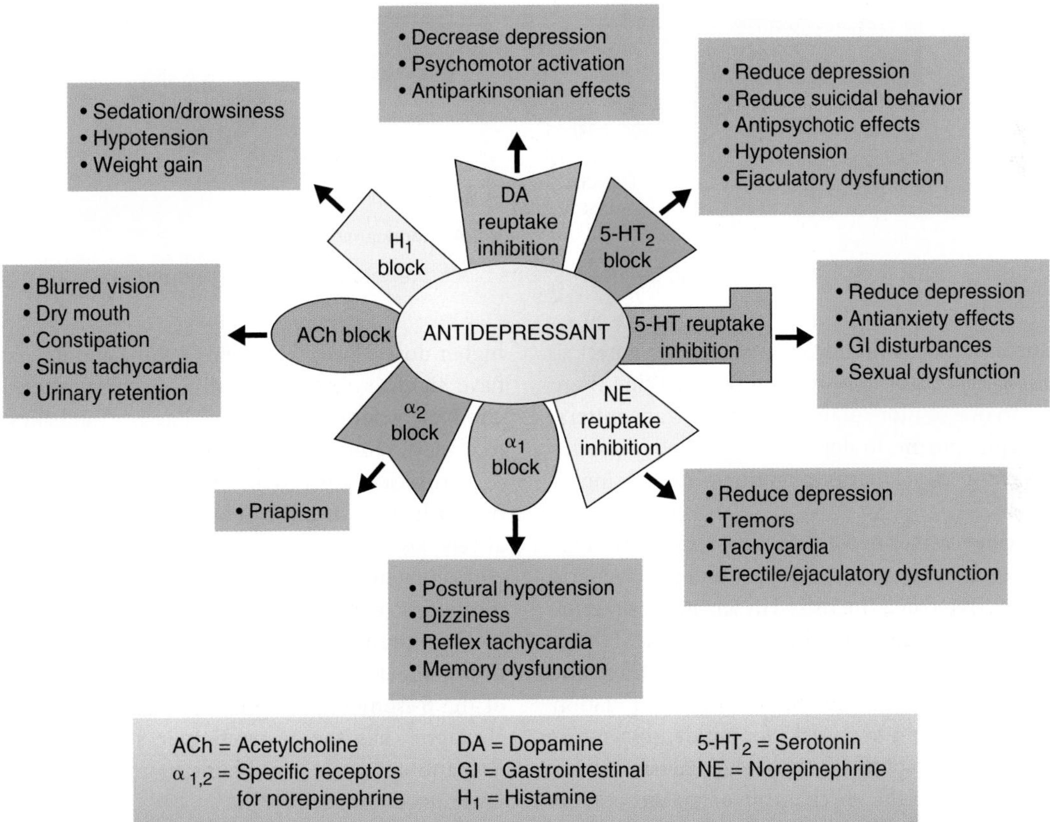

FIG. 3.12 Possible effects of receptor binding of the antidepressant medications.

serotonin reuptake inhibitors (SSRIs) are often used to treat obsessive-compulsive disorder (OCD), social anxiety disorder (SAD), generalized anxiety disorder (GAD), panic disorder (PD), and posttraumatic stress disorder (PTSD). The selective serotonin norepinephrine reuptake inhibitor (SNRI), venlafaxine (Effexor XR), is used to treat GAD, SAD, and PD. Another drug in that classification, duloxetine (Cymbalta), has FDA approval for GAD.

Antidepressant Drugs

Our understanding of the neurophysiological basis of mood disorders is far from complete. However, a great deal of evidence indicates that the neurotransmitters norepinephrine and serotonin play a major role in regulating mood. A transmission deficiency of one or both of these monoamines within the limbic system may underlie depression. One piece of evidence is that all of the drugs that demonstrate efficacy in the treatment of depression increase the synaptic level of one or both of these neurotransmitters. Fig. 3.12 identifies the side effects of specific neurotransmitters being blocked or activated. Fig. 3.13 illustrates the normal release, reuptake, and destruction of the monoamine neurotransmitters. A grasp of this underlying physiology is essential for understanding how the antidepressant drugs act.

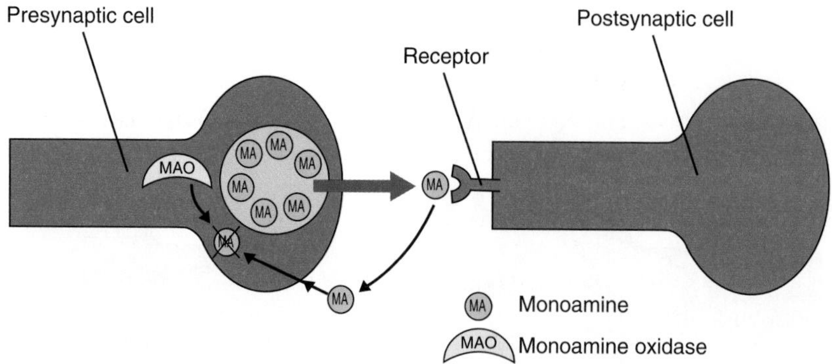

FIG. 3.13 Normal release, reuptake, and destruction of the monoamine neurotransmitters.

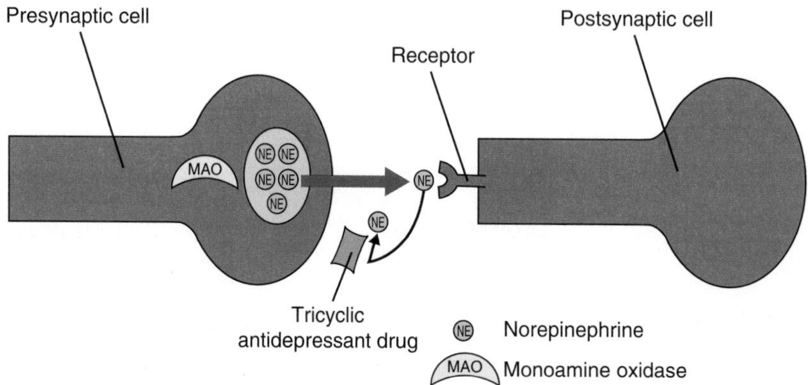

FIG. 3.14 How the tricyclic antidepressants block the reuptake of norepinephrine.

Hypotheses of antidepressants' mechanism of action are:

1. The *monoamine hypothesis of depression* suggests that there is a deficiency in one or more of the three neurotransmitters: serotonin, norepinephrine, or dopamine. The theory implies that by increasing these neurotransmitters depression is alleviated.

   The *monoamine receptor hypothesis of depression* also suggests that low levels of neurotransmitters cause postsynaptic receptors to be up-regulated (increased in sensitivity or number). Increasing neurotransmitters by antidepressants results in down-regulation (desensitization) of key neurotransmitter receptors. Delayed length of time for down-regulation may explain why it takes 4 to 6 weeks for antidepressants to work, especially if they rapidly increase neurotransmitters.
2. Another hypothesis for the mechanism of antidepressant drugs suggests that with prolonged use they increase production of neurotrophic factors. These factors regulate the survival of neurons and enhance the sprouting of axons to form new synaptic connections (Stahl, 2013).

Selective Serotonin Reuptake Inhibitors

As the name implies, the **selective serotonin reuptake inhibitors (SSRIs)**, such as fluoxetine (Prozac), sertraline (Zoloft), paroxetine (Paxil), citalopram (Celexa), escitalopram (Lexapro), and fluvoxamine (Luvox), block the reuptake of serotonin thereby making more of this neurotransmitter available. However, they each have slightly different effects.

Fluoxetine (Prozac) is a serotonin (5-HT_{2C}) antagonist, which can lead to the anorexic and antibulimic effects of fluoxetine at higher doses. Both sertraline (Zoloft) and fluvoxamine (Luvox) have sigma-1 receptor binding property. Researchers do not completely understand sigma-1 action but believe it contributes to anxiety-reducing and antipsychotic actions.

Paroxetine (Paxil) is the most anticholinergic among the SSRIs due to its muscarinic-1 antagonist property. Although it is relatively less anticholinergic than the tricyclic antidepressants, paroxetine may not be the best choice for patients with contraindications to anticholinergic agents (e.g., narrow angle glaucoma).

Citalopram (Celexa) has R- and S-enantiomers. At lower doses, the R-isomer may inhibit the increased 5-HT effects of the S-isomer leading to inconsistent efficacy. Escitalopram (Lexapro) has the S-enantiomer structure only without the R-enantiomer, which explains its more predictable efficacy at lower doses (Stahl, 2013).

As a class, SSRIs have less ability to block the muscarinic and histamine receptors than do the tricyclic antidepressants. As a result of their more selective action, they seem to show comparable efficacy without causing the anticholinergic and sedating side effects. However, SSRIs have other side effects resulting from stimulation of different serotonin receptors. Stimulation of the 5-HT_{2A} and 5-HT_{2C} receptors in the spinal cord may inhibit the spinal reflexes of orgasm. Stimulation of the 5-HT_{2A} receptors in the mesocortical area may decrease dopamine activity in this area, leading to apathy and low libido. Stimulation of the 5-HT_3 receptors in the hypothalamus or brainstem may cause nausea or vomiting while gastrointestinal (GI) side effects are secondary to the 5-HT_3 and/or 5-HT_4 receptors in the GI tract (Stahl, 2013; Fig. 3.14).

Norepinephrine and Serotonin Specific Antidepressant

The class of drugs known as the norepinephrine and serotonin specific antidepressant (NaSSA) is represented by only one drug, mirtazapine (Remeron), which increases norepinephrine and serotonin transmission by antagonizing (blocking) presynaptic alpha-2 adrenergic autoreceptors. Mirtazapine offers both antianxiety and antidepressant effects with minimal sexual dysfunction and improved sleep. This antidepressant causes fewer GI symptoms. The most common side effects are sedation, appetite stimulation, and weight gain.

Norepinephrine Dopamine Reuptake Inhibitor

Bupropion (Wellbutrin) is an antidepressant also used for smoking cessation (Zyban). It seems to act as a norepinephrine-dopamine reuptake inhibitor (NDRI). With no serotonergic activities, it does not cause sexual dysfunction side effects. Side effects include insomnia, tremor, anorexia, and weight loss. It is contraindicated in patients with a seizure disorder, in patients with a current or prior diagnosis of bulimia or anorexia nervosa, and in patients undergoing abrupt discontinuation of alcohol or sedatives (including benzodiazepines) due to the potential of seizures.

Serotonin Antagonist and Reuptake Inhibitors

Nefazodone, formerly sold as Serzone, is a novel drug indicated only for depression. It is a serotonin antagonist and reuptake inhibitor (SARI) that works by blocking serotonin receptors and weakly inhibiting the reuptake of norepinephrine and serotonin. The most common side effects are sedation, headache, fatigue, dry mouth, nausea, constipation, dizziness, and blurred vision. Weight gain and sexual dysfunction are minimal. This drug should be used with caution due to life-threatening liver failure and should never be given to people with pre-existing liver problems.

Trazodone, formerly sold under the trade name Desyrel, was not used for antidepressant treatment for many years. It was often given, along with another agent, for the treatment of insomnia as sedation is one of its common side effects. A trademarked version, Oleptro, has FDA approval as an extended-release drug indicated for the use of major depressive disorder in adults. Its antidepressant effects are due to its action as a 5-HT reuptake inhibitor and 5-$HT_{2A/2C}$ antagonist.

Common side effects of trazodone are sedation, dizziness, and orthostatic hypotension. Potent alpha-1 antagonists with little anticholinergic effects, such as trazodone, can lead to priapism, a painful prolonged erection caused by the inability for detumescence (subsidence of erection).

Brexpiprazole (Rexulti) was introduced in 2015. It has FDA approval as a treatment for the depression that accompanies schizophrenia. It works as a partial agonist at serotonin 5-HT_{1A} and dopamine D_2 receptors and antagonist activity at serotonin 5-HT_{2A} receptors. Due to dopamine effects, it may result in akathisia. Weight gain is also a side effect of this drug.

Serotonin Modulator and Stimulator

Vortioxetine (Trintellix) is a serotonin modulator and stimulator. It affects many different serotonin receptors by inhibiting serotonin reuptake like the SSRIs, agonizing the 5-HT_{1A} receptor like buspirone, partially agonizing the 5-HT_{1B} receptor, and antagonizing the 5-HT_3, 5-HT_{1D}, and 5-HT_7 receptors. Geriatric patients may experience an improvement of cognitive deficits independent of its antidepressant properties. Common side effects include constipation, nausea, and vomiting. More serious side effects are hyponatremia and, rarely, induction of hypomania/mania.

Serotonin Norepinephrine Reuptake Inhibitors

Serotonin norepinephrine reuptake inhibitors (SNRIs) increase both serotonin and norepinephrine. Venlafaxine (Effexor) acts more like a serotonergic agent at lower therapeutic doses and promotes norepinephrine reuptake blockade at higher doses, leading to the dual SNRI action. Hypertension may be induced in about 5% of patients and is a dose-dependent effect based on norepinephrine reuptake blockade. Doses greater than 150 mg/day can increase diastolic blood pressure by approximately 7 to 10 mm Hg.

Desvenlafaxine (Pristiq) is the primary active metabolite of venlafaxine. When people take venlafaxine, the majority of the benefit comes from venlafaxine being metabolized into desvenlafaxine. Therefore the mechanism of action and effects of the two antidepressants are similar.

Duloxetine (Cymbalta) is an SNRI indicated for both depression and GAD, as well as diabetic peripheral neuropathy, fibromyalgia, and chronic musculoskeletal pain.

Like the tricyclic antidepressants, many of the SNRIs also have therapeutic effects on neuropathic pain. The common underlying mechanism of neuropathic pain is nerve injury or dysfunction. The mechanism by which tricyclic antidepressants and SNRIs reduce neuropathic pain is activating the descending norepinephrine and 5-HT pathways to the spinal cord, thereby limiting pain signals from reaching the brain.

The previously discussed SNRIs inhibit serotonin reuptake more than they inhibit norepinephrine reuptake. Levomilnacipran (Fetzima) is an SNRI with a greater effect on norepinephrine reuptake than any of the other SNRIs available for treating depression. Increasing norepinephrine may be responsible for observed increases in heart rate and blood pressure in some patients.

Serotonin Partial Agonist and Reuptake Inhibitor

Vilazodone (Viibryd) is an antidepressant approved by the FDA in 2011. It enhances the release of serotonin by inhibiting the serotonin transporter (similar to SSRIs) and by stimulating serotonin (5-HT_{1A}) receptors through partial agonism (similar to the antianxiety medication buspirone). With this dual activity, vilazodone is considered to be a serotonin partial agonist and reuptake inhibitor (SPARI). Commonly observed adverse reactions during clinical trials include diarrhea, nausea, insomnia, and vomiting. Patients should take this antidepressant with food for better bioavailability, and avoid nighttime doses due to insomnia.

Tricyclic Antidepressants

Tricyclic antidepressants (TCAs) were widely used before the development of SSRIs. They are no longer considered first-line

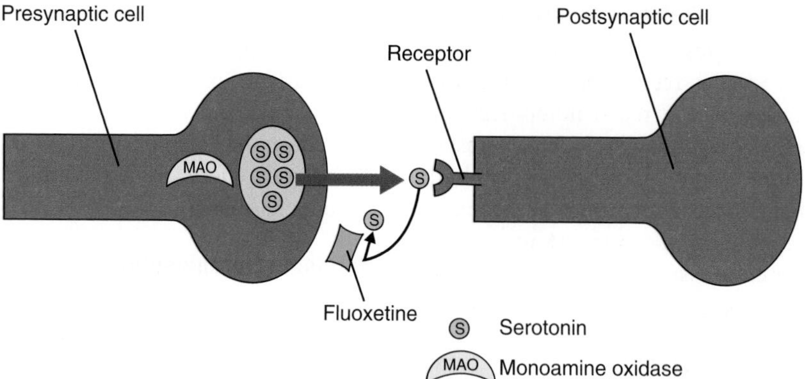

FIG. 3.15 How the selective serotonin reuptake inhibitors work.

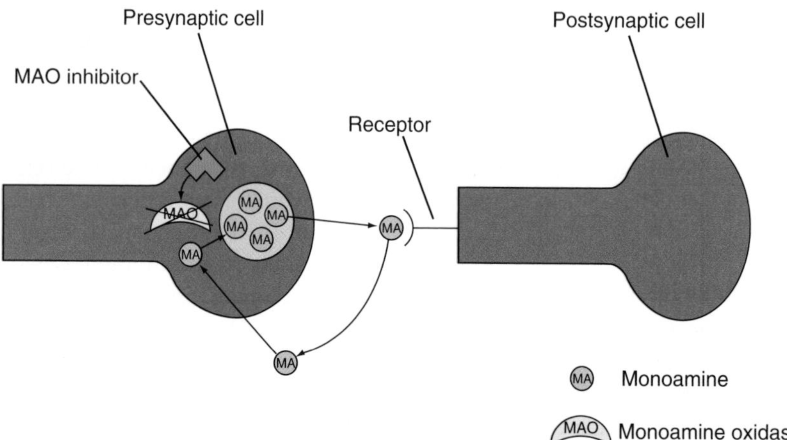

FIG. 3.16 Blocking of monoamine oxidase (MAO) by inhibiting agents (MAOIs), which prevents the breakdown of monoamine by MAO.

medications since they have more side effects, take longer to reach an optimal therapeutic dose, and are far more lethal in overdose. The TCAs act primarily by blocking the reuptake of norepinephrine for the secondary amines (e.g., nortriptyline [Pamelor]) and both norepinephrine and serotonin for the tertiary amines (e.g., amitriptyline, imipramine [Tofranil]). As shown in Fig. 3.15, this blockade prevents norepinephrine from coming into contact with its degrading enzyme, MAO, increasing the level of norepinephrine at the synapse. Similarly, the tertiary TCAs block the reuptake and destruction of serotonin and increase the synaptic level of this neurotransmitter.

To varying degrees, many of the tricyclic drugs also block the muscarinic acetylcholine receptors. As discussed in the previous section, this blockade leads to anticholinergic effects such as blurred vision, dry mouth, tachycardia, urinary retention, and constipation. These adverse effects can be troubling to patients and limit their adherence to the regimen.

Depending on the individual drug, these agents can also block histamine 1 (H_1) receptors in the brain. Blockade of these receptors by any drug causes sedation and drowsiness, an unwelcome symptom in daily use (see Fig. 3.12). Persons taking TCAs often have adherence issues because of their adverse reactions. TCA overdose can be fatal secondary to cardiac conduction disturbances from excessive sodium channel blockade.

Monoamine Oxidase Inhibitors

Monoamine oxidase inhibitors (MAOIs) are a class of antidepressant drugs that can have a desired effect in the brain while exerting potentially dangerous effects elsewhere. To understand the action of these drugs, keep in mind the following definitions:

- Monoamines are organic compounds.
- Monoamines include the neurotransmitters norepinephrine, epinephrine, dopamine, serotonin, and many different food substances and drugs.
- MAO is an enzyme that destroys monoamines.
- MAOIs are drugs that inhibit the action of MAO to prevent the destruction of monoamines.
- MAOIs increase the synaptic level of neurotransmitters resulting in the antidepressant effects of these drugs (Fig. 3.16).
- Examples of MAOIs include isocarboxazid (Marplan), phenelzine (Nardil), selegiline (EMSAM), and tranylcypromine (Parnate).

There is a problem with inhibiting MAO. The liver uses these enzymes to degrade monoamine substances that enter the body from food. One monoamine, tyramine, is present in most protein-based foods. However, some foods are extremely rich in tyramine. They include aged cheeses, pickled or smoked fish, and wine. If the liver cannot break down the tyramine from these substances, tyramine can produce significant vasoconstriction.

This vasoconstriction results in an elevation in blood pressure and the threat of a hypertensive crisis.

In addition to food, a number of drugs, such as other antidepressants and sympathomimetic drugs, can result in serious reactions. In a patient taking drugs to inhibit MAO, the blood level of monoamine drugs can reach high levels and cause serious toxicity. Any drug that amplifies serotonin (e.g., an antidepressant) or norepinephrine (e.g., amphetamines) is at risk for a hypertensive crisis due to an excess supply of these neurotransmitters. For example, paroxetine (Paxil) inhibits the reuptake of serotonin, making more serotonin available. At the same time, if MAO is inhibited and is not degrading the serotonin as quickly, dangerous levels of serotonin can occur. Patients should avoid using some over-the-counter products with sympathomimetic properties (e.g., oral decongestants) or serotonergic properties (e.g., dextromethorphan).

Because of the dangers that result from inhibition of hepatic and intestinal MAO, patients taking MAOIs must be given a list of foods and drugs to avoid. Chapter 14 discusses the treatment of depression and contains a list of foods to avoid and foods to be taken in moderation along with nursing measures and instructions for patient education.

Mood Stabilizers

Lithium

Although **lithium** (Eskalith, Lithobid) has been used as a **mood stabilizer** in patients with bipolar (manic-depressive) disorder for many years, we do not understand its mechanism of action. As a positively charged cation, similar in structure to sodium and potassium, lithium may well act by affecting electrical conductivity in neurons.

As discussed earlier, an electrical impulse consists of the inward, depolarizing flow of sodium followed by an outward, repolarizing flow of potassium. These electrical charges are propagated along the neuron so that, if they are initiated at one end of the neuron, they will pass to the other end. Once they reach the end of a neuron, a neurotransmitter is released.

It may be that an overexcitement of neurons in the brain underlies bipolar disorder and lithium interacts in some complex way with sodium and potassium at the cell membrane to stabilize electrical activity. Furthermore, lithium may reduce the excitatory neurotransmitter glutamate and exert an antimanic effect. Another mechanism by which lithium functions to regulate mood includes the noncompetitive inhibition of the enzyme inositol monophosphatase. Inhibition of 5-HT autoreceptors by lithium is more related to lithium's antidepressant effects rather than its antimanic effects.

While we do not know exactly how lithium works, we are certain that its influence on electrical conductivity results in adverse effects and toxicity. By altering electrical conductivity, lithium represents a potential threat to all body functions regulated by electrical currents, especially cardiac contraction. Lithium can induce, although not commonly, sinus bradycardia. Extreme alteration of cerebral conductivity with overdose can lead to convulsions. Alteration in nerve and muscle conduction can commonly lead to tremor at therapeutic doses or more extreme motor dysfunction with overdose.

TABLE 3.3 Adverse Effects of Lithium

System	Adverse Effects
Nervous and muscular	Tremor, ataxia, confusion, convulsions
Digestive	Nausea, vomiting, diarrhea
Cardiac	Arrhythmias
Fluid and electrolyte	Polyuria, polydipsia, edema
Endocrine	Goiter and hypothyroidism

Sodium and potassium play a strong role in regulating fluid balance, and the distribution of fluid in various body compartments explains the disturbances in fluid balance that lithium can cause. These include polyuria (the output of large volumes of urine) and edema (the accumulation of fluid in the interstitial space). Long-term use of lithium can cause hypothyroidism in some patients, which is secondary to interfering with the iodine molecules affecting the formation and conversion to its active form (T3) thyroid hormone. In addition, hyponatremia can increase the risk of lithium toxicity because increased renal reabsorption of sodium leads to increased reabsorption of lithium as well.

Primarily because of its effects on electrical conductivity, lithium has a low therapeutic index. The **therapeutic index** represents the ratio of the lethal dose to the effective dose and is a measure of overall drug safety in regard to the possibility of overdose or toxicity. A low therapeutic index means that the blood level of a drug that can cause death is not far above the blood level required for drug effectiveness. Lithium blood levels need to be monitored on a regular basis to ensure that the drug is not accumulating and rising to dangerous levels. Table 3.3 lists some of the adverse effects of lithium. Chapter 13 considers lithium treatment in more depth and discusses specific dosage-related adverse and toxic effects, nursing implications, and the patient teaching plan.

Anticonvulsant Drugs

Valproate (available as divalproex sodium [Depakote] and valproic acid [Depakene]), carbamazepine (Tegretol), and lamotrigine (Lamictal) are useful in the treatment of bipolar disorders. Their anticonvulsant properties derive from the alteration of electrical conductivity in membranes. In particular, they reduce the firing rate of very-high-frequency neurons in the brain. It is possible that this membrane-stabilizing effect accounts for the ability of these drugs to reduce the mood swings that occur in patients with bipolar disorders. Other proposed mechanisms as mood stabilizers are glutamate antagonists and GABA agonist.

Valproate

Valproate (Depakote, Depakene) is structurally different from other anticonvulsants and psychiatric drugs that show efficacy in the treatment of bipolar disorder. Valproate is recommended for mixed episodes and has been found useful for rapid cycling. Common side effects include tremor, weight gain, and sedation. Occasional serious side effects are thrombocytopenia, pancreatitis, hepatic failure, and birth defects.

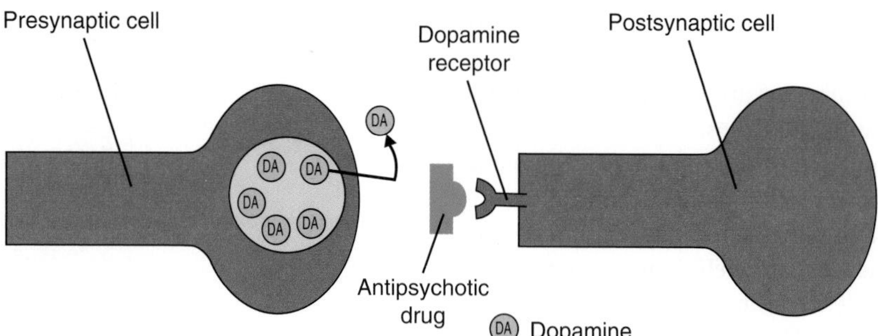

FIG. 3.17 How the first-generation antipsychotics block dopamine receptors.

Baseline levels are measured for liver function tests and complete blood count (CBC) before an individual is initiated on this medication and laboratory monitoring is repeated periodically. In addition, the therapeutic blood level of the drug is monitored.

Carbamazepine

Carbamazepine (Equetro, Tegretol) is useful in treating acute mania. It reduces the firing rate of overexcited neurons by reducing the activity of sodium channels. Baseline liver function tests, CBC, electrocardiogram, and electrolyte levels should be obtained. Blood levels are monitored to avoid toxicity (>12 mcg/mL), but there are no established therapeutic blood levels for carbamazepine in the treatment of bipolar disorder.

Common effects include anticholinergic side effects (e.g., dry mouth, constipation, urinary retention, blurred vision), orthostasis, sedation, and ataxia. A rash may occur in about 10% of patients during the first 20 weeks of treatment. This potentially serious side effect should be reported immediately because it could progress to a life-threatening exfoliative dermatitis or Stevens-Johnson syndrome. The FDA requires genetic testing before this drug is used in people of Asian descent.

Lamotrigine

The FDA approved lamotrigine (Lamictal) for maintenance therapy in bipolar disorder, but it is not effective in acute mania. Lamotrigine works well in treating the depression of bipolar disorder. It modulates the release of glutamate and aspartate. Patients should promptly report any rashes, which could be a sign of life-threatening Stevens-Johnson syndrome. This adverse drug reaction can be minimized by slowly increasing to therapeutic doses. Concurrent use with valproate may double the blood levels of lamotrigine and increase the risk of Stevens-Johnson syndrome.

Refer to Chapter 13 for more detailed discussion on mood stabilizers.

Antipsychotic Drugs

First-Generation Antipsychotics

First-generation antipsychotics are also referred to as conventional antipsychotics and typical antipsychotics. An overactivity of the dopamine system in the mesolimbic system may be responsible for at least some of the symptoms of schizophrenia. These drugs are strong **antagonists** (blocking the action) of the D_2 receptors for dopamine. By binding to these receptors and blocking the attachment of dopamine, they reduce dopaminergic stimulation. These drugs may be most effective on the "positive" symptoms of schizophrenia, such as delusions (e.g., paranoid and grandiose ideas) and hallucinations (e.g., hearing or seeing things not present in reality). Refer to Chapter 12 for a more detailed discussion of schizophrenia and its symptoms.

These drugs are also antagonists—to varying degrees—of the muscarinic receptors for acetylcholine, α_1 receptors for norepinephrine, and (H_1) receptors for histamine. Although it is unclear if this antagonism plays a role in the beneficial effects of the drugs, it is certain that antagonism is responsible for some of their major side effects.

Fig. 3.17 illustrates the proposed mechanism of action of the first-generation antipsychotics, which include the phenothiazines, thioxanthenes, butyrophenones, and pharmacologically related agents. As summarized in Fig. 3.18, many of the unpleasant side effects are logical given their receptor-blocking activity. For example, because dopamine (D_2) in the basal ganglia plays a major role in the regulation of movement, it is not surprising that dopamine blockade can lead to motor abnormalities known as extrapyramidal symptoms (EPS). These EPS include acute dystonic reactions, parkinsonism, akathisia, and tardive dyskinesia.

Nurses and physicians often monitor patients for evidence of involuntary movements after administration of the first-generation antipsychotic agents. One popular scale is called the Abnormal Involuntary Movement Scale (AIMS). Refer to Chapter 12 for an example of AIMS and a discussion of the clinical use of antipsychotic drugs, side effects, specific nursing interventions, and patient teaching strategies.

An important physiological function of dopamine is that it acts as the hypothalamic factor that inhibits the release of prolactin from the anterior pituitary gland. Therefore blockade of dopamine transmission can lead to increased pituitary secretion of prolactin. In women, this hyperprolactinemia can result in amenorrhea (absence of the menses) or galactorrhea (excessive or inappropriate breast milk production), and in men, it can lead to gynecomastia (development of the male mammary glands) and galactorrhea.

Acetylcholine is a neurotransmitter that attaches to muscarinic receptors and helps regulate internal function. Blockade of the muscarinic receptors by phenothiazines and a wide variety

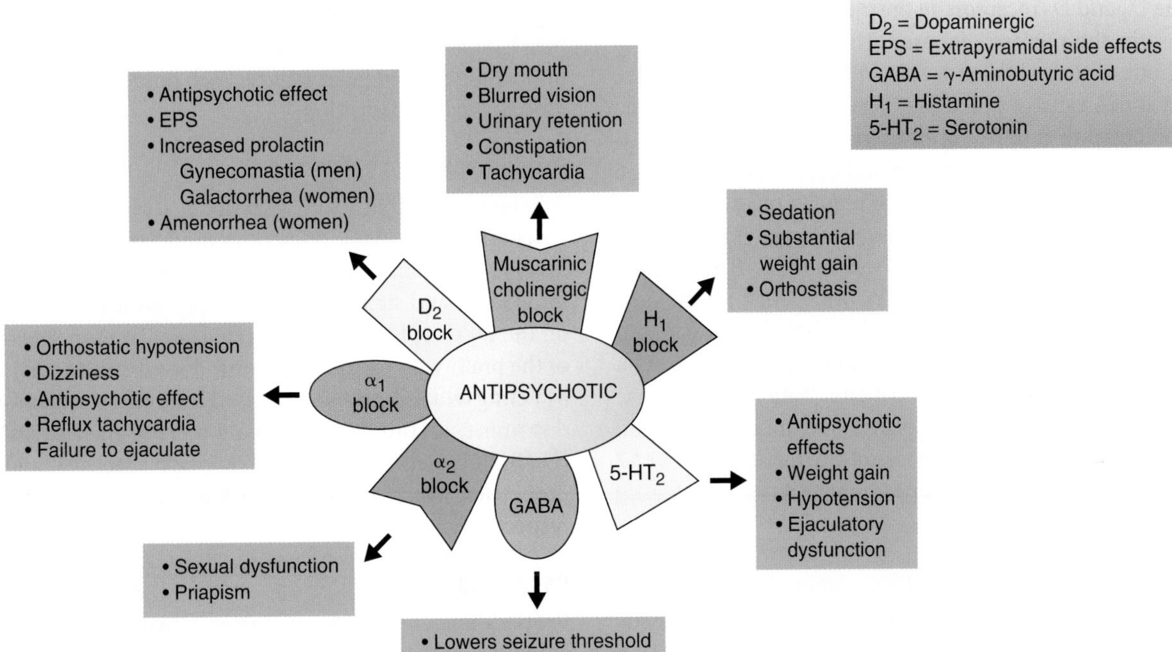

FIG. 3.18 Adverse effects of receptor blockage of antipsychotic agents. (From Varcarolis, E. [2004]. *Manual of psychiatric nursing care plans* [2nd ed.]. St. Louis, MO: Elsevier.)

of other psychiatric drugs can lead to a constellation of adverse effects. These side effects usually involve blurred vision, dry mouth, constipation, and urinary hesitancy. These drugs can also impair memory since acetylcholine is important for memory function.

Many of the first-generation antipsychotic drugs also act as antagonists for norepinephrine. These receptors are found on smooth muscle cells that contract in response to norepinephrine from sympathetic nerves. For example, the ability of sympathetic nerves to constrict blood vessels is dependent on the attachment of norepinephrine to α_1 receptors. Therefore blockade of these receptors can bring about vasodilatation and a consequent drop in blood pressure. Vasoconstriction mediated by the sympathetic nervous system is essential for maintaining normal blood pressure when the body is in the upright position; blockade of the α_1 receptors can lead to orthostatic hypotension.

Finally, many of these first-generation antipsychotic agents, as well as a variety of other psychiatric drugs, block the H_1 receptors for histamine. The two most significant side effects of blocking these receptors are sedation and substantial weight gain. Sedation may be beneficial in severely agitated patients. Nonadherence to the medication regimen is a significant issue because of these troublesome side effects.

Second-Generation Antipsychotics

Second-generation antipsychotics are also known as atypical antipsychotics. These drugs produce fewer EPS and target both the negative and positive symptoms of schizophrenia (Chapter 12). These newer agents are often chosen as first-line treatments over the first-generation antipsychotics due a more favorable side effect profile.

Most of the available second-generation antipsychotics, however, can increase the risk of metabolic syndrome with increased weight, blood glucose, and triglycerides. The simultaneous blockade of receptors 5-HT_{2C} and H_1 is associated with weight gain from increased appetite stimulation via the hypothalamic eating centers. Strong anti-muscarinic properties at the M3 receptor on the pancreatic beta cells can cause insulin resistance leading to hyperglycemia. The receptor responsible for elevated triglycerides is currently unknown (Stahl, 2013). Clozapine and olanzapine have the highest risk of causing metabolic syndrome, while aripiprazole and ziprasidone are among the lowest risk in this classification.

The second-generation antipsychotics are predominantly D_2 (dopamine) and 5-HT_{2A} (serotonin) antagonists (blockers). The blockade at the mesolimbic dopamine pathway decreases psychosis, similar to the way the first-generation antipsychotics work. Decreasing D_2 stimulation can decrease psychosis, but cause adverse effects in the:

- Nigrostriatal area, which can cause the movement side effects of EPS.
- Mesocortical area, which can worsen cognitive and negative symptoms of schizophrenia.
- Tuberoinfundibular area, which can increase the hormone prolactin leading to gynecomastia, galactorrhea, amenorrhea, and low libido.

Most second-generation antipsychotics have more 5-HT_{2A} than D_2 antagonist effects. Blocking the 5-HT_{2A} receptors increases dopamine and norepinephrine. This may explain why the second-generation antipsychotics have less effect on causing EPS, cognitive impairment, and prolactin effects.

Clozapine

Clozapine (Clozaril) is an antipsychotic drug that is relatively free of the motor side effects of the phenothiazines and other second-generation antipsychotics. Clozapine preferentially blocks the D_1 and D_2 receptors in the mesolimbic system rather than those in the nigrostriatal area. This allows it to exert an antipsychotic action without leading to difficulties with EPS. However, it can cause a potentially fatal side effect. Clozapine has the potential to suppress bone marrow and induce agranulocytosis. Any deficiency in white blood cells renders a person prone to serious infection. Therefore regular measurement of absolute neutrophil count (ANC) is necessary. Typically, the count is measured weekly for the first 6 months. If results are normal, counts will be measured every other week for the next 6 months and every month thereafter.

Clozapine has the potential for inducing convulsions, a dose-related side effect, in 3.5% of patients. Patients should use caution with other drugs that can increase the concentration of clozapine. Note that smoking cessation reduces CYP 1A2 enzymes and can increase clozapine's concentration.

Risperidone

Risperidone (Risperdal) has a low potential for inducing agranulocytosis or convulsions. However, high therapeutic dosages (>6 mg/day) may lead to motor difficulties. As a potent D_2 antagonist, it has the highest risk of EPS among the second-generation antipsychotics and may increase prolactin, which may lead to sexual dysfunction. Because risperidone blocks α_1 and H_1 receptors, it can cause orthostatic hypotension and sedation, respectively. Keep in mind that orthostatic hypotension can lead to falls, which are a serious problem among older adults.

Weight gain, sedation, and sexual dysfunction are adverse effects that may affect adherence to the medication regimen and should be discussed with patients. Risperdal Consta is an injectable form of the drug that is administered every 2 weeks, providing an alternative to the depot form of first-generation antipsychotics.

Quetiapine

Quetiapine (Seroquel) has a broad receptor-binding profile. Its strong blockade of H_1 receptors accounts for the high sedation. The combination of H_1 and 5-HT_{2C} blockade leads to the weight gain associated with use of this drug and also to a moderate risk for metabolic syndrome. It causes moderate blockade of α_1 receptors and associated orthostasis. Quetiapine has a low risk for EPS or prolactin elevation from low D_2 binding due to rapid dissociation at D_2 receptors. This drug is too commonly prescribed for sleep problems when other drugs should be considered.

Olanzapine

Olanzapine (Zyprexa) is similar to clozapine in chemical structure. It is an antagonist of 5-HT_2, D_2, H_1, alpha-1, and muscarinic receptors. Side effects include sedation, weight gain, hyperglycemia with new-onset type 2 diabetes, and higher risk for metabolic syndrome. Olanzapine is also available in a long-acting intramuscular agent under the trade name of Zyprexa Relprevv.

Ziprasidone

Ziprasidone (Geodon) is a serotonin-norepinephrine reuptake inhibitor at multiple receptors: 5-HT_2, D_2, alpha-1, and H_{1D}. Ziprasidone is contraindicated in patients with a known history of QT interval prolongation, recent acute myocardial infarction, or uncompensated heart failure. Each dose should be taken with food to enable absorption.

Aripiprazole

Aripiprazole (Abilify) is a unique second-generation antipsychotic known as a dopamine modulator in addition to its 5-HT_{2A} antagonist activity. Depending on endogenous dopamine levels and signaling status, aripiprazole has varying effects on the D_2 receptor due to its partial agonist properties. In areas of the brain with excess dopamine, it lowers the dopamine level by acting as a receptor antagonist. However, in regions with low dopamine, it stimulates receptors to raise the dopamine level (De Bartolomeis et al., 2015). Aripiprazole lacks H_1 and 5-HT_{2C} properties, which explains its lack of sedation and weight gain, respectively.

Paliperidone

Paliperidone (Invega) is the major active metabolite of risperidone. It has similar side effects with regard to prolactin elevation. Other than the D_2 and 5-HT_{2A} antagonistic properties as an antipsychotic, paliperidone is also an antagonist at alpha-1 receptors and H_1 receptors, which explains the side effects of orthostasis and sedation, respectively. The Osmotic Release Oral System (OROS) provides consistent 24-hour release of the medication, leading to minimal peaks and troughs in plasma concentrations. It also has two long-acting injectable formulations: Invega Sustenna (every month) and Invega Trinza (every 3 months).

Iloperidone

Iloperidone (Fanapt) possesses minimal binding affinity for H_1 receptors and has minimal affinity for cholinergic muscarinic receptors. A common adverse effect is orthostatic hypotension from the α_1 blockade, which necessitates a slow dosage titration over the first few days to minimize orthostatic hypotension. There was a significant increase in the mean QT interval, although no deaths or serious arrhythmias were noted in the clinical trials. Another limitation of this medication is the risk of orthostatic hypotension (Holmes & Zacher, 2012).

Lurasidone

Lurasidone (Latuda) has high affinity for 5-HT_{2A} and D_2 receptors in addition to other serotonergic receptors such as 5-HT_{1A}. Lurasidone has similar pharmacological properties to the tetracyclic antidepressant mirtazapine. Lurasidone has high affinity for serotonergic (such as $5HT_{2A}$ and $5HT_{2C}$), noradrenergic, and dopaminergic receptors (D_3 and D_4). There is minimal muscarinic receptor activity. Each dose must be taken with 350 calories to ensure optimal absorption.

Asenapine

Asenapine (Saphris) is unique among the antipsychotics as being administered in a sublingual formulation, which enhances its direct absorption. Therefore it avoids much of the hepatic metabolism that restricts its availability when administered orally. Bioavailability of asenapine is reduced from 35% with sublingual administration to less than 2% with oral administration. Patients should avoid food and water for 10 minutes after sublingual administration (Holmes & Zacher, 2012). It has a higher affinity for 5-HT_{2A} receptors than D_2 receptors. It also has antagonistic activity at alpha-1 receptor that accounts for the orthostatic hypotension, and H_1 antagonistic activity, which causes sedation. Chapter 12 discusses the first- and second-generation antipsychotic drugs in detail including the indications for use, adverse reactions, nursing implications, and patient and family teaching.

Drug Treatment for Attention-Deficit/Hyperactivity Disorder

Children and adults with attention-deficit/hyperactivity disorder (ADHD) show symptoms of short attention span, impulsivity, and overactivity. Paradoxically, psychostimulant drugs are the mainstay of treatment for this condition in children and increasingly in adults. Both methylphenidate (Ritalin, Daytrana—a transdermal system) and dextroamphetamine (Adderall, Vyvanse) are helpful in these conditions. They are sympathomimetic amines and have been shown to function as direct and indirect agonists at adrenergic receptor sites. Psychostimulants act by blocking the reuptake of norepinephrine and dopamine into the presynaptic neuron and increasing the release of these monoamines into the synapse. How this translates into clinical efficacy is far from understood, but it is thought that the monoamines may inhibit an overactive part of the limbic system.

Among many concerns with the use of psychostimulant drugs are side effects of agitation, exacerbation of psychotic thought processes, hypertension, and growth suppression, as well as their potential for abuse. The FDA has approved three nonstimulants for the treatment of ADHD: atomoxetine (Strattera), guanfacine (Intuniv), and clonidine (Kapvay). Atomoxetine is a norepinephrine reuptake inhibitor approved for use in children 6 years and older. Common side effects include decreased appetite and weight loss, fatigue, and dizziness. It is contraindicated for patients with severe cardiovascular disease due to its potential to increase blood pressure and heart rate.

Guanfacine and clonidine are centrally acting alpha-2 adrenergic agonists that have traditionally been used for hypertension. The FDA-approved forms for ADHD are used in children ages 6 to 17. Both should be increased slowly and should not be discontinued abruptly. Guanfacine's most common side effects include sleepiness, low blood pressure, nausea, stomach pain, and dizziness. The drug's effectiveness with teenagers is questionable, and it probably works best in preteens. Clonidine extended-release tablets can be used alone or in addition to other ADHD drugs. Common side effects include fatigue, irritability, throat pain, insomnia, nightmares, emotional disorder, constipation, increased body temperature, dry mouth, and ear pain.

Drug Treatment for Alzheimer's Disease

The insidious and progressive loss of memory and other higher brain functions brought about by Alzheimer's disease is a great individual, family, and social tragedy. Because the disease seems to involve progressive structural degeneration of the brain, there are two major pharmacological directions in its treatment. The first is to attempt to prevent or slow the structural degeneration. Although actively pursued, this approach has been unsuccessful so far. The second is to attempt to maintain normal brain function for as long as possible.

Much of the memory loss in this disease has been attributed to insufficient acetylcholine, a neurotransmitter essential for learning, memory, and mood and behavior regulation. One class of drugs for Alzheimer's disease, **cholinesterase inhibitors**, shows some efficacy in slowing the rate of memory loss and even improving memory. They work by inactivating the enzyme that breaks down acetylcholine, cholinesterase, leading to less destruction of acetylcholine and, therefore, a higher concentration at the synapse.

Four of the FDA-approved drugs for treatment of Alzheimer's disease are cholinesterase inhibitors: tacrine (Cognex), donepezil (Aricept), galantamine (Razadyne, formerly named Reminyl), and rivastigmine (Exelon, Exelon Patch). Tacrine is no longer used extensively because of the risk of hepatic toxicity. All of these drugs are used for mild to moderate Alzheimer's disease. Donepezil and the Exelon Patch are for the mild to severe form of the disease. All of them become less effective as the brain produces less acetylcholine.

Glutamate, an abundant excitatory neurotransmitter, plays an important role in memory function. However, too much glutamate can be destructive to neurons. A fifth agent approved by the FDA for treatment of Alzheimer's disease is memantine, or Namenda and Namenda XR (an extended-release formulation), named for the receptor it blocks from glutamate, *N*-methyl-D-aspartate (NMDA). Normally, when glutamate binds to NMDA receptors, calcium flows freely and is essential to cell communication. However, pathological gray tangles of amyloid protein that build up in Alzheimer's brains, or amyloid plaques, are associated with excess glutamate. This excess receptor stimulation by glutamate results in excess calcium, which becomes toxic to surrounding brain cells. Memantine fills some of the NMDA receptor sites, reduces glutamate binding and calcium excess, and reduces damage. Memantine has been effective in the treatment of moderate to severe Alzheimer's disease. Since memantine has a very different mechanism of action than the cholinesterase inhibitors, they can be taken at the same time.

Refer to Chapter 23 for a more detailed discussion of these drugs, as well as their nursing considerations, and patient and family teaching.

Herbal Treatments

There are a variety of factors that drive the growing interest in medicinal herbs. Many people believe that herbal treatments are safer because they are "natural" or that they may have fewer side effects than more costly traditional medications.

Herbal treatments have been researched to understand their mechanisms of action and have also been used in clinical trials to determine their safety and efficacy. This is especially true of St. John's wort. Many medicinal herbs have been found to be nontherapeutic and some even deadly if taken over long periods of time or in combination with other chemical substances and prescription drugs. The risk of bleeding may be increased in patients taking ginkgo biloba and warfarin, and kava may increase the risk of hepatotoxicity. Chapter 36 covers complementary and integrative approaches in more detail.

KEY POINTS TO REMEMBER

- All actions of the brain—sensory, motor, and intellectual—are carried out physiologically through the interactions of nerve cells. These interactions involve impulse conduction, neurotransmitter release, and receptor response. Alterations in these basic processes can lead to mental disturbances and physical manifestations.
- In particular, it seems that excess activity of dopamine is involved in the thought disturbances of schizophrenia, and deficiencies of norepinephrine, serotonin, or both underlie depression and anxiety. Insufficient activity of GABA also plays a role in anxiety.
- Pharmacological treatment of mental disturbances is directed at the suspected neurotransmitter-receptor problem. Thus antipsychotic drugs decrease dopamine, antidepressant drugs increase synaptic levels of norepinephrine and/or serotonin, and antianxiety drugs increase the effectiveness of GABA or increase serotonin and/or norepinephrine.
- Because the immediate target activity of a drug can result in many downstream alterations in neuronal activity, drugs with a variety of chemical actions may show efficacy in treating the same clinical condition. Newer drugs with novel mechanisms of action are thus being used in the treatment of schizophrenia, depression, and anxiety.
- Unfortunately, agents used to treat psychiatric disorders can cause various undesired effects. Prominent among these are sedation or excitement, motor disturbances, muscarinic blockage, alpha antagonism, sexual dysfunction, and weight gain. There is a continuing effort to develop new drugs that are effective, safe, and well tolerated.

CRITICAL THINKING

1. Knowing that no matter where you practice nursing, many individuals under your care will be taking one psychotropic drug or another, how important is it for you to understand normal brain structure and function as they relate to mental disturbances and psychotropic drugs? Include the following in your answer:
   - **a.** How nurses can use the knowledge about how normal brain function (control of peripheral nerves, skeletal muscles, the autonomic nervous system, hormones, and circadian rhythms) can be affected by either psychotropic drugs or psychiatric illness
   - **b.** How brain imaging can help in understanding and treating people with mental disorders
   - **c.** How your understanding of neurotransmitters may affect your ability to assess your patients' responses to specific medications
2. What specific information would you include in medication teaching based on your understanding of symptoms that may occur when the following neurotransmitters are altered?
   - **a.** Dopamine D_2 (as with use of antipsychotic drugs)
   - **b.** Blockage of muscarinic receptors (as with use of phenothiazines and other drugs)
   - **c.** Alpha-1 receptors (as with use of phenothiazines and other drugs)
   - **d.** Histamine (as with use of phenothiazines and other drugs)
   - **e.** MAO (as with use of an MAOI)
   - **f.** GABA (as with use of benzodiazepines)
   - **g.** Serotonin (as with the use of SSRIs and other drugs)
   - **h.** Norepinephrine (as with the use of SNRIs)

CHAPTER REVIEW

Questions

1. Besides antianxiety agents, which classification of drugs is also commonly given to treat anxiety and anxiety disorders?
   - **a.** Antipsychotics
   - **b.** Mood stabilizers
   - **c.** Antidepressants
   - **d.** Cholinesterase inhibitors
2. What assessment question will provide the nurse with information regarding the effects of a woman's circadian rhythms on her quality of life?
   - **a.** "How much sleep do you usually get each night?"
   - **b.** "Does your heart ever seem to skip a beat?"
   - **c.** "When was the last time you had a fever?"
   - **d.** "Do you have problems urinating?"
3. You realize that your patient who is being treated for a major depressive disorder requires more teaching when she makes the following statement:
   - **a.** "I have been on this antidepressant for 3 days. I realize that the full effect may not happen for a period of weeks."
   - **b.** "I am going to ask my nurse practitioner to discontinue my Prozac today and let me start taking a monoamine oxidase inhibitor tomorrow."
   - **c.** "I may ask to have my medication changed to Wellbutrin due to the problems I am having being romantic with my wife."
   - **d.** "I realize that there are many antidepressants and it might take a while until we find the one that works best for me."

4. A patient being treated for insomnia is prescribed ramelteon (Rozerem). Which comorbid mental health condition would make this medication the hypnotic of choice for this particular patient?
   a. Obsessive-compulsive disorder
   b. Generalized anxiety disorder
   c. Persistent depressive disorder
   d. Substance use disorder
5. Which statement made by a patient prescribed bupropion (Wellbutrin) demonstrates that the medication education the patient received was effective? *Select all that apply.*
   a. "I hope Wellbutrin will help my depression and also help me to finally quit smoking."
   b. "I'm happy to hear that I won't need to worry too much about weight gain."
   c. "It's okay to take Wellbutrin since I haven't had a seizure in 6 months."
   d. "I need to be careful about driving since the medication could make me drowsy."
   e. "My partner and I have discussed the possible effects this medication could have on our sex life."
6. Which drug group calls for nursing assessment for development of abnormal movement disorders among individuals who take therapeutic dosages?
   a. SSRIs
   b. antipsychotics
   c. benzodiazepines
   d. tricyclic antidepressants
7. A nurse reviews an order for a CYP450 test. He explains to his patient from Thailand that the test will determine how the antidepressant will be:
   a. Metabolized
   b. Absorbed
   c. Administered
   d. Excreted
8. Psychotropic drugs have been used for more than half a century. What statement regarding their current status is true?
   a. Only one classification of psychotropic drugs exists.
   b. The Food and Drug Administration no longer approves new antidepressants.
   c. We do not know exactly how they work.
   d. Chlorpromazine (Thorazine), the first psychotropic, continues to be the treatment of choice with hallucinations.
9. The nurse administers each of the following drugs to various patients. The patient who should be most carefully assessed for fluid and electrolyte imbalance is the one receiving:
   a. lithium (Eskalith)
   b. clozapine (Clozaril)
   c. diazepam (Valium)
   d. amitriptyline
10. A psychiatric nurse is reviewing prescriptions for a patient with major depression at the county clinic. Since the patient has a mild intellectual disability, the nurse would question which classification of antidepressant drugs:
   a. Selective serotonin reuptake inhibitors
   b. Monoamine oxidase inhibitors
   c. Serotonin and norepinephrine reuptake inhibitors
   d. All of the above

Answers

1. **c**; 2. **a**; 3. **b**; 4. **d**; 5. **a, b**; 6. **b**; 7. **a**; 8. **c**; 9. **a**; 10. **b**

Visit the Evolve website for a posttest on the content in this chapter: http://evolve.elsevier.com/Varcarolis

Post-Test interactive review

REFERENCES

De Bartolomeis, A., Tomasetti, C., & Iasevoli, F. (2015). Update on the mechanism of action of aripiprazole: Translational insights into antipsychotic strategies beyond dopamine receptor antagonism. *CNS Drugs, 29*, 773–799.

Hamilton, S. P. (2015). The promise of psychiatric pharmacogenomics. *Biological Psychiatry, 77*, 29–35.

Holmes, J. C., & Zacher, J. L. (2012). Second-generation antipsychotics: A review of recently-approved agents and drugs in the pipeline. *Formulary, 47*, 106–121.

Howes, O., McCutcheon, R., & Stone, J. (2015). Glutamate and dopamine in schizophrenia: An update for the 21st century. *Journal of Psychopharmacology, 29*(2), 97–115.

Stahl, S. W. (2013). *Stahl's essential psychopharmacology* (4th ed.). New York, NY: Cambridge University Press.

4

Treatment Settings

Monica J. Halter, Christine M. Tebaldi

Visit the Evolve website for a pretest on the content in this chapter: http://evolve.elsevier.com/Varcarolis Pre-Test interactive review

OBJECTIVES

1. Analyze the continuum of psychiatric care and the variety of care options available.
2. Describe the role of the primary care provider and the psychiatric specialist in treating psychiatric disorders.
3. Explain the purpose of patient-centered medical homes and implications for holistically treating individuals with psychiatric disorders.
4. Identify key components and benefits of community-based care such as psychiatric home care.
5. Discuss other community-based care providers including assertive community treatment (ACT) teams, partial hospitalization programs, and alternate delivery of care methods such as telepsychiatry.
6. Describe the role of the nurse as it pertains to outpatient settings.
7. Identify the main types of inpatient care and the functions of each.
8. Discuss the purpose of identifying the rights of hospitalized psychiatric patients.
9. Define the therapeutic milieu.
10. Describe the role of the nurse as it pertains to inpatient settings.

OUTLINE

KEY TERMS AND CONCEPTS

assertive community treatment (ACT)
clinical pathway
community mental health centers
continuum of psychiatric-mental healthcare
decompensation
elopement
least restrictive environment
milieu
patient-centered medical home
prevention
psychiatric case management
recovery
stabilization
stigma
triage

Obtaining traditional healthcare is fairly straightforward. For example, if you wake up with a sore throat, you know what to do and basically what will happen. It is likely that if you feel bad enough, you will see your primary care provider to be examined, and maybe get a throat culture to diagnose the problem. If the cause is bacterial, you will probably be prescribed an antibiotic. If you do not improve in a certain length of time, your primary care provider may order more tests or recommend that you see an ear, nose, and throat specialist.

Compared with obtaining treatment for other physical disorders, entry into the healthcare system for the treatment of psychiatric problems can be a mystery. Challenges in accessing and navigating this care system exist for several reasons. One reason is that we just do not have much of a frame of reference. We are unlikely to benefit from the experience of others because having a psychiatric illness is often hidden as a result of embarrassment or concern over the **stigma** or a sense of responsibility, shame, and being flawed associated with these disorders (refer to Chapter 2 for more on stigma). You may know that when your grandmother had heart disease, she saw a cardiac specialist and had a coronary artery bypass. However, you may be unaware that she was also treated for depression by a psychiatrist.

Seeking treatment for mental health problems is also complicated by the very nature of mental illness. At the most extreme, disorders with a psychotic component may disorganize thoughts and impede a person's ability to recognize the need for care. There is even a word for this inability: anosognosia (try saying this: uh-no-sog-NOH-zee-uh). Major depression, a common psychiatric disorder, may interfere with motivation to seek care because the illness often causes feelings of apathy, hopelessness, and anergia (lack of energy).

Mental health symptoms are also confused with other problems. For example, anxiety disorders often manifest in somatic symptoms such as racing heartbeat, sweaty palms, and dizziness, which could be symptoms of cardiac problems. Prudence would dictate ruling out other causes, such as physical illness, particularly because diagnosing psychiatric illness is largely based on symptoms and not on objective measurements such as electrocardiograms (ECGs) and blood counts. Unfortunately, this necessary process of ruling out other illnesses often results in a troublesome treatment delay.

Further complicating treatment for mental illness is the unique nature of the system of care, which is rooted in the public and private sectors. The purpose of this chapter is to provide an overview of this system, briefly examine the evolution of mental healthcare, and explore different venues by which people receive treatment for mental health problems. Treatment options are presented in order of acuteness, beginning with those in the **least restrictive environment**, that is, the setting that provides the necessary care while allowing the greatest personal freedom.

BACKGROUND

Psychiatric care in the United States has its roots in asylums created in most existing states before the Civil War. These asylums were created with good intentions and a belief that states had a special responsibility to care for the "insane." Effective treatments were not yet developed, and community care was virtually nonexistent. By the early 1950s, there were only two real options for psychiatric care—a private psychiatrist's office or a mental hospital. At that time, there were 550,000 patients in state hospitals. A majority were individuals with disabling conditions who had become stuck in the asylums.

The number of people in state-managed psychiatric hospitals began to decrease with the creation of Medicare and Medicaid during the 1960s Great Society reform period. Medicaid had an especially potent effect because it paid for short-term hospitalization in general hospitals and medical centers and for long-term care in nursing homes. It did not, however, cover care for most patients in psychiatric hospitals. These incentives stimulated development of general hospital psychiatric units and also led states to transfer geriatric patients from 100% state-paid psychiatric hospitals to Medicaid-reimbursed nursing facilities.

In the 1999 Olmstead decision, the Supreme Court decreed that keeping people in psychiatric hospitals was "unjustified isolation." The opinion of the court was that mental illness is a disability, that institutionalization is in violation of the Americans with Disabilities Act, and that all people with disabilities have a right to live in the community.

These forces led to the creation of state- and county-financed community care systems to complement, and largely replace, functions of the state hospitals. The population in state hospitals dropped dramatically and many of these institutions were closed. The number of state psychiatric hospitals continues to be cut and has been reduced from 322 in 1950 to 195 in 2016 (National Association of State Mental Health Program Directors, 2016).

BOX 4.1 Policy and Politics of the Provision of Psychiatric Care

Mental health advocates develop policies to create an ideal image of what we should be striving for in our healthcare delivery system. Organizations such as the World Health Organization (WHO) work hard at strategically planning policies that help direct the government's goals for healthcare. Improvements in mental health policy across the world are needed and impact how people with mental illness are treated. Policies can address various issues including availability and accessibility of care, discrimination, and basic human rights (WHO, 2012).

Grassroots organizations such as the National Alliance on Mental Illness (NAMI) along with groups specific to each state advocate for better mental healthcare. These organizations are able to share information with legislators about special interest issues. Nurses are encouraged to contact their legislators and work collaboratively on legislation that may positively impact patient care and the profession of psychiatric-mental health nursing. This is a special advocacy role for a nurse to engage in and provides a way to be involved in policymaking.

Related to the shift from hospital to community care were the pharmacological breakthroughs in the mid-20th century that resulted in dramatic changes in the provision of psychiatric care. The introduction of chlorpromazine (Thorazine), the first antipsychotic medication, in the early 1950s contributed to hospital discharges. Gradually, more psychopharmacological agents were added to treat psychosis, depression, anxiety, and other disorders. Treatment provision expanded beyond specialists in psychiatry, as general practitioners began to feel more comfortable prescribing medication and managing symptoms.

Our current system of psychiatric care includes outpatient and inpatient settings. Decisions for level of care tend to be based on the condition being treated and the acuteness of the problem. However, these are not the only criteria. Levels of care may be influenced by such factors as a concurrent psychiatric or substance use problem, medical problems, acceptance of treatment, social supports, disease chronicity, or potential for relapse (Box 4.1).

CONTINUUM OF CARE

What if you, your friend, or a family member needed psychiatric treatment or care? What would you do or recommend? Fig. 4.1 presents a **continuum of psychiatric-mental healthcare** that may help you to make a decision.

Movement along the continuum is fluid and can go in either direction. For example, patients discharged from the most acute levels of care (e.g., hospitalization) may need intensive services to maintain their initial gains. Failure to follow up with outpatient treatment increases the likelihood of rehospitalization and other adverse outcomes. Patients may also reverse direction on the treatment continuum. That is, if symptoms do not improve, professionals from a lower-intensity service may refer the patient to a higher level of care to prevent **decompensation** (deterioration of mental health) and hospitalization.

Differences in characteristics, treatment outcomes, and interventions between inpatient and outpatient settings are identified in Table 4.1.

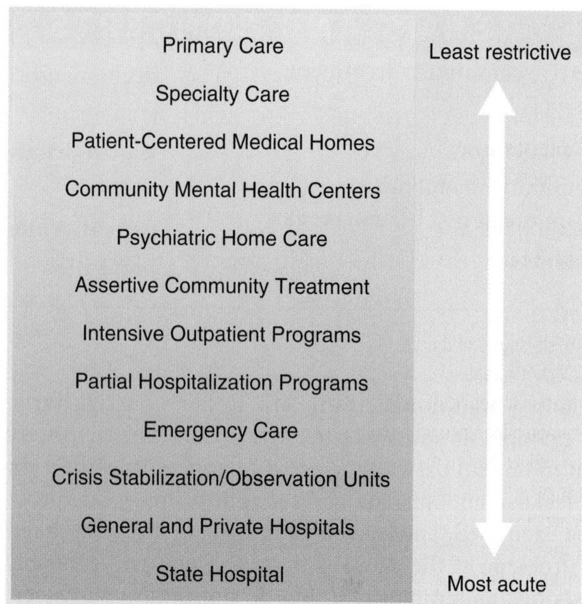

FIG. 4.1 The continuum of psychiatric-mental health treatment.

OUTPATIENT CARE SETTINGS

Primary Care Providers

Primary care providers are the first choice for most people when they are ill, but what about psychiatric symptoms? Imagine that you are feeling depressed, so depressed in fact that you are miserable and cannot carry out your normal activities. You recall that a friend who was depressed saw a psychiatrist (or was that a psychologist?), but that seems too drastic. You do not feel *that* bad. Perhaps you are coming down with something like a cold or flu. After all, you have been tired and you are not eating very well. You decide to visit your primary care provider, a general healthcare provider who may be a physician, an advanced practice nurse, or a physician assistant in an office, clinic, or hospital.

This is not an unusual choice. Seeking help for mental health problems from primary care providers rather than from mental health specialists is common and similar to seeking help for other medical disorders. This is especially true because most psychiatric disorders are accompanied by unexplained physical symptoms such as headaches, backaches, and digestive problems. Most people treated for psychiatric disorders will not go beyond this level of care and may feel more comfortable being treated in a familiar setting. Being treated in primary care rather than in the mental health system may also lessen the degree of stigma, self-perceived or societally, attached to getting psychiatric care.

Disadvantages to being treated by primary care providers include time constraints, because a 15-minute appointment is usually inadequate for a mental and physical assessment. Additionally, primary care providers typically have limited training in psychiatry and may lack expertise in the diagnosis and treatment of psychiatric disorders. These professionals may refer people to specialty mental healthcare.

TABLE 4.1 Characteristics, Treatment Outcomes, and Interventions by Setting

Outpatient/Community Mental Health Setting	Inpatient Setting
Characteristics	
Intermittent supervision	24-hour supervision
Independent living environment with self-care, safety risks	Therapeutic milieu with hospital/staff supported healing environment
Treatment Outcomes	
Stable or improved level of functioning in community	Stabilization of symptoms and return to community
Interventions	
Establish long-term therapeutic relationship	Develop short-term therapeutic relationship
Develop comprehensive plan of care with patient and support system, with attention to sociocultural needs and maintenance of community living	Develop comprehensive plan of care, with attention to sociocultural needs of patient and focus on reintegration into the community
Encourage adherence with medication regimen	Administer medication
Teach and support adequate nutrition and self-care with referrals as needed	Monitor nutrition and self-care with assistance as needed
Assist patient in self-assessment, with referrals for health needs in community as needed	Provide health assessment and intervention as needed
Use creative strategies to refer patient to positive social activities	Offer structured socialization activities
Communicate regularly with family/support system to assess and improve level of functioning	Plan for discharge with family/significant other with regard to housing and follow-up treatment

VIGNETTE: Josh Miller is a registered nurse at a primary care office where he works with a nurse practitioner. He greets his next patient, Mr. Newton, a 56-year-old male whom Josh has known for years and has established a solid rapport.

While taking vital signs, he notices that Mr. Newton isn't his usual self. His affect is dull and his eye contact is poor. He vaguely responds with short answers. Mr. Newton reports that within the past couple of months he has been increasingly tired, doesn't enjoy anything, aches constantly, and has been eating mostly carbohydrates.

After documenting his findings Josh leans forward slightly on his stool and states in a caring tone, "Mr. Newton, I've known you for a while. The change in your behavior has me concerned. Is there anything going on in your life that you'd like to talk about?" Mr. Newton hesitates but then tells Josh that he was demoted at work last year and that he hasn't felt right since then.

Josh shares his assessment with the nurse practitioner who subsequently diagnoses Mr. Newton with major depressive disorder. The nurse practitioner prescribes fluoxetine (Prozac) 20 mg daily and educates him about his diagnosis and new medication. Josh reinforces this teaching and provides him with written educational material. He also provides him with referrals for therapy and support groups.

Specialized Psychiatric Care Providers

Most primary care providers feel comfortable in treating common psychiatric illnesses such as uncomplicated depression. However, they may feel less comfortable when suicide ideation is present or with more severe disorders such as schizophrenia.

Specialized psychiatric care providers have an educational background and experience in care of psychiatric problems and mental health. These providers include psychiatrists, psychiatric-mental health advanced practice registered nurses (nurse practitioners or clinical nurse specialists), psychologists, social workers, counselors, and other licensed therapists. Many primary care practices are partnering with specialty psychiatric providers who work in the same location allowing for rapid access to care and effective triage and screening.

Specialized care providers can provide numerous services. Psychiatrists can prescribe medications. Depending on the state, advanced practice psychiatric nurses and physician assistants can prescribe medications with some restrictions. Most specialized care providers are educated to use individual psychotherapy (talk therapy) and lead group therapy. These providers may have subspecialties such as a provider who specializes in working with veterans with posttraumatic stress disorder (PTSD).

How do you locate one of these specialized psychiatric care providers? One of the first steps is to inquire with a local care organization such as a primary care office, hospital, clinic, or therapy practice. Other ways to find specialty care include asking peers, seeking help through support organizations, or contacting one's insurance company for a list of covered providers. Electronic searches are also good options. Reputable websites, particularly those with state or federal funding, can provide a wealth of information designed to point consumers in the proper direction. Reviews of the care provider on these websites can be helpful in making your decision.

Patient-Centered Medical Homes

Patient-centered medical homes (PCMHs) or primary care medical homes received strong support from the Affordable Care Act of 2010 under President Barack Obama. These health homes were developed in response to fragmented care that result in some services never being delivered while others are duplicated. The focus of care is patient-centered and provides access to physical health, behavioral health, and supportive community and social services. Patients are provided with a range of support for preventive care, acute care, chronic disease management, and end-of-life issues. According to the Agency for Healthcare Research and Quality (2015), these homes have five key characteristics:

1. Patient-centered—Care is relationship-based with the patient and takes into account the unique needs of the whole person. The patient is a core member of the team.
2. Comprehensive care—All levels (preventive, acute, and chronic) of mental and physical care are addressed. Physicians

or advanced practice nurses lead teams that include nurses, physician assistants, pharmacists, nutritionists, social workers, educators, and care coordinators.

3. Coordination of care—Care is coordinated with the broader health system such as hospitals, specialty care, and home health.
4. Improved access—Patients are not limited to Monday through Friday from 9 a.m. to 5 p.m. to get the care they need. In addition to extended hours of service, these homes provide e-mail and phone support.
5. Systems approach—Evidence-based care is provided with a continuous feedback loop of evaluation and quality improvement.

The treatment of psychiatric disorders and mental health alterations can be addressed as part of a comprehensive approach to care. Electronic communication (e.g., follow-up e-mails and reminders) and record keeping are viewed as essential aspects of this process.

Community Mental Health Centers

Beginning in the 1960s, patients with severe mental illness were diverted from state-funded psychiatric hospitals to federally funded **community mental health centers**. Since that time these centers have become the mainstay for those who lack funding for mental healthcare. They offer free or low-cost sliding scale care.

Community mental health centers provide emergency services, community/home-based services, and outpatient services across the lifespan. Common treatments include medication prescribing and administration, individual therapy, psychoeducational and therapy groups, family therapy, and dual-diagnosis (mental health and substance use) treatment. A clinic may also be aligned with a structured program that offers rehabilitation, vocational services, and residential services. Some community mental health centers have an associated intensive **psychiatric case management** service to assist patients in finding housing or obtaining entitlements.

Community mental health centers also utilize multidisciplinary teams. Psychiatric-mental health registered nurses are key members of these teams. Nurses provide medication administration and mental health education to help individuals continue treatment and reach an optima level of functioning. Advanced practice psychiatric registered nurses hold a significant role in community mental health centers by conducting patient intakes, psychotherapy, and medication management.

> **VIGNETTE:** Ashley Morton is a registered nurse at a community mental health center. She is on the adult team and carries a caseload of patients diagnosed with chronic mental illness. An advanced practice registered nurse supervises her. Ashley's responsibilities include responding to crisis calls, seeing patients for regular assessment, administering medications, leading psychoeducation groups, and participating in staff meetings.
>
> Today, Ashley's first patient is Ms. Enright, a 35-year-old woman diagnosed with schizophrenia. She has been in the psychosocial rehabilitation program for 10 years on a daily basis. She has a history of grandiose delusions.
>
> During their 30-minute counseling session, Ashley assesses Ms. Enright for exacerbation (worsening) of psychotic symptoms and eating and sleep habits. Ashley administers Ms. Enright's long-acting injectable (LAI) antipsychotic medication and schedules a return appointment for a month from now.

Psychiatric Home Care

Psychiatric home care is a community-based treatment modality. Medicare requires that four elements be met in order for these services to be reimbursed: (1) homebound status of the patient, (2) presence of a psychiatric diagnosis, (3) need for the skills of a psychiatric registered nurse, and (4) development of a plan of care under orders of a physician or advanced practice registered nurse. Reimbursement and guidelines for psychiatric home care by other payers besides Medicare vary greatly.

Homebound refers to the patient's inability to leave home independently due to physical or mental conditions. Patients may be referred for psychiatric home care after an acute inpatient hospitalization episode of care or to prevent hospitalization.

Medicare allows two groups of healthcare providers to be involved in psychiatric home care. They are social workers with a master's degree and psychiatric registered nurses. Social workers provide counseling and medical social services such as linking people with necessary healthcare and services.

Psychiatric registered nurses provide evaluation, therapy, and teaching. Typically, the nurse visits the patient one to three times per week for a limited period of time. By going to the patient's home, the nurse is better able to address the concerns of access to services and adherence with treatment. Nurses working in the home have to be especially adept at assessing anxiety, agitation, and the potential for violence in this nonclinical setting.

> **VIGNETTE:** Emma Castillo is a registered nurse employed by a home care agency in a rural county. She visits patients living in a radius of 50 miles from her home and has daily telephone contact with her supervisor. She stops by the office weekly to drop off paperwork and attends a team meeting once a month. The team includes her team leader, other field nurses, a psychiatrist consultant, and a social worker. Emma makes her visits from 8:00 a.m. until 3:30 p.m. and then completes her documentation.
>
> Emma spends an hour with Mr. Johnson, a 66-year-old man with a diagnosis of major depression after a stroke. His primary care provider referred him because of suicidal ideation. Emma has met with Mr. Johnson and his wife 3 times a week for the past 2 weeks. He denies suicidal ideation, plan, or intent and has been adherent with his antidepressant regimen. Today, she teaches the couple about stress-management techniques. Case-management responsibilities for Mr. Johnson include supervision of the home health aide, who helps him with hygiene, and coordination with the physical and occupational therapists who also provide care.

Assertive Community Treatment

Assertive community treatment (ACT) is an intensive type of case management developed in the 1970s. This treatment was in response to the hard-to-engage, community-living needs of people with serious, persistent psychiatric symptoms. Due to the severity of their symptoms, they are often unable or unwilling to participate in traditional forms of treatment. As a result, this population has unnecessary and expensive repeat hospitalizations for services such as emergency room and inpatient care.

ACT teams work intensively with patients in their homes or in agencies, hospitals, and clinics—whatever settings patients find themselves in. Creative problem solving and interventions are hallmarks of care provided by mobile teams. The ACT concept takes into account that people need support and resources after 5 p.m. Therefore, teams are on call 24 hours a day.

ACT teams are multidisciplinary and typically composed of psychiatric-mental health registered nurses, social workers, psychologists, advanced practice registered nurses, and psychiatrists. One of these professionals (often the registered nurse) serves as the case manager and may have a caseload of patients who require visits three to five times per week. An advanced practice registered nurse or a psychiatrist usually supervises the case manager. Length of treatment may extend to years until the patient is more stabilized or ready to accept transfer to a more structured site for care.

Intensive Outpatient Programs and Partial Hospitalization Programs

Intensive outpatient programs (IOPs) and partial hospitalization programs (PHPs) function as intermediate steps between inpatient and outpatient care. The primary difference between the two groups is the amount of time that patients spend in them. Both groups tend to be Monday through Friday, but IOPs are usually half a day while PHPs are longer (about 6 hours because they are "partially hospitalized"). They provide structured activities along with nursing and medical supervision, intervention, and treatment. These programs tend to be located within general hospitals, in psychiatric hospitals, or as part of a community mental health.

A multidisciplinary team facilitates group therapy, individual therapy, other therapies (e.g., art and occupational), and pharmacological management. Coping strategies learned during the program can be applied and practiced in the outside world then later explored and discussed. Patients admitted to IOPs and PHPs are closely monitored in case of need for readmission to inpatient care.

Other Outpatient Venues for Psychiatric Care

Mobile mental health units have been developed in some service areas. In a growing number of communities, mental health programs are collaborating with other health or community services to provide integrated approaches to treatment. A prime example of this is the growth of dual-diagnosis programming at both mental health and substance use disorders clinics.

Telephone crisis counseling, telephone outreach, and the internet are being used to enhance access to mental health services. Although face-to-face interaction is still preferred, the new forms of treatment through technology, such as telepsychiatry, have shown immense patient satisfaction and no evidence of complications (Garcia-Lizana & Munoz-Mayorga, 2010). Access and overall health quality and outcomes are expected to improve as models of care that include telehealth and other innovative practices advance (Deslich et al., 2013).

Emergency Care

Patients and families seeking emergency care range from the worried well to those with acute symptoms. The primary goal in emergency services is to perform **triage** and **stabilization**. Triage refers to determining the severity of the problem and the urgency of a response. Stabilization is the resolution of the immediate crisis. Emergency department care often provides a bridge from the community to more intensive psychiatric services such as inpatient care.

Individuals may seek emergency care voluntarily. However, there are times when family, friends, treatment providers, schools, emergency medical personnel, or even law enforcement may suggest or require an individual to undergo emergency evaluation. When emergency evaluation and stabilization are needed, psychiatric clinicians, including psychiatric-mental health nurses, will determine the correct interventions and level of care required. Refer to Chapter 6 for a more detailed discussion about involuntary treatment.

Emergency psychiatric care varies across the nation due to differences in state mental health system design, access to care, and workforce. Despite these differences, emergency psychiatric care can be categorized into three major models:

1. **Comprehensive emergency service model** is often affiliated with a full-service emergency department (ED) in a hospital or medical center setting. Typically, there is dedicated clinical space with specialty staffing. Psychiatric-mental health nurses, psychiatric technicians, mental health specialists, social workers, mental health counselors, and psychiatrists generally make up the multidisciplinary workforce. The concepts of triage and stabilization are incorporated into the individualized care plan for each patient.
2. **Hospital-based consultant model** utilizes the concepts of the comprehensive model by incorporating triage and stabilization. However, there is generally no dedicated clinical space or comprehensive separate staffing. Psychiatric clinical staff members are assigned to a specific hospital and are on-site or on-call, serving as part of the emergency department staff. Psychiatric clinicians manage emergency psychiatric evaluations as requested. Clinicians complete a "level of care" assessment, attempt to stabilize patients, and arrange for discharge or transfer. The emergency department staff maintain responsibility for all immediate care needs.
3. **Mobile crisis team model** is considered for stabilization in the field.

The teams meet face to face with the person in crisis to assess and de-escalate the situation. While the teams vary in composition, psychiatric-mental health nurses, social workers, and counselors, in collaboration with a psychiatrist and/or an advanced practice nurse, often make up the care team.

EVIDENCE-BASED PRACTICE

Patients Wait Longer for Psychiatric Care in Emergency Departments

Problem

Thousands of people in need of psychiatric care are seen in emergency departments. Patients with acute psychiatric disorders may wait for psychiatric evaluation for hours or even days.

Purpose of Study

Researchers sought to understand the individual patient factors and hospital factors that contribute to prolonged emergency department lengths of stay. They also looked at how those same factors contributed to where the patients were ultimately sent.

Methods

Hospital emergency department visits between 2001 and 2011 were analyzed. Visits that were for substance use problems and psychiatric disorders were categorized as mental health, and all other problems as medical.

Findings

- More psychiatric patients (23%) compared to medical patients (10%) stayed in the emergency department more than 6 hours.
- More psychiatric patients (7%) compared to medical patients (2.3%) stayed in the emergency department for more than 12 hours.
- Admission to the hospital happened more frequently with psychiatric patients (21%) compared to medical patients (13.5%).
- Transfers to another facility were more common in psychiatric patients (11%) compared to medical patients (1.4%).

Why should nurses be interested in this study?

Patients who are experiencing the emotional pain, confusion, or need for substance use treatment are being subjected to the additional stress and indignity of being held in this demanding atmosphere. Overly long stays also crowd this already congested department.

As patient advocates, nurses who work in this area can help to facilitate the timely disposition of these patients. Psychiatric nurses can help patients being discharged to link up with assertive community treatment teams or case management. All nurses can help to advise people who are experiencing psychiatric symptoms to seek treatment at alternate crisis service centers or even primary care.

Lippert, S.C., Jain, N., Nesper, A., Fahimi, J., Pirrotta, E., & Wang, N.E. (2016). Waiting for care: Differences in emergency department length of stay and disposition between medical and psychiatric patients. *Annals of Emergency Medicine, 68*(4), S97.

PREVENTION IN OUTPATIENT CARE

A distinct concept in the healthcare literature is that of treatment based on a public health model that takes a community approach to **prevention**. Primary, secondary, and tertiary prevention are levels at which interventions are directed.

Primary Prevention

Primary prevention occurs before any problem manifests and seeks to reduce the incidence or rate of new cases. Primary prevention may prevent or delay the onset of symptoms in genetically or otherwise predisposed individuals. Coping strategies and psychosocial support for vulnerable young people are effective interventions in preventing mood and anxiety disorders.

Secondary Prevention

Secondary prevention is also aimed at reducing the prevalence of psychiatric disorders. Early identification of problems, screening, and prompt and effective treatment are hallmarks of this level. While it does not stop the actual disorder from beginning, it is intended to delay or avert progression.

Tertiary Prevention

Tertiary prevention is the treatment of disease with a focus on preventing the progression to a severe course, disability, or even death. Tertiary prevention is closely related to rehabilitation, which aims to preserve or restore functional ability. In the case of treating major depression, the aim is to avoid loss of employment, reduce disruption of family processes, and prevent suicide.

OUTPATIENT PSYCHIATRIC NURSING CARE

Psychiatric-mental health nursing in the outpatient or community setting requires strong problem solving and clinical skills, cultural competence, flexibility, solid knowledge of community resources, and comfort in functioning more autonomously than acute care nurses. Patients need assistance with problems related to individual psychiatric symptoms, family and support systems, and basic living needs, such as housing and financial support.

Psychiatric-mental health nurses can be leaders in transforming an illness-driven and dependency-oriented system into a system that emphasizes recovery and empowerment. Nurses are adept at understanding the system and coordinating care. Further, nurses are respected members of the interdisciplinary team. They serve not only in lead clinical roles but also as advocates for the inclusion of patient-centered and trauma-informed care models (American Nurses Association [ANA] et al., 2014).

The role of the outpatient or community psychiatric-mental health registered nurse ideally includes service provision in a variety of these treatment settings. For example, psychiatric needs are well known in the criminal justice system and the homeless population. Individuals suffering from a mental illness tend to cycle through the correctional systems and generally comprise 50% of the incarcerated population, and from that number, 20% have a serious mental illness (American Psychological Association, 2014). The nurse's role is not only to provide care to individuals as they leave the criminal justice system and re-enter the community but also to educate police officers and justice staff in how to work with individuals entering the criminal system.

Table 4.2 describes the educational preparation for a variety of outpatient and community roles.

Promoting Recovery and Continuation of Treatment

In the not too distant past, treatment for mental illness consisted of patients being told what medications to take and what treatments to accept. Good patients were those who were compliant. A newer model of recovery promotes

TABLE 4.2 **Roles Relevant to Educational Preparation in Outpatient and Community Settings**

Role	Basic Practice (Diploma, AD, BS)	Advanced Practice (MS, DNP, PHD)
Practice	Provide nursing care; assist with medication management as prescribed, under direct supervision	Nurse practitioner or clinical nurse specialist; manage consumer care and prescribe or recommend interventions independently
Consultation	Consult with staff about care planning and work with nurse practitioner or physician to promote health and mental healthcare; collaborate with staff from other agencies	Consultant to staff about plan of care, to consumer and family about options for care; collaborate with community agencies about service coordination and planning processes
Administration	Take leadership role within mental health treatment team	Administrative or contract consultant role within mental health agencies or mental health authority
Research and education	Participate in research at agency or mental health authority; serve as preceptor to undergraduate nursing students	Role as educator or researcher within agency or mental health authority

self-involvement in care. Recovery is "a process of change through which individuals improve their health and wellness, live a self-directed life, and strive to reach their full potential" (Substance Abuse Mental Health Services Administration [SAMHSA], 2015).

Nurses are real assets in supporting patients in the recovery process, especially with medication management. Nurses are in a position to help the patient recognize side effects and be aware of interactions among medications prescribed for both physical illness and mental illness. This knowledge increases the individual's ability to self-advocate. Patient-family education and behavioral strategies, in the context of a therapeutic relationship with the nurse, promote adherence with a medication regimen.

Patient-centered care, also referred to as person-centered care, supports values in the recovery model. It is respectful and responsive care that incorporates patients' preferences, needs, and values. This concept is essential for ensuring that the patient's wishes and values are the guiding principle for care management and shared decision making.

INPATIENT CARE SETTINGS

Hospitalization is available for the treatment of acute symptoms or safety concerns for patients with mental disorders and emotional crises. In fact, 2.4 million adult patients were treated in hospitals in 2014 with a mental illness (SAMHSA, 2015). The top five mental health diagnoses treated were mood disorders, substance use disorders, neurocognitive disorders, anxiety disorders, and schizophrenia. Admission is commonly reserved for those people who are suicidal, homicidal, or extremely disabled and in need of acute care.

Crisis Stabilization/Observation Units

Care models that prioritize rapid stabilization and short length of stay have become more prevalent in medical and psychiatric settings. Overnight short-term observation, often 1 to 3 days, are designed for individuals who have symptoms that are expected to remit in 72 hours or less. This observation is also helpful for individuals who have a psychosocial stressor that can be addressed in that time frame, maximizing their stability and allowing them to rapidly return to a community treatment setting.

General Hospital and Private Hospital

Acute care hospital psychiatric units tend to be housed on a floor or floors of a general hospital. Private psychiatric hospitals are freestanding facilities. As noted, the dramatic growth of acute care psychiatric hospitals and hospital units is the result of a shift away from institutionalization in state-managed hospitals. Since that time, reduced reimbursement increased managed care, enhanced outpatient options, and expanded availability of outpatient and partial hospitalization programs have resulted in the steady decline of these facilities.

State Hospital

Although the quality of care in state hospitals has improved dramatically, today's state-operated psychiatric hospitals are an extension of what remains of the old system. The clinical role of state hospitals is to serve the most seriously ill patients. However, this role varies widely, depending on available levels of community care and on payments by state Medicaid programs. In some states, these hospitals primarily provide intermediate treatment for patients unable to be stabilized in short-term general hospital units and long-term care for individuals judged too ill for community care. In other states, the emphasis is on acute care that is reflective of gaps in the private sector, especially for the uninsured or for those who have exhausted limited insurance benefits.

In most states, the state hospitals provide forensic (court-related) care and monitoring as part of their function. The state or county system also advises the courts as to defendants' sanity who may be judged to have been so ill when they committed the criminal act that they cannot be held responsible but require treatment instead. These judgments are not guilty by reason of insanity (NGRI). One tragic example is that of Andrea Yates, the Texas woman who, in 2001, drowned her five young children under the delusional belief she was saving them from their sinfulness. She was found NGRI and was committed to a Texas state psychiatric facility.

CONSIDERATIONS FOR INPATIENT CARE

Entry to Acute Inpatient Care

Some patients are admitted directly to inpatient care based on a specialized care provider or primary care provider referral.

However, the majority of patients receiving inpatient acute psychiatric care are admitted through an emergency department or crisis intervention service. Of the 12 million emergency department visits in the United States, nearly 13% are due to mental health and/or substance use conditions (Agency for Healthcare Research and Quality, 2010).

Patients may be admitted voluntarily or involuntarily (see Chapter 6). Units may be unlocked or locked. Locked units provide privacy and prevent **elopement**—leaving before being discharged (also referred to as being away without leave or AWOL). There may also be psychiatric intensive care units (PICUs) within the general psychiatric units to provide better monitoring of those who display an increased risk for danger to self or others.

> **VIGNETTE:** Mr. Reese is a 22-year-old male who was brought to the emergency room by police after expressing thoughts of suicide. He is restless and irritable. When approached, he becomes agitated and threatening to the nurses and physicians. He states that his mother and brother, who are only trying to have him admitted so they can take his money, tricked him. He is exhibiting poor judgment, insight, and impulse control. He stopped taking his antipsychotic medication 3 weeks ago because of side effects.
>
> The psychiatric nurse, Morgan, in the emergency department approaches Mr. Reese in a nonthreatening manner. She calmly asks him if he'd be more comfortable sitting while they speak with one another. Mr. Reese chooses to sit on the gurney, and the nurse sits on a chair near the door. Mr. Reese already appears calmer after accepting a cold drink and nods as the nurse observes that he seems anxious. When asked if any medication ever helps him with feeling anxious, he responds that he has taken lorazepam (Ativan) before and it helps. Morgan obtains an order for the medication and provides Mr. Reese with education about lorazepam.

Rights of the Hospitalized Patient

Patients admitted to any psychiatric unit retain rights as citizens, which vary from state to state, and are entitled to certain privileges. Laws and regulatory standards require that patients' rights be provided in a timely fashion after an individual has been admitted to the hospital, and that the treatment team must always be aware of these rights. Any infringement by the team during the patient's hospitalization—such as a failure to protect patient safety—must be documented, and actions must be justifiable. All mental health facilities must provide a written statement of patients' rights often with copies of applicable state laws attached. Box 4.2 provides a sample list of patients' rights.

BOX 4.2 Typical Items Included in Hospital Statements of Patients' Rights

- Right to be treated with dignity
- Right to be involved in treatment planning and decisions
- Right to refuse treatment, including medications
- Right to request to leave the hospital, even against medical advice
- Right to be protected against harming oneself or others
- Right to a timely evaluation in the event of involuntary hospitalization
- Right to legal counsel
- Right to vote
- Right to communicate privately by telephone and in person
- Right to informed consent
- Right to confidentiality regarding one's disorder and treatment
- Right to choose or refuse visitors
- Right to be informed of research and to refuse to participate
- Right to the least restrictive means of treatment
- Right to send and receive mail and to be present during any inspection of packages received
- Right to keep personal belongings unless they are dangerous
- Right to lodge a complaint through a plainly publicized procedure
- Right to participate in religious worship

Teamwork and Collaboration

Psychiatric-mental health nurses are core members of a team of professionals and nonprofessionals who work together to provide care (Box 4.3). The team (including the patient) generally formulates a full treatment plan. The nurse's role in this process is often to lead the planning meeting. This nursing leadership reflects the holistic nature of nursing, as well as the fact that nursing is the discipline that is represented on the unit at all times. Nurses are in a unique position to contribute valuable information such as continuous assessment findings, the patient's adjustment to the unit, any health concerns, psychoeducational needs, and deficits in the patient's self-care. Additionally, nurses have an integral function to facilitate a patient's achievement of therapeutic goals by offering education and support in an individual or group format.

Ultimately, the treatment plan will be the guideline for the patient's care during the hospital stay. It is based on goals for the hospitalization and defines how achievement of the goals will be measured. Input from the patient and family (if available and desirable) is critical in formulating goals. Incorporating the patient's feedback in developing the treatment plan goals increases the likelihood of the success of the outcomes.

Members of each discipline are responsible for gathering data and participating in the planning of care. Newly admitted patients may find multiple professionals asking them similar questions to be extremely stressful or threatening. The urgency of the need for data should be weighed against the patient's ability to tolerate assessment. Often, assessments made by the intake team and the nurse provide the basis for care. In most settings, the psychiatrist or advanced practice nurse evaluates the patient and provides orders within a limited time frame. Medical problems are usually referred to a medical consultant service often consisting of physicians and advanced practice nurses who assess the patient and consult with the unit clinical team.

To provide standardization in treatment and improve outcomes, inpatient units use **clinical pathways**. These task-oriented plans detail the essential steps in the care of patients with specific clinical problems based on the usual and expected clinical course. These tools provide an essential link between evidence-based knowledge and clinical practice. The treatment plan is revised if the patient's progress differs from the expected

BOX 4.3 Members of the Multidisciplinary Treatment Team

Psychiatric-mental health registered nurses: Licensed registered nurses whose focus is on mental health and mental illness and who may or may not be certified in psychiatric-mental health nursing. The registered nurse is typically the only 24-hours-a-day, 7-days-a-week professional working in acute care. Among the responsibilities of the registered nurse are diagnosing and treating responses to psychiatric disorders, coordinating care, counseling, giving medication and evaluating responses, and providing education.

Psychiatric-mental health advanced practice registered nurses: Licensed registered nurses who are prepared at the master's or doctoral level and hold specialty certification as either clinical nurse specialists or nurse practitioners. These nurses are qualified for clinical functions such as diagnosing psychiatric conditions, prescribing psychotropic medications and integrative therapy, and conducting psychotherapy. They are also involved in case management, consulting, education, and research.

Psychiatrists: Psychiatrists prescribe medication for psychiatric symptoms. They may also provide psychotherapy. As physicians, psychiatrists may be employed by the hospital or may hold practice privileges in the facility.

Psychologists: In keeping with their doctoral or doctorate degree preparation, psychologists conduct psychological testing, provide consultation for the team, and offer direct services such as specialized individual, family, or marital therapies.

Social workers: Basic level social workers help the patient prepare a support system that will promote mental health on discharge from the hospital. This includes contacts with day treatment centers, employers, sources of financial aid, and landlords. Licensed clinical social workers undergo training in individual, family, and group therapies.

Counselors: Counselors prepared in disciplines such as psychology, rehabilitation counseling, and addiction counseling may augment the treatment plan by co-leading groups, providing basic supportive counseling, or assisting in psychoeducational and recreational activities.

Occupational, recreational, art, music, and dance therapists: Based on their specialist preparation, these therapists assist patients in gaining skills that help them cope more effectively, gain or retain employment, use leisure time to the benefit of their mental health, and express themselves in healthy ways.

Medical advanced practice nurses, medical doctors, and physician assistants: Medical professionals provide diagnoses and treatments on a consultation basis. Occasionally, a medical professional who is trained as an addiction specialist may play a more direct role on a unit that offers treatment for addictive disease.

Mental health workers (mental health specialists/psychiatric technicians): Mental health workers, including nursing assistants, function under the direction and supervision of registered nurses. They provide assistance to patients in meeting basic needs and also help the community to remain supportive, safe, and healthy.

Pharmacists: In view of the intricacies of prescribing, coordinating, and administering combinations of psychotropic and other medications, the consulting pharmacist can offer a valuable safeguard. Physicians and nurses collaborate with the pharmacist regarding new medications, which are proliferating at a steady rate.

outcomes. Clinical pathways result in decreased costs, length of stay, and complications while improving outcomes.

Therapeutic Milieu

Milieu (mil'yōō) is a word of French origin (mi "middle" + lieu "place") and refers to surroundings and physical environment. In a therapeutic context, it refers to the overall environment and interactions within that environment. Peplau (1989) referred to this as the therapeutic milieu. It is an all-inclusive term that recognizes the people (patients and staff), the setting, the structure, and the emotional climate as important to healing. Regardless of whether the setting involves treatment of psychotic children, adult patients in a psychiatric hospital, substance users in a residential treatment center, or psychiatric patients in a day treatment program, a well-managed milieu offers patients a sense of security and promotes healing. Structured aspects of the milieu include activities, rules, reality orientation practices, and environment.

Managing Behavioral Crises

Behavioral crises can lead to patient violence toward self or others and usually, but not always, escalate through fairly predictable stages. Staff members in most mental health facilities practice crisis prevention and management techniques. Training generally consists of a full-day course learning the skills to recognize and avoid crisis and de-escalate behavioral emergencies. Hands-on techniques, which are only used as a last resort, are also taught. At minimum, annual training is recommended to maintain competency.

Some facilities have special teams of nurses, psychiatric technicians, mental health specialists, and other professionals who respond to psychiatric emergencies called codes. Each member of the team takes part in the team effort to defuse a crisis in its early stages. If preventive measures fail and imminent risk of harm to self or others persists, each member of the team participates in a rapid, organized plan to safely manage the situation. The nurse is most often this team's leader not only in organizing the plan but also in timing the actions and managing the concurrent administration of medications.

Seclusion, restraint, and emergency medication are actions of last resort. The trend is to reduce or completely eliminate these practices whenever safely possible. The nurse can initiate such an intervention in the absence of a physician in most places, but must secure a physician's order for restraint or seclusion within a specified time. Refer to Chapters 6 and 27 for further discussions and protocols for use of restraints and seclusion. The concept of trauma-informed care is a guiding principle for clinical interventions and unit philosophy and is addressed more comprehensively in Chapter 16.

Safety

A safe environment is an essential component of any inpatient setting. Protecting the patient is essential, but equally important is the safety of the staff and other patients. Safety needs are identified, and individualized interventions begin on admission. Staff members check all personal property and clothing to prevent any potentially harmful items (e.g., medication, alcohol, or sharp objects) from being taken onto the unit or left in their immediate possession. Some patients are at greater risk for suicide than others, and psychiatric-mental health nurses are skillful in evaluating this risk through questions and observations.

The Joint Commission, an agency that accredits hospitals, developed National Patient Safety Goals (2015) specific to

TABLE 4.3 National Patient Safety Goals in Behavioral Healthcare

Goal	Process	Example
Identify patients correctly	Use at least two identifiers when providing care, treatment, or services.	Use the patient's name *and* date of birth for identification before drawing blood.
Use medicines safely	Maintain and communicate accurate medication information for the individual served.	Find out what medications the patient is taking and compare them to newly ordered medications.
Prevent infection	Use the hand cleaning guidelines from either the Centers for Disease Control and Prevention or the World Health Organization.	Wet hands first; apply an amount of product recommended by the manufacturer to hands, and rub hands together for at least 15 seconds, covering all surfaces of the hands and fingers. Rinse with water and dry thoroughly with a disposable towel. Use towel to turn off the faucet.
Identify patient safety risk	Determine which patients are most likely to attempt suicide	Routinely administer a screening tool such as the Beck Scale for Suicidal Ideation, a 21-item tool that takes 5–10 minutes to complete.

From the Joint Commission. (2015). *Behavioral health care: 2016 national patient safety goals.* Retrieved from http://www.jointcommission.org/assets/1/6/2016_NPSG_BHC.pdf.

specialty areas within hospitals to promote patient safety. Table 4.3 lists safety goals specific to behavioral healthcare. Centers for Medicare and Medicaid Services also emphasize safety and have identified several preventable hospital-acquired injuries for which they will not provide reimbursement. For example, they will not compensate healthcare organizations when a patient falls and fractures a hip as nearly all falls are preventable. It is likely that other health insurance providers will also begin to limit payment for preventable injuries under the regulatory concept of pay for performance.

Tracking patients' whereabouts and activities is done periodically or continuously, depending upon patients' risk for harming themselves or others. For patients with active suicidal thoughts, continuous in-person observation is essential because even checking on a patient every 15 minutes may not prevent a suicide that takes only several minutes.

Monitoring visitation is an important aspect of patient well-being and safety. Although visitors can contribute to patients' healing, visits may be overwhelming or distressing. Also, visitors may unwittingly or purposefully provide patients with unsafe items. Staff should inspect bags and packages. Sometimes, the unsafe items take the form of comfort foods from home or a favorite restaurant and should be monitored because they may be incompatible with diets or medications.

Intimate relationships between patients are prohibited. There are risks for sexually transmitted diseases, pregnancy, and emotional distress at a time when patients are vulnerable and may lack the capacity for consent.

Unit Design

The goal in designing psychiatric units is to provide a therapeutic and aesthetically pleasing environment while balancing the need for safety since patients on inpatient psychiatric units may be at risk for suicide or violence. Full compliance with regulatory and accrediting bodies should be required for each clinical setting. Promoting an environment of safety and empowering patients to partner with clinical staff and take ownership of their own health and safety is critical.

Safety precautions are taken into account in each area of the unit. For example, closets may be equipped with breakaway bars or hooks designed to hold a minimal amount of weight to prevent strangulation by hanging. Windows are locked and are made of safety glass, and safety mirrors are typically used. Showers may have non–weight-bearing or nonlooping designed showerheads. Beds are often platforms rather than mechanical hospital beds, which can be dangerous because of their crushing potential, looping hazard, and cords. However, standard hospital beds may be indicated, depending on patient physical health needs. Other important design elements on inpatient psychiatric units include:

- Doors that open out instead of in to prevent patients from barricading themselves in their rooms.
- Continuous hinges on doors rather than three butt hinges to prevent hanging risk.
- Furniture that is anchored in place with the exception of a desk chair to prevent their use as a weapon or barricade.
- Drapes that are mounted on a track firmly anchored to the ceiling rather than curtain rods.
- Mini blinds contained within window glass provide significantly more safety than those whose mountings are accessible.
- Plumbing fixtures that are boxed in.

INPATIENT PSYCHIATRIC NURSING CARE

Management of these acute care units, ideally, is by nurses who have backgrounds in psychiatric-mental health nursing, preferably with advanced practice degrees. Staff nurses tend to be nurse generalists, that is, nurses who have basic training as registered nurses. Some registered nurses achieve national certification in psychiatric-mental health nursing through the American Nurses Credentialing Center. The staff psychiatric registered nurse carries out the following nursing responsibilities:

- Completing comprehensive data collection that includes the patient, family, and other healthcare workers
- Developing, implementing, and evaluating plans of care

TABLE 4.4 Sample Nursing Diagnoses Outcomes and Interventions for Patients In Acute Care Settings

Nursing Diagnoses	Outcomes	Interventions
Risk for self-directed violence: Vulnerable to behaviors in which an individual demonstrates that he or she can be physically, emotionally, and/or sexually harmful to self	*Suicide self-restraint:* Personal actions to refrain from gestures and attempts at killing self	*Suicide prevention:* Reducing the risk for self-inflicted harm with intent to end life
Risk for other-directed violence: Vulnerable to behaviors in which an individual demonstrates that he or she can be physically, emotionally, and/or sexually harmful to others	*Aggression self-control:* Personal actions to refrain from assaultive, combative, or destructive behaviors toward others	*Violence prevention:* Monitoring and manipulation of the physical environment to decrease the potential for violent behavior directed toward, self-others, or environment
Impaired mood regulation: A mental state characterized by shifts in mood or affect ... [with] affective, cognitive, somatic, and/or physiological manifestations	*Mood equilibrium:* Appropriate adjustment of prevailing emotional tone in response to circumstances	*Mood management:* Providing for safety, stabilization, recovery, and maintenance of a patient who is experiencing dysfunctionally depressed or elevated mood

Data from Herdman, T. H., & Kamitsuru, S. (2014). *NANDA nursing diagnoses: Definitions and classification 2015-17.* Philadelphia, PA: Author; Moorhead, S., Johnson, M., Maas, M., & Swanson, E. (Eds.). (2013). *Nursing outcomes classification (NOC)* (5th ed.). St. Louis, MO: Mosby; Bulechek, G. M., Butcher, H. K., Dochterman, J. M., & Wagner, C. (Eds.). (2013). *Nursing interventions classification (NIC)* (6th ed.). St. Louis, MO: Mosby.

- Assisting or supervising mental healthcare workers (e.g., nursing assistants with or without additional training in working with people who have mental illnesses)
- Maintaining a safe and therapeutic environment
- Facilitating health promotion through teaching
- Monitoring behavior, affect, and mood
- Maintaining oversight of restraint and seclusion
- Coordinating care by the treatment team

Medication management is an essential skill for psychiatric nurses. In this specialty area, nurses often exert a strong influence on medication decisions. This influence is due to continual observation of the expected, interactive effects and adverse effects of medications provides the data necessary for medication adjustment. For example, feedback about a patient's excessive sedation or increased agitation may lead to a decision to decrease or increase the dosage of an antipsychotic medication.

A common misperception regarding psychiatric nurses is that, because they "just talk," they lose their skills for physical tasks such as starting and maintaining intravenous (IV) lines and changing dressings. In fact, most psychiatric nurses provide some degree of physical care. Patients on psychiatric units are not limited to psychiatric disorders and often have complex healthcare needs. For example, an older adult male with brittle diabetes and a recent foot amputation may become actively suicidal. In this case, it is likely he will be transferred to the psychiatric unit where his blood glucose level will be monitored and wound care provided

Table 4.4 provides sample nursing diagnoses, outcomes, and interventions for patients during admission to the acute care setting.

SPECIALTY TREATMENT SETTINGS

Treatment options are available that provide specialized care for specific groups of people. These options include inpatient, outpatient, and residential care.

Pediatric Psychiatric Care

Children with mental illnesses have the same range of treatment options as do adults but receive them apart from adults in pediatric settings. Inpatient care may be necessary if the child's symptoms become severe. Parental or guardian—including the Department of Children and Families—involvement in the plan of care is integral so that they understand the illness, treatment, and the family's role in supporting the child. Additionally, hospitalized children, if able, attend school several hours a day.

Geriatric Psychiatric Care

The older adult population may be treated in specialized mental health settings that take into account the effects of aging on psychiatric symptoms. Physical illness and loss of independence can be strong precipitants in the development of depression and anxiety. Dementia is a particularly common problem encountered in geriatric psychiatry. Treatment is aimed at careful evaluation of the interaction of mind and body and provision of care that optimizes strengths, promotes independence, and focuses on safety.

Veterans Administration Centers

Active military personnel and veterans who were honorably discharged may receive federally funded inpatient or outpatient care and medication for psychiatric and alcohol or substance use disorders. One of the greatest challenges veterans face is dealing with the after effects of the traumas of active combat. During Civil War times, these late effects were termed "soldier's heart." After World War I, soldiers had "shell shock," and after World War II, it was termed "battle fatigue." Currently, mental health services are being inundated by people suffering from PTSD. There is a prevalence of PTSD in the general population of about 7% and nearly 14% for veterans of the wars in Iraq and Afghanistan. This creates a tremendous need for strong psychiatric services for this population (Gradus, 2010).

Forensic Psychiatric Care

Incarcerated populations, both adult and juvenile, have higher than average incidences of mental disorders or substance use disorders. Researchers estimate that there are more people with mental illness in prisons than in hospitals (Torrey et al., 2010). Treatment may be provided within the prison system where inmates are often separated from the general prison population. State hospitals also treat forensic patients. Most facilities provide psychotherapy, group counseling, medication management, and assistance with transition to the community.

Alcohol and Drug Use Disorder Treatment

All the mental health settings that were previously described may provide treatment for alcohol and substance use disorders, although specialized treatment centers exist apart from the mental healthcare system. More than 22 million individuals aged 12 or older needed treatment in 2013 for illicit drug or alcohol use problems. Only 2.5 million received specialized care (Substance Abuse and Mental Health Services Administration [SAMHSA], 2014). This treatment is typically outpatient and includes counseling, education, medication management, and 12-step programs. Because alcohol detoxification and other substance withdrawal can be life threatening, inpatient care may be required for medical management.

Self-Help Options

Obtaining sufficient sleep, meditating, eating right, exercising, abstaining from smoking, and limiting the use of alcohol are healthy responses to a variety of illnesses such as diabetes and hypertension. As with other medical conditions, lifestyle choices and self-help responses can have a profound influence on the quality of life and the course, progression, and outcome of psychiatric disorders. If we accept the notion that psychiatric disorders are usually a combination of biochemical interactions, genetics, and environment, then it stands to reason that, by providing a healthy living situation, we are likely to fare better. If, for example, a person has a family history of anxiety and has demonstrated symptoms of anxiety, then a good first step (or an adjunct to psychiatric treatment) could be to learn yoga and balance the amounts of life's obligations with relaxation.

A voluntary network of self-help groups operates outside the formal mental healthcare system to provide education, contacts, and support. Since the introduction of Alcoholics Anonymous in the early 20th century, self-help groups have multiplied and have proven to be effective in the treatment and support of psychiatric problems. Groups specific to anxiety, depression, loss, caretakers' issues, bipolar disorder, PTSD, and almost every other psychiatric issue are widely available in most communities.

Consumers, people who use mental health services, and their family members have successfully united to shape the delivery of mental healthcare. Nonprofit organizations such as the National Alliance on Mental Illness (NAMI) encourage self-help and promote the concept of recovery, or the self-management of mental illness. These grassroots groups also confront social stigma, influence policies, and support the rights of people experiencing mental illness.

KEY POINTS TO REMEMBER

- Entry into the mental health system can be a bewildering process due to people's reluctance to share their own experiences, cognitive changes from the disorders themselves, and confusion over physical versus mental symptoms.
- Treatment options should be based on the least restrictive environment, that is, the setting that provides the necessary care while allowing the greatest personal freedom.
- Psychiatric care settings evolved during the 20th century from mass institutionalization to a variety of outpatient and inpatient settings.
- A continuum of care model helps differentiate between levels of acuity within treatment settings.
- Primary care providers have an increasingly important role in identifying and treating mental disorders. This treatment choice may feel familiar and reduce stigma. Time limitations may impact a complete mental assessment and training limitations may make some providers uncomfortable.
- Specialty care providers possess an educational and experiential background in psychiatric and mental health.
- Patient-centered medical homes with multiple services and an array of providers are becoming increasingly popular as a way to integrate mental and other physical care.
- Community mental health centers provide a wide range of mental health services for individuals who lack funding for care.
- Registered nurses and social workers provide psychiatric home care for individuals who are homebound.
- Assertive community treatment (ACT) is an intensive case management for people who are unable or unwilling to participate in traditional treatment. ACT teams are composed of a variety of professionals who provide 24-hour, 7-days-a-week support.
- Intensive outpatient and partial hospitalization programs are available as a step down from inpatient care or as a step up from other less restrictive treatment settings.
- Emergency psychiatric care and crisis stabilization is available in emergency rooms and from emergency teams.
- Primary, secondary, and tertiary prevention are aimed at reducing the effects of mental illness by preventing its occurrence, preventing its progression, or by restoring functional ability.
- Inpatient settings include crisis stabilization units, general hospital and private hospital acute care, and a state-funded acute care system.
- Inpatient psychiatric-mental health nursing requires strong skills in management, communication, and collaboration.
- Basic level inpatient nursing interventions include admission, providing a safe environment, psychiatric and physical assessments, milieu management, documentation, medication administration, and preparation for discharge to the community.

CRITICAL THINKING

1. You are a nurse working at a local community mental health center. During an assessment of a 45-year-old single, male patient, he reports that he has not been sleeping and that his thoughts seem to be "all tangled up." Although he does not admit directly to being suicidal, he remarks, "I hope that this helps today because I don't know how much longer I can go on like this."

   He is disheveled and has been sleeping in homeless shelters. He has little contact with his family and becomes agitated when you suggest that it might be helpful to contact them. He reports a recent hospitalization at the local veterans' hospital and previous treatment at a dual-diagnosis facility, yet he denies substance use. When asked about his physical condition, he says that he has tested positive for hepatitis C and is "supposed to take" multiple medications that he cannot name.
   - **a.** List your concerns about this patient in order of priority.
   - **b.** Which of these concerns must be addressed before he leaves the clinic today?
   - **c.** Do you feel there is an immediate need to consult with any other members of the multidisciplinary team today about this patient?
   - **d.** Keeping in mind the concept of patient-centered care, how will you develop trust with the patient to increase his involvement with the treatment plan?
2. Imagine that you were asked for your opinion with regard to your patient's ability to make everyday decisions independently. What sort of things would you consider as you weighed safety versus autonomy and personal rights?
3. If nurses function as equal members of the multidisciplinary mental health team, what differentiates the nurse from the other members of the team?

CHAPTER REVIEW

Questions

1. A patient needs supportive care for the maintenance treatment of bipolar disorder. The new nurse demonstrates an understanding of the services provided by the various members of the patient's mental healthcare team when he makes which statement:
   - **a.** "Your social worker will help you learn to budget your money effectively."
   - **b.** "Your counselor asked me to remind you of the group session on critical thinking at 2:00 today."
   - **c.** "The mental health technician on staff today will administer the medication that you require."
   - **d.** "Remember to ask the occupational therapist about sources of financial help that you are qualified for."
2. A patient has been voluntarily admitted to a mental health facility after an unsuccessful attempt to harm himself. Which statement demonstrates a need to better educate the patient on his patient's rights?
   - **a.** "I understand why I was restrained when I was out of control."
   - **b.** "You can't tell my boss about the suicide attempt without my permission."
   - **c.** "I have a right to know what all of you are planning to do to me."
   - **d.** "I can hurt myself if I want too. It's none of your business."
3. Which intervention demonstrates an attempt by nursing staff to meet the goals identified by the Joint Commission as National Patient Safety Goals? *Select all that apply.*
   - **a.** Identifying patients using both name and date of birth before drawing blood.
   - **b.** Sitting with the patient diagnosed with an eating disorder during meals.
   - **c.** Administering the Beck Scale on each patient at the time of admission.
   - **d.** Performing a medication history assessment on each new patient.
   - **e.** Using appropriate hand washing technique at all times.
4. The mental health team is determining treatment options for a male patient who is experiencing psychotic symptoms. Which question(s) should the team answer to determine whether a community outpatient or inpatient setting is most appropriate? *Select all that apply.*
   - **a.** "Is the patient expressing suicidal thoughts?"
   - **b.** "Does the patient have intact judgment and insight into his situation?"
   - **c.** "Does the patient have experiences with either community or inpatient mental healthcare facilities?"
   - **d.** "Does the patient require a therapeutic environment to support the management of psychotic symptoms?"
   - **e.** "Does the patient require the regular involvement of their family/significant other in planning and executing the plan of care?"
5. The nurse frequently includes daily sessions involving relaxation techniques. Which assessment data would most indicate a need for this intervention to be included in the initial plan of care for a patient?
   - **a.** Family history of anxiety and symptoms of anxiety
   - **b.** Significant other has a chronic health issue
   - **c.** Hopes to retire in 6 months
   - **d.** Recently adopted infant twins
6. A newly divorced 36-year-old mother of three has difficulty sleeping. When she shares this information to her gynecologist, she suggests which of the following services as appropriate for her patient's needs?
   - **a.** Assertive community treatment
   - **b.** Patients-centered medical home
   - **c.** Psychiatric home care
   - **d.** Primary care provider

7. A Gulf War veteran has been homeless since being discharged from military service. He is now diagnosed with schizophrenia. The nurse practitioner recognizes that assertive community treatment (ACT) is a good option for this patient since ACT provides:
   a. Psychiatric home care
   b. Care for hard-to-engage, seriously ill patients
   c. Outpatient community mental health center care
   d. A comprehensive emergency service model
8. An adolescent female is readmitted for inpatient care after a suicide attempt. What is the most important nursing intervention to accomplish upon admission?
   a. Allowing the patient to return to her previous room so that she will feel safe
   b. Orienting the patient to the unit and introduce her to patients and staff
   c. Building trust through therapeutic communication
   d. Checking the patient's belongings for dangerous items
9. Emma is a 40-year-old married female who has found it increasingly difficult to leave her home due to agoraphobia. Emma's family is appropriately concerned and suggests that she seek psychiatric care. After investigating her options, Emma decides to try:
   a. Telepsychiatry
   b. Assertive community treatment
   c. Psychiatric home care
   d. Outpatient psychiatric care
10. Pablo is a homeless adult who has no family connection. Pablo passed out on the street and emergency medical services took him to the hospital where he expresses a wish to die. The physician recognizes evidence of substance use problems and mental health issues and recommends inpatient treatment for Pablo. What is the rationale for this treatment choice? *Select all that apply.*
   a. Intermittent supervision is available in inpatient settings.
   b. He requires stabilization of multiple symptoms.
   c. He has nutritional and self-care needs.
   d. Medication adherence will be mandated.
   e. He is in imminent danger of harming himself.

Answers

1. **b**; 2. **d**; 3. **a, c, d, e**; 4. **a, b, d, e**; 5. **a**; 6. **d**; 7. **b**; 8. **d**; 9. **a**; 10. **b, c, e**

Visit the Evolve website for a posttest on the content in this chapter: http://evolve.elsevier.com/Varcarolis

Post-Test interactive review

REFERENCES

Agency for Healthcare Research and Quality. (2010). *Statistical brief #92*. Retrieved from http://www.hcup-us.ahrq.gov/reports/statbriefs/sb92.pdf.

Agency for Healthcare Research and Quality. (2015). *Defining the PCMH*. Retrieved from http://www.pcmh.ahrq.gov/page/defining-pcmh.

American Nurses Association, American Psychiatric Nurses Association & International Society of Psychiatric-Mental Health Nurses. (2014). *Psychiatric-mental health nursing: Scope and standards of practice*. Silver Spring, MD: NurseBooks.org.

American Psychological Association. (2014). Incarceration nation. *Monitor on Psychology, 45*(9). Retrieved from http://www.apa.org/monitor/2014/10/incarceration.aspx.

Deslich, S., Stec, B., Tomblin, S., & Coustasse, A. (2013). *Telepsychiatry in the 21st century:* Transforming healthcare with technology. *Perspectives in Health Information Management, 10*(summer). Retrieved from http://www.ncbi.nlm.nih.gov/pmc/articles/PMC3709879/.

Garcia-Lizana, F., & Munoz-Mayorga, I. (2010). What about telepsychiatry? A systematic review. *The Primary Care Companion to the Journal of Clinical Psychiatry, 12*(2).

Gradus, J. L. (2010). Epidemiology of PTSD. In *United States Department of Veterans Affairs*. Retrieved from www.ptsd.va.gov/professional/pages/epidemiological-facts-ptsd.asp.

The Joint Commission. (2015). *Behavioral health care: 2016 national patient safety goals*. Retrieved from http://www.jointcommission.org/bhc_2016_npsgs/.

National Association of State Mental Health Directors. (2016). *State hospital organizations*. Retrieved from http://www.nasmhpd.org/content/state-hospital-organizations.

Peplau, H. E. (1989). Interpersonal constructs for nursing practice. In A. W. O'Toole & S. R. Welt (Eds.), *Interpersonal theory in nursing practice: Selected works of Hildegard E. Peplau* (pp. 42–55). New York, NY: Putnam.

Substance Abuse and Mental Health Services Administration. (2014). *The NSDUH Report: Substance use and mental health Estimates from the 2013 National Survey on Drug Use and Health*. Retrieved from http://www.samhsa.gov/data/sites/default/files/NSDUH-SR200-RecoveryMonth-2014/NSDUH-SR200-RecoveryMonth-2014.htm.

Substance Abuse and Mental Health Services Administration (SAMHSA). (2015). *Recovery and recovery support*. Retrieved from http://www.samhsa.gov/recovery.

Torrey, E. F., Kennard, A. D., Eslinger, D., Lamb, R., & Pavle, J. (2010). *More mentally ill persons are in jails and prisons than hospitals: A survey of the states*. Retrieved from http://74.125.155.132/scholar?q=cache:_ulTyMxYGAsJ:scholar.google.com/+percent+of+prison+population+with+a+mental+disorder&hl=en&as_sdt=0,36&as_ylo=2009.

World Health Organization. (2012). *Mental health policy, planning and service department*. Retrieved from http://www.who.int/mental_health/policy/services/en/index.html.

5

Cultural Implications

Rick Zoucha, Kimberly Wolf

Visit the Evolve website for a pretest on the content in this chapter: http://evolve.elsevier.com/Varcarolis Pre-Test interactive review

OBJECTIVES

1. Explain the importance of culturally relevant care in psychiatric-mental health nursing practice.
2. Discuss potential problems in applying Western methods of care to patients of other cultures.
3. Compare and contrast Western nursing beliefs, values, and practices with the beliefs, values, and practices of patients from diverse cultures.
4. Perform culturally sensitive assessments that include risk factors and barriers to quality mental healthcare that culturally diverse patients frequently encounter.
5. Develop culturally appropriate nursing care plans for patients of diverse cultures.

OUTLINE

KEY TERMS AND CONCEPTS

acculturation
assimilation
cultural competence
cultural concepts of distress
cultural explanations
cultural idioms of distress
cultural norms
cultural syndromes
culture
Eastern tradition
enculturation
ethnicity
ethnocentrism
indigenous culture
minority status
pharmacogenetics
race
refugee
somatization
stereotyping
Western tradition
worldview

How a society views mental health and mental illness has a tremendous impact on how mental health resources are allocated and how mental healthcare is funded. Societal attitudes also impact whether individuals are agreeable to accessing mental healthcare and the type of treatments they engage in. Stigma—negative attitudes toward mental illness and its treatment—is a phenomenon found across cultures globally. Fortunately, the United States has a relatively enlightened view regarding mental healthcare.

While we tend to consider psychiatric disorders and their treatment from the perspective of the dominant majority culture, not all racial/ethnic groups in the United States think the same way about these issues. According to a Substance Abuse and Mental Health Services Administration report (SAMHSA, 2015), discrepancies in the use of mental health services among racial/ethnic groups are a national problem.

Psychiatric nurses can help address these discrepancies by practicing culturally relevant nursing that meets the needs of culturally diverse patients. All mental health providers should strive to provide care as congruent as possible with patients' cultural beliefs, values, and practices—keeping in mind that certain cultural practices (e.g., sweat lodges, sun ceremonies, witchcraft) may be impractical, harmful, or even illegal.

This chapter focuses on culture and how it affects the mental health and care of patients with mental illness. In this chapter, you will learn about:

- Culture, race, ethnicity, minority status, and how they are related
- Demographic shifts, which make it essential that mental health nurses know how to provide culturally competent care
- The impact of cultural worldviews on mental health nursing
- Variations in cultural beliefs, values, and practices that affect mental health and care of patients with mental health problems
- Barriers to providing quality mental health services to culturally diverse patients
- Culturally diverse populations at increased risk of developing mental illness
- Techniques for providing culturally competent care to diverse populations

MINORITY STATUS, RACE, ETHNICITY, AND CULTURE

Let's begin by clarifying some key terms related to culture. Although the definitions of these terms distinguish them from one another, they are related.

Minority Status

Minority status is a subset of people who think of themselves, and are thought of by others, as a differentiated group. They may be different from mainstream society based on race, nationality, religion, or language. Typically, minority groups are socially and economically disadvantaged. Relatively speaking, they are lacking in power. Due to this lack of power, they may be treated differently and discriminated against. Adding to the problem of discrimination is the tendency to self-segregate from within the group.

A minority is not necessarily a smaller group of people living among a larger group. People from different countries, various religions, races, or languages can live in the same communities for generations without considering themselves different. To confer minority status to a group, cultures must socially define them as differentiated.

Race

Race can be defined biologically, anthropologically, or genetically. Racial groups can be distinguished visually from one another based on physical characteristics. For the purpose of this chapter we will use the federal government's operational definition of race that is socially defined. When the government conducts a national census it allows individuals to self-identify the race with which they are associated.

Ethnicity

Ethnic groups have a common heritage and history, which is referred to as **ethnicity**. These groups share a **worldview**, a system for thinking about how the world works and how people should act, especially in relationship to one another. From this worldview, they develop beliefs, values, and practices that guide members of the group in how they should think and act in different situations.

Culture

Culture is the shared beliefs, values, and practices that guide a group's members in patterned ways of thinking and acting. Culture includes religious, geographic, socioeconomic, occupational, ability- or disability-related, and sexual orientation–related beliefs and behaviors. Each group has cultural beliefs, values, and practices that guide its members in ways of thinking and acting.

Cultural norms refers to attitudes and behaviors considered normal, typical, or average within that group. They help members of the group make sense of the world around them and make decisions about appropriate ways to relate and behave. Because cultural norms prescribe what is normal and abnormal, culture helps develop concepts of mental health and illness.

As nurses, *culture* rather than race or ethnicity should guide our patient care and help us to make better decisions on their behalf. Culture is a blueprint for guiding actions that impact care, health, and well-being (McFarland & Wehbe-Alamah, 2015).

Measuring Race and Ethnicity in the United States

Acknowledging the inadequacy of describing minority groups according to a single biological race, the US Census Bureau (2010) used the combined race/ethnicity categorization system for the 2010 census. Respondents were first asked whether they were of Hispanic, Latino, or Spanish origin. If not, they were asked to further identify their race from 14 choices. Respondents who did not identify with any of the predefined categories were provided with blank spaces to classify their race (Fig. 5.1).

Is Person 1 of Hispanic, Latino, or Spanish origin?

- ☐ No, not of Hispanic, Latino, or Spanish origin
- ☐ Yes, Mexican, Mexican Am., Chicano
- ☐ Yes, Puerto Rican
- ☐ Yes, Cuban
- ☐ Yes, another Hispanic, Latino, or Spanish origin — *Print origin, for example, Argentinean, Colombian, Dominican, Nicaraguan, Salvadoran, Spaniard, and so on.*

A

What is Person 1's race? *Mark ☒ one or more boxes.*

- ☐ White
- ☐ Black, African Am., or Negro
- ☐ American Indian or Alaska Native — *Print name of enrolled or principal tribe.*
- ☐ Asian Indian
- ☐ Japanese
- ☐ Native Hawaiian
- ☐ Chinese
- ☐ Korean
- ☐ Guamanian or Chamorro
- ☐ Filipino
- ☐ Vietnamese
- ☐ Samoan
- ☐ Other Asian — *Print race, for example, Hmong, Laotian, Thai, Pakistani, Cambodian, and so on.*
- ☐ Other Pacific Islander — *Print race, for example, Fijian, Tongan, and so on.*
- ☐ Some other race — *Print race.*

B

FIG. 5.1 Race-ethnicity categorizations included in the 2010 US Census. **(A)** Respondents were first asked if they were of Hispanic, Latino, or Spanish origin. **(B)** Respondents were asked to further identify their race.

One purpose of categorizing individuals according to racial-ethnic descriptions is to help the government understand the needs of its citizens. The census helps identify disparities in healthcare along racial-ethnic lines. Recording these classifications also helps determine when and how the healthcare needs of these populations are being met.

Despite the benefits, classifying groups of people can be confusing, confounding, and offensive. Consider the following:

- Each racial group contains multiple ethnic cultures. There are more than 560 Native American and Alaskan tribes and more than 40 countries in Asia and the Pacific Islands. The cultural norms of blacks or African Americans whose ancestors were brought to the United States centuries ago as slaves are very different from the norms of those who have recently immigrated from Africa or the Caribbean. Americans of European origin are a diverse group, some of whom have been in the United States for hundreds of years and some of whom are new immigrants.
- The Latino-Hispanic group is a cultural group based on a shared language, but all of its members are also members of a racial group or groups (white, black, and/or Native American). They may include Mexican Americans, Puerto Ricans, and Cuban Americans.
- Persons from the Middle East and the Arabian subcontinent are considered white in the classification system.
- Although children of multiracial, multicultural, and multiheritage marriages fall into more than one category, their unique identity is not distinguished and sometimes viewed as invisible.

TABLE 5.1 Year 2060 Population Projections (Percentage of Total Population)*

	2012	2060
White, non-Hispanic	63	43
Black, non-Hispanic	13	15
Hispanic (of any race)	17	31
Asian	5	8
All other races	2	3

*Population percentages are rounded to the nearest 1%.
Data from US Census Bureau. (2012). *Population by race and Hispanic origin: 2012 and 2060.* Retrieved from http://www.census.gov/newsroom/releases/img/racehispanic_graph.jpg.

The difficulty of describing minority groups continues to be an issue. The National Census Bureau's 2015 mid-decade National Content Test was implemented to improve the 2020 census (US Census Bureau, 2015a). The goals of this test were to evaluate questionnaire content and response rates from the internet.

DEMOGRAPHIC SHIFTS IN THE UNITED STATES

In 2043 the US population is projected for the first time to become a majority-minority nation. That is, no one group will make up the majority or make up 51% of the population (US Census Bureau, 2012). However, non-Hispanic whites will continue to remain the largest single group. The Hispanic and Asian populations are growing at the fastest rates. A comparison of population composition in 2012 and the projected population for 2060 is shown in Table 5.1.

BASIC WORLDVIEWS

Western Tradition

Nursing theories, psychological theories, and the understanding of mental health and illness used by nurses in the United States have been derived from a Western philosophical and scientific framework. This framework is based on Western cultural ideals, beliefs, and values. Because psychiatric-mental health nursing is grounded in Western culture, nurses should consider how their core assumptions about personality development, emotional expression, ego boundaries, culture, and interpersonal relationships affect the nursing care of any patient.

A long history of Western science and European American norms for mental health has shaped present-day American beliefs and values about people. Our understanding of how a person relates to the world and to other people is based on Greek, Roman, and Judeo-Christian thought. Other Western scientists and philosophers, such as Descartes (credited with the Western concept of body-mind dualism), have contributed to the Western scientific tradition.

In the **Western tradition**, a person finds identity in individuality. Individuality is accompanied by the values of autonomy, independence, and self-reliance. Mind and body are two separate entities. Because they are separate, different practitioners treat disorders of the mind and the body. Disease has a

TABLE 5.2 Worldviews

Western (Science)	Eastern (Balance)	Indigenous (Harmony)
Roman, Greek, Judeo-Christian; the Enlightenment; Descartes	Chinese and Indian philosophers: Buddha, Confucius, Lao-tse	Deep relationship with nature
The "real" has form and essence; reality tends to be stable	The "real" is a force or energy; reality is always changing	The "real" is multidimensional; reality transcends time and space
Cartesian dualism: body and mind-spirit	Mind-body-spirit unity	Mind, body, and spirit are united; there may not be words to indicate them as distinct entities
Self is starting point for identity	Family is starting point for identity	Community is starting point for identity; a person is only an entity in relation to others; may be no concept of person or personal ownership
Time is linear	Time is circular, flexible	Time is focused on the present
Wisdom: preparation for the future	Wisdom: acceptance of what is	Wisdom: knowledge of nature
Disease has a cause (e.g., pathogen, toxin) that creates the effect; disease can be observed and measured	Disease is caused by a lack of balance in energy forces (e.g., yin-yang, hot-cold); imbalance between daily routine, diet, and constitutional type	Disease is caused by a lack of personal, interpersonal, environmental, or spiritual harmony; thoughts and words can shape reality; evil spirits exist
Ethics of rights and obligations: Based on the individual's right *Value given to:* Right to decide, right to be informed, open communication, truthfulness	*Ethics of care:* Based on promoting positive relationships *Value given to:* Sympathy, compassion, fidelity, discernment; action on behalf of those with whom one has a relationship; persons in need of healthcare considered to be vulnerable and require protection from cruel truth	*Ethics of community:* Based on needs of the community *Value given to:* Contribution to community

specific, measurable, and observable cause, and care providers focus treatment on eliminating the cause. Time is seen as linear, always moving forward, and waiting for no one. Success in life is obtained by preparing for the future.

Eastern Tradition

The **Eastern tradition** of Asia is based on the philosophical thought of Chinese and Indian philosophers and the spiritual traditions of Confucianism, Taoism, Buddhism, and Hinduism. Native Americans, African tribes, Australian and New Zealand aborigines, and tribal peoples on other continents frequently include rich cultural traditions based on deep personal connections to the natural world and the tribe.

Eastern tradition and some Western collective cultures see the family as the basis for one's identity, so that family interdependence and group decision making are the norm. The body, mind, and spirit are considered a single entity. Therefore there is no sense of separation between a physical illness and a psychological one (Camann, 2013). Time is circular and recurring and consistent with a belief in reincarnation. One is born into an unchangeable fate, with which one has a duty to comply. For the Chinese, fluctuations in opposing forces—the yin-yang energies—cause disease.

Indigenous Culture

The term **indigenous culture** refers to the culture of those people who have inhabited a country for thousands of years and includes such groups as the New Zealand Maoris, Australian aborigines, American natives, and native Hawaiians. These groups place special significance on the place of humans in the natural world and frequently manifest a more dramatic difference from Western views. Frequently, the basis of one's identity is the tribe. There may be no concept of person. Instead, a person is an entity only in relation to others. The holism of body-mind-spirit may be so complete that there may be no adequate words in the language to describe them as separate entities. Disease is frequently a lack of harmony of the individual with others or the environment.

World cultures have grown out of different worldviews and philosophical traditions. Worldview shapes how cultures perceive reality, the person, and the person in relation to the world and to others. Worldview also shapes perceptions about time, health and illness, and rights and obligations in society. Table 5.2 provides an overview of Western, Eastern, and indigenous culture. The three worldviews compared here are broad categories and generalizations created to contrast some of the themes found in diverse world cultures. They do not necessarily fit any particular cultural group.

IMPACT OF CULTURE

Diverse cultures have evolved from the three broad categories of worldview described in the previous section. Cultures developed norms consistent with their worldviews and adapted to their own historical experiences and the influences of the outside world. Cultures are not static. They change and adjust, although usually very slowly.

Nonverbal Communication. Each culture has different patterns of nonverbal communication (Table 5.3). For instance, in American culture, eye contact is a sign of respectful attention, but in many other cultures, it is considered arrogant and intrusive. In Western culture, emotional expressiveness is valued, but in many other cultures, it may be a sign of immaturity.

Etiquette. People tend to feel offended when their rules for polite behavior are violated. However, the rules for polite behavior vary greatly from one culture to another. Unless we are aware of cultural differences in etiquette norms, we could infer rudeness on the part of a patient who is operating from a

TABLE 5.3 Selected Nonverbal Communication Patterns

Nonverbal Communication Pattern	Predominant Patterns in the United States	Patterns Seen in Other Cultures
Eye contact	Eye contact is associated with attentiveness, politeness, respect, honesty, and self-confidence.	Eye contact is avoided as a sign of rudeness, arrogance, challenge, or sexual interest.
Personal space	*Intimate space:* 0-1½ ft *Personal space:* 1½-3 ft In a personal conversation, if a person enters into the intimate space of the other, the person is perceived as aggressive, overbearing, and offensive. If a person stays more distant than expected, the person is perceived as aloof.	Personal space is significantly closer or more distant than in US culture. *Closer*—Middle Eastern, Southern European, and Latin American cultures *Farther*—Asian cultures When closer is the norm, standing very close frequently indicates acceptance of the other.
Touch	Moderate touch indicates personal warmth and conveys caring.	Touch norms vary. *Low-touch cultures*—Touch may be considered an overt sexual gesture capable of "stealing the spirit" of another or taboo between women and men. *High-touch cultures*—People touch one another as frequently as possible (e.g., linking arms when walking or holding a hand or arm when talking).
Facial expressions and gestures	A nod means "yes." Smiling and nodding means "I agree." Thumbs up means "good job." Rolling one's eyes while another is talking is an insult.	Raising eyebrows or rolling the head from side to side means "yes." Smiling and nodding means "I respect you." Thumbs up is an obscene gesture. Pointing one's foot at another is an insult.

BOX 5.1 Norms of Etiquette

Norms of etiquette that vary across cultures include:

- Whether "promptness" is expected and how important it is to be on time
- How formal one should be in addressing others
- Which people deserve recognition and honor and how respect is shown
- Whether shaking hands and other forms of social touch are appropriate
- Whether or not shoes can be worn in the home
- How much clothing should be worn to be modest
- What it means to accept or reject offers of food or drink and other gestures of hospitality
- What importance is given to small talk and how long it should continue before getting down to business
- Whether communication should be direct and forthright or circuitous and subtle
- What the tone of voice and pace of the conversation should be
- Which topics are considered taboo
- Whether or not the children in the home can be touched and admired

different set of cultural norms and believes his or her behavior is respectful. Box 5.1 identifies norms for etiquette that may be different based on the prevailing culture.

Beliefs and Values. As we have discussed, cultural beliefs and values that are dominant in the United States are often in contrast with those that are common in various other world cultures. Table 5.4 identifies patterns and concepts in the United States and other cultures. Beliefs and values and health and illness are contrasted in Table 5.5.

The culture's worldview, beliefs, values, and practices are transmitted to its members in a process called **enculturation**. As children, we learn from our parents which behaviors, beliefs, values, and actions are right and which are wrong. The individual is free to make choices, but the culture expects these choices to be made from its acceptable range of options.

Deviance from cultural expectations is a problem and frequently may be defined by the cultural group as illness. Mental health is often the degree to which a person fulfills the expectations of the culture. The culture defines which differences are still within the range of normal (mentally healthy) and which are outside the range of normal (mentally ill).

The same thoughts and behaviors considered mentally healthy in one culture can indicate mental illness in another. For example, some religious traditions view speaking in tongues as mentally healthy and a gift from God, whereas a different cultural group might consider this same behavior as psychosis and a sign of mental illness.

All people are raised to view the world and everything in it through their own cultural lens, and nurses are no exception. We are products of our culture of professional socialization. Nurses may think that the only good care is the care they have learned to believe in, value, and practice. This sort of thinking can lead to **ethnocentrism**, the universal tendency of humans to think their way of thinking and behaving is the only correct and natural way (Purnell, 2014).

CULTURAL BARRIERS TO MENTAL HEALTH SERVICES

The first part of this chapter focused on the impact of culture on mental health and illness in a theoretical way. The following sections present practice issues that nurses are likely to encounter when providing care to culturally diverse patients along with suggestions to overcome these barriers.

Communication Barriers

Communication is a key aspect of caring for patients, yet healthcare providers and patients may not even speak the same

TABLE 5.4 Cultural Belief and Value Systems

Predominant Culture Patterns and Concepts in the United States	Patterns and Concepts in Various Other Cultures
Individualism	Familism
Independence, self-reliance	Interdependence of family
Autonomy, autonomous decision making	Interconnectedness
	Family decision making
Egalitarians: Everyone has an equal voice and deserves equal opportunities.	Social hierarchy: Some deserve more honor or power than others because of their age, gender, occupation, or role in the family; family hierarchies can be patriarchal or matriarchal.
Youth	Age
Physical beauty	Wisdom
Competition	Cooperation
Achievement	Relationships
Materialistic orientation	Metaphysical orientation
Possessions	Spirituality, nature
Reason and logic	Meditation and intuition
Doing and activity	Being and receptivity
Mastery over nature	Harmony with nature
Latest technology	Natural, traditional ways
Master of one's fate: "I am the master of my destiny."	Fate is one's master: "Fate is responsible for my destiny."
Optimism	Fatalism
Internal locus of control: Life events and circumstances are the result of one's actions.	External locus of control: Life events and circumstances are beyond one's own control and rest in the hands of fate, chance, other people, or God.
Future orientation: "He who prepares for tomorrow will be successful."	Present orientation: "Live for today and let tomorrow take care of itself."
	Past orientation: Tradition
Punctuality ("clock time"): "Time waits for no one." "Time flies." "Time is money."	"People time": Time is flexible, indefinite; "Time starts when the group gathers." "Time walks."
Being on time is a sign of courtesy and responsibility.	Being on time can be a sign of compulsiveness and disregard for the people one was with before the appointment time.

TABLE 5.5 Cultural Beliefs and Values About Health and Illness

	Western Biomedical Perspective	Perspective of Various Other Cultures
Health	Absence of disease	Being in a state of balance
	Ability to function at a high level	Being in a state of harmony
		Ability to perform family roles
Disease causation	Measurable, observable cause that leads to measurable, observable effect	Frequently intangible, immeasurable cause
		Lack of balance (yin and yang)
	Pathogens, mutant cells, toxins, poor diet	Lack of harmony with environment
Location of disorder	Body	Whole entity: mind, body, and spirit are merged
	Mind	Disorder causing disease in the person may be in the family or environment
Decisions about care	Made by patient or holder of power of attorney	Made by the whole family or family head
	Goals are autonomy and confidentiality	Goals are protection and support of patient
	Truth telling required so patient has information to make decisions	Hope should be preserved; patient should be protected from painful truth
Sick role	Sick people should be as independent and self-reliant as possible	Sick people should be as passive as possible
	Self-care is encouraged; one gets better by getting up and getting going	Family members should take care of and "do for" the sick person
		Passivity stimulates recovery
Best treatments	Physician-prescribed drugs and treatments	Regaining of lost balance or harmony by counteracting negative forces with positive ones and vice versa
	Advanced medical technology	Treatment by folk healers and traditional remedies
Pain	Stoicism valued	Pain expressed vocally and dramatically
	Pain described quantitatively	Use of quantitative scales to measure pain is difficult
	Able to pinpoint location of pain	Pain experienced globally
	Pain may be kept as silent as possible in Northern European, Asian, and Native American	More dramatic pain expression is expected: Southern European, African, Middle Eastern
Ethics	Based on bioethical principles of autonomy, beneficence, justice, and confidentiality	Based on virtue or community needs
		Hope should be preserved, painful truth hidden
	Informed consent requires truthfulness	Support and care should be provided
		Emphasis is on greatest good for the greatest number

language. The US Department of Health and Human Services (HHS) Office of Minority Health (2013) states that healthcare organizations should offer and provide language assistance services, including an interpreter, at all points of contact and in a timely manner during all hours of operation and service. These services should be provided at no cost to each patient who has limited English proficiency. Patients with limited English proficiency are those who cannot speak English or do not speak English well enough to meet their communication needs. The HHS asserts that providing language services benefits patients, providers, and facilities alike.

A professional interpreter should match the patient as closely as possible in gender, age, social status, and religion. In addition to interpreting the language, the interpreter can provide information regarding nonverbal communication patterns and cultural norms that are relevant to the encounter. In this way, the interpreter acts as a cultural broker, interpreting not only the language but also the culture.

Especially important in psychiatric settings, interpreters should not be relatives or friends of the patient. The stigma of mental illness may prevent the openness needed during the encounter. Also, those close to the patient may not have the language skills necessary to meet the demands of interpretation, which is a complex task. Languages frequently cannot be translated word for word. The literal translations of words in one language can carry many different connotations in the other language, and certain concepts are so culturally linked that an adequate translation is difficult.

Even people who speak English well may have difficulty communicating emotional nuances in English. Certain terms may be more accessible to patients in their own languages. Idioms and figures of speech can be extremely confusing. For instance the terms *feeling blue* or *feeling down* may have no meaning at all in the patient's literal understanding of English.

In addition to interpreters, translators can be critically important in the healthcare setting, since a translation error can be a matter of life and death. Translators can provide patients with materials written in the language that they understand.

Stigma of Mental Illness

Mental illnesses are stigmatized disorders, and this stigma presents significant barriers to treatment. Many people in all sectors of society in the United States associate mental illness with moral weakness. Others express fear of, or bias against, those with mental health problems. However, in many cultural groups, the stigma of mental illness is more severe and prevalent than it generally is in the United States.

In cultural groups that emphasize the interdependence and harmony of the family, mental illness is perceived as a failure of the family. In such groups, the pressures on both the individual with the mental illness and the family are increased. Both the individual and the whole family are ill, and the illness reflects badly on the character of all family members. Stigma and shame can lead to reluctance to seek help, so members of these cultural groups may enter the mental healthcare system at an advanced stage when the family has exhausted its ability to cope with the problem.

Misdiagnosis

Another barrier to mental healthcare is misdiagnosis. Studies indicate that blacks and African Americans, Afro-Caribbean, and Latino-Hispanic Americans run a significant risk of being misdiagnosed with schizophrenia when the true diagnosis is bipolar disease or an affective disorder (Schwartz et al., 2014). Why does this happen? One reason for misdiagnosis is the use of culturally inappropriate assessment tools. Experts have validated most of the available tools using subjects of European origin. Marsella (2011) asserts that the use of standardized Western assessment instruments may result in inaccuracy of diagnosis when applied to non-Western patients.

In cultures where the body and mind are considered one entity, or in cultures in which there is a high degree of stigma associated with mental health problems, individuals frequently somatize their feelings of psychological distress. In **somatization**, psychological distress is experienced as physical problems. For example, a Cambodian woman may describe feelings of back pain, fatigue, and dizziness and say nothing about feelings of sadness or hopelessness (Henderson et al., 2016).

Somatization is just one example of how psychological distress is manifested in a way that seems different. Because of this, using psychiatric diagnostic criteria that were developed based on studies with predominantly white American samples are often invalid when applied to other cultures. The impact of cultural concepts on a psychiatric diagnosis has been included in the American Psychiatric Association's (APA, 2013a) diagnostic criteria for the fifth edition of the *Diagnostic and Statistical Manual of Mental Disorders (DSM-5)*.

Furthermore, the *DSM-5* includes a standardized tool for taking into account cultural variations during the assessment phase of patient care. The Cultural Formulation Interview (APA, 2013b) is a 14-question inventory that helps clinicians plan for care based on orientation, values, and assumptions that originate from particular cultures. It takes into consideration the meaning of the illness for the patient, the role of family and others as support, the patient's attempts to cope with previous illness, and expectations of current care.

Cultural Concepts of Distress

Cultural concepts of distress take into account the way that groups experience, understand, and communicate problematic behaviors, suffering, or troubling emotions and thoughts (APA, 2013a). All forms of distress are local constructs including the disorders described in the *DSM-5*. There are three specific types of cultural concepts:

1. **Cultural syndromes**, or culture-bound syndromes, exist when clusters of symptoms occur in specific groups and are recognized by these groups as a known pattern of experience. These syndromes are typically given a distinct name.
2. **Cultural idioms of distress** are specific ways of expressing distress that people in particular cultures understand. In the United States, saying, "I am depressed" or "I'm a nervous wreck" may refer to a variety of problems and not a specific disorder.
3. **Cultural explanations** refer to explanations for symptoms, illness, or distress understood within the context of the particular culture.

Cultural syndromes may seem exotic or irrational to nurses who have been trained within a Western medical framework. The symptoms may be shocking, and other-culture explanations regarding causation and treatment may be mystifying. These illnesses, however, are usually well understood by the people within the cultural group. They know the name of the problem, its etiology, its course, and the way it should be treated. Frequently, when these illnesses are treated in culturally prescribed ways, the remedies are quite effective.

There are many cultural syndromes. Some of these syndromes seem to be mental health problems manifested in somatic ways. *Hwa-byung* and *neurasthenia* have many similarities to depression and do not carry the degree of stigma associated with a mental disorder. Because the somatic complaints are so prominent, and because patients frequently deny feelings of sadness or depression, they may not fit the *DSM-5* diagnostic criteria for depression.

Ataque de nervios and *ghost sickness* belong to another group of culture-based illnesses characterized by abnormal behaviors. These types of illnesses seem to be culturally acceptable ways for patients to express that they can no longer endure the stressors in their lives. People in the culture understand the patient is ill and provide support using culturally prescribed treatments, which often relieve the symptoms. A list of some of the syndromes that psychiatric nurses may see is provided in Box 5.2.

We tend to think of cultural syndromes as strange or exotic, yet there are disorders listed in the *DSM-5* that may seem unusual to others. Consider anorexia nervosa, bulimia nervosa, and binge-eating disorder. These problems are bound to Western culture apparently because other cultures do not value the thinness so prized by European and North American cultural groups.

When we consider culture in diagnosis and treatment, we are more likely to see culturally different behavior as normal. For example, in African American churches, it is common to refer to spiritual experiences in terms such as "I was talking to Jesus this morning." Rather than considering the speaker to be delusional, the care provider understands that he was praying. If a Vietnamese father says he tried to take the wind illness out of his child by vigorously rubbing a coin down her back, the care provider realizes that the father is not a potential threat to the child.

BOX 5.2 Examples of Cultural Syndromes and Explanations

Because there are so many cultural syndromes, they cannot all be described in this chapter. However, the list here includes some of the syndromes the psychiatric-mental health nurse might encounter.

Ataque de nervios: Latin American. Characterized by a sudden attack of trembling, palpitations, dyspnea, dizziness, and loss of consciousness. Thought to be caused by an evil spirit and related to intolerable stress. Treated by an espiritista (spiritual healer) and by the support of the family and community who provide aid to the patient and consider the patient to be calling for help in a culturally acceptable way.

Ghost sickness: Navajo. Characterized by "being out of one's mind," dyspnea, weakness, and bad dreams. Thought to be caused by an evil spirit. Treated by overcoming the evil spirit with a stronger spiritual force the healer, a "singer," calls forth through a powerful healing ritual.

Hwa-byung: Korean. Characterized by epigastric pain, anorexia, palpitations, dyspnea, and muscle aches and pains. Thought to be caused by a lack of harmony in the body or in interpersonal relationships. Treated by reestablishing harmony. Some researchers feel that it is closely related to depression.

"Jin" possession: Somalian. Symptoms of psychological distress and anxiety. Thought to be caused by possession by a Jin, an invisible being that is angry with the human. Intermittent, involuntary, abnormal body movements occur along with the psychological distress. Treatment consists of an exorcism by a religious leader, such as an Imam, who will ask the Jin what the person has done to anger it so that the person can apologize and make amends. (Somali inpatient psychiatric nurse, personal communication, March 8, 2012.)

Neurasthenia: Chinese. Characterized by somatic symptoms of depression such as anorexia, weight loss, fatigue, weakness, trouble concentrating, and insomnia. Feelings of sadness or depression are denied. Thought to be related to a lack of yin-yang balance. Traditional treatment includes eating healthier, exercise, massage, rest, and lifestyle adjustment. Antidepressant therapy is now common.

Susto: Latin American. Characterized by a broad range of somatic and psychological symptoms similar to posttraumatic stress disorder. Precipitated by a traumatic incident or fright that caused the patient's soul to leave the body. Treated by an espiritista (spiritual healer).

Wind illness: Chinese, Vietnamese. Characterized by a fear of cold, wind, or drafts. Derived from the belief that yin-yang and hot-cold elements must be in balance in the body or illness occurs. Treated by keeping warm and avoiding foods, drinks, and herbs that are cold or considered to have a cold quality, as well as cold colors, emotions, and activities. Also treated by pulling the "cold wind" out of the patient by coining (vigorously rubbing a coin over the body) or cupping (applying a heated cup to the skin, creating a vacuum).

Genetic Variation in Pharmacodynamics

Another clinical practice issue that presents a barrier to quality mental health services for some groups is genetic variation in drug responses. There is a growing realization that many drugs vary in their action and effects along genetic and psychosocial lines (Lehne, 2013). In most clinical trials a high percentage of participants are white while other racial subgroups are underrepresented. This is a real problem since what is found true in drug studies primarily performed with subjects of European origin may not be true in racially and ethnically diverse populations.

The relatively new field of **pharmacogenetics** focuses on how genes affect individual responses to medicines (National Institutes of Health, 2014). Genes carry "recipes" for making specific protein molecules. Medications interact with thousands of proteins, and the smallest difference in the quantities or composition of these molecules can make a big difference in how they work. By understanding how genes influence drug responses, we hope to one day prescribe drugs that are best suited for each person.

Genetic variations in drug metabolism have been documented for several classifications of drugs, including antidepressants and antipsychotics. An important variation that impacts the ability to metabolize drugs relates to the more than 20 cytochrome P-450 (CYP) enzymes present in human beings (Henderson et al., 2016). Genetic variations in these enzymes may alter drug metabolism, and these variations tend to be propagated through racial/ethnic populations.

CYP enzymes metabolize most antidepressants and antipsychotics. Some genetic variations result in rapid metabolism, and if the body metabolizes medications too quickly, serum levels become too low, minimizing therapeutic effects. Other variations may result in poor metabolism. If the body metabolizes medications too slowly, serum levels become too high, increasing the risk of intolerable side effects. Care providers are utilizing genetic testing to determine correct medications and dosages with fairly good success (Brennan et al., 2015).

POPULATIONS AT RISK FOR MENTAL ILLNESS AND INADEQUATE CARE

Many people of the nondominant cultures in the United States are subject to experiences that challenge their mental health in ways that members of the majority group do not have to face. Among these challenges are issues related to the experience of being an immigrant and the socioeconomic disadvantages of minority status.

Immigrants

Immigrants face many unknowns. Upon arriving in the United States, they may not speak English, yet they need to learn how to navigate new economic, political, legal, educational, transportation, and healthcare systems. Many who had status and skills in their homeland—jobs as teachers, physicians, or other professional positions—find that, because of certification requirements or limited English skills, only menial jobs are open to them.

After immigration, family roles may be upset with wives finding jobs before their husbands. Immigrant families may find the struggle to live successfully in America arduous and wearisome. Long-honored cultural values and traditions, which once provided stability, are challenged by new cultural norms. During the period of adjustment, many immigrants find that the hope they felt on first immigrating turns into anxiety and depression.

Immigrants and their families embark on a process of **acculturation**—learning the beliefs, values, and practices of their new cultural setting—that sometimes takes several generations. Some immigrants adapt to the new culture quickly, absorbing the new worldview, beliefs, values, and practices rapidly until they are more natural than the ones they learned in their homeland. This process of adaptation is called **assimilation**. Others attempt to maintain their traditional cultural ways. Some may become bicultural—able to move in and out of their traditional culture and their new culture, depending on where they are and with whom they associate. Some immigrants may suffer culture shock, finding the new norms disconcerting or offensive because they contrast so deeply with their traditional beliefs, values, and practices.

Not surprisingly, children tend to assimilate the new culture at a rapid pace, whereas the elders maintain their traditional cultural beliefs, values, and practices. This sets the stage for intergenerational conflict. Children who are assimilating different values about family may challenge the traditional status of elders in a hierarchical family. Some children may feel lost between two cultures and unsure of where to place their cultural identity.

Refugees

A **refugee** is a special kind of immigrant. Whereas the immigrant generally values the new culture and wishes to enjoy a change in life circumstances, the refugee has left his or her own homeland to escape intolerable conditions and would have preferred to stay in the culture if that had been possible. Refugees do not perceive entry into the new culture as an active choice and may experience the stress of adjusting as imposed on them against their will.

Many refugees from the Middle East, Southeast Asia, Central America, and Africa have been traumatized by war, genocide, torture, starvation, and other catastrophic events. Many have lost family members, a way of life, and a homeland to which they can never return. The degree of trauma and loss they have experienced may make them particularly vulnerable to a variety of psychiatric disorders including major depressive disorder and posttraumatic stress disorder.

Cultural Minorities

Individuals who are considered minorities (non-whites or whites of non-European heritage) may be vulnerable to a variety of disadvantages including poverty and limited opportunities for education and jobs. Cultural minority groups are frequent victims of bias, discrimination, and racism—subtle but pervasive forms of rejection that diminish self-esteem and self-efficacy and leave victims feeling excluded and marginalized.

In the United States the prevalence of psychiatric disorders among cultural and racial minority groups is similar to that of whites *if* you exclude the poor and other vulnerable populations (e.g., homeless, institutionalized, children in foster care, and victims of trauma) within the minority groups. The higher incidence of mental health problems is related to poverty not race/ethnicity.

People who live in poverty are two to three times more likely to develop mental illness than those who live above the poverty line. In 2014, about 10% of non-Hispanic whites, 12% of Asian, 23% of Latino-Hispanic Americans, and 26% of blacks lived below the poverty level (US Census Bureau, 2015b). Poverty is associated with other disadvantages, such as scarce educational and economic opportunities, which in turn are associated with substance abuse and violent crime. Persons who are poor are subject to a daily struggle for survival, and this takes its toll on mental health.

Individuals from cultural minorities may perceive bias and experience culturally uncomfortable care from healthcare providers. These perceptions and experiences may make them less likely to seek medical services in the future. Bias and discrimination taint the healthcare system, resulting in further stresses on the mental health of those in minority groups instead of delivering the help they need.

CULTURALLY COMPETENT CARE

So far, this chapter has explained why the nursing needs of culturally diverse patient populations are so varied. Mental health and illness are biological, psychological, social, spiritual, and *cultural* processes. Cultural competence is required of nurses if they are to assist patients in achieving mental health and well-being. How, exactly, are psychiatric-mental health nurses to practice culturally competent care? The remainder of this chapter suggests techniques that address this question.

The HHS (2017) describes cultural competence as the ability to work effectively in cross-cultural situations and provide the best possible service to patients from various racial/ethnic backgrounds and who speak different languages. Cultural and linguistic competence is a set of congruent behaviors, attitudes, and policies that come together in a system, agency, or among professionals to enable effective work in cross-cultural situations. **Cultural competence** means that nurses adjust their practices to meet their patients' cultural beliefs, practices, needs, and preferences. Having cultural sensitivity or awareness is an essential component of cultural competence.

Campinha-Bacote (2008) provides a blueprint for psychiatric-mental health nurses in providing culturally effective care. This model is called the Process of Cultural Competence in the Delivery of Healthcare Services. In this model, nurses view themselves as *becoming* culturally competent rather than *being* culturally competent. This model suggests that nurses should constantly see themselves as learners throughout their careers—always open to, and learning from, the immense cultural diversity they will see among their patients. The model consists of five constructs that promote the process and journey of cultural competence:

1. Cultural awareness
2. Cultural knowledge
3. Cultural encounters
4. Cultural skill
5. Cultural desire

Cultural Awareness

Through cultural awareness, the nurse recognizes the enormous impact culture makes on patients' health values and practices. Culture also impacts how and when patients decide they are ill and need care, and what treatments they will seek when illness occurs.

Cultural awareness allows nurses to first acknowledge themselves as cultural beings so close to the norms of their own ethnic and professional cultures that these norms seem "right" (ethnocentrism). Through cultural awareness nurses often discover that many of their norms are cultural, few are universal, and that they have an obligation to be open to and respectful of patients' cultural norms.

By practicing cultural awareness, nurses also examine their cultural assumptions and expectations about what constitutes mental health, a healthy self-concept, a healthy family, and the right way to behave in society. They also examine assumptions and expectations about how people manifest psychological distress. The culturally aware nurse understands that evidence-based practice guidelines may not be applicable to all people since they are derived from studies involving people of primarily European origins.

A culturally aware nurse recognizes that three cultures are intersecting during any encounter with a patient: the culture of the patient, the culture of the nurse, and the culture of the setting (e.g., agency, clinic, hospital). As patient advocates, our job is to negotiate and support the patient's cultural needs and preferences.

Cultural Knowledge

Nurses can enhance their cultural knowledge in various ways. They can attend cultural events and programs, develop friendships with members of diverse cultural groups, and participate in in-service programs where members of diverse groups talk about their cultural norms. Another way to obtain cultural knowledge is to study online resources designed for healthcare providers.

Cultural knowledge can assist in understanding behaviors that might otherwise be misinterpreted. It helps nurses establish rapport, ask the right questions, avoid misunderstandings, and identify cultural variables to consider when planning nursing care. A summary of cultural knowledge, some of which we have already discussed, includes the following:

- Worldview, beliefs, and values that permeate the culture
- Nonverbal communication patterns such as the meaning of eye contact, facial expressions, gestures, and touch
- Etiquette norms such as the importance of punctuality, the pace of conversation, and the way respect and hospitality are shown
- Family roles and psychosocial norms such as the way decisions are made and the degree of independence versus interdependence of family members
- Cultural views about mental health and illness such as the degree of stigma and the nature of the "sick role"
- Patterns related to health and illness including cultural syndromes, pharmacogenetic variations, and folk and herbal treatments frequently used within the culture

Cultural Encounters

Although obtaining cultural knowledge sets a foundation, cultural guides cannot tell us anything about a particular patient or reduce stereotyping. **Stereotyping** is the tendency to believe that every member of a group is like all other members. According to Campinha-Bacote (2011), multiple cultural encounters with diverse patients deter us from stereotyping. We recognize that, although there are patterns that characterize a culture, individual members of the culture adhere to the culture's norms in diverse ways.

Cultural encounters help nurses develop confidence in cross-cultural interactions. Every nurse is likely to make cultural blunders and will need to recover from cultural mistakes. Cultural encounters help us to develop the skill of recognizing, avoiding, and reducing the cultural pain that can occur when nursing care causes the patient discomfort or offense by a failure to be sensitive to cultural norms. Every nurse can learn to recognize signs of cultural pain, such as a patient's discomfort or alienation, and take measures to recover trust and rapport by asking what has caused the offense, apologizing for any lack of sensitivity, and expressing willingness to learn from the patient.

Cultural Skill

Cultural skill is the ability to perform a cultural assessment in a sensitive way (Campinha-Bacote, 2011). The first step is to ensure that meaningful communication can occur. If the patient is not proficient in English, a professional medical interpreter should be engaged.

Many cultural assessment tools are available (Andrews & Boyle, 2016; Giger, 2016; Leininger, 2002; Purnell, 2013; Spector, 2012). An appendix in the *DSM-5* (APA, 2013), "Outline for Cultural Formulation," recommends cultural assessment areas. A useful mental health assessment tool is the classic set of questions proposed by Kleinman and colleagues (1978):

- What do you call this illness? *(diagnosis)*
- When did it start? Why then? *(onset)*
- What do you think caused it? *(etiology)*
- How does the illness work? What does it do to you? *(course)*
- How long will it last? Is it serious? *(prognosis)*
- How have you treated the illness? How do you think it should be treated? *(treatment)*

These questions allow the patient to feel heard and understood. They also help in eliciting cultural syndromes. You can expand on this list to include questions such as:

- What kind of problems has this illness has caused you?
- What do you fear most about this illness? Do you think it is curable?
- Do you know others who have had this problem? What happened to them? Do you think this will happen to you?

Approaching these questions conversationally is generally more effective than using a direct, formal approach. One indirect technique is to ask the patient what another family member thinks is causing the problem. The nurse can ask, "What does your family think is wrong? Why do they think it started? What do they think you should do about it?" After the patient describes what the family thinks, the nurse can simply ask if the patient agrees.

Another technique for promoting openness is to make a declaratory statement before asking the questions. For instance, before asking about cultural treatments the patient has tried, the nurse can first say, "People have remedies they find helpful when they are ill. Are there any special healers or treatments you have used or that you think might be helpful to you?"

There are some areas that deserve special attention during an assessment interview:

- Ethnicity, religious affiliation, and degree of acculturation to Western medical culture
- Spiritual practices that are important to preserving or regaining health
- Degree of proficiency in speaking and reading English
- Dietary patterns including foods prescribed for sick people
- Attitudes about pain and experiences with pain in a Western medical setting
- Attitudes about and experience with Western medications
- Cultural remedies such as healers, herbs, and practices the patient may find helpful
- Whom the patient considers "family," who should receive health information, and how decisions are made in the family
- Cultural customs the patient feels are essential to preserve and is fearful will be violated in the mental health setting

The purpose of a culturally sensitive assessment is to develop a therapeutic plan that is mutually agreeable, culturally acceptable, and potentially productive of positive outcomes. While gathering assessment data, you should identify cultural patterns that may support or interfere with the patient's health and recovery process. You can use your professional knowledge to categorize the patient's cultural norms into three different groups:

1. Those that facilitate the patient's health and recovery from the Western medical perspective
2. Those that are neither helpful nor harmful from the Western medical perspective
3. Those that are harmful to the patient's health and well-being from the Western medical perspective

McFarland and Wehbe-Alamah (2015) suggest a preservation/maintenance, accommodate/negotiate, repatterning/restructuring framework for care planning. Using this framework, effective nursing care preserves the aspects of the patient's culture that, from a Western perspective, promote health and well-being—such as a strong family support system and traditional values such as cooperation and emphasis on relationships.

You can accommodate for cultural values and practices that are neither helpful nor harmful or negotiate as needed. You may encourage the patient's use of neutral values and practices such as folk remedies and healers. Including these culture-specific interventions in nursing care builds on the patient's own coping and healing systems. For example, Native Americans with substance abuse problems may find tribal healing ceremonies helpful as a complement to the therapeutic program.

Finally, when you have determined that cultural patterns are harmful, make attempts to repattern and restructure them. For instance, if a patient is taking an herb that interferes with the prescription medication regimen, educate and negotiate with the patient until you have developed a mutually agreeable therapeutic program.

Cultural Desire

The final construct in Campinha-Bacote's cultural competence model for psychiatric-mental health nurses is cultural desire. Cultural desire indicates that the nurse is not acting out of a sense of duty but from a sincere and genuine concern for patients' welfare. This concern ideally leads to attempts to truly understand each patient's viewpoint. Nurses exhibit cultural desire through patience, consideration, and empathy. Giving the impression that you are willing to learn from the patient is the hallmark of cultural desire as opposed to behaving as if you know what is best and are going to impose the "correct" treatment on the patient.

Cultural desire inspires openness and flexibility in applying nursing principles to meet the patient's cultural needs. Although it may be easier to establish a therapeutic relationship with someone who comes from a similar cultural background, cultural desire enables the nurse to achieve good outcomes with culturally diverse patients.

KEY POINTS TO REMEMBER

- As the diversity of the world and the United States increases, psychiatric-mental health nurses will be caring for more and more people from diverse cultural groups.
- Nurses should learn to deliver culturally competent care, meaning culturally sensitive and attentive assessments and culturally congruent interventions.
- *Culture* is the shared beliefs, values, and practices of a group. It shapes the group's thinking and behavior in patterned ways. Cultural groups share these norms with new members of the group through *enculturation.*
- A group's culture influences its members' worldview, nonverbal communication patterns, etiquette norms, and ways of viewing the person, the family, and the right way to think and behave in society.
- The concept of mental health is formed within a culture, and other members of the group may define deviance from cultural expectations as illness.
- Psychiatric-mental health nursing is based on personality and developmental theories advanced by Europeans and Americans and grounded in Western cultural ideals and values.
- Nurses are as influenced by their own professional and ethnic cultures as patients are by theirs. Nurses should guard against ethnocentric tendencies when caring for patients.
- Barriers to quality mental healthcare include communication barriers, genetic variations in psychotropic drug metabolism, and misdiagnoses caused by culturally inappropriate diagnostic tools.
- Immigrants (especially refugees) and minority groups suffering from the effects of low socioeconomic status, including poverty and discrimination, are at particular risk for mental illness.
- Cultural competence consists of five constructs: cultural awareness, cultural knowledge, cultural encounters, cultural skill, and cultural desire.
- Through cultural awareness, nurses recognize that they, as well as patients, have cultural beliefs, values, and practices.
- Nurses obtain cultural knowledge by seeking cultural information from friends, participating in in-service programs, immersing oneself in the culture, or consulting print and online sources.
- Nurses experience intra-ethnic diversity through multiple cultural encounters, which prevents nurses from stereotyping their patients.
- Nurses demonstrate cultural skill by performing culturally sensitive assessment interviews and adapting care to meet patients' cultural needs and preferences.
- Cultural desire is a genuine interest in the patient's unique perspective; it enables nurses to provide considerate, flexible, and respectful care to patients of all cultures.

CRITICAL THINKING

1. Describe the cultural factors that have influenced the development of Western psychiatric-mental health nursing practice. Contrast these Western influences with the cultural factors that influence patients who come from Eastern, indigenous, or collective cultures.
2. What do you think about the claim that mental illness, such as schizophrenia, is a cultural phenomenon and that individuals are judged to be mentally ill if they do not fit within the social definition of normal? What implications (good or bad) does a diagnosis of a mental illness have?
3. Analyze the effects cultural competence (or incompetence) can have on psychiatric-mental health nurses and their patients.
4. How can barriers such as cultural imposition, misdiagnosis, and communication problems impede the promotion of competent psychiatric-mental healthcare? What can the members of the healthcare team do to overcome such barriers?

CHAPTER REVIEW

Questions

1. Which intervention demonstrates the nurse's understanding of what guides effective nursing care with a diverse patient population?
   - **a.** Treating all patients the same to avoid prejudicial actions.
   - **b.** Identifying the cultural norms of the population being served.
   - **c.** Recognizing that race and ethnicity result in specific illness management views.
   - **d.** Addressing the physical and emotional needs that originate from genetic factors.
2. Which statement indicates the beliefs and values that tend to be representative of a member of an indigenous culture? *Select all that apply.*
   - **a.** "I've reinforced the importance of taking medications at the time they are prescribed."
   - **b.** "The patient believes that illness is a result of being out of harmony with nature."
   - **c.** "Spending money on medicine for his diabetes is not a comfortable concept for my patient."
   - **d.** "The patient refuses treatment."
   - **e.** "We discussed the patient's needs regarding warding off evil spirits before her surgery."
3. Which assessment questions will support effective communication with a patient who recently emigrated from an Asian country? *Select all that apply.*
   - **a.** "What do you call this kind of pain?"
   - **b.** "What do you think is causing your pain?"
   - **c.** "How do you think your pain should be treated?"
   - **d.** "Do you consider this kind of pain a serious problem?"
   - **e.** "Do you think American medicine will help your pain?"

4. When considering culturally competent care for a Muslim patient diagnosed with cardiac problems, which intervention is particularly important to implement initially when a low fat diet is prescribed?
   a. Requesting a dietary consult
   b. Identifying dietary considerations
   c. Explaining the importance of a low fat diet
   d. Including the family in conversation about food preparation
5. Which statement by the nurse demonstrates ethnocentrism toward the Hispanic patient?
   a. "What do you want us to do to help your symptoms?"
   b. "Tell me more about what you think is causing these symptoms."
   c. "I'm sure we can do something to make your symptoms more manageable."
   d. "How much have these symptoms made it more difficult for you to go to work?"
6. Ling has a nursing diagnosis of risk for other-directed violence. Ling's Eastern culture family is having difficulty coping with the illness due to their beliefs. A favorable therapeutic modality for this patient might include:
   a. Outpatient therapy
   b. Family therapy
   c. Long-term inpatient care
   d. Assimilation therapy
7. A nurse practitioner is interviewing a female patient from Southeast Asia. She complains of stomach pain and chest discomfort. Knowing that the patient's adult son died in a car accident last month, the nurse suspects:
   a. Vulnerability
   b. Acid reflux
   c. Somatization
   d. Transference
8. Which nursing intervention can assist a Hindu patient in maintaining his religious practice?
   a. Assisting the patient to choose his own food from the menu
   b. Contacting the hospital pastor for a visit
   c. Showing him which side of the room faces east
   d. Offering a Torah to the patient
9. Intergenerational conflict may arise in immigrant families because the process of acculturation may be:
   a. Ignored due to cultural beliefs
   b. Filled with traumatic experiences
   c. Easier for children
   d. A function of assimilation
10. Which nursing actions demonstrate cultural competence? *Select all that apply.*
   a. Planning mealtime around the patient's prayer schedule
   b. Helping a patient to visit with the hospital chaplain
   c. Researching foods that a lacto-ovo-vegetarian patient will eat
   d. Providing time for a patient's spiritual healer to visit
   e. Ordering standard meal trays to be delivered three times daily

Answers

1. **b;** 2. **a, b, c, e;** 3. **a, b, c, d;** 4. **b;** 5. **c;** 6. **b;** 7. **c;** 8. **a;** 9. **c;** 10. **a, b, c, d**

Visit the Evolve website for a posttest on the content in this chapter: http://evolve.elsevier.com/Varcarolis

Post-Test interactive review

REFERENCES

American Psychiatric Association. (2013a). *Diagnostic and statistical manual of mental disorders* (5th ed.). Washington, DC: APA.

American Psychiatric Association. (2013b). *DSM-5 cultural formulation interview*. Retrieved from http://www.dsm5.org/proposedrevision/Pages/Cult.aspx.

Andrews, M., & Boyle, J. (2016). *Transcultural concepts in nursing care* (8th ed.). Philadelphia, PA: Wolters.

Brennan, F. X., Gardner, K. R., Lombard, J., Perlis, R. H., Fava, M., Harris, H. W., & Scott, R. (2015). A naturalistic study of the effectiveness of pharmacogenetic testing to guide treatment in psychiatric patients with mood and anxiety disorders. *Primary Care Companion for CNS Disorders, 17*(2). Retrieved from http://www.ncbi.nlm.nih.gov/pmc/articles/PMC4560190/.

Camann, M. A. (2013). Global perspectives in mental health. In C. Holtz (Ed.), *Global health care: Issues and policies* (2nd ed.) (pp. 385–408). Burlington, MA: Jones and Bartlett.

Campinha-Bacote, J. (2008). Cultural desire: 'Caught' or 'taught'? *Contemporary Nurse: Advances in Contemporary Transcultural Nursing, 28*(1–2), 141–148.

Campinha-Bacote, J. (2011). Delivering patient-centered care in the midst of a cultural conflict: The role of cultural competence. *Online Journal of Issues in Nursing, 16*(2).

Giger, J. N. (2016). *Transcultural nursing: Assessment and intervention* (7th ed.). St. Louis, MO: Elsevier.

Henderson, D. C., Vincenzi, B., Yeung, A. S., & Fricchione, G. L. (2016). Culture and psychiatry. In T. A. Stern, M. Fava, T. E. Wilens, & J. F. Rosenbaum (Eds.), *Massachusetts General Hospital Comprehensive Clinical Psychiatry* (pp. 718–725). St. Louis, MO: Elsevier.

Kleinman, A., Eisenberg, L., & Good, B. (1978). Culture, illness and care: Clinical lessons from anthropologic and cross-cultural research. *Annals of Internal Medicine, 88*, 251–258.

Lehne, R. A. (2013). Individual variation in drug responses. In R. A. Lehne (Ed.), *Pharmacology for nursing care* (pp. 79–87). St. Louis, MO: Elsevier.

Leininger, M. (2002). Culture care assessments for congruent competency practices. In M. Leininger & M. McFarland (Eds.), *Transcultural nursing: Concepts, theories, research and practice* (pp. 117–144). New York, NY: McGraw-Hill.

Marsella, A. J. (2011). *Twelve critical issues for mental health professionals working with ethno-culturally diverse populations. American Psychological Association*. Retrieved from http://www.apa.org/international/pi/2011/10/critical-issues.aspx.

McFarland, M., & Wehbe-Alamah, H. (2015). *Leininger's culture care diversity and universality: A worldwide nursing theory* (3rd ed.). Burlington, MA: Jones & Bartlett.

National Institutes of Health. (2014). *Frequently asked questions about pharmacogenetics*. Retrieved from https://www.genome.gov/27530645.

Purnell, L. D. (2013). Transcultural diversity and health care. In L. D. Purnell & B. J. Paulanka (Eds.), *Transcultural health care* (4th ed.) (pp. 1–15). Philadelphia, PA: Davis.

Purnell, L. D. (2014). *Guide to culturally competent health care* (3rd ed.). Philadelphia, PA: F. A. Davis Company.

Spector, R. E. (2012). *Cultural diversity in health and illness* (8th ed.). Upper Saddle River, NJ: Prentice-Hall.

Schwartz, R. C., & Blankenship, D. M. (2014). Racial disparities in psychotic disorder diagnosis: A review oxf empirical literature. *World Journal of Psychiatry*, *4*(4), 133–140.

Substance Abuse and Mental Health Services Administration. (2015). *Racial/ethnic differences in mental health service use among adults*. HHS Publication No. SMA-15-4906. Rockville, MD: Author. Retrieved from http://www.samhsa.gov/data/sites/default/files/MHServicesUseAmongAdults/MHServices UseAmongAdults.pdf.

United States Census Bureau. (2010). *Overview of race and Hispanic origin*. 2010. Retrieved from http://www.census.gov/prod/cen2010/briefs/c2010br-02.pdf.

United States Census Bureau. (2012). *US Census Bureau projections show a slower growing, older, more diverse nation in a half century from now*. Retrieved from http://www.census.gov/newsroom/releases/archives/population/cb12-243.html.

United States Census Bureau. (2015a). *2015 National Content Test: Preparing for the 2020 census*. Retrieved from http://www.census.gov/content/dam/Census/programs-surveys/decennial/2020-census/2015_census_tests/nct/2015-nct-factsheet.pdf.

United States Census Bureau. (2015b). *Income, poverty and health insurance coverage in the United States, 2014*. Retrieved from http://www.census.gov/hhes/www/poverty/data/incpovhlth/2014/table3.pdf.

United States Department of Health and Human Services Office of Minority Health. (2013). *National standards on culturally and linguistically appropriate services in health and healthcare*. Retrieved from https://www.thinkculturalhealth.hhs.gov/pdfs/EnhancedCLASStandardsBlueprint.pdf.

United States Department of Health and Human Services Office of Minority Health. (2017). *Cultural and linguistic competency*. Retrieved from https://minorityhealth.hhs.gov/omh/browse.aspx?lvl=1&lvlid=6.

6

Legal and Ethical Considerations

Margaret Jordan Halter, Diane K. Kjervik

Visit the Evolve website for a pretest on the content in this chapter: http://evolve.elsevier.com/Varcarolis Pre-Test interactive review

OBJECTIVES

1. Differentiate the terms ethics and bioethics.
2. Describe five ethical principles central to bioethics.
3. Describe the legal process for admissions and discharges.
4. Discuss patient's rights including the patient's right to treatment, refuse treatment, and informed consent.
5. Describe patient's rights and legal concerns with regard to restraint and seclusion.
6. Explain the importance of confidentiality in psychiatric care.
7. Identify situations in which healthcare professionals have a duty to break patient confidentiality.
8. Define laws (e.g., torts, negligence, malpractice) relevant to psychiatric nursing.
9. Discuss the basic standards by which nurses are held including nurse practice acts, professional associations, organizational policies and procedures, and customary practice.
10. Identify the steps nurses are advised to take if they suspect negligence or illegal activity in the provision of healthcare.
11. Discuss the importance of clear and thorough documentation.
12. Identify healthcare workers' legal protection from violence in the healthcare setting.

OUTLINE

KEY TERMS AND CONCEPTS

assault
assisted outpatient treatment
battery
bioethics
competency
conditional release
confidentiality
duty to protect
duty to warn
emergency commitment
ethical dilemma
ethics
false imprisonment
Health Insurance Portability and Accountability Act (HIPAA)
implied consent
informal admission
informed consent
intentional torts
involuntary commitment
least restrictive alternative doctrine
malpractice
negligence
parity
right to privacy
right to refuse treatment
right to treatment
tort
unconditional release
unintentional torts
voluntary admission
writ of habeas corpus

While a basic understanding of legal and ethical issues is important in every healthcare setting, the nature of the problems in psychiatric care elevates the significance of these issues. Patients in this population experience alterations in thought, mood, and behavior that may render them less capable of making appropriate decisions regarding their care. On the other hand, individuals with mental illness may need their rights protected through the legal system. This chapter introduces ethical concepts and legal issues you may encounter in the practice of psychiatric-mental health nursing.

ETHICAL CONCEPTS

No legal chapter would be complete without first discussing ethics because laws tend to reflect the ethical values of society. Ethics is the study of philosophical beliefs about what is right or wrong in a society. When you consider ethics, you are considering hard questions. For example, one big ethical issue that Americans have been asking is "Is healthcare a right or a privilege?" in response to mandated insurance coverage for all Americans. Recently, countries were faced with the Ebola crisis where providers asked, "How should resources be allocated and to whom?" Ethics provide a framework for answering these questions.

The term bioethics is the study of specific ethical questions that arise in healthcare. The five basic ethical principles important to bioethics are:

1. **Beneficence**: The duty to act to benefit or promote the good of others (e.g., spending extra time to help calm an anxious patient).
2. **Autonomy**: Respecting the rights of others to make their own decisions (e.g., acknowledging the patient's right to refuse medication supports autonomy).
3. **Justice**: The duty to distribute resources or care equally, regardless of personal attributes (e.g., an intensive care unit nurse devotes equal attention to someone who has attempted suicide as to someone who suffered a brain aneurysm).
4. **Fidelity** (nonmaleficence): Maintaining loyalty and commitment to the patient and doing no wrong to the patient (e.g., maintaining expertise in nursing skill through continuing nurse education).
5. **Veracity**: The duty to communicate truthfully (e.g., describing the purpose and side effects of psychotropic medications in a truthful and nonmisleading way).

An ethical dilemma results when there is a conflict between two or more courses of action, each carrying favorable and unfavorable consequences. The response to these dilemmas is based partly on morals (beliefs of right or wrong) and values. Suppose you are caring for a pregnant woman with schizophrenia who wants to have the baby but whose family insists she get an abortion. To promote fetal safety, her antipsychotic medication would need to be reduced, putting her at risk of exacerbating the psychiatric illness. Furthermore, there is a question as to whether she can safely care for the child. If you rely on the ethical principle of autonomy, you may conclude that she has the right to decide. Would other ethical principles be in conflict with autonomy in this case?

At times, your values may be in conflict with the value system of the organization where you work. This situation further complicates the decision-making process and necessitates careful consideration of the patient's desires and rights. For example, you may experience a conflict of values in a setting where older adults are routinely sedated to a degree to which you do not feel comfortable. When your value system is challenged, this increases stress. Some nurses respond proactively by working to change the system or even advocate for legislation related to some particular issue.

An ethical nursing practice has a profound impact on patient safety and quality of care. In recognition of that impact, the American Nurses Association (ANA, 2015a) designated 2015 as the "Year of Ethics" and released a revised *Code of Ethics for Nurses* for the profession. The revision was driven by the changing dynamics in healthcare and issues facing contemporary nursing. The code provides the professional ethical foundation for registered nurses in the United States (Box 6.1).

BOX 6.1 Code of Ethics for Nurses

1. The nurse, in all professional relationships, practices with compassion and respect for the inherent dignity, worth, and uniqueness of every individual, unrestricted by considerations of social or economic status, personal attributes, or the nature of health problems.
2. The nurse's primary commitment is to the patient, whether an individual, family, group, or community.
3. The nurse promotes, advocates for, and strives to protect the rights, health, and safety of the patient.
4. The nurse has authority, accountability, and responsibility for nursing practice; makes decisions; and takes action consistent with the obligation to promote health and provide optimal care.
5. The nurse owes the same duties to self as to others, including the responsibility to promote health and safety, preserve wholeness of character and integrity, maintain competence, and continue personal and professional growth.
6. The nurse, through individual and collective effort, establishes, maintains, and improves the ethical environment of the work setting and conditions of employment that are conducive to safe, quality care.
7. The nurse, in all roles and settings, advances the profession through research and scholarly inquiry, professional standards development, and the generation of both nursing and health policy.
8. The nurse collaborates with other health professionals and the public to protect human rights, promote health diplomacy, and reduce health disparities.
9. The profession of nursing, collectively through its professional organizations, must articulate nursing values, maintain the integrity of the profession, and integrate principles of social justice into nursing and health policy.

From American Nurses Association. (2015). *Code of ethics for nurses with interpretive statements*. Washington, DC: American Nurses Publishing.

MENTAL HEALTH LAWS

Federal and state legislatures have enacted laws to regulate the care and treatment of people with mentally illness. Mental health laws—or statutes—vary from state to state. Therefore you are encouraged to review your state's code to better understand the legal climate in which you will be practicing. You can accomplish this by visiting the web page of your state's mental health department or by doing an internet search using the keywords "mental + health + statutes + (your state)."

Many of the state laws underwent substantial revision after the landmark Community Mental Health Centers Act of 1963 enacted under President John F. Kennedy (refer to Chapter 4) that promoted deinstitutionalization of the mentally ill. The changes reflect a shift in emphasis from institutional care of people with psychiatric disorders to community-based care. There was an increasing awareness of the need to provide the mentally ill with humane care that respects their civil rights. Widespread, progressive use of psychotropic drugs in the treatment of mental illness enabled many patients to integrate more readily into the larger community.

Additionally, the legal system has adopted a more therapeutic approach to persons with substance use disorders and mental health disorders. There are now drug courts where the emphasis is more on rehabilitation than punishment. Similarly, mental health courts handle criminal charges against the mentally ill by diverting them to community resources to prevent reoffending by, among other things, monitoring medication adherence.

Federal legislation providing equality for the mentally ill with other patients in terms of payments for services from health insurance plans also improves access to treatment. This equal payment is called **parity**. The Paul Wellstone and Pete Domenici Mental Health Parity and Addiction Equity Act, which went into effect in July 2010, and the Affordable Care Act, also enacted in 2010, provide for insurance funding for mental illness (Bazelton Center for Mental Health Law, 2012).

ADMISSION AND DISCHARGE PROCEDURES

Admission Procedures

The following sections discuss several types of admissions, all of which must be based on several fundamental guidelines:

- Neither voluntary admission nor involuntary commitment determines a patient's ability to make informed decisions about personal healthcare.
- Care providers must establish a well-defined psychiatric problem, based on current illness classifications in the *Diagnostic and Statistical Manual of Mental Disorders, Fifth Edition* (*DSM-5*; American Psychiatric Association [APA], 2013).
- The presenting illness should be of such a nature that it causes an immediate crisis situation or that other less-restrictive alternatives (i.e., outpatient care) are inadequate or unavailable.
- There must be a reasonable expectation that the hospitalization and treatment will improve the presenting problems.

You are encouraged to become familiar with the laws in your state and provisions for admissions, discharges, patients' rights, and informed consent. The admissions described in the following paragraphs provide a general overview of the standards and process.

Voluntary Admissions

Informal Admission

Informal admission is the least restrictive of all admissions. It is similar to any general hospital admission in which there is no formal application. The person does not pose a substantial threat of harm to self or others. Under this model, the normal caregiver-patient relationship exists, and the patient is free to stay or leave, even against medical advice.

Voluntary admissions occur when patients apply in writing for admission to the facility. The person must understand the need for treatment and be willing to be admitted. If the person is under 16, the parent, legal guardian, custodian, or next of kin may have authority to apply on the person's behalf. If a person is between 16 and 18, he or she may seek admission independently or on the application of an authorized individual or agency.

Voluntarily admitted patients have the right to request and obtain release. Before being released, reevaluation may be necessary. Reevaluation can result in a decision on the part of the care provider to initiate an involuntary commitment according to criteria established by state law.

Involuntary Commitment

Involuntary commitment, also known as assisted inpatient psychiatric treatment, is a court-ordered admission to a facility without the patient's consent. State laws vary, but they address both the criteria for commitment and the process for commitment. The criteria for commitment are the legal standards under which the court decides whether admission is necessary. These standards include a person who is:

1. Mentally ill
2. Posing a danger to self or others
3. Gravely disabled (unable to provide for basic necessities such as food, clothing, and shelter)
4. In need of treatment, and the mental illness prevents help-seeking on a voluntary basis

The process for commitment has evolved. Many years ago, it was fairly easy to have someone committed. For example, a common problem in 1930s Maine was husbands getting rid of wives through psychiatric commitment (Curtis, 2001). Legislation was enacted to penalize husbands who brought false testimony. One startling chief complaint listed on an actual admitting record was, "Patient does not do her housework." Forced hospitalization was also considered appropriate for "treating" homosexuality.

In reaction to abusive practices of the past, the pendulum has swung and forced hospitalization is far less common. We currently have a very complex system for involuntary commitment.

Generally, involuntary commitment begins with someone who is familiar with the individual and believes that treatment is necessary. Often, when things become unbearable, a call is made to the police or local mental health facility, "I can't take it anymore, he's not himself, can you help us?" This person making the call might be a family member, legal guardian, custodian, or someone who lives with the individual. It could also be a healthcare professional. At this point, the individual begins a formal application for admission. To support the application, a specified number of physicians (usually two), or a combination of other mental health professionals, certify that a person's mental health status justifies detention and treatment.

Patients have the right of access to legal counsel and the right to take their case before a judge who may order a release. If they are not released, patients can be kept involuntarily for a state-specified number of days with interim court appearances. After that time, a panel of professionals that includes psychiatrists, medical doctors, lawyers, and private citizens reviews their cases.

A patient who believes that he or she is being held without just cause can file a petition for a **writ of habeas corpus**, which means a "formal written order" to "free the person." The writ of habeas corpus is the procedural mechanism used to challenge unlawful detention by the government. The hospital must immediately submit the document to the court. The court must then decide if the patient has been denied due process of law.

Patients can also challenge the hospitalization based on the **least restrictive alternative doctrine**. The least restrictive alternative doctrine mandates that care providers must take the least drastic action to achieve a specific purpose. For example, if you can treat someone safely for depression on an outpatient basis, hospitalization would be too restrictive and unnecessarily disruptive.

> **VIGNETTE:** Elizabeth is a 50-year-old woman with a long history of admissions to psychiatric hospitals. During previous hospitalizations, she was diagnosed with paranoid schizophrenia. She has refused visits from her caseworker, quit taking medication, and her young-adult children have become increasingly concerned about her behavior. When they stop to visit, she is typically unkempt and smells bad and her apartment is filthy and filled with cats. There is no food in the refrigerator except for ketchup and an old container of yogurt, and she is not paying her bills.
>
> Elizabeth accuses her children of spying on her. She believes they are in collusion with the government to get secrets of mind control and oil-rationing plans. She is making vague threats to the local officials, claiming that people who have caused the problems need to be "taken care of." Her daughter contacts her psychiatrist with this information, and they make a decision to begin emergency involuntary commitment proceedings.

Emergency commitment. **Emergency commitment** is also known as a temporary admission or emergency hospitalization. Emergency commitment is used (1) for people who are so confused they cannot make decisions on their own or (2) for people who are so ill they need emergency admission. In some states, anyone can initiate these proceedings through the court system. Other states require that care providers, such as a physician, advanced practice psychiatric nurses, a social worker, or an officer of the law initiate a temporary admission. Generally, a psychiatrist employed by the facility must confirm the need for hospitalization.

The primary purpose of this type of hospitalization is observation, diagnosis, and treatment of those who have mental illness or pose a danger to themselves or others. The length of time that patients can be held in this temporary admission ranges from 24 to 96 hours depending on the state. A court hearing is held and a decision is made for discharge, voluntary admission, or involuntary commitment.

Assisted outpatient treatment. **Assisted outpatient treatment** is also known as court-ordered outpatient treatment and more than 20 other names throughout the United States. This type of involuntary outpatient commitment arose in the 1990s when states began to pass legislation that permitted court-ordered outpatient treatment as an alternative to forced inpatient treatment. As of 2014, only five states—Connecticut, Massachusetts, Maryland, New Mexico, and Tennessee—had not adopted this model of less restrictive care.

Assisted outpatient treatment can be a preventive measure, allowing a court order before the onset of a psychiatric crisis that would result in an inpatient admission. The order for involuntary outpatient care is usually tied to receipt of goods and services provided by social welfare agencies, including disability benefits and housing. To access these goods and services, the patient must participate in treatment and may face inpatient admission for failing to participate in treatment.

Discharge Procedures

Release from hospitalization depends on the patient's admission status. As previously discussed, voluntarily admitted patients have the right to request and receive release. Some states, however, do provide for conditional release of voluntary patients, which enables the treating physician or administrator to order continued treatment on an outpatient basis if the patient needs further care.

Conditional Release

Conditional release usually requires outpatient treatment for a specified period to determine if the patient follows the medication regimen, can meet basic needs, and is able to reintegrate into the community. Generally, a voluntarily admitted patient who is conditionally released can only be involuntarily admitted through the usual methods described earlier. However, an involuntarily admitted patient who is conditionally released may be reinstitutionalized, although the commitment is still in effect without recommencement of formal admission procedures.

Unconditional Release

Unconditional release is the termination of a patient-institution relationship. This release may be court-ordered or administratively ordered by the institution's officials. Generally, the administrative officer of an institution has the discretion to discharge patients.

Release against Medical Advice (AMA)

In some cases, there is a disagreement between the mental healthcare providers and the patient as to whether continued hospitalization is necessary. In cases where treatment seems beneficial but there is no compelling reason (e.g., danger to self or others) to seek an involuntary continuance of stay, patients may be released against medical advice.

PATIENTS' RIGHTS UNDER THE LAW

Psychiatric facilities usually provide patients with a written list of basic rights derived from a variety of sources, especially legislation that came out of the 1960s. Since that time, rights have been modified to some degree, but most lists share commonalities described in the following sections.

Right to Treatment

One of the most fundamental rights of a patient admitted for psychiatric care is the right to *quality* care. We refer to this as the right to treatment. Particularly in the case of involuntary commitment, how can we deny a person's liberty and then not provide treatment?

Based on the decisions of a number of early court cases, patients have specific rights to treatment. They include:

- The right to be free from excessive or unnecessary medication
- The right to privacy and dignity
- The right to the least restrictive environment
- The right to an attorney, clergy, and private care providers
- The right to not be subjected to lobotomies, electroconvulsive treatments, and other treatments without fully informed consent

Right to Refuse Treatment

Just as patients have the right to receive treatment, they also have the right to refuse it. Patients may withhold consent or withdraw consent at any time, even if they are involuntarily committed. Patients can also retract consent previously given, and care providers must respect this whether it is a verbal or written retraction. However, the patient's right to refuse treatment with psychotropic drugs has been debated in the courts. This debate is based partly on the issue of patients' mental ability to give or withhold consent to treatment and their status under the civil commitment statutes.

Early cases—initiated by state hospital patients—considered medical, legal, and ethical considerations such as basic treatment problems, the doctrine of informed consent, and the bioethical principle of autonomy. Tables 6.1 and 6.2 summarize the evolution of two landmark sets of cases regarding the patient's right to refuse treatment.

In an emergency to prevent a person from causing serious and imminent harm to self or others, institutions can medicate a

TABLE 6.1 Right to Refuse Treatment: Evolution from Massachusetts Case Law to Present Law

Case	Court	Decision
Rogers v. Okin, 478 F. Supp. 1342 (D. Mass. 1979)	Federal district court	Ruled that involuntarily hospitalized patients with mental illness are competent and have the right to make treatment decisions. Forcible administration of medication is justified in an emergency if needed to prevent violence and if other alternatives have been ruled out. A guardian may make treatment decisions for an incompetent patient.
Rogers v. Okin, 634 F.2nd 650 (1st Cir. 1980)	Federal court of appeals	Affirmed that involuntarily hospitalized patients with mental illness are competent and have the right to make treatment decisions. The staff has substantial discretion in an emergency. Forcible medication is also justified to prevent the patient's deterioration. A patient's rights must be protected by judicial determination of competency or incompetency.
Mills v. Rogers, 457 U.S. 291 (1982)	US Supreme Court	Set aside the judgment of the court of appeals with instructions to consider the effect of an intervening state court case.
Rogers v. Commissioner of the Department of Mental Health, 458 N.E.2d 308 (Mass. 1983)	Massachusetts Supreme Judicial Court answering questions certified by federal court of appeals	Ruled that involuntarily hospitalized patients are competent and have the right to make treatment decisions unless they are judicially determined to be incompetent.

TABLE 6.2 Right to Refuse Treatment: Evolution from New Jersey Case Law to Present Law

Case	Court	Decision
Rennie v. Klein, 476 F. Supp. 1292 (D. N.J. 1979)	Federal district court	Ruled that involuntarily hospitalized patients with mental illness have a qualified constitutional right to refuse treatment with antipsychotic drugs. Voluntarily hospitalized patients have an absolute right to refuse treatment with antipsychotic drugs under New Jersey law.
Rennie v. Klein, 653 F.2d 836 (3d Cir. 1981)	Federal court of appeals	Ruled that involuntarily hospitalized patients with mental illness have a constitutional right to refuse antipsychotic drug treatment. The state may override a patient's right when the patient poses a danger to self or others. Due process protections must be complied with before forcible medication of patients in nonemergency situations.
Rennie v. Klein, 454 U.S. 1078 (1982)	US Supreme Court	Set aside the judgment of the court of appeals, with instructions to consider the case in light of the US Supreme Court decision in *Youngberg v. Romeo*.
Rennie v. Klein, 720 F.2d 266 (3d Cir. 1983)	Federal court of appeals	Ruled that involuntarily hospitalized patients with mental illness have the right to refuse treatment with antipsychotic medications. Decisions to forcibly medicate must be based on accepted professional judgment and must comply with due process requirements of the New Jersey regulations.

person without a court hearing. After a court hearing, a person can be medicated if all of the following criteria are met:

1. The person has a serious mental illness
2. The person's ability to function is deteriorating or he or she is suffering or exhibiting threatening behavior
3. The benefits of treatment outweigh the harm
4. The person lacks the capacity to make a reasoned decision about the treatment
5. Less-restrictive services have been found inappropriate

Right to Informed Consent

Informed consent is a legal term that means the patient has been provided with basic information regarding risks, benefits, and alternatives of treatment. The person must be voluntarily accepting the treatments. While registered nurses may provide education about treatment, typically, it is the prescriber who is legally responsible for securing informed consent.

The principle of informed consent is based on a person's right to self-determination as described in the landmark case of *Canterbury v. Spence* (1972):

> *The root premise is the concept, fundamental in American jurisprudence, that every human being of adult years and sound mind has a right to determine what shall be done with his own body…True consent to what happens to one's self is the informed exercise of choice, and that entails an opportunity to evaluate knowledgeably the options available and the risks attendant on each. (p. 780)*

Consent must be secured for surgery, electroconvulsive treatment, or the use of experimental drugs or procedures. Some state institutions require consent for each medication addition or change. Patients have the right to refuse participation in experimental treatments or research and the right to voice grievances and recommend changes in policies or services offered by the facility, without fear of punishment or reprisal.

Patients must be informed of the following elements:

- The nature of the problem or condition
- The nature and purpose of a proposed treatment
- The risks and benefits of that treatment
- The alternative treatment options
- The probability that the proposed treatment will be successful
- The risks of not consenting to treatment

Implied Consent

Many procedures nurses perform carry an element of **implied consent**. For example, if you approach the patient with a medication in hand, and the patient indicates a willingness to receive the medication, implied consent has occurred. Many institutions—particularly state psychiatric hospitals—have a requirement to obtain informed consent for every medication given.

A general rule for you to consider is that the more intrusive or risky the procedure, the greater the need for you to obtain informed consent. While you may not have a legal duty to inform the patient of the associated risks and benefits of a particular medical procedure, morally and ethically you are bound to clarify the procedure to the patient and ensure expressed or implied consent. If after attempting to clarify with the patient, you believe he or she really does not understand what is happening, the next step is to notify the prescriber of your concerns.

Capacity and Competency

For an individual to provide informed consent, as previously mentioned, he or she must have the capacity to understand. Therefore capacity is a person's ability to make an informed decision. Capacity is a fluid concept and individuals may possess capacity one minute and lack capacity in another. Mental health providers may provide opinions about capacity. For example, "Does the patient have the capacity to consent for electroconvulsive therapy?"

Competency is a different, but closely related term to capacity. **Competency** is a legal term and not a medical determination related to the degree of mental soundness a person has to make decisions or to carry out specific acts. Like the phrase, "Innocent until proven guilty," patients are considered competent until they have been declared incompetent. If found incompetent through a formal legal proceeding, the patient may be appointed a legal guardian or representative who is responsible for giving or refusing consent for the patient, while always considering the patient's wishes.

Guardians are typically selected from among family members. The order of selection is usually (1) spouse, (2) adult children or grandchildren, (3) parents, (4) adult siblings, and (5) adult nieces and nephews. In the event a family member is either unavailable or unwilling to serve as in this role, the court may also appoint a court-trained volunteer guardian.

Rights Regarding Psychiatric Advance Directives

Patients who have experienced an episode of severe mental illness have the opportunity to express their treatment preferences in a psychiatric advance directive. This document is prepared when the individual is well and identifies, in detail, his or her wishes and treatment choices.

These directives vary somewhat from state to state, but generally cover the same basic areas. The following choices are addressed in Ohio's Declaration for Mental Health Treatment:

- Designation of preferred physician and therapists
- Appointment of someone to make mental health treatment decisions
- Preferences regarding medications to take or not take
- Consent or lack of consent for electroconvulsive therapy
- Consent or lack of consent for admission to a psychiatric facility
- Preferred facilities and unacceptable facilities
- Individuals who should not visit

Rights Regarding Restraint and Seclusion

The history of restraint and seclusion is marked by abuse, overuse, and even a tendency to use restraint as punishment. This was especially true before the 1950s when there were no effective chemical treatments. In the book *The Shame of the States*, Deutsch (1949) wrote that in 1948 one out of every four patients was restrained during the day. The practice of restraining patients rose to one in three patients at night.

Legislation and accreditation requirements have dramatically reduced this problem by mandating strict guidelines. In fact, the pendulum has swung so far from the days of rampant use of restraint and seclusion that these methods have been referred to disparagingly as *therapeutic assault*.

The American Psychiatric Nurses Association (APNA) promotes a culture that minimizes and eventually eliminates the use of seclusion and restraint (APNA, 2014). As previously mentioned, the use of the least restrictive means of restraint for the shortest duration is always the general rule. According to the Centers for Medicare and Medicaid Services (CMS, 2008), in emergency situations, less-restrictive measures do not necessarily have to be tried, they only need to be considered ineffective in the staff's professional judgment.

Sometimes agitation, confusion, and combative behavior can have physical origins. Drug interaction, drug side effects, temperature elevation, hypoglycemia, hypoxia, and electrolyte imbalances can all result in behavioral disturbances. Addressing these problems can reduce or eliminate the need for restraint or seclusion. Nurses should consider the following before using seclusion and restraint:

- Verbally intervening (e.g., asking the patient for cooperation)
- Reducing stimulation
- Actively listening
- Providing diversion
- Offering as needed (PRN) medications

While we tend to think of classical restraining devices, a restraint can actually be any mechanical or physical device, equipment, or material that prevents or reduces movement of the patient's legs, arms, body, or head. Even side rails are a restraint if you use them to prevent the patient from exiting the bed.

Restricting a patient's movement by holding is also a restraint. These so-called *therapeutic holds* have resulted in the deaths of many people. A 16-year-old boy in a residential treatment center for disturbed youth in New York died after being placed in a therapeutic hold by several staff members (Bernstein, 2012). According to witnesses, the boy had complained he could not breathe then became unresponsive.

A restraint may be chemical. Chemical restraints are medications or doses of medication that are not being used for the patient's condition. Chemical interventions are usually less restrictive than physical or mechanical interventions. However, they can have a greater impact on the patient's ability to relate to the environment due to their effect on levels of awareness and their side effects. Medication can be extremely effective and helpful as an alternative to physical methods of restraint.

Seclusion is confining a patient alone in an area or a room and preventing the patient from leaving. It is used only when a patient is demonstrating violent or self-destructive behavior that jeopardizes the safety of others or the patient. Even if the door is not locked, making threats if the patient tries to leave the room is still considered secluding. However, a person who is physically restrained in an open room is not considered to be in seclusion.

Seclusion should be distinguished from timeout. This is an intervention in which a patient chooses to spend time alone in a specific area for a certain amount of time. The patient can leave the timeout area at any point.

Orders and Documentation with Restraint and Seclusion

In an emergency, a nurse may place a patient in seclusion or restraint but must obtain a written or verbal order as soon as possible thereafter. Orders for restraint or seclusion are never written as an as needed or as a standing order. These orders to manage self-destructive or violent behavior may be renewed for a total of 24 hours with limits depending upon the patient's age (CMS, 2008). Adults 18 years or older are limited to 4 hours; children and adolescents 9 to 17 years old are limited to 2 hours; and children under 9 years old have a 1 hour limit. After 24 hours, a physician or other licensed person responsible for the patient's care must personally assess the patient. Restraint or seclusion must be discontinued as soon as safer and quieter behavior begins. Once a patient is removed from restraints or seclusion, a new order is required to reinstitute the intervention.

The nurse should carefully document restraint or seclusion in the treatment plan or plan of care. The documentation should include the specific behaviors leading to restraint or seclusion, and the time the patient is placed in and released from restraint. The patient must be monitored through continuous observation. You must assess the patient in restraint at regular and frequent intervals such as every 15 to 30 minutes for physical needs (e.g., food, hydration, and toileting), safety, and comfort. You will also document these observations every 15 to 30 minutes. While in restraints, the patient must be protected from all sources of harm.

Rights Regarding Confidentiality

Confidentiality is an ethical responsibility of healthcare professionals that prohibits the disclosure of privileged information without the patient's consent. Confidentiality of care and treatment remains an important right for all patients, particularly psychiatric patients. Only the patient can waive the legal privilege of confidentiality.

Discussions about a patient in public places such as elevators and the cafeteria should be completely avoided. Even if the patient's name is not mentioned, such discussions can lead to disclosures of confidential information and liability for you and the facility. Your paperwork should never contain full patient identifiers.

> **VIGNETTE:** During the psychiatric rotation in her senior year, Lori learned that her mother's best friend, Sandy, was a patient. In the report the nurse shared that Sandy was diagnosed with major depressive disorder, is going through a painful divorce, and that she has breast cancer.
>
> Though she was uncomfortable and uncertain, Lori approached Sandy on the unit, gave her a hug, and asked how she's doing. To Lori's relief, Sandy seemed to take comfort in having a familiar person around and openly shared what was happening.
>
> When Lori suggests that Sandy call her mom so that she can visit, Sandy's eyes widen, she shakes her head, and adamantly says, "I don't want anyone to know I'm here. I'm so ashamed." As a friend, Lori believes that her mom would be hurt if she didn't know, and more importantly, she could also provide strong social support. As a future nurse, Lori knows that she must maintain confidentiality and never mentions the encounter.

Health Insurance Portability and Accountability Act

The **Health Insurance Portability and Accountability Act (HIPAA)**, enacted in 1996, legally protects the psychiatric patient's right to receive treatment and to have medical records kept confidential. Generally, your legal duty to maintain confidentiality is to protect the patient's **right to privacy.**

According to the 2003 HIPAA Privacy Rule, you may not, without the patient's consent, disclose information obtained from the patient or the medical record to anyone except those persons for whom it is necessary for implementation of the patient's treatment plan. HIPAA also gives special protection to notes taken during psychotherapy that are kept separate from the patient's health information.

Confidentiality and Social Media

It is essential that people working in mental health understand the legal implications of social media and the internet. The internet is not confidential and is open to legal subpoenas. Some mental health workers have blogged about patients, thinking that they had disguised the identity. People in these posts have been identified and lawsuits have followed.

Even what seems to be a fairly innocent electronic transmission can be disastrous. Consider the nursing students in Kansas who posted a picture of a placenta on social media. Standing next to the placenta were four smiling nursing students wearing lab coats and surgical gloves. What they considered to be victimless fun resulted in these students being expelled from nursing school. Fortunately for them, a federal judge ruled for reinstatement of one of the students. Subsequently, the other three were also allowed back in school.

Confidentiality After Death

A person's reputation can be damaged even after death. It is important that you do not divulge information after a person's death that you could not legally share before the death. In the courtroom setting, the Dead Man's Statute protects confidential information about individuals when they are not alive to speak for themselves. About half the states have such a law, and again, these laws vary from state to state.

Confidentiality of Professional Communications

A legal privilege exists as a result of specific laws to protect the confidentiality of certain professional communications (e.g., nurse-patient [in some states], physician-patient, attorney-patient). The theory behind providing a privilege is to ensure that patients will speak frankly and be willing to disclose personal information because they know that care providers will not repeat or distribute confidential conversations.

In 12 states, the legal privilege of confidentiality has been extended to registered nurses and advanced practice nurses (Pierce, 2014). In the remaining states, nurses must answer a court's questions regarding the patient, even if this information implicates the patient in a crime. In these states, the confidentiality of communications cannot be guaranteed.

Exceptions to the Rule

Duty to warn and protect third parties. The California Supreme Court in its 1974 landmark decision *Tarasoff v. Regents of University of California* ruled that a therapist has a duty to warn a patient's potential victim of potential harm. This **duty to warn** is an obligation to warn third parties when they may be in danger from a patient.

This ruling came about as a result of a tragic case. Prosenjit Poddar, a university student who was being counseled at the University of California, was despondent over a rejection by Tatiana Tarasoff, whom he had once kissed. The psychologist notified police verbally and in writing that the young man might pose a danger to Tarasoff. The police questioned the student, found him to be rational, and he promised to stay away from his love interest. Subsequently, he stalked and fatally stabbed Tarasoff 2 months later.

This case created much controversy and confusion in the psychiatric and medical communities over issues concerning (1) breach of patient confidentiality and its impact on the therapeutic relationship in psychiatric care and (2) the ability of the therapist to predict when a patient is truly dangerous. The court found the patient-therapist relationship sufficient to create a duty of the therapist to aid the victim.

When a therapist determines that a patient presents a serious danger of violence to another, the therapist has the duty to protect that other person. In fulfilling this duty, the therapist may be required to call and warn the intended victim, the victim's family, or the police or to take whatever steps are reasonably necessary under the circumstances.

Most states have similar laws regarding the duty to protect third parties of potential life threats. The duty to protect usually includes the following:

- Assessing and predicting the patient's danger of violence toward another
- Identifying the specific persons being threatened
- Taking appropriate action to protect the identified victims

Implications for psychiatric-mental health nursing. Staff nurses are obligated to report a patient's threats of harm against specified victims or classes of victims to other members of the treatment team. Advanced practice psychiatric-mental health nurses in private practice who engage in individual therapy are obligated to warn the endangered party themselves.

Statutes for reporting child and elder abuse. All 50 states and the District of Columbia have child abuse reporting statutes. Although these statutes differ from state to state, they generally include a definition of child abuse, a list of persons required or encouraged to report abuse, and the governmental agency designated to receive and investigate the reports. Most statutes include civil penalties for failure to report. Many states specifically require nurses to report cases of suspected abuse.

There is a conflict between federal and state laws with respect to child abuse reporting. This conflict occurs when the healthcare professional discovers child abuse or neglect during the suspected abuser's alcohol or drug treatment. Federal laws and regulations governing confidentiality of patient records, which apply to almost all drug abuse and alcohol treatment providers, prohibit any disclosure without a court order. In this case, federal law supersedes state reporting laws, although compliance with the state law may be maintained under the following circumstances:

- If a court order is obtained
- If a report can be made without identifying the abuser as a patient in an alcohol or drug treatment program
- If the report is made anonymously (some states, to protect the rights of the accused, do not allow anonymous reporting)

States may require health professionals to report other kinds of abuse. Most states have enacted elder abuse reporting statutes, which require registered nurses and others to report cases of abuse of adults 65 and older. Agencies that receive federal funding (e.g., Medicare or Medicaid) must follow strict guidelines for reporting and preventing elder abuse.

These laws also apply to dependent or disabled adults. These are adults between the ages of 18 and 64 whose physical or mental limitations restrict their ability to carry out normal activities or to protect themselves. Under most state laws, failure to report suspected abuse, neglect, or exploitation of a disabled adult may be guilty of a misdemeanor crime. Most state statutes protect one who makes a report in good faith by providing immunity from civil liability. **Because state laws vary, students should become familiar with the requirements of their states.**

Failure to Protect Patients

Another common legal issue in psychiatric-mental health nursing concerns the failure to protect the safety of patients. For example, if a suicidal patient is left alone with the means of self-harm, the nurse who has a duty to protect the patient will be held responsible for any resultant injuries. Leaving a suicidal patient alone in a room on the sixth floor with an open window is an example of unreasonable judgment on the part of a nurse.

Miscommunications and medication errors are common in all areas of nursing including psychiatric care. Because most psychiatric patients are ambulatory, carefully checking identification before medicating is essential.

Another common area of liability in psychiatry arises from the abuse of the therapist-patient relationship. Issues of sexual misconduct during the therapeutic relationship have been a source of concern in the psychiatric community. This is particularly significant given the connection that exists between care providers and patients and the power differential between them.

The nurse must also take precautions to prevent harm whenever a patient is restrained, as there is a risk of strangulation from the restraints. They may even be at risk from other patients given the vulnerable state of being restrained. Incidents of rape while patients are restrained have occurred.

Even without restraints, you need to protect patients from other patients. One patient sued a hospital when she was beaten unconscious by another patient who entered her room looking for a fight. Her lawsuit alleged that there was inadequate staffing to monitor and supervise the patients under the hospital's care.

Potential threats from the patient's family or friends present another source of concern for patient safety. Patients may come from families where domestic violence is common. The nurse may witness controlling behavior by these family members that is based in fear, anxiety, and possibly guilt. The nurse can promote safety by remaining calm, listening carefully, and assuring family members of the importance of their contributions to the patient's welfare. If a patient reports domestic violence to the nurse or the nurse witnesses it, objective documentation of the information or event is also necessary and for reporting to authorities.

LAWS RELEVANT TO PSYCHIATRIC NURSING

Tort Law

When a person wrongfully harms another, the injured party (the plaintiff) can seek money for damages from the responsible party (the defendant). We call this wrongful harm a tort. The injury can be to person, property, or reputation.

Intentional Torts

The nurse in the psychiatric setting should understand intentional torts, which are willful or intentional acts that violate

BOX 6.2 Workplace Bullying: *Raess v. Doescher*

Daniel Raess was a cardiovascular surgeon at a hospital near Indianapolis. According to testimony, Raess got into a verbal confrontation with Joseph Doescher, an operating room perfusionist (a professional who manages the heart-lung machine during surgeries). According to the testimony of Doescher, Raess was angry because he had complained to the hospital's administration about the surgeon's treatment of perfusionists. There was evidence, some of it inadmissible, that Raess had a history of hostile acts toward the hospital staff.

On the day in question, Raess approached Doescher outside the operating room. He was described as having clenched fists, piercing eyes, a red face, and popping veins. As Raess screamed and cursed at him, Doescher backed up against a wall and raised his hands in a defensive stance, believing he was going to be struck.

Doescher (the plaintiff) filed a lawsuit against Raess (the defendant). A jury found in his favor and awarded a judgment of $325,000 against the surgeon. The Indiana Supreme Court reviewed the traditional legal components of assault and determined that there was sufficient evidence to support the jury's conclusion that an assault had occurred, that the defendant acted with intent, and that the plaintiff acted reasonably under the circumstances.

another person's rights or property. Examples of intentional torts include **assault**, **battery**, and **false imprisonment**.

Assault is the intentional threat designed to make another personal fearful that you will cause them harm. Verbal threats such as "You'll never get out of here" or pretending to hit a patient are both examples of assault that can occur in a healthcare setting. Assault can even occur in the context of workplace bullying, as shown in Box 6.2.

Battery, on the other hand, is the actual harmful or offensive touching of another person. Shoving a patient from behind to hurry them up is an example of battery. Often assault and battery occur together when a threat is made and then carried out.

False imprisonment occurs when a person is confined in a limited area or within an institution. A charge of false imprisonment may be made after a person is placed in restraints or seclusion. Medications that result in chemical restraint may also fit in this category of tort.

Other types of intentional torts may hurt a person's sense of self. **Invasion of privacy** in healthcare has to do with breaking a person's confidences or taking photographs without explicit permission. An interesting example of invasion of privacy occurred when a psychology firm in New Jersey attempted to collect on past due bills by suing 24 former patients (Ornstein, 2015). These publicly available lawsuits included patient names, diagnoses, and listings of their treatments. Philip, a lawyer and patient of the psychology firm, believed that his professional life could be negatively impacted and countersued for invasion of privacy.

In the context of healthcare, defamation of character occurs when a provider makes a false statement that causes some degree of harm, usually to the reputation of the patient. Defamation includes slander (verbal), such as talking about patients on the elevator with others around, and libel (printed), where written information about the patient is shared with people outside the professional setting.

Unintentional Torts

Unintentional torts are unintended acts against another person that produce injury or harm. **Negligence** is the most common unintentional tort. It is defined as the failure to use ordinary care in any professional or personal situation when you have a duty to do so. Failure to question a physician's order, failure to protect a patient from self-harm, and failure to provide patient teaching are all examples of negligence.

Malpractice is a special type of professional negligence. The five elements required to prove negligence are:

1. Duty
2. Breach of duty
3. Cause in fact
4. Proximate cause
5. Damages

Duty. When nurses represent themselves as being capable of caring for psychiatric patients and accept employment, a duty of care has been assumed. As a nurse, you have the duty to understand the theory and medications used in the specialty care of psychiatric patients. The staff nurse assigned to a psychiatric unit must be knowledgeable enough to assume a reasonable duty of care for the patients. Persons who represent themselves as possessing superior knowledge and skill, such as advanced practice psychiatric nurses, are held to a higher standard of care in the practice of their profession.

Breach of duty. If you do not meet the standard of care that other nurses would be expected to supply under similar circumstances, you have breached the duty of care. A breach of duty occurs if the nursing performance falls below the standard of care and exposes the patient to an unreasonable risk of harm. This breach of duty includes doing something that results in harm (an act of *commission*) or failing to do something that results in harm (an act of *omission*).

Cause in fact and ***proximate cause.*** Cause in fact may be evaluated by asking the question, "If it were not for what this nurse did (or failed to do), would this injury have occurred?" Proximate cause, or legal cause, is determined by whether there were any intervening actions or persons that were, in fact, the causes of harm to the patient.

Damages. These include actual damages (e.g., loss of earnings, medical expenses, and property damage), as well as pain and suffering. They also include incidental or consequential damages. For example, giving a patient the wrong medication may have actual damage of a complicated hospital stay, but it also may result in permanent disability, requiring such things as special education needs and special accommodations in the home. Furthermore, incidental damages may deprive others of the benefits of the injured person, such as losing a normal relationship with a spouse or parent.

Foreseeability of harm evaluates the likelihood of the outcome under the circumstances. If the average, reasonable nurse could foresee that injury would result from the action or inaction, then the injury was foreseeable.

Table 6.3 summarizes laws relevant to psychiatric nursing and provides examples of each.

Box 6.3 describes of a case of false imprisonment, negligence, and malpractice.

TABLE 6.3 Common Liability Issues

Issue	Examples
Patient safety	Failure to notice or take action on suicide risks
	Failure to use restraints properly or monitor the patient
	Miscommunication
	Medication errors
	Violation of boundaries (e.g., sexual misconduct)
	Misdiagnosis
Intentional torts	Voluntary acts intended to bring a physical or mental consequence
May carry criminal penalties	Purposeful acts
Punitive damages may be awarded	Recklessness
	Not obtaining patient consent
Not covered by malpractice insurance	*Note:* Self-defense or protection of others may serve as a defense to charges of an intentional tort.
Negligence/malpractice	Carelessness
	Foreseeability of harm
Assault and battery	Person apprehensive (assault) of harmful/offensive touching (battery)
	Threat to use force (words alone are not enough) with opportunity and ability
	Treatment without patient's consent
False imprisonment	Intent to confine to a specific area
	Indefensible use of seclusion or restraints
	Detention of voluntarily admitted patient, with no agency or legal policies to support detaining
Invasion of privacy	Notifying parents of a 21-year-old that she is being treated on a psychiatric unit
Defamation of character	Telling friends that your patient is a local mayor
Slander	Telling your Facebook friends that your patient is a local mayor
Libel	
Unintentional torts	Unintended acts against another person that produce injury or harm.
Negligence	Leaving an unlocked car running in front of a high school
Malpractice	Failure to follow up with patient teaching after finding orthostatic hypotension

STANDARDS FOR NURSING CARE

Nurses are held to a basic standard of care. This standard is based on what other nurses who possess the same degree of skill or knowledge in the same or similar circumstances would do.

State boards of nursing, professional associations, policies and procedures from various institutions, and even historical customs influence how nurses practice. They contribute standards by which nurses are measured and are important in determining legal responsibility and liability.

State Boards of Nursing

Nursing boards are state governmental agencies that regulate nursing practice and whose primary goal is to protect the health of the public by overseeing the safe practice of nursing. They have the authority to license nurses who meet a minimum competency score on board examinations and also the power to revoke licenses. Each state has its own Nurse Practice Act that identifies the qualifications for registered nurses, identifies the titles that registered nurses will use, defines what nurses are legally allowed to do (scope of practice), and describes the actions that are followed if nurses do not follow the nursing law.

BOX 6.3 False Imprisonment, Negligence, and Malpractice: *Plumadore v. State of New York* (1980)

Delilah Plumadore was admitted to Saranac Lake General Hospital for a gallbladder condition. During her medical workup, she confessed that marital problems had resulted in suicide attempts several years before her admission. After a series of consultations and tests, the attending surgeon scheduled gallbladder surgery for later that day. After the surgeon's visit, a consulting psychiatrist who examined Mrs. Plumadore told her to dress and pack her belongings because she was going to be admitted to a state hospital at Ogdensburg.

Subsequently, two uniformed state troopers handcuffed Mrs. Plumadore and strapped her into the back seat of a patrol car and transported her to the state hospital. On arrival, the admitting psychiatrist realized that the referring psychiatrist lacked the authority to order this involuntary commitment. He therefore requested that Mrs. Plumadore sign a voluntary admission form, which she refused to do.

Despite Mrs. Plumadore's protests regarding her admission to the state hospital, the psychiatrist assigned her to a ward without physical or psychiatric examination. She did not even have the opportunity to contact her family or her medical doctor and remained in the hospital for the weekend.

The court awarded $40,000 to Mrs. Plumadore for malpractice and false imprisonment on the part of healthcare professionals and negligence on the part of the troopers. This settlement was greatly influenced by the fact that she had an acute medical illness that was left untreated for days due to being locked in a psychiatric ward.

Professional Associations

As a profession, nursing also self-regulates through professional associations. A professional association's primary focus is to elevate the practice of its members by setting standards of excellence.

Two of the main nursing associations that influence psychiatric nursing are the ANA and the APNA, each with individual state chapters. The ANA fosters high standards of nursing practice. The ANA's *Nursing: Scope and Standards of Practice* (2015b) provides parameters for nursing practice through 16 standards and outlines the role of nurses regardless of level, setting, or specialty area.

APNA is a professional association that is organized to advance the science and education of psychiatric-mental health nursing. More specific guidelines for psychiatric nursing practice are provided in *Psychiatric-Mental Health Nursing: Scope and Standards of Practice* (2014). This publication is a joint effort of the ANA, APNA, and the International Society of Psychiatric-Mental Health Nurses.

Institutional Policies and Procedures

Institutional policies and procedures define criteria for care, and these criteria can be used during legal proceedings to prove that a nurse met or failed to meet them. A weakness of this method is that the hospital's policy may be substandard. For example, an institution may determine that patients can be kept in seclusion for up to 6 hours based on the original physician's order, but state licensing laws for institutions might set a limit of 4 hours. Substandard institutional policies may put nurses at risk of liability, so be sure to follow laws and professional standards of nursing care. As advocates for patients and the profession, nurses should address questionable policies and bring about positive change.

Custom as a Standard of Care

Custom can also be used as evidence of a standard of care. In the absence of a written policy on the use of restraint, testimony might be offered regarding the customary use of restraint in emergency situations in which the combative, violent, or confused patient poses a threat of harm to self or others.

Using custom to establish a standard of care may have the same weakness as in using hospital policies and procedures. After all, customs may not comply with the laws, recommendations of the accrediting body, or other recognized standards of care. Custom must be carefully and regularly evaluated to ensure that substandard routines have not developed. Substandard customs do not protect you when a psychiatric patient charges that a right has been violated or that harm has been caused by the staff's common practices.

ACTING ON QUESTIONABLE PRACTICE

Negligence, Irresponsibility, or Impairment

In your professional life, you may suspect negligence on the part of a peer. In most states, you have a legal duty to intervene and to report such risks of harm to the patient. It is important to document the evidence clearly and accurately before making serious accusations against a peer.

Imagine that you are working with Doreen, a nurse on the night shift on a busy medical floor. She shows up for work disheveled, angry, and uncommunicative. As the shift progresses, her mood lightens. You notice that she keeps a bottle of soda close by and regularly drinks from it. You realize with horror that she is slurring a bit. Thinking back on previous shifts, you realize that this behavior is not new.

How should you respond? In less dangerous situations, the first step might be to communicate directly with your colleague. However, in this case you have an obligation to immediately communicate your concerns to a supervisor. The supervisor should then intervene to protect the patient's rights and well-being. If the supervisor is unavailable or unresponsive, you have no choice but to act to protect the patient's life. If you do not intervene, the patient may be injured, and you may be liable for these injuries.

Some problems are not life-threatening but are troubling—*maybe* something bad could happen. Who do you tell? The answer is, "It depends." It depends on which state you live in. State laws vary in the following ways:

- Some states require that nurses report incompetence or impairment to the state board of nursing but not to the institution.
- Some states require that nurses report *themselves* for incompetence, negligence, unethical or unprofessional conduct, or physical, mental, or chemical impairment.
- Some states require that nurses treating patients who are also nurses, report them for problems that constitute a public danger.
- Some states allow a nurse to report a colleague to a peer assistance program rather than the state board of nursing.
- Most states do not require a nurse to report an impaired member of a different profession.

The problem of reporting impaired colleagues causes deep concerns, especially if you have not observed direct harm to a patient. Nurses may feel protective of other nurses due to concerns for professional reputations and personal privacy. The ANA (2015a, p. 12) identifies "acting on questionable practice" as being part of a nurse's professional responsibility. As a patient advocate, the nurse should be alert and take proper actions in cases of impaired colleagues.

The issues are less complex when a professional colleague's conduct (including that of a student nurse) is criminally unlawful. Specific examples include the diversion of drugs from the hospital and sexual misconduct with patients. These are criminal behaviors and must be immediately reported.

VIGNETTE: Amanda recently completed the hospital and unit orientations and has begun to care for patients independently. As she prepares to give the 5 p.m. medications, Amanda notices that Greg Thorn, a 55-year-old man admitted after a suicide attempt, has been ordered the antidepressant sertraline (Zoloft). Amanda remembers that Mr. Thorn had been taking phenelzine (Nardil) before his admission. She seems to recall something dangerous about mixing these two classifications of medications.

She looks the antidepressants up in her drug guide. She relearns that Nardil is a monoamine oxidase inhibitor (MAOI) and the other is a selective serotonin reuptake inhibitor (SSRI) antidepressant. Beginning the new medication within 2 weeks of discontinuing the Nardil could result in severe side effects and a potentially lethal response.

After clarifying with Mr. Thorn that he had been on Nardil and discussing the issue with another nurse, Amanda puts the Zoloft on hold and contacts Mr. Thorn's psychiatrist, Dr. Cruz, by phone. Amanda begins by saying, "I see that Mr. Thorn has been ordered Zoloft. His nursing admission assessment says that he had been taking Nardil up until a few days ago. However, I don't see it listed on the assessment that was done by the medical resident."

First Possible Outcome

Dr. Cruz responds, "Really? Wow, thanks for calling that to my attention. When I make rounds in the morning, I'll decide what to do with his medications. For now, I definitely agree that we hold the Zoloft." Amanda clarifies what Dr. Cruz has said, writes the order, and documents what happened in the nurses notes.

Second Possible Outcome

Dr. Cruz responds, "It sounds like you must have earned a medical degree. Listen, if the medication wasn't listed on my resident's assessment, then he wasn't taking it. Probably another nursing error. I wrote an order for Zoloft. Give it to him." The doctor hangs up on Amanda, who then documents the exchange. She determines that the safest and most appropriate response is to continue to hold the medication and contacts her nursing supervisor. The supervisor supports her decision and follows up with the chief of psychiatry.

When the nurse is given an assignment to care for a patient, the nurse must provide the care or ensure that the patient is safely reassigned to another nurse. Abandonment, a legal concept, occurs if a nurse does not deliver a patient safely to another health professional before discontinuing treatment. Abandonment issues arise when a nurse does not provide accurate, timely, and thorough reporting or when follow-through of patient care, on which the patient is relying, has not occurred.

The same principles apply for the psychiatric-mental health nurse working in a community setting. For example, if a suicidal patient refuses to come to the hospital for treatment, you must take the necessary steps to ensure the patient's safety. These actions may include enlisting the assistance of the law in involuntarily admitting the patient on a temporary basis.

DOCUMENTATION OF CARE

The purposes of the medical record are to provide accurate and complete information about the care and treatment of patients and to give healthcare personnel a means of communicating with one another, allowing continuity of care. A record's usefulness is determined by how accurately and completely it portrays the patient's behavioral status at the time it was written. The patient has the right to see the medical record, but it belongs to the institution. The patient must follow appropriate protocol to view personal records.

For example, if a psychiatric patient describes intent to harm him- or herself or another person and the nurse fails to document the information—including the need to protect the patient or the identified victim—the information will be lost when the nurse leaves work. If the patient's plan is carried out, the harm caused could be linked directly to the nurse's failure to communicate the patient's intent. Even though documentation takes time away from patient care, its importance in communicating and preserving the nurse's assessment and memory cannot be overemphasized.

Medical Records and Quality Improvement

The medical record has many other uses aside from providing information on the course of the patient's care and treatment by healthcare professionals. According to the Institute of Medicine (2011), quality improvement is a key goal for the future of nursing and healthcare. A retrospective medical record review provides valuable information to the facility on the quality of care provided and on ways to improve that care.

A facility may also conduct reviews for risk management purposes. These reviews help to determine areas of potential liability for the facility and to evaluate methods used to reduce the facility's exposure to liability. For example, risk managers often review documentation of the use of restraints and seclusion for psychiatric patients. Accordingly, risk managers may use the medical record to evaluate care for quality assurance or peer review. Utilization review analysts evaluate the medical record to determine appropriate use of hospital and staff resources consistent with reimbursement schedules. Insurance companies and other reimbursement agencies rely on the medical record in determining which payments they will make on the patient's behalf.

Medical Records as Evidence

From a legal perspective, the medical record is a recording of data and opinions made in the normal course of the patient's hospital care. Courts consider it good evidence because it is presumed to be true, honest, and untainted by memory lapses. Accordingly, the medical record finds its way into a variety of legal cases for a variety of reasons.

Medical records help to determine:

1. The extent of the patient's damages and pain and suffering in personal injury cases such as when a psychiatric patient attempts suicide while under the protective care of a hospital.
2. The nature and extent of injuries in child abuse or elder abuse cases.
3. The nature and extent of physical or mental disability in disability cases.
4. The nature and extent of injury and rehabilitative potential in workers' compensation cases.

Medical records may also be used in police investigations, civil conservatorship proceedings, competency hearings, and involuntary commitment procedures. In states that mandate mental health legal services or a patients' rights advocacy program, audits may be performed to determine the facility's compliance with state laws or violation of patients' rights. Finally, medical records may be used in professional and hospital negligence cases.

Guidelines for Electronic Documentation

Informatics provides the healthcare system with essential technology to manage knowledge, communicate, reduce error, and facilitate decision making (Quality and Safety Education for Nurses, 2012). However, electronic record keeping creates challenges for protecting the confidentiality of the records of psychiatric patients. Sensitive information regarding treatment for mental illness can adversely impact patients seeking employment, insurance, and credit.

Federal laws address concerns for the privacy of patients' records and provide guidelines for agencies that use electronic documentation. Only staff members who have a legitimate need to know about the patient are authorized to access a patient's electronic medical record. There are penalties, including termination of employment, if a staff member enters a record without authorization.

You are responsible for all entries into records using your password. As a result, your password should remain private and should be changed periodically. In the event a documentation error is made, the various systems allow specific time frames to make medical record corrections.

Institutions should encourage documentation methods that improve communication between care providers. Courts assume that nurses and physicians read each other's notes on patient progress. They also assume that if care is not documented, it did not occur. Your notes may serve as a valuable memory refresher if the patient sues years after the care is rendered.

FORENSIC NURSING

The evolving specialty of forensic nursing includes the application of nursing principles in a court of law to assist in reaching a decision on a contested issue. The nurse often educates the

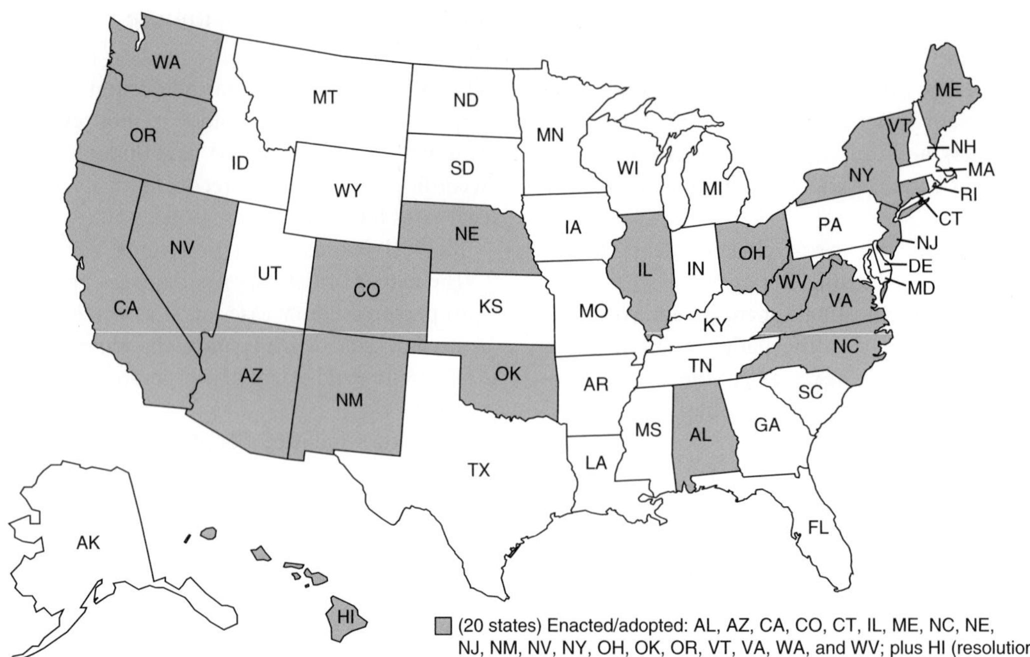

FIG. 6.1 The American Nurses Association's Nationwide State Legislative Agenda, which identifies states with workplace violence legislation. (Reprinted with permission from the American Nurses Association. Retrieved from http://nursingworld.org/MainMenuCategories/Policy-Advocacy/State/Legislative-Agenda-Reports/State-WorkplaceViolence/WorkplaceViolenceMap.pdf.) *(This 2014 map is a snapshot from the status in January 2014 and the current status can be found at: http://lghttp.48653.nexcesscdn.net/80223CF/springer-static/media/samplechapters/9780826198914/mobile/9780826198914_Chapter1.html)*

court about the science of nursing. The witness applies nursing knowledge to the facts in the lawsuit and may provide opinions using appropriate nursing standards.

Some situations in which a psychiatric-mental health nurse may be helpful include testimony related to patient competency, fitness to stand trial, involuntary commitment, or responsibility for a crime. Forensic nurses may also focus on victims and perpetrators of crime and violence, the collection of evidence, and the provision of healthcare in prison settings. Refer to Chapter 33 for a complete discussion of forensic nursing.

VIOLENCE IN THE PSYCHIATRIC SETTING

Between the years of 2011 and 2013, healthcare workers in the United States suffered 15,000 to 20,000 workplace violence-related injuries each year (United States Bureau of Labor Statistics, 2013). These injuries required workers to take time off work for treatment and recovery. The number of healthcare injuries accounts for nearly as many injuries as in all other industries combined. Although emergency room nurses are more likely to be assaulted, psychiatric nurses also have fairly high rates.

In a survey of 3,765 nurses and nursing students, 21% reported being physically assaulted during a 1-year period (ANA, 2015c). Over 50% of this sample reported being verbally abused.

Nurses, as citizens, have the same rights as patients not to be threatened or harmed. In recent years, nurses have actively sought workplace violence legislation. New laws enhance criminal charges and penalties for striking nurses and other healthcare workers in the course of duty. Usually, a prosecutor will not bring charges against disoriented, delirious, psychotic, or otherwise mentally impaired patients. However, violent patients, friends of patients, and family members who are aware of their actions can be charged with serious crimes. Fig. 6.1 identifies states with workplace violence legislation (ANA, 2015).

KEY POINTS TO REMEMBER

- Psychiatric-mental health nurses frequently encounter problems requiring ethical choices. Understanding ethical principles and applying them to ethical dilemmas can help in making choices.
- Mental health laws protect both patients and caregivers.
- Psychiatric admissions are either voluntary or involuntary.
- State laws vary in how involuntary commitments are handled. In general, a significant mental health problem exists that interferes with a person's safe functioning. Psychiatric professionals confirm this problem and courts are responsible for determining competency and continuing involuntary treatment.

- Patients have the right to quality treatment, the right to refuse treatment, and the right to informed consent (i.e., knowing their treatment options and voluntarily accepting treatment).
- Restraint and seclusion abuses in the past have resulted in strict laws concerning their use and documentation of their use.
- Confidentiality is one of the most important legal concepts in psychiatry. Only patients can waive the right to confidentiality.
- Exceptions to the confidentiality rule include warning third parties of threats by patients and in cases of suspected child and elder abuse.
- The nurse's privilege to practice carries with it the responsibility to practice safely, competently, and in a manner consistent with state and federal laws.
- Important laws for psychiatric nurses include intentional torts such as assault, battery, false imprisonment, invasion of privacy, and defamation of character.
- Unintentional torts are a type of negligence called malpractice where professionals fail to act in accordance with professional standards. They fail to foresee consequences of their action or inaction at the level that would be expected of someone with similar training and experience.
- Knowledge of the law, professional association standards, organizational policies and procedures, and customs are essential for providing safe, effective nursing care.

CRITICAL THINKING

1. As Joe, a registered nurse, prepares the medication for the evening shift, he notices that two of his patients' medications are missing. Both are bedtime Ativan (lorazepam). When he phones the pharmacy to send up the missing medications, the pharmacist responds, "You people need to watch your carts more carefully because this has become a pattern."

   Shortly after, another patient complains to Joe that he did not receive his 5 p.m. Xanax (alprazolam). On the medication administration record, Beth has recorded that she has given the drugs. Joe suspects that Beth may be diverting the drugs.
   a. Should Joe confront Beth with his suspicions?
   b. If Beth admits that she has been diverting the drugs, should Joe's next step be to report Beth to the supervisor or to the board of nursing?
   c. When Joe talks to the nursing supervisor, should he identify Beth or should he state his suspicions in general terms?
2. One day, Linda arrives at work on the behavioral care unit. She is informed that the staffing office has requested that a nurse from the psychiatric unit report to the intensive care unit (ICU). They need help in caring for an agitated car accident victim with a history of schizophrenia.

   Linda goes to the ICU and joins a nurse named Corey in providing care for the patient. Eventually, the patient is stabilized and goes to sleep, and Corey leaves the unit for a break. Because Linda is unfamiliar with the telemetry equipment, she fails to recognize that the patient is having an arrhythmia, and the patient experiences a cardiopulmonary arrest. Although he is successfully resuscitated, he suffers permanent brain damage.
   a. Can Linda legally practice in this situation? (That is, does her RN license permit her to practice in the intensive care unit?)
   b. Does the ability to practice legally in an area differ from the ability to practice competently in that area?
   c. Did Linda have any legal or ethical grounds to refuse the assignment to the intensive care unit?
   d. What are the risks in accepting an assignment in an area of specialty in which you are professionally unprepared to practice?
   e. Would there have been any way for Linda to minimize the risk of retaliation by the employer had she refused the assignment?
   f. If Linda is negligent, is the hospital liable for any harm to the patient caused by her?
3. A 40-year-old man is admitted to the emergency department for a severe nosebleed and has both of his nostrils packed. Because of a history of alcoholism and the possibility for developing withdrawal symptoms, the patient is transferred to the psychiatric unit. His physician orders a private room, restraints, continuous monitoring, and 15-minute checks of vital signs and other indicators. At the next 15-minute check, the nurse discovers that the patient does not have a pulse or respiration. The patient had apparently inhaled the nasal packing and suffocated.
   a. Does it sound as if the nurse was responsible for the patient's death?
   b. Was the order for the restraint appropriate for this type of patient?
   c. What factors did you consider in making your determination?

CHAPTER REVIEW

Questions

1. Which statement made by the nurse concerning ethics demonstrates the best understanding of the concept?
   a. "It isn't right to deny someone healthcare because they can't pay for it."
   b. "I never discuss my patient's refusal of treatment."
   c. "The hospital needs to buy more respirators so we always have one available."
   d. "Not all ICU patients have the right to unbiased attention from the staff."

2. Which nursing intervention demonstrates the ethical principle of beneficence?
   a. Refusing to administer a placebo to a patient.
   b. Attending an in-service on the operation of the new IV infusion pumps
   c. Providing frequent updates to the family of a patient currently in surgery
   d. Respecting the right of the patient to make decisions about whether or not to have electroconvulsive therapy
3. How can a newly hired nurse best attain information concerning the state's mental health laws and statutes?
   a. Discuss the issue with the facility's compliance officer
   b. Conduct an internet search using the keywords "mental + health + statutes + (your state)"
   c. Consult the American Nurses Association's (ANA) *Code of Ethics for Nurses*
   d. Review the facility's latest edition of the policies manual
4. When considering facility admissions for mental healthcare, what characteristic is unique to a voluntary admission?
   a. The patient poses no substantial threat to themselves or to others
   b. The patient has the right to seek legal counsel
   c. A request in writing is required before admission
   d. A mental illness has been previously diagnosed
5. Which situations demonstrate liable behavior on the part of the staff? *Select all that apply.*
   a. Forgetting to obtain consent for electroconvulsive therapy for a cognitively impaired patient
   b. Leaving a patient with suicidal thoughts alone in the bathroom to shower
   c. Promising to restrain a patient who stole from another patient on the unit
   d. Reassuring a patient with paranoia that his antipsychotic medication was not tampered with
   e. Placing a patient who has repeatedly threatened to assault staff in seclusion
6. A nurse makes a post on a social media page about his peer taking care of a patient with a crime-related gunshot wound in the emergency department. He does not use the name of the patient. The nurse:
   a. Has not violated confidentiality laws because he did not use the patient's name.
   b. Cannot be held liable for violating confidentiality laws because he was not the primary nurse for the patient.
   c. Has violated confidentiality laws and can be held liable.
   d. Cannot be held liable because postings on a social media site are excluded from confidentiality laws.
7. In providing care for patients of a mental health unit, Li recognizes the importance of standards of care. When Li notices that some policies fall short of the state licensing laws, which of the following statements represents the most appropriate standard of care pathway?
   a. Professional association, customary care, facility policy
   b. State board of nursing, facility policy, customary care
   c. Facility policy, professional associations, state board of nursing
   d. State board of nursing, professional association, facility policy
8. Lucas has completed his inpatient psychiatric treatment, which was ordered by the court system. Which statement reveals that Lucas does not understand the concept of conditional release?
   a. "I will continue treatment in an outpatient treatment center."
   b. "My nurse practitioner has recommended group therapy."
   c. "I am finally free, no more therapy."
   d. "Attending therapy and taking my meds are a part of this conditional release."
9. Implied consent occurs when no verbal or written agreement takes place prior to a caregiver delivering treatment. Which of the following examples represents implied consent?
   a. The mother of an unconscious patient saying okay to surgery
   b. Care given to a heroin overdose victim
   c. Immobilizing a patient who has refused to take medication
   d. Signing general intake paperwork with specific parameters
10. Based on Maslow's hierarchy of needs, physiological needs for a restrained patient include: *Select all that apply.*
   a. Private toileting, oral hydration
   b. Checking the tightness of the restraints
   c. Therapeutic communication
   d. Maintaining a patent airway

Answers

1. **a**; 2. **c**; 3. **b**; 4. **c**; 5. **a, b, c**; 6. **c**; 7. **d**; 8. **c**; 9. **b**; 10. **a, b, d**

Visit the Evolve website for a posttest on the content in this chapter: http://evolve.elsevier.com/Varcarolis

Post-Test interactive review

REFERENCES

American Nurses Association. (2015a). *Code of ethics for nurses with interpretive statements.* Washington, DC: American Nurses Publishing.

American Nurses Association. (2015b). *Nursing: Scope and standards of practice* (3rd ed.). Silver Springs, MD: NursesBooks.org.

American Nurses Association. (2015c). *Health risk appraisal.* Retrieved from http://www.nursingworld.org/HRA-Executive-Summary.

American Nurses Association, American Psychiatric-Mental Health Nurses Association, & International Society of Psychiatric-Mental Health Nurses. (2014). *Psychiatric-mental health nursing: Scope and standards of practice.* Silver Spring, MD: American Nurses Association.

American Psychiatric Association. (2013). *Diagnostic and statistical manual of mental disorders (DSM-5).* (5th ed.). Washington, DC: Author.

American Psychiatric Nurses Association. (2014). *APNA position statement on the use of seclusion and restraint.* Retrieved from http://www.apna.org/i4a/pages/index.cfm?pageid=3728.

Bazelton Center for Mental Health Law. (2012). *Where we stand: Mental health parity.* Retrieved from http://www.bazelton.org/Where-We-Stand?Access-to-Services/Mental-Health-Parity.aspx.

Bernstein, N. (2012). Restrained youth's death in Yonkers is investigated. *New York Times.* Retrieved from http://www.nytimes.com/2012/04/21/nyregion/death-of-youth-at-leake-watts-center-in-yonkers-is-investigated.html?_r=0.

Canterbury v. Spence, 464 F.2d 722 (D.C. Cir. 1972), quoting Schloendorf v. Society of N.Y. Hosp., 211 N.Y. 125 105 N.E.2d 92, 93 (1914).

Centers for Medicare and Medicaid Services. (2008). *Hospitals—Restraint/seclusion interpretive guidelines and updated state operations manual.* Retrieved from http://www.cms.gov/Medicare/Provider-Enrollment-and-Certification/SurveyCertificationGenInfo/downloads/SCLetter08-18.pdf.

Curtis, A. (2001). *Involuntary commitment.* Retrieved from http://psychrights.org/states/Maine/InvoluntaryCommitmentbyAliciaCurtis.htm.

Deutsch, A. (1949). *The shame of the states.* New York, NY: Harcourt Brace.

Health Insurance Portability and Accountability Act, U.S.C.45C.F.R § 164.501 (2003).

Institute of Medicine (IOM). (2011). *The future of nursing: Focus on education.* Retrieved from http://www.iom.edu/Reports/2010/The-Future-of-Nursing-Leading-Change-Advancing-Health/Report-Brief-Education.aspx.

Ornstein, C. (2015, December 23). A patient is sued, and his mental health diagnosis becomes public. *New York Times.* Retrieved from http://www.nytimes.com/2015/12/24/nyregion/a-patient-is-sued-and-his-mental-health-diagnosis-becomes-public.html.

Pierce, R. (2014). *Statutory solutions for a common law defect: Advancing the nurse practitioner-patient privilege.* Retrieved from http://repository.jmls.edu/cgi/viewcontent.cgi?article=1961&context=lawreview.

Plumadore v. State of New York. (1980). 427 N.Y.S.2d 90.

Quality and Safety Education for Nurses. (2012). *Competency knowledge, skills, and attitudes.* Retrieved from http://www.qsen.org/ksas_prelicensure.php#informatics.

Raess v. Doescher, 883 N.E.2d 790 (Indiana 2008)

Tarasoff v. Regents of University of California (1974). 529 P.2d 553, 118 Cal Rptr 129.

United States Bureau of Labor Statistics. (2013). *Illnesses, injuries, and fatalities.* Retrieved from http://www.bls.gov/iif/.

7

The Nursing Process and Standards of Care

Elizabeth M. Varcarolis

Visit the Evolve website for a pretest on the content in this chapter:
http://evolve.elsevier.com/Varcarolis Pre-Test interactive review

OBJECTIVES

1. Compare the different approaches you would consider when performing an assessment with a child, an adolescent, and an older adult.
2. Differentiate between the use of an interpreter and a translator when performing an assessment with a non–English-speaking patient.
3. Conduct a mental status examination (MSE).
4. Perform a psychosocial assessment including brief cultural and spiritual components.
5. Explain three principles a nurse follows in planning actions to reach agreed-upon outcome criteria.
6. Construct a plan of care for a patient with a mental health problem.
7. Identify three advanced practice psychiatric-mental health nursing interventions.
8. Demonstrate basic nursing interventions and evaluation of care following the American Nurses Association's (ANA) Standards of Practice.
9. Compare and contrast *Nursing Interventions Classification (NIC)*, *Nursing Outcomes Classification (NOC)*, and evidence-based practice (EBP).

OUTLINE

KEY TERMS AND CONCEPTS

evidence-based practice (EBP)
health teaching
mental status examination (MSE)
milieu therapy
Nursing Interventions Classification (NIC)
Nursing Outcomes Classification (NOC)
objective data
outcome criteria
psychosocial assessment
self-care activities
subjective data

The nursing process is a six-step, problem-solving approach. It is intended to facilitate and identify appropriate, safe, culturally competent, developmentally relevant, quality care for individuals, families, groups, or communities. Psychiatric-mental health nurses base judgments and behaviors on this accepted theoretical framework (Fig. 7.1). Whenever possible, scientific theories support interventions as we apply evidence-based research to our nursing plans and actions of care.

The nursing process is also the foundation of the standards of practice as presented in *Psychiatric-Mental Health Nursing: Scope*

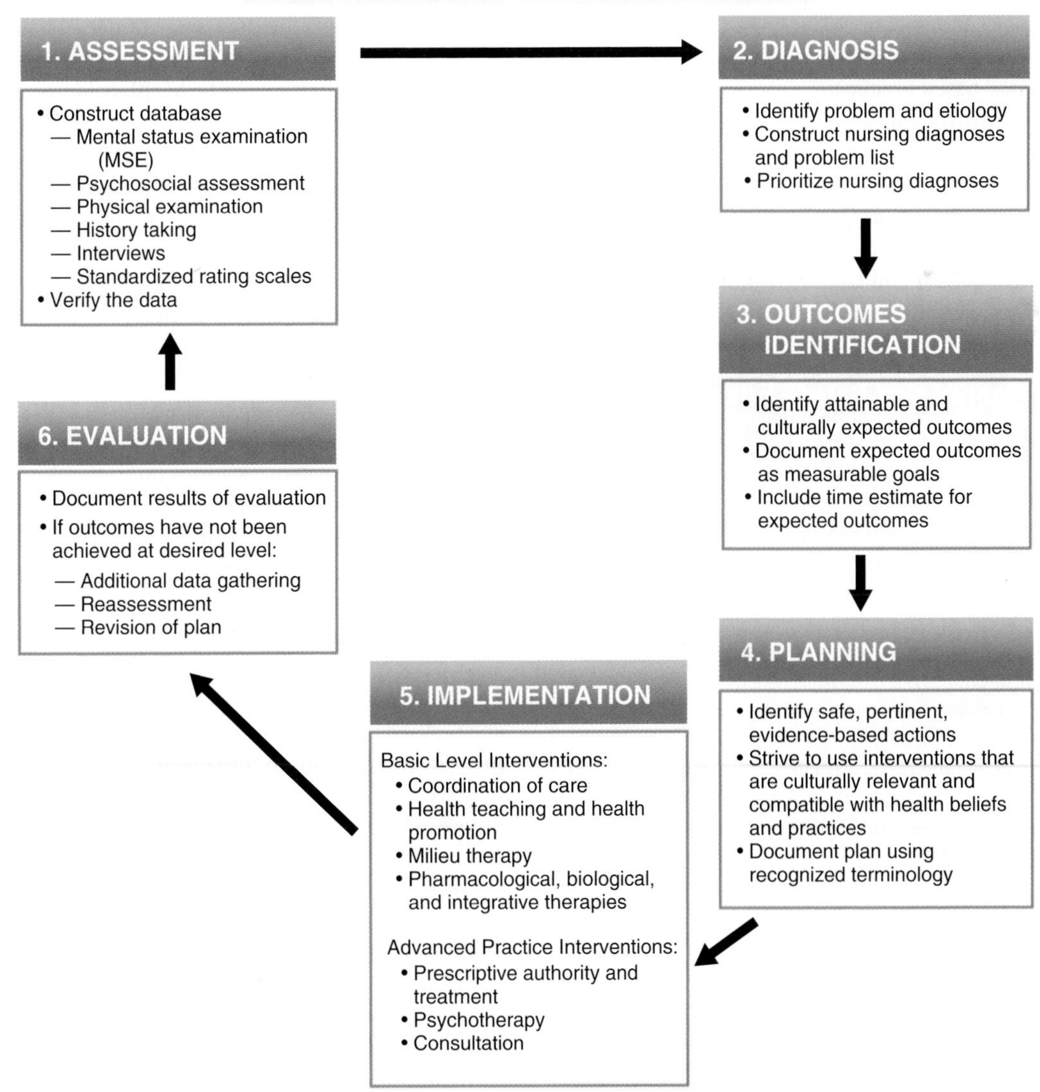

FIG. 7.1 The nursing process in psychiatric-mental health nursing.

and Standards of Practice, second edition (American Nurses Association [ANA] et al., 2014). The word scope in the book's title answers the following questions about psychiatric nursing: what do they do, where do they do it, when do they do it, why do they do it, and how do they do it? The book also provides a historical description of psychiatric nursing, current issues and trends, and levels of practice (i.e., registered nurses and advanced practice registered nurses).

The standards of practice are statements that identify the duties and obligations for which psychiatric-mental health nurses are held accountable. These standards provide the basis for:

- Certification criteria
- Legal definition of psychiatric-mental health nursing
- National Council of State Boards of Nursing Licensure Examination (NCLEX-RN®) questions

Quality and Safety Education in Nursing

Safety and quality care for patients has become an essential focus for nursing education. In the late 1990s, the Institute of Medicine (IOM)* and other organizations sought to improve the quality of patient care and safety. The competencies mandated by the National Academy of Sciences require a change in the way that all healthcare professionals are educated. According to the IOM (2003), healthcare workers in the 21st century should possess the ability to:

1. Provide patient-centered care
2. Work in interdisciplinary teams
3. Employ evidence-based practice
4. Apply quality improvement
5. Utilize informatics

A group of faculty adapted these competencies for nursing students in an initiative known as *Quality and Safety Education in Nursing (QSEN)*. They developed definitions that describe essential features of a competent and respected nurse. These competency definitions provide the basis for statements regarding the knowledge, skills, and attitudes (KSAs) that should be developed in nursing education (Cronenwett et al., 2007). The six QSEN competencies reflect the IOM's competencies with the addition of safety as a separate competency. These competencies are integrated into this chapter and throughout the textbook (Box 7.1).

Suggestions for the use of QSEN competencies in nursing education can be found in "Competency Knowledge, Skills, Attitudes (KSAs) (Pre-Licensure)" at the website www.qsen.org/competencies/pre-licensure-ksas/.

BOX 7.1 Quality and Safety Education for Nurses (QSEN) Competencies

Patient-centered care: Recognize the patient or designee as the source of control and full partner in providing compassionate and coordinated care based on respect for the patient's preferences, values, and needs.

Quality improvement: Use data to monitor the outcomes of care processes and use improvement methods to design and test changes to continuously improve the quality and safety of healthcare systems.

Safety: Minimize risk of harm to patients and provide optimal healthcare through both system effectiveness and individual performance.

Informatics: Use information and technology to communicate, manage knowledge, mitigate error, and support decision making.

Teamwork and collaboration: Function effectively within nursing and interprofessional teams, fostering open communication, mutual respect, and shared decision making to achieve quality patient care.

Evidence-based practice (EBP): Integrate best current evidence with clinical expertise and patient/family preferences and values for delivery of optimal healthcare.

From Cronenwett, L., Sherwood, G., Barnsteiner, J., Disch, J., Johnson, J., Mitchell, P., Sullivan, D., & Warren, J. (2007). *Quality and safety education for nurses. Nursing Outlook, 55*(3), 122–131.

Standards of Practice in Psychiatric-Mental Health Nursing

The following sections describe the standards of practice for psychiatric-mental health nursing. These standards describe care that is provided by a competent psychiatric-mental health nurse.

STANDARDS OF PRACTICE FOR PSYCHIATRIC-MENTAL HEALTH NURSING: STANDARD 1: ASSESSMENT

The psychiatric-mental health registered nurse collects and synthesizes comprehensive health data pertinent to the healthcare consumer's health and/or situation (ANA et al., 2014, p. 44).

A view of the individual as a complex blend of many parts is consistent with nurses' holistic approach to care. Nurses who work in the psychiatric-mental health field need to assess or have access to the past and present medical history, a recent physical examination, and knowledge of any physical complaints, as well as document any observable physical conditions or behaviors (e.g., unsteady gait, abnormal breathing patterns, wincing as if in pain, doubling over to relieve discomfort).

The assessment process begins with the initial patient encounter and continues throughout the care of the patient. To develop a basis for the plan of care and in preparation for discharge, every patient should have a thorough, formal nursing assessment upon entering treatment.

Subsequent to the formal assessment, the nurse collects data continually and systematically as the patient's condition changes and—hopefully—improves. Perhaps the patient came into treatment actively suicidal, and the initial focus of care was on protection from injury. Through regular assessment, the nurse may determine that although suicidal ideation has diminished, negative thinking may still be a problem.

A variety of professionals conduct assessments, including nurses, psychiatrists, social workers, dietitians, and other therapists. Virtually all facilities have standardized nursing assessment forms to aid in organization and consistency among reviewers. These forms may be paper or electronic versions, according to the resources and preferences of the institution.

The time required for the nursing interview varies, depending on the assessment form. Longer interviews may be required based on the patient's response pattern (e.g., a patient whose responses are lengthy or rambling, a patient who has tangential thoughts or memory disturbances, or a patient who gives markedly slowed responses). Refer to Chapter 9 for guidelines for setting up and conducting a clinical interview.

In all situations, the patient must receive a copy of the Health Insurance Portability and Accountability Act (HIPAA) guidelines.

*Now known as the Health and Medicine Division of the National Academy of Medicine.

Essentially, the purpose of the HIPAA privacy rule is to ensure that an individual's health information is protected while at the same time allowing healthcare providers to obtain personal health information for the purpose of providing and promoting high-quality healthcare (US Department of Health and Human Services, 2003). Chapter 7 has a more detailed discussion of HIPAA.

In patient-centered care, the nurse's *primary source* for data collection is the patient. However, there may be times when it is necessary to supplement or rely completely on another for the assessment information. These *secondary sources* are essential when caring for a patient experiencing psychosis, muteness, agitation, or catatonia. Such secondary sources include members of the family, friends, neighbors, police, healthcare workers, and medical records.

Age Considerations

Assessment of Children

Although the child is the best source in determining inner feelings and emotions, the caregivers (parents or guardians) often can best describe the behavior, performance, and conduct of the child. Caregivers also are helpful in interpreting the child's words and responses, but a separate interview is advisable when a child is reluctant to share information, especially in cases of suspected abuse (Arnold & Boggs, 2016).

Consider developmental levels in the evaluation of children. One of the hallmarks of psychiatric disorders in children is the tendency to regress (i.e., return to a previous level of development). For example, although it is developmentally appropriate for toddlers to suck their thumbs, such a gesture is unusual in an older child.

You should assess children through a combination of interview and observation. Watching children at play provides important clues to their functioning. Play is a safe area for children to act out thoughts and emotions. Asking the child to tell a story, draw a picture, or engage in specific therapeutic games can be useful, particularly when the child is having difficulty expressing him- or herself in words. Usually, a clinician with special training in child and adolescent psychiatry works with young children.

Assessment of Adolescents

Adolescents are especially concerned with confidentiality and may fear that you will repeat what they say to their parents. This is a difficult area. In the eyes of the law, parents must give consent for treatment and therefore have a right to know how their child will be treated. Clinically and ethically nurses should understand that certain zones of privacy exist even for adolescents. Use of your best judgment is appropriate. You may need to consult with your clinical instructor or supervisor when in doubt.

The adolescent and the adolescent's family should be provided with an overview of how information sharing will work, what information will be shared, with whom, and when. Adolescents should receive an explanation on the role of the treatment team in providing care and the need to share certain information. Threats of suicide, homicide, sexual abuse, or behaviors that put the patient or others at risk for harm must be shared with other professionals, as well as with the parents.

Identifying risk factors is one of the key objectives when assessing adolescents. It is helpful to use a brief, structured interview technique such as the HEADSSS interview (Box 7.2).

BOX 7.2 The HEADSSS Psychosocial Interview Technique

H Home environment (e.g., relations with parents and siblings)
E Education and employment (e.g., school performance)
A Activities (e.g., sports participation, after-school activities, peer relations)
D Drug, alcohol, or tobacco use
S Sexuality (e.g., whether the patient is sexually active, practices safe sex, or uses contraception)
S Suicide risk or symptoms of depression or other mental disorder
S Safety (e.g., how safe does the patient feel at home and school, wear a safety belt, or engage in dangerous or risky activities)

From Reif, C. J. & Elster, A. B. (1998). Adolescent preventive services. *Primary Care: Clinics in Office Practice, 25*(1), 1-21.

Assessment of Older Adults

As we get older, our five senses (taste, touch, sight, hearing, and smell) and brain function begin to diminish, but the extent to which this affects each person varies. Your patient may be a spry and alert 80-year-old or a frail and confused 60-year-old. Therefore it is important not to stereotype older adults and expect them to be physically and mentally deficient.

On the other hand, many older adults need special attention. The nurse needs to be aware of any physical limitations. They may be sensory (difficulty seeing or hearing), motor (difficulty walking or maintaining balance), or medical (back pain, cardiac or pulmonary deficits). All of these problems can cause increased anxiety, stress, or physical discomfort.

It is wise to identify any physical deficits at the onset of the assessment and make accommodations for them. If the patient is hard of hearing, speak a little more slowly in clear, louder tones (but not too loud). Without invading his personal space, seat the patient close to you. Often, a voice that is lower in pitch is easier for older adults to hear. Refer to Chapter 31 for more on assessing and communicating with the older adult.

Language Barriers

Psychiatric-mental health nurses can best serve their patients if they understand the complex cultural and social factors that influence health and illness. Awareness of individual cultural beliefs and healthcare practices can help nurses minimize stereotyped assumptions that can lead to ineffective care. There are many opportunities for misunderstandings when assessing a patient from a different cultural or social background from your own. This is particularly problematic when the patient does not speak the same language as the caregiver.

Often healthcare professionals require an interpreter or a translator to understand the patient's history and healthcare needs. An interpreter is someone who interprets the spoken words of a foreign language speaking person or someone who uses American Sign Language (ASL). A translator is an individual who speaks one or more languages in addition to English who translates the written word. Healthcare providers who receive federal funding are required by law to provide interpreters and translators to limited English proficient patients free of charge. Typically interpreters are on staff, although they may be telephone-based, particularly with less common languages.

The use of untrained interpreters such as family members, friends, and neighbors may be tempting, especially because they are more convenient and there is no charge involved. However, the cost of even one malpractice lawsuit brought on by incorrect interpretations can be devastating to organizations, not to mention the consequences to the patient. Unpaid, nonprofessionals may censor or omit certain content (e.g., profanity, psychotic thoughts, and sexual topics) due to a desire to protect the patient. They can also make subjective interpretations based on their own feelings, share confidential details with outsiders, or leave out traumatic topics because they are too familiar or painful for them.

Psychiatric-Mental Health Nursing Assessment

The purpose of the psychiatric-mental health nursing assessment is to:

- Establish rapport
- Obtain an understanding of the current problem or chief complaint
- Review physical status and obtain baseline vital signs
- Assess for risk factors affecting the safety of the patient or others
- Perform a mental status examination
- Assess psychosocial status
- Identify mutual goals for treatment
- Formulate a plan of care
- Document data in a retrievable format

Gathering Data

Review of systems. The mind-body connection is significant in the understanding and treatment of psychiatric disorders. An advanced care provider such as a physician, a nurse practitioner, or a physician assistant typically conducts a physical examination on patients who are admitted for treatment of psychiatric conditions. A complete physical examination may be deferred depending on the setting or the condition of the patient. Registered nurses gather a baseline set of vital statistics, a historical and current review of body systems, and a documentation of allergic responses.

Several medical conditions and physical illnesses may mimic psychiatric illnesses (Box 7.3). Therefore it important to rule out or address physical causes of symptoms. Conversely, psychiatric disorders can result in physical or somatic symptoms such as stomachaches, headaches, lethargy, insomnia, intense fatigue, and even pain. When depression is secondary to a known medical condition, it often goes unrecognized and thus untreated.

Some people with certain physical conditions may be more prone to psychiatric disorders such as depression. Multiple sclerosis, Parkinson's disease, or other autoimmune disorders may actually bring about depression. Other problems typically associated with depression are coronary artery disease, diabetes, and stroke. Women with both depression and diabetes have a significantly higher risk for mortality and cardiovascular disease than do women with either depression or diabetes alone (Brauser & Barclay, 2011). Individuals need to be evaluated for medical origins of depression or anxiety.

Laboratory data. Hypothyroidism may have the clinical appearance of depression, and hyperthyroidism may appear to be a manic phase of bipolar disorder. A simple blood test can usually differentiate between a mood disorder and thyroid problems, although a person could certainly have both. Abnormal liver enzyme levels can explain irritability, depression, and lethargy. People who have chronic renal disease often suffer from the same symptoms when their blood urea nitrogen and electrolyte levels are abnormal. Results of a toxicology screen for the presence of either prescription or illegal drugs also may provide explanations of unusual psychiatric signs and symptoms.

Mental status examination. Fundamental to the psychiatric-mental health nursing assessment is a **mental status examination (MSE)**. In fact, an MSE is part of the assessment in all areas of medicine. The MSE in psychiatry is analogous to the physical examination in general medicine, and the purpose is to evaluate an individual's current cognitive processes. Box 7.4 is an example of a basic MSE.

The MSE aids in collecting and organizing objective information. **Objective data** refers to all things that nurses observe about the patient with five senses. The nurse observes the patient's physical behavior, nonverbal communication, appearance, speech patterns, mood and affect, thought content, perceptions, cognitive ability, and insight and judgment. Objective data also includes all measurable information such as body weight, blood pressure, and oxygen saturation.

Psychosocial assessment. A **psychosocial assessment** provides additional information from which to develop a plan of care. This type of assessment always begins by asking the patient to describe how treatment became necessary. This is known as the chief complaint and should be documented verbatim, that is, in the patient's own words.

The patient's psychosocial history is the subjective part of the assessment. **Subjective data** refers to all information that you gather from a patient and from people who may accompany the patient. The focus of the history is the *patient's perceptions and recollections* of current lifestyle and life in general. Support, such as family and friends, education, work experience, coping styles, and spiritual and cultural beliefs, is typically discussed during a psychosocial history.

To conduct such an assessment, the nurse should have fundamental knowledge of growth and development, basic cultural and religious practices, pathophysiology, psychopathology, and pharmacology. Box 7.5 identifies items that are usually included in a basic psychosocial assessment tool.

Spiritual/religious assessment. The importance of spirituality and religious beliefs is an often overlooked element of patient care. It is overlooked despite evidence that suggests being part of a spiritual community is helpful to people coping with illness and recovering from surgery (Kling, 2011). Spirituality and religious beliefs have the potential to exert an influence on how people understand meaning and purpose in their lives and how they use critical judgment to solve problems (e.g., crises of illness).

The terms spirituality and religion are different, but not mutually exclusive. Spirituality refers to how we find meaning, hope, purpose, and a sense of peace in our lives. Spirituality is more of an internal phenomenon centering on universal personal questions and needs. It is the part of us that seeks to understand life. A person's spiritual beliefs may or may not be connected with the community or with religious rituals.

BOX 7.3 Some Medical Conditions that May Mimic Psychiatric Illness

Depression

Neurological Disorders
- Cerebrovascular accident (stroke)
- Alzheimer's disease
- Brain tumor
- Huntington's disease
- Epilepsy
- Multiple sclerosis
- Parkinson's disease

Infections
- Mononucleosis
- Encephalitis
- Hepatitis
- Neurosyphilis
- Human immunodeficiency virus (HIV)

Endocrine Disorders
- Hypothyroidism and hyperthyroidism
- Cushing's syndrome
- Addison's disease
- Parathyroid disease

Gastrointestinal Disorders
- Liver cirrhosis
- Pancreatitis

Cardiovascular Disorders
- Hypoxia
- Congestive heart failure

Respiratory Disorders
- Sleep apnea

Nutritional Disorders
- Thiamine deficiency
- Protein deficiency
- B_{12} deficiency
- B_6 deficiency
- Folate deficiency

Collagen Vascular Diseases
- Lupus erythematosus
- Rheumatoid arthritis

Cancer

Anxiety

Neurological Disorders
- Alzheimer's disease
- Brain tumor
- Stroke
- Huntington's disease

Infections:
- Encephalitis
- Meningitis
- Neurosyphilis
- Septicemia

Endocrine Disorders
- Hypothyroidism and hyperthyroidism
- Hypoparathyroidism
- Hypoglycemia
- Pheochromocytoma
- Carcinoid

Metabolic Disorders
- Low calcium
- Low potassium
- Acute intermittent porphyria
- Liver failure

Cardiovascular Disorders
- Angina
- Congestive heart failure
- Pulmonary embolus

Respiratory Disorders
- Pneumothorax
- Acute asthma
- Emphysema

Drug Effects
- Stimulants
- Sedatives (withdrawal)
- Lead, mercury poisoning

Psychosis

Medical Conditions
- Temporal lobe epilepsy
- Migraine headaches
- Temporal arteritis
- Occipital tumors
- Narcolepsy
- Encephalitis
- Hypothyroidism
- Addison's disease
- Human immunodeficiency virus (HIV)

Drug Effects:
- Hallucinogens (e.g., LSD)
- Phencyclidine
- Alcohol withdrawal
- Stimulants
- Cocaine
- Corticosteroids

In contrast, **religion** is an external system that includes beliefs, patterns of worship, and symbols. An individual connects personal and spiritual beliefs with a larger organized group or institution. Belonging to a religious community can provide support during difficult times. Although religion is often concerned with spirituality, religious groups are social entities and are characterized by other nonspiritual goals (cultural, economic, political, social).

Spiritual and religious practices enhance healthy behaviors. For example, many major religions place a taboo on unhealthy practices such as smoking and drinking, thereby reducing these behaviors. Spirituality and religiosity also provide social support and a

BOX 7.4 Mental Status Examination

Appearance
- Grooming and dress
- Level of hygiene
- Pupil dilation or constriction
- Facial expression
- Height, weight, nutritional status
- Presence of body piercing or tattoos, scars, etc.
- Relationship between appearance and age

Behavior
- Excessive or reduced body movements
- Peculiar body movements (e.g., scanning of the environment, odd or repetitive gestures, level of consciousness, balance, and gait)
- Abnormal movements (e.g., tardive dyskinesia, tremors)
- Level of eye contact (keep cultural differences in mind)

Speech
- Rate: slow, rapid, normal
- Volume: loud, soft, normal
- Disturbances (e.g., articulation problems, slurring, stuttering, mumbling)

Mood
- Affect: flat, bland, animated, angry, withdrawn, appropriate to context
- Mood: sad, labile, euphoric

Disorders of the Form of Thought
- Thought process (e.g., disorganized, coherent, flight of ideas, neologisms, thought blocking, circumstantiality)
- Thought content (e.g., delusions, obsessions)

Perceptual Disturbances
- Hallucinations (e.g., auditory, visual)
- Illusions

Cognition
- Orientation: time, place, person
- Level of consciousness (e.g., alert, confused, clouded, stuporous, unconscious, comatose)
- Memory: remote, recent, immediate
- Fund of knowledge
- Attention: performance on serial sevens, digit span tests
- Abstraction: performance on tests involving similarities, proverbs
- Insight
- Judgment

Ideas of Harming Self or Others
- Suicidal or homicidal history and current thoughts
- Presence of a plan
- Means to carry out the plan
- Opportunity to carry out the plan

sense of meaning in people's lives. These behaviors, support, and meaning are linked to decreased mental and physical stress. This, in turn, relates to a decreased incidence of illness in many people.

The following questions may be included in a spiritual or religious assessment:

- Who or what supplies you with strength and hope?
- Do you have a religious affiliation?
- Do you practice any spiritual activities (e.g., yoga, tai chi, meditation)?
- Do you participate in any religious activities?
- What role does religion or spiritual practice play in your life?
- Does your faith help you in stressful situations?
- Do you pray or meditate?
- Has your illness affected your religious/spiritual practices?
- Would you like to have someone from your church/synagogue/temple or from our facility visit?

Cultural and social assessment. Nursing assessments, diagnoses, and subsequent care should be planned around the unique cultural healthcare beliefs, values, and practices of each patient. Chapter 5 provides a detailed discussion of the cultural implications for psychiatric-mental health nursing and how to conduct a cultural and social assessment.

Some questions we can ask to help with a cultural and social assessment are:

- What is your primary language? Would you like an interpreter?
- How would you describe your cultural background?
- Who are you close to?
- Who do you seek in times of crisis?
- Who do you live with?
- How is your family responding to your treatment?
- Who do you seek when you are medically ill? Mentally upset or concerned?
- What do you do to get better when you have physical problems?
- What are the attitudes toward mental illness in your culture?
- How is your current problem viewed by your culture? Is it seen as a problem that can be fixed? A disease? A taboo? A fault or curse?
- Are there special foods that you eat?
- Are there special healthcare practices within your culture that address your particular mental or emotional health problem?
- Are there any special cultural beliefs about your illness that might help me give you better care?

After the cultural and social assessment, it is useful to summarize pertinent data with the patient. This summary provides patients with reassurance that they have been heard and gives them the opportunity to clarify any misinformation. The patient should be told what will happen next. For example, if the initial assessment takes place in the hospital, you should tell the patient who else will require a meeting. Tell the patient when and how often he or she will meet with the nurse to work on the patient's problems. If you believe a referral—such as talking with a dietician—is necessary, discuss this with the patient.

Validating the Assessment

To gain a clearer understanding of your patient, it is helpful to look to outside sources. Ideally, patients will have electronic medical records where all healthcare information is available. Emergency department records can be a valuable resource in understanding an individual's presenting behavior and problems. Police reports may be available in cases in which hostility and legal altercations occurred. Old medical records, most now accessible by computer, are a great help in validating information you already have or in adding new information

BOX 7.5 Psychosocial Assessment

Previous hospitalizations
Educational background
Occupational background
- Employed? Where? What length of time?
- Special skills

Social patterns
- Describe family.
- Describe friends.
- With whom does the patient live?
- To whom does the patient go in time of crisis?
- Describe a typical day.

Sexual patterns
- Sexually active? Practices safe sex? Practices birth control?
- Sexual orientation
- Sexual difficulties

Interests and abilities
- What does the patient do in his or her spare time?
- What sport, hobby, or leisure activity is the patient good at?
- What gives the patient pleasure?

Substance use and abuse
- What medications does the patient take? How often? How much?
- What herbal or over-the-counter drugs does the patient take (caffeine, cough medicines, St. John's wort)? How often? How much?
- What psychotropic drugs does the patient take? How often? How much?
- How many drinks of alcohol does the patient take per day? Per week?
- What recreational drugs does the patient use (club drugs, marijuana, psychedelics, steroids)? How often? How much?
- Does the patient overuse prescription drugs (benzodiazepines, pain medications)?
- Does the patient identify the use of drugs as a problem?

Coping abilities
- What does the patient do when he or she gets upset?
- To whom can the patient talk?
- What usually helps relieve stress?
- What did the patient try this time?

Spiritual assessment
- What importance does religion or spirituality have in the patient's life?
- Do the patient's religious or spiritual beliefs relate to self-care practices? How?
- Does the patient's faith help the patient in stressful situations?
- Whom does the patient see when he or she is medically ill? Mentally upset?
- Are there special healthcare practices within the patient's culture that address his or her particular mental problem?

to your database. If the patient was admitted to a psychiatric unit in the past, information about the patient's previous level of functioning and behavior gives you a baseline for making clinical judgments. Consent forms usually have to be signed by the patient or an appropriate relative to obtain access to records.

Using Rating Scales

A number of standardized rating scales are useful for psychiatric evaluation and monitoring. A clinician often administers rating scales, but many are self-administered. These rating scales highlight important areas in psychiatric assessment. Because many of the answers are subjective, experienced clinicians use these tools as a guide when planning care and also draw on their knowledge of their patients.

The American Psychiatric Association provides online measures that are available to clinicians (and you!) at https://www.psychiatry.org/psychiatrists/practice/dsm/dsm-5/online-assessment-measures. Table 7.1 lists some of the common tools in use. Many of the clinical chapters in this book include a rating scale.

STANDARDS OF PRACTICE FOR PSYCHIATRIC-MENTAL HEALTH NURSING: STANDARD 2: DIAGNOSIS

The psychiatric-mental health registered nurse analyzes the assessment data to determine diagnoses, problems, and areas of focus for care and treatment including level of risk (ANA et al., 2014, p. 46).

A nursing diagnosis is a clinical judgment about a patient's response, needs, actual and potential psychiatric disorders, mental health problems, and potential comorbid physical illnesses. An accurate, clear, and standardized nursing diagnosis is the basis for selecting therapeutic outcomes and interventions.

NANDA International, Inc. (NANDA-I) provides evidence-based diagnoses for nursing care (Herdman & Kamitsuru, 2014). See the appendix for a list of NANDA-I 2015–2017–approved nursing diagnoses and definitions.

Diagnostic Statements

Nursing diagnostic statements are made up of the following structural components:

1. Problem/potential problem
2. Related factors
3. Defining characteristics

The **problem**, or unmet need, describes the state of the patient at present. Problems that are within the nurse's domain to treat are termed *nursing diagnoses*. The nursing diagnostic label indicates what should change.

Related factors are linked to the diagnostic label with the words *related to*. Related factors are always used with problem-focused diagnoses (to be discussed later). The related factors usually indicate what needs to be addressed to effect change through nursing interventions. In the case of *hopelessness related to long-term stress*, the nurse would work with the patient to reduce or prevent the negative impacts of stress. However, in the case of *hopelessness related to abandonment*, there may be nothing the nurse can do to change the abandonment. In that case, the focus would be on symptom management by addressing the defining characteristics.

Defining characteristics include signs (objective and measurable) and symptoms (subjective and reported by the patient). All types of nursing diagnoses use defining characteristics. They may be linked to the diagnosis with the words *as evidenced by*. The previous example would then become: *Hopelessness related to abandonment as evidenced by stating, "Nothing will change," lack of involvement with family and friends, and inattention to self-care for self.*

Types of Nursing Diagnoses

In **problem-focused diagnoses,** we make a judgment about undesirable human responses to a health condition or life

TABLE 7.1 Standardized Rating Scales*

USE	Scale
Depression	Beck Inventory
	Brief Patient Health Questionnaire (Brief PHQ)
	Geriatric Depression Scale (GDS)
	Hamilton Depression Scale
	Zung Self-Report Inventory
	Patient Health Questionnaire-9 (PHQ-9)
	Patient Health Questionnaire for Adolescents (PHQ-A)
Anxiety	Brief Patient Health Questionnaire (Brief PHQ)
	Generalized Anxiety Disorder–7 (GAD-7)
	Modified Spielberger State Anxiety Scale
	Hamilton Anxiety Scale
	Severity Measure for Generalized Anxiety Disorder Child (11–17)
Substance use disorders	Addiction Severity Index (ASI)
	Recovery Attitude and Treatment Evaluator (RAATE)
	Brief Drug Abuse Screen Test (B-DAST)
Obsessive-compulsive behavior	Yale-Brown Obsessive-Compulsive Scale (Y-BOCS)
Mania	Mania Rating Scale
Schizophrenia	Scale for Assessment of Negative Symptoms (SANS)
	Brief Psychiatric Rating Scale (BPRS)
Abnormal movements	Abnormal Involuntary Movement Scale (AIMS)
	Simpson Neurological Rating Scale
General psychiatric assessment	Brief Psychiatric Rating Scale (BPRS)
	Global Assessment of Functioning Scale (GAF)
Cognitive function	Mini-Mental State Examination (MMSE)
	St. Louis University Mental Status Examination (SLUMS)
	Cognitive Capacity Screening Examination (CCSE)
	Alzheimer's Disease Rating Scale (ADRS)
	Memory and Behavior Problem Checklist
	Functional Assessment Screening Tool (FAST)
	Global Deterioration Scale (GDS)
Family assessment	McMaster Family Assessment Device
Eating disorders	Eating Disorders Inventory (EDI)
	Body Attitude Test
	Diagnostic Survey for Eating Disorders

* These rating scales highlight important areas in psychiatric assessment. Because many of the answers are subjective, experienced clinicians use these tools as a guide when planning care and also draw on their knowledge of their patients.

process. This category of nursing diagnosis is accompanied by related factors and evidence. An example of a problem-focused diagnosis is: Anxiety related to losing employment and financial burdens as evidenced by stating "I can't concentrate," crying, restlessness, and insomnia (Formula: Problem + Related Factors + Defining Characteristics).

In a **health promotion diagnosis**, a motivation and desire to improve is diagnosed. Related factors are not used in this problem statement because they would always be the same, that is, motivated to improve health standing. Defining characteristics support this type of diagnosis. Health promotion diagnoses always begin with the phrase "Readiness for enhanced…" An example of this type of diagnosis is *Readiness for enhanced coping as evidenced by seeking social support and knowledge of new strategies* (Formula: Problem + Defining Characteristics).

Risk diagnoses pertain to vulnerability that carries a high probability of developing problematic experiences or responses. Common problems in this category include preventable occurrences such as falls, self-injury, pressure ulcers, and infection. These problems are directly linked with quality improvement and patient safety (QSEN).

This category of diagnosis always begins with the phrase "risk for," followed by the problem. Because the problem has not yet happened, we cannot cite causation in the form of related factors. An example of a risk diagnosis is: *Risk for self-mutilation as evidenced by impulsivity, inadequate coping, isolation, and unstable self-esteem* (Formula: Problem + Defining Characteristics/Risk Factors).

STANDARDS OF PRACTICE FOR PSYCHIATRIC-MENTAL HEALTH NURSING: STANDARD 3: OUTCOMES IDENTIFICATION

The psychiatric-mental health registered nurse identifies expected outcomes and the healthcare consumer's goals for a plan individualized to the healthcare consumer or to the situation (ANA et al., 2014, p. 48).

Outcome criteria are the hoped-for outcomes that reflect the maximum level of patient health that the patient can realistically achieve through nursing interventions. Whereas nursing diagnoses identify nursing problems, outcomes reflect the desired change. The expected outcomes provide direction for continuity of care (ANA et al., 2014).

Moorhead and colleagues (2013) have compiled a standardized list of nursing outcomes in *Nursing Outcomes Classification (NOC)*. Outcomes for each NANDA-I diagnosis are included. *NOC* gives us a way to evaluate the effect of nursing interventions. Each outcome has an associated group of indicators used to determine patient status in relation to the outcome. Table 7.2 provides suggested *NOC* indicators for the outcome of *Suicide self-restraint*, along with the Likert scale that quantifies the achievement from 1 (never demonstrated) to 5 (consistently demonstrated).

All outcomes (goals) are written in positive terms. The clinical chapters in this book will include these short- and long-term outcomes. Table 7.3 shows how to state specific outcome criteria for a suicidal individual with a nursing diagnosis of *Risk for suicide related to depression and suicide attempt*.

STANDARDS OF PRACTICE FOR PSYCHIATRIC-MENTAL HEALTH NURSING: STANDARD 4: PLANNING

The psychiatric–mental health registered nurse develops a plan that prescribes strategies and alternatives to assist the healthcare consumer in attainment of expected outcomes (ANA et al., 2014, p. 50).

Once you have done an assessment and formulated nursing diagnoses, it is time to prioritize them. Maslow's hierarchy of needs (see Chapter 2) provides a useful framework for doing so. Physiological needs and safety always come first because they have the potential for the most serious harm. Then the higher order needs can be addressed including love and belonging and self-esteem can be the focus. For each nursing diagnosis, measurable goals are set and interventions for attaining the goals are selected.

TABLE 7.2 *Nursing Outcomes Classification* Indicators for Suicide Self-Restraint

Definition: Personal actions to refrain from gestures and attempts at killing self

Outcome target rating: Maintain at ________ Increase to ________

Suicide Self-Restraint Overall Rating	Never Demonstrated 1	Rarely Demonstrated 2	Sometimes Demonstrated 3	Often Demonstrated 4	Consistently Demonstrated 5	
Expresses feelings	1	2	3	4	5	NA
Expresses sense of hope	1	2	3	4	5	NA
Maintains connectedness in relationships	1	2	3	4	5	NA
Obtains assistance as needed	1	2	3	4	5	NA
Verbalizes suicidal ideas	1	2	3	4	5	NA
Controls impulses	1	2	3	4	5	NA
Refrains from gathering means for suicide	1	2	3	4	5	NA
Refrains from giving away possessions	1	2	3	4	5	NA
Refrains from inflicting serious injury	1	2	3	4	5	NA
Refrains from using unprescribed mood-altering substances	1	2	3	4	5	NA
Discloses plan for suicide if present	1	2	3	4	5	NA
Upholds suicide contract	1	2	3	4	5	NA
Maintains self-control without supervision	1	2	3	4	5	NA
Refrains from attempting suicide	1	2	3	4	5	NA
Obtains treatment for depression	1	2	3	4	5	NA
Obtains treatment for substance abuse	1	2	3	4	5	NA
Reports adequate pain control for chronic pain	1	2	3	4	5	NA
Uses suicide prevention resources	1	2	3	4	5	NA
Uses social support group	1	2	3	4	5	NA
Uses available mental healthcare services	1	2	3	4	5	NA
Plans for future	1	2	3	4	5	NA

Modified from Moorhead, S., Johnson, M., Maas, M., & Swanson, E. (2013). *Nursing outcomes classification (NOC)* (5th ed.). St. Louis, MO: Elsevier.

TABLE 7.3 Examples of Long- and Short-Term Goals for a Suicidal Patient

Long-Term Goals or Outcomes	Short-Term Goals or Outcomes
Patient will remain free from injury throughout the hospital stay.	Patient will identify the rationale and procedure of the unit's protocol for suicide precautions shortly after admission. Patient will seek out staff when feeling overwhelmed or self-destructive during hospitalization.
By discharge, patient will express hope and a desire to live and identify at least two people to contact if suicidal thoughts arise.	Patient will meet with social worker to find supportive resources in the community before discharge and work on trigger issues (e.g., housing, job). By discharge, patient will state the purpose of medication, time and dose, adverse effects, and whom to call for questions or concerns. Patient will have the written name and telephone numbers of at least two people to turn to if feeling overwhelmed or self-destructive. Patient will have a follow-up appointment to meet with a mental health professional by discharge.

The nurse considers the following specific principles when planning interventions:

- **Safe:** Interventions must be safe for the patient, as well as for other patients, staff, and family.
- **Compatible and appropriate:** Interventions must be compatible with other therapies and with the patient's personal goals and cultural values, as well as with institutional rules.
- **Realistic and individualized:** Interventions should be (1) within the patient's capabilities, given the patient's age, physical strength, condition, and willingness to change; (2) based on the number of staff available; (3) reflective of the actual available community resources; and (4) within the student's or nurse's capabilities.
- **Evidence-based:** Interventions should be based on scientific evidence and principles when available.

Evidence-based interventions and treatments is the gold standard in healthcare. Evidence-based practice (EBP) for nurses is a combination of clinical skill and the use of clinically relevant research in the delivery of effective patient-centered care. Using the best available research, incorporating patient preferences, and making sound clinical judgment and skills provide an optimal patient-centered nurse-patient relationship.

The *Nursing Interventions Classification (NIC)* (Bulechek et al., 2013) is a research-based, standardized listing of interventions .These interventions are linked to NOC outcomes and represent the third level in unifying the nursing process through NANDA-I, NOC, and NIC.

This evidence-based approach to care is consistent with QSEN standards. Nurses in all settings can use *NIC* to support quality patient care and incorporate evidence-based nursing actions. Although many safe and appropriate interventions may not be included in *NIC*, it is a useful guide for standardized care. Individualizing interventions to meet a patient's special needs should always be part of the planning.

STANDARDS OF PRACTICE FOR PSYCHIATRIC-MENTAL HEALTH NURSING: STANDARD 5: IMPLEMENTATION

The psychiatric-mental health registered nurse implements the identified plan (ANA et al., 2014, p. 52).

The psychiatric-mental health registered nurse accomplishes patient care through the nurse-patient partnership and the use of therapeutic intervention skills. The nurse implements the plan using evidence-based interventions whenever possible, utilizing community resources, and collaborating with nursing colleagues. Provision of care implies that interventions are age appropriate and culturally and ethnically sensitive.

The psychiatric-mental health registered nurse has passed a state board examination to practice at the basic level of intervention. The psychiatric-mental health advanced practice registered nurse (psychiatric-mental health advanced practice registered nurse) is prepared at the master's or doctorate level and is prepared to function as at an advanced level. Most of the interventions that follow apply only to all levels of nurses, although a few apply only to the advanced practice role.

Standard 5A. Coordination of Care

The psychiatric-mental health registered nurse coordinates care delivery (ANA et al., 2014, p. 54).

One of the most important jobs that a registered nurse does is to coordinate care. The nurse is generally in the most contact with the patient and communicates patient status, needs, and goals with the interprofessional team. Nurses also tend to be the families' advocates and help them to navigate an often-bewildering healthcare system at a difficult time in their lives. Documentation of the coordination of care is an essential aspect of this standard.

Standard 5B. Health Teaching and Health Promotion

The psychiatric-mental health registered nurse employs strategies to promote health and safe environment (ANA et al., 2014, p. 55).

Psychiatric-mental health nurses use a variety of health teaching methods adaptive to the patient's special needs (age, culture, ability to learn, readiness) and recovery goals. Healthcare teaching includes coping skills, self-care activities, stress management, problem-solving skills, relapse prevention, conflict management, and interpersonal relationships. A vital part of health promotion is identifying resources for services in the community.

Standard 5C. Consultation

The psychiatric-mental health advanced practice registered nurse provides consultation to influence the identified plan, enhance the abilities of other clinicians to promote services for healthcare consumers, and effect change (ANA et al., 2014, 57).

Consultation is an advanced practice role. Consultation involves assisting other registered nurses and members of the interprofessional team in addressing complex clinical and other situations. Evidence-based information, clinical data, and theoretical frameworks provide the foundation nurse consultants.

Standard 5D. Prescriptive Authority and Treatment

The psychiatric-mental health advanced practice registered nurse uses prescriptive authority, procedures, referrals, treatments, and therapies in accordance with state and federal law and regulation (ANA et al., 2014, p. 58).

Another advanced practice role, prescribing is accomplished by using evidence-based treatments, procedures, and therapies for healthcare consumers. Medication is prescribed in collaboration with the patient based on clinical symptoms and the results of diagnostic and laboratory tests. Evaluation of the therapeutic benefit and adverse effects of pharmacology is assisted by using standard symptom measurements along with the healthcare consumer's appraisal.

Standard 5E. Pharmacological, Biological, and Integrative Therapies

The psychiatric-mental health registered nurse incorporates knowledge of pharmacological, biological, and complementary interventions with applied clinical skills to restore the healthcare consumer's health and prevent further disability (APA et al., 2014, p. 59).

Nurses are knowledgeable regarding the current research findings, intended action, therapeutic dosage, adverse reactions, and safe blood levels of medications being administered. Monitoring the patient for any negative effects protects the patient from unnecessary harm. The nurse communicates this assessment of the patient's response to psychobiological interventions to other members of the mental health team.

Standard 5F. Milieu Therapy

The psychiatric-mental health registered nurse provides, structures, and maintains a safe, therapeutic, recovery-oriented environment in collaboration with healthcare consumers, families, and other healthcare clinicians (ANA et al., 2014, p. 60).

Milieu refers to a physical and social environment. Milieu therapy is a psychiatric philosophy that involves a secure environment including people, settings, structure, and emotional climate to effect positive change. Milieu therapy takes naturally occurring events in the environment and uses them as rich learning opportunities for patients. A consistent routine and structure is maintained to provide predictability and trust.

Milieu management includes orienting patients to their rights and responsibilities. Milieu management takes into consideration the need for culturally sensitive care. The nurse selects activities (both individual and group) that meet the patient's physical and mental health needs. The nurse always maintains patients in the least restrictive environment.

Standard 5G. Therapeutic Relationship and Counseling

The psychiatric-mental health registered nurse uses the therapeutic relationship and counseling interventions to assist healthcare consumers in their individual recovery journeys by improving and regaining their previous coping abilities, fostering mental health, and preventing mental disorder and disability (ANA et al., 2014, p. 62).

The therapeutic relationship is the basis of interactions between the nurse and patient. While medications and other treatments are important for recovery from a psychiatric disorder, nurses are vital in providing presence and being a sounding board. In an individual or group setting, you can reinforce healthy behavior and help the patient to recognize maladaptive behaviors, identify positive coping methods, and try out the new coping methods

Standard 5H. Psychotherapy

The psychiatric-mental health advanced practice registered nurse conducts individual, couples, group, and family psychotherapy using evidence-based psychotherapeutic frameworks and nurse-patient therapeutic relationships (ANA et al., 2014, p. 63).

The practice of psychotherapy is an advanced practice skill that is built upon principles of therapeutic communication. Evidence-based therapies are chosen in order to meet the needs of healthcare consumers who are encouraged to be active participants in treatment. When possible, standardized tools are used to evaluate effectiveness of interventions.

STANDARDS OF PRACTICE FOR PSYCHIATRIC-MENTAL HEALTH NURSING: STANDARD 6: EVALUATION

The psychiatric-mental registered nurse evaluates progress toward attainment of expected outcomes (ANA et al., 2014, p. 65).

Unfortunately, nurses often neglect evaluation of patient outcomes during the nursing process. Evaluation of the individual's response to treatment should be systematic, ongoing, and criteria-based. You should include supporting data to clarify the evaluation. Ongoing assessment of data allows for revisions of nursing diagnoses, changes to more realistic outcomes, or identification of more appropriate interventions when outcomes are not met.

DOCUMENTATION

Documentation has been called the seventh step in the nursing process. Keep in mind that medical records are legal documents and may be used in a court of law. Besides the evaluation of stated outcomes, the medical record should include changes in patient condition, informed consents (for medications and treatments), reaction to medication, documentation of symptoms (verbatim when appropriate), concerns of the patient, and any problematic incidents in the healthcare setting. Documentation of patient progress is the responsibility of the entire mental health team.

Communication among team members and coordination of services are the primary goals when choosing a system for documentation. Information must be in a format that is retrievable for quality improvement monitoring, utilization management, peer review, and research. Documentation—using the nursing process as a guide—is reflected in two of the formats commonly used in healthcare settings and described in Table 7.4.

Informatics, in general, and electronic medical records, specifically, are the preferred formats in both inpatient and outpatient settings. Nurses need to be trained to use these technologies in the medical setting. We should also be prepared to provide further training for nurses in the use of terminology, progress notes relating to needs assessment, nursing interventions, and nursing diagnoses. Whatever format is used, documentation must be focused, organized, pertinent, and conform to certain legal and other generally accepted principles (Box 7.6).

Documentation of "Nonadherence"

When patients do not follow medication and treatment plans, they are often labeled as "noncompliant." Applied to patients, the term noncompliant often has negative connotations because compliance traditionally referred to the extent that a patient obediently and faithfully followed healthcare providers' instructions. "That patient is noncompliant" often translates into the patient being bad or lazy, subjecting the patient to blame and criticism. The term noncompliant is invariably judgmental. A much more useful term is nonadherent. This term encourages healthcare providers to find out what is going on in the patient's life and explore barriers to taking the medication.

Crane (2012) also emphasizes that under the Affordable Care Act, documenting "noncompliance" no longer protects the physician, nurse, manager, or hospital for bad outcomes, which have led to further illness or injury. A finding of noncompliance may void Medicaid or Medicare reimbursements, which can lead to financial losses for the institution and damage to the facility's reputation (Scudder, 2013).

Furthermore, "patient did not comply" does not protect nurses, physicians, or healthcare workers from malpractice lawsuits. Meticulous records that document the reason for interventions, clear explanation and teaching, and the patient's response support healthcare workers in the event of lawsuits. Probably the biggest problem in a malpractice lawsuit is whether the patient understood the instructions given by the healthcare provider. Even if the patient was given instructions or printed information sheets, it is possible that the patient did not understand the instructions or didn't realize how important the treatment (e.g., medication, a follow-up) was to his or her health.

TABLE 7.4 Narrative Versus Problem-Oriented Charting

	Narrative Charting	Problem-Oriented Charting: SOAPIE
Characteristics	A descriptive statement of patient status written in chronological order throughout a shift. Used to support assessment findings from a flow sheet. In charting by exception, narrative notes are used to indicate significant symptoms, behaviors, or events that are exceptions to norms identified on an assessment flow sheet.	Developed in the 1960s for physicians to reduce inefficient documentation. Intended to be accompanied by a problem list. Originally SOAP, with IE added later. The emphasis is on problem identification, process, and outcome. S: Subjective data (patient statement) O: Objective data (nurse observations) A: Assessment (nurse interprets *S* and *O* and describes either a problem or a nursing diagnosis) P: Plan (proposed intervention) I: Interventions (nurse's response to problem) E: Evaluation (patient outcome)
Example	(Date/time/discipline) Patient was agitated in the morning and pacing in the hallway. Blinked eyes, muttered to self, and looked off to the side. Stated heard voices. Verbally hostile to another patient. Offered 2 mg haloperidol (Haldol) PRN and sat with staff in quiet area for 20 minutes. Patient returned to community lounge and was able to sit and watch television.	(Date/time/discipline) S: "I'm so stupid. Get away, get away." "I hear the devil telling me bad things." O: Patient paced the hall, mumbling to self, and looking off to the side. Shouted insulting comments when approached by another patient. Watched walls and ceiling closely. A: Patient was having auditory hallucinations and increased agitation. P: Offered patient haloperidol PRN. Redirected patient to less stimulating environment. I: Patient received 2 mg haloperidol PO PRN. Sat with patient in quiet room for 20 minutes. E: Patient calmer. Returned to community lounge, sat, and watched television.
Advantages	Uses a common form of expression (narrative writing) Can address any event or behavior Explains flow-sheet findings Provides multidisciplinary ease of use	Structured Provides consistent organization of data Facilitates retrieval of data for quality assurance and utilization management Contains all elements of the nursing process Minimizes inclusion of unnecessary data Provides multidisciplinary ease of use
Disadvantages	Unstructured May result in different organization of information from note to note Makes it difficult to retrieve quality assurance and utilization management data Frequently leads to omission of elements of the nursing process Commonly results in inclusion of unnecessary and subjective information	Requires time and effort to structure the information Limits entries to problems May result in loss of data about progress Not chronological Carries negative connotation

BOX 7.6 Legal Considerations for Documentation of Care

Do

- Chart in a timely manner all pertinent and factual information.
- Be familiar with the nursing documentation policy in your facility and make your charting conform to this standard. The policy generally states the method, frequency, and pertinent assessments, interventions, and outcomes to be recorded. If your agency's policies and procedures do not encourage or allow for quality documentation, bring the need for change to the administration's attention.
- Be familiar with the electronic charting in your institution.
- Chart facts fully, descriptively, and accurately.
- Chart what you see, hear, feel, and smell.
- Chart pertinent observations: psychosocial observations, physical symptoms pertinent to the medical diagnosis, and behaviors pertinent to the nursing diagnosis.
- Chart follow-up care provided when a problem has been identified in earlier documentation. For example, if a patient has fallen and injured a leg, describe how the wound is healing.
- Chart fully the facts surrounding unusual occurrences and incidents.
- Chart *all* nursing interventions, treatments, and outcomes (including teaching efforts and patient responses) and safety and patient-protection interventions.
- Chart the patient's expressed subjective feelings.
- Chart each time you notify a physician and record the reason for notification, the information that was communicated, the accurate time, the physician's instructions or orders, and the follow-up activity.
- Chart physicians' visits and treatments.
- Chart discharge medications and instructions given for use, as well as all discharge teaching performed, and note which family members were included in the process.

Do Not

- Do *not* chart opinions that are not supported by facts.
- Do *not* defame patients by calling them names or making derogatory statements about them (e.g., "an unlikable patient who is demanding unnecessary attention").
- Do *not* chart before an event occurs.
- Do *not* chart generalizations, suppositions, or pat phrases (e.g., "patient in good spirits").
- Do *not* obliterate, erase, alter, or destroy a record. If an error is made, draw one line through the error, write "mistaken entry," the date, and initial. Follow your agency's guidelines closely.
- Do *not* leave blank spaces for chronological notes. If you must chart out of sequence, chart "late entry." Identify the time and date of the entry and the time and date of the occurrence.
- If an incident report is filed, *do not note in the chart that one was filed.* This form is generally a privileged communication between the hospital and the hospital's attorney. Describing it in the chart may destroy the privileged nature of the communication.

KEY POINTS TO REMEMBER

- The nursing process is a six-step, problem-solving approach to patient care.
- The Institute of Medicine (IOM) and Quality and Safety Education for Nurses (QSEN) faculty have established mandates to prepare future nurses with the knowledge, skills, and attitudes (KSAs) necessary for achieving quality and safety as they engage in the six competencies of nursing: patient-centered care, teamwork and collaboration, evidence-based practice (EBP), quality improvement (QI), safety, and informatics.
- The *primary source* of assessment is the patient. *Secondary sources* of information include family members, neighbors, friends, police, and other members of the health team.
- A professional interpreter is required by law to prevent serious misunderstandings during assessment, treatment, and evaluation with limited English proficient patients or American Sign Language–using patients. Translators are used to transcribe written documents into English.
- The assessment interview includes mental or emotional status and psychosocial assessment.
- Medical examination, history, and systems review round out a complete assessment.
- Assessment tools and standardized rating scales may be used to evaluate and monitor a patient's progress.
- Determination of the nursing diagnosis (NANDA-I) defines the practice of nursing, improves communication between staff members, and assists in accountability of care.
- Nursing diagnoses always include a problem. Depending upon the type of diagnosis (e.g., actual or risk), related factors and defining characteristics are included in the diagnostic statement.
- Outcomes are measurable and positively stated in terms that reflect a patient's actual state. *NOC* provides standardized outcomes. Planning involves determining desired outcomes.
- Behavioral goals support outcomes. Goals are short, specific, and measurable; indicate the desired patient behavior(s); and include a set time for achievement.
- Planning nursing actions (using *NIC* or other sources) to achieve outcomes includes the use of specific principles. The plan should be (1) safe, (2) compatible with and appropriate for implementation with other therapies, (3) realistic and individualized, and (4) evidence-based whenever possible.
- Psychiatric-mental health nursing practice includes four basic-level interventions: coordination of care, health teaching and health promotion, milieu therapy, and pharmacological, biological, and integrative therapies.
- Nurses certified for advanced practice psychiatric-mental health nursing can prescribe psychiatric medications, practice psychotherapy, and perform consulting work.
- The evaluation of care is a continual process of determining to what extent the outcome criteria have been achieved. The plan of care may be revised based on the evaluation.
- Documentation of patient progress through evaluation of the outcome criteria is crucial. The medical record is a legal document and should accurately reflect the patient's condition, medications, treatment, tests, responses, and any untoward incidents.

CRITICAL THINKING

Pedro Gonzales, a 37-year-old Hispanic man, arrives by ambulance from a supermarket where he had fallen. On his arrival to the emergency department (ED), his breath smells "fruity." He appears confused and anxious, saying that "they put the evil eye on me, they want me to die, they are drying out my body…it's draining me dry…they are yelling, they are yelling…no, no, I'm not bad…oh, God, don't let them get me!" When his mother arrives in the ED, she tells the staff, through the use of an interpreter, that Pedro is a severe diabetic, has a diagnosis of paranoid schizophrenia, and this happens when he doesn't take his medications. In a group or in collaboration with a classmate, respond to the following:

1. A number of nursing diagnoses are possible in this scenario. Given the provided information, formulate at least two nursing diagnoses (problems) and include "related to" and "as evidenced by" as appropriate.
2. For each of your nursing diagnoses, write out one long-term outcome (the problem, what should change, etc.). Include a time frame, desired change, and three criteria that will help you evaluate whether the outcome has been met, not met, or partially met.
3. What specific needs might you take into account when planning nursing care for Mr. Gonzales?
4. Using the SOAPIE format (see Table 7.4), formulate an initial nurse's note for Mr. Gonzales.

CHAPTER REVIEW

Questions

1. What is the purpose of the Health Insurance Portability and Accountability Act (HIPAA)? *Select all that apply.*
   - **a.** Ensuring that an individual's health information is protected
   - **b.** Providing third-party players with access to patient's medical records
   - **c.** Facilitating the movement of a patient's medical information to the interested parties
   - **d.** Guaranteeing that all those in need of healthcare coverage have options to obtain it
   - **e.** Allowing healthcare providers to obtain personal health to provide high-quality healthcare.
2. Which intervention demonstrates a nurse's understanding of the initial action associated with the assessment of a patient's spiritual beliefs?
   - **a.** Offering to pray with the patient

b. Providing a consult with the facility's chaplain
c. Asking the patient what role spirituality plays in his or her daily life
d. Arranging for care to be provided with respect to religious practices

3. Which nursing interventions best demonstrate an understanding of the Quality and Safety Education in Nursing (QSEN) competences? *Select all that apply.*
a. Asking the patient what he or she expects from the treatment he or she is receiving
b. Seeking recertification for cardiopulmonary resuscitation (CPR)
c. Accessing the internet to monitor social media related to opinions on healthcare
d. Consulting with a dietician to discuss a patient's cultural food preferences and restrictions
e. Reviewing the literature regarding the best way to monitor the patient for a fluid imbalance

4. Which disadvantage is inherent to the problem-oriented charting system (SOAPIE)?
a. Does not support a universal organizational system
b. Commonly allows for the inclusion of subjective information
c. Documentation is not listed in chronological order
d. Does not support the nursing process as a format

5. Which standardized rating scale will the nurse specifically include in the assessment of a newly admitted patient diagnosed with major depressive disorder?
a. Mini-Mental State Examination (MMSE)
b. Body Attitude Test
c. Global Assessment of Functioning Scale (GAF)
d. Beck Inventory

6. A 13-year-old boy is undergoing a mental health assessment. The nurse practitioner assures him that his medical records are protected and private. The nurse recognizes that this promise cannot be kept when the youth divulges:
a. "I lost my virginity last year."
b. "I am angry with my parents most of the time."
c. "I have thoughts of being in love with boys."
d. "My parents do not know that I hit my grandpa."

7. During an interview with a non–English-speaking middle-aged woman recently diagnosed with major depression, the patient's husband states, "She is happy now and doing very well." The patient, however, sits motionless, looking at the floor, and wringing her hands. A professional interpreter would provide better information due to the fact that a family member in the interpreter role may: *Select all that apply.*
a. Be too close to accurately capture the meaning of the patient's mood.
b. Censor the patient's thoughts or words.
c. Avoid interpretation.
d. Leave out unsavory details.

8. A nurse identified a nursing diagnosis of *self-mutilation* for a female diagnosed with borderline personality disorder. The patient has multiple self-inflicted cuts on her forearms and inner thighs. What is the most important patient outcome for this nursing diagnosis?
a. Identify triggers to self-mutilation
b. Demonstrate a decrease in frequency and intensity of cutting
c. Describe strategies in increase socialization on the unit
d. Describe two strategies to increase self-care

9. Medical records are considered legal documents. Proper documentation needs to reflect patient condition along with changes. It should also be based on professional standards designated by the state board of nursing, regulatory agencies, and reimbursement requirements. Proper documentation can be enhanced by:
a. Only using objective data
b. Using the nursing process as a guide
c. Using language the specific patient can understand
d. Avoiding legal jargon

10. Amadi is a 40-year-old African national being treated in a psychiatric outpatient setting due to a court order. Amadi's medical record is limited in scope, so where can Renata, his registered nurse, obtain more data on Amadi's condition within legal parameters? *Select all that apply.*
a. Emergency department records
b. Police records related to the offense resulting in the court order for treatment
c. Calling his family in Africa for details about Amadi's mental health
d. Past medical records in the current facility

Answers

1. **a, e;** 2. **c;** 3. **a, b, d, e;** 4. **c;** 5. **d;** 6. **d;** 7. **b;** 8. **a;** 9. **b;** 10. **a, b, d**

ⓔ Visit the Evolve website for a posttest on the content in this chapter: http://evolve.elsevier.com/Varcarolis

Post-Test interactive review

REFERENCES

American Nurses Association (ANA), American Psychiatric Nurses Association, & International Society of Psychiatric–Mental Health Nurses. (2014). *Psychiatric–mental health nursing: Scope and standards of practice* (2nd ed.). Washington, DC: Nursebooks.org. © 2014 American Psychiatric Nurses Association & International Society of Psychiatric-Mental Health Nurses. Reproduced with permission.

Arnold, E. C., & Boggs, K. U. (2016). *Interpersonal relationships: Professional communication skills for nurses* (6th ed.). St. Louis, MO: Saunders.

Brauser, D., & Barclay, X. (2011). Deadly combination of depression and diabetes doubles mortality risk. *Medscape Nurses Education.* Retrieved from http://www.medscape.org/viewarticle/735714.

Bulechek, G. M., Butcher, H. K., McCloskey, Dochterman, J. M., & Wagner, C. (2013). *Nursing interventions classification (NIC)* (6th ed.). St. Louis, MO: Mosby.

Crane, M. (2012). *Documenting noncompliance won't protect you anymore.* Retrieved from www.Medscape.com/viewarticle/773918.

Cronenwett, L., Sherwood, G., Barnsteiner, J., Disch, J., Johnson, J., Mitchell, P., et al. (2007). Quality and safety education for nurses. *Nursing Outlook*, *55*(3), 122–131.

Herdman, T. H., & Kamitsuru, S. (Eds.). (2014). *NANDA International nursing diagnoses: Definitions and classification 2015–2017*. Oxford, UK: Wiley-Blackwell.

Institute of Medicine. (2003). *Health professions education*. Washington, DC: National Academies Press.

Kling, J. (2011). Spirituality an important component of patient care. *Medscape Nurses News*. Retrieved from http://www.medscape.com/viewarticle/738237.

Moorhead, S., Johnson, M., Maas, M. L., & Swanson, E. (2013). *Nursing outcomes classification (NOC)* (5th ed.). St. Louis, MO: Mosby.

Scudder, L. (2013). *Nurses and noncompliance: A primer*. Retrieved March 18, 2013, from www.medscape.com/viewarticle/779149_.

United States Department of Health and Human Services. (2003). *Summary of HIPAA privacy rule*. Retrieved from http://www.hhs.gov/sites/default/files/ocr/privacy/hipaa/understanding/summary/privacysummary.pdf.

8

Therapeutic Relationships

Elizabeth M. Varcarolis

Visit the Evolve website for a pretest on the content in this chapter: http://evolve.elsevier.com/Varcarolis Pre-Test interactive review

OBJECTIVES

1. Compare and contrast a social relationship and a therapeutic relationship regarding purpose, focus, communications style, and goals.
2. Explore qualities that foster a therapeutic nurse-patient relationship and qualities that contribute to a nontherapeutic relationship.
3. Analyze the meaning of boundaries and the influence of transference and countertransference on boundary blurring.
4. Discuss the influences of disparate values and cultural beliefs on the therapeutic relationship.
5. Explain Peplau's four phases of the nurse-patient relationship.
6. Define and discuss the roles of genuineness, empathy, and positive regard on the part of the nurse in a nurse-patient relationship.
7. Identify the use of attending behaviors (e.g., eye contact, body language, and vocal qualities).

OUTLINE

KEY TERMS AND CONCEPTS

clinical supervision
contract
counseling
countertransference
empathy
genuineness
orientation phase
patient-centered care
preorientation phase
psychotherapy
rapport
social relationship
termination phase
therapeutic encounter
therapeutic relationship
therapeutic use of self
transference
values
working phase

Psychiatric-mental health nursing is in many ways based on principles of *science*. A background in anatomy, physiology, and chemistry is the basis for providing safe and effective biological treatments. Knowledge of pharmacology—a medication's mechanism of action, indications for use, and adverse effects based on evidence-based studies and trials—is vital to nursing practice. However, it is the caring relationship and the development of the interpersonal skills needed to enhance and maintain such a relationship that make up the *art* of psychiatric nursing. A therapeutic relationship creates a space where caring and healing can occur.

CONCEPTS OF THE NURSE-PATIENT RELATIONSHIP

The healthcare community accepts the concept of **patient-centered care** as the gold standard. The core concepts of patient- and family-centered care consist of (1) dignity and respect, (2) information sharing, (3) patient and family participation, and (4) collaboration in policy and program development (Institute for Patient- and Family-Centered Care, 2010). These tenets are familiar to members of the nursing profession as the nurse-patient relationship.

The nurse-patient relationship is the basis of all psychiatric-mental health nursing treatment approaches, regardless of the specific goals. The very first connections between nurse and patient are to establish an understanding that the nurse is safe, confidential, reliable, and consistent and that the relationship will occur within appropriate and clear boundaries.

Virtually all psychiatric disorders, including schizophrenia, bipolar disorder, and major depression, have biochemical and genetic components. However, many accompanying emotional problems such as poor self-image, low self-esteem, and difficulties with adherence to a treatment regimen can be significantly improved through a therapeutic nurse-patient relationship. All too often, patients entering treatment have taxed or exhausted their familial and social resources and find themselves isolated and in need of emotional support.

We all have distinct gifts—unique personality traits and talents—that we can learn to use creatively to form positive bonds with others. The use of these gifts to promote healing in others is referred to as the **therapeutic use of self**. A positive therapeutic alliance, which is collaborative and respectful, is one of the best predictors of positive outcomes in therapy (Gordon & Beresin, 2016).

Importance of Talk Therapy

A formalized approach to talk therapy that is based on theoretical models is called **psychotherapy**. Healthcare providers with advanced degrees and specialized knowledge, including psychiatric-mental health advanced practice registered nurses, psychiatrists, and psychologists, are licensed to practice psychotherapy. Evidence suggests that psychotherapy within a therapeutic partnership actually changes brain chemistry in much the same way as medication. Thus the best treatment for most psychiatric problems (less so with psychotic disorders) is a combination of medication and psychotherapy.

Basic level psychiatric-mental health nurses do not practice psychotherapy as this is an advanced skill. They do, however, use counseling techniques in the context of the therapeutic relationship. **Counseling** is a supportive face-to-face process that helps individuals problem-solve, resolve personal conflicts, and feel supported.

Goals and Functions

The nurse-patient relationship is often loosely defined, but a therapeutic nurse-patient relationship has specific goals and functions including the following:

- Facilitating communication of distressing thoughts and feelings
- Assisting patients with problem solving to help facilitate activities of daily living
- Helping patients examine self-defeating behaviors and test alternatives
- Promoting self-care and independence
- Providing education about medications and symptom management
- Promoting recovery

Social Versus Therapeutic

A relationship is an interpersonal process that involves two or more people. Throughout life, we meet people in a variety of settings and share an array of experiences. With some individuals, we develop long-term relationships. With others, the relationship lasts only a short time. Naturally, the kinds of relationships we enter vary from person to person and from situation to situation.

Generally, relationships are *intimate*, *social*, or *therapeutic*. Intimate relationships occur between people who have an emotional commitment to each other. Within intimate relationships, mutual needs are met and intimate desires and hopes are shared. Morally, legally, and ethically nurses and nursing students do not have intimate relationships with patients. Therefore for the purpose of this chapter, we will limit our exploration to clarifying the differences between social and therapeutic relationships.

Social Relationships

A **social relationship** is primarily initiated for the purpose of friendship, socialization, enjoyment, or accomplishment of a task. Mutual needs are met during social interaction (e.g., participants share ideas, feelings, and experiences). Communication skills may include giving advice and sometimes meeting basic dependency needs such as lending money and helping with jobs. Often, the content of the communication is superficial.

During social interactions, roles may shift such as being the listener one day and being listened to the next. Within a social relationship, there is little emphasis on the evaluation of the interaction. In the following example, notice the casual friend-like tone of the nurse:

Patient: "Oh, I just hate to be alone. It's getting me down, and sometimes it hurts so much."

Nurse: "I know how you feel. I don't like being alone either. What I do is get on Facebook and see if anyone wants to do something. Maybe you should try this?" *(In this response, the nurse is minimizing the patient's feelings and giving advice prematurely.)*

Patient: "I don't get on Facebook. Anyway, I usually don't even feel like going out. I just sit at home feeling lonely and empty."

Nurse: "Most of us feel like that at one time or another. Maybe if you took a class or joined a group you could meet more people. I know of some great groups you could join. *(Again, the nurse is not "hearing" the patient's distress and is minimizing her pain and isolation. The nurse goes on to give the patient unwanted and unhelpful advice, thus closing off the patient's feelings and experience.)*

Therapeutic Relationships

In a **therapeutic relationship**, the nurse maximizes communication skills, understanding of human behaviors, and personal strengths to enhance the patient's growth. Patients more easily engage in the relationship when the clinician's interactions address their concerns, respect patients as partners in decision making, and use straightforward language. These interactions are evidence that the focus of the relationship is on the patient's ideas, experiences, and feelings.

Inherent in a therapeutic relationship is the nurse's addressing issues introduced by the patient during the initial nursing assessment or in subsequent meetings. The nurse and the patient identify areas that need exploration and periodically evaluate the degree of progress of the patient.

Although the nurse may assume a variety of roles (e.g., teacher, counselor, socializing agent, liaison), the relationship is consistently focused on the patient's problem and needs. Nurses' needs are met outside the relationship. Nurses who want the patient to "like me," "do as I suggest," or "give me recognition," undercut the needs of the patient.

Nursing students have the opportunity to develop a therapeutic relationship with patients while having the support of both clinical faculty and nursing staff. This **clinical supervision** is a mentoring relationship characterized by feedback and evaluation. Typically, students experience a gradual increase in autonomy and responsibility.

Communication skills and knowledge of the stages and phenomena in a therapeutic relationship are crucial tools in the formation and maintenance of that relationship. Within the context of a therapeutic relationship, the nurse will:

- Identify the needs of the patient and explore them
- Establish clear boundaries
- Encourage alternate problem-solving approaches
- Help the patient develop new coping skills
- Support behavioral change

Just like staff nurses, nursing students may struggle with the boundaries between social and therapeutic relationships because there is a fine line between the two. In fact, students often feel more comfortable being a friend because it is a more familiar role, especially with patients close to their own age. When this occurs, the student needs to make it clear (to themselves and the patient) that the relationship is a therapeutic one.

This does *not* mean that the nurse is not friendly toward the patient, and it does *not* mean that talking about everyday topics (e.g., television, weather, and children's pictures) is forbidden. In fact, a small amount of self-disclosure on the nurse's part may strengthen the therapeutic relationship. For example, your patient is about 24 years old (your age) and asks you about nursing school and what the hardest parts are. Briefly sharing your views on nursing school will increase the trust in the relationship. Can you imagine saying, "We won't be talking about me"? On the other hand, multiple questions about your dating life by a sexually preoccupied patient should result in redirection and clarification of roles.

In a therapeutic relationship, the patient's problems and concerns are explored. Both patient and nurse discuss potential solutions. The patient, as in the following example, implements the solutions:

Patient: "Oh, I just hate to be alone. It's getting me down, and sometimes it hurts so much."

Nurse: "Loneliness can be painful. What is going on now that you are feeling so alone?"

Patient: "Well, my mom died 2 years ago, and last month, my—oh, I am so scared." *(Patient takes a deep breath, looks down, and looks as if she might cry.)*

Nurse: *(Sits in silence while the patient recovers)* "Go on."

Patient: "My boyfriend left for Afghanistan. I haven't heard from him, and they say he's missing. He was my best friend, and we were going to get married. If he dies, I don't want to live."

Nurse: *(Leans in slightly, nodding gently)* "That must be scary not knowing what is going on with your boyfriend. Have you thought of killing yourself?"

Patient: "Well, if he dies, I will. I can't live without him."

Nurse: "Have you ever felt like this before?"

Patient: "Yes, when my mom died. I was depressed for about a year until I met my boyfriend."

Nurse: "It sounds as if you're going through a very painful and scary time. Perhaps you and I can talk some more and come up with some ways for you to feel less anxious, scared, and overwhelmed. Would you be willing to work on this together?"

Sometimes the relationship may be informal and not extensive such as when the nurse and patient meet for only a few sessions. Even though it is brief, the relationship may be substantial, useful, and important for the patient. This limited relationship is referred to as a **therapeutic encounter**. When the nurse shows genuine concern for another's circumstances (has positive regard and empathy), even a short encounter can have a powerful effect.

At other times, the encounters may be longer and more formal such as in inpatient settings, community mental health centers, crisis centers, and freestanding psychiatric facilities. This longer timespan allows the therapeutic nurse-patient relationship to be more fully developed.

Relationship Boundaries and Roles

Establishing Boundaries

Professional boundaries exist to protect patients. Boundaries are the expected and accepted social, physical, and psychological boundaries that separate nurses from patients. This separation is essential considering the power differential between the nurse and the patient. This differential also exists between you and the patient, even if you do not feel powerful. You have

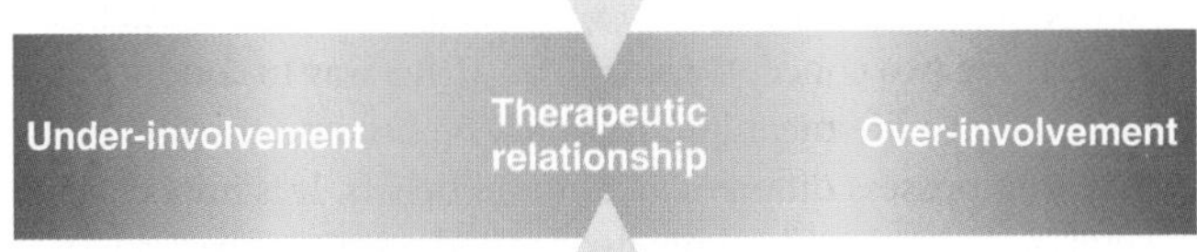

FIG. 8.1 Continuum of therapeutic involvement

read the patient's chart, you are there to help, you are close to becoming a registered nurse, and you are not a patient. These qualities put nursing students in a position of some authority, particularly from the patient's perspective.

Nurses and other healthcare workers should seek a level of involvement that is healthy. A well-defined therapeutic nurse-patient relationship allows the establishment of clear boundaries. These boundaries provide a safe space in which the patient can explore feelings and treatment concerns. Fig. 8.1 illustrates the balance of involvement in a therapeutic relationship.

Blurring of Boundaries

Boundaries are always at risk for becoming blurred. Two common circumstances in which boundaries are blurred are (1) when the relationship slips into a social context and (2) when the nurse's needs (for attention, affection, and emotional support) are met at the expense of the patient's needs.

Boundaries are necessary to protect the patient. The most extreme boundary violations are those of a sexual nature. This type of violation results in high levels of malpractice actions and the loss of professional licensure on the part of the nurse. Consider the case of the 48-year-old psychiatric nurse who had, in his words, a "loving and sexual relationship" with a 19-year old patient after she was discharged (BBC News, 2014). The licensing board determined that his actions could have resulted in harm due to her clear vulnerability. The board also stated that this serious misconduct was abuse due to the special position of trust he held. The nurse lost his job and his license.

Other boundary issues are not as obvious. Table 8.1 illustrates some examples of patient and nurse behaviors that reflect blurred boundaries.

TABLE 8.1 Patient and Nurse Behaviors that Reflect Blurred Boundaries

When the Nurse is not Involved	When the Nurse is Overly Involved
Patient's increased verbal or physical expression of isolation (depression)	More frequent requests by the patient for assistance, which causes increased dependency on the nurse
Lack of mutually agreed-upon goals	Inability of the patient to perform tasks of which he or she is known to be capable prior to the nurse's help, which causes regression
Lack of progress toward goals	Unwillingness on the part of the patient to maintain performance or progress in the nurse's absence
Nurse's avoidance of spending time with the patient	Expressions of anger by other staff who do not agree with the nurse's interventions or perceptions of the patient
Failure of the nurse to follow through on agreed-upon interventions	Nurse's keeping of secrets about the nurse-patient relationship

Data from Pilette, P. C., Berck, C. B., & Achber, L. C. (1995). Therapeutic management of helping boundaries. *Journal of Psychosocial Nursing and Mental Health Services, 33*(1), 40–47.

Blurring of Roles

Blurring of roles in the nurse-patient relationship is often a result of unrecognized transference or countertransference.

Transference. Sigmund Freud originally identified transference as a phenomenon when he used psychoanalysis to treat patients. **Transference** occurs when the patient unconsciously and inappropriately displaces (transfers) onto the nurse feelings and behaviors related to significant figures in the patient's past. The patient may even say, "You remind me of my [mother, sister, father, brother, etc.]."

Patient: "Oh, you are so high and mighty. Did anyone ever tell you that you are a cold, unfeeling machine, just like others I know?"

Nurse: "Let's talk about a person who is or was cold and unfeeling toward you." *(In this example, the patient is experiencing the nurse in the same way she experienced significant other[s] during her formative years. In this case, the patient's mother was aloof, leaving the patient with feelings of isolation, worthlessness, and anger.)*

Although transference occurs in all relationships, it seems to be intensified in relationships where one person is in authority. This may occur because parental figures were the original figures of authority. Nurses, physicians, and social workers all are potential objects of transference.

This transference may be positive or negative. If a patient is motivated to work with you, completes assignments between sessions, and shares feelings openly, it is likely the patient is experiencing positive transference.

Positive transference does not need to be addressed with the patient. However, the nurse may need to explore negative transference that threatens the nurse-patient relationship. Common forms of transference include the desire for affection or respect and the gratification of dependency needs. Other transferential feelings are hostility, jealousy, competitiveness, and love.

Sometimes patients experience positive or negative thoughts, feelings, and reactions that are realistic and appropriate and *not* a result of transference onto the healthcare worker. For example, if a nurse makes promises to the patient that are not kept, such as not showing up for a meeting, the patient may feel resentment and mistrust toward the nurse.

Countertransference. **Countertransference** is transference in reverse. It occurs when the nurse unconsciously displaces feelings related to significant figures in the nurse's past onto the patient. Frequently, the intense emotions of transference on the part of the patient bring out countertransference in the nurse. For example, you remind your patient of his much loved older sister and he works very hard to please you. In response to this idealization and caring, you experience feelings of tenderness toward the patient and spend extra time with him each day.

Countertransference often results in overinvolvement and impairs the therapeutic relationship. Patients are experienced not as individuals but rather as extensions of ourselves. Example:

Patient: "Well I decided not to go to that dumb group. 'Hi, I'm so-and-so, and I'm an alcoholic.' Who cares?"*(Patient sits slumped in a chair chewing gum, and nonchalantly looking around.)*

Nurse: *(In an impassioned tone)* "You seem to always sabotage your chances. You need AA to get in control of your life. Last week you were going to go, and now you've disappointed everyone."*(In this case, the patient reminds the nurse of her mother, who was an alcoholic. The nurse took it as a personal failure that her mother never sought recovery. The nurse sorts her feelings and realizes the feelings of disappointment and failure belonged with her mother and not the patient. She starts out the next session with the following approach.)*

Nurse: "Look, I was thinking about yesterday, and I realize the decision to go to AA or find other help is solely up to you. Let's talk about what happened to change your mind about going to the meeting."

If the nurse feels either a strongly positive or a strongly negative reaction to a patient, the feeling most often signals countertransference. One common sign is overidentification with the patient. In this situation, the nurse may have difficulty recognizing or objectively seeing patient problems that are similar to the nurse's own. For example, a nurse who is struggling with a depressed family member may feel disinterested, cold, or disgusted toward a depressed patient. Other indicators of countertransference are when the nurse gets involved in power struggles, competition, or arguments with the patient. Table 8.2 lists some common countertransference reactions.

Identifying and working through transference and countertransference issues is crucial in accomplishing professional growth and in helping the patient meet his or her goals. No matter how hard clinicians try to examine their responses objectively, professional support and help are extremely helpful. Supervision by peers or by the therapeutic team can help work through transference and countertransference, as well as numerous other issues. Regularly scheduled supervision sessions provide the nurse with the opportunity to increase self-awareness, clinical skills, and growth, as well as allow for continued growth of the patient.

Self-Check on Boundaries

It is useful for all of us to take time out to be reflective and aware of our thoughts and actions with patients, as well as with colleagues, friends, and family. Fig. 8.2 is a helpful boundary self-test you can use throughout your career, no matter what area of nursing you choose.

A FOCUS ON SELF-AWARENESS

While nurses routinely perform clinical assessments on patients, they are not usually trained to know and understand themselves. In psychiatric nursing, self-awareness is a key component to forming a therapeutic relationship. We all have likes (e.g., sweets or salty food) and areas of interest (e.g., sports and reality shows). We are usually aware of those aspects of our personality and it is fairly simple not to let a difference in what we like interfere with our ability to provide care.

More sacred to us than likes or dislikes are our values and beliefs. These two concepts provide us with a way to conduct ourselves and give life meaning. It is easy to become threatened by others who possess different values and beliefs. It is important to develop awareness and acknowledge then monitor our responses to patients who possess different values and beliefs.

Values are abstract standards and represent an ideal, either positive or negative. It is your judgment of what is important in life. Examples of values are self-reliance, honesty, cleanliness, organization, justice, respect, and a healthy lifestyle. You can probably list those things that you find most personally important and valuable.

Beliefs are another area of self-awareness. They are defined in several different ways. Each of the definitions has relevance to the practice of psychiatric nursing and the therapeutic relationship.

1. An opinion or conviction, something that you hold to be true. For example, "Healthcare is a right for everyone, just like having paved roads." This type of belief may be rational (the earth is round) or irrational or delusional (my brain is being monitored).
2. Confidence, trust, or faith. For example, "I believe that my doctor is the best in her field."
3. Religious tenets, creed, or faith. For example, "It's fine if you celebrate birthdays, but in my religion, we don't."

When working with patients, it is important for nurses to understand that our values and beliefs are not necessarily right and certainly are not right for everyone. It is helpful to realize that our values and beliefs (1) reflect our own culture or subculture, (2) are derived from a range of choices, and (3) are those we have *chosen* for ourselves from a variety of influences and role models. These chosen values stem from religious, cultural, and societal forces. Our values guide us in making decisions and taking actions that we hope will make our lives meaningful, rewarding, and fulfilled.

Working with others whose values and beliefs are radically different from our own can be a challenge. Topics that cause controversy in society in general—including religion, gender roles, abortion, war, politics, money, drugs, alcohol, sex, and corporal punishment—also can cause conflict between nurses and patients. What happens when the nurse's values and beliefs are very different from those of a patient? Consider the following examples of possible conflicts:

- The patient is planning to have an abortion, which is against the nurse's belief that life begins at conception.
- The nurse values cleanliness while the patient believes that showering more than once a week wastes water and harms the environment.
- The nurse believes in feminism and values women's rights. She resents her female patient who wears a hijab (head covering) for religious reasons.
- The patient makes disparaging remarks and uses insulting language about a certain race of people.
- The nurse has a strong religious belief system and thinks that everyone needs the support of a church, whereas the patient does not believe in organized religion.

Self-awareness requires that we understand what we value and those beliefs that guide our behavior. Being self-aware helps us to accept the uniqueness and differences in others.

TABLE 8.2 Common Countertransference Reactions

As a nurse, you will sometimes experience countertransference feelings. Once you are aware of them, use them for self-analysis to understand those feelings that may inhibit productive nurse-patient communication.

Reaction to Patient	Behaviors Characteristic of the Reaction	Self-Analysis	Solution
Boredom (indifference)	Showing inattention. Frequently asking the patient to repeat statements. Making inappropriate responses.	Is the content of what the patient presents uninteresting? Or is it the style of communication? Does the patient exhibit an offensive style of communication? Have you anything else on your mind that may be distracting you from the patient's needs? Is the patient discussing an issue that makes you anxious?	Redirect the patient if he or she provides more information than you need or goes "off track." Clarify information with the patient. Confront ineffective modes of communication.
Rescue	Reaching for unattainable goals. Resisting peer feedback and supervisory recommendations. Giving advice.	What behavior stimulates your perceived need to rescue the patient? Has anyone evoked such feelings in you in the past? What are your fears or fantasies about failing to meet the patient's needs? Why do you want to rescue this patient?	Avoid secret alliances. Develop realistic goals. Do not alter meeting schedule. Let the patient guide interaction. Facilitate patient problem solving.
Overinvolvement	Coming to work early, leaving late. Ignoring peer suggestions, resisting assistance. Buying the patient clothes or other gifts. Accepting the patient's gifts. Behaving judgmentally at family interventions. Keeping secrets. Calling the patient when off duty.	What particular patient characteristics are attractive? Does the patient remind you of someone? Who? Does your current behavior differ from your treatment of similar patients in the past? What are you getting out of this situation? What needs of yours are being met?	Establish firm treatment boundaries, goals, and nursing expectations. Avoid self-disclosure. Avoid calling the patient when off duty.
Overidentification	Having special agenda, keeping secrets. Increasing self-disclosure. Feeling omnipotent. Experiencing physical attraction.	With which of the patient's physical, emotional, cognitive, or situational characteristics do you identify? Recall similar circumstances in your own life. How did you deal with the issues now being created by the patient?	Allow the patient to direct issues. Encourage a problem-solving approach from the patient's perspective. Avoid self-disclosure.
Misuse of honesty	Withholding information. Lying.	Why are you protecting the patient? What are your fears about the patient's learning the truth?	Be clear in your responses and aware of your hesitation; do not hedge. If you can provide information, tell the patient and give your rationale. Avoid keeping secrets. Reinforce the patient with regard to the multidisciplinary nature of treatment.
Anger	Withdrawing. Speaking loudly. Using profanity. Asking to be taken off the case.	What patient behaviors are offensive to you? What dynamic from your past may this patient be re-creating?	Determine the origin of the anger (nurse, patient, or both). Explore the roots of patient anger. Avoid contact with the patient if the anger is not understood.
Helplessness or hopelessness	Feeling sadness.	Which patient behaviors evoke these feelings in you? Has anyone evoked similar feelings in the past? Who? What past expectations were placed on you (verbally and nonverbally) by this patient?	Maintain therapeutic involvement. Explore and focus on the patient's experience rather than on your own.

Data from Aromando, L. (1995). *Mental health and psychiatric nursing* (2nd ed.). Springhouse, PA: Springhouse.

PEPLAU'S MODEL OF THE NURSE-PATIENT RELATIONSHIP

Hildegard Peplau introduced the concept of the nurse-patient relationship in 1952 in her groundbreaking book *Interpersonal Relations in Nursing*. This model of the nurse-patient relationship is well accepted in the United States and Canada as an important tool for all nursing practice. A **professional nurse-patient relationship** consists of a nurse who has skills and expertise and a patient who wants to alleviate suffering, find solutions to problems, explore different avenues to increased quality of life, or find an advocate.

Peplau (1952) proposed that the nurse-patient relationship "facilitates forward movement" for both the nurse and the

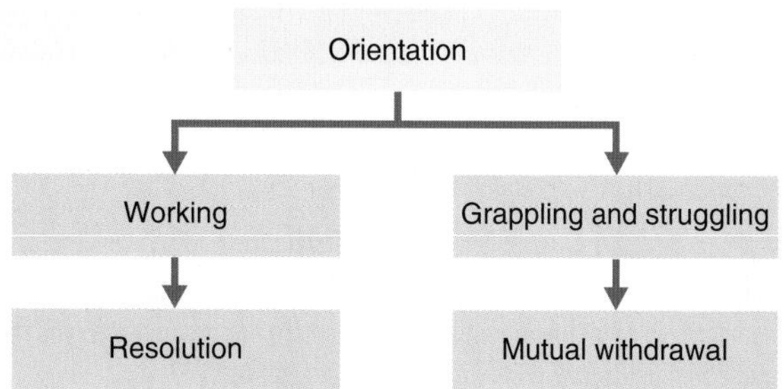

FIG. 8.2 Phases of therapeutic and nontherapeutic relationships. (From Forchuk, C., Westwell, J., Martin, M., Bamber-Azzapardi, W., Kosterewa-Tolman, D., & Hux, M. [2000]. The developing nurse-client relationship: Nurses' perspectives. *Journal of the American Psychiatric Nurses Association, 6*[1], 3–10.)

patient (p. 12). This interactive nurse-patient process is designed to facilitate the patient's boundary management, independent problem solving, and decision making that promotes autonomy.

Peplau (1952, 1999) described the nurse-patient relationship as evolving through three distinct interlocking and overlapping phases. An additional preorientation phase, during which the nurse prepares for the orientation phase, is included. The four phases are as follows:

1. Preorientation phase
2. Orientation phase
3. Working phase
4. Termination phase

Most likely, you will not have time to develop all phases of the nurse-patient relationship in your brief psychiatric-mental health nursing rotation. However, it is important to be aware of these phases to recognize and use them later.

Preorientation Phase

The **preorientation phase** begins with preparing for your assignment. The chart is a rich source of information including mental and physical evaluation, progress notes, and patient orders. You will probably be required to research your patient's condition, learn about prescribed medications, and understand laboratory results. Staff may be available to share more anecdotal information or provide you with tips on how to best interact with your patient.

Another task before meeting your patient is recognizing your own thoughts and feelings regarding this first meeting. Nursing students usually have many concerns and experience anxiety on their first clinical day. These universal concerns include being afraid of persons with psychiatric problems, of saying "the wrong thing," and of not knowing what to do in response to certain patient behaviors. Table 8.3 identifies patient behaviors (e.g., crying, asking the nurse to keep a secret, threatening to commit suicide, giving a gift, or wanting physical contact) and gives examples of possible reactions and suggested responses.

Experienced faculty and staff monitor the unit atmosphere and have a sixth sense for behaviors that indicate escalating tension. They are trained in crisis interventions, and formal security is often available on-site to give the staff support. Your instructor will set the ground rules for safety during the first clinical day. These rules may include not going into a patient's room alone, staying where others are around in an open area, and reporting signs and symptoms of escalating anxiety.

Orientation Phase

The **orientation phase** can last for a few meetings or extend over a longer period. It is the first time the nurse and the patient meet and is the phase in which the nurse conducts the initial interview (refer to Chapter 9). During the orientation phase, the patient may begin to express thoughts and feelings, identify problems, and discuss realistic goals. Specific tasks of the orientation phase follow.

Introductions

The first task of the orientation phase is introductions. The patient needs to know about the nurse (who the nurse is and the nurse's background) and the purpose of the meetings. For example, a student might furnish the following information:

Student: "Hello, Ms. Chang, I am Bob Jacobs, I'm a registered nursing student from Fairlawn University. I am in my psychiatric rotation and will be coming here for the next six Thursdays. I would like to spend time with you on Thursdays until you are discharged. I'm here to be a support person for you as you work on your treatment goals."

Knowing what the patient would like to be called is also essential—names and titles are meaningful to most people. In the previous example, the student began by using a formal title of Ms. Chang. After checking the patient's identification band and reading it out loud, "Dorothy Chang" ask, "What would you like to be called?"

Establishing rapport. A major emphasis during the first few encounters with the patient is on providing an atmosphere in which trust and understanding, or rapport, can grow. As in any relationship, you can nurture **rapport** by demonstrating genuineness, empathy, and unconditional positive regard. Being consistent, offering assistance in problem solving, and providing support are also essential aspects of establishing and maintaining rapport.

Specifying a contract. A contract emphasizes the patient's participation and responsibility because it shows that the nurse does something *with* the patient rather than *for* the patient. The **contract**, either stated or written, contains the place, time, date, and duration of the meetings. You should also discuss termination of the relationship.

Student: "Ms. Chang, we will meet at 10 a.m. each Thursday in the consultation room. We have 45 minutes to discuss the feelings that you have identified. We will also discuss your diagnosis and symptom management, and review your medications. Like I said earlier, we will be able to work together until you are discharged."

Explaining confidentiality. The patient has a right to know (1) who else will be given the information shared with the nurse and (2) that the information may be shared with specific people such as a clinical supervisor, the physician, the staff, or other students in conference. The patient also needs to know that the information will not be shared with relatives, friends, or

TABLE 8.3 Patient Behaviors, Possible Nurse Reactions, and Suggested Nurse Responses

Possible Reactions	Useful Responses
IF THE PATIENT THREATENS SUICIDE	
The nurse may feel overwhelmed or responsible for "talking the patient out of it." The nurse may pick up some of the patient's feelings of hopelessness.	The nurse assesses whether the patient has a plan and the lethality of the plan. The nurse tells the patient that this is serious, that the nurse does not want harm to come to the patient, and that this information needs to be shared with other staff: "This is very serious, Mr. Lamb. I don't want any harm to come to you. I'll have to share this with the other staff." The nurse can then discuss with the patient the feelings and circumstances that led up to this decision. (Refer to Chapter 25 for strategies in suicide intervention.)
IF THE PATIENT ASKS THE NURSE TO KEEP A SECRET	
The nurse may feel conflict because the nurse wants the patient to share important information but is unsure about making such a promise.	The nurse *cannot* make such a promise. The information may be important to the health or safety of the patient or others: "I cannot make that promise. It might be important for me to share it with other staff." The patient then decides whether to share the information.
IF THE PATIENT ASKS THE NURSE A PERSONAL QUESTION	
The nurse may think that it is rude not to answer the patient's question. A new nurse may feel relieved to put off having to start the interview. The nurse may feel put on the spot and want to leave the situation. New nurses are often manipulated by a patient into changing roles. This keeps the focus off the patient and prevents the building of a relationship.	The nurse may or may not answer the patient's query. If the nurse decides to answer a natural question, he or she answers in a word or two, then refocuses back on the patient: **Patient:** Are you married? **Nurse:** Yes. Do you have a spouse? **Patient:** Do you have any children? **Nurse:** This time is for you. Tell me about yourself. **Patient:** You can just tell me if you have any children. **Nurse:** This is your time to focus on your concerns. Tell me something about your family.
IF THE PATIENT MAKES SEXUAL ADVANCES	
The nurse feels uncomfortable but may feel conflicted about "rejecting" the patient or making him or her feel "unattractive" or "not good enough."	The nurse needs to set clear limits on expected behavior: "I'm not comfortable having you touch (kiss) me. This time is for you to focus on your problems and concerns." Frequently restating the nurse's role throughout the relationship can help maintain boundaries. If the patient doesn't stop, the nurse might say: "If you can't stop this behavior, I'll have to leave. I'll be back at [time] to spend time with you then." Leaving gives the patient time to gain control. The nurse returns at the stated time.
IF THE PATIENT CRIES	
The nurse may feel uncomfortable and experience increased anxiety or feel somehow responsible for making the person cry.	The nurse should stay with the patient and reinforce that it is all right to cry. Often it is at that time that feelings are closest to the surface and can be best identified: "You seem ready to cry." "You are still upset about your brother's death." "What are you thinking right now?" The nurse offers tissues when appropriate.
IF THE PATIENT LEAVES BEFORE THE SESSION IS OVER	
The nurse may feel rejected, thinking it was something that he or she did. The nurse may experience increased anxiety or feel abandoned by the patient.	Some patients are not able to relate for long periods without experiencing an increase in anxiety. On the other hand, the patient may be testing the nurse: "I'll wait for you here for 15 minutes, until our time is up." During this time, the nurse does not engage in conversation with any other patient or even with the staff. When the time is up, the nurse approaches the patient, says the time is up, and restates the day and time the nurse will see the patient again.
IF THE PATIENT DOES NOT WANT TO TALK	
The nurse new to this situation may feel rejected or ineffectual.	At first, the nurse might say something to this effect: "It's all right. I would like to spend time with you. We don't have to talk." The nurse might spend short, frequent periods (e.g., 5 minutes) with the patient throughout the day: "Our 5 minutes is up. I'll be back at 10 a.m. and stay with you 5 more minutes." This gives the patient the opportunity to understand that the nurse means what he or she says and is back on time consistently. It also gives the patient time between visits to assess how he or she feels, what he or she thinks about the nurse, and perhaps to feel less threatened.

Continued

TABLE 8.3 Patient Behaviors, Possible Nurse Reactions, and Suggested Nurse Responses—cont'd

Possible Reactions	Useful Responses
IF THE PATIENT GIVES THE NURSE A PRESENT	
The nurse may feel uncomfortable when offered a gift. The meaning needs to be examined. Is the gift (1) a way of getting better care, (2) a way to maintain self-esteem, (3) a way of making the nurse feel guilty, (4) a sincere expression of thanks, or (5) a cultural expectation?	Possible guidelines: If the gift is expensive, the only policy is to graciously refuse. If it is inexpensive, then (1) if it is given at the end of hospitalization when a relationship has developed, graciously accept; (2) if it is given at the beginning of the relationship, graciously refuse and explore the meaning behind the present: "Thank you, but it is our job to care for our patients. Are you concerned that some aspect of your care will be overlooked?" If the gift is money, it is always graciously refused.
IF ANOTHER PATIENT INTERRUPTS DURING TIME WITH YOUR CURRENT PATIENT	
The nurse may feel a conflict. The nurse does not want to appear rude. Sometimes the nurse tries to engage both patients in conversation.	The time the nurse had contracted with a selected patient is that patient's time. By keeping his or her part of the contract, the nurse demonstrates that the nurse means what he or she says and views the sessions as important: "I am with Mr. Rob for the next 20 minutes. At 10 a.m., after our time is up, I can talk to you for 5 minutes."

others outside the treatment team, except in extreme situations. Extreme situations include child or elder abuse and threats of self-harm or harm to others

The nurse must be aware of the patient's right to confidentiality and must not violate that right. Safeguarding the privacy and confidentiality of patients is not only an ethical obligation but a legal responsibility as well.

Working Phase

A strong working relationship allows the patient to safely experience increased levels of anxiety and recognize dysfunctional responses. New and more adaptive coping behaviors can be practiced within the context of the **working phase**. Specific tasks for the nurse in this phase include:

- Gathering further data
- Identifying problem-solving skills and self-esteem
- Providing education about the disorder
- Promoting symptom management
- Providing medication education
- Evaluating progress

During the working phase, the nurse and patient identify and explore areas that are causing problems in the patient's life. Often, the patient's coping methods were developed to survive in a chaotic and dysfunctional family environment. Although coping methods may have worked for the patient at an earlier age, they may now interfere with the patient's functioning and interpersonal relationships.

An important aspect of this working relationship is patient education. In order to facilitate this education you need to become familiar with biological factors (e.g., genetic, biochemical) and also with psychological factors (e.g., cognitive distortions, learned helplessness) that may be the basis of your patients' psychiatric disorders. Understanding psychotropic medication, laboratory work and results, and other treatments is also essential. This knowledge prepares you to help your patients to learn, which in turn prepares them to take an active role in their own care and eventual recovery.

Termination Phase

The **termination phase** is the final, integral phase of the nurse-patient relationship. You discuss termination during the first interview and again during the working stage at appropriate times. Termination may occur when the patient is discharged or when the student's clinical rotation ends. Basically, the tasks of termination include the following:

- Summarizing the goals and objectives achieved in the relationship
- Discussing ways for the patient to incorporate into daily life any new coping strategies learned
- Reviewing situations that occurred during the nurse-patient relationship
- Exchanging memories, which can help validate the experience for both nurse and patient and facilitate closure of that relationship

Termination often awakens strong feelings in both the nurse and patient. Termination of the relationship signifies a loss for both, although the intensity and meaning of termination may be different for each. If a patient has unresolved feelings of abandonment, loneliness, or rejection, these feelings may be reawakened during the termination process. This process can be an opportunity for the patient to express these feelings, perhaps for the first time.

If a nurse has been working with a patient for a while, it is important for the nurse to recognize that separation may be difficult for the patient. A general question—such as "How do you feel about being discharged?"—may provide the opening necessary for the patient to describe feelings.

Part of the termination process is to discuss the patient's plans for the future. If the termination is the result of a discharge, part of these plans have usually been discussed by the psychiatrist or advanced practice nurse including follow-up care and referrals. Registered nurses generally reinforce those plans and emphasize understanding of medications and recognizing when symptoms are getting out of control. Self-help groups can also be encouraged.

FACTORS THAT PROMOTE PATIENTS' GROWTH

Rogers and Truax (1967) identified three personal characteristics of the nurse that help promote change and growth in patients—factors still valued today as vital components for establishing a therapeutic relationship: (1) genuineness, (2) empathy, and (3) positive regard. These are some of the intangibles that are at the heart of the art of nursing and patient-centered care.

Genuineness

Genuineness refers to the nurse's ability to be open, honest, and authentic in interactions with patients. Being genuine is a key ingredient in building trust. When a person is genuine, one gets the sense that what is displayed on the outside of the person is congruent with who the person is on the inside. Nurses convey genuineness by listening to and communicating clearly with patients. Being genuine in a therapeutic relationship implies the ability to use therapeutic communication tools in an appropriately spontaneous manner rather than rigidly or in a parrot-like fashion.

Empathy

Empathy occurs when the helping person attempts to understand the world from the patient's perspective. Essentially it means "temporarily living in the other's life, moving about in it delicately without making judgments" (Rogers, 1980, p. 142).

Ward and colleagues (2012) state that empathy is consistent with improved patient outcomes and increased patient satisfaction with care. However, it does not seem that we are doing a great job of instilling empathy in nursing students. In a study of 214 undergraduate nursing students, empathy actually declined over the course of a year in which students were practicing in the clinical years. These findings are consistent with those of medical students as they progress through years of school. It may be that these once-empathetic students are following the cue of other nurses. What do you think would cause students to demonstrate less empathy?

Researchers have wondered whether empathy can be taught. Chaffin (2010) demonstrated that simulation exercises might help students increase their range and depth of understanding another's experience. Students were asked to listen to a CD with headphones that simulated the voices heard by a person with schizophrenia. These distracting voices were present while their lab partners were performing a mental status exam on them. During this exam, students were annoyed, distracted, frustrated, angry, and overwhelmed.

Students who were subjected to this experiment seemed to empathize more with psychotic patients. After this experience, students were:

- Choosing to interact with more patients on a 1:1 basis
- More willing to wait for patients to answer
- Desiring a therapeutic relationship with patients
- More understanding, focused, and caring

Can the use of clinical simulation provide more depth in understanding and a more lasting impression of patient experience? From this study and others, the answer seems to be yes.

Empathy Versus Sympathy

You may wonder how empathy differs from sympathy. A simple way to distinguish them is that in empathy, we *understand* the feelings of others, and in sympathy, we *feel* pity or sorrow for others. Although these are considered nurturing human traits, they may not be particularly useful in a therapeutic relationship.

The following examples clarify the distinction between empathy and sympathy. A friend tells you that her mother was just diagnosed with inoperable cancer. Your friend then begins to cry and pounds the table with her fist.

Sympathetic response: "I feel so bad for you *(tearing up)*. I know how close you are to your mom. She is such an amazing person. Oh, I am so sorry." *(You hug your friend.)*

Empathetic response: "This must be devastating for you *(silence)*. It must seem so unfair. What thoughts and feelings are you having?" *(You stay with your patient and listen.)*

Empathy is not a technique but rather an attitude that conveys respect, acceptance, and validation of the patient's strengths. Empathy may be one of the most important qualities that a psychiatric-mental health nurse can possess.

Positive Regard

Positive regard implies respect. It is the ability to view another person as being worthy of caring about and as someone who has strengths and achievement potential. Positive regard is usually communicated indirectly by attitudes and actions rather than directly by words.

Attitudes

One attitude that might convey positive regard, or respect, is willingness to work with the patient. That is, the nurse takes the patient and the relationship seriously. The experience is viewed not as "a job," or "part of a course," but as an opportunity to work with patients to help them develop personal resources and actualize more of their potential in living.

Actions

Some actions that manifest an attitude of respect are attending, suspending value judgments, and helping patients develop their own resources.

Attending. Attending behavior is the foundation of a therapeutic relationship. To succeed, nurses must pay attention to their patients in culturally and individually appropriate ways. *Attending* is a special kind of listening that refers to an intensity of presence or being with the patient. At times, simply being with another person during a painful time can make a difference.

Posture, eye contact, and body language are nonverbal behaviors that reflect the degree of attending and are highly culturally influenced. Refer to Chapter 9 for a more detailed discussion of the cultural implications of nonverbal communication.

Suspending value judgments. As previously discussed, we all have values and beliefs. Using our own value systems to judge patients' thoughts, feelings, or behaviors is not helpful or productive. For example, if a patient is taking drugs or is involved in risky sexual behavior, the nurse recognizes that these behaviors are unhealthy. However, labeling these activities as bad or good is not useful. Rather, the nurse should help the patient explore the thoughts and feelings that influence this behavior. Judgment on the part of the nurse will most likely interfere with further exploration.

The first steps in eliminating judgmental thinking and behaviors are to (1) recognize their presence, (2) identify how or where you learned these responses, and (3) construct alternative ways to view the patient's thinking and behavior. Denying judgmental thinking will only compound the problem.

Patient: "I guess you could consider me an addictive personality. I love to gamble when I have money and spend most of my time in the casino. It seems like I'm hooking up with a different woman every time I'm there, and it always ends in sex."

A judgmental response would be:

Nurse A: "So your compulsive gambling and promiscuous sexual behaviors really haven't brought you much happiness, have they? You're running away from your problems and could end up with an STD and broke."

A more helpful response would be:

Nurse B: "So your sexual and gambling activities are part of the picture also. How do these activities impact your life?"

In this example, Nurse B focuses on the patient's behaviors and how they affect his life. Nurse B does not introduce personal value statements or prejudices regarding the promiscuous behaviors, as does Nurse A.

Helping patients develop resources. It is important that patients remain as independent as possible to develop new resources for problem solving. The nurse does not do the work the patient should be doing unless it is absolutely necessary and then only as a step toward helping them act on their own. The following are examples of helping the patient to develop independence:

Patient: "This medication makes my mouth so dry. Could you get me something to drink?"

Nurse: "There is juice in the refrigerator. I'll wait here for you until you get back." *or* "I'll walk with you while you get some juice from the refrigerator."

Patient: "Could you ask the doctor to let me have a pass for the weekend?"

Nurse: "Your doctor will be on the unit this afternoon. I'll let her know that you want to speak with her."

Consistently encouraging patients to use their own resources helps minimize the patients' feelings of helplessness and dependency. It also validates their ability to bring about change.

KEY POINTS TO REMEMBER

- The nurse-patient relationship is the basis of all psychiatric-mental health nursing treatment approaches, regardless of the specific goals.
- Using unique personality traits and talents to promote healing in others is referred to as the therapeutic use of self.
- Counseling is used by psychiatric-mental health registered nurses as a supportive face-to-face process that helps individuals problem-solve, resolve personal conflicts, and feel supported.
- Psychotherapy refers to a group of theoretically based therapies that are used by psychiatric-mental health advanced practice registered nurses.
- A social relationship is a relationship for the purpose of friendship, socialization, enjoyment, or accomplishment of a task. A therapeutic nurse-patient relationship focuses on the patient's needs, thoughts, feelings, and goals.
- Professional boundaries protect patients. Boundaries are the expected and accepted social, physical, and psychological boundaries that separate nurses from patients.
- Boundary blurring may occur on an unconscious level. Transference and countertransference phenomena are operating when boundaries are blurred.
- Values and beliefs influence our conduct and give life meaning. It is important to develop awareness, acknowledge, and then monitor our responses to patients who possess different values and beliefs.
- Peplau's phases of the nurse-patient relationship provide a framework to structure care. They are the preorientation, orientation, working, and termination phases.
- Factors vital for establishing a therapeutic relationship include genuineness, empathy, and positive regard.

CRITICAL THINKING

1. On your first clinical day, you are assigned to work with an older adult, Ms. Schneider, who is depressed. Your first impression is, "Oh, my, she looks like my rude Aunt Elaine. She even dresses like her." You approach her with a vague feeling of uneasiness and say, "Hello, Ms. Schneider. My name is Alisha. I am a nursing student, and I will be working with you today." She tells you that "a student" could never understand what she is going through.
   a. Identify transference and countertransference issues in this situation. What is your most important course of action?
   b. What other information will you give Ms. Schneider during this first clinical encounter? Be specific.
   c. What are some useful responses you could give Ms. Schneider regarding her concern about whether you could understand what she was going through?
2. You are interviewing Tom Stone, a 17-year-old who was admitted to a psychiatric unit after a suicide attempt. How would you best respond to each of the following patient requests and behaviors?
   a. "I would feel so much better if you would sit closer to me and hold my hand."
   b. "I will tell you if I still feel like killing myself, but you have to promise not to tell anyone else. If you do, I can't trust you, ever."
   c. "I don't want to talk to you. I have absolutely nothing to say."
   d. "I will be going home tomorrow, and you have been so helpful and good to me. I want you to have my watch to remember me by."
   e. Tom breaks down and starts sobbing.

CHAPTER REVIEW

Questions

1. Which statement made by either the nurse or the patient demonstrates an ineffective patient-nurse relationship?
   a. "I've given a lot of thought about what triggers me to be so angry."
   b. "Why do you think it's acceptable for you to be so disrespectful to staff?"
   c. "Will your spouse be available to attend tomorrow's family group session?"
   d. "I wanted you to know that the medication seems to be helping me fell less anxious."
2. The patient expresses sadness at "being all alone with no one to share my life with." Which response by the nurse demonstrates the existence of a therapeutic relationship?
   a. "Loneliness can be a very painful and difficult emotion."
   b. "Let's talk and see if you and I have any interests in common."
   c. "I use Facebook to find people who share my love of cooking."
   d. "Loneliness is managed by getting involved with people."
3. Which patient outcome is directly associated with the goals of a therapeutic nurse-patient relationship?
   a. Patient will be respectful of other patients on the unit.
   b. Patient will identify suicidal feelings to staff whenever they occur.
   c. Patient will engage in at least one social interaction with the unit population daily.
   d. Patient will consume a daily diet to meet both nutritional and hydration needs.
4. What is the greatest trigger for the development of a patient's nurse focused transference?
   a. The similarity between the nurse and someone the patient already dislikes
   b. The nature of the patient's diagnosed mental illness
   c. The history the patient has with their parents
   d. The degree of authority the nurse has over the patient
5. Which patient statement demonstrates a value held regarding children?
   a. "Nothing is more important to me than the safety of my children."
   b. "I believe my spouse wants to leave both me and our children."
   c. "I don't think my child's success depends on going to college."
   d. "I know my children will help me through my hard times."
6. Mary is a 39-year-old attending a psychiatric outpatient clinic. Mary believes that her husband, sister, and son cause her problems. Listening to Mary describe the problems the nurse displays therapeutic communication in which response?
   a. "I understand you are in a difficult situation."
   b. "Thinking about being wronged repeatedly does more harm than good."
   c. "I feel bad about your situation, and I am so sorry it is happening to you and your family."
   d. "It must be so difficult to live with uncaring people."
7. A registered nurse is caring for an older male who reports depressive symptoms since his wife of 54 years died suddenly. He cries, maintains closed body posture, and avoids eye contact. Which nursing action describes attending behavior?
   a. Reminding the patient gently that he will "feel better over time"
   b. Using a soft tone of voice for questioning
   c. Sitting with the patient and taking cues for when to talk or when to remain silent
   d. Offering medication and bereavement services
8. A male patient frequently inquires about the female student nurse's boyfriend, social activities, and school experiences. Which is the best *initial* response by the student?
   a. The student requests assignment to a patient of the same gender as the student.
   b. She limits sharing personal information and stresses the patient-centered focus of the conversation.
   c. The student shares information to make the therapeutic relationship more equal.
   d. She explains that if he persists in focusing on her, she cannot work with him.
9. Morgan is a third-year nursing student in her psychiatric clinical rotation. She is assigned to an 80-year-old widow admitted for major depressive disorder. The patient describes many losses and sadness. Morgan becomes teary and says meaningfully, "I am so sorry for you." Morgan's instructor overhears the conversation and says, "I understand that getting tearful is a human response. Yet, sympathy isn't helpful in this field." The instructor urges Morgan to focus on:
   a. "Adopting the patient's sorrow as your own."
   b. "Maintaining pure objectivity."
   c. "Using empathy to demonstrate respect and validation of the patient's feelings."
   d. "Using touch to let her know that everything is going to be alright."
10. Emily is a 28-year-old nurse who works on a psychiatric unit. She is assigned to work with Jenna, a 27-year-old who was admitted with major depressive disorder. Emily and Jenna realize that they graduated from the same high school and each has a 2-year-old daughter. Emily and Jenna discuss getting together for a play date with their daughters after Jenna is discharged. This situation reflects:
    a. Successful termination
    b. Promoting interdependence
    c. Boundary blurring
    d. A strong therapeutic relationship

Answers

1. **b**; 2. **a**; 3. **b**; 4. **d**; 5. **a**; 6. **a**; 7. **c**; 8. **b**; 9. **c**; 10. **c**

Visit the Evolve website for a posttest on the content in this chapter: http://evolve.elsevier.com/Varcarolis

Post-Test interactive review

REFERENCES

BBC News. (2014). *Bodmin Hospital nurse struck off.* BBC News. Retrieved from http://www.bbc.com/news/uk-england-cornwall-25596856.

Chaffin, A. J. (2010). *Use of a psychiatric nursing skills lab simulation to develop empathy in nursing students.* Retrieved from http://www.cinhc.org/wordpress/wp-content/uploads/2009/09/23-Use-of-a-Psychiatric-Nursing-Chaffin.pdf.

Gordon, C., & Bereson, E. V. (2016). The doctor-patient relationship. In T. A. Stern, M. Fava, T. E. Wilens, & J. F. Rosenbaum (Eds.), *Massachusetts General Hospital comprehensive clinical psychiatry* (2nd ed.) (pp. 1–7). Philadelphia, PA: Saunders.

Institute for Patient- and Family-Centered Care. (2010). *Frequently asked questions.* Retrieved from http://www.ipfcc.org/faq.html.

Peplau, H. E. (1952). *Interpersonal relations in nursing: A conceptual frame of reference for psychodynamic nursing.* New York, NY: Putnam.

Peplau, H. E. (1999). *Interpersonal relations in nursing: A conceptual frame of reference for psychodynamic nursing.* New York, NY: Springer.

Rogers, C. R. (1980). *A way of being.* Boston, MA: Houghton Mifflin.

Rogers, C. R., & Truax, C. B. (1967). The therapeutic conditions antecedent to change: A theoretical view. In C. R. Rogers (Ed.), *The therapeutic relationship and its impact.* Madison, WI: University of Wisconsin Press.

Ward, J., Cody, J., Schaal, M., & Hojat, M. (2012). The empathy enigma: An empirical study of decline in empathy among undergraduate nursing students. *Journal of Professional Nursing, 28*, 34–40.

9

Therapeutic Communication

Elizabeth M. Varcarolis

Visit the Evolve website for a pretest on the content in this chapter:
http://evolve.elsevier.com/Varcarolis Pre-Test interactive review

OBJECTIVES

1. Describe the communication process.
2. Identify two personal and two environmental factors that can interfere with communication.
3. Discuss the differences between verbal and nonverbal communication.
4. Identify two attending behaviors the nurse might focus on to increase communication skills.
5. Discuss verbal and nonverbal communication of different cultural groups in the areas of communication style, eye contact, and touch.
6. Relate problems that can arise when nurses are insensitive to cultural influences on patients' communication styles.
7. Identify four techniques that can *enhance* communication, highlighting what makes them *effective.*
8. Identify four techniques that can *obstruct* communication, highlighting what makes them *ineffective.*
9. Summarize the best setting, seating arrangement, and methods for engaging in the nurse-patient interaction.
10. Describe the importance of clinical supervision.
11. Identify the advantages of information communication technologies and some of the concerns.

OUTLINE

KEY TERMS AND CONCEPTS

active listening
closed-ended questions
cultural filters
double-bind messages
feedback
information communication technology
mobile medical applications
nontherapeutic communication techniques
nonverbal behaviors
nonverbal communication
open-ended questions
patient-centered
personal space
telehealth technologies
therapeutic communication techniques
verbal communication

INTRODUCTION

Humans have a built-in need to relate to others. Our advanced ability to communicate with others gives substance and meaning to our lives. All our actions, words, and facial expressions convey meaning to others. It has been said that we cannot *not* communicate. Even silence can convey acceptance, anger, or thoughtfulness. Strong communication is the foundation for happy and productive relationships. On the other hand, ineffective communication within a relationship often results in stress and negative feelings.

In the provision of nursing care, communication takes on a new emphasis. Just as social relationships are different from therapeutic relationships, *basic communication* is different from patient-centered, goal-directed, and scientifically based *therapeutic communication.*

The ability to form patient-centered therapeutic relationships is fundamental and essential to effective nursing care. **Patient-centered** refers to the patient as a full partner in care whose values, preferences, and needs are respected (Quality and Safety Education for Nurses, 2012). Therapeutic communication is crucial to the formation of patient-centered therapeutic relationships. Determining levels of pain in the postoperative patient, listening as parents express feelings of fear concerning their child's diagnosis, or understanding, without words, the needs of the intubated patient in the intensive care unit are essential skills in providing quality nursing care.

Ideally, therapeutic communication is a professional ability you learn and practice early in your nursing curriculum. But in psychiatric-mental health nursing, communication skills take on a different and new emphasis. Psychiatric disorders cause physical symptoms (e.g., fatigue, loss of appetite, insomnia) and also emotional symptoms (e.g., sadness, anger, hopelessness, euphoria) that affect a patient's ability to relate to others.

It is often during the psychiatric rotation that students discover the usefulness of therapeutic communication and begin to rely on techniques they may have once considered artificial. For example, restating sounds so simplistic, you may hesitate to use it:

Patient: "At the moment they told me my daughter would never be able to walk like her twin sister, I felt like I couldn't go on."

Student: *(Restates the patient's words after a short silence)* "You felt like you couldn't go on."

The technique, and the empathy it conveys, is supportive in such a situation. Developing therapeutic communication skills takes time, and with continued practice, you will find your own style and rhythm. Eventually, these techniques will become a part of the way you instinctively communicate with others in the clinical setting.

Saying the Wrong Thing

Nursing students are often concerned that they may say the wrong thing, especially when learning to apply therapeutic techniques Will you say the "wrong thing"? Yes, you probably will. That is how we all learn to find more useful and effective ways of helping individuals reach their goals. The challenge is to recover from your mistakes and use them for learning and growth (Sommers-Flanagan & Sommers-Flanagan, 2013).

Will saying the wrong thing be harmful to the patient? Consider that symptoms of psychiatric disorders—irritability, agitation, negativity, little communication, or being hypertalkative—often frustrate and alienate friends and family. It is likely that the interactions the patient had been having were not always pleasant. Patients tend to appreciate a well-meaning person who conveys genuine acceptance, respect, and concern for their situation. Even if you make mistakes in communication or when you say the "wrong thing," there is little chance that the comments will do actual harm.

Benefits of Therapeutic Communication

Just as social relationships are different from therapeutic relationships, basic communication is different from the professional and goal-directed communication we call therapeutic communication. Research supports the use of this type of communication. Benefits include feeling safer and protected, being more satisfied with the care, increased recovery rates, and improved adherence to treatment (Neese, 2015).

Conversely, poor communication can create serious problems. According to Patient Safety America (2013), as many as 440,000 people die each year from preventable medical errors, representing the third leading cause of death in the United States. The Joint Commission (2012) estimates that 80% of these deaths involve either miscommunication or poor communication techniques. This impaired communication is particularly problematic during patient hand-offs such as change of shift reports.

THE COMMUNICATION PROCESS

Communication is an interactive process between two or more persons who send and receive messages to one another. The following is a simplified model of communication (Berlo, 1960):

1. **Stimulus.** One person has a need to communicate with another for information, comfort, or advice.

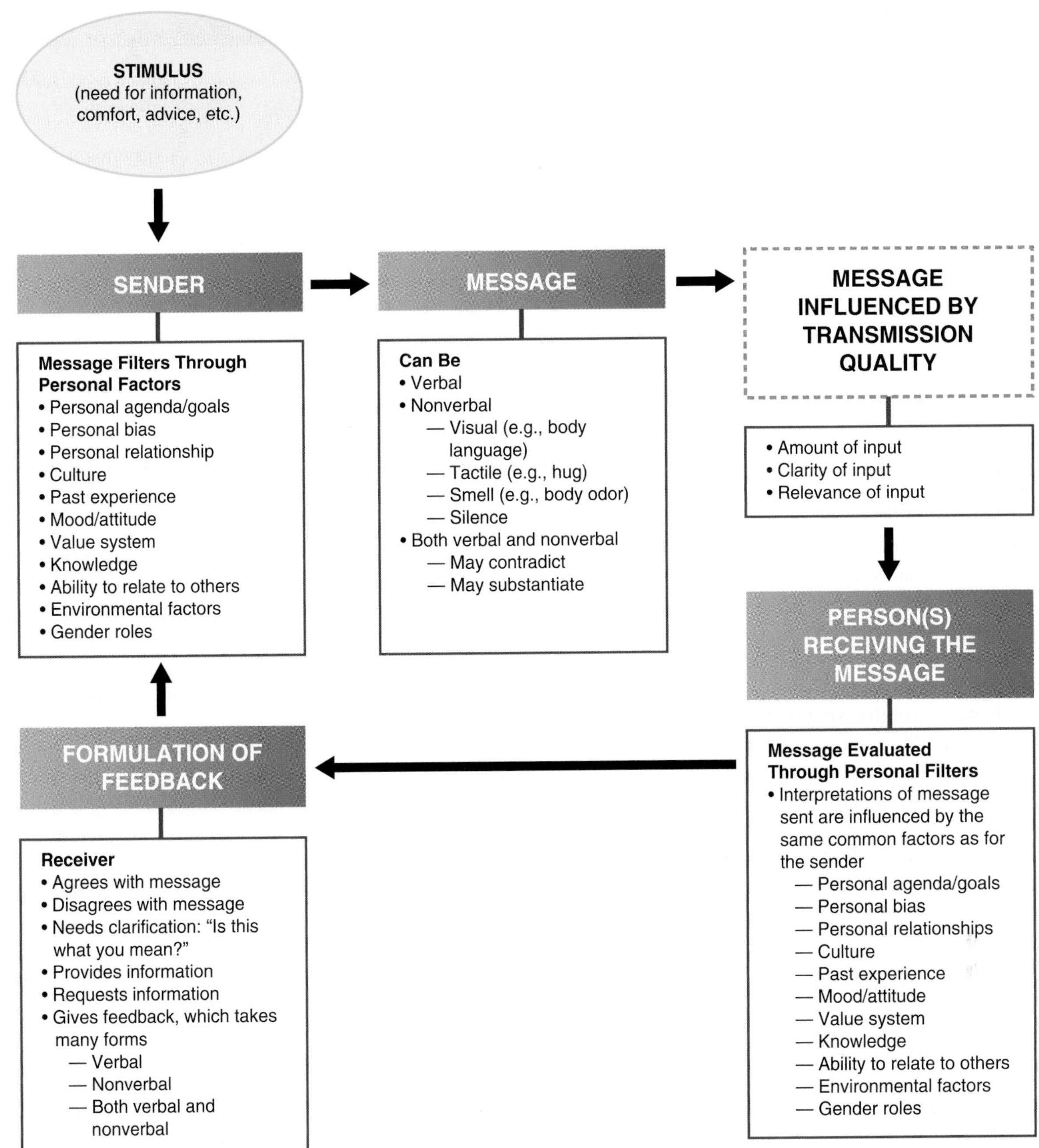

FIG. 9.1 Operational definition of communication. (Data from Ellis, R., & McClintock, A. [1990]. *If you take my meaning*. London, UK: Arnold.)

2. **Sender.** The person sending the message initiates interpersonal contact.
3. **Message.** The message is the information sent or expressed to another. The clearest messages are those that are well-organized and expressed in a manner familiar to the receiver.
4. **Channel.** The message can be sent through a variety of channels, including auditory (hearing), visual (seeing), tactile (touch), olfactory (smell), or any combination of these.
5. **Receiver.** The person receiving the message then interprets the message and responds to the sender by providing **feedback.**

Feedback that validates the accuracy of the sender's message is extremely important. The nature of the feedback often indicates whether the receiver has correctly interpreted the meaning of the message sent. You can check accuracy by simply asking the sender, "Is this what you mean?" or "I notice you turn away when we talk about your going back to college. Is there a conflict there?"

Fig. 9.1 shows this simple model of communication along with some of the many factors that affect it.

Peplau (1952) identified two main principles that can guide the communication process: (1) clarity, which ensures that the meaning of the message is accurately understood by both parties "as the result of joint and sustained effort of all parties concerned," and (2) continuity, which promotes connections among ideas "and the feelings, events, or themes conveyed in those ideas" (p. 290).

TABLE 9.1 Nonverbal Behaviors

Behavior	Possible Nonverbal Cues	Example
Body behaviors	Posture, body movements, gestures, gait	The patient is slumped in a chair, puts her face in her hands, and occasionally taps her right foot.
Facial expressions	Frowns, smiles, grimaces, raised eyebrows, pursed lips, licking of lips, tongue movements	The patient grimaces when speaking to the nurse; when alone, he smiles and giggles to himself.
Eye expression and gaze behavior	Lowering brows, intimidating gaze	The patient's eyes harden with suspicion.
Voice-related behaviors	Tone, pitch, level, intensity, inflection, stuttering, pauses, silences, fluency	The patient talks in a loud sing-song voice.
Observable autonomic physiological responses	Increase in respirations, diaphoresis, pupil dilation, blushing, paleness	When the patient mentions discharge, she becomes pale, her respirations increase, and her face becomes diaphoretic.
Personal appearance	Grooming, dress, hygiene	The patient is dressed in a wrinkled shirt, his pants are stained, his socks are dirty, and he is unshaven.
Physical characteristics	Height, weight, physique, complexion	The patient is grossly overweight, and his muscles appear flabby.

FACTORS THAT AFFECT COMMUNICATION

Personal Factors

Personal factors can impede accurate transmission or interpretation of messages. Patients may have difficulty communicating due to a psychiatric disorder. For example, depression may result in slow thinking and reduced communication, anxiety can cause lack of concentration, and mania creates an inability to focus for any length of time.

Even with an interpreter, language barriers will reduce the normal flow of communication. Cultural differences such as gender-related beliefs (i.e., the role of women in caring for male patients) can negatively impact communication.

Cognitive factors have to be considered when communicating and providing education. Problem-solving ability, knowledge level, and language use are reduced in intellectual development disability, neurocognitive disorders, and psychotic states.

Environmental Factors

Environmental factors within a healthcare setting that may affect communication include physical factors. Background noise, lack of privacy, and uncomfortable accommodations are not conducive to a smooth flow of communication. While units are not as crowded and noisy as they once were, it may still be difficult to carry on a private conversation in the day hall or other common area.

Relationship Factors

For the purpose of this discussion, relationship factors refer to the level of equality within the relationship. When the two participants are equal, such as friends or colleagues, the relationship is symmetrical. However, when there is a difference in status or power, such as between nurse and patient or teacher and student, the relationship is characterized by inequality. One participant has more control. This is called a *complementary* relationship. Usually, the inequality decreases as the patient recovers and as the student progresses and graduates. Complementary relationships also exist based on social status, age or developmental differences, gender differences, and educational differences.

VERBAL AND NONVERBAL COMMUNICATION

Verbal Communication

Verbal communication consists of all the words a person speaks. We live in a society of symbols, and our main social symbols are words. Words are the symbols for emotions and mental images. Talking is our link to one another and the primary instrument of instruction. Talking is a need, an art, and one of the most personal aspects of our private lives. When we speak, we:

- Communicate our beliefs and values
- Communicate perceptions and meanings
- Convey interest and understanding *or* insult and judgment
- Convey messages clearly *or* convey conflicting or implied messages
- Convey clear, honest feelings *or* disguised, distorted feelings

Nonverbal Communication

It is said, "It's not what you say but how you say it." In other words, it is the **nonverbal behaviors** that may be sending the real message through. The tone of voice, emphasis on certain words, and the manner in which a person paces speech are examples of **nonverbal communication**. Other common examples of nonverbal communication are physical appearance, body posture, eye contact, hand gestures, sighs, fidgeting, and yawning. Table 9.1 identifies examples of nonverbal behaviors.

Facial expression is extremely important in terms of nonverbal communication. The eyes and the mouth seem to hold the biggest clues into how people are feeling through emotional decoding. Eisenbarth and Alpers (2011) tracked how long participants looked at various parts of the face in response to different emotions. Participants focused on the eyes more frequently when looking at a sad face. They focused on the mouth more frequently when looking at a happy face. Like sadness, anger was more frequently decoded in the eyes. When presented with either a fearful or neutral expression, there was an equal amount of attention given to both the eyes and the mouth.

Interaction of Verbal and Nonverbal Communication

Many of us may think of communication primarily in terms of what is said. Yet, classic communication research by Mehrabian

(1972) indicates that nonverbal cues are a better predictor of attitudes and feelings than are words. Therefore it comes as no surprise that nonverbal behaviors and cues drastically influence communication. Effective communicators pay attention to verbal and nonverbal cues.

Spoken words represent our public selves and can be straightforward or used to distort, conceal, deny, or disguise true feelings. Nonverbal behaviors include a wide range of human activities, from body movements to facial expressions to physical reactions to messages from others. How a person listens and uses silence and sense of touch may also convey important information about the private self that is not available from conversation alone, especially in consideration of cultural norms.

Some elements of nonverbal communication, such as facial expressions, seem to be inborn and are similar across cultures (Matsumoto & Hwang, 2011). Some cultural groups (e.g., Japanese, Russians) may control their facial expressions in public while others (e.g., Americans) tend to be open with facial expressions. Gender also plays a role in facial expressions. Men are more likely to hide surprise and fear while women control disgust, contempt, and anger.

Other types of nonverbal behaviors, such as how close people stand to each other when speaking, depend on cultural conventions. Some nonverbal communication is formalized and has specific meanings (e.g., the military salute, the Japanese bow).

Messages are not always simple. They can appear to be one thing when in fact they are another. Often, persons have greater conscious awareness of their verbal messages than their nonverbal behaviors. The verbal message is sometimes referred to as the *content* of the message (what is said), and the nonverbal behavior is called the *process* of the message (nonverbal cues a person gives to substantiate or contradict the verbal message).

When the content is congruent with the process, the communication is more clearly understood and is considered healthy. For example, if a student says, "It's important that I get good grades in this class," that is *content*. If the student has bought the books, takes good notes, and has a study buddy, that is *process*. Therefore the content and process are congruent and straightforward, and there is a healthy message. If, however, the verbal message is not reinforced or is in fact contradicted by the nonverbal behavior, the message is confusing. If a student says, "It's important that I get good grades in this class" and does not have the books, skips classes, and does not study, the content and process do not match. The student's verbal and nonverbal behaviors are incongruent.

Messages are sent to create meaning, but people can also use them to hide what is actually going on or to mask their feelings either consciously or unconsciously. One way a nurse can respond to verbal and nonverbal incongruity is to reflect and validate the patient's feelings. For example, the nurse could say, "You say you are upset you did not pass this semester, but I notice you look relaxed. What do you see as some of the pros and cons of not passing the course this semester?"

Bateson and colleagues (1956) coined the term **double-bind messages**. They are characterized by two or more mutually contradictory messages given by a person in power. Opting for either choice will result in displeasure of the person in power. Such messages may be a mix of content (what is said) and process (what is conveyed nonverbally) that has both nurturing and hurtful aspects. The following vignette gives an example.

> **VIGNETTE:** A 21-year-old female who lives at home with her chronically ill mother wants to go out for an evening with her friends. She is told by her frail but not helpless mother: "Oh, go ahead, have fun. I'll just sit here by myself, and I can always call 911 if I don't feel well. You go ahead and have fun." The mother says this while looking sad, eyes downcast, slumped in her chair, and letting her cane drop to the floor.

The recipient of this double-bind message is caught inside contradictory statements, so she cannot decide what is right. If she goes, the implication is that she is being selfish by leaving her sick mother alone, but if she stays, the mother could say, "I told you to go have fun." If she does go, the chances are she will not have much fun, so the daughter is trapped in a no-win situation.

With experience in making observations, nurses become increasingly aware of the verbal and nonverbal communication of the patient. Nurses can compare patients' dialogue with their nonverbal behaviors to gain important clues about the real message. What individuals do may either express and reinforce or contradict what they say. Like the saying "actions speak louder than words," *actions* often reveal the true meaning of a person's intent, whether the intent is conscious or unconscious.

COMMUNICATION SKILLS FOR NURSES

Therapeutic Communication Techniques

Once you have established a therapeutic relationship, you and your patient can identify specific needs and problems. You can then begin to work with the patient on increasing problem-solving skills, learning new coping behaviors, and experiencing more appropriate and satisfying ways of relating to others. Strong communication skills will facilitate your work. These skills are called **therapeutic communication techniques** and include words and actions that help to achieve health-related goals. Some useful techniques for nurses when communicating with their patients are (1) silence, (2) active listening, (3) clarifying techniques, and (4) questions.

Using Silence

Students and practicing nurses alike may find that, when the flow of words stops, they become uncomfortable. They may rush to fill the void with questions or chatter. This response may cut off important thoughts and feelings the patient might be taking time to think about. Silence is not the absence of communication but a specific channel for transmitting and receiving messages. Therefore the practitioner needs to understand that silence is a significant means of influencing and being influenced by others.

In the initial interview, patients may be reluctant to speak because of the newness of the situation and the fact that the nurse is a stranger. Some patients may also be profoundly depressed, distrustful, self-consciousness, embarrassed, or shy. The nurse must recognize and respect individual differences in styles and tempos of responding.

Although there is no universal rule concerning how much silence is too much, silence is worthwhile only as long as it is serving some function and not frightening the patient. Knowing when to speak during the interview largely depends on the nurse's perception about what is being conveyed through the silence. Icy silence may be an expression of anger and hostility.

Silence may provide meaningful moments of reflection for both participants. It provides an opportunity to contemplate thoughtfully what has been said and felt, weigh alternatives, formulate new ideas, and gain a new perspective. If the nurse waits to speak and allows the patient to break the silence, the patient may share thoughts and feelings that would otherwise have been withheld.

It is crucial to recognize that some psychiatric disorders, such as major depression and schizophrenia, and medications may cause an overall slowing of thought processes. This slowing may be so severe that it may seem like an eternity before the patient responds. Patience and gentle prompting can help patients gather their thoughts. For example, "You were saying that you would like to get a pass this weekend to visit your niece."

Conversely, silence is not always therapeutic. Prolonged and frequent silences by the nurse may hinder an interview that requires verbal articulation. Although a less-talkative nurse may be comfortable with silence, this mode of communication may make the patient feel uncomfortable and withhold information. Moreover, without feedback, patients have no way of knowing whether what they said was understood. It is important to point out that children and adolescents in particular tend to feel uncomfortable with silence.

Active Listening

People want more than just a physical presence in human communication. Most people want the other person to be there for them psychologically, socially, and emotionally. In **active listening**, nurses fully concentrate, understand, respond, and remember what the patient is saying verbally and nonverbally.

By giving the patient undivided attention, the nurse communicates that the patient is not alone. This kind of intervention enhances self-esteem and encourages the patient to direct energy toward finding ways to deal with problems. Active listening helps strengthen the patient's ability to solve problems. Serving as a sounding board, the nurse listens as the patient tests thoughts by voicing them aloud. This form of interpersonal interaction often enables the patient to clarify thinking, link ideas, and tentatively decide what should be done and how best to do it.

Clarifying Techniques

Understanding depends on clear communication, which is aided by verifying the nurse's interpretation of the patient's messages. The nurse can request feedback on the accuracy of the message received from verbal and nonverbal cues.

Paraphrasing. Paraphrasing occurs when you restate the basic content of a patient's message in different, usually fewer, words. Using simple, precise, and culturally relevant terms, the nurse may confirm an interpretation of the patient's message before the interview continues. Prefacing statements with a phrase such as "I'm not sure I understand" or "You seem to be saying…" helps the nurse to understand the message in what may be a bewildering mass of details. It helps the patient to feel heard and may provide greater focus. The patient may confirm or deny the perceptions nonverbally by nodding or looking bewildered, or by direct responses, "Yes, that is what I was trying to say" or "No, I meant…"

Restating. Restating is an active listening strategy that helps the nurse to understand what the patient is saying. It also lets the patient know he is being heard. Restating differs from paraphrasing in that it involves repeating the same key words the patient has just spoken. If a patient remarks, "My life is empty…it has no meaning," additional information may be gained by restating, "Your life has no meaning?"

While this is a valuable technique, it should be used sparingly. Patients may interpret frequent and indiscriminate use of restating as inattention or disinterest. Overuse makes restating sound mechanical. To avoid overuse of restating, the nurse can combine restatements with direct questions that encourage descriptions: "What does your life lack?" "What kind of meaning is missing?" "Describe a day in your life that appears empty to you."

Reflecting. Reflection is a means of assisting patients to better understand their own thoughts and feelings. Reflecting may take the form of a question or a simple statement that conveys the nurse's observations of the patient when discussing sensitive issues. The nurse might then describe briefly to the patient the apparent meaning of the emotional tone of the patient's verbal and nonverbal behaviors. For example, to reflect a patient's feelings about his or her life, a good beginning might be, "You sound as if you have had many disappointments."

When you reflect, you make the patient aware of inner feelings and encourage the patient to own them. For example, you may say to a patient, "You look sad." Perceiving your concern may allow the patient to spontaneously share feelings. The use of a question in response to the patient's question is another reflective technique (Arnold & Boggs, 2016). For example:

Patient: "Nurse, do you think I really need to be hospitalized?"

Nurse: "What do you think, Kelly?"

Patient: "I don't know. That's why I'm asking you."

Nurse: "I'll be willing to share my impression with you at the end of this first session. However, you've probably thought about hospitalization and have some feelings about it. I wonder what they are."

Exploring. A technique that enables the nurse to examine important ideas, experiences, or relationships more fully is exploring. For example, if a patient tells you he does not get along well with his wife, you will want to further explore this area. Possible openers include the following:

"*Tell me more* about your relationship with your wife."

"*Describe* your relationship with your wife."

"Give me an example of how you and your wife don't get along."
Asking for an example can greatly clarify a vague or generic statement made by a patient.

Patient: "No one likes me."

Nurse: "Give me an example of one person who doesn't like you."

or

Patient: "Everything I do is wrong."

Nurse: "Let's talk about one thing you do that you think is wrong."

Table 9.2 lists more examples of therapeutic communication techniques.

Questions

Open-ended questions. **Open-ended questions** encourage patients to share information about experiences, perceptions, or responses to a situation. For example:

- "What do you perceive as your biggest problem right now?"
- "What is an example of some of the stresses you are under right now?"
- "How would you describe your relationship with your wife?"

Because open-ended questions are not intrusive and do not put the patient on the defensive, they help the clinician elicit information. This technique is especially useful in the beginning of an interview or when a patient is guarded or resistant to answering questions. They are particularly useful when establishing rapport with a person.

Closed-ended questions. Nurses are usually urged to ask open-ended questions to elicit more than a "yes" or "no" response. However, **closed-ended questions**, when used sparingly, can give you specific and needed information. Closed-ended questions are most useful during an initial assessment or intake interview or to ascertain results as in "Are the medications helping you?" "When did you start hearing voices?" "Did you seek therapy after your first suicide attempt?"

Projective questions. Projective questions usually start with a *"what if"* to help people articulate, explore, and identify thoughts and feelings. They are surprisingly strong in their ability to facilitate a patient's thinking about problems differently and

TABLE 9.2 Therapeutic Communication Techniques

Therapeutic Technique	Description	Example
Silence	Gives the person time to collect thoughts or think through a point.	Encouraging a person to talk by waiting for the answers.
Accepting	Indicates that the person has been understood. An accepting statement does not necessarily indicate agreement but is nonjudgmental.	"Yes." "Uh-huh." "I follow what you say."
Giving recognition	Indicates awareness of change and personal efforts. Does not imply good or bad, right or wrong.	"Good morning, Mr. James." "You've combed your hair today." "I see you've eaten your whole lunch."
Offering self	Offers presence, interest, and a desire to understand. Is not offered to get the person to talk or behave in a specific way.	"I would like to spend time with you." "I'll stay here and sit with you a while."
Offering general leads	Allows the other person to take direction in the discussion. Indicates that the nurse is interested in what comes next.	"Go on." "And then?" "Tell me about it."
Giving broad openings	Clarifies that the lead is to be taken by the patient. However, the nurse discourages pleasantries and small talk.	"Where would you like to begin?" "What are you thinking about?" "What would you like to discuss?"
Placing the events in time or sequence	Puts events and actions in better perspective. Notes cause-and-effect relationships and identifies patterns of interpersonal difficulties.	"What happened before?" "When did this happen?"
Making observations	Calls attention to the person's behavior (e.g., trembling, nail biting, restless mannerisms). Encourages patient to notice the behavior and describe thoughts and feelings for mutual understanding. Helpful with mute and withdrawn people.	"You appear tense." "I notice you're biting your lips." "You appear nervous whenever John enters the room."
Encouraging description of perception	Increases the nurse's understanding of the patient's perceptions. Talking about feelings and difficulties can lessen the need to act them out inappropriately.	"What do these voices seem to be saying?" "What is happening now?" "Tell me when you feel anxious."
Encouraging comparison	Brings out recurring themes in experiences or interpersonal relationships. Helps the person clarify similarities and differences.	"Has this ever happened before?" "Is this how you felt ...?" "Was it something like...?"
Restating	Repeats the main idea expressed. Gives the patient an idea of what has been communicated. If the message has been misunderstood, the patient can clarify it.	*Patient:* "I can't sleep. I stay awake all night." *Nurse:* "You have difficulty sleeping?" *or* *Patient:* "I don't know...he always has some excuse for not coming over or keeping our appointments." *Nurse:* "You think he no longer wants to see you?"

Continued

TABLE 9.2 **Therapeutic Communication Techniques—cont'd**

Therapeutic Technique	Description	Example
Reflecting	Directs questions, feelings, and ideas back to the patient. Encourages the patient to accept his or her own ideas and feelings. Acknowledges the patient's right to have opinions and make decisions and encourages the patient to think of self as a capable person.	*Patient:* "What should I do about my husband's affair?" *Nurse:* "What do you think you should do?" *or* *Patient:* "My brother spends all of my money and then has the nerve to ask for more." *Nurse:* "You feel angry when this happens?"
Focusing	Concentrates attention on a single point. It is especially useful when the patient jumps from topic to topic. If a person is experiencing a severe or panic level of anxiety, the nurse should not persist until the anxiety lessens.	"This point you are making about leaving school seems worth looking at more closely." "You've mentioned many things. Let's go back to your thinking of 'ending it all.'"
Exploring	Examines certain ideas, experiences, or relationships more fully. If the patient chooses not to elaborate by answering no, the nurse does not probe or pry. In such a case, the nurse respects the patient's wishes.	"Tell me more about that." "Would you describe it more fully?" "Could you talk about how it was that you learned your mom was dying of cancer?"
Giving information	Makes facts the person needs available. Supplies knowledge from which decisions can be made or conclusions drawn. For example, the patient needs to know the role of the nurse, the purpose of the nurse-patient relationship, and the time, place, and duration of the meetings.	"My purpose for being here is…" "This medication is for…" "The test will determine…"
Seeking clarification	Helps patients clarify their own thoughts and maximize mutual understanding between nurse and patient.	"I am not sure I follow you." "What would you say is the main point of what you just said?" "Give an example of a time you thought everyone hated you."
Presenting reality	Indicates what is real. The nurse does not argue or try to convince the patient, just describes personal perceptions or facts in the situation.	"That was Dr. Todd, not a man from the Mafia." "That was the sound of a car backfiring." "Your mother is not here; I am a nurse."
Voicing doubt	Expressing uncertainty regarding the reality of the patient's perceptions or conclusions especially in hallucinations and delusions.	"Isn't that unusual?" "Really?" "That's hard to believe."
Seeking consensual validation	Clarifies that both the nurse and patient share mutual understanding of communications. Helps the patient become clearer about what he or she is thinking.	"Tell me whether my understanding agrees with yours."
Verbalizing the implied	Puts into concrete terms what the patient implies, making the patient's communication more explicit.	*Patient:* "I can't talk to you or anyone else. It's a waste of time." *Nurse:* "Do you feel that no one understands?"
Encouraging evaluation	Aids the patient in considering other persons and events from the perspective of the patient's own set of values.	"How do you feel about…?" "What did it mean to you when he said he couldn't stay?"
Attempting to translate into feelings	Responds to the feelings expressed, not just the content. Often termed *decoding.*	*Patient:* "I am dead inside." *Nurse:* "Are you saying that you feel lifeless? Does life seem meaningless to you?"
Suggesting collaboration	Emphasizes working with the patient, not doing things for the patient. Encourages the view that change is possible through collaboration.	"Perhaps you and I can discover what produces your anxiety." "Perhaps by working together, we can come up with some ideas that might improve your communications with your spouse."
Summarizing	Brings together important points of discussion to enhance understanding. Also allows the opportunity to clarify communications so that both nurse and patient leave the interview with the same ideas in mind.	"Have I got this straight?" "You said that…" "During the past hour, you and I have discussed…"
Encouraging formulation of a plan of action	Allows the patient to identify alternative actions for interpersonal situations the patient finds disturbing (e.g., when anger or anxiety is provoked).	"What could you do to let anger out harmlessly?" "The next time this comes up, what might you do to handle it?" "What are some other ways you can approach your boss?"

Adapted from Hays, J. S., & Larson, K. (1963). *Interacting with patients.* New York, NY: Macmillan.

to identify priorities. Projective questions can also help people imagine thoughts, feelings, and behaviors they might have in certain situations (Sommers-Flanagan & Sommers-Flanagan, 2013, p. 5):

- If you had three wishes, what would you wish for?
- What if you could go back and change how you acted in (a situation/significant life event); what would you do differently now?
- What would you do if you were given $1 million, no strings attached?

The miracle question. The miracle question is a goal-setting question that helps patients to see what the future would look like if a particular problem were to vanish. The question should be asked deliberately and dramatically. Here is a sample script from de Shazer (1988, p. 5):

> Now, I want to ask you a strange question. Suppose that while you are sleeping tonight…a miracle happens. The miracle is that the problem that brought you here is solved… When you wake up tomorrow morning, what will be different that will tell you that a miracle has happened?

You can use the miracle question to identify goals that the patient may be motivated to pursue. This very basic question often gets to the source of the most important issues in a person's thinking and life. Try this question out on yourself and see if you find any surprises.

Nontherapeutic Communication Techniques

Although people may use "nontherapeutic" or ineffective communication techniques in their daily lives, they can cause problems for nurses because they tend to impede or shut down nurse-patient interaction. Table 9.3 describes **nontherapeutic communication techniques** and suggests more helpful responses.

Excessive Questioning

Excessive questioning—asking multiple questions (particularly closed-ended) consecutively or rapidly—casts the nurse in the role of interrogator who demands information without respect for the patient's willingness or readiness to respond. This approach conveys a lack of respect for and sensitivity to the patient's needs. Excessive questioning controls the range and nature of the responses, can easily result in a therapeutic stall, or may completely shut down an interview. It is a controlling tactic and may reflect the interviewer's lack of security in letting the patient tell his or her own story. It is better to ask more open-ended questions and follow the patient's lead. For example:

Excessive questioning: "Why did you leave your wife? Did you feel angry with her? What did she do to you? Are you going back to her?"

More therapeutic approach: "Tell me about the situation between you and your wife."

Giving Approval or Disapproval

"You look great in that dress." "I'm proud of the way you controlled your temper at lunch." What could be bad about giving someone a pat on the back once in a while? Nothing, if it is done without conveying a positive or negative judgment. We often give our friends and family approval when they do something well, but giving praise and approval becomes much more complex in a nurse-patient relationship.

A patient may be feeling overwhelmed, experiencing low self-esteem, feeling unsure of where his or her life is going, and desperate for recognition, approval, and attention. Yet when people are feeling vulnerable, a value comment might be misinterpreted. For example:

Giving approval: "You did a great job in group telling John just what you thought about how rudely he treated you."

This message implies that the nurse was pleased by the manner in which the patient talked to John. The patient then sees such a response as a way to please the nurse by doing the right thing. To continue to please the nurse and get approval, the patient may continue the behavior. The behavior might be useful for the patient, but when the patient is doing a behavior to please another person, it is not coming from the individual's own conviction. Also, when the other person the patient needs to please is not around, the motivation for the new behavior might not be there either. Thus the new response really is not a change in behavior as much as an act to win approval and acceptance from another.

Giving approval also cuts off further communication.

More therapeutic approach: "I noticed that you spoke up to John in group yesterday about his rude behavior. How did it feel to be more assertive?"

This opens the way for finding out if the patient was scared, was comfortable, or wants to work more on assertiveness. It also suggests that this was a self-choice the patient made. The nurse gives the patient recognition for the change in behavior and also opens the topic for further discussion.

Giving disapproval implies that the nurse has the *right* to judge the patient's thoughts or feelings. Again, an observation should be made instead.

Giving disapproval: "You really should not cheat on exams even if you think everyone else is doing it."

More therapeutic approach: "Can you give me two examples of how cheating could negatively affect your goal of graduating?"

Giving Advice

We ask for and give advice all the time. Yet, when a nurse gives advice to a patient, the nurse is interfering with the patient's ability to make personal decisions. When a nurse offers the patient solutions, the patient eventually begins to think the nurse does not view him or her as capable of making effective decisions. People often feel inadequate when they are given no choices over decisions in their lives. Giving advice to patients also can foster dependency ("I'll have to ask the nurse what to do about…") and undermine the patient's sense of competence and adequacy.

However, people do need information to make informed decisions. Often, you can help a patient define a problem and identify what information might be needed to come to an informed decision. A useful approach would be to ask, "What do you see as some possible actions you can take?" It is much more constructive to encourage problem solving by

TABLE 9.3 Nontherapeutic Communication Techniques

Nontherapeutic Technique	Description	Example	More Helpful Response
Giving premature advice	Assumes the nurse knows best and the patient can't think for self. Inhibits problem solving and fosters dependency.	"Get out of this situation immediately."	**Encouraging problem solving**: "What are the pros and cons of your situation?" "What were some of the actions you thought you might take?" "What are some of the ways you have thought of to meet your goals?"
Minimizing feelings	Indicates that the nurse is unable to understand or empathize with the patient. Here the patient's feelings or experiences are being belittled, which can cause the patient to feel small or insignificant.	*Patient:* "I wish I were dead." *Nurse:* "Everyone gets down in the dumps." "I know what you mean." "You should feel happy you're getting better." "Things get worse before they get better."	**Empathizing and exploring**: "You must be feeling very upset. Are you thinking of hurting yourself?"
Falsely reassuring	Underrates a person's feelings and belittles a person's concerns. May cause the patient to stop sharing feelings if the patient thinks he or she will be ridiculed or not taken seriously.	"I wouldn't worry about that." "Everything will be all right." "You will do just fine, you'll see."	**Clarifying the patient's message:** "What specifically are you worried about?" "What do you think could go wrong?" "What are you concerned might happen?"
Making value judgments	Prevents problem solving. Can make the patient feel guilty, angry, misunderstood, not supported, or anxious to leave.	"How come you still smoke when your wife has lung cancer?"	**Making observations:** "I notice you are still smoking even though your wife has lung cancer. Is this a problem?"
Asking "why" questions	Implies criticism; often has the effect of making the patient feel defensive.	"Why did you stop taking your medication?"	**Asking open-ended questions; giving a broad opening:** "Tell me some of the reasons that led up to your not taking your medications."
Asking excessive questions	Results in the patient's not knowing which question to answer and possibly being confused about what is being asked.	*Nurse:* "How's your appetite? Are you losing weight? Are you eating enough?" *Patient:* "No."	**Clarifying:** "Tell me about your eating habits since you've been depressed."
Giving approval, agreeing	Implies the patient is doing the *right* thing—and that not doing it is wrong. May lead the patient to focus on pleasing the nurse or clinician; denies the patient the opportunity to change his or her mind or decision.	"I'm proud of you for applying for that job." "I agree with your decision."	**Making observations:** "I noticed that you applied for that job." "What factors will lead up to your changing your mind?" **Asking open-ended questions; giving a broad opening**: "What led to that decision?"
Disapproving, disagreeing	Can make a person defensive.	"You really should have shown up for the medication group." "I disagree with that."	**Exploring**: "What was going through your mind when you decided not to come to your medication group?" "That's one point of view. How did you arrive at that conclusion?"
Changing the subject	May invalidate the patient's feelings and needs. Can leave the patient feeling alienated and isolated and increase feelings of hopelessness.	*Patient:* "I'd like to die." *Nurse:* "Did you go to Alcoholics Anonymous like we discussed?"	**Validating and exploring:** *Patient:* "I'd like to die." *Nurse:* "This sounds serious. Have you thought of harming yourself?"

Adapted from Hays, J. S., & Larson, K. (1963). *Interacting with patients*. New York, NY: Macmillan. Copyright © 1963 by Macmillan Publishing Company.

the patient. At times you might suggest several alternatives a patient might consider (e.g., "Have you ever thought of telling your friend about the incident?"). The patient is then free to give you a yes or no answer and make a decision from among the suggestions.

Asking "Why" Questions

"Why" demands an explanation and implies wrong doing. Think of the last time someone asked you why: "Why did you come late?" "Why didn't you go to the funeral?" "Why didn't you study for the exam?" Such questions imply criticism. We may ask our friends or family such questions, and in the context of a solid relationship, the *why* may be understood more as "What happened?" With people we do not know—especially those who may be anxious or overwhelmed—a *why* question from a person in authority (e.g., nurse, physician, and teacher) can be experienced as intrusive and judgmental, which serves only to make the person defensive.

It is much more useful to ask what is happening rather than why it is happening. Questions that focus on who, what, where, and when often elicit important information that can facilitate problem solving and further the communication process. See Table 9.3 for additional ineffective communication techniques and statements that would better facilitate interaction and patient comfort.

Cultural Considerations

Communicating across culture poses many challenges for healthcare workers. We all need a frame of reference to help us function in our world. The trick is to understand that other people use many other frames of reference to help them function in their worlds. Acknowledging that others view the world quite differently and trying to understand other people's ways of experiencing and living in the world can minimize our personal distortions in listening. Building acceptance and understanding of those culturally different from ourselves is a skill, too.

The US Census Bureau announced that, in 2014, there were more than 20 million children under 5 years old living in the United States, and slightly more than 50% of them were minorities. Healthcare professionals need to be familiar with the cultural meaning of certain verbal and nonverbal communications. Cultural awareness in initial face-to-face encounters with a patient can lead to the formation of positive therapeutic alliances with members of a diverse society. Always assess the patient's ability to speak and understand English well and provide an interpreter when needed.

Unrecognized differences in cultural identities can result in assessment and interventions that are not optimally respectful of the patient and can be inadvertently biased or prejudiced. Healthcare workers need to have knowledge of various patients' cultures and also awareness of their own cultural identities. Nurses' attitudes and beliefs derived from their own cultural background toward those from ethnically diverse populations and subcultures (e.g., alternate lifestyles, different socioeconomic groups, those with disabilities, different ethnic backgrounds, lifestyle differences, the elderly) can greatly impact their ability to be effective healers. Four areas that may prove problematic for the nurse interpreting specific verbal and nonverbal messages of the patient include the following:

1. Communication style
2. Use of eye contact
3. Perception of touch
4. Cultural filters

There is no quick and easy-to-use reference guide for culturally based behaviors, and lists of cultural dos and don'ts are ineffective. Even if it were possible to assemble a truly comprehensive list of facts for each culture, memorizing such information and keeping it straight is unrealistic. The following paragraphs provide useful guidelines. It is important to recognize that there are varying degrees of diversity among and within cultural groups.

Communication Style

Some people may consider it normal to use dramatic body language when describing emotional problems, and others may perceive such behavior as being out of control or reflective of some degree of pathology. For example, within the Hispanic community, intensely emotional styles of communication are often culturally appropriate and expected (Ehrmin, 2015). French and Italian Americans typically show animated facial expressions and expressive hand gestures during communication, which others can easily misinterpret.

In other cultures, a calm facade may mask severe distress. For example, in many Asian cultures, expression of positive or negative emotions is a private affair, and open expression of them is considered to be in bad taste and possibly a weakness. A quiet smile by an Asian American may express joy, an apology, stoicism in the face of difficulty, or even anger. In general, Asian individuals exercise emotional restraint, and interpersonal conflicts are not directly addressed or even allowed (Arnold & Boggs, 2016). German and British individuals also tend to highly value the concept of self-control and may show little facial emotion in the presence of great distress or emotional turmoil.

Eye Contact

Culture also influences the presence or absence of eye contact. Cultural norms dictate a person's comfort or lack of comfort with direct eye contact. Therefore do not use the amount of eye contact to assess attentiveness, judge truthfulness, or make assumptions on the degree of engagement one has with a patient.

Some cultures consider direct eye contact disrespectful and improper. For example, Hispanic individuals have traditionally been taught to avoid eye contact with authority figures such as nurses, physicians, and other healthcare professionals. Avoidance of direct eye contact is a sign of respect to those in authority, but it could be misinterpreted as disinterest or even as a lack of respect.

In Japan, direct eye contact shows a lack of respect and is a personal insult. The preference is for shifting or downcast eyes or focus on the speaker's neck. With many Chinese, gazing around and looking to one side when listening to another is polite. However, when speaking to an older adult, direct eye contact is used (Ehrmin, 2015). Filipino Americans may try to avoid eye contact. However, once it is established, it is important to return and maintain eye contact. In some Middle Eastern cultures, for a woman to make direct eye contact with a man may imply a sexual interest or even promiscuity.

Many Native Americans also believe it is disrespectful or even a sign of aggression to engage in direct eye contact, especially if the speaker is younger. Direct eye contact by members of the dominant culture in the healthcare system can and does cause discomfort for some patients and is considered a sign of disrespect, while listening is considered a sign of respect and essential to learning about the other individual (Ehrmin, 2015).

On the other hand, among German Americans, direct and sustained eye contact indicates that the person listens or trusts, is somewhat aggressive, or, in some situations, is sexually interested. Russians also find direct, sustained eye contact the norm for social interactions (Giger, 2017). In Haiti, it is customary to hold eye contact with everyone but the poor (Ehrmin, 2015). French, British, and many African Americans maintain eye contact during conversation. These cultures may interpret avoidance of eye contact by another person as being disinterested, not telling the truth, or avoiding the sharing of important information. In Greece, staring in public is acceptable (Ehrmin, 2015).

Touch

The therapeutic use of touch is a basic aspect of the nurse-patient relationship and is generally considered a gesture of warmth, support, and consolation. However, the degree to which a patient is comfortable with the use of touch is often culturally determined. People from some cultures, Hispanic for example, are accustomed to frequent physical contact. Holding a patient's hand in response to a distressing situation or giving the patient a reassuring pat on the shoulder may be experienced as supportive and thus help facilitate openness (Ehrmin, 2015). People from Italian and French backgrounds may also be accustomed to frequent touching during conversation, and in the Russian culture, touch is an important part of nonverbal communication, used freely with intimate and close friends (Giger, 2017).

However, some may perceive personal touch within the context of an interview as an invasion of privacy or it may be experienced as patronizing, intrusive, aggressive, or sexually inviting in other cultures. Among German, Swedish, and British Americans, touch practices are infrequent, although a handshake may be common at the beginning and end of an interaction. Chinese Americans may not like to be touched by strangers.

Even among people from similar cultures, the use of touch has different interpretations and rules regarding gender and class. Students are urged to find out if their facility has a "no touch" policy, particularly with adolescents and children who have experienced inappropriate touch and may not know how to interpret therapeutic touch from the healthcare worker.

Cultural Filters

It is important to recognize that it is impossible to listen to people in an unbiased way. In the process of socialization, we develop **cultural filters** through which we listen to the world around us (Egan, 2013). Cultural filters are a form of cultural bias or cultural prejudice that determines what we pay attention to and what we ignore. These cultural filters provide structure for our lives and help us interpret and interact with the world. However, these filters also unavoidably introduce various forms of bias into our communication, because they are bound to influence our personal, professional, familial, and sociological values and interpretations.

We all need a frame of reference to help us function in our world, but the trick is to understand that other people use many other frames of reference to help them function in their worlds. Acknowledging that everyone views the world differently and understanding that these various views impact each person's beliefs and behaviors can go a long way toward minimizing our personal distortions in listening. Building acceptance and understanding of cultural diversity is a skill that you can learn. Chapter 5 has a more in-depth discussion of cultural considerations in nursing.

Information Communication Technologies

Telehealth is the use of electronic information and telecommunication technologies to support long-distance clinical healthcare. It is used primarily to eliminate barriers from the delivery of healthcare services. **Telehealth technologies** include video conferencing, the internet, phone consultation and counseling, image transmission, and interactive video sessions.

Technology does create new challenges. "Particular attention must be directed to confidentiality, informed consent, documentation, maintenance of records, and the integrity of the transmitted information" (American Nurses Association et al., 2014, p. 37).

Telehealth technologies are used as a live interactive mechanism, as a way to track clinical data, and to provide access to people who otherwise might not receive good medical or psychosocial help. These people include those in rural areas and chronically ill, homebound, and underserved individuals.

Information communication technology is a valuable tool for consumers and practitioners to access current psychiatric and medical breakthroughs, diagnoses, and treatment options (Arnold & Boggs, 2016). As information communication technologies advance, it is possible that electronic house calls, internet support groups, and virtual health examination may well be the wave of the future, eliminating office visits altogether.

The use of telehealth technologies allows nurses to monitor patients' vital signs, including lung sounds, and to identify changes in patients' physiological states. Clinicians can conduct remote physical assessment and consults, which are especially helpful in facilities that have limited nursing resources including schools, prisons, health clinics, or rural hospitals.

Technology is being adopted for psychiatric and mental healthcare. Telehealth can be of tremendous value for people with mental health concerns. Often, these mental health issues are not addressed due to fear of stigma, scarcity of mental health providers in remote areas, or lack of transportation. These technologies can be used for telepsychiatric appointments ranging from treating posttraumatic stress disorder and depression to providing wellness and resiliency interventions, especially in rural areas.

FACILITATIVE SKILLS CHECKLIST

Instructions: Periodically during your clinical experience, use this checklist to identify areas where growth is needed and progress has been made. Think of your clinical client experiences. Indicate the extent of your agreement with each of the following statements by marking the scale: *SA,* strongly agree; *A,* agree; *NS,* not sure; *D,* disagree; *SD,* strongly disagree.

1. I maintain good eye contact.	SA	A	NS	D	SD
2. Most of my verbal comments follow the lead of the other person.	SA	A	NS	D	SD
3. I encourage others to talk about feelings.	SA	A	NS	D	SD
4. I am able to ask open-ended questions.	SA	A	NS	D	SD
5. I can restate and clarify a person's ideas.	SA	A	NS	D	SD
6. I can summarize in a few words the basic ideas of a long statement made by a person.	SA	A	NS	D	SD
7. I can make statements that reflect the person's feelings.	SA	A	NS	D	SD
8. I can share my feelings relevant to the discussion when appropriate to do so.	SA	A	NS	D	SD
9. I am able to give feedback.	SA	A	NS	D	SD
10. At least 75% or more of my responses help enhance and facilitate communication.	SA	A	NS	D	SD
11. I can assist the person to list some alternatives available.	SA	A	NS	D	SD
12. I can assist the person to identify some goals that are specific and observable.	SA	A	NS	D	SD
13. I can assist the person to specify at least one next step that might be taken toward the goal.	SA	A	NS	D	SD

FIG. 9.2 Facilitative skills checklist. (Adapted from Myrick, D., & Erney, T. [2000]. *Caring and sharing* [2nd ed., p. 168]. Copyright © 2000 by Educational Media Corporation, Minneapolis, MN.)

Mobile Applications

Mobile phones have been the most rapidly adopted consumer technology in human history (Peek, 2015). In 2014 about 58% of the US population owned a smartphone. Clinicians are increasingly drawn to **mobile medical applications** (apps) as tools to monitor, diagnose, treat, and communicate with patients.

The Substance Abuse and Mental Health Services Administration (SAMHSA) has introduced a line of free apps that can help address some of the toughest mental health and substance use challenges. Three of these apps are:

- **Suicide Safe** helps healthcare providers integrate suicide prevention strategies into their practice and addresses suicide risk among their patients.
- **KnowBullying** provides information and guidance on ways to prevent bullying and build resilience in children. A great tool for parents and educators, KnowBullying is for kids ages 3 to 18.
- **Talk. They Hear You** is an interactive game that can help parents and caregivers prepare for one of the more important conversations they may ever have with children—underage drinking.

Mobile apps are evolving quickly and concerns about privacy and confidentiality issues, lack of data for efficacy and safety, as well and liability issues have been raised. Research is needed to evaluate the risks versus the benefits of these apps. Professional organizations will need to develop professional and ethical guidelines for the use of apps.

Evaluation of Communication Skills

After you have had some introductory clinical experience, you may find the facilitative skills checklist in Fig. 9.2 useful for evaluating your progress in developing interviewing skills. Note that some of the items might not be relevant for some of your patients (e.g., numbers 11 through 13 may not be possible when a patient is experiencing psychosis [disordered thought, delusions, and/or hallucinations]). Self-evaluation of clinical skills is a way to focus on therapeutic improvement. Role-playing can help prepare you for clinical experience and to practice effective and professional communication skills.

THE CLINICAL INTERVIEW

Ideally, the patient decides and leads the content and direction of the clinical interview. The nurse employs communication skills and active listening to better understand the patient's situation.

Preparing for the Interview

Pace

Helping a person with an emotional or medical problem is rarely a straightforward task, and the goal of assisting a patient to regain psychological or physiological stability can be difficult to achieve. Extremely important to any kind of counseling is permitting the patient to set the pace of the interview, no matter how slow or halting the progress may be.

Setting

Effective communication can take place almost anywhere. However, the quality of the interaction—whether in a clinic, a clinical unit, an office, or the patient's home—depends on the degree to which the nurse and patient feel safe. Establishing a setting that enhances feelings of security is important to the therapeutic relationship. A healthcare setting, a conference room, or a quiet part of the unit that has relative privacy but is within view of others is ideal, but when the interview takes place in the patient's home, it offers the nurse a valuable opportunity to assess the patient in the context of everyday life.

Seating

In all settings, arrange chairs so that conversation can take place in normal tones of voice and so that eye contact can be comfortably maintained or avoided. A nonthreatening physical environment for both nurse and patient would involve:

- Assuming the same height, either both sitting or both standing.
- Avoiding a face-to-face arrangement when possible; a 90- to 120-degree angle or side-by-side position may be less intense, and patient and nurse can look away from each other without discomfort.
- Providing safety and psychological comfort in terms of exiting the room. Do not position the patient between the nurse and the door, nor should you position yourself in such a way that the patient feels trapped in the room.
- Avoiding a desk barrier between the nurse and the patient.

Introductions

In the orientation phase, students tell the patient who they are, what the purpose of the meeting is, and how long and at what time they will be meeting with the patient. Bring up the issue of confidentiality during the initial interview. Remember that all healthcare professionals must respect the private, personal, and confidential nature of the patient's communication except in the specific situations outlined earlier (e.g., harm to self or others, child abuse, elder abuse). Do not discuss what is discussed with staff and your clinical group in conference outside with others, no matter who they are (e.g., patient's relatives, news media, friends, etc.). The patient needs to know that whatever is discussed will stay confidential unless permission is given for it to be disclosed. Refer to Chapter 8 to review the nurse's responsibilities in the orientation phase.

Ask the patient how he or she would like to be addressed. This question conveys respect and gives the patient direct control over an important ego issue. Some patients like to be called by their last names while others prefer being on a first-name basis with the nurse.

Initiating the Interview

Once you have made introductions, you can turn the interview over to the patient by using one of a number of open-ended questions or statements:

- "Where should we start?"
- "Tell me a little about what has been going on with you."
- "What are some of the stresses you have been coping with recently?"
- "Tell me a little about what has been happening in the past couple of weeks."
- "Perhaps you can begin by letting me know what some of your concerns have been recently."
- "Tell me about your difficulties."

You can facilitate communication by appropriately offering leads (e.g., "Go on"), making statements of acceptance (e.g., "Uh-huh"), or otherwise conveying interest.

Tactics to Avoid

Certain behaviors are counterproductive and should be avoided. For example:

DO NOT:	TRY TO:
Argue with, minimize, or challenge the patient.	Keep focus on facts and the patient's perceptions.
Give false reassurance.	Make observations of the patient's behavior: "Change is always possible."
Interpret to the patient or speculate on the dynamics.	Listen attentively, use silence, and try to clarify the patient's problem.
Question or probe patients about sensitive areas they do not wish to discuss.	Pay attention to nonverbal communication. Strive to keep the patient's anxiety to a minimum.
Try to sell the patient on accepting treatment.	Encourage the patient to look at pros and cons.
Join in attacks patients launch on their mates, parents, friends, or associates.	Focus on facts and the patient's perceptions. Be aware of nonverbal communication.
Participate in criticism of another nurse or any other staff member.	Focus on facts and the patient's perceptions. Check out serious accusations with the other nurse or staff member. Have the patient meet with the nurse or staff member in question in the presence of a senior staff member/clinician and clarify perceptions.

Helpful Guidelines

Guidelines for conducting the initial interview are suggested by Meier and Davis (2010). In the interview:

- Speak briefly.
- When you do not know what to say, say nothing.
- When in doubt, focus on feelings.
- Avoid advice.
- Avoid relying on questions.
- Pay attention to nonverbal cues.
- Keep the focus on the patient.

Attending Behaviors: The Foundation of Interviewing

Engaging in attending behaviors and actively listening are two key principles of counseling on which almost everyone can agree (Sommers-Flanagan & Sommers-Flanagan, 2013). Positive attending behaviors serve to open up communication and encourage free expression, whereas negative attending behaviors are more likely to inhibit expression. All behaviors must be evaluated in terms of cultural patterns and past experiences of both the interviewer and the interviewee.

Eye Contact

As previously discussed, cultural and individual variations influence a patient's comfort with eye contact. For some patients and interviewers, sustained eye contact is normal and comfortable. For others, it may be more comfortable and natural to make brief eye contact but look away or down much of the time. A general rule of communication and eye contact is that it is appropriate for nurses to maintain more eye contact when the patient speaks and less constant eye contact when the nurse speaks.

Body Language

Body language involves two elements: kinesics and proxemics. *Kinesics* is associated with physical characteristics such as body movements and postures. Facial expressions, eye contact or lack thereof, the way someone holds the head, legs, and shoulders, and so on convey a multitude of messages. A person who slumps in a chair, rolls the eyes, and sits with arms crossed in front of the chest can be perceived as resistant and unreceptive. On the other hand, a person who leans in slightly toward the speaker, maintains a relaxed and attentive posture, makes appropriate eye contact, makes hand gestures that are unobtrusive and smooth while minimizing the number of other movements, and who matches facial expressions to personal feelings or to the patient's feelings can be perceived as open to and respectful of the communication.

Proxemics refers to the study of personal space and the significance of the physical distance between individuals. Proxemics takes into account that these distances may be different for different cultural groups.

- **Intimate distance** in the United States is up to 18 inches and is reserved for those we trust most and with whom we feel most safe.
- **Personal distance** (18 to 40 inches) is for personal communications such as those with friends or colleagues.
- **Social distance** (4 to 12 feet) applies to strangers or acquaintances, often in public places or formal social gatherings.
- **Public distance** (12 feet or more) relates to public space (e.g., public speaking). In public space, one may hail another, and the parties may move about while communicating.

Vocal Quality

Vocal quality, or paralinguistics, encompasses voice loudness, pitch, rate, and fluency. Sommers-Flanagan and Sommers-Flanagan (2013) report that vocal qualities can improve rapport, demonstrate empathy and interest, and add emphasis to words or concepts. Speaking in soft and gentle tones is apt to encourage a person to share thoughts and feelings, whereas speaking in a rapid, high-pitched tone may convey anxiety and create it in the patient. Consider, for example, how tonal quality can affect communication in a simple sentence like "I will see you tonight."

1. "*I* will see you tonight." (I will be the one who sees you tonight.)
2. "I *will* see you tonight." (No matter what happens, or whether you like it or not, I will see you tonight.)
3. "I will see *you* tonight." (Even though others are present, it is you I want to see.)
4. "I will see you *tonight*." (It is definite, tonight is the night we will meet.)

Clinical Supervision and Debriefing

Communication and interviewing techniques are acquired skills. You will learn to increase these abilities through practice and clinical supervision. In clinical supervision, the focus is on your skills within the context of the nurse-patient relationship. The student and clinical faculty have opportunities to examine and analyze the nurse's feelings and reactions to the patient and the way they affect the relationship. Clinical supervision can occur in a one-to-one conversation or as part of a group discussion in postconference.

An increasingly popular method of providing clinical supervision is through debriefing. According to the National League of Nursing (2015), debriefing is such an excellent learning method that it should be incorporated into all clinical experiences. **Debriefing** refers to a critical conversation and reflection regarding an experience that results in growth and learning. Debriefing supports essential learning along a continuum of "knowing what" to "knowing how" and "knowing why."

Process Recordings

A good way to increase communication and interviewing skills is to review your clinical interactions exactly as they occur. This process offers the opportunity to identify themes and patterns in both your own and your patients' communications. As students, clinical review helps you learn to deal with the variety of situations that arise in the clinical interview.

Process recordings are written records of a segment of the nurse-patient session that reflect as closely as possible the verbal and nonverbal behaviors of both patient and nurse. Process recordings have some disadvantages because they rely on memory and are subject to distortions. However, you may find them to be useful in identifying communication patterns.

Sometimes an observing clinician takes notes during the interview, but this practice may be distracting for both interviewer and patient. Some patients (especially those with a paranoid disorder) may resent or misunderstand the student's intent.

Assigning process recordings is becoming less common in schools of nursing. Videotaping clinical simulations in a laboratory setting and subsequent debriefing are becoming the mainstay in nursing education. Psychiatric-mental health simulation experiences are used for students to practice therapeutic communication along with other psychiatric nursing skills such as crisis management and medication administration. A wide range of patient problems such as alcohol and drug use problems, hallucinations, delusions, aggression, and cognitive impairment can be simulated safely in a laboratory setting. After the simulation, debriefing helps students realize what went right and what may have gone wrong.

Table 9.4 gives an example of a process recording.

TABLE 9.4 Example of a Process Recording

Nurse	Patient	Communication Technique	Student's Thoughts and Feelings
"Good morning, Mr. Long."		**Therapeutic.** Giving recognition. Acknowledging a patient by name can enhance self-esteem and communicates that the patient is viewed as an individual by the nurse.	I was feeling nervous. He had attempted suicide, and I didn't know if I could help him. Initially I was feeling somewhat overwhelmed.
	"Who are you, and where the devil am I?" Gazes around with a confused look on his face—quickly sits on the edge of the bed.		
"I am Ms. Rodriguez. I am a student nurse from the college, and you are at Mount Sinai Hospital. I would like to spend some time with you today."		**Therapeutic.** Giving information. Informing the patient of facts needed to make decisions or come to realistic conclusions. **Therapeutic.** Offering self. Making oneself available to the patient.	
	"What am I doing here? How did I get here?" *(Spoken in a loud, demanding voice.)*		I felt a bit intimidated when he raised his voice.
"You were brought in by your wife last night after swallowing a bottle of aspirin. You had to have your stomach pumped."		**Therapeutic.** Giving information. Giving needed facts so that the patient can orient himself and better evaluate his situation.	
	"Oh…yeah." Silence for 2 minutes. Shoulders slumped, Mr. Long stares at the floor and drops his head and eyes.		I was uncomfortable with the silence, but because I didn't have anything useful to say, I stayed with him in silence for the 2 minutes.
"You seem upset, Mr. Long. What are you thinking about?"		**Therapeutic.** Making observations. He looks sad. **Therapeutic.** Giving broad openings in an attempt to get at his feelings.	I began to feel sorry for him; he looked so sad and helpless.
	"Yeah, I just remembered…I wanted to kill myself." *(Said in a low tone almost to himself.)*		
"Oh, Mr. Long, you have so much to live for. You have such a loving family."		**Nontherapeutic.** Defending. **Nontherapeutic.** Introducing an unrelated topic.	I felt overwhelmed. I didn't know what to say—his talking about killing himself made me nervous. I could have said, "You must be very upset" *(verbalizing the implied)* or "Tell me more about this" *(exploring)*.
	"What do you know about my life? You want to know about my family?...My wife is leaving me, that's what." *(Faces the nurse with an angry expression on his face and speaks in loud tones.)*		Again, I felt intimidated by his anger, but now I linked it with his wife's leaving him, so I didn't take it as personally as I did the first time.
"I didn't know. You must be terribly upset by her leaving."		**Therapeutic.** Reflective. Observing the angry tone and content of the patient's message and reflecting back the patient's feelings.	I really felt for him, and now I thought that encouraging him to talk more about this could be useful for him.

KEY POINTS TO REMEMBER

- Knowledge of communication and interviewing techniques is the foundation for developing any nurse-patient relationship. Goal-directed professional communication is referred to as *therapeutic communication.*
- Communication is a complex process. Our communication model has five parts: stimulus, sender, message, medium, and receiver. Feedback is a vital component of the communication process for validating the accuracy of the sender's message.
- A number of factors can minimize, enhance, or otherwise influence the communication process: culture, language, knowledge level, noise, lack of privacy, presence of others, and expectations.

- There are verbal and nonverbal elements in communication. Verbal communication consists of all the words a person speaks. Nonverbal communication consists of the behaviors displayed by an individual, in addition to the actual content of speech. Nonverbal communication is particularly useful in understand feelings and attitudes.
- Communication has two levels: the content level (verbal speech) and the process level (nonverbal behavior). When content is congruent with process, the communication is said to be *healthy.* When the verbal message is incongruent with the communicator's actions, the message is ambiguous.
- Cultural background (as well as individual differences) has a great deal to do with what nonverbal behavior means to different individuals. The degree of eye contact and the use of touch are two nonverbal behaviors that can differ depending on cultures.
- There are a number of therapeutic communication techniques nurses can use to enhance their nursing practices.
- There are also a number of nontherapeutic communication techniques that nurses can learn to avoid to enhance their effectiveness with people.
- Most nurses are most effective when they use nonthreatening and open-ended communication techniques.
- Effective communication is a skill that develops over time and is integral to the establishment and maintenance of a therapeutic relationship.
- Effective/therapeutic communication in nursing points to improved recovery rates, facilitates a sense of protection and safety, improves patient satisfaction, and results in greater treatment adherence.
- The clinical interview is a key component of psychiatric-mental health nursing, and the nurse must establish a safe setting and plan for appropriate seating, introductions, and initiation of the interview.
- Attending behaviors (e.g., eye contact, body language, and vocal qualities) are key elements in effective communication.
- A meaningful therapeutic relationship is facilitated when values and cultural influences are considered. It is the nurse's responsibility to seek to understand the patient's perceptions.
- The application of telehealth information communication technologies in the psychosocial sciences is relatively new but viewed as a valuable tool for helping people with mental health and issues in behavioral health and medicine.

CRITICAL THINKING

1. Keep a written log of a conversation you have with a patient. In your log, identify the therapeutic and nontherapeutic techniques you noticed yourself using. Rewrite the nontherapeutic communications and replace them with statements that would better facilitate discussion of thoughts and feelings. Share your log and discuss the changes you are working on with one classmate.
2. Role-play with a classmate at least five nonverbal communications and have your partner identify the message he or she received.
3. With the other students in your class watching, plan and role-play a nurse-patient conversation that lasts about three minutes. Use both therapeutic and nontherapeutic techniques. When you are finished, have your other classmates try to identify the techniques that you used.
4. Demonstrate how the nurse would use touch and eye contact when working with patients from three different cultural groups.

CHAPTER REVIEW

Questions

1. Which statement made by the nurse demonstrates the best understanding of nonverbal communication?
   a. "The patient's verbal and nonverbal communication is often different."
   b. "When my patient responds to my question, I check for congruence between verbal and nonverbal communication to help validate the response."
   c. "If a patient is slumped in the chair, I can be sure he's angry or depressed."
   d. "It's easier to understand verbal communication that nonverbal communication."
2. Which nursing statement is an example of reflection?
   a. "I think this feeling will pass."
   b. "So you are saying that life has no meaning."
   c. "I'm not sure I understand what you mean."
   d. "You look sad."
3. When should a nurse be most alert to the possibility of communication errors resulting in harm to the patient?
   a. Change of shift report
   b. Admission interviews
   c. One-to-one conversations with patients
   d. Conversations with patient families
4. During an admission assessment and interview, which channels of information communication should the nurse be monitoring? *Select all that apply.*
   a. Auditory
   b. Visual
   c. Written
   d. Tactile
   e. Olfactory
5. What principle about nurse-patient communication should guide a nurse's fear about "saying the wrong thing" to a patient?
   a. Patients tend to appreciate a well-meaning person who conveys genuine acceptance, respect, and concern for their situation.
   b. The patient is more interested in talking to you than listening to what you have to say and so is not likely to be offended.

c. Considering the patient's history, there is little chance that the comment will do any actual harm.
d. Most people with a mentally illness have by necessity developed a high tolerance of forgiveness.

6. You have been working closely with a patient for the past month. Today he tells you he is looking forward to meeting with his new psychiatrist but frowns and avoids eye contact while reporting this to you. Which of the following responses would most likely be therapeutic?
   a. "A new psychiatrist is a chance to start fresh; I'm sure it will go well for you."
   b. "You say you look forward to the meeting, but you appear anxious or unhappy."
   c. "I notice that you frowned and avoided eye contact just now. Don't you feel well?"
   d. "I get the impression you don't really want to see your psychiatrist—can you tell me why?"
7. Which student behavior is consistent with therapeutic communication?
   a. Offering your opinion when asked to convey support.
   b. Summarizing the essence of the patient's comments in your own words.
   c. Interrupting periods of silence before they become awkward for the patient.
   d. Telling the patient he did well when you approve of his statements or actions.
8. James is a 42-year-old patient with schizophrenia. He approaches you as you arrive for day shift and anxiously reports, "Last night, demons came to my room and tried to rape me." Which response would be most therapeutic?
   a. "There are no such things as demons. What you saw were hallucinations."
   b. "It is not possible for anyone to enter your room at night. You are safe here."
   c. "You seem very upset. Please tell me more about what you experienced last night."
   d. "That must have been very frightening, but we'll check on you at night and you'll be safe."
9. Therapeutic communication is the foundation of a patient-centered interview. Which of the following techniques is not considered therapeutic?
   a. Restating
   b. Encouraging description of perception
   c. Summarizing
   d. Asking "why" questions
10. Carolina is surprised when her patient does not show for a regularly scheduled appointment. When contacted, the patient states, "I don't need to come see you anymore. I have found a therapy app on my phone that I love." How should Carolina respond to this news?
    a. "That sounds exciting, would you be willing to visit and show me the app?"
    b. "At this time, there is no real evidence that the app can replace our therapy."
    c. "I am not sure that is a good idea right now, we are so close to progress."
    d. "Why would you think that is a better option than meeting with me?"

Answers

1. **b**; 2. **d**; 3. **a**; 4. **a, b, d, e**; 5. **a**; 6. **b**; 7. **b**; 8. **c**; 9. **d**; 10. **a**

Visit the Evolve website for a posttest on the content in this chapter: http://evolve.elsevier.com/Varcarolis

Post-Test interactive review

REFERENCES

American Nurses Association (ANA), American Psychiatric Nurses Association, & International Society of Psychiatric–Mental Health Nurses. (2014). *Psychiatric–mental health nursing: Scope and standards of practice*. Washington, DC: Nursebooks.org.

Arnold, E. C., & Boggs, K. U. (2016). *Interpersonal relationships: Professional communication skills for nurses* (7th ed.). St. Louis, MO: Saunders.

Bateson, G., Jackson, D., & Haley, J. (1956). Toward a theory of schizophrenia. *Behavioral Sciences, 1*(4), 251–264.

Berlo, D. K. (1960). *The process of communication*. San Francisco, CA: Reinhart Press.

de Shazer, S. (1988). *Clues: investigating solutions in brief therapy*. New York, NY: Norton.

Egan, G. (2013). *The skilled helper: A problem-management approach and opportunity-development approach to helping* (10th ed.). Belmont, CA: Brooks/Cole, Cengage Learning.

Ehrmin, J. T. (2015). Transcultural perspectives in mental health nursing. In M. M. Andrews & J. S. Boyle (Eds.), *Transcultural concepts in nursing care* (7th ed.) (pp. 272–316). Philadelphia, PA: Lippincott Williams & Wilkins.

Eisenbarth, H., & Halpers, G. W. (2011). Happy mouth and sad eyes: Scanning emotional facial expressions. *Emotion, 11*(4), 860–865.

Giger, J. N. (2017). *Transcultural nursing: Assessment and intervention* (7th ed.). St. Louis, MO: Mosby.

Joint Commission. (2012). *Joint Commission Center for Transforming Healthcare releases targeted solutions tool for hand-off communication*. Retrieved from http://www.jointcommission.org/assets/1/6/tst_hoc_persp_08_12.pdf.

Matsumoto, D., & Hwang, H. S. (2011). *Reading facial expressions of emotion. Psychological Science Agenda*. Retrieved from http://www.apa.org/science/about/psa/2011/05/facial-expressions.aspx.

Mehrabian, A. (1972). *Nonverbal communication*. Chicago, IL: Aldine-Atherton.

Meier, S. T., & Davis, S. R. (2010). *The elements of counseling* (7th ed.). Pacific Grove, CA: Brooks/Cole.

National League for Nursing. (2015). *Debriefing across the curriculum*. Retrieved from http://www.nln.org/docs/default-source/about/nln-vision-series-(position-statements)/nln-vision-debriefing-across-the-curriculum.pdf?sfvrsn=0.

Neese, B. (2015). *Effective communication in nursing: Theory and best practices*. Retrieved from http://online.seu.edu/effective-communication-in-nursing/#sthash.hNHpFiV3.dpuf.

Patient Safety America. (2013). A new, evidence-based estimate of patient harms associated with hospital care. *Journal of Patient Safety*, *9*(3), 122–128.

Peek, H. (2015). *Evolving potential of mobile psychiatry: Current barriers and future solutions*. Retrieved from http://www.psychiatrictimes.com/telepsychiatry/technology-psychiatry-year-review?GUID=67CBCF91-8666-442D-9DDD-0FED4DF8E580&rememberme=1&ts=26122015#sthash.0Yr4YTpt.dpuf.

Peplau, H. E. (1952). *Interpersonal relations in nursing: A conceptual frame of reference for psychodynamic nursing*. New York, NY: Putnam.

Quality and Safety Education for Nurses. (2012). *Patient centered care*. Retrieved from http://www.qsen.org/definition.php?id=1.

Sommers-Flanagan, J., & Sommers-Flanagan, R. (2013). *Clinical interviewing* (5th ed.). Hoboken, NJ: Wiley.

Substance Abuse and Mental Health Services Administration. (n.d.). *Get connected with SAMHSA's free mobile apps*. Retrieved from http://www.store.samhsa.gov/apps/.

United States Census Bureau. (2014). *American fact finder*. Retrieved from http://factfinder.census.gov/faces/nav/jsf/pages/index.xhtml.

10

Stress Responses and Stress Management

Margaret Jordan Halter

Visit the Evolve website for a pretest on the content in this chapter: http://evolve.elsevier.com/Varcarolis Pre-Test interactive review

OBJECTIVES

1. Recognize the short- and long-term physiological consequences of stress.
2. Compare and contrast Cannon's (fight-or-flight) and Selye's (general adaptation syndrome) models of stress.
3. Describe how responses to stress are mediated through perception, personality, social support, culture, and spirituality.
4. Assess stress level using the Recent Life Changes Questionnaire.
5. Identify and describe holistic approaches to stress management.
6. Teach a classmate or patient a relaxation technique to help lower stress and anxiety.
7. Explain how cognitive techniques can help increase a person's tolerance for stressful events.

OUTLINE

KEY TERMS AND CONCEPTS

biofeedback
cognitive reframing
coping styles
deep breathing exercises
distress
eustress
fight-or-flight response
general adaptation syndrome (GAS)
guided imagery
humor
journaling
meditation
mindfulness
physiological stressors
progressive relaxation
psychological stressors
relaxation response
stressors

Before turning our attention to the clinical disorders in the chapters that follow, we will explore the important subject of stress. According to the National Institute of Mental Health (2016), stress is simply the brain's response to any demand. Stress is natural, and humans have evolved with a capacity to respond to internal and external demands.

Stress and responses to it are central to understanding psychiatric disorders and providing mental healthcare. The interplay between stress, the development of psychiatric disorders, and the exacerbation (worsening) of psychiatric symptoms has been widely researched.

The old adage "what doesn't kill you will make you stronger" does not hold true with the development of psychiatric disorders. In fact, early exposure to stressful events actually sensitizes people to stress in later life. In other words, we know that people who are exposed to high levels of stress as children—especially during stress-sensitive developmental periods—have a greater incidence of all mental illnesses as adults (Taylor, 2010).

We do not know if severe stress causes a vulnerability to mental illness, or if vulnerability to mental illness influences the likelihood of adverse stress responses. It is most important to recognize that severe stress is unhealthy and can weaken biological resistance to psychiatric pathology in any individual. However, stress is especially harmful for those who have a genetic predisposition to these disorders.

Fig. 10.1 illustrates stress and health across the life span. The model first takes into account nurture (environment) and nature (inborn qualities), responses to stressors (biological and psychological), resultant physiological responses to stressors, and, finally, mental and physical health risks.

While an understanding of the connection between stress and mental illness is essential in the psychiatric setting, it is also important when caring for any patient, in any setting, with any diagnosis. Imagine having an appendectomy and being served with an eviction notice on the same day. How well could you cope with either situation, let alone both simultaneously? The nurse's role is to intervene to reduce stress by promoting a healing environment, facilitating successful coping, and developing future coping strategies. In this chapter, we will explore how we are equipped to respond to stress, what can go wrong with the stress response, and how to care for our patients and even ourselves during times of stress.

RESPONSES TO AND EFFECTS OF STRESS

Early Stress Response Theories

Fight-or-Flight Response

The earliest research into the stress response (Fig. 10.2) began as a result of observations that stressors increased the incidence of physical disorders and made existing conditions worse. **Stressors** are any psychological or physical stimuli or events that provoke a stress response in an organism. Stressors can be acute or chronic and may be external or internal.

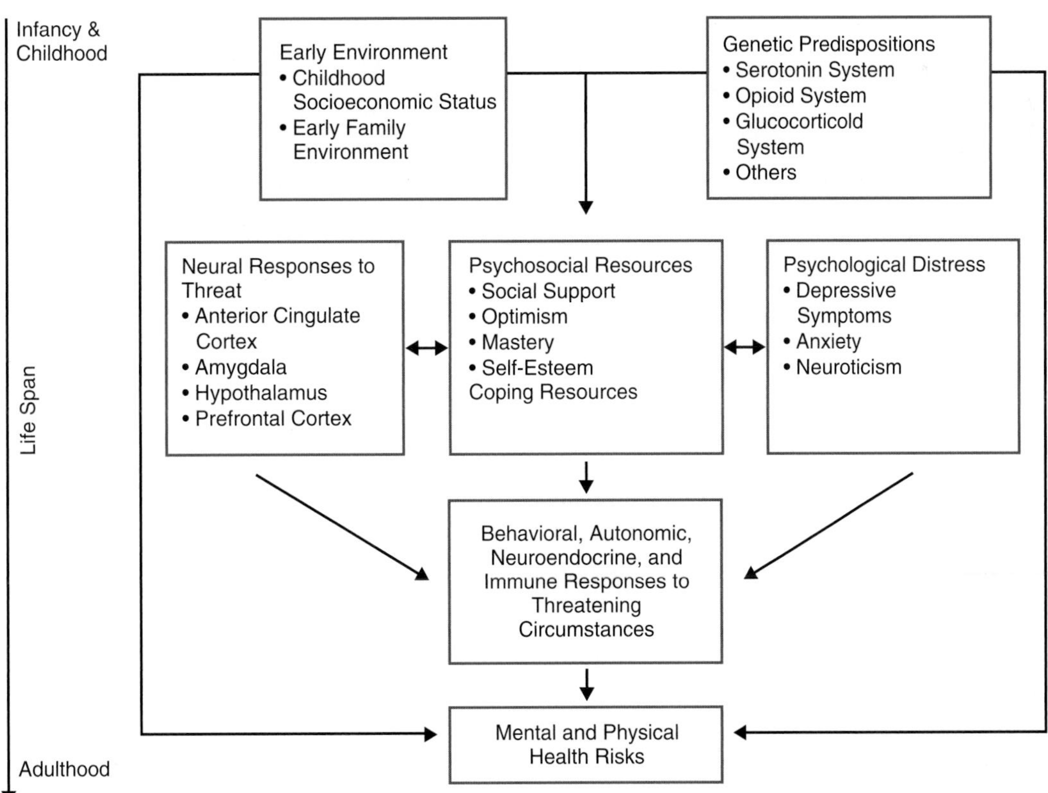

FIG. 10.1 Early life stress and adult mental health outcomes. (From Taylor. S. [2010]. *Mechanisms linking early life stress to adult health outcomes.* Proceedings of the National Academy of Sciences of the United States of America.

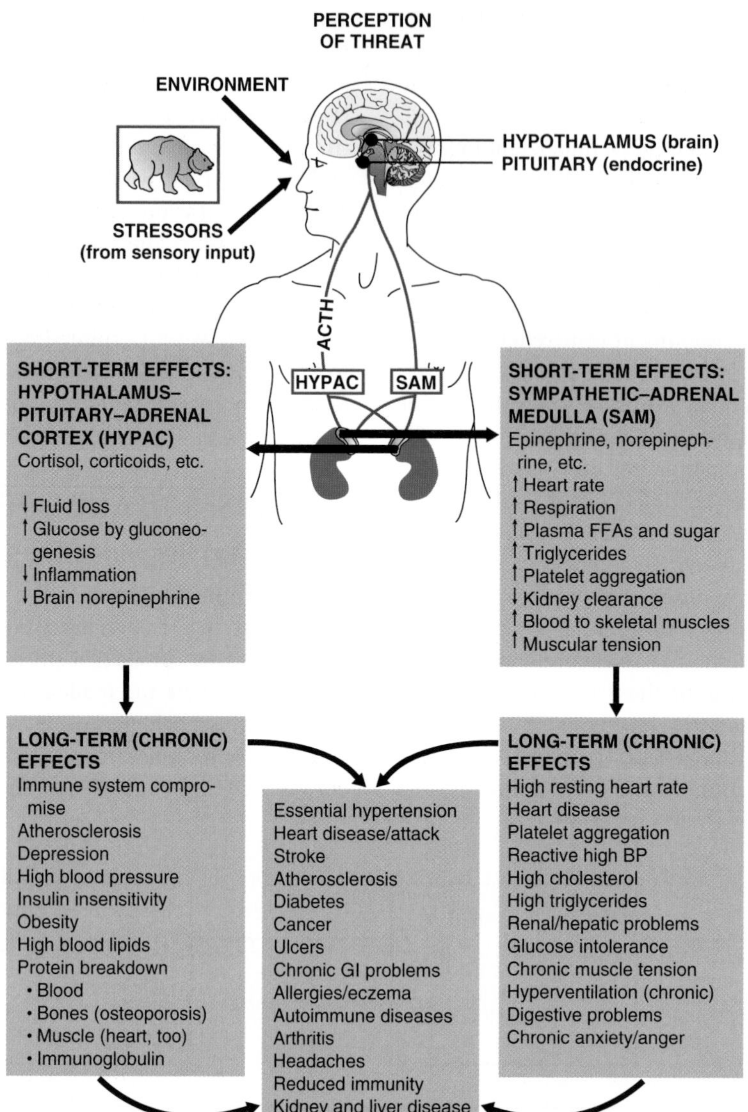

FIG. 10.2 The stress response. *ACTH*, Adrenocorticotropic hormone; *BP*, blood pressure; *FFAs*, free fatty acids; *GI*, gastrointestinal. (From Brigham, D. D. [1994]. *Imagery for getting well: Clinical applications of behavioral medicine.* New York, NY: W. W. Norton.)

Walter Cannon (1871–1945) methodically investigated the sympathetic nervous system in animals in response to stressors. His worked revealed a phenomenon he referred to as an acute stress response, now commonly described with the words *fight* (aggression) *and flight* (withdrawal). The well-known **fight-or-flight response** is the body's way of preparing for a situation an individual perceives as a threat to survival. This response results in increased blood pressure, heart rate, respirations, and cardiac output.

While groundbreaking, Cannon's theory has been criticized for being simplistic, as not all animals or people respond by fighting or fleeing. In the face of danger, some animals become frozen (think of a deer in the headlights) to avoid being noticed or to observe the environment in a state of heightened awareness. Freezing may also happen when you are not sure whether you should fight or flee.

General Adaptation Syndrome

Hans Selye (1907–1982) was another pioneer in stress research who introduced the concept of stress into both the scientific and popular literature. Selye (1936) defined stress as "a nonspecific response of the body to any demand for change." He incorporated Cannon's fight or flight response into an expanded theory of stress known as the **general adaptation syndrome (GAS)**. According to Selye (1974), the GAS occurs in three stages (Fig. 10.3):

1. The *alarm* stage is the initial, brief, and adaptive response (fight or flight) to the stressor. It begins with the eyes or ears sending information such as a car running a light or the sound of a fire alarm to the brain's amygdala. If the amygdala, which processes emotional data, interprets the event as dangerous, it sounds the alarm to the hypothalamus, which responds in two ways:

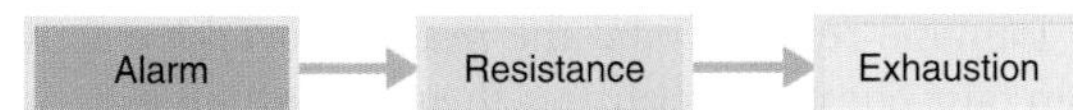

FIG. 10.3 Stages of the general adaptation syndrome.

- *Sympathetic.* The hypothalamus signals through the autonomic nerves to the adrenal glands. The adrenals then pump the catecholamine epinephrine (also known as adrenaline) into the blood stream, thereby activating the sympathetic nervous system. This results in a faster heart rate and increased blood pressure that pushes blood to muscles and the heart. Breathing becomes more rapid and the lungs expand more fully. Extra oxygen is sent to the brain to aid in cognitive processing. All senses including sight (pupils dilate for a broad view of the environment) and hearing become sharper. Glucose is dumped in the bloodstream to supply additional energy. Blood is shunted away from the digestive tract (resulting in a dry mouth) and kidneys to more essential organs.

All of this happens so quickly that most people are not aware of the full scope of the threat. This is why you can jump out of the way of oncoming car before you really realize what is happening.

- *Hypothalamic-Pituitary-Adrenal (HPA) Axis.* As the initial surge of epinephrine subsides, the HPA axis, which is comprised of the hypothalamus, the pituitary, and the adrenal gland, is activated. You can conceptualize this axis as the gas pedal of the system that keeps the system on high alert.

The hypothalamus secretes corticotropin-releasing hormone that stimulates the pituitary to release adrenocorticotropic hormone (ACTH). ACTH travels through the bloodstream to the adrenal cortex. The adrenal cortex then produces extra cortisol to increase blood glucose and muscle endurance. At the same time, other nonessential functions (e.g., digestion) are decreased. Unfortunately, cortisol also impacts the immune system and memory.

The alarm stage is extremely intense, and no organism can sustain this level of reactivity and excitement for long. If the threat subsides, the other part of the autonomic nervous system, the parasympathetic nervous system, slowly puts on the brakes. It allows the body to rest and digest (versus fight or flight) and dampens the stress response. However, if the threat continues, the resistance stage follows.

2. The *resistance* stage could also be called the *adaptation stage* because it is during this time sustained and optimal resistance to the stressor occurs. Usually, stressors are successfully overcome. Recovery, repair, and renewal may occur. At this point individuals have used up valuable resources and have reduced defenses and adaptive energy. If stressors continue, the body remains in a state of arousal and may transition to the final stage of the syndrome.
3. The *exhaustion* stage occurs when attempts to resist the stressor prove futile. At this point, resources are depleted, and the stress may become chronic. The impact of long-term overexposure to cortisol renders people more vulnerable to all kinds of illness.

Bad Stress Versus Good Stress?

Selye also noted that individuals become energized by both negative and positive events. These reactions are *distress* and *eustress:*

- **Distress** is a negative draining energy that results in anxiety, depression, confusion, helplessness, hopelessness, and fatigue. Stressors such as a death in the family, financial overload, or school/work demands may cause distress.
- **Eustress** ("*eu*" is Greek for well or good) is a positive beneficial energy that motivates and results in feelings of happiness, hopefulness, and purposeful movement. Eustress is the result of a positive perception toward a stressor. Examples of eustress are a much-needed vacation, playing a favorite sport, the birth of a baby, or the challenge of a new job. Because the same physiological responses are in play with stress and eustress, eustress can still tax the system, and downtime is important.

Critique of the GAS

Selye's GAS remains a popular theory, but it has been expanded and reinterpreted since the 1950s. Some researchers question the notion of "nonspecific responses" and believe that different types of stressors bring about different patterns of responses and that it is the *degree* of stress that is important (Koolhaas et al., 2011).

Furthermore, the GAS is most accurate in the description of how males respond when threatened. Females do not typically respond to stress by fighting or fleeing but rather by "tending and befriending," a survival strategy that emphasizes the protection of the young and a reliance on the social network for support. Women are more vulnerable to stress-related disorders. This may be due to females being more sensitive to even low levels of corticotropin-releasing hormone, a peptide hormone released from the hypothalamus in response to stress (Bangasser et al., 2010).

Increased understanding of the exhaustion stage of the GAS has revealed that illness results not only from the depletion of reserves but also the stress mediators themselves. For example, people experiencing chronic distress have wounds that heal more slowly. Table 10.1 describes some reactions to acute and prolonged (chronic) stress.

Neurotransmitter Stress Responses

Serotonin is a brain catecholamine that plays an important role in mood, sleep, sexuality, appetite, and metabolism. It is one of the main neurotransmitters implicated in depression, and many medications used to treat depression do so by increasing the availability of serotonin.

During times of stress, serotonin production becomes more active. This stress-activated turnover of serotonin is at least partially mediated by the corticosteroids. Researchers believe this activation may dysregulate or impair serotonin receptor sites and the brain's ability to use serotonin.

Immune System Stress Responses

Cannon and Selye focused on the physical and mental responses of the nervous and endocrine systems to acute and chronic

TABLE 10.1 Some Reactions to Acute and Prolonged (Chronic) Stress

Acute Stress Can Cause	Prolonged (Chronic) Stress Can Cause
Uneasiness and concern	Anxiety and panic attacks
Sadness	Depression
Loss of appetite	Anorexia or overeating
Suppression of the immune system	Lowered resistance to infections, leading to increase in opportunistic viral and bacterial infections
Increased metabolism and use of body fats	Insulin-resistant diabetes
Hypertension	
Infertility	Amenorrhea or loss of sex drive
Impotence, anovulation	
Increased energy mobilization and use	Increased fatigue and irritability
Decreased memory and learning	
Increased cardiovascular tone	Increased risk for cardiac events (e.g., heart attack, angina, and sudden heart-related death)
Increased risk of blood clots and stroke	
Increased cardiopulmonary tone	Increased respiratory problems

stress. Later work revealed that there was also an interaction between the nervous system and the immune system that occurs during the alarm phase of the GAS.

In one study, rats were given saccharine, an artificial sweetener, along with a drug that reduces the immune system (Ader & Cohen, 1975). Afterward, when given *only* the saccharine, the rats continued to have decreased immune responses, contracted bacterial and viral infections, and often died. The taste of the sweetener by itself was sufficient to bring about neural signals in the rats' brains that suppressed their immune systems. This research contradicted the notion that the immune system functioned autonomously, and pointed to a brain-immune system connection.

Researchers continue to find evidence that stress, through the hypothalamic-pituitary-adrenal and sympathetic-adrenal medullary axes, can induce changes in the immune system. This model helps explain what many researchers and clinicians have believed and witnessed for centuries: There are links among stress (biopsychosocial), the immune system, and disease—a clear mind-body connection that may alter health outcomes. Stress may result in malfunctions in the immune system that are implicated in autoimmune disorders, immunodeficiency, and hypersensitivities.

Stress influences the immune system in several complex ways. Stress can enhance the immune system and prepare the body to initially respond to injury by fighting infections and healing wounds. Immune cells normally release cytokines, which are proteins and glycoproteins used for communication between cells, when a pathogen is detected. Cytokines activate and recruit other immune cells. During times of stress, these cytokines are released, and the immune system is activated. The activation is limited because the cytokines stimulate further release of corticosteroids, which inhibits the immune system.

The immune response and the resulting cytokine activity in the brain raise questions regarding their connection with psychological and cognitive states such as depression. Researchers have found significantly higher concentrations of cytokines that cause systemic inflammation in depressed subjects compared with control subjects (Dahl et al., 2014). Recovery from depression is associated with reduction to normal levels of most of the cytokines.

Cancer patients are often treated with cytokine molecules known as *interleukins*. Unfortunately, but understandably, these chemotherapy drugs tend to cause or increase depression (National Cancer Institute, 2015).

Research in this field is promising. Investigators are examining how psychosocial factors, such as optimism and social support, moderate the stress response. They are mapping the biological and cellular mechanisms by which stress affects the immune system and are testing new theories.

Fig. 10.4 illustrates the effects of stress on the body.

MEDIATORS OF THE STRESS RESPONSE

Stressors

Many situations such as emotional arousal, fatigue, fear, humiliation, loss of blood, extreme happiness, or unexpected success are capable of producing stress and triggering the stress response (Selye, 1993). Stressors can be divided into two broad categories: physiological and psychological.

Physiological stressors include environmental conditions (e.g., trauma and excessive cold or heat) and physical conditions (e.g., infection, hemorrhage, hunger, and pain). **Psychological stressors** include such events as divorce, loss of a job, unmanageable debt, the death of a loved one, retirement, and fear of a terrorist attack. Psychological stressors also include changes we consider positive such as marriage, the arrival of a new baby, or unexpected success.

Perception

Have you ever noticed that something that upsets your friend doesn't bother you at all? Or that your professor's habit of going over the scheduled class time drives you up a wall, yet (to your annoyance) your best friend doesn't seem to notice? It is not always the stressor itself that determines a response, but it is the *perception* of the stressor that determines the person's emotional and psychological reactions to it.

The way that we perceive stressors is affected by factors such as age, gender, culture, life experience, and lifestyle. All of these factors may work to either lessen or increase the degree of emotional or physical influence and the sequelae (consequence or result) of stress. For example, a man in his 40s who has a new baby, a new home, and gets laid off may feel more stress than a man in his 60s who is financially secure and is asked to take an early retirement.

Individual Temperament

As mentioned earlier, part of the response to stressors is based on our own individual perceptions. These perceptions are colored by a variety of factors including genetic structure and vulnerability, childhood experiences, coping strategies, and

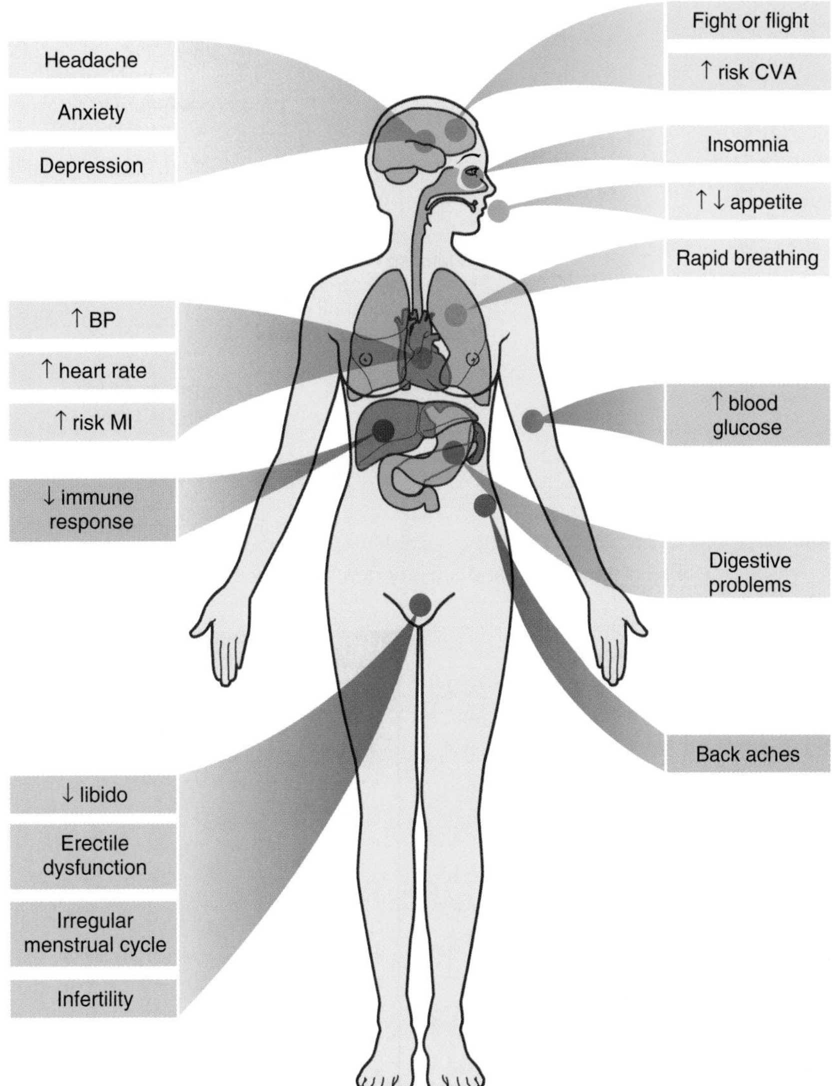

FIG. 10.4 Effects of stress on the body.

personal outlook on life and the world. All these factors combine to form a unique personality with specific strengths and vulnerabilities.

Social Support

The benefit of social support cannot be emphasized enough, whether it is for you or for your patients. Humans once lived in close communities with extended family sharing the same living quarters. Essentially, neighbors were the therapists of the past. Suburban life often results in isolated living spaces where neighbors interact sporadically. In fact, you may not even know your neighbors. People in crowded cities may also live in isolation where eye contact and communication may be considered an invasion of privacy.

Strong social support from significant others can enhance mental and physical health and act as a substantial buffer against distress. A shared identity—whether with a family, social network, religious group, or colleagues—helps people overcome stressors more adaptively. Researchers have found a strong correlation between lower mortality rates and intact support systems (Cruces et al., 2014). People, and even animals, without social companionship risk early death and have higher rates of illness.

Support Groups

The proliferation of self-help groups attests to the need for social supports. Many of the support groups currently available are for people going through similar stressful life events: Alcoholics Anonymous (a prototype for 12-step programs), Gamblers Anonymous, Reach for Recovery (for cancer patients), and Parents Without Partners to note a few. Online support groups provide cost-effective, anonymous, and easily accessible self-help for people with every disorder imaginable. A Google search for online + support + groups yielded nearly 60 million hits. There has to be a group out there for everyone, although quality and fit are always factors to be considered.

Culture

Each culture not only emphasizes certain problems of living more than others but also interprets emotional problems differently. Although Western European and North American

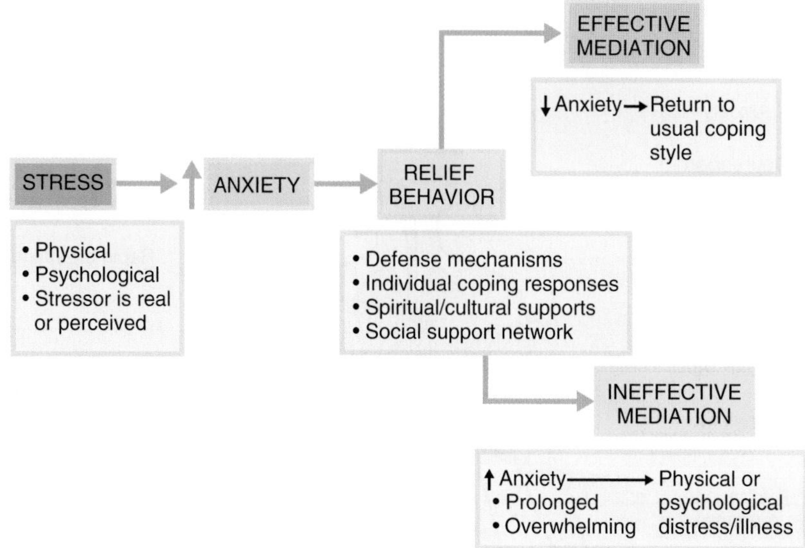

FIG. 10.5 Stress and anxiety operationally defined.

cultures tend to subscribe to a psychophysiological view of stress and somatic distress, this is not the dominant view in other cultures. The overwhelming majority of Asians, Africans, and Central Americans tend to express distress in somatic terms and actually experience it physically.

Spirituality and Religion

Spirituality and religious affiliation help people cope with stress. Studies have demonstrated that spiritual practices can even enhance the immune system and sense of well-being (Koenig et al., 2012). Spiritual well-being helps people deal with health issues, primarily because spiritual beliefs help people cope with issues of living. People who include spiritual solutions to physical or mental distress often gain a sense of comfort and support that can aid in healing and lowering stress. Even prayer, in and of itself, can elicit the relaxation response (discussed later in this chapter) known to reduce stress physically and emotionally and to reduce the impact of stress on the immune system.

For many people, religious beliefs promote hope and optimism. Organized religious groups provide structure and may promote a feeling of belonging. Beyond coming together as a congregation to listen to a sermon or take part in religious rites, religious groups are an important social outlet. As we discussed earlier, social support is an essential mediator to the stress response.

Fig. 10.5 operationally defines the process of stress and the positive or negative results of attempts to relieve stress, and Box 10.1 identifies several stress busters that can be incorporated into our lives with little effort.

NURSING MANAGEMENT OF STRESS RESPONSES

Measuring Stress

In 1967, psychiatrists Holmes and Rahe developed the Social Readjustment Scale. This life-change scale measures positive or

BOX 10.1 Effective Stress Busters

Sleep
- 7 to 9 hours of sleep is recommended.
- Try going to sleep 30 to 60 minutes early each night for a few weeks.
- Sleeping later in the morning is not helpful and can disrupt body rhythms.
- Invest in a tracker that can monitor sleep and make adjustments based on the data it provides.

Exercise (Aerobic)
- 150 minutes a week (about 20 minutes a day) of moderate intensity aerobic activity such as walking is recommended.
- Reduces chronic and acute stress.
- Decreases levels of anxiety, depression, and sensitivity to stress.
- Decreases muscle tension and increases endorphin levels.
- Exercise at least 3 hours before bedtime to prevent sleep disruption.

Reduction or Cessation of Caffeine Intake
- No more than four cups of coffee or colas are recommended for anyone.
- Overuse or sensitivity may cause insomnia, nervousness, restlessness, irritability, stomach upset, rapid heartbeat, muscle tremors, and shakiness.
- Slowly wean off coffee, tea, colas, and chocolate drinks.

Music
- Listening to familiar music promotes relaxation.
- Rates of healing may be improved with music.
- Music can decrease agitation and confusion in older adults.
- Quality of life in hospice settings is enhanced by music.

Pets
- Can bring joy and reduce stress.
- May provide real social support.
- Alleviate medical problems aggravated by stress.

Massage
- Slows the heart rate and relaxes the body.
- Improves alertness by reducing anxiety.

TABLE 10.2 Perception of Life Stressors in 1967 and 2007

Life Change Event	1967	2007
Death of spouse	100	80
Death of family member	63	70
Divorce/separation	73/65	66
Job lay off or firing	47	62
Birth of child/pregnancy	40	60
Death of friend	50	50
Marriage	50	50
Retirement	45	49
Marital reconciliation	45	48
Change job field	36	47
Child leaves home	29	43

Data from First30Days. (2008). *Making changes today considered more difficult to handle than 40 years ago.* Retrieved from http://www.first30days.com/pages/press_changereport.html.

negative life events. Each life-change event is assigned a weight depending on its severity. For example, the death of a child was rated significantly higher than attending college. The purpose of the scale is to assess the person's vulnerability to stress-related disorders.

Since the scale was developed in 1967, perceptions of stress changed. To more accurately measure life change events, 1306 online participants were collected and then compared with data collected in the original study (First30Days, 2008). Although some life-change events were viewed as more stressful in 1967, most events were viewed as more stressful in 2007 (Table 10.2).

Take a few minutes to assess your stress level for the past 6 or 12 months using the Recent Life Changes Questionnaire, a revised version of the Social Readjustment Scale (Table 10.3). A 6-month score of 300 or more, or a year score of 500 or more,

TABLE 10.3 Recent Life Changes Questionnaire

Life-Changing Event	Life Change Unit*
Health	
An injury or illness that:	
Kept you in bed a week or more or sent you to the hospital	74
Was less serious than above	44
Major dental work	26
Major change in eating habits	27
Major change in sleeping habits	26
Major change in your usual type and/or amount of recreation	28
Work	
Change to a new type of work	51
Change in your work hours or conditions	35
Change in your responsibilities at work:	
More responsibilities	29
Fewer responsibilities	21
Promotion	31
Demotion	42
Transfer	32
Troubles at work:	
With your boss	29
With co-workers	35
With persons under your supervision	35
Other work troubles	28
Major business adjustment	60
Retirement	52
Loss of job:	
Laid off from work	68
Fired from work	79
Correspondence course to help you in your work	18
Home and Family	
Major change in living conditions	42
Change in residence:	
Move within the same town or city	25
Move to a different town, city, or state	47
Change in family get-togethers	25
Major change in health or behavior of family member	55
Marriage	50
Pregnancy	67
Miscarriage or abortion	65
Gain of a new family member:	
Birth of a child	66
Adoption of a child	65
A relative moving in with you	59
Spouse beginning or ending work	46
Child leaving home:	
To attend college	41
Due to marriage	41
For other reasons	45
Change in arguments with spouse	50
In-law problems	38
Change in the marital status of your parents:	
Divorce	59
Remarriage	50
Separation from spouse:	
Due to work	53
Due to marital problems	76
Divorce	96
Birth of grandchild	43
Death of spouse	119
Death of other family member:	
Child	123
Brother or sister	102
Parent	100

Continued

TABLE 10.3 Recent Life Changes Questionnaire—cont'd

Life-Changing Event	Life Change Unit*	Life-Changing Event	Life Change Unit*
Personal and Social		Being held in jail	75
Change in personal habits	26	Death of a close friend	70
Beginning or ending of school or college	38	Major decision regarding your immediate future	51
Change of school or college	35	Major personal achievement	36
Change in political beliefs	24		
Change in religious beliefs	29	**Financial**	
Change in social activities	27	**Major change in finances:**	
Vacation	24	Increase in income	38
New close personal relationship	37	Decrease in income	60
Engagement to marry	45	Investment and/or credit difficulties	56
Girlfriend or boyfriend problems	39	Loss or damage of personal property	43
Sexual differences	44	Moderate purchase	20
"Falling out" of a close personal relationship	47	Major purchase	37
An accident	48	Foreclosure on a mortgage or loan	58
Minor violation of the law	20		

*One-year totals ≥ 500 life change units are considered indications of high recent life stress.
From Miller, M. A., & Rahe, R. H. (1997). Life changes scaling for the 1990s. *Journal of Psychosomatic Research, 43*(3), 279–292.

indicates high stress. When you self-administer the questionnaire, take into account the following:

- Not all events are perceived to have the same degree of intensity or disruptiveness.
- Culture may dictate whether or not an event is stressful or how stressful it is.
- Different people may have different thresholds beyond which disruptions occur.
- The questionnaire equates change with stress.

Other stress scales that may be useful to nursing students have been developed. You might want to try the Perceived Stress Scale, a popular scale that measures perceived stress (Fig. 10.6). Although there are no absolute scores, this scale measures how relatively uncontrollable, unpredictable, and overloaded you find your life. You might try this scale alone or suggest that it be used in a clinical post-conference for comparison and discussion.

Assessing Coping Styles

People cope with life stressors in a variety of ways, and a number of factors can act as effective mediators to decrease stress in our lives. Four personal attributes (**coping styles**) people can develop to help manage stress:

1. Health-sustaining habits (e.g., medical compliance, proper diet, relaxation, pacing one's energy)
2. Life satisfactions (e.g., work, family, hobbies, humor, spiritual solace, arts, nature)
3. Social supports
4. Effective and healthy responses to stress

Examining these four coping categories can help nurses identify areas to target for improving their patients' responses to stress.

Managing Stress through Relaxation Techniques

Poor management of stress has been correlated with an increased incidence of a number of physical and emotional conditions such as cardiac disease, poor diabetes control, chronic pain, and significant emotional distress. There is now considerable evidence that many mind-body therapies can be used as effective adjuncts to conventional medical treatment for a number of common clinical conditions.

Nurses should be aware of the conditions that can benefit from stress- and anxiety-reduction techniques. Psychiatric problems that are known to benefit from relaxation techniques include anxiety, depression, insomnia, and nightmares (National Center for Complementary and Alternative Medicine, 2014). Stress- and anxiety-reduction techniques may also have benefits for some other conditions including asthma, childbirth, epilepsy, fibromyalgia, headache, irritable bowel syndrome, cardiac disease and cardiac symptoms, menopause symptoms, menstruation, nausea, and pain. Although the results are not clear, there is some evidence to indicate that stress-reduction techniques may aid in smoking cessation and may improve temporomandibular disorder, ringing in the ears, and overactive bladder.

Because no single stress-management technique feels right for everyone, employing a mixture of techniques brings the best results. Essentially, there are stress-reducing techniques for every personality type, situation, and level of stress. Give them a try. Practicing relaxation techniques will help you to help your patients reduce their stress levels and also help you manage your own physical responses to stressors.

Biofeedback

Through the use of sensitive instrumentation, **biofeedback** provides immediate and exact information regarding muscle activity, brain waves, skin temperature, heart rate, blood pressure, and other bodily functions. Indicators of the particular internal physiological process are detected and amplified by a sensitive recording device. An individual can achieve greater voluntary control over phenomena once considered to be exclusively involuntary if he or she knows instantaneously, through an

Perceived Stress Scale–10 Item (PSS-10)

Instructions: The questions in this scale ask you about your feelings and thoughts during the last month. In each case, please indicate with a check how often you felt or thought a certain way.

1. In the last month, how often have you been upset because of something that happened unexpectedly?
   ___0 never ___1 almost never ___2 sometimes ___3 fairly often ___4 very often
2. In the last month, how often have you felt that you were unable to control the important things in your life?
   ___0 never ___1 almost never ___2 sometimes ___3 fairly often ___4 very often
3. In the last month, how often have you felt nervous and "stressed"?
   ___0 never ___1 almost never ___2 sometimes ___3 fairly often ___4 very often
4. In the last month, how often have you felt confident about your ability to handle your personal problems?
   ___0 never ___1 almost never ___2 sometimes ___3 fairly often ___4 very often
5. In the last month, how often have you felt that things were going your way?
   ___0 never ___1 almost never ___2 sometimes ___3 fairly often ___4 very often
6. In the last month, how often have you found that you could not cope with all the things that you had to do?
   ___0 never ___1 almost never ___2 sometimes ___3 fairly often ___4 very often
7. In the last month, how often have you been able to control irritations in your life?
   ___0 never ___1 almost never ___2 sometimes ___3 fairly often ___4 very often
8. In the last month, how often have you felt that you were on top of things?
   ___0 never ___1 almost never ___2 sometimes ___3 fairly often ___4 very often
9. In the last month, how often have you been angered because of things that were outside of your control?
   ___0 never ___1 almost never ___2 sometimes ___3 fairly often ___4 very often
10. In the last month, how often have you felt difficulties were piling up so high that you could not overcome them?
   ___0 never ___1 almost never ___2 sometimes ___3 fairly often ___4 very often

Perceived stress scale scoring

Items 4, 5, 7, and 8 are the positively stated items. PSS-10 scores are obtained by reversing the scores on the positive items, e.g., 0=4, 1=3, 2=2, etc. and then adding all 10 items.

FIG. 10.6 Perceived Stress Scale–10 Item (PSS-10). (Modified from Cohen S and Williamson G: Perceived stress in a probability sample of the US. In Spacepan S and Oskamp S (eds): *The Social Psychology of Health: Claremont Symposium on Applied Social Psychology,* Newbury Park, CA: Sage.)

auditory or visual signal, whether a somatic activity is increasing or decreasing.

The use of biofeedback was once reserved for clinicians with specialized training. Now, with increasingly sophisticated technology most people can use some form of biofeedback themselves. Exercise trackers and smart watches provide us with the ability to track sleep patterns and heart rates. One high-tech gadget is a clip-on device that tracks respiration changes that indicates tension; a companion application (app) suggests relaxation techniques such as meditation. A hand-held device that measures electrodermal changes that indicate stress, also comes with an app that teaches calming techniques.

Deep Breathing Exercises

The US Department of Health and Human Services (2015) conducted a study and found that the most common relaxation technique used in the United States was **deep breathing exercises**. About a third of respondents used this technique as a mainstay or a quick fix to calm down. Breathing exercises are simple and easy to remember, even when anxiety begins to escalate. This technique involves focusing on taking slow, deep, and even breaths.

One breathing exercise that has proved helpful for many people coping with anxiety and anxiety disorders has two parts (Box 10.2). The first part focuses on abdominal breathing while the second part helps patients interrupt trains of thought, thereby quieting mental noise. With increasing skill, breathing becomes a tool for dampening the cognitive processes likely to induce stress and anxiety reactions.

BOX 10.2 Deep Breathing Exercise

- Find a comfortable position.
- Relax your shoulders and chest; let your body relax.
- Shift to relaxed, abdominal breathing. Take a deep breath through your nose, expanding the abdomen. Hold it for 3 seconds and then exhale slowly through the mouth; exhale completely, telling yourself to relax.
- With every breath, turn attention to the muscular sensations that accompany the expansion of the belly.
- As you concentrate on your breathing, you will start to feel focused.
- Repeat this exercise for 2 to 5 minutes.

BOX 10.3 Script For Guided Imagery

- Imagine releasing all the tension in your body...letting it go.
- Now, with every breath you take, feel your body drifting down deeper and deeper into relaxation...floating down...deeper and deeper.
- Imagine a peaceful scene. You are sitting beside a clear, blue mountain stream. You are barefoot, and you feel the sun-warmed rock under your feet. You hear the sound of the stream tumbling over the rocks. The sound is hypnotic, and you relax more and more. You see the tall pine trees on the opposite shore bending in the gentle breeze. Breathe the clean, scented air, with each breath moving you deeper and deeper into relaxation. The sun warms your face.
- You are very comfortable. There is nothing to disturb you. You are experiencing a feeling of well-being.
- Come back to this peaceful scene by taking time to relax. The positive feelings can grow stronger and stronger each time you choose to relax.
- You can return to your activities now, feeling relaxed and refreshed.

Guided Imagery

Long before we learn to speak, our experience is based on mental images. With **guided imagery** people are taught to focus on pleasant images to replace negative or stressful feelings. Guided imagery may be self-directed or led by a practitioner or a recording.

Imagery techniques are a useful tool in the management of medical conditions and are an effective means of relieving pain for some people. Inducing muscle relaxation and focusing the mind away from the pain reduce pain. For some, imagery techniques are healing exercises in that they not only relieve the pain but also, in some cases, diminish the source of the pain. Cancer patients use guided imagery to help reduce high levels of cortisol, epinephrine, and catecholamines—which prevent the immune system from functioning effectively—and to produce β-endorphins—which increase pain thresholds and enhance lymphocyte proliferation.

Often, audio recordings are made specifically for patients and their particular situations. Many generic guided-imagery CDs and MP3s are available to patients and healthcare workers online. See Box 10.3 for a sample script for guided imagery.

Progressive Relaxation

In 1938 Edmund Jacobson, a Harvard-educated physician, developed a rather simple procedure that elicits a **relaxation response**, which he coined **progressive relaxation** or progressive muscle relaxation. This technique can be done without any external gauges or feedback and can be practiced almost anywhere by anyone.

The premise behind progressive relaxation is that, because anxiety results in tense muscles, one way to decrease anxiety is to nearly eliminate muscle contraction. This is accomplished by deliberately tensing groups of muscles (beginning with feet and ending with face or vice versa) as tightly as possible for about 8 seconds and then releasing the tension you have created.

Considerable research supports the use of progressive relaxation as helpful for a number of medical conditions, such as tension headaches. People with depression and posttraumatic stress disorder have been found to benefit from this relaxation technique (Bryan, 2013).

BOX 10.4 Short Progressive Muscle Relaxation

Find a quiet, comfortable place to sit. A reclining chair is ideal. Take five slow, deep breaths before you begin. Now tense and relax each area listed below. Tighten your muscles only until you feel tension, not pain.

- First, let's focus on your neck and shoulders. Raise your shoulders up toward your head . . . tighten the muscles there... hold... feel the tension there...and now release. Let your shoulders drop to a lower, more comfortable position.
- Now let's move to your hands. Tighten your hands into fists. Very tight...as if you are squeezing a tennis ball tightly in each hand...hold...feel the tension in your hands and forearms...and now release. Shake your hands gently, shaking out the tension. Feel how much more relaxed your hands are now.
- Now, your forehead: Raise your eyebrows, feeling the tight muscles in your forehead. Hold that tension. Now tightly lower your eyebrows and scrunch your eyes closed, feeling the tension in your forehead and eyes. Hold it tightly. And now, relax...let your forehead be relaxed and smooth, your eyelids gently resting.
- Your jaw is the next key area: Tightly close your mouth, clamping your jaw shut, very tightly. Your lips will also be tight and tense across the front of your teeth. Feel the tension in your jaws. Hold...and now relax. Release all of the tension. Let your mouth and jaw be loose and relaxed.
- There is only one more key area to relax, and that is your breathing: Breathe in deeply, and hold that breath. Feel the tension as you hold the air in. Hold...and now relax. Let the air be released through your mouth. Breathe out all the air.
- Once more, breathe in...and now hold the breath. Hold...and relax. Release the air, feeling your entire body relax. Breathe in...and out...in... and out...
- Continue to breathe regular breaths.
- You have relaxed some of the key areas where tension can build up. Remember to relax these areas a few times each day, using this quick progressive muscle relaxation script, to prevent stress symptoms.

There are many free progressive relaxation scripts, audios, and videos on the internet and some of them can be quite lengthy. An abbreviated example of a script that focuses on key muscle tension areas is listed in Box 10.4. Many people prefer to hear their own voice reciting the script, so you may want to make a tape of yourself.

Meditation

Meditation follows the basic guidelines described for the relaxation response. It is a discipline for training the mind to develop greater calm and then using that calm to bring penetrative insight into one's experience. Meditation can be used to help people to tap into their deep inner resources for healing, calm their minds, and help them operate more efficiently in the world. It can help people develop strategies to cope with stress, make sensible adaptive choices under pressure, and feel more engaged in life.

Meditation elicits a relaxation response by creating a hypometabolic state of quieting the sympathetic nervous system. Some people meditate using a visual object or a sound to help them focus. Others may find it useful to concentrate on their breathing while meditating. Meditation is easy to practice anywhere. Some students find that meditating before a test helps them focus and lessens anxiety. Keep in mind that meditation, like most other techniques, becomes better with practice.

Mindfulness, a centuries-old form of meditation that dates back to Buddhist tradition, has received increased attention among healthcare professionals. Mindfulness is based on two ways our brains work. One is a default network that includes the medial prefrontal cortex and memory regions such as the hippocampus. In this state we operate on a sort of mental autopilot or "mind wandering." You are thinking about what to make for dinner or how your hair looks and are continually compiling the narrative of your life and people you know. This type of thinking tends to be dominant.

The other network is the direct experience network that is the focus of mindfulness. Several areas of the brain are activated in this state. The insular cortex is active and makes us aware of bodily sensation and a sense of self. The anterior cingulate cortex is active and is central to attention and focuses us on what is happening around us. In this state you are in tune with your environment, live in the moment, and take a break from planning, strategizing, and setting goals.

Being mindful includes being in the moment by paying attention to what is going on around you—what you are seeing, feeling, hearing. Imagine how much you miss during an ordinary walk to class if you spend it staring straight ahead as your mind wanders from one concern to the next. You miss the pattern of sunlight filtered through the leaves, the warmth of the sunshine on your skin, and the sounds of birds calling out to one another. By focusing on the here and now, rather than past and future, you are practicing mindfulness.

With practice, people can gradually learn to let go of internal dialogue and reactiveness. Practicing mindfulness can be done at any time, and proponents suggest that it should become a way of life. One mindfulness technique can be found in Box 10.5.

BOX 10.5 A Mindfulness Technique

Creating space to come down from the worried mind and back into the present moment has been shown to be enormously helpful to people. When we are present, we have a firmer grasp of all our options and resources that often make us feel better. Next time you find your mind racing with stress, try the acronym STOP.

S – Stop what you are doing; put things down for a minute.

T – Take a breath. Breathe normally and naturally and follow your breath coming in and out of your nose. You can even say to yourself "in" as you're breathing in and "out" as you're breathing out if that helps with concentration.

O – Observe your thoughts, feelings, and emotions. You can reflect about what is on your mind and also notice that thoughts are not facts, and they are not permanent. If the thought arises that you are inadequate, just notice the thought, let it be, and continue on. Notice any emotions that are there and just name them. Just naming your emotions can have a calming effect. Then notice your body. Are you standing or sitting? How is your posture? Any aches and pains?

P – Proceed with something that is important to you in the moment, whether that is talking with a friend, appreciating your children, or walking while paying attention to the world.

From Goldstein, E. (2012). *The now effect.* New York, NY: Atria Books.

OTHER WAYS TO RELAX

Physical Exercise

Physical exercise can lead to protection from the harmful effects of stress on both physical and mental states. Researchers have been particularly interested in the influence exercise has over depression. Exercise is associated with a reduction in depressive symptoms (Cooney et al., 2014). Blumenthal and colleagues (2007) found that patients who had either 4 months of treatment with a selective serotonin reuptake inhibitor antidepressant or with aerobic exercise had similar relief of depression. Older adults who engage in regular physical activity have some protection from anxiety and depressive disorder (Pasco et al., 2011).

Yoga, an ancient form of exercise, has been found to be helpful for depression when used in conjunction with medication (Cramer et al., 2013). Other popular forms of exercise that can decrease stress and improve well-being are walking, tai chi, dancing, cycling, aerobics, and water exercise.

Cognitive Reframing

Cognitive reframing stems from an evidenced-based practice known as cognitive-behavioral therapy. The goal of **cognitive reframing** (also known as *cognitive restructuring*) is to change the individual's perceptions of stress by reassessing a situation and replacing irrational beliefs. For example the thought "I can't pass this course" is replaced with a more positive self-statement, "If I choose to study for this course, I will increase my chances of success." We can learn from most situations by asking ourselves the following:

- "What positive things came out of this situation or experience?"
- "What did I learn in this situation?"
- "What would I do in a different way?"

The desired result is to reframe a disturbing event or experience as less disturbing and to give the patient a sense of control over the situation. When the perception of the disturbing event is changed, there is less stimulation to the sympathetic nervous system, which in turn reduces the secretion of cortisol and catecholamines that destroy the balance of the immune system.

Cognitive distortions often include overgeneralizations ("He always…" or "I'll never…") and "should" statements ("I should have done better" or "He shouldn't have said that"). Table 10.4 shows some examples of cognitive reframing of anxiety-producing thoughts. Often cognitive reframing is used along with progressive muscle relaxation, mindfulness, and guided imagery to reduce stress.

Journaling

Writing in a journal (**journaling**) is an extremely useful and surprisingly simple method of identifying stressors. It is a technique that can ease worry and obsession, help identify hopes and fears, increase energy levels and confidence, and facilitate

TABLE 10.4 Cognitive Reframing of Irrational Thoughts

Irrational Thought	Positive Statements
"I'll never be happy until I am loved by someone I really care about."	"If I do not get love from one person, I can still get it from others and find happiness that way." "If someone I deeply care for rejects me, that will seem unfortunate, but I will hardly die." "If the only person I truly care for does not return my love, I can devote more time and energy to winning someone else's love and probably find someone better for me." "If no one I care for ever cares for me, I can still find enjoyment in friendships, in work, in books, and in other things."
"He should treat me better after all I do for him."	"I would like him to do certain things to show that he cares. If he chooses to continue to do things that hurt me after he understands what those things are, I am free to make choices about leaving or staying in this hurtful relationship."

Adapted from Ellis, A., & Harper, R. A. (1975). *A new guide to rational living.* North Hollywood, CA: Wilshire.

the grieving process. Keeping an informal diary of daily events and activities can reveal surprising information on sources of daily stress. Simply noting which activities put a strain on energy and time, which trigger anger or anxiety, and which precipitate a negative physical experience (e.g., headache, backache, fatigue) can be an important first step in stress reduction. Writing down thoughts and feelings is helpful not only in dealing with stress and stressful events but also in healing both physically and emotionally.

Humor

The use of **humor** as a cognitive approach is a good example of how a stressful situation can be "turned upside down." The intensity attached to a stressful thought or situation can be dissipated when it is made to appear absurd or comical. Essentially, the bee loses its sting.

KEY POINTS TO REMEMBER

- Stress is a universal experience and an important concept when caring for any patient in any setting.
- The body responds similarly whether stressors are real or perceived and whether the stressor is negative or positive.
- Physiologically, the body reacts to anxiety and fear by arousal of the sympathetic nervous system. Specific symptoms include rapid heart rate, increased blood pressure, diaphoresis, peripheral vasoconstriction, restlessness, repetitive questioning, feelings of frustration, and difficulty concentrating.
- Cannon introduced the fight-or-flight model of stress, and Selye introduced the widely known general adaptation syndrome (GAS).
- Prolonged stress can lead to chronic psychological and physiological responses when not mitigated at an early stage.
- There are basically two categories of stressors: physiological (e.g., heat, hunger, cold, noise, trauma) and psychological (e.g., death of a loved one, loss of job, schoolwork, humiliation).
- Age, gender, culture, life experience, and lifestyle all are important in identifying the degree of stress a person is experiencing.
- Lowering the effects of chronic stress can alter the course of many physical conditions; decrease the need for some medications; diminish or eliminate the urge for unhealthy and destructive behaviors such as smoking, insomnia, and drug addiction; and increase a person's cognitive functioning.
- An extremely important factor to assess is a person's support system. Studies have shown that high-quality social and intimate supports can go a long way toward minimizing the long-term effects of stress.
- Cultural differences exist in the extent to which people perceive an event as stressful and in the behaviors they consider appropriate to deal with a stressful event.
- Spiritual practices have been found to lead to an enhanced immune system and a sense of well-being.
- A variety of relaxation techniques are available to reduce the stress response and elicit the relaxation response, which results in improved physiological and psychological functioning.

CRITICAL THINKING

1. Assess your level of stress using the Recent Life Changes Questionnaire found in Table 10.3, and evaluate your potential for illness in the coming year. Identify stress-reduction techniques you think would be useful to learn.
2. Teach a classmate the deep-breathing exercise identified in this chapter (see Box 10.2).
3. Assess a classmate's coping styles and have the same classmate assess yours. Discuss the relevance of your findings.
4. Using Fig. 10.2, explain to a classmate the short-term effects of stress on the sympathetic–adrenal medulla system, and identify three long-term effects if the stress is not relieved. How would you use this information to provide patient teaching? If your classmate were the patient, how would his or her response indicate that effective learning had taken place?
5. Using Fig. 10.2, have a classmate explain to you the short-term effects of stress on the hypothalamus–pituitary–adrenal

cortex and the eventual long-term effects if the stress becomes chronic. Summarize to your classmate your understanding of what was presented. Using your knowledge of the short-term effects of stress on the hypothalamus–pituitary–adrenal cortex and the long-term effects of stress, develop and present a patient education model related to stress for your clinical group.

6. In postconference discuss a patient you have cared for who had one of the stress-related effects identified in Fig. 10.2. See if you can identify some stressors in the patient's life and possible ways to lower chronic stress levels.

CHAPTER REVIEW

Questions

1. What assessment question is focused on identifying a long-term consequence of chronic stress on physical health?
   a. "Do you have any problems with sleeping well?"
   b. "How many infections have you experienced in the past 6 months?"
   c. "How much moderate exercise do you engage in on a regular basis?"
   d. "What management techniques to you regularly use to manage your stress?"
2. Which nursing assessments are directed at monitoring a patient's fight-or-flight response? *Select all that apply.*
   a. Blood pressure
   b. Heart rate
   c. Respiratory rate
   d. Abdominal pain
   e. Dilated pupils
3. The patient you are assigned unexpectedly suffers a cardiac arrest. During this emergency situation, your body will produce a large amount of:
   a. carbon dioxide.
   b. growth hormone.
   c. epinephrine
   d. aldosterone
4. Which question is focused on the assessment of an individual's personal ability to manage stress? *Select all that apply.*
   a. "Have you ever been diagnosed with cancer?"
   b. "Do you engage in any hobbies now that you have retired?"
   c. "Have you been taking your antihypertensive medication as it is prescribed?"
   d. "Who can you rely on if you need help after you're discharged from the hospital?"
   e. "What do you do to help manage the demands of parenting a 4-year-old and a newborn?"
5. When considering stress, what is the primary goal of making daily entries into a personal journal?
   a. Providing a distraction from the daily stress
   b. Expressing emotions to manage stress
   c. Identifying stress triggers
   d. Focusing on one's stress
6. Jackson has suffered from migraine headaches all of his life. Fatima, his nurse practitioner, suspects muscle tension as a trigger for his headaches. Fatima teaches him a technique that promotes relaxation by using:
   a. Biofeedback
   b. Guided imagery
   c. Deep breathing
   d. Progressive muscle relaxation
7. Hugo is 21 and diagnosed with schizophrenia. His history includes significant turmoil as child and adolescent. Hugo reports his father was abusive and routinely beat him, all of his siblings, and his mother. Hugo's early exposure to stress most likely:
   a. Made him resilient to stressful situations
   b. Increased his future vulnerability to psychiatric disorders
   c. Developed strong survival skills
   d. Shaped his nurturing nature
8. Hugo has a fraternal twin named Franco who is unaffected by mental illness even though they were raised in the same dysfunctional household. Franco asks the nurse, "Why Hugo and not me?" The nurse replies:
   a. "Your father was probably less abusive to you."
   b. "Hugo likely has a genetic vulnerability."
   c. "You probably ignored the situation."
   d. "Hugo responded to perceived threats by focusing on an internal world."
9. First responders and emergency department healthcare providers often use dark humor in an effort to:
   a. Reduce stress and anxiety
   b. Relive the experience
   c. Rectify moral distress
   d. Alert others to the stress
10. Your 39-year-old patient, Samantha, who was admitted with anxiety, asks you what the stress-relieving technique of mindfulness is. The best response is:
    a. Mindfulness is focusing on an object and repeating a word or phrase while deep breathing
    b. Mindfulness is progressively tensing, then relaxing, body muscles
    c. Mindfulness is focusing on the here and now, not the past or future, and paying attention to what is going on around you
    d. Mindfulness is a memory system to assist you in short-term memory recall

Answers

1. **b**; 2. **a, b, c, e**; 3. **c**; 4. **b, d, e**; 5. **c**; 6. **d**; 7. **b**; 8. **b**; 9. **a**; 10. **c**

Visit the Evolve website for a posttest on the content in this chapter: http://evolve.elsevier.com/Varcarolis

Post-Test interactive review

REFERENCES

Ader, R., & Cohen, N. (1975). Behaviorally conditioned immunosuppression. *Psychosomatic Medicine, 37*(4), 333–340.

Bangasser, A., Curtis, A., Reyes, B. A. S., Bethea, T. T., Parastatidis, I., Ischiropoulos, H., & Valentino, R. J. (2010). Sex differences in corticotropin-releasing factor receptor signaling and trafficking: Potential role in female vulnerability to stress-related psychopathology. *Molecular Psychiatry, 15*(9), 896–904.

Blumenthal, J. A., Babyak, M. A., Doraiswamy, P. M., Watkins, L., Hoffman, B. M., Barbour, K. A., & Sherwood, A. (2007). Exercise and pharmacotherapy in the treatment of major depressive disorder. *Psychosomatic Medicine, 69*, 587–596.

Bryan, D. (2013). *Progressive muscle relaxation as a CAM*. Retrieved from http://www.camcommons.org/progressive-muscle-relaxation-as-an-evidence-based-cam-treatment.html.

Cooney, G., Dwan, K., & Mead, G. (2014). Exercise for depression. *Journal of the American Medical Association, 311*(23), 2432–2433.

Cramer, H., Lauche, R., Langhorst, J., & Dobos, J. (2013). Yoga for depression: A systematic review and meta-analysis. *Depression and Anxiety, 30*(11), 1068–1083.

Cruces, J., Venero, C., Pereda-Perez, I., & De la Fuente, M. (2014). The effect of psychological stress and social isolation on neuroimmunoendocrine communication. *Current Pharmaceutical Design, 20*(29), 4608–4628.

Dahl, J., Ormstad, H., Aas, H. C. D., Malt, U. F., Bendz, L. T., Sandvik, L., & Brundin, L. (2014). The plasma levels of various cytokines are increased during ongoing depression and are reduced to normal levels after recovery. *Psychoneuroendicronology, 45*, 77–86.

First30Days. (2008). *First30days' the change report: Making changes today considered more difficult to handle than 40 years ago*. Retrieved from http://www.first30days.com/pages/press_changereport.html.

Holmes, T. H., & Rahe, R. H. (1967). The social readjustment rating scale. *Journal of Psychosomatic Research, 11*(2), 213.

Koenig, H. G., King, D. E., & Carson, V. B. (2012). *Handbook of religion and health* (2nd ed.). New York, NY: Oxford University Press.

Koolhaas, J. M., Bartolomucci, A., Buwalda, B., de Boer, S. F., Flugge, G., Korte, S. M., & Fuchs, E. (2011). Stress revisited: A critical evaluation of the stress concept. *Neuroscience & Biobehavioral Reviews, 35*(5), 1291–1301.

National Cancer Institute. (2015). *Depression*. Retrieved from http://www.cancer.gov/cancertopics/pdq/supportivecare/depression/HealthProfessional/page2#Reference2.3.

National Center for Complementary and Alternative Medicine. (2014). *Relaxation techniques for health*. Retrieved from https://nccih.nih.gov/health/stress/relaxation.htm.

National Institute of Mental Health. (2016). *Fact sheet on stress*. Retrieved from http://www.nimh.nih.gov/health/publications/stress/index.shtml.

Pasco, J. A., Williams, L. J., Jacka, F. N., et al. (2011). Habitual physical activity and the risk for depressive and anxiety disorders among older men and women. *International Psychogeriatrics, 23*(2), 292–298.

Selye, H. (1936). A syndrome produced by diverse nocuous agents. *Nature, 138*(32).

Selye, H. (1974). *Stress without distress*. Philadelphia, PA: Lippincott.

Selye, H. (1993). History of the stress concept. In L. Goldberger & S. Breznitz (Eds.), *Handbook of stress: Theoretical and clinical aspects* (pp. 7–17). New York, NY: Free Press.

Taylor, S. (2010). Mechanisms linking early life stress to adult health outcomes. *Proceedings of the National Academy of Sciences of the United States of America, 107*(19), 8507–8512.

US Department of Health and Human Services. (2015). Trends in the use of complementary health approaches among adults. *United States, 2002–2012.*

11

Childhood and Neurodevelopmental Disorders

Cindy Parsons

Visit the Evolve website for a pretest on the content in this chapter: http://evolve.elsevier.com/Varcarolis Pre-Test interactive review

OBJECTIVES

1. Identify the prevalence and significance of psychiatric disorders in children and adolescents.
2. Examine factors and influences contributing to neurodevelopmental disorders.
3. Identify characteristics of mental health and factors that promote resilience in children and adolescents.
4. Describe the specialty area of psychiatric-mental health nursing.
5. Discuss the assessment of a child or adolescent.
6. Compare and contrast at least six treatment modalities for children and adolescents with neurodevelopmental disorders.
7. Describe clinical features and behaviors of at least three childhood neurodevelopmental disorders.
8. Formulate one nursing diagnosis, stating patient outcomes and interventions for patients with intellectual disability, autism spectrum disorder, and attention-deficit/hyperactivity disorder.

OUTLINE

KEY TERMS AND CONCEPTS

attention-deficit/hyperactivity disorder
autism spectrum disorder
bibliotherapy
communication disorders
early intervention programs
intellectual disability
play therapy
principle of least restrictive intervention
resilience
specific learning disorders
temperament
therapeutic games

We tend to think of mental illness as a phenomenon of adulthood, yet research shows that more than half of all lifetime cases began before the patient was age 14. About 20% of children and adolescents in the United States suffer from a psychiatric disorder that causes significant impairment at home, at school, with peers, and in the community (McGorry et al., 2011).

Because of the timing of onset, these disorders can disrupt the normal pattern of childhood development. They may result in devastating consequences for academic, social, and psychological functioning. The symptoms of these disorders can also can cause significant distress for families and disrupt family functioning. Fear of stigma can cause patients and families to attempt to conceal the conditions or even limit help seeking and professional care.

Younger children are more difficult to diagnose than older children because of limited language skills and cognitive and emotional development. Additionally, children undergo more rapid psychological, neurological, and physiological changes over a briefer period than adults.

Clinicians and parents often wait to see whether symptoms are the result of a developmental lag or trauma response that will eventually correct itself. Unfortunately, this wait and see approach means that helpful early interventions do not always happen. Other barriers to assessment and treatment include (1) lack of consensus for screening children, (2) lack of coordination among multiple systems, (3) lack of community-based resources and long waiting lists for services, (4) lack of mental health providers, and (5) cost and inadequate reimbursement (Children's Defense Fund, 2014).

Fortunately, changes in the accessibility and availability of health insurance have created opportunities to improve funding, access to care, and research to understand the reasons for underutilization and early termination of services. The Substance Abuse and Mental Health Services Administration (SAMHSA, 2015) has revised and updated its 3-year strategic plan to improve the use of resources in the prevention, early detection, treatment, and recovery services for individuals with mental or substance abuse disorders.

The White House Conference on Mental Health in 2013 brought together community, state, and national representatives with national stakeholders. This group was charged to develop an initiative to bring about greater awareness to the mental health needs of all Americans, especially those more vulnerable populations. The "Now is the Time" campaign followed and provided SAMSHA (2014) with increased funding for access to children's mental health services and community awareness efforts.

In this chapter, we begin with an overview of the risk factors for psychiatric disorders in children and adolescents, overall assessments, and general interventions. You will learn about the specialty of child-adolescent psychiatric nursing. Several neurodevelopmental disorders—communication disorder, learning disorder, and motor disorder—will be summarized. A few specific disorders—intellectual disability, autism spectrum disorder, and attention-deficit/hyperactivity disorder (ADHD)—will be discussed in greater depth.

EVIDENCE-BASED PRACTICE

Parents' Experience with a Child Admitted for Psychiatric Care

Problem

When a young person is admitted to acute inpatient care for a mental illness, it is a crisis for both the patient and the patient's family. Families are often traumatized by the hospitalization and the fragmented communication and exclusion they experience during the hospital stay.

Purpose of Study

This study evaluated the effect of an Early Psychosis Education Program. This program is designed to support parents of children with new diagnoses of mental illness and first admission to a psychiatric hospital.

Methods

Four participants were male and six were female with an age range of 34 to 56. Parents were invited to participate in a 2-hour-a-week educational program for 4 weeks. Pretests and posttests with open-ended questions were used to evaluate parents' perceptions and feelings regarding their children's admission, knowledge of diagnosis, understanding of the recovery process, and general knowledge of mental illness, drugs, and alcohol.

Key Findings

Pretests indicated that parents:

- Shared two recurring themes: "We didn't see it coming" and "Hopelessness/Helplessness."

EVIDENCE-BASED PRACTICE—cont'd

Parents' Experience with a Child Admitted for Psychiatric Care

- Lacked knowledge regarding mental illness, psychiatric care, and the recovery process.
- Lacked understanding of the medications prescribed and treatment options available.
- Felt guilt, anger, and responsibility for their child's illness.

Posttests indicated that parents:

- Demonstrated improved overall level of knowledge.
- Continued to experience feelings of hopelessness, helplessness, inadequacy, and lack of confidence regarding the future and their child's recovery.

The Early Psychosis Education Program was evaluated as valuable and worthwhile. The researched concluded that it would have been more helpful to have the training before their child's admission.

Implications for Nursing Practice

The findings indicate a significant need for mental health awareness and education among the general public. Programs like EPEP should be implemented at admission to help support and educate the families throughout the process. Nurses play a critical role in supporting and educating the families throughout the process.

Ward, L., & Gwinner, K. (2014). It broke our heart: Understanding parents lived experiences of their child's admission to an acute mental health care facility. *Journal of Psychosocial Nursing and Mental Health services, (52)7*, 24–29.

RISK FACTORS

Biological Factors

Genetic

Hereditary factors are implicated in numerous childhood-onset psychiatric disorders. Because not all genetically vulnerable children develop mental disorders, researchers assume that factors such as resilience, intelligence, and a supportive environment aid in avoiding the development of mental disorders.

Neurobiological

Dramatic changes occur in the brain during childhood and adolescence, including a declining number of synapses (they peak at age 5), changes in the relative volume and activity level in different brain regions, and interactions of hormones (Menzies et al., 2015). Myelination of brain fibers increases the speed of information processing, improves the conduction speed of nerve impulses, and enables faster reactions to occur.

Changes in the frontal and prefrontal cortex regions occur during the teen years. This leads to improvements in executive functions, organization and planning skills, and inhibiting responses. These changes, including cerebellum maturation and hormonal changes, reflect the emotional and behavioral fluctuations characteristic of adolescence. Early adolescence is typically characterized by low emotional regulation and intolerance for frustration. Emotional and behavioral control usually increases over the course of adolescence.

Psychological Factors

Temperament

Temperament refers to the usual attitude, mood, or behavior that a child habitually uses to cope with the demands and expectations of the environment. This style is present in infancy, is modified somewhat with maturation, and develops in the context of the social environment. All people have temperaments, and the fit between the child's and parent's temperament is critical to the child's development. If there is incongruence between parent and child temperament and the caregiver is unable to respond positively to the child, there is a risk of insecure attachment, developmental problems, and future mental disorders.

Temperament and behavioral traits can be powerful predictors of future problems. Traits such as shyness, aggressiveness, and rebelliousness, for example, may increase the risk for substance use problems. External risk factors for using illicit substances include peer or parental substance use and involvement in legal problems such as truancy or vandalism. Protective factors that shield some children from drug use include self-control, parental monitoring, academic achievement, antidrug-use policies, and strong neighborhood attachment.

Resilience

Despite risk factors for the development of psychiatric disorders, many children and adolescents develop normally. This is likely due to resilience. The phenomenon of **resilience** is the relationship between a person's inborn strengths and success in handling stressful environmental factors (Hoffman, 2010). Internal and external factors such as self-concept, future expectations, social competence, problem-solving skills, family, and school and community interactions all influence resilience. According to Zoloski and Bullock (2012), the *resilient child* has the following characteristics:

1. Adaptability to changes in the environment
2. Ability to form nurturing relationships with other adults when the parent is not available
3. Ability to distance self from emotional chaos
4. Social intelligence
5. Good problem-solving skills
6. Ability to perceive a long-term future

Environmental Factors

To a far greater degree than adults, children are dependent on others. During childhood, the main context is the family. Parents model behavior and provide the child with a view of the world. If parents are abusive, rejecting, or overly controlling, the child may suffer detrimental effects at the developmental point(s) at which the trauma occurs (Shonkoff et al., 2009). Some familial risk factors correlate with child psychiatric disorders. These risk factors include severe marital discord, low socioeconomic status, large families and overcrowding, parental criminality, maternal psychiatric disorders, and foster-care placement.

Trauma in childhood is strongly associated with adult dysfunction. The Centers for Disease Control and Prevention (CDC)-Kaiser Permanente Adverse Childhood Experiences (ACE) study is one of the largest studies of childhood and adolescent abuse and neglect and subsequent adult health and well-being (CDC, 2016). ACEs include abuse (emotional, physical, sexual), neglect, and household challenges such as mental illness, spousal abuse, and substance use. The original study had more than 17,000 participants and was published in 1998. As the number of ACEs increase, so do the following:

- Alcohol use disorder
- Cardiac problems
- Fetal death
- Financial stress
- Intimate partner violence
- Liver disease
- Major depressive disorder
- Multiple sexual partners
- Poor academic performance
- Poor work performance
- Pregnancies (unintended)
- Sexual activity at a young age
- Sexually transmitted disease
- Smoking
- Suicide attempts

The CDC continues to monitor ACEs by assessing the medical status of the study participants.

Neglect is the most prevalent form of child abuse in the United States. According to the US Department of Health and Human Services (2016), 75% of all abuse victims were neglected, 17% were physically abused, and about 8% were sexually abused.

Girls are more frequently the victims of sexual abuse. Boys are also sexually abused, but the numbers are likely underreported due to shame and stigma. Sexual abuse varies from fondling to forcing a child to observe lewd acts to sexual intercourse. All instances of sexual abuse are devastating to a child who lacks the mental capacity or emotional maturation to consent to this type of a relationship. Nurses are required to report suspected abuse of a minor child to the local child protective services.

Witnessing violence is traumatizing and a well-documented risk factor for many mental health problems. Children who have experienced abuse are at risk for identifying with their aggressor and may act out, bully others, become abusers, or develop dysfunctional interpersonal relationships in adulthood.

HEALTH POLICY

HEALTH POLICY BOX

E-Cigarettes: A Rising Trend Among Youth

E-cigarettes have become part of the American teenage culture. The number of middle school and high school students who used the devices tripled from 2013 to 2014 (Centers for Disease Prevention and Control, 2015). Thirteen percent of high school students smoke e-cigarettes; this is more than those who smoke traditional cigarettes.

The general population, and likely the youth, believes that e-cigarettes are harmless. Yet e-cigarettes can cause nicotine addiction, nicotine overdose, and toxicity. They may also be gateway drugs into riskier substances. E-cigarettes have resulted in hospitalization for illnesses such as:

- Pneumonia
- Congestive heart failure
- Disorientation
- Seizures
- Hypotension

E-cigarettes can be easily accessed online, in malls, gas stations, and even grocery stores. E-cigarette marketing is targeting the youth by offering flavors such as candy, fruit, and coffee flavors. Advertisements include claims that this practice makes you more modern, popular, and more romantically attractive. Celebrity endorsements are also used as draws.

In May 2016 the FDA finalized a rule extending its authority to cover these unregulated tobacco products. This rule aims at restricting youth access with the following provisions:

- Not allowing products to be sold to people under the age of 18 years (both in person and online);
- Requiring age verification by photo ID;
- Not allowing the selling of covered tobacco products in vending machines (unless in an adult-only facility); and
- Not allowing the distribution of free samples.

Healthcare providers and educators should support these tighter regulations and policy regarding the manufacture, distribution, and marketing of e-cigarettes. Nursing students can be instrumental in providing education to patients and serving as role models for younger peers.

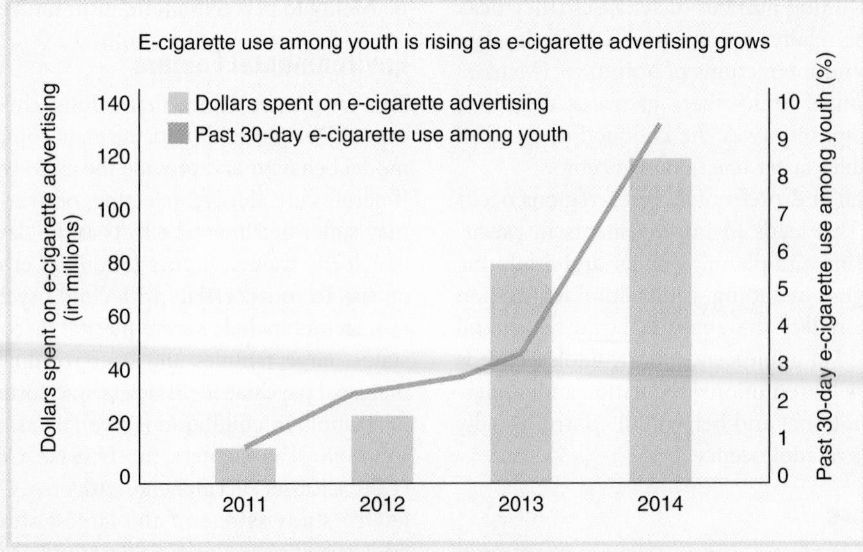

Centers for Disease Control and Prevention. (2015). *E-cigarette use triples among middle and high school students in just one year.* Retrieved from http://www.cdc.gov/media/releases/2015/p0416-e-cigarette-use.html; US Food and Drug Administration. (2016). Vaporizers, e-cigarettes, and other electronic nicotine delivery systems. Retrieved from http://www.fda.gov/TobaccoProducts/Labeling/ProductsIngredientsComponents/ucm456610.htm

Cultural

Differences in cultural expectations, presence of stressors, and lack of support by the dominant culture may have profound effects on children and adolescents. Working with patients from diverse backgrounds requires an increased awareness of one's own biases and the patient's needs. Nurses should consider the social and cultural context of the patient including factors such as age, ethnicity, gender, sexual orientation, worldview, religiosity, and socioeconomic status when assessing and planning care.

CONSIDERING CULTURE

Addressing Child Psychiatric Problems in Developing Countries

Child and adolescent mental health services are limited throughout the world. In developing countries, such as Bangladesh, this deficiency is especially pronounced. Compounding the problem is a cultural tendency toward somatization of psychiatric symptoms. Also, due to fear of being stigmatized, families tend to seek help by general practitioners rather than in specialty care.

Researchers sought to gain a clearer picture of the prevalence of psychiatric disorders in children and adolescents. A sample of 240 patients ages 5-16 were evaluated in an outpatient clinic.

Psychiatric disorders were found in 18% of the sample. Overall disorders were identified as: emotional disorders (e.g., depression, anxiety) 15%, behavioral disorders (e.g., conduct disorder, oppositional defiant disorder) 9%, hyperkinetic disorder (i.e., attention-deficit/hyperactivity disorder) 5%, and developmental disorders (e.g., learning disorders, intellectual disability) 0.4%. Autism spectrum disorder was nearly absent from the sample.

Overall, the prevalence of psychiatric disorders among this Bangladesh population was lower than Western estimates. The authors speculate that this difference is due to cultural variation and other factors such as lack of awareness and social stigma. They recommend improving early identification of psychiatric problems through screening, referral, and management.

Jesmin, A., Mullick, M. S. I., Rahman, K. M. Z., & Muntasir, M. M. (2016). Psychiatric disorders in children and adolescents attending pediatric out patient departments of tertiary hospitals. *Oman Medical Journal, 31*(4), 258–262.

CHILD AND ADOLESCENT PSYCHIATRIC-MENTAL HEALTH NURSING

In 2014 the American Nurses Association (ANA), along with the American Psychiatric Nurses Association (APNA) and International Society of Psychiatric-Mental Health Nurses (ISPN), defined the functions of nurses in the *Psychiatric-Mental Health Nursing: Scope and Standards of Practice.* According to this document, psychiatric-mental health nurses utilize evidence-based psychiatric practices to provide care responsive to the patient's and family's specific problems, strengths, personality, sociocultural context, and preferences.

Nurses who work in psychiatric-mental health settings may focus on specific populations such as pediatric, adolescent, adult, and geriatric patients. All of these nurses are referred to as psychiatric-mental health registered nurses regardless of the population. Formal recognition of the role occurs through certification at either the basic or advanced practice level.

APPLICATION OF THE NURSING PROCESS

ASSESSMENT

The type of data collected to assess mental health depends on the setting, the severity of the presenting problem, and the availability of resources. Box 11.1 identifies essential assessment data including history of the present illness; medical, developmental, and family history; mental status; and neurological developmental characteristics. Agency policies determine which data are collected, but a nurse should be prepared to make an independent judgment about what to assess and how to assess it. In all cases, a physical examination is part of a complete assessment for children and adolescents with serious mental problems who require hospitalization.

Data Collection

Methods of collecting data include interviewing, screening, testing (neurological, psychological, intelligence), observing, and interacting with the child or adolescent. In addition to the patient, ideally, data will be taken from multiple sources, including parents, teachers, and other caregivers. Parents and

BOX 11.1 Types of Assessment Data

History of Present Illness
- Chief complaint
- Development and duration of problems
- Help sought and results
- Effect of problem on child's life at home and school
- Effect of problem on family and siblings' lives

Developmental History
- Pregnancy, birth, neonatal data
- Developmental milestones
- Description of eating, sleeping, and elimination habits and routines
- Attachment behaviors
- Types of play
- Social skills and friendships
- Sexual activity

Developmental Assessment
- Psychomotor skills
- Language skills
- Cognitive skills
- Interpersonal and social skills
- Academic achievement
- Behavior (response to stress, to changes in environment)
- Problem-solving and coping skills (impulse control, delay of gratification)
- Energy level and motivation

Neurological Assessment
- Cerebral functions
- Cerebellar functions
- Sensory functions
- Reflexes

Continued

BOX 11.1 Types of Assessment Data—cont'd

NOTE: Functions can be observed during developmental assessment and while playing games involving a specific ability (e.g., "Simon says, 'Touch your nose.'")

Medical History
- Review of body systems
- Traumas, hospitalizations, operations, and child's response
- Illnesses or injuries affecting central nervous system
- Medications (past and current)
- Allergies

Family History
- Illnesses in related family members (e.g., seizures, mental disorders, intellectual disability, hyperactivity, drug and alcohol abuse, diabetes, cancer)
- Background of family members (occupation, education, social activities, religion)
- Family relationships (separation, divorce, deaths, contact with extended family, support system)

Mental Status Assessment
- General appearance
- Activity level
- Coordination and motor function
- Affect
- Speech
- Manner of relating
- Intellectual functions
- Thought processes and content
- Characteristics of play

teachers can complete structured questionnaires and behavior checklists. A family diagram, called a genogram, can illustrate family composition, history, and relationships (refer to Chapter 35). Numerous assessment tools and rating scales are available, and with training, nurses can use them to effectively monitor symptoms, behavioral change, and response to treatment.

The initial interview is key to observing interactions among the child, caregiver, and siblings (if available) and building trust and rapport. The observation-interaction part of a mental health assessment begins with a semi-structured interview in which the nurse asks the young person about the home environment, parents, and siblings and the school environment, teachers, and peers. In this format, the patient is encouraged to describe current problems and give information about developmental history. Nurses use play activities such as **therapeutic games**, drawings, and puppets for younger children who have difficulty responding to a direct approach.

Mental Status Examination

Assessment of mental status of children and adolescents is similar to that of adults. The main difference is that assessment is adapted to be appropriate for the child's developmental stage, cognitive capabilities, and verbal skills. It provides information about the mental state at the time of the examination and identifies problems with thinking, feeling, and behaving. Broad categories to assess include safety, general appearance, socialization, activity level, speech, coordination and motor function, affect, manner of relating, intellectual function, thought processes and content, and characteristics of play.

Developmental Assessment

A child or adolescent who does not have a psychiatric disorder matures with only minor regressions, coping with the stressors and developmental tasks of life. Learning and adapting to the environment and bonding with others in a mutually satisfying way are signs of mental health (Box 11.2).

BOX 11.2 Characteristics of a Mentally Healthy Child or Adolescent

- Trusts others and sees his or her world as being safe and supportive
- Correctly interprets reality and makes accurate perceptions of the environment and one's ability to influence it through actions (e.g., self-determination)
- Behaves in a way that is developmentally appropriate and does not violate social norms
- Has a positive realistic self-concept and developing identity
- Adapts to and copes with anxiety and stress using age-appropriate behavior
- Can learn and master developmental tasks and new situations
- Expresses self in spontaneous and creative ways
- Develops and maintains satisfying relationships

The developmental assessment provides information about the child or adolescent's maturational level. These data are then reviewed in relation to the chronological age to identify developmental strengths or deficits. The Denver II Developmental Screening Test is a popular assessment tool with 125 items. This tool covers four areas: social/personal, fine motor function, language, and gross motor function.

Abnormal findings in the developmental and mental status assessments may be related to stress and adjustment problems or to more serious disorders. Nurses need to evaluate behaviors brought on by stress, as well as those of more serious psychopathology, and identify the need for further evaluation or referral. Stress-related behaviors or minor regressions may be managed by working with parents. Serious psychopathology requires evaluation by an advanced practice nurse in collaboration with clinicians from other specialty disciplines.

General Interventions for Children and Adolescents

You can use the interventions described in this section in a variety of settings: inpatient, residential, outpatient, day treatment, outreach programs in schools, and home visits. Many of the modalities can encompass activities of daily living, learning activities, multiple forms of play and recreational activities, and interactions with adults and peers.

Behavioral Interventions

Behavioral interventions reward desired behavior to reduce maladaptive behaviors. Most child and adolescent treatment settings use a structured program that includes a behavioral program to motivate and reward age-appropriate behaviors. One popular method is the point system in which care providers award points for desired behaviors. Specific behaviors have specific points. Privileges are awarded based on the points that are recorded each day.

Play Therapy

Play is often described as the work of childhood. Through play children develop their physical, intellectual, emotional, social, and moral capacities. **Play therapy** is a type of intervention that allows children to express feelings such as anxiety, self-doubt, and fear through the natural use of play. It is also useful in helping young patients to access and work through painful memories. Trauma is often stuck in the nonverbal parts of the brain—amygdala, thalamus, hippocampus, or brainstem. Playing out memories helps move them to verbal frontal lobes.

> **VIGNETTE:** Seth, a 6-year-old male, was walking home from the store with his grandmother when an out of control car charged toward them on the sidewalk. Seth's grandmother was able to push him to safety, but she was struck and died at the scene. Since that time he has become withdrawn, anxious, and has frequent nightmares. He is inconsolable when his mother goes to work or takes him to school. Seth and his mother were referred to a play therapist.
>
> During play therapy the therapist used dolls and toy vehicles to help Seth work through his anxiety and distress related to the accident. He even reenacted the tragic event and said he was very mad at the driver. After four sessions he begins to talk about positive memories of his grandmother and his mother reports that his anxiety is decreasing.

Bibliotherapy

Bibliotherapy involves using literature to help the child express feelings in a supportive environment, gain insight into feelings and behavior, and learn new ways to cope with difficult situations. When children listen to or read a story, they unconsciously identify with the characters and experience a catharsis of feelings. You should select stories and books that reflect the situations or feelings the child is experiencing. Also take into consideration the child's cognitive and developmental level and emotional readiness for the particular topic.

Expressive Arts Therapy

The therapeutic use of art provides a nonverbal means of expressing difficult or confusing emotions. Drawing, painting, and sculpting are a few of the commonly used mediums. Creating something may help young people express the thoughts, feelings, and tensions that they cannot express verbally, are unaware of, or are denying. Children who have experienced trauma will often show the traumatic event in their drawing when asked to draw whatever they wish.

Journaling

Another effective technique when working with younger people, particularly teenagers, is using a journal. Journaling is a tangible way of recording and viewing emotions and may be a way to begin a dialogue with others. The use of a daily journal is also effective in setting goals and evaluating progress.

Music Therapy

The healing power of music has been recognized for centuries. Music therapy is an evidence-based approach to accomplish therapeutic goals within the context of a therapeutic relationship. Music can be used to improve physical, psychological, cognitive, behavioral, and social functioning. It is a nonthreatening approach that engages multiple senses. Children and adolescents can be involved in music by listening, singing, playing, moving, and other creative activities.

Family Interventions

The family is critical to improving the functional capacity of a young person with a psychiatric illness. Family counseling is often a key component of treatment. Nurses can help family members develop specific goals, identify ways to improve, and work to achieve the goals for the family or subunits within the family (e.g., parental, sibling).

Homework assignments are often used for family members to practice new skills outside the therapeutic environment. Sometimes families are taught in groups. Group education may be useful for (1) learning how other families solve problems and build on strengths, (2) developing insight and improved judgment about their own family, and (3) learning and sharing new information.

Psychopharmacology

The treatment of psychiatric disorders in young people requires a multimodal approach, which may include the use of medication. Medication typically works best when combined with another treatment such as cognitive-behavioral therapy (CBT). Medications that target specific symptoms can make a real difference in a family's ability to cope and improve quality of life, while enhancing the child's or adolescent's potential for growth.

Teamwork and Safety

Children and adolescents with neurodevelopmental disorders may require intensive teamwork to promote safety in inpatient units, long-term residential care, or intensive outpatient care. Nurses collaborate with other healthcare providers in structuring and maintaining the therapeutic environment to provide physical safety and psychological security and improve coping.

The nurse provides leadership to the nursing team in planning, implementing, and delivering safe, effective, quality care to maintain the therapeutic milieu and safety of all patients. The multidisciplinary team shares and articulates a philosophy regarding how to provide physical and psychological security, promote personal growth, and work with problematic behaviors.

Disruptive Behavior Management

To ensure that the civil and legal rights of individuals are maintained, techniques are selected according to the **principle of least** restrictive intervention. This principle requires that you use more restrictive interventions *only* after attempting less restrictive interventions that have been unsuccessful to manage the behavior. Less restrictive interventions include verbal (e.g., asking if the patient would like to talk about his anger), offering medication to help him gain control, and suggesting a time-out (e.g., his room or other quiet area). Finally, as a last resort, seclusion or restraint may be considered. In general, seclusion is viewed as less restrictive than restraint, where all movement is constrained.

Time-out. Asking or directing a child or adolescent to take a time-out from an activity is an excellent intervention that promotes self-reflection and encourages self-control. It is a less restrictive alternative to seclusion and restraint. Taking a time-out may involve going to a designated room or sitting on the periphery of an activity until self-control is regained. This technique may be an integral part of the treatment plan, and the child's and family's input are considered in including this modality.

Quiet room. A unit may have an unlocked room for a child who needs an area with decreased stimulation for regaining and maintaining self-control. The types of quiet rooms include the feelings room, which is carpeted and supplied with soft objects that can be punched and thrown, and the sensory room, which contains items for relaxation and meditation such as music and yoga mats. The child is encouraged to express freely and work through feelings of anger or sadness in privacy and with staff support.

VIGNETTE: Isabelle, a school-aged child, was admitted to the hospital from her foster home placement. She has been in foster care since her mother died from a drug overdose. Her father is incarcerated for armed robbery and drug-related offenses. Isabelle has a history of self-injurious behavior that includes biting and pinching herself and hitting her head against the wall when she is frustrated. The nurse and activity therapist have taught Isabelle to request time in the sensory room when she begins to feel upset or anxious. She has been able to identify certain triggers and to request time in the sensory room, decreasing episodes of self-injury over the past week.

Seclusion and restraint. Evidence suggests that both seclusion and restraint are psychologically harmful and can be physically dangerous. Deaths have resulted, primarily by asphyxiation due to physical holds during the use of restraints. However, a child's or adolescent's behavior may be so destructive or dangerous that physical restraint or seclusion is required for the safety of all. Members of the treatment team who use locked seclusion or physical restraint of children and adolescents must receive training to decrease the risk of injury to the young person and themselves.

The registered nurse assigned to the patient is often the one to make the decision to restrain or seclude a child. A physician, nurse practitioner, or other advanced level practitioner must authorize this action according to facility policy and state regulation. The patient's family should be notified of any incident of seclusion or restraint.

Patients in seclusion or restraints must be monitored constantly and not be left alone. Vital signs and range of motion in extremities must be monitored at a set interval. Hydration, elimination, comfort, and other psychological and physical needs should be monitored and addressed as needed. Policy and regulations should provide guidelines as to the appropriate physical monitoring and care.

Children are released as soon as they are no longer dangerous. Once the child is calm, the staff should include the child in a debriefing and discuss the events leading up to and including the restrictive interventions with the patient. Debriefings provide an opportunity for staff members to discuss the event and explore ways it may have been prevented, evaluate their emotional responses, review the plan of care, and enhance their clinical skills.

Advanced Practice Interventions

Group Therapy

Advanced practice nurses are trained at the graduate level and qualified to conduct group therapy. Groups are effective when dealing with specific issues in a child's life such as bereavement, physical abuse, or chronic illnesses such as juvenile diabetes. Group therapy for younger children uses play to introduce ideas and work through issues. For grade-school children, it combines play, learning skills, and talking about the activity. The child learns to identify feelings and improve impulse control and social skills by taking turns and sharing with peers.

For teens, this modality offers them the opportunity to see how their peers are coping with or have managed similar problems and can be a means for developing a positive source of peer support. For adolescents, group therapy involves identifying emotions, modifying responses, learning skills and talking, focusing largely on peer relationships, and addressing specific problems. Adolescent group therapy might use a popular media event or personality as the basis for a group discussion.

Cognitive-Behavioral Therapy

CBT is an evidence-based treatment approach for a number of psychiatric diagnoses. It is based on the premise that negative and self-defeating thoughts lead to psychiatric pathology. Learning to replace these thoughts with more realistic and accurate appraisals results in improved functioning.

NEURODEVELOPMENTAL DISORDERS: CLINICAL PICTURE

According to the American Psychiatric Association (APA, 2013), the following disorders are considered neurodevelopmental disorders and will be discussed now:

- Communication disorders
- Motor disorders
- Specific learning disorder
- Intellectual disability
- Autism spectrum disorder
- Attention-deficit/hyperactivity disorder

COMMUNICATION DISORDERS

Communication disorders are a deficit in language skills acquisition that creates impairments in academic achievement, socialization, or self-care. Broadly, we consider speech and language as two separate categories for evaluating communication.

Speech disorders have to do with problems in making sounds. They may distort, add, or omit sounds. Children may have trouble making certain sounds such as "no" for "snow" or "wabbit" for "rabbit."

Another aspect of speech that may be disturbed is fluency. Child-onset fluency disorder, also known as stuttering, is manifested by hesitations and repetition. While all children may have mild and transient symptoms of speech problems, speech disorders significantly impact a child's ability to communicate.

Children may have a **receptive language disorder** where they experience difficulty understanding or are unable to follow directions. Children may have an **expressive language disorder** that results in difficulty in finding the right words and forming clear sentences. The child demonstrates difficulty learning words or an inability to speak in complete coherent sentences. Some children have a mixed receptive-expressive mixture of both problems and can neither understand others nor communicate properly. These disorders range from mild to severe and tend to show up prior to the age of 4 (National Institute on Deafness and Other Communication Disorders, 2015).

While some children have no problem with language and no problem speaking, they may have problems relating with other people. In **social communication disorder,** children have problems using verbal and nonverbal means for interacting socially with others. Impairments are also evident in written communication when the child is trying to relate to others. Prior to 2013 this disorder did not exist and many children with communication problems were diagnosed with Asperger's disorder, a disorder that has since been retired. Autism spectrum disorder needs to be ruled out to receive a diagnosis of social communication disorder (APA, 2013).

About 6% of children have some sort of communication disorder. Language disorders may be present from birth or may occur later in life. Causes include hearing loss, neurological disorders, intellectual disabilities, drug abuse, brain injury, physical problems such as cleft palate or lip, and vocal abuse or misuse. Frequently, the cause is unknown.

The Disabilities Education Act provides for early intervention services in every state for toddlers up to age 3. Service providers will meet with the family to develop a treatment plan. Special education and services are also available for individuals ages 3 to 21. Typically, the first step in the plan is a hearing test.

MOTOR DISORDERS

Developmental Coordination Disorder

A key feature of growth and development is the acquisition of fine and gross motor skills and coordination. **Developmental coordination disorder** is based on (1) impairments in motor skill development, (2) coordination below the child's developmental age, and (3) problems interfere with academic achievement or activities of daily living. Symptoms include delayed sitting or walking or difficulty jumping or performing tasks such as tying shoelaces.

Serious impairments in skills development or coordination are usually obvious. Children with less severe impairments may be less noticeable. They may be identified by their avoidance of certain tasks or activities. These children typically make comments like, "I hate to draw" or "I don't like it when we have to play kickball."

Early diagnosis, treatment, and education are essential to prevent frustration and unnecessary problems in adult life. Physical therapy and occupational therapy are the treatments of choice for developmental coordination disorder.

Stereotypic Movement Disorder

Stereotypic movement disorder is manifested by repetitive purposeless movements such as hand waving, rocking, head banging, nail biting, and teeth grinding for a period of 4 weeks or more (APA, 2013). This disorder is more common in boys than in girls. Intellectual disability is a risk factor for these repetitive movements with up to 16% of this population affected.

Interventions for stereotypic movement disorder focus on safety and prevention of injury. Helmets may be required for children who have the potential for head injury. Behavioral therapy includes habit-reversal techniques such as folding the arms when the urge to hand-wave begins. Naltrexone, an opioid receptor antagonist, may block euphoric responses from these behaviors, thereby reducing their occurrence.

TIC DISORDERS

Tics are sudden, nonrhythmic, and rapid motor movements or vocalizations. Motor tics usually involve the head, torso, or limbs, and they change in location, frequency, and severity over time. Other motor tics are tongue protrusion, touching, squatting, hopping, skipping, retracing steps, and twirling when walking. Vocal tics are spontaneous production of words unrelated to conscious communication and sounds such as sniffs, barks, coughs, or grunts.

According to the APA (2013), there are three types of tic disorders listed from least to most severe:

1. **Provisional tic disorder**—Single or multiple motor and or vocal tics for less than 1 year.
2. **Persistent motor or vocal tic disorder**—Single or multiple motor or vocal tics but not both for more than 1 year.
3. **Tourette's disorder**—Multiple motor tics and at least one vocal tic for more than 1 year.

All of these problems occur before age 18 with the typical age of onset between 4 and 6 years. Symptoms tend to peak in early adolescence and diminish into adulthood.

The comical Hollywood characterization of Tourette's disorder is a person with a foul mouth. In reality, coprolalia (uttering of obscenities) occurs in fewer than 10% of cases. A child or adolescent with tics may have low self-esteem as a result of feeling ashamed, self-conscious, and rejected by peers and may severely limit public appearances for fear of displaying tics.

A familial pattern exists in about 90% of cases. Tourette's disorder often coexists with depression, obsessive-compulsive disorder, and ADHD (Tamara, 2013). Central nervous system stimulants increase severity of tics, so medications must be carefully monitored in children with coexisting ADHD.

Behavioral techniques can reduce tic expression (McGuire et al., 2014). They are referred to as habit reversal, and the most promising form is called comprehensive behavior intervention for tics (CBITS). It works by helping the patient become aware of the building up of a tic urge then using a muscular response in competition to or incompatible with the tic.

Drugs with FDA approval for treating tics are the first-generation antipsychotics haloperidol (Haldol) and pimozide (Orap) and the second-generation antipsychotic aripiprazole (Abilify). Another second-generation drug, risperidone (Risperdal), does not have FDA approval, but is commonly used for tic disorders.

Clonidine hydrochloride (Catapres), an alpha 2-adrenergic agonist used to treat hypertension, is also prescribed for tics. While less effective and far slower acting than the antipsychotics, it has fewer side effects. The antianxiety drug clonazepam (Klonopin) is used as a supplement to other medications. It may work by reducing anxiety and resultant tics. Botulinum toxin type A (Botox) injections are used to calm the muscle(s) associated with tics.

A sort of pacemaker for the brain, deep brain stimulation (DBS) is used when more conservative treatments fail. A fine wire is threaded into affected areas of the brain and connected to a small device implanted under the collarbone that delivers electrical impulses. Users of DBS can turn the device on to control tics or shut it off when they go to sleep.

SPECIFIC LEARNING DISORDER

Children with **specific learning disorders** are identified during the school years. A specific learning disorder is diagnosed when a child demonstrates persistent difficulty in reading (dyslexia), mathematics (dyscalculia), and/or written expression (dysgraphia). With any of these problems their performance is well below the expected performance of their peers. Diagnosis of a learning disorder is made through multiple assessments, including formal psychological evaluations.

Screening for learning disorders is essential so that crucial early interventions may be put in place. Most students with this type of disability are eligible for assistance at a school that is supported by the Disabilities Education Improvement Act. This assistance involves an individualized treatment plan for each child, careful monitoring of progress, special education intervention, and the establishment of an Individualized Education Program (IEP).

According to the Child Trends Databank (2014), the prevalence of learning disorders is about 8% and has remained consistent at this rate for the past two decades. Compared with general learning disorders, specific learning disorders affect children with special health needs at more than 25% compared with about 5% in average developing children. Some factors associated with this problem are lower family education, poverty, and male gender.

Long-term outcomes for children with learning disorders can vary. The rate of enrollment in postsecondary education has risen significantly in the past 15 years. Without educational, social, and psychiatric interventions, low self-esteem, poor social skills, higher rates of school dropout, difficulties with attaining and maintaining employment, and poorer social adjustment may result (Cortiella & Horowitz, 2014).

INTELLECTUAL DISABILITY

Intellectual disability is characterized by deficits in three areas:

- *Intellectual functioning.* Deficits in reasoning, problem solving, planning, judgment, abstract thinking, and academic ability.
- *Social functioning.* Impaired communication and language, interpreting and acting on social cues, and regulating emotions.
- *Daily functioning.* Practical aspects of daily life are impacted by a deficit in managing age-appropriate activities of daily living, functioning at school or work, and performing self-care.

Impairments begin during childhood development, range from mild to severe, and include the consideration of the person's level of dependence on others for ongoing care and support (Taua et al., 2012). The incidence of intellectual disability is estimated at about 1% of the population (APA, 2013).

The etiology of intellectual disability may be heredity, problems with pregnancy or perinatal development, environmental influences, or a direct result of a medical condition. Hereditary factors can include chromosomal disorders such as Fragile X, Down or Klinefelter's syndrome, inborn errors of metabolism such as phenylketonuria, or genetic abnormalities.

Approximately 10% of affected individuals results from problems during pregnancy or birth and include malnutrition, chronic maternal substance abuse, and maternal infection. Complications of pregnancy such as toxemia, placenta previa, or trauma to the head during birth are also implicated. In addition, up to 20% of cases are attributed to environmental or social neglect that does not foster the development of social or linguistic skills or a lack of a nurturing relationship. Intellectual disabilities can also be associated with other mental disorders such as autism spectrum disorder.

APPLICATION OF THE NURSING PROCESS

ASSESSMENT

ASSESSMENT GUIDELINES

Intellectual Disability

1. Assess for delays in cognitive and physical development or lack of ability to perform tasks or achieve milestones in relation to peers. Gather information from family, caregivers, or others actively involved in the child's life.
2. Assess for delays in cognitive, social, or personal functioning, focusing on strengths and abilities.
3. Assess for areas of independent functioning and the need for support/assistance to meet requirements of daily living (examples are hygiene, dressing, or feeding).
4. Assess for physical and emotional signs of potential neglect or abuse. Be aware that children with behavioral and developmental problems are at risk for abuse.
5. Assess for need of community resources or programs that can provide resources and support the child's need for intellectual and social development and the family's need for education and emotional support.

DIAGNOSIS

The child with an intellectual disability has impairments in conceptual, social, and practical functioning, ranging from mild to severe. The severity of impairment is demonstrated in the ability to communicate effectively, meet one's self-care and safety needs, and socialize in an age-appropriate manner. Due to the increased need for supervision and assistance with daily living and the chronic nature of the disorder, families or caregivers may experience significant stress and be at risk for impaired family functioning. Table 11.1 lists potential nursing diagnoses.

TABLE 11.1 Signs and Symptoms and Nursing Diagnoses Neurodevelopmental Disorders

Signs and Symptoms	Nursing Diagnosis
Lack of responsiveness or interest in others, empathy, or sharing	*Impaired social interaction* *Risk for impaired attachment* *Risk for impaired parenting* *Risk for social isolation*
Lack of cooperation or imaginative play with peers	*Activity intolerance* *Situational low self-esteem* *Impaired social interaction*
Language delay or absence, stereotyped, or repetitive use of language	*Impaired verbal communication*
Inability to feed, bathe, dress, or toilet self at age-appropriate level	*Delayed growth and development* *Dressing, toileting, bathing self-care deficit*
Head banging, face slapping, hand biting	*Ineffective impulse control* *Risk for injury* *Risk for trauma* *Self-mutilation*
Frequent disregard for bodily needs	*Bathing or toileting* *Risk for situational low self-esteem* *Self-care deficit*
Failure to follow age-appropriate social norms	*Ineffective coping* *Ineffective role performance* *Risk for ineffective relationships*
Depression	*Risk for self-directed violence* *Stress overload* *Spiritual distress*
Refusal to attend school	*Ineffective coping* *Ineffective role performance* *Readiness for enhanced parenting*
Inability to concentrate, withdrawal, difficulty in functioning, feeling down, change in vegetative symptoms	*Risk for suicide* *Anxiety* *Risk for situational low self-esteem*
Family reports insufficient knowledge about child's disorder, overprotectiveness interferes with child's autonomy, parental anxiety	*Compromised family coping* *Risk for impaired attachment*

Herdman, T. H., & Kamitsuru, S. (Eds.). *Nursing diagnoses—Definitions and classification 2015-2017* (10th ed.). Copyright © 2015, 1994–2017 by NANDA International. Used by arrangement with John Wiley & Sons Limited.

OUTCOMES IDENTIFICATION

Nursing Outcomes Classification (NOC) (Moorhead et al., 2013) identifies a number of outcomes appropriate for the child with an intellectual disability:

- Uses spoken language to make or respond to requests.
- Engages in simple social interactions and accepts assistance or feedback regarding behavior without frustration.
- Tolerates social interaction for short periods of time without becoming disruptive or frustrated.
- Refrains from acting impulsively toward self or others when frustrated.

Additionally, the family may be in denial over the diagnosis. An outcome would be for the family to acknowledge the existence of impairment and its potential to alter family routines.

IMPLEMENTATION

Psychosocial Interventions

Nurses provide services to children with intellectual disabilities in a variety of settings. Children with intellectual disabilities are cared for in the community through early intervention programs or public school programs as they reach school age. Federal legislation, the Individuals with Disabilities in Education Act (IDEA), requires that public schools provide services to assist children with emotional or developmental disorders to participate in school (APA, 2015). Individuals may also require short-term hospitalization related to socially impaired behaviors such as aggression, self-harm, or severe self-care deficits.

Treatment plans should be individualized and realistic. Although the care plan is developed for the child, family members or caregivers and school personnel should be included in the process. Supportive education should be ongoing regarding the scope and nature of the illness; conceptual, social, and practical deficits; and realistic assessment of the child's potential. Long-term planning should include consideration of continuing care needs as the child ages and matures into adulthood.

EVALUATION

In evaluating the child and family with an intellectual disability, it is important for nurses to use a strength-based perspective. In the assessment, we identify both the areas of need and capabilities, focusing on how to maximize the family resources and link to services where need exists. Specific areas to evaluate relate to making a connection with service providers. Are the child and family receiving timely and efficient services? Is the care patient- and family-centered, allowing for the family to take a lead role in directing the plan of care?

While the individual may be the direct recipient of care, the family system is also disrupted. Families may require a great deal of education and ongoing reinforcement to accept realistic expectations for the child. Families and individuals with intellectual disabilities require lifelong support, so evaluations will focus on both short- and long-term goals. Long-term planning should include a goal of transitioning the child to a level of supervised or assisted care as he or she ages into adulthood.

AUTISM SPECTRUM DISORDER

Autism spectrum disorder is a complex neurobiological and developmental disability that typically appears during a child's first 3 years of life. Autism spectrum disorder affects the normal development of social interaction and communication skills. It ranges in severity from mild to moderate to severe.

Symptoms associated with autism spectrum disorder include deficits in social relatedness, which are manifested in disturbances in developing and maintaining relationships. Other behaviors include stereotypical repetitive speech, obsessive focus on specific objects, overadherence to routines or rituals, hyperreactivity or hyporeactivity to sensory input, and extreme resistance to change. The symptoms will first occur in childhood and cause impairments in everyday functioning. The *DSM-5* box provides diagnostic criteria for autism spectrum disorder.

DSM-5 CRITERIA FOR AUTISM SPECTRUM DISORDER

A. Persistent deficits in social communication and social interaction across multiple contexts, as manifested by the following, currently or by history (examples are illustrative, not exhaustive):
   1. Deficits in social-emotional reciprocity, ranging, for example, from abnormal social approach and failure of normal back-and-forth conversation; to reduced sharing of interests, emotions, or affect; to failure to initiate or respond to social interactions.
   2. Deficits in nonverbal communicative behaviors used for social interaction, ranging, for example, from poorly integrated verbal and nonverbal communication; to abnormalities in eye contact and body language or deficits in understanding and use of gestures; to total lack of facial expressions or nonverbal communication.
   3. Deficits in developing, maintaining, and understanding relationships, ranging, for example, from difficulties adjusting behavior to suit various social contexts; to difficulties in sharing imaginative play or in making friends; to an absence of interest in peers.

Specify current severity:

Severity is based on social communication impairments and restricted repetitive patterns of behavior.

B. Restricted, repetitive patterns of behavior, interests, or activities as manifested by at least two of the following, currently or by history (examples are illustrative, not exhaustive):
   1. Stereotyped or repetitive motor movements, use of objects, or speech (e.g., simple motor stereotypies, lining up toys or flipping objects, echolalia, idiosyncratic phrases).
   2. Insistence on sameness, excessive adherence to routines, or ritualized patterns of verbal or nonverbal behavior (e.g., extreme distress at small changes, difficulties with transitions, rigid thinking patterns, greeting rituals, need to take same route or eat food every day).
   3. Highly restricted, fixated interests that are abnormal in intensity or focus (e.g., strong attachment to or preoccupation with unusual objects, excessively circumscribed or perseverative interests).
   4. Hyperreactivity or hyporeactivity to sensory input or unusual interest in sensory aspects of the environment (e.g., apparent indifference to pain/temperature, adverse response to specific sounds or textures, excessive smelling or touching of objects, visual fascination with lights or movement).

Specify current severity:

Severity is based on social communication impairments and restricted repetitive patterns of behavior.

C. Symptoms must be present in the early developmental period (but may not become fully manifest until social demands exceed limited capacities, or may be masked by learned strategies in later life).

D. Symptoms together limit and impair everyday functioning.

E. These disturbances are not better explained by intellectual disability (intellectual developmental disorder) or global developmental delay. Intellectual disability and autism spectrum disorder frequently co-occur; to make comorbid diagnoses of autism spectrum disorder and intellectual disability, social communication should be below that expected for general developmental level.

Specify if:

With or without accompanying intellectual impairment

With or without accompanying language impairment

Associated with a known medical or genetic condition or environmental factor

Associated with another neurodevelopmental, mental, or behavioral disorder

With catatonia

American Psychiatric Association. (2013). *Diagnostic and statistical manual of mental disorders* (5th ed.). Washington, DC: Author.

There is a genetic component to autism spectrum disorder. The concordance rate for monozygotic (identical) twins is 70% to 90%, meaning that most of the time if one twin is affected so is the other. Autism spectrum disorder is four times more common in boys than girls (Devlin & Scherer, 2012). Autism spectrum disorder has no racial, ethnic, or social boundaries and is not influenced by family income, educational levels, or lifestyles.

Without intensive intervention, individuals with severe autism spectrum disorder may not be able to live and work independently. Only about one-third achieve partial independence with restricted interests and activities. Early intervention for children with autism spectrum disorder can greatly enhance their potential for a full, productive life. Unfortunately, many families with a child with an autism spectrum disorder may not seek help early.

Often, symptoms are first noticed when the infant fails to be interested in others or to be socially responsive through eye contact and facial expressions. Some children show improvement during development, but puberty can be a turning point toward either improvement or deterioration.

Some individuals with autism spectrum disorder may have low IQs yet are brilliant in specific areas. These areas include musical, visual-spatial, or intellectual abilities such as the ability to complete complex mathematical calculations or photographic memory recall. This is a condition known as savant syndrome.

APPLICATION OF THE NURSING PROCESS

ASSESSMENT

ASSESSMENT GUIDELINES

Autism Spectrum Disorder

1. Assess for developmental delays, uneven development, or loss of acquired abilities. Use baby books and diaries, photographs, videotapes, or anecdotal reports from nonfamily caregivers.
2. Assess the child's communication skills (verbal and nonverbal), sensory, social and behavioral skills (including presence of any aggressive or self-injurious behaviors)
3. Assess the parent-child relationship for evidence of bonding, anxiety, tension, and fit of temperaments.
4. Assess for physical and emotional signs of possible abuse. Be aware that children with behavioral and developmental problems are at risk for abuse.
5. Ensure that screening for comorbid intellectual disability has been completed.
6. Assess the need for community programs with support services for parents and children including parent education, counseling, and after-school programs.

DIAGNOSIS

The child with autism spectrum disorder has severe impairments in social interactions and communication skills, often accompanied by stereotypical behavior, interests, and activities. At least half of those diagnosed with autism spectrum disorder will have some intellectual disability (IQ <85), which will impact their academic performance as well. The stress on the family can be severe, due to the chronic nature of the disease. The severity of the impairment is evident in the degree of responsiveness to or interest in others, the presence of associated behavioral problems (e.g., head banging), and the ability to bond with peers. Table 11.1 lists potential nursing diagnoses.

OUTCOMES IDENTIFICATION

NOC (Moorhead et al., 2013) identifies a number of outcomes appropriate for the child with autism spectrum disorder and the family. Outcomes for social interaction skills include cooperating with others, exhibiting consideration, and exhibiting sensitivity to others. Communication skills outcomes include accurately interpreting messages and accurately exchanging messages. Family normalization is associated with adapting to the challenges of a child with autism spectrum disorder and using community support.

IMPLEMENTATION

Psychosocial Interventions

Children with autism spectrum disorder should be referred to **early intervention programs** once communication and behavioral symptoms are identified, typically in the second or third year of life. Through case management and coordination of care, they may be treated in therapeutic nursery schools, day treatment programs, and special education classes in public or specialized private schools. Their education and treatment with therapeutic modalities are mandated under the Children with Disabilities Act.

Treatment plans include behavior management with a reward system, teaching parents to provide structure, rewards, consistency in rules, and expectations at home to shape and modify behavior and foster the development of socially appropriate skills. Children with autism spectrum disorder may receive physical, occupational, and speech therapy as part of the plan of care.

It is important that the nurse recognize and capitalize on the individual's and family's strengths. Also, the family's goals and priorities should influence the plan of care. The multidisciplinary team serves to guide and support the family in making realistic goals for their child.

Psychobiological Interventions

Pharmacological

Pharmacological agents target specific symptoms and may be used to improve relatedness and decrease anxiety, compulsive behaviors, or agitation. The second-generation antipsychotics risperidone (Risperdal) and aripiprazole (Abilify) have FDA approval for treating children 5 and 6 years of age and older, respectively. These drugs improve irritability that is expressed in severe temper tantrums, aggression, and self-injurious behavior.

The SSRIs are the most popular medication used in this population. They improve mood and reduce anxiety, which provides the patient with a higher degree of tolerance for new situations. Stimulant medications may be used to target hyperactivity, impulsivity, or inattention.

EVALUATION

Autism spectrum disorder causes deficits in communication and social skills in the individual with a range of individual severity. The *DSM-5* (APA, 2013) classifies autism spectrum disorder in three levels depending on the degree of assistance and support the individual requires:

- Level 1 requires support
- Level 2 requires substantial support
- Level 3 requires very substantial support

For children with milder forms of autism spectrum disorder it is reasonable to expect greater participation and input from the child. For individuals with more severe impairments, there will be greater reliance on the family. Family members must have clear and realistic expectations of the long-term needs of their child and be linked with the appropriate resources to assist with care and long-term planning.

Evaluation should target the family's awareness of how to advocate for appropriate service provision. Has the early intervention program been accessed? How are the child and family coordinating appointments? For the school-aged child, is the early intervention plan reflective of realistic educational goals?

The nurse should monitor both the individual and the family for the effects of stress. Increased stress may interfere with the family's ability to utilize resources, or family members may find the coordination and integration of services to be overwhelming.

ATTENTION-DEFICIT/HYPERACTIVITY DISORDER

Individuals with **attention-deficit/hyperactivity disorder** (ADHD) show an inappropriate degree of inattention, impulsiveness, and hyperactivity. Some children are inattentive, but not hyperactive. In this case the diagnosis is attention-deficit disorder (ADD). To diagnose a child with ADHD symptoms must be present in at least two settings (e.g., at home and school) and occur before age 12. The disorder is most often detected when the child has difficulty adjusting to elementary school. Attention problems and hyperactivity contribute to low frustration tolerance, temper outbursts, labile moods, poor school performance, peer rejection, and low self-esteem.

The behaviors and symptoms associated with ADHD can include hyperactivity and impulsivity. Peer relationships are strained due to difficulty taking turns, poor social boundaries, intrusive behaviors, and interrupting others. Those with inattentive type of ADHD may exhibit high degrees of distractibility and disorganization. They may be unable to complete challenging or tedious tasks, become easily bored, lose things frequently, or require frequent prompts to complete tasks. The *DSM-5* box provides diagnostic criteria for ADHD.

DSM-5 CRITERIA FOR ATTENTION-DEFICIT/HYPERACTIVITY DISORDER

A. A persistent pattern of inattention and/or hyperactivity-impulsivity that interferes with functioning or development, as characterized by (1) and/or (2):
   1. **Inattention:** Six (or more) of the following symptoms have persisted for at least 6 months to a degree inconsistent with developmental level and that negatively impacts directly on social and academic/occupational activities:
   Note: The symptoms are not solely a manifestation of oppositional behavior, defiance, hostility, or failure to understand tasks or instructions. For older adolescents and adults (age 17 and older), at least five symptoms are required.
      a. Often fails to give close attention to details or makes careless mistakes in schoolwork, at work, or during other activities (e.g., overlooks or misses details, work is inaccurate).
      b. Often has difficulty sustaining attention in tasks or play activities (e.g., has difficulty remaining focused during lectures, conversations, or lengthy reading).
      c. Often does not seem to listen when spoken to directly (e.g., mind seems elsewhere, even in the absence of any obvious distraction).
      d. Often does not follow through on instructions and fails to finish schoolwork, chores, or duties in the workplace (e.g., starts task but quickly loses focus and is easily sidetracked).
      e. Often has difficulty organizing tasks and activities (e.g., difficulty managing sequential tasks, difficulty keeping materials and belongings in order, messy disorganized work, has poor time management, fails to meet deadlines).
      f. Often avoids, dislikes, or is reluctant to engage in tasks that require sustained mental effort (e.g., schoolwork or homework; for older adolescents and adults, preparing reports, completing forms, reviewing lengthy papers).
      g. Often loses things necessary for tasks or activities (e.g., school materials, pencils, books, tools, wallets, keys, paperwork, eyeglasses, mobile telephones).
      h. Is often easily distracted by extraneous stimuli (for older adolescents and adults, may include unrelated thoughts).
      i. Is often forgetful in daily activities (e.g., doing chores, running errands; for older adolescents and adults, returning calls, paying bills, keeping appointments).
   2. **Hyperactivity and impulsivity:** Six (or more) of the following symptoms have persisted for at least 6 months to a degree inconsistent with development level and that negatively impacts directly on social and academic/occupational activities:
   Note: The symptoms are not solely a manifestation of oppositional behavior, defiance, hostility, or a failure to understand tasks or instructions. For older adolescents and adults (age 17 and older), at least five symptoms are required.
      a. Often fidgets with or taps hands or feet or squirms in seat.
      b. Often leaves seat in situations when remaining seated is expected (e.g., leaves his or her place in the classroom, in the office or other workplace, or in situations that require remaining in place).
      c. Often runs about or climbs in situations where it is inappropriate. (**Note:** In adolescents or adults, may be limited to feeling restless.)
      d. Often unable to play or engage in leisure activities quietly.
      e. Is often "on the go," acting as if "driven by a motor" (e.g., is unable to be or uncomfortable being still for extended time, as in restaurants, meetings; may be experienced by others as being restless or difficult to keep up with).
      f. Often talks excessively.
      g. Often blurts out an answer before a question has been completed (e.g., completes people's sentences; cannot wait for turn in conversation).
      h. Often has difficulty waiting for his or her turn (e.g., while waiting in line).
      i. Often interrupts or intrudes on others (e.g., butts into conversations, games, or activities; may start using other people's things without asking or receiving permission; for adolescents and adults, may intrude into or take over what others are doing).

B. Several inattentive or hyperactive-impulsive symptoms were present before age 12 years.

C. Several inattentive or hyperactive-impulsive symptoms are present in two or more settings (e.g., at home, school, or work; with friends or relatives; in other activities).

D. There is clear evidence that the symptoms interfere with, or reduce the quality of, social, academic, or occupational functioning.

E. The symptoms do not occur exclusively during the course of schizophrenia or another psychotic disorder and are not better explained by another mental disorder (e.g., mood disorder, anxiety disorder, dissociative disorder, personality disorder, substance intoxication or withdrawal).

Specify if: **In partial remission:** When full criteria were previously met, fewer than the full criteria have been met for the past 6 months, and the symptoms still result in impairment in social, academic, or occupational functioning.

American Psychiatric Association. (2013). *Diagnostic and statistical manual of mental disorders* (5th ed.). Washington, DC: Author.

About 10% of children and adolescents between the ages of 5 and 17 have ADHD. It affects about 14% of boys and about 6% of girls in that same age range (CDC, 2016). Children in poor health are more than twice as likely to have ADHD (21% versus 8%). The median age of onset is 7 years old. However, some people may go undiagnosed until functional impairments become noticeable in adulthood.

Children with ADHD are often diagnosed with comorbid disorders such as oppositional defiant disorder or conduct disorder. Other comorbid disorders include conduct disorder, disruptive mood dysregulation disorder, and specific learning disorder.

APPLICATION OF THE NURSING PROCESS

ASSESSMENT

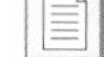

ASSESSMENT GUIDELINES

Attention-Deficit/Hyperactivity Disorder

1. Gather data from parents, caregivers, teachers, or other adults involved with the child. Ask about level of physical activity, span, talkativeness, frustration tolerance, impulse control, and the ability to follow directions and complete tasks. Also, assess these areas through your own observations and note any developmental variance in these behaviors.
2. Assess social skills, friendship history, problem-solving skills, and school performance. Gather this data from the family or caregiver and one or two additional sources.

ASSESSMENT GUIDELINES—cont'd

Attention-Deficit/Hyperactivity Disorder

3. Assess for comorbidities such as anxiety and depression.
4. Assess for any indicators of learning disorders, autism spectrum disorder, or intellectual disabilities.
5. Gather data on eating and sleeping patterns and monitor these regularly for the child treated with stimulants.

DIAGNOSIS

Children and adolescents with ADHD can be overactive and may display disruptive behaviors that are impulsive, angry, aggressive, and often dangerous. They may have difficulty with maintaining attention in situations that require sustained attention. In addition, their behaviors negatively impact their ability to develop fulfilling peer and family relationships. They are often in conflict with others, are noncompliant, do not follow age-appropriate social norms, and may use inappropriate ways to meet their needs. Refer to Table 11.1 for potential nursing diagnoses.

OUTCOMES IDENTIFICATION

NOC (Bulechek et al., 2013) identifies a number of outcomes appropriate for the child with ADHD. *NOC* outcomes target hyperactivity, impulse self-control, freedom from injury, improved social relationships, the development of self-identity and self-esteem, positive coping skills, and family functioning.

IMPLEMENTATION

Psychosocial Interventions

Interventions for patients with ADHD focus on recognizing ineffective coping mechanisms, such as blaming others and denial of responsibility for their actions. Children and adolescents can be helped to adopt adaptive coping mechanisms and pro-social goals.

Treatment may include hospitalization for those who present an imminent danger to self or others. Typically, treatment is provided on an outpatient basis, using individual, group, and family therapy, with an emphasis on parenting issues. Children whose behavior requires longer-term intensive treatment may be referred to intensive outpatient programs and specialized charter schools. Residential treatment or group home placement may even be an option.

CBT is used to change the pattern of misconduct by fostering the development of internal controls and working with the family to improve coping and support. Development of problem solving, conflict resolution, empathy, and social skills is an important component of the treatment program.

Families are actively engaged in therapy and given support in using parenting skills to provide nurturance and set consistent limits. They are taught techniques for modifying behavior, monitoring medication for effects, collaborating with teachers to foster academic success, and setting up a home environment that is consistent, structured, and nurturing and that promotes achievement of normal developmental milestones. If families are abusive, drug dependent, or highly disorganized, the child may require out-of-home placement.

Box 11.3 lists techniques for managing disruptive behaviors.

Psychobiological Interventions

Psychopharmacology

Paradoxically, we treat the symptoms of ADHD with stimulant drugs. Responses to these drugs are often dramatic and can quickly increase attention and task-directed behavior while reducing impulsivity, restlessness, and distractibility (Lehne, 2016). Methylphenidate (Ritalin and others) and the

BOX 11.3 Techniques for Managing Disruptive Behaviors

Behavioral contract: A verbal or written agreement between the patient and nurse or other parties (e.g., family, treatment team, teacher) about behaviors, expectations, and needs. The contract is periodically evaluated and reviewed and typically coupled with rewards and other contingencies, positive and negative.

Collaborative and proactive solutions: A therapeutic intervention used with parents and children designed to help both identify and define problematic behaviors, specific triggers, and develop a collaborative method for creating mutually agreeable solutions to the specific situation or trigger.

Counseling: Verbal interactions, role playing, and modeling to teach, coach, or maintain adaptive behavior and provide positive reinforcement. Best used with motivated youth and those with well-developed communication and self-reflective skills.

Modeling: A method of learning behaviors or skills by observation and imitation that can be used in a wide variety of situations. It is enhanced when the modeler is perceived to be similar (e.g., age, interests) and attending to the task is required.

Role playing: A counseling technique in which the nurse, the patient, or a group of youngsters acts out a specified script or role to enhance their understanding of that role, learn and practice new behaviors or skills, and practice specific situations. It requires well-developed expressive and receptive language skills.

Planned ignoring: When behaviors are determined by staff to be attention seeking and not dangerous, they may be ignored. Additional interventions may be used in conjunction (e.g., positive reinforcement for on-task actions).

Use of signals or gestures: Use a word, a gesture, or eye contact to remind the child to use self-control. To help promote behavioral change, this may be used in conjunction with a behavioral contract and a reward system. An example is placing your finger to your lips and making eye contact with a child who is talking during a quiet drawing activity.

Physical distance and touch control: Moving closer to the child for a calming effect, perhaps putting an arm around the child (with permission). Evaluate the effect of this because some children may find this more agitating and may need more space and less physical closeness. It also may involve putting the nurse or a staff member between certain children who have a history of conflict.

Redirection: A technique used after an undesirable or inappropriate behavior to engage or re-engage an individual in an appropriate activity. It may involve the use of verbal directives (e.g., setting firm limits), gestures, or physical prompts.

Additional affection: Involves giving a child planned emotional support for a specific problem or engaging in an enjoyable activity. It can be used to redirect a child away from an undesirable activity as well. This shows acceptance of the child while ignoring the behavior and can increase rapport in the nurse-patient relationship.

Continued

BOX 11.3 Techniques for Managing Disruptive Behaviors—cont'd

Use of humor: Use well-timed appropriate kidding about some external nonpersonal (to the child) event as a diversion to help the child save face and relieve feelings of guilt or fear.

Clarification as intervention: Breaking down a problem situation that a child experiences can help the child understand the situation, the roles of others, and his or her own motivation for the behavior. This can be done verbally and using worksheets depending on the age and functional level of the child.

Restructuring: Changing an activity in a way that will decrease the stimulation or frustration (e.g., shorten a story or change to a physical activity). This requires flexibility and planning and an alternative if the activity is not going well.

Limit setting: Involves giving direction, stating an expectation, or telling a child what to do or where to go. Caregivers should do this firmly, calmly, without judgment or anger, preferably in advance of any problem behavior occurring, and all staff should do this consistently in a treatment setting. An example would be, "I would like for you to stop turning the light on and off."

Simple restitution: Refers to a procedure in which an individual is required or expected to correct the adverse environmental or relational effects of his or her misbehavior by restoring the environment to its prior state, making a plan to correct his or her actions with the nurse, and implementing the plan (e.g., apologizing to the people harmed, fixing the chairs that are upturned).

Physical restraint: Using mechanical means to control and protect the child from impulses to act out and hurt self or others.

mixed amphetamine salts (Adderall) are the most widely used stimulants because of their relative safety and simplicity of use. As with any controlled substance, however, there is a risk of abuse and misuse such as the sale of the medication on the street or the use by people for whom the medication was not intended.

Not surprisingly, insomnia is a common side effect while taking stimulant medications. Treating with the minimum effective dose is essential. Administering the medication no later than 4:00 in the afternoon or lowering the last dose of the day helps. The extended-release formulations of these medications have improved dosing and scheduling. The long-acting versions allow for a morning administration with sustained release of the medication over the course of the day and with a decreased incidence of insomnia. Other common side effects include appetite suppression, headache, abdominal pain, and lethargy.

A nonstimulant selective norepinephrine reuptake inhibitor, atomoxetine (Strattera), is approved for childhood and adult ADHD. Therapeutic responses develop slowly, and it may take up to 6 weeks for full improvement. This medication is preferable for individuals whose anxiety is increased with stimulants. It is also useful for those with comorbid anxiety, active substance use disorders, or tics.

The most common side effects of atomoxetine are gastrointestinal disturbances, reduced appetite, weight loss, urinary retention, dizziness, fatigue, and insomnia. It may also cause liver injury in some patients and a small increase in blood pressure and heart rate. Ongoing monitoring of vital signs and regular screening of liver function are key aspects of assessment. Rarely, serious allergic reactions occur. Patients and their families should be clearly educated on the risks and benefits of treatment before starting this medication. Atomoxetine should be used with extreme caution in those patients with comorbid depression since its use has been associated with an increased suicidal ideation. See Table 11.2 for a summary of the FDA approved medications used to treat ADHD.

Two centrally acting alpha-2 adrenergic agonists, clonidine (Kapvay) and guanfacine (Intuniv), are FDA approved for the treatment of ADHD. They may be used alone or in conjunction with other ADHDA medications. Of the two drugs, clonidine carries more side effects: somnolence, fatigue, insomnia, nightmares, irritability, constipation, respiratory symptoms, dry mouth, and ear pain. The most common side effects of guanfacine are somnolence, lethargy, fatigue, insomnia, nausea, dizziness, hypotension, and abdominal pain.

Medication for Aggressive Behaviors

To control aggressive behaviors, pharmacological agents including stimulants, mood stabilizers, alpha-adrenergic agonists, and antipsychotics are used. Stimulants have a dose-dependent effect. Low doses stimulate aggressive behaviors while moderate to high doses suppress aggression. Mood stabilizers such as lithium and anticonvulsants reduce aggressive behavior and are recommended for impulsivity, explosive temper, and mood lability.

Due to the side effects of fatigue and somnolence, clonidine and guanfacine are helpful in reducing agitation and rage and in increasing frustration tolerance. Antipsychotic medications have reduced violent behavior, hyperactivity, and social unresponsiveness. Due to the risk of tardive dyskinesia associated with long-term use, antipsychotic medications are only recommended for severely aggressive behavior.

EVALUATION

For the family and child with ADHD, evaluation will focus on the symptom patterns and severity. For those with ADHD, inattentive type, the focus of evaluation will be academic performance, activities of daily living, social relationships, and personal perception. For those with ADHD, hyperactive-impulsive type, or combined type, the focus will be on academic performance, social skills and relationships, impulse control, and behavioral responses.

Evaluation of the response to pharmacotherapy is important. Stimulant medications are quite effective in symptom management yet can cause troublesome side effects. Monitoring and managing the timing and administration of medication are dependent on ongoing evaluation of efficacy or side effects. As the individual and family members become familiar with the use of the medication, they begin to recognize when a need for medication adjustment is required.

TABLE 11.2 FDA Approved Drugs for ADHD

Generic Name	Trade Name	Indications	Duration	Schedule
Stimulants				
Amphetamine	Adzenys XR-ODT	Ages 6 and older	12 hours	Once a day
	Dyanavel XR	Ages 6 and older	12 hours	Once a day
Dexmethylphenidate	Focalin	Ages 6 and older	4-5 hours	Two times a day
	Focalin XR	Ages 6 and older	8-12 hours	Once a day
Dextroamphetamine	Dexedrine	Ages 3 to 16	4-6 hours	Two or three times a day
Lisdexamfetamine dimesylate	Vyvanse	Ages 6 and older	10-12 hours	Once a day
Methamphetamine	Desoxyn	Ages 6 and older	6-8 hours	One or two times a day
Methylphenidate HCL	Concerta	Ages 6 to 65	10-12 hours	Once a day
	Daytrana (transdermal patch)	Ages 6 to 17	10-12 hours (up to 3 hours after removal)	Once a day
	Metadate ER	Ages 6 to 15	6-8 hours	One or two times a day
	Metadate CD	Ages 6 to 15	6-8 hours	Once a day
	Methylin ER	Ages 6 and older	6-8 hours	Once a day
	Quillichew ER	Ages 6 and older	12 hours	Once a day
	Quillivant XR	Ages 6 to 12	12 hours	Once a day
	Ritalin	Ages 6 to 12	6-8 hours	One or two times a day
	Ritalin LA	Ages 6 to 12	7-9 hours	Once a day
	Ritalin SR	Ages 6 to 12	6-8 hours	One or two times a day
Mixed salts of a single entity amphetamine product	Adderall	Ages 6 and older	4-6 hours	Two times a day
	Adderall–XR	Ages 6 and older	10-12 hours	One or two times a day
Nonstimulants				
Atomoxetine	Strattera	Ages 6 to 65	24 hours	One or two times a day
Clonidine	Kapvay	Ages 6 to 17	24 hours	Two times a day
Guanfacine	Intuniv	Ages 6 to 17	24 hours	Once a day

Food and Drug Administration. (2016). FDA online label repository. Retrieved from http://labels.fda.gov/; Howland, R. (2016). FDA-approved drugs to treat ADHD. *Journal of Psychosocial Nursing, 54*(3), 22–23.

For all children with neurobiological disorders, safety is a major emphasis and an important subject of evaluation. Young people who have ADHD can have difficulties in assessing the environment or realistically assessing risks of danger. When aggressive or disruptive behaviors are present there is always the potential for harm.

At the family system level the nurse will assess the degree of understanding of symptoms and symptom management by family members. Unrealistic expectations can result in frustration for both the individual and family and yield unfulfilling or negative interpersonal relationships. What is the family's perception of the problem? What type of services do they need to support their attempts in implementing effective behavioral plans? Has the family system stabilized?

Finally, long-term planning and goal setting should be a core evaluation measure. ADHD is chronic and unremitting, and symptoms frequently persist into adulthood. Are the patient and family setting realistic expectations as the child prepares to transition to postsecondary education or a vocation? Has the patient assumed primary responsibility for treatment planning and symptom management? Supporting the patient and family in the decision-making process and linking them with any additional resources can assist in a smooth transition.

QUALITY IMPROVEMENT

Improving the quality and effectiveness of nursing care for children with psychiatric disorders is a continuous process. Currently, there is a lack of reliable quality measures designed for child and adolescent mental health. However, the Center for Quality Assessment and Improvement in Mental Health (2015) identify the following measures for improving child and adolescent mental healthcare:

- Access to child specialty care for treatment of depression
- Family involvement in the treatment of ADHD
- Stimulant medication treatment for ADHD
- Antipsychotic treatment for childhood psychoses
- Completion of treatment for substance use disorders
- Referral to postdetoxification treatment services

The Mental Health Quality Measures, Child Healthcare toolbox (Agency for Healthcare Research and Quality, 2014) promotes the use of two assessment tools. They help to identify high-risk and problem-prone child populations, knowledge deficits in parenting, gaps in access, new evidence-based interventions and effective treatment. Psychiatric-mental health nurses can play a key role in assisting with this through the use of tools and involvement in quality assessment and measurement activities in the wide variety of work settings where child and adolescent mental health services are delivered.

KEY POINTS TO REMEMBER

- One in five children and adolescents in the United States suffers from a major mental illness that causes significant impairments at home, at school, with peers, and in the community.
- Factors known to affect the development of mental and emotional problems in children and adolescents include genetic influences, biochemical (prenatal and postnatal) factors, temperament, psychosocial developmental factors, social and environmental factors, and cultural influences.
- The characteristics of a resilient child include an adaptable temperament, the ability to form nurturing relationships with surrogate parental figures, the ability to distance the self from emotional chaos in parents and family, good social intelligence, the ability to perceive a future, and problem-solving skills.
- Use seclusion and restraint as last resorts after less restrictive interventions have failed and only in the case of dangerous behavior toward self or others. Seclusion and restraint require continuous monitoring by trained staff and must not be used as a punishment. Notify parents/guardians if such measures are used.
- Communication disorders are a deficit in language skills acquisition that creates impairments in academic achievement, socialization, or getting self-care.
- Motor disorders are manifested by impairments in gross and fine motor skill acquisition. They can range from mild to profound in severity. Purposeless, repetitive movements that interfere with daily living activities characterize stereotypic movement disorders.
- Tics are sudden, nonrhythmic, and rapid motor movements or vocalizations. Tic disorders vary in severity and degree of interference with the child's social and academic functioning.
- Learning disorders may be in the areas of reading, mathematics, or written expression with performance in those areas below the level expected for the age and cognitive level. Interventions are designated in an Individualized Education Program (IEP) and provided through special education in public schools.
- Autism spectrum disorder typically occurs within the first 3 years of life, yielding deficits in social interaction and communication skills. Children with autism spectrum disorder are referred to early intervention programs and continue to receive school-based services as they enter the public education system.
- Attention-deficit/hyperactivity disorders are evidenced by symptoms of inattentiveness and/or hyperactivity and impulsivity that are developmentally inappropriate. These disorders cause the child problems in a number of settings, such as home, school, and community. ADHD is treated primarily with stimulant medications and behavioral therapies.
- Treatment of childhood and adolescent disorders requires a multimodal approach in almost all instances, and family involvement is seen as critical to improvement in outcomes.
- Nurses can be important advocates for children with severe emotional and behavioral disorders.

CRITICAL THINKING

1. Bettina, a 12-year-old girl, has been diagnosed with autism spectrum disorder, moderate severity. She has an individualized education program (IEP) that includes remedial reading, social skills group, and occupational therapy to assist with her skills in feeding, dressing, and safety and attends a weekly social skills group to improve relational and communication skills.
   a. Describe the specific behavioral data you would find on assessment in terms of (1) communication, (2) social interactions, and (3) behaviors and activities.
   b. Name a minimum of three specific measurable and behavioral nursing outcomes for a child with autism spectrum disorder.
   c. Which nursing and behavioral interventions do you think are the most important for a pre-adolescent with autism spectrum disorder? Identify at least six.
   d. List three types of community-based resources to which the family should be referred.
2. Carlos is a 6-year-old boy in the first grade diagnosed with attention-deficit/hyperactivity disorder (ADHD), combined type.
   a. Create a concept map of clinical behaviors he might be exhibiting at home and in the classroom. Identify specific behavioral examples of his (1) inattention, (2) hyperactivity, and (3) impulsivity and the correlated neurotransmitter involved.
   b. Develop a nursing care plan with two priority nursing diagnoses.
   c. Identify at least six intervention strategies one might use for him including a discussion of the use of medication management. Identify at least two different medications that could be used, and identify their intended effect, potential side effects, and key patient teaching information.
   d. Describe the concept of redirecting and planned ignoring and how it could be used therapeutically with Carlos.
3. Melissa is a 15-year-old girl who has been diagnosed with intellectual disability and has been biting her arms and hitting her peers when frustrated.
   a. Explain to one of your classmates the assessment data that would be relevant in terms of (1) school performance, (2) socialization with peers, (3) activities of daily living, and (4) coping with frustration.
   b. What are the normal maturational developmental milestones for a 15-year-old child? What developmental issues will be a priority concern with Melissa? Create an individual and family education plan to address sexuality and sexual health for this teenager.
   c. What are three nursing interventions you could use to support Melissa's parents? List two or three resources within your own community that you could refer the family to for emotional and caregiving/respite support.

CHAPTER REVIEW

Questions

1. Which statement demonstrates a well-structured attempt at limit setting?
   a. "Hitting me when you are angry is unacceptable."
   b. "I expect you to behave yourself during dinner."
   c. "Come here, right now!"
   d. "Good boys don't bite."
2. Which activity is most appropriate for a child with ADHD?
   a. Reading an adventure novel
   b. Monopoly
   c. Checkers
   d. Tennis
3. Cognitive-behavioral therapy is going well when a 12-year-old patient in therapy reports to the nurse practitioner:
   a. "I was so mad I wanted to hit my mother."
   b. "I thought that everyone at school hated me. That's not true. Most people like me and I have a friend named Todd."
   c. "I forgot that you told me to breathe when I become angry."
   d. "I scream as loud as I can when the train goes by the house."
4. What assessment question should the nurse ask when attempting to determine a teenager's mental health resilience? *Select all that apply.*
   a. "How did you cope when your father deployed with the Army for a year in Iraq?"
   b. "Who did you go to for advice while your father was away for a year in Iraq?"
   c. "How do you feel about talking to a mental health counselor?"
   d. "Where do you see yourself in 10 years?"
   e. "Do you like the school you go to?"
5. Which factors tend to increase the difficulty of diagnosing young children who demonstrate behaviors associated with mental illness? *Select all that apply.*
   a. Limited language skills
   b. Level of cognitive development
   c. Level of emotional development
   d. Parental denial that a problem exists
   e. Severity of the typical mental illnesses observed in young children
6. Pam, the nurse educator, is teaching a new nurse about seclusion and restraint. Order the following interventions from least (1) to most (5) restrictive:
   a. With the patient identify the behaviors that are unacceptable and consequences associated with harmful behaviors
   b. Placing the patient in physical restraints
   c. Allowing the patient to take a time-out and sit in his or her room
   d. Offering a PRN medication by mouth
   e. Placing the patient in a locked seclusion room
7. In pediatric mental health there is a lack of sufficient numbers of community-based resources and providers, and there are long waiting lists for services. This has resulted in: *Select all that apply.*
   a. Children of color and poor economic conditions being underserved
   b. Increased stress in the family unit
   c. Markedly increased funding
   d. Premature termination of services
8. Child protective services have removed 10-year-old Christopher from his parents' home due to neglect. Christopher reveals to the nurse that he considers the woman next door his "nice" mom, that he loves school, and gets above average grades. The strongest explanation of this response is:
   a. Temperament
   b. Genetic factors
   c. Resilience
   d. Paradoxical effects of neglect
9. April, a 10-year-old admitted to inpatient pediatric care, has been getting more and more wound up and is losing self-control in the day room. Time-out does not appear to be an effective tool for April to engage in self-reflection. April's mother admits to putting her in time-out up to 20 times a day. The nurse recognizes that:
   a. Time-out is an important part of April's baseline discipline.
   b. Time-out is no longer an effective therapeutic measure.
   c. April enjoys time-out, and acts out to get some alone time.
   d. Time-out will need to be replaced with seclusion and restraint.
10. Adolescents often display fluctuations in mood along with undeveloped emotional regulation and poor tolerance for frustration. Emotional and behavioral control usually increases over the course of adolescence due to:
    a. Limited executive function
    b. Cerebellum maturation
    c. Cerebral stasis and hormonal changes
    d. A slight reduction in brain volume

Answers

1. **a;** 2. **d;** 3. **b, e;** 4. **a, b, d;** 5. **a, b, c;** 6. **a-1, b-5, c-3, d-2, e-4;** 7. **a, b, d;** 8. **c;** 9. **b;** 10. **b**

ⓔ Visit the Evolve website for a posttest on the content in this chapter: http://evolve.elsevier.com/Varcarolis

Post-Test interactive review

REFERENCES

Agency for Healthcare Research and Quality. (2014). *Mental health quality measures.* Retrieved from http://www.ahrq.gov/professionals/quality-patient-safety/quality-resources/tools/chtoolbx/measures/measure9.html.

American Nurses Association [ANA]. (2014). American Psychiatric-Mental Health Nurses Association [APNA], & International Society of Psychiatric-Mental Health Nurses [ISPN]. In *Psychiatric mental health nursing: Scope and standards of practice.* Silver Spring, MD: American Nurses Association.

American Psychiatric Association. (2013). *Diagnostic and statistical manual (DSM-5). Diagnostic and statistical manual of mental disorders* (5th ed.). Washington, DC: Author.

American Psychiatric Association. (2015). *Individuals with Disabilities in Education Act.* Retrieved from http://www.apa.org/about/gr/issues/disability/idea.aspx.

Bulechek, G. M., Butcher, H. K., Dochterman, J. M., & Wagner, C. (2013). *Nursing interventions classification (NIC)* (6th ed.). St. Louis: Mosby.

Center for Quality Assessment and Improvement in Mental Health. (2015). *Quality measure inventory.* Retrieved from http://www.cqaimh.org/index.html.

Centers for Disease Control and Prevention. (2016). *About the CDC-Kaiser ACE study.* Retrieved from https://www.cdc.gov/violenceprevention/acestudy/about.html.

Centers for Disease Control and Prevention. (2016). *Health, United States, 2015.* Retrieved from http://www.cdc.gov/nchs/data/hus/hus15.pdf#035.

Child Trends Databank. (2014). *Learning disabilities.* Retrieved from http://www.childtrends.org/wp-content/uploads/2012/09/65_Learning_Disabilities.pdf.

Children's Defense Fund. (2014). *Action strategies and resource guide: Promoting children's mental health screens and assessment.* Washington, DC: Author.

Cortiella, C., & Horowitz, S. H. (2014). *The state of learning disabilities: Facts, trends and emerging issues.* New York: National Center for Learning Disabilities.

Devlin, B., & Scherer, S. W. (2012). Genetic architecture in autism spectrum disorder. *Current Opinion in Genetic Development, 22,* 229–237.

Hoffman, D. (2010). Risky Investments: Parenting and the production of the "resilient" child. Health. *Risk and Society, 12*(4), 385–394.

Lehne, R. A. (2016). *Pharmacology for nursing care* (9th ed.). Philadelphia, PA: Saunders.

McGorry, P. D., Purcell, R., Goldstone, S., & Amminger, G. P. (2011). Age of onset and timing of treatment for mental and substance use disorders: Implications for preventative intervention strategies and models of care. *Current Opinion in Psychiatry, 24*(4), 301–306.

McGuire, J. F., Piacentini, J., Brennan, E. A., Lewin, A. B., Murphy, T. K., Small, B., & J.Viner, R. M. (2015). The effects of puberty on white matter development. *Developmental Cognitive Neuroscience, 11,* 116–128.

Menzies, L., Goddings, A., Whitaker, K. J., Blakemore, S. J., &Viner, R. M. (2015). The effects of puberty on white matter development in boys. *Developmental Cognitive Neuroscience, 11,* 116–128.

Moorhead, S., Johnson, M., Maas, M. L., & Swanson, E. (2013). *Nursing outcomes classification (NOC)* (5th ed.). St Louis: Mosby.

National Institute on Deafness and Other Communication Disorders. (2015). *Speech and language disorders.* Retrieved from http://www.nidcd.nih.gov/health/voice/pages/specific-language-impairment.aspx.

Shonkoff, J. P., Boyce, W. T., & McEwen, B. S. (2009). Neuroscience, molecular biology, and the childhood roots of health disparities. *Journal of the American Medical Association, 301,* 2252–2259.

Substance Abuse Mental Health Administration. (2015). *Leading change 2.0: Advancing the behavioral health of the nation.* Retrieved from http://www.samhsa.gov/about-us/strategic-initiatives.

Tamara, P. (2013). Tourette syndrome and other disorders of childhood. In M. J. Aminoff, F. Boller, & D. F. Swobb (Eds.), *Handbook of clinical neurology* (3rd ed.) (pp. 853–856). St. Louis: Elsevier.

Taua, C., Hepworth, J., & Neville, C. (2012). Nurses' role in caring for people with comorbidity of mental illness and intellectual disability: A literature review. *International Journal of Mental Health Nursing, 21*(2), 163–174.

US Department of Health & Human Services. (2016). *Child maltreatment 2014.* Retrieved from http://www.acf.hhs.gov/sites/default/files/cb/cm2014.pdf.

Zoloski, S., & Bullock, l. (2012). Resilience in children and youth: A review. *Children and Youth Services Review, 4*(12), 2295–2303.

12

Schizophrenia Spectrum Disorders

Edward A. Herzog

Visit the Evolve website for a pretest on the content in this chapter: http://evolve.elsevier.com/Varcarolis Pre-Test interactive review

OBJECTIVES

1. Identify the schizophrenia spectrum disorders.
2. Discuss at least three of the neurobiological findings that indicate that schizophrenia is a brain disorder.
3. Differentiate among the positive and negative symptoms of schizophrenia in terms of treatment and effect on quality of life.
4. Discuss how to deal with common reactions the nurse may experience while working with a patient with schizophrenia.
5. Develop teaching plans for patients taking first-generation and second-generation antipsychotic drugs.
6. Create a nursing care plan incorporating evidence-based interventions for symptoms of psychosis, including hallucinations, delusions, paranoia, cognitive disorganization, anosognosia, and impaired self-care.
7. Demonstrate or role-play interventions for a patient who is hallucinating, delusional, and exhibiting disorganized thinking.

OUTLINE

KEY TERMS AND CONCEPTS

acute dystonia
affect
affective symptoms
akathisia
anosognosia
anticholinergic toxicity
antipsychotic medication
associative looseness
clang association
cognitive symptoms
command hallucination
concrete thinking
delusions
depersonalization
derealization
echolalia
echopraxia
executive functioning
extrapyramidal side effects
hallucinations
illusions
long-acting injectable
metabolic syndrome
negative symptoms
neologism
neuroleptic malignant syndrome
paranoia
positive symptoms
prodromal phase
pseudoparkinsonism
psychosis
reality testing
recovery model
tardive dyskinesia
word salad

Schizophrenia spectrum disorders are disorders that share features with schizophrenia. These disorders are characterized by psychosis, which refers to altered cognition, altered perception, and/or an impaired ability to determine what is or is not real. This chapter begins with an overview of schizophrenia spectrum disorders and then focuses on schizophrenia and associated nursing care.

DELUSIONAL DISORDER

Delusional disorder is characterized by delusions that have lasted 1 month or longer. The delusions tend to have a general theme that includes grandiose, persecutory, somatic, and referential delusions. These delusions are usually not severe enough to impair occupational or daily functioning. Individuals with this personality disorder do not tend to behave strangely or bizarrely. The lifetime prevalence of delusional disorder is fairly low at around 0.2%

BRIEF PSYCHOTIC DISORDER

Brief psychotic disorder is characterized by the sudden onset of at least one of the following: delusions, hallucinations, disorganized speech, and disorganized or catatonic (severely decreased motor activity) behavior. The symptoms must last longer than 1 day, but no longer than 1 month with the expectation of a return to normal functioning. Brief psychotic disorder accounts for about 9% of all first-time psychoses and is twice as common in females.

SCHIZOPHRENIFORM DISORDER

The essential features of this disorder are exactly like those of schizophrenia, except that symptoms last a much shorter period of time (less than 6 months). Also, impaired social or occupational functioning during some part of the illness is not apparent (although it might occur). It is difficult to know the prognosis of a schizophreniform disorder because some individuals return to their previous level of functioning, while others have a more difficulties in moving forward.

SCHIZOAFFECTIVE DISORDER

This disorder is characterized by an uninterrupted period of illness during which there is a major depressive, manic, or mixed episode, concurrent with symptoms that meet the criteria for schizophrenia. The symptoms must not be caused by any substance use or abuse or general medical condition. It is about one-third as common as schizophrenia with a lifetime prevalence of 0.3%.

SUBSTANCE INDUCED PSYCHOTIC DISORDER AND PSYCHOTIC DISORDER DUE TO ANOTHER MEDICAL CONDITION

Substances such as drugs, alcohol, medications, or toxin exposure can induce delusions and/or hallucinations. Hallucinations or delusions can also be caused by a general medical condition such as delirium, neurological problems, alterations, hepatic or renal diseases, and many more. Substance use and medical conditions should always be ruled out before a primary diagnosis of schizophrenia or other psychotic disorder is made.

SCHIZOPHRENIA

CLINICAL PICTURE

In about 75% of those with schizophrenia the disorder develops gradually, usually presenting between 15 and 25 years of age (Dean et al., 2016). However, there are also child-onset (before 15 years) and late-onset (after 40 years) forms as well. People who later develop schizophrenia often experience a prodromal phase during which some milder symptoms of the disorder develop, often months or years before the disorder becomes fully apparent (Miller, 2016). During the prodromal phase the person may do less well in school than his or her peers, be less socially engaged or adept, and demonstrate memory impairment, suspiciousness, and/or disorganization or oddities in speech or thought.

All people diagnosed with schizophrenia have at least one psychotic symptom such as hallucinations, delusions, and/or disorganized speech or thought. The symptoms are severe enough to disrupt normal activities such as school, work, family and social interaction, and self-care; in children and young adults they often delay or halt achievement of age-appropriate milestones. Basic needs such as hygiene, nutrition, and healthcare are often neglected, and socialization and relationships are often disrupted. The full criteria for schizophrenia are listed in the *DSM-5* box.

DSM-5 CRITERIA FOR SCHIZOPHRENIA

A. Two or more of the following, each present for a significant portion of time during a 1-month period (or less if successfully treated). At least one of these must be (1), (2), or (3):
  1. Delusions.
  2. Hallucinations.
  3. Disorganized speech (e.g., frequent derailment or incoherence).
  4. Grossly disorganized or catatonic behavior.
  5. Negative symptoms (i.e., diminished emotional expression or avolition).

B. For a significant portion of the time since the onset of the disturbance, level of functioning in one or more major areas, such as work, interpersonal relations, or self-care, is markedly below the level achieved before the onset (or when the onset is in childhood or adolescence, there is failure to achieve expected level of interpersonal, academic, or occupational functioning).

C. Continuous signs of the disturbance persist for at least 6 months. This 6-month period must include at least 1 month of symptoms (or less if successfully treated) that meet Criterion A (i.e., active-phase symptoms) and may include periods of prodromal or residual symptoms. During these prodromal or residual periods, the signs of the disturbance may be manifested by only negative symptoms or by two or more symptoms listed in Criterion A present in an attenuated form (e.g., odd beliefs, unusual perceptual experiences).

D. Schizoaffective disorder and depressive or bipolar disorder with psychotic features have been ruled out because either (1) no major depressive or manic episodes have occurred concurrently with the active-phase symptoms, or (2) if mood episodes have occurred during active-phase symptoms, they have been present for a minority of the total duration of the active and residual periods of the illness.

E. The disturbance is not attributable to the physiological effects of a substance (e.g., a drug of abuse, a medication) or another medical condition.

F. If there is a history of autism spectrum disorder or a communication disorder of childhood onset, the additional diagnosis of schizophrenia is made only if prominent delusions or hallucinations, in addition to the other required symptoms of schizophrenia, are also present for at least 1 month (or less if successfully treated).

Specify if: The following course specifiers are only to be used after a 1-year duration of the disorder and if they are not in contradiction to the diagnostic course criteria.

First episode, currently in acute episode: First manifestation of the disorder meeting the defining diagnostic symptom and time criteria. An *acute episode* is a time period in which the symptom criteria are fulfilled.

First episode, currently in partial remission: *Partial remission* is a period of time during which an improvement after a previous episode is maintained and in which the defining criteria of the disorder are only partially fulfilled.

First episode, currently in full remission: *Full remission* is a period of time after a previous episode during which no disorder-specific symptoms are present.

Multiple episodes, currently in acute episode: Multiple episodes may be determined after a minimum of two episodes (i.e., after a first episode, a remission and a minimum of one relapse).

Multiple episodes, currently in partial remission

Multiple episodes, currently in full remission

Continuous: Symptoms fulfilling the diagnostic symptom criteria of the disorder are remaining for the majority of the illness course with subthreshold symptom periods being very brief relative to the overall course.

Unspecified

Specify if: **With catatonia**

Specify current severity: Severity is rated by a quantitative assessment of the primary symptoms of psychosis, including delusions, hallucinations, disorganized speech, abnormal psychomotor behavior, and negative symptoms. Each of these symptoms may be rated for its current severity (most severe in the last 7 days) on a 5-point scale ranging from 0 (not present) to 4 (present and severe).

From American Psychiatric Association. (2013). *Diagnostic and statistical manual of mental disorders* (5th ed.). Washington, DC: Author.

EPIDEMIOLOGY

The prevalence of childhood-onset schizophrenia is about 1 in 40,000 children. It affects individuals of all races and cultures equally. It is diagnosed more frequently in males (1.4:1) and among individuals growing up in urban areas (Haddad et al., 2015). Onset in males is usually between the ages of 15 and 25 years and is associated with poorer functioning and more structural abnormality in the brain. The onset tends to be somewhat later in women (ages 25 to 35 years), who tend to have a better prognosis and experience less structural changes in the brain.

COMORBIDITY

Substance use disorders, particularly alcohol and marijuana, occur in nearly half of affected individuals. Substance use is associated with higher rates of treatment nonadherence, relapse, incarceration, homelessness, violence, suicide, and a poorer prognosis (Marquez-Arrico et al., 2015). About 60% of individuals with schizophrenia use nicotine, possibly due to genetically mediated causes or as a form of coping with cognitive impairment or anxiety (Akbarian & Kundakovic, 2015). Smoking doubles the risk of cancer and contributes to cardiovascular and respiratory disorders.

Anxiety, depression, and **suicide** co-occur frequently in schizophrenia. At least 20% of people with schizophrenia attempt suicide while 5% to 10% die by suicide, a rate five times that of the general population. Suicide attempts are more common within 3 years of diagnosis and especially upon discharge after the first episode of the schizophrenia but can occur at any point in the illness (American Psychiatric Association, 2013).

Physical illnesses are more common among people with schizophrenia than in the general population. The risk of premature death due to medical illness is 3.5 times greater than that in the general population, and on average, patients with schizophrenia die more than 20 years prematurely (Rao et al., 2015).

Individuals with psychotic disorders may be at greater risk of poor health maintenance behaviors, poor nutrition, substance use, medication effects, poverty, limited access to healthcare, and reduced ability to recognize or respond to signs of illness.

They may also receive poorer quality healthcare due to poverty, stigma, impaired ability to express their needs, or stereotyping (e.g., emergency room staff assuming that chest pain is imaginary or not serious).

Polydipsia is compulsive drinking of excess fluids. It occurs in up to 20% of individuals with schizophrenia and causes hyponatremia (also known as *water intoxication*) in 2% to 5%. Symptoms include confusion, delirium, hallucinations, worsening of existing psychotic symptoms, and ultimately coma. Contributing factors include antipsychotic medication (causes dry mouth), compulsive behavior (present in some with schizophrenia), and neuroendocrine abnormalities (Goldman, 2009). One should consider the possibility of hyponatremia when there is a sudden increase in psychotic symptoms, particularly if delirium (e.g., disorientation, restlessness, fluctuating vital signs) is also present.

RISK FACTORS

What has traditionally been called *schizophrenia* is now believed to be a group of disorders with common overlapping etiologies. People with schizophrenia demonstrate differences in brain chemistry, structure, and neurotransmission. This variation in etiologies makes it difficult to identify reliable neurostructural or neurochemical variations that could be used to identify individuals at high risk for developing schizophrenia.

The diathesis-stress model is probably the best explanation for the existence of this disorder (Berry & Cirulli, 2016). Schizophrenia occurs when multiple inherited gene abnormalities combine with nongenetic factors. These factors include viral infections, birth injuries, environmental stressors, prenatal malnutrition, and abnormal neural pruning that alters brain development or function and/or injure the brain directly.

Biological Factors

Genetic

Schizophrenia-spectrum disorders are inherited. About 80% of the risk of schizophrenia comes from genetic and epigenetic factors (factors such as toxins or psychological trauma that affect the expression of genes). Over 100 loci in the human genome are associated with an increased risk of schizophrenia (Castellani et al., 2015). Concordance rates (i.e., the percentage of a shared disorder in twins) are about 50% for identical twins and about 15% for fraternal twins. Evidence suggests that multiple genes on different chromosomes interact with one another in complex ways to create vulnerability for schizophrenia.

Neurobiological

Dopamine theory. The first antipsychotic drugs, known as **first-generation (typical) antipsychotics,** (e.g., haloperidol and chlorpromazine), block the activity of dopamine-2 (D_2) receptors in the brain and reduce symptoms such as hallucinations and delusions. Symptom reduction suggested that dopamine plays a significant role in psychosis.

Amphetamines and cocaine can induce psychosis in people without schizophrenia and can also bring on the disorder. Almost any drug of abuse, particularly marijuana, can increase the risk of schizophrenia in biologically vulnerable individuals (Morgan et al., 2016). However, because medications that reduce dopamine activity do not alleviate all the symptoms of schizophrenia, it seems likely that other neurotransmitters or other factors are involved as well.

Other neurochemical hypotheses. **Second-generation (atypical) antipsychotics** block serotonin (5-hydroxytryptamine 2A, or 5-HT_{2A}) and dopamine, which suggests that serotonin may play a role in schizophrenia as well.

Phencyclidine (PCP) induces a state that resembles schizophrenia. This observation led to interest in the *N*-methyl-D-aspartate (NMDA) receptor complex and the possible role of glutamate in the pathophysiology of schizophrenia. Glutamate, dopamine, and serotonin act synergistically in neurotransmission and thus glutamate may also play a role in causing psychosis (Andreou et al., 2015). Neurotransmission by another calming neurotransmitter, gamma-aminobutyric acid (GABA), is also impaired in schizophrenia (Frankle et al., 2015). Acetylcholine, active in the muscarinic system, may play a role in psychosis.

Brain Structure Abnormalities

It is possible that structural abnormalities cause disruption in communication within the brain. Structural differences may be due to errors in neurodevelopment or errors in the normal pruning of neuronal tissue that happens in late adolescence and early adulthood. Inflammation or neurotoxic effects from factors such as oxidative stress, infection, or autoimmune dysfunction may also alter the brain's structure (Sekar et al., 2016).

Using brain imaging techniques—computed tomography (CT), magnetic resonance imaging (MRI), functional MRI (fMRI), and positron emission tomography (PET)—researchers (Dean et al., 2016) demonstrated structural brain abnormalities including:

- Reduced volume in the right anterior insula (may contribute to negative symptoms)
- Reduced volume and changes in the shape of the hippocampus
- Accelerated age-related decline in cortical thickness
- Gray matter deficits in the dorsolateral prefrontal cortex area, thalamus, and anterior cingulate cortex, as well as in the frontotemporal, thalamocortical, and subcortical-limbic circuits
- Reduced connectivity among various brain regions
- Neuronal overgrowth in some areas, possibly due to inflammation or inadequate neural pruning
- Widespread white matter abnormalities (e.g., in the corpus callosum)

PET scans also show a lowered rate of blood flow and glucose metabolism in the prefrontal cortex. This executive functioning part of the brain governs planning, abstract thinking, social adjustment, and decision making. Fig. 3.5 in Chapter 3 shows a PET scan demonstrating reduced brain activity in the frontal lobe of a patient with schizophrenia. Such structural and functional changes may worsen as the disorder continues. Postmortem studies show a reduced volume of gray matter, especially in the temporal and frontal lobes. People with the most tissue loss had the worst symptoms.

Psychological and Environmental Factors

A number of biological, chemical, and environmental stressors are believed to combine with genetic vulnerabilities to produce schizophrenia.

Neurobiology of Schizophrenia and the Effects of Antipsychotics

The antipsychotics affect a number of neurotransmitters including dopamine, noradrenaline/norepinephrine, serotonin, and GABA. An excess of serotonin may contribute to both the positive and negative symptoms of schizophrenia. GABA regulates dopamine activity and in some people with schizophrenia, there is a loss of GABAergic neurons in the hippocampus, potentially causing hyperactivity of dopamine. Since dopamine is the most studied and most prominent of the neurotransmitters (D_1, D_2, D_3, D_4, and D_5) in schizophrenia, the role of dopamine is presented here.

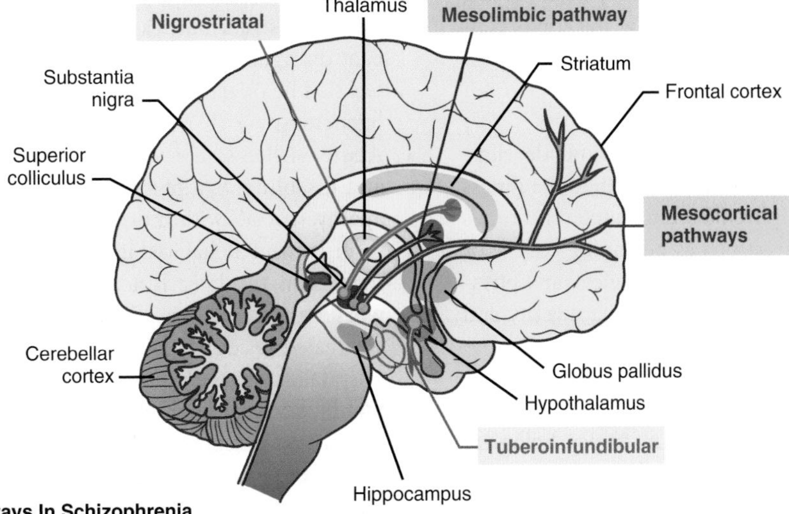

Dopamine Pathways In Schizophrenia

Mesolimbic pathway: reward motivation, emotions and positive symptoms of schizophrenia.

Mesocortical pathways: relevant to cognitive function and executive function and negative symptoms of schizophrenia.

Nigrostriatal: normally responsible for purposeful movement.

Tuberoinfundibular: normally responsible for regulation of prolactin.

First-generation antipsychotic (FGA) drugs are potent antagonists/blockers of D_2.

Second-generation antipsychotics (SGA) have less affinity for D_2 receptors, and tend to bind with D_3 and D_4 receptors. Since the expression of D_3 and D_4 is limited to the neurons of the limbic system and cerebral cortex, the action of these drugs are limited to areas involved in the pathology of schizophrenia. Second-generation drugs also inhibit the serotonin (5HT) receptors. Since serotonin inhibits the release of dopamine, the dopaminergic transmission is affected.

The potential serious effects of the SGA's (metabolic effects: weight gain, diabetes, and dyslipidemia) come from the blockade of noradrenaline/norepinephrine (alpha-1), histamine, and acetylcholine.

Dopamine Pathways and Antipsychotic Responses

Dopamine Pathway	Abnormality in Schizophrenia	Responses to Antipsychotic Drugs
Mesolimbic pathway connects the VTA to the nucleus accumbens Associated with reward, motivation, and emotion	Hyperactive in schizophrenia Associated with positive symptoms (hallucinations, delusions, disorganized thought)	**FGA** - D_2 blockage results in reduction in positive symptoms **SGA** - D_3 and D_4 antagonism results in reduction of positive symptoms
Mesocortical pathway made up of dopaminergic neurons that project from the ventral tegmental area to the prefrontal cortex Relevant to cognition, executive function, emotions, and affect	Hypofunction in schizophrenia results in cognitive impairment and negative symptoms (apathy, anhedonia, lack of motivation)	**FGA** - D_2 blockage may result in a worsening of these symptoms **SGA** - Since there are more serotonin (5HT) receptors than D_2 receptors in this area, blockage of 5HT is more profound. Blockage of 5HT may help improve negative symptoms
Tuberoinfundibular pathway consists of dopaminergic projections from the hypothalamus to the pituitary gland Inhibits prolactin release	Unaffected	**FGA** (to a less degree SGA) - Blockade of D_2 receptors increases prolactin levels resulting in hyperprolactinemia and lactation
Nigrostriatal pathway-substantial nigra to basal ganglia Responsible for purposeful movement	Unaffected	**FGA** (to a lesser degree SGA) - Long-term blockade of D_2 receptors can cause upregulation (increase response to a stimulus) to those receptors, which may lead to extrapyramidal side effects e.g., tardive dyskinesia (TD)

Prenatal Stressors

Infection during pregnancy increases the risk of mental illness in the child. Prenatal infections in the mother also increase the risk of infection in the child after birth, and those infections in the children also can make them more vulnerable to mental illness (Blomström et al., 2016). Other factors associated with an increased risk of schizophrenia include a father older than 35 at the child's conception and a child's being born during late winter or early spring.

Psychological Stressors

Stress increases cortisol levels, impeding hypothalamic development and causing other changes that may precipitate the illness in vulnerable individuals. Schizophrenia often manifests at times of developmental and family stress such as beginning college or moving away from one's family. Social, psychological, and physical stressors may play a significant role in both the severity and course of the disorder and the person's quality of life.

Other risk factors include childhood sexual abuse, exposure to social adversity (e.g., chronic poverty), migration to or growing up in a foreign culture, and exposure to psychological trauma or social defeat (Evans et al., 2015). These factors may cause structural changes in the brain via epigenetic changes to the genome. Even psychological trauma in a parent or grandparent may cause epigenetic changes that increase vulnerability, and this increased risk can be passed on to one's descendants.

Environmental Stressors

Environmental factors such as toxins, including the solvent tetrachloroethylene (used in dry cleaning, to line water pipes, and sometimes found in drinking water), are also believed to contribute to the development of schizophrenia in vulnerable people (Aschengrau et al., 2012). Living in urban areas or high-crime environments is also believed to increase the risk of schizophrenia (Haddad et al., 2015).

Prognostic Considerations

For most individuals symptoms improve with medications and psychosocial interventions. As a result, many people with schizophrenia experience a good quality of life and success within their families, occupations, and other roles.

In many cases, schizophrenia does not respond fully to treatments, leaving mild to severe residual symptoms and varying degrees of dysfunction or disability. A minority of individuals requires repeated or lengthy inpatient care or institutionalization. Factors associated with a less positive prognosis include a slow onset (e.g., more than 2 to 3 years), younger age at onset, longer duration between first symptoms and first treatment, longer periods of untreated illness, and more negative symptoms. Reducing the frequency, intensity, and duration of relapse (when previously controlled symptoms return) is believed to improve the long-term prognosis.

Phases of Schizophrenia

Schizophrenia usually progresses through predictable phases, although the presenting symptoms during a given phase and the length of the phase can vary widely. These phases are:

- **Prodromal**—Mild changes in thinking, reality testing, and mood, insufficient to meet the diagnostic criteria for schizophrenia. Symptoms appear a month to more than a year before the first full-blown episode of the illness. During this phase speech and thought may be odd or eccentric. Anxiety, obsessive thoughts, and compulsive behaviors may be present. Deterioration in concentration, school or job performance, and social functioning are accompanied by distressing thoughts, suspiciousness, memory impairment, and significant disorganization in speech or behavior. The person may feel that he or she is "not right" or that "something strange" is happening.
- **Acute**—Later symptoms vary, from few and mild to many and disabling. Symptoms such as hallucinations, delusions, apathy, social withdrawal, diminished affect, anhedonia, disorganized behavior, impaired judgment, and cognitive regression result in functional impairment. As symptoms worsen the person has difficulty coping, and symptoms once concealed become apparent to others. Increased support or hospitalization may be required.
- **Stabilization**—Symptoms are stabilizing and diminishing, and there is movement toward a previous level of functioning (baseline). Care in an outpatient mental health center or partial hospitalization program (which includes many of the services offered in inpatient mental health units, but without an overnight stay in the hospital) may be needed. The person may receive care in a residential crisis center (similar to a mental health unit but based in the community and less restrictive in nature) or a staff-supervised residential group home or apartment.
- **Maintenance or Residual**—The condition has stabilized and a new baseline is established. Positive symptoms (which will be described later) are usually absent or significantly diminished, but negative and cognitive symptoms continue to be a concern. Ideally, recovery with few or no residual symptoms will occur, and the patient is again able to live independently or with family.

A pattern of recurrent exacerbations (worsening of symptoms) separated by periods of reduced or dormant symptoms is common. Some people have several episodes and none thereafter. For most patients, however, schizophrenia is a chronic disorder that, like diabetes or heart disease, is managed with ongoing treatment.

APPLICATION OF THE NURSING PROCESS

ASSESSMENT

Assessment involves interviewing the patient and observing behavior and other manifestations of the disorder. Information from others who know the patient is also important as patients may conceal or minimize symptoms. Assessment should include a mental status examination along with review of spiritual, cultural, biological, psychological, social, and environmental elements that might be affecting the presentation. Trust, a therapeutic nurse-patient relationship, sound therapeutic communication skills, and an understanding of the disorder and what patients may be experiencing all strengthen the assessment.

Prodromal Phase

Early assessment plays a key role in improving the prognosis for individuals with schizophrenia. Intervening at this early stage to reduce risk factors such as high levels of stress and substance abuse, coupled with enhancing social and coping skills, can reduce the risk of developing schizophrenia in biologically vulnerable people. Box 12.1 identifies other schizophrenia prevention strategies during this phase.

BOX 12.1 Can Schizophrenia Be Prevented?

Malnutrition, infection, and tobacco use during pregnancy, and marijuana and drug use in biologically vulnerable people increase the risk of developing schizophrenia. Primary prevention aims at avoiding these factors. However, not all risk factors can be avoided. Avoiding triggers, such as environmental stressors, and interventions to promote resiliency and coping in children and families, are helpful. Two additional options are (1) early treatment with antipsychotic medications and (2) supplemental essential fatty acids.

Assessment tools help to identify prodromal (early) symptoms such as eccentric or magical thinking, cognitive disorganization, or quasi-hallucinations. Once at-risk symptoms are identified, antipsychotic medications may reduce the development or severity of schizophrenia. Controversially, only one-third of those deemed at risk for schizophrenia actually develop the disorder. Prophylactic antipsychotic use can unnecessarily expose people to significant side effect risks.

More promising is the use of omega-3 and omega-6 polyunsaturated fatty acids found in fish oils and oily fish such as tuna, salmon, and sardines. These fats are abnormally low in the brains of people with schizophrenia. They reduce inflammation and free radicals in the brain and contribute to ACH and serotonin stability. Preliminary evidence suggests that fatty acid supplements reduce rates of conversion from "at risk" to actually having schizophrenia from 27% to 5%.

Kohler, C., Borgmann-Winter, K. E., Hurford, I., Neustadter, E., Yi, J., & Calkins, M. E. (2014). Is prevention a realistic goal for schizophrenia? *Current Psychiatry Reports*, 6, 439.

General Assessment

Not all people with schizophrenia have the same symptoms, and some of the symptoms of schizophrenia are also found in other disorders. Fig. 12.1 describes the four main symptom categories in schizophrenia:

1. *Positive symptoms:* The presence of something that should not be present. Positive symptoms include hallucinations, delusions, paranoia, or disorganized or bizarre thoughts, behavior, or speech.
2. *Negative symptoms:* The absence of something that should be present. Negative symptoms include the inability to enjoy activities, social discomfort, or lack of goal-directed behavior.
3. *Cognitive symptoms:* Subtle or obvious impairment in memory, attention, thinking (e.g., disorganized or irrational thoughts), judgment, or problem solving.
4. *Affective symptoms:* Symptoms involving emotions and their expression.

Positive Symptoms

The positive symptoms usually appear early. Their dramatic nature captures our attention and is often what precipitates treatment. These symptoms are what most individuals associate with mental illness, making schizophrenia the classic "crazy" disorder. Positive symptoms include:

Alterations in Reality Testing. We all experience thoughts that are irrational or distorted, yet we can usually catch and correct the error by using reality testing. **Reality testing** is the automatic and unconscious process by which we determine what is and is not real. You might think you hear a voice but you see that no one is present. You conclude you are mistaken—it wasn't real. With impaired reality testing the person believes that hallucinations or delusions *are* real.

Delusions are false beliefs held despite a lack evidence to support them. The most common delusions involve persecutory, grandiose,

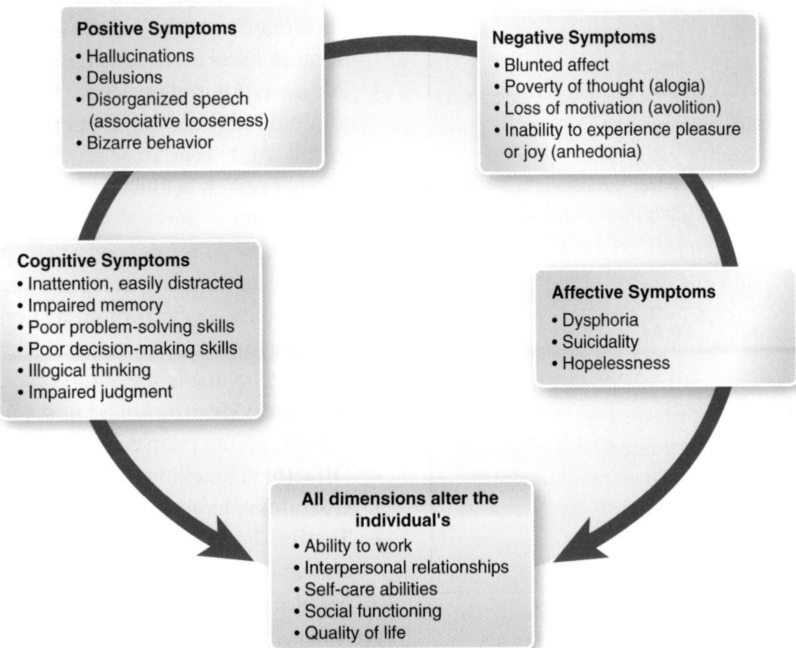

FIG. 12.1 Four main symptom groups of schizophrenia.

or religious ideas. Table 12.1 provides definitions and examples of types of delusions. Delusions can reflect underlying issues or needs (e.g., a person with poor self-esteem may believe he is Beethoven or God, possibly driven by a need to feel more beloved or powerful).

Just because someone has a mental illness does not mean that every story that sounds improbable is delusional. One patient repeatedly told the staff that the Mafia was out to kill him. The staff later learned that he had been selling drugs and had not paid his drug sources, and that drug dealers *were* trying to harm him.

Alterations in Speech. A striking positive symptom of schizophrenia spectrum disorders is the use of unusual speech patterns. One of the most common, **associative looseness**, or looseness of association, results from haphazard and illogical thinking where concentration is poor and individuals loosely associate their thoughts. For example: "I need to get a Band-Aid. My friend was talking about AIDS. Friends talk about French fries but how can you trust the French?" A **word salad**, the most extreme form of associative looseness, is a jumble of words that is meaningless to the listener (e.g., "throat hoarse strength of policy highlighters on a boat reigning supreme").

Clang association is choosing words based on their sound rather than their meaning and often involves words that rhyme or have a similar beginning sound ("On the track...have a Big Mac" or "Click, clack, clutch, close").

TABLE 12.1 Types of Delusions*

Delusion	Definition	Example
Persecutory	Believing that one is being singled out for harm, or prevented from making progress, by others	Shannon believes that her food is poisoned; therefore, she eats only prepackaged food. John believes co-workers plot to prevent his promotion.
Referential	A belief that events or circumstances that have no connection to you are somehow related to you	Barbara believes that the birds sing songs to cheer her up. Andrea believes songs on the radio are chosen to send her a message.
Grandiose	Believing that one is a very powerful or important person	Brianna believes she is a famous playwright.
Erotomanic	Believing that another person desires you romantically	Although he barely knows her, Patty insists that Eric would marry her if only his current wife would stop interfering.
Nihlistic	The conviction that a major catastrophe will occur	Larry gives away all his belongings since they won't be of any use when the comet hits.
Somatic	Believing that the body is changing in unusual ways	Chris says her heart is dead and rotting away.
Control	Believing that another person, group of individuals, or external force controls thoughts, feelings, impulses, or behavior	Brian covered his apartment walls with aluminum foil to block aliens' efforts to control his thoughts.

*A false belief held regardless of evidence to the contrary. Note that unusual beliefs that stem from one's culture or subculture are not considered delusions.

Neologisms are words that have meaning for the patient but a different or nonexistent meaning to others. A person may use a known word differently than others understand it or can create a completely new word that others do not understand (e.g., "His *mannerologies* are poor").

Echolalia is the pathological repeating of another's words, occurring perhaps because the patient's thought processes are so impaired that he is unable to generate speech of his own.

Nurse: Mary, come get your medication.

Mary: Come get your medication.

Other pathological speech patterns are:

- **Circumstantiality:** Including unnecessary and often tedious details in conversation but eventually reaching the point.
- **Tangentiality:** Wandering off topic or going off on tangents and never reaching the point.
- **Cognitive retardation:** Generalized slowing of thinking, which is represented by delays in responding to questions or difficulty finishing thoughts.
- **Pressured speech:** Urgent or intense speech; resists allowing comments from others.
- **Flight of ideas:** Moving rapidly from one thought to the next, often making it difficult for others to follow the conversation.
- **Symbolic speech:** Using symbols instead of direct communication. For example, a patient reports "demons are sticking needles in me" when what he means is that he is experiencing a sharp pain (symbolized by "needles").
- **Thought blocking:** A reduction or stoppage of thought. Interruption of thought by hallucinations can cause this.
- **Thought insertion:** The uncomfortable belief that someone else has inserted thoughts into the brain.
- **Thought deletion:** A belief that thoughts have been taken or are missing.

Other positive symptoms manifested in disorders of thought include:

- **Magical thinking:** Believing that thoughts or actions affect others. This is common and usually nonpathological in children (e.g., wearing pajamas inside out to make it snow, or because I was mad at him, he fell down).
- **Paranoia**: An irrational fear, ranging from mild (wary, guarded) to profound (believing irrationally that another person intends to kill you). Fear may result in defensive actions, harming another person before that person can harm the patient.

Alterations in perception. Alterations in perception involve errors in how one interprets perceptions or perceives reality. The most common perceptual errors are **hallucinations**. Hallucinations occur when a person perceives a sensory experience for which no external stimulus exists (e.g., hearing a voice when no one is speaking). Types of hallucination include:

- **Auditory:** Hearing voices or sounds
- **Visual:** Seeing people or things
- **Olfactory:** Smelling odors
- **Gustatory:** Experiencing tastes
- **Tactile:** Feeling bodily sensations (e.g., feeling an insect crawling on one's skin)

Auditory hallucinations, the most common form in schizophrenia, are experienced by more than 60% of people with schizophrenia (Waters, 2014). They may be vague sounds or indistinct or clear "voices." Hallucinations seem to come from outside the person's head. Auditory processing areas of the brain are activated during these hallucinations just as they are when a genuine sound is heard.

John Nash, the world-renowned mathematician with schizophrenia portrayed in the film *A Beautiful Mind* (2001), describes his hallucinations:

> *I thought of the voices as…something a little different from aliens. I thought of them more like angels…It's really my subconscious talking; it was really that, I know that now.*

Internal voices may be single or multiple, distinct or indistinct, and can be attributed to specific sources (e.g., God, a family member) or unrecognized. They may be supportive and pleasant or derogatory and frightening. They can be subtle and unobtrusive or intrusive and highly distressing. Hallucinations commenting on the person's behavior or conversing with the person are common. Indications that a person is hallucinating include tracking motions (turning one's head in the direction of the perceived sound), lips moving silently, talking as if to another when no one is present, and otherwise unexplained changes in affect (e.g., suddenly laughing without apparent reason).

A person who hears voices struggles to understand the experience, sometimes developing related delusions to explain the voices (e.g., believing the voices are from God or due to a device implanted by the CIA). Patients may attempt to cope by drowning out auditory hallucinations with loud music or by competing with them by talking loudly, humming, or singing. Such auditory competition may, in fact, reduce hallucinations and serve as a recommended intervention.

A **command hallucination** is a particularly disturbing symptom that directs the person to take an action. This type of hallucination must be monitored carefully because they may be dangerous, for example, telling a patient to "jump out the window" or "hit that nurse." Command hallucinations are often frightening and may be a warning flag for a psychiatric emergency. It is essential to assess *what* the patient hears, the ability to *recognize the hallucination as "not real,"* and the patient's ability to resist any commands.

Visual hallucinations are the second most common form in schizophrenia. They may involve distortion of visual stimuli or can be formed and realistic images. Seeing individuals and animals are most common.

Olfactory, tactile, or gustatory hallucinations are unusual in mental illness. When present, other causes should be investigated.

Other alterations in perception are:

- **Illusions**: Misperceptions or misinterpretations of a real experience. For example, a man sees a coat on a shadowy coat rack and believes it is a bear.
- **Depersonalization**: A feeling of being unreal or having lost identity. Body parts do not belong or the body has drastically changed (e.g., a patient may see the fingers as being smaller or not theirs).
- **Derealization**: A feeling that the environment has changed (e.g., everything seems bigger or smaller or familiar surroundings seem somehow strange and unfamiliar).

Alterations in Behavior. Alterations in behavior involve changes in the speed of movement and behaviors that are illogical or inappropriate including:

- **Catatonia:** A pronounced increase or decrease in the rate and amount of movement. Excessive motor activity is purposeless and accompanied by echolalia (repeating others' words) and echopraxia (mimicking others' movements). The most common form of catatonia is when the person moves little or not at all. Muscular rigidity, or **catalepsy**, may be so severe that the limbs remain in whatever position they are placed. Freezing in place may result in problems such as exhaustion, pneumonia, blood clotting, malnutrition, or dehydration.
- **Waxy flexibility:** Maintaining a given posture inappropriately, usually seen in catatonia. For example, when the nurse raises the arm, the patient continues to hold this position in a statue-like manner.
- **Motor retardation:** A pronounced slowing of movement.
- **Motor agitation:** Excited behavior such as running or pacing rapidly, often in response to internal or external stimuli. The agitation can put the patient at risk (e.g., exhaustion, running into traffic) or others at risk (being knocked down).
- **Stereotyped behaviors:** Repetitive behaviors that do not serve a logical purpose.
- **Echopraxia:** The mimicking of movements of another.
- **Negativism:** A tendency to resist or oppose the requests or wishes of others.
- **Impaired impulse control:** A reduced ability to resist one's impulses. Examples include interrupting in the group setting or throwing unwanted food on the floor. It can increase the risk of assault.
- **Gesturing or posturing:** Assuming unusual and illogical expressions (often grimaces) or positions.
- **Boundary impairment:** An impaired ability to sense where one's body or influence ends and another's begins. For example, a patient might stand too close to others or might drink another's beverage, believing that because it is near, it is theirs.

Negative Symptoms

Positive symptoms are so attention-getting, they make treatment seem more urgent than negative symptoms. Yet negative symptoms are serious problems for people with schizophrenia because they are the absence of essential human qualities. Treating negative symptoms is more difficult than treating positive symptoms.

Negative symptoms include the following six symptoms that all start with the letter A:

- **Anhedonia** (*an* = without + *hedonia* = pleasure): A reduced ability or inability to experience pleasure in everyday life.
- **Avolition** (*a* = without + *volition* = making a decision): Loss of motivation; difficulty beginning and sustaining goal-directed activities; reduction in motivation or goal-directed behavior.
- **Asociality:** Decreased desire for, or comfort during, social interaction.
- **Affective blunting:** Reduced or constricted affect.
- **Apathy:** A decreased interest in, or attention to, activities or beliefs that would otherwise be interesting or important.
- **Alogia:** Reduction in speech, sometimes called *poverty of speech.*

These symptoms can contribute to poor social functioning and social withdrawal. They can impede a person's ability to initiate and maintain conversations and relationships or succeed in school or work. Apathy and avolition result in deficits in basic activities such as maintaining adequate hygiene, grooming, and other activities of daily living

Affect, an additional "A" word, is the external expression of a person's internal emotional state. In schizophrenia, affect may be diminished or not coincide with inner emotions. Some antipsychotics can also cause diminished affect. Affect in schizophrenia can usually be categorized in one of four ways:

- **Flat:** Immobile or blank facial expression
- **Blunted:** Reduced or minimal emotional response
- **Constricted:** Reduced in range or intensity (e.g., shows sadness or anger but no other moods)
- **Inappropriate:** Incongruent with the actual emotional state or situation (e.g., laughing in response to a tragedy)
- **Bizarre:** Odd, illogical, inappropriate, or unfounded; includes grimacing

Cognitive Symptoms

Cognitive symptoms represent the third symptom group and are evident in most patients with schizophrenia. These impairments can lead to poor judgment and leave the patient less able to cope, learn, manage health, or succeed in school or work. Cognitive symptoms include the following.

Concrete thinking is an impaired ability to think abstractly, resulting in interpreting or perceiving things in a literal manner. For example, a nurse might ask what brought the patient to the hospital, and the patient answers "a cab" rather than explaining a suicide attempt. Interpreting proverbs can be used to assess abstract thought. An abstract interpretation of "The grass is always greener on the other side of the fence" is that it always seems we would be happier given other circumstances. A concrete interpretation could be "That side gets more sun, so it's greener there." Concreteness reduces one's ability to understand and respond to concepts requiring abstract reasoning such as love or humor.

Concreteness, especially when combined with an impaired ability to recognize variations in affect or tone of voice, can also make it difficult to recognize social cues such as sarcasm. For example, a patient who had forgotten his wallet asked a store clerk if he could pay later for a bag of chips. When the clerk sarcastically replied, "Oh sure, we let our customers pay whenever they want," the patient took this literally. The patient was distressed when police arrested him for theft despite his protests that he had permission not to pay.

Impaired memory impacts short-term memory and the ability to learn. Repetition and verbal or visual cues may help the patient to learn and recall needed information (e.g., a picture of a toothbrush on the patient's wall as a reminder to brush his or her teeth).

Impaired information processing can lead to problems such as delayed responses, misperceptions, or difficulty understanding others. Patients may lose the ability to screen out insignificant stimuli such as background sounds or objects in one's peripheral vision. This can lead to overstimulation.

Impaired executive functioning includes difficulty with reasoning, setting priorities, comparing options, placing things in logical order or groups, anticipation and planning, and inhibiting undesirable impulses or actions. Impaired executive functioning interferes with problem solving and can contribute to inappropriateness in social situations.

Affective Symptoms

Affective symptoms are those that involve the experience and expression of emotions. They are common and increase patients' suffering. Mood may be unstable, erratic, labile (changing rapidly and easily), or incongruent (not what would be expected for the circumstances).

A serious affective change often seen in schizophrenia is depression. Depression may occur as part of a shared inflammatory reaction affecting the brain or may simply be a reaction to the stress and despair that can come from living with a chronic illness. Assessment for depression is crucial because it may indicate an impending relapse, further impair functioning, and increase risk of substance use disorders. Most importantly, depression puts people at increased suicide risk.

Self-Assessment

People with schizophrenia often experience anosognosia (uh-no-sog-NOH-zee-uh), an inability to realize they are ill caused by the illness itself. Anosognosia may result in the patient resisting or stopping treatment, making care challenging and frustrating to staff. The inability to recognize the illness along with paranoia creates a situation in which requesting or even accepting help is impossible.

Working with individuals who have schizophrenia can bring about anxiety or fear. Discussing your feelings with staff, faculty, and peers may help. Examining whether one's expectations of patients are realistic, learning more about the nature of the illness, and seeking new more effective ways of helping patients can help staff overcome feelings of helplessness and reduce countertransference.

ASSESSMENT GUIDELINES

Schizophrenia and Other Psychotic Disorders

1. Ensure that the patient has had a medical workup. Concurrent medical disorders are common and patients may have experienced recent trauma or illness that has affected their mental status.
2. Assess for indications of medical problems that might mimic psychosis (e.g., digitalis or anticholinergic toxicity, brain trauma, drug intoxication, delirium, fever).
3. Assess for substance or alcohol-use disorders.
4. Complete a mental status examination (MSE) including insight, reality testing, judgment, cognitive abilities (memory, concentration, abstract reasoning), knowledge of the illness, relationships and support systems, other coping resources, and strengths and need.
5. Assess for hallucinations:
   - Do not imply that the perceptions are real (e.g., ask: "What do you hear?" not "What are the voices saying?").
   - Assess when the hallucinations began, their content, how the patient experiences them (e.g., supportive or distressing, in the background or intrusive), what makes them worse or better, how the patient is responding, and what the patient does to cope.

ASSESSMENT GUIDELINES—cont'd

Schizophrenia and Other Psychotic Disorders

- Questions should include: "Are you hearing a voice that is telling you to do something?" "Do you believe what you hear is real?" Any "yes" suggests an increased risk that the patient will act on the commands and, if they involve dangerous behavior, create a risk to self or others.

7. Assess for delusions:
   - If present, are they firmly held? Is the patient able to reality test (determine what is real)?
   - Does the patient believe that there is danger (e.g., is paranoia present)? Does the patient believe that acting against a person or organization will provide protection or vengeance? A "yes" to either of these questions poses an increased risk of danger to others.
8. Assess for suicide risk (refer to Chapter 25).
9. Assess for ability to ensure personal safety and health:
   - Maintain adequate food and fluid intake? (e.g., patients may make poor nutritional choices or experience a risk of choking due to medication side effects impairing swallowing)
   - Achieve adequate sleep and rest?
   - Complete hygiene and self-care?
   - Move about safely? (e.g., fall risk, distractibility that leads to walking into traffic)
   - Control impulses and make sound safe decisions?
   - Dress safely for weather conditions? (e.g., hypothermia and hyperthermia—patients with schizophrenia are at risk of heat-related emergencies)
   - Meet health needs? (e.g., recognize onset or worsening of medical illnesses, adhere to treatment for concurrent medical conditions)
10. Assess prescribed medications, whether and how they are taken, effectiveness, side effects, and what factors (e.g., costs, mistrust of staff, stigma) are affecting adherence.
11. Determine the impact of symptoms and side effects on functioning (e.g., hygiene, caring for health needs, socialization).
12. Assess the family's knowledge of and response to the patient's illness and symptoms. Are family members overprotective? Hostile? Anxious? Are they familiar with and using family support groups and respite resources?

CONSIDERING CULTURE

Stigma of Schizophrenia in Chinese Families

Mrs. Chou, a young Chinese-American woman, learned that her mother died from pneumonia. Mrs. Chou commented that her mother would not have become ill if she had been a better daughter and that she brought evil upon her family.

After the funeral Mrs. Chou became increasingly lethargic, staring into space and mumbling to herself. When Mr. Chou asked to whom she was talking, she answered, "My mother." Mr. Chou knew something was wrong with his wife but was reluctant to seek help. In his culture there is strong stigma against mental illness, and it is often perceived as a punishment.

When Mrs. Chou quit eating and taking care of herself, Mr. Chou took her to an herbalist. The herbalist convinced Mr. Chou to take her to a hospital. During her admission, the unkempt, dehydrated, and pale Mrs. Chou sat motionless and mute.

Mr. Chou apologized for burdening others with her care and asked that her treatment be kept secret. Staff helped Mr. Chou recognize that Mrs. Chou had a physical illness of her brain that affected her thinking and behavior, and that treatment was comparable to treatment for heart disease or diabetes. They also stressed that seeking help for brain illness is accepted in the American culture.

Mr. Chou calmed down as he realized he did not need to feel shame and that others would help. As Mrs. Chou improved, she and Mr. Chou came to attribute the illness to grief, reducing their guilt. They met with a Chinese healer who assisted them to integrate their beliefs with the beliefs and resources of their adopted culture.

DIAGNOSIS

Patients with schizophrenia have multiple distressing and often disabling symptoms. They require a multifaceted approach to care and treatment of both the patient and the family. Table 12.2 lists signs and symptoms and potential nursing diagnoses for a person with schizophrenia.

OUTCOMES IDENTIFICATION

Nursing Outcomes Classification (NOC; Moorhead et al., 2013) is one useful guide for developing outcomes. Outcomes should focus on illness knowledge, management, coping, and quality of life. Outcomes should be consistent with the **recovery model** (refer to Chapter 32), which stresses hope, living a full and productive life, and eventual recovery rather than focusing on controlling symptoms and adapting to disability. Desired outcomes vary with the phase of the illness.

Phase I: Acute

For the acute phase of schizophrenia, the overall goal is **patient safety and stabilization**. If the patient is a risk to self or others,

TABLE 12.2 Signs and Symptoms and Nursing Diagnoses for Schizophrenia

Signs and Symptoms	Nursing Diagnoses
Positive Symptoms	
Hears voices that others do not *(auditory hallucinations)*	*Disturbed sensory perception: auditory/visual*
Hears voices telling him or her to hurt self or others *(command hallucinations)*	*Risk for self-directed/other-directed violence*
Delusions	*Disturbed belief system* *Altered thought processes**
Shows loose association of ideas *(associative looseness)*	*Impaired verbal communication*
Conversation is derailed by unnecessary and tedious details *(circumstantiality)*	*Altered thought processes**
Negative Symptoms	
Uncommunicative, withdrawn	*Social isolation*
Expresses feelings of rejection or aloneness (lies in bed all day, positions back to door)	*Impaired verbal communication* *Impaired social interaction* *Risk for loneliness*
Talks about self as "bad" or "no good"	*Chronic low self-esteem*
Feels guilty because of "bad thoughts"; extremely sensitive to real or perceived slights	*Risk for self-directed violence*
Shows lack of energy *(anergia)*	*Ineffective coping*
Shows lack of motivation *(avolition)*, unable to initiate tasks (social contact, grooming, and other aspects of daily living)	*Self-care deficit (bathing/hygiene, dressing/grooming)*
Other	
Families and significant others become confused or overwhelmed, lack knowledge about disorder or treatment, feel powerless in coping with patient	*Compromised family coping* *Caregiver role strain* *Deficient knowledge*

*Non-NANDA diagnosis

Herdman, T. H., & Kamitsuru, S. (Eds.) (2014). *NANDA International nursing diagnoses: Definitions and classification, 2015–2017*. Oxford, UK: Wiley-Blackwell.

initial outcome criteria address such safety issues (e.g., patient refrains from self-injury, hyponatremia is prevented). Another example of a desired outcome is a patient who consistently labels hallucinations as "not real—a symptom of an illness."

Phase II: Stabilization

Outcome criteria during phase II focus on patient understanding of the illness and treatment, achieving an optimal medication and psychosocial treatment regimen, and controlling and/or coping with symptoms and side effects. The outcomes target the negative and cognitive symptoms as these tend to respond less well to initial treatment than do positive symptoms and may reduce treatment success.

Phase III: Maintenance

Outcome criteria for phase III focus on maintaining and increasing symptom control and insight. Measures during the maintenance phase include adhering to treatment, preventing relapse, maintaining and increasing independence, and achieving a satisfactory quality of life.

PLANNING

Again, the planning of appropriate interventions is guided by the phase of the illness and the strengths and needs of the patient. Cultural considerations, available resources, and patient preferences influence planning.

Phase I: Acute

Hospitalization is indicated if the patient is considered a danger to self or others (e.g., refuses to eat or is too disorganized to function safely in the community). It may also be needed to clarify and confirm the diagnosis. Planning focuses on selecting the best strategies to ensure patient safety and control symptoms.

Phase II: Stabilization and Phase III: Maintenance

Planning during the stabilization and maintenance phases focuses on providing patient and family education, support, and skills training. Planning incorporates interpersonal, functional, coping, healthcare, shelter, educational and vocational strengths and needs, and addresses how and where these needs can best be met within the community.

Relapse prevention efforts (Box 12.2) are vital. Each relapse of psychosis may increase residual dysfunction and deterioration and can contribute to despair, hopelessness, and suicide risk. Recognition of the early warning signs of relapse—such as reduced sleep, social withdrawal, and worsening concentration—followed by close monitoring and intensification of treatment is essential to minimize the duration of psychotic episodes and resulting disruption to the patient's life.

BOX 12.2 Relapse Prevention

A. Know the early warning signs of relapse: sleep disturbances, troubling thoughts, difficulty thinking or remembering, being unsure of what is real, hearing voices, and becoming more uncomfortable around others.

B. Let your treatment team know right away if you begin to have symptoms of relapse. Make a list of whom to call, what to do, and where to go for help. Keep it with you.

C. Find people you can trust who will help you and listen to them if they tell you that your illness seems to be becoming worse.

D. Remember that relapse is part of the illness. It is not a sign of failure, and it does not mean that your illness won't get better.

E. Develop a relapse prevention plan: not using drugs or alcohol, taking medications, managing stress through stress avoidance and relaxation techniques, seeking support when upset or in crisis, avoid conflict with others, do not become isolated, and get enough sleep.

F. Participate in family, group, and individual therapy as needed or suggested by staff.

G. Learn new ways to act and new coping skills to help handle family, work, and other stress. Get information from your nurse, case manager, doctor, support groups, community mental health groups, or a hospital. Everyone needs a place to talk about fears and losses and to learn new ways of coping.

H. Have a written plan of how to cope with especially stressful times: go for a walk, pet the dog, distract yourself with a book, or talk with a friend. One resource is the Wellness Recovery Action Plan at http://mentalhealthrecovery.com/getting-started-with-wrap/.

I. Adhere to treatment. We know that individuals who stay on their medication and follow other treatments that work for them are more likely to get better and stay better. Patients and families should remember that:
   1. Stopping medication or keeping side effects a secret can make it harder for you to have the life you want.
   2. Engaging in struggles over adherence does not help but tying adherence to the patient's own goals does. "Staying in treatment will help you keep your job and stay out of the hospital."
   3. Share concerns about troubling side effects or treatment such as sexual problems, weight gain, or "feeling funny" with your nurse, case manager, doctor, or social worker. Most side effects can be managed.

J. Avoid alcohol and/or drugs; they can act on the brain in ways that cause a relapse. Learn other ways to feel better or deal with stress.

IMPLEMENTATION

Phase I: Acute

Settings

In general, during the acute phase of schizophrenia, 24-hour support is required to prevent harm to self or others. Hospitalization provides external structure and support (e.g., others guiding the patient's activities). As previously discussed, anosognosia is a symptom of schizophrenia that may impair a person's ability to recognize that he or she is ill. In this case, court-ordered hospitalization might be required.

While a minority of patients require extended inpatient care (more than 1 month), the length of hospitalization or other intensive treatment during the acute phase is typically short (days to weeks), ending when acute symptoms have been stabilized. However, this does not necessarily take into account the extended time needed for full recovery from serious mental illness, making continued engagement and care in the community all the more important after discharge. Community-based services provide such care during the stabilization and maintenance phases.

Interventions

Structure within the therapeutic milieu provides a feeling of safety and security for patients who have been experiencing severe anxiety. Patients are monitored for suicide risk and intervene promptly to address risk factors such as despair or hopelessness and provide for the patient's safety (see Chapter 25).

Virtually all people with psychotic disorders will be given pharmacological treatments to manage positive and negative symptoms. Medication response is monitored and side effects will be addressed. For example, fluid intake and weight can be assessed to identify polydipsia. Registered nurses provide support, psychoeducation, and guidance regarding the nature of the illness and its treatment. Psychoeducation promotes patient-centered care by helping the patient to recognize and self-manage symptoms such as anxiety, impaired concentration, social withdrawal, impaired rest or nutrition, impaired cognition, and hallucinations and delusions

Working with an Aggressive Patient

A small percentage of patients with schizophrenia, especially during the acute phase, may exhibit a risk for physical violence. Violence may be in response to hallucinations (especially command hallucinations), delusions, paranoia, and impaired judgment or impulse control. Interpersonal conflict, fear, desperation, and conflicts (e.g., about unit rules) also increase the risk of aggression. Assessment and periodic reassessment for risk of violence are essential. When the potential for violence exists, measures to protect the patient and others become a priority. Refer to Table 12.3 and Chapter 27 for more information on caring for the aggressive or potentially violent patient.

Phase II: Stabilization and Phase III: Maintenance

Effective long-term care of patients with schizophrenia relies on a four-pronged approach:

1. Medication
2. Treatment adherence
3. Relationships with trusted care providers and support people
4. Community-based therapeutic services

All care is geared toward the patient's strengths, culture, personal preferences, and needs. Communication, continuity in care, and trusting relationships with care providers are essential for optimum recovery and relapse prevention.

Postdischarge care typically includes group and individual psychotherapy and psychoeducation (e.g., social or coping skills), medication and case management, and structured activities such as day programs and recreational activities. Community mental health centers usually provide medication services, day treatment, case management, and 24/7 crisis and psychiatric emergency services. Community mental healthcare can also provide housing support, allied physical health services, employment programs. Peer-led services are available in most communities. These services include drop-in centers, sometimes called *clubhouses*, that offer socialization, activities, and sometimes employment opportunities.

Hospital staff must be aware of such community services and ideally should directly connect patients and families with these resources before discharge. Support groups are also very helpful and patients and family members should be connected to these (e.g., the National Alliance on Mental Illness [NAMI, www.nami.org]).

Nurses provide essential family psychoeducation about the illness and how best to help the patient. Education can be provided even if the patient does not provide consent *if* the family initiates the request *and* the information is provided in a way that does not divulge confidential health information about the patient. Alternately, the family can be connected to other resources for information. NAMI's "Family-to-Family" program educates families about severe mental illnesses and their treatment. Support and respite for caregivers are also important.

A sample care plan can be found in the Case Study and Nursing Care Plan box. Additional nursing interventions often helpful in caring for individuals with schizophrenia are provided in Table 12.3.

CASE STUDY AND NURSING CARE PLAN

Schizophrenia

Don, 42, a patient in a Veterans Administration hospital, has been in and out of hospitals for 13 years. A former Marine, auditory hallucinations began at age 19 while serving in the Gulf War. He subsequently received a medical discharge. He has been separated from his wife and four children for 3 years. He does not sleep much because "the voices get worse at night."

Don uses marijuana and sometimes cocaine, which he knows increases his paranoia. "It makes me feel good, and not much else does."

This hospitalization was precipitated by auditory hallucinations and paranoia that was worsened by drug abuse. "I thought people were following me. The voices tell me people hate me and I should die. People say that it happens because I don't take my medications...but they make me tired, and I can't have sex."

He has had two previous episodes of suicidal ideation when the voices were telling him to jump off a building. During a previous admission he assaulted a peer who he thought planned to kill him.

Sarah is Don's nurse. During the first interview, Don rarely makes eye contact and speaks in a soft monotone. At times, he glances about the room as if distracted, mumbles to himself, and appears upset.

Nurse: Don, my name is Sarah. I will be your nurse while you're in the hospital. If it is okay with you, we will meet every day for 20 minutes. We can talk about anything that concerns you.

Don: Well...don't believe what they say about me. I want to start...Are you married?

Nurse: This time is for you to talk about your concerns.

Don: (scans the room, then lowers his eyes) I think someone is trying to kill me...

Nurse: You seem to be focusing on something other than our conversation.

Don: Voices tell me things...I should die...

Nurse: That must be very upsetting. Tell me what is happening, and I will try to help you.

After acknowledging his distress, Sarah keeps the 1:1 with Don short, focusing on the here and now and on his security. As Don gradually attends more to the conversation, his thoughts become more connected and he appears less distracted.

Self-Assessment

In a previous admission and again during this admission, Don assaulted peers he thought wanted to kill him, once reporting, "God told me it was me or him."

This frightens Sarah. She is worried that Don may hurt her. An experienced nurse suggests that Sarah meet with Don in public areas on the unit with other staff nearby until he is more stabile. Sarah feels more secure knowing that other staff are nearby. After 5 days Don is calmer and relates well with Sarah.

Continued

CASE STUDY AND NURSING CARE PLAN—cont'd

Schizophrenia

Assessment

Subjective Data (Patient)

- "The voices get worse at night, and I can't sleep."
- "Someone is trying to kill me."
- "I hear voices...telling me I don't deserve to live"
- "Medications make me tired, and I can't have sex."
- "[Drugs] make me feel good...not much else does."

Subjective Data (Other Sources)

- Separated from wife and children
- History of drug abuse (cocaine, marijuana)
- First hospitalized at age 19; has not worked since leaving military
- Has had suicidal impulses twice, both associated with command hallucinations
- Assaulted a peer in the hospital and attributed the assault to paranoid ideation

Objective Data

1. Speaks in soft monotone
2. Poor eye contact
3. Impaired reality testing
4. Appears internally stimulated
5. Thoughts scattered when anxious

Nursing Diagnosis 1

- *Altered thought processes** related to neurological dysfunction as evidenced by persecutory hallucinations and paranoid delusions that he perceives as real:
  - "The voices get worse at night, and I can't sleep."
  - Voices have told him "You should die" and "Someone is trying to kill you."
  - Although they increase his paranoia, he abuses cocaine and marijuana—"they make me feel good."

*Non-NANDA diagnosis

Outcomes Identification

1. Don refrains from acting upon auditory hallucinations and delusions.
2. Don and others remain safe.

Short-Term Goal	Intervention	Rationale	Evaluation
1. By (date), Don will report when he has hallucinations and identify one or more contributing factors (e.g., telling his nurse what preceded the hallucinations).	1a. Engage with Don several times each day to establish trust and rapport. 1b. Explore those times when voices are most threatening and disturbing, noting the circumstances that preceded them (triggers). 1c. Encourage use of competing auditory stimulation such as humming or music	1a. Short consistent meetings help decrease anxiety and establish trust. 1b. Identifies events that increase anxiety and trigger voices; by learning to avoid or manage triggers, hallucinations can be reduced. 1c. Competing reality-based auditory stimulation reduce patient's subjective distress from hallucinations.	**GOAL MET** By the end of the first week, Don tells the nurse when he is experiencing hallucinations and reports that "music helps."
2. By (date), Don will recognize hallucinations as "not real" and ascribe them to his illness	2a. Explore content of hallucinations with Don to identify possible command hallucinations. 2b. Educate Don about the nature of hallucinations and ways to determine if auditory hallucinations are real (e.g., encourage Don to compare his experiences with others' to determine if his are real).	2a. Identifies risks (e.g., suicidal or aggressive themes, command hallucinations). 2b. Improves Don's reality testing and helps him begin to attribute his experiences to schizophrenia; helps him realize that voices are not real and that any commands can be safely ignored.	**GOAL MET** Don identifies that the auditory hallucinations tell him he is a loser and that "someone is after me." He notes that others do not seem to hear what he hears and also states that smoking marijuana and taking cocaine produce very threatening voices.
3. By discharge, Don consistently reports a decrease in hallucinations, recognizes that they are not real, and reports that he will not act on any commands he hears.	3a. Explore with Don possible actions that can minimize anxiety and/or reduce hallucinations such as relaxation exercises and engaging in reality-based activities. 3b. Guide Don to recognize that hallucinations are helped by medication and other techniques he has mastered.	3a. Offers means to lower anxiety level. 3b. Helps Don exert a measure of control over his hallucinations, reducing powerlessness.	**GOAL MET** Don states that he is hearing internal voices less, and they are less threatening to him. Don identifies that if he whistles or sings, he stays calm and can control the voices. Don has not assaulted others even when command hallucinations occurred.

Note: Additional interventions for hallucinations are found in Box 12.3.

Nursing Diagnosis 2

- *Nonadherence** to medication related to side effects as evidenced by verbalization of nonadherence and persistence of symptoms:
  - Doesn't take prescribed medications because "They make me tired, and I can't have sex."
  - History of recurrent relapses.

Outcome Identification

1. Don consistently adheres to treatment.

*Non-NANDA diagnosis

CASE STUDY AND NURSING CARE PLAN—cont'd

Schizophrenia

1. By the end of week 1, Don will discuss his concerns about medication side effects with staff.	1a. Evaluate medication response and side-effect issues. 1b. Convey empathy and support while educating Don regarding how to manage side effects so that they are less disruptive. 1c. Discuss possible medication change with Don's medication prescriber.	1a. Identify drugs and dosages that have increased therapeutic value and decreased side effects. 1b. Reduces patient distress and resulting resistance caused by side effects, increasing patient's sense of control. 1c. Olanzapine causes no known sexual difficulties.	**GOAL MET** Don identifies the reasons for stopping his medication. He agrees to try olanzapine because he trusts staff's assurances that the side effects will be reduced. Don states that he sleeps better at night but is still tired during the day.
2. By the end of week 2, Don identifies advantages of taking medications.	2a. Connect Don with the local National Alliance of Mentally Ill (NAMI) support group. 2b. Guide Don to see areas where medications help him meet his goals (e.g., eliminate tormenting hallucinations).	2a. Provides peer support and a chance to hear from others further along in recovery how medications can be helpful and side effects can be managed. NAMI members can also offer suggestions for dealing with his loneliness and other problems. 2b. Seeing that medication helps him to achieve his goals he will increase motivation for treatment.	**GOAL MET** Week 1: Don attends meeting at the hospital. Week 2: He speaks in the group about "not feeling good." Several group members say they understand and supportively and helpfully. Peers describe how taking medication has helped them.

At discharge, Don reports that the medicines help him feel better and think more clearly. He voices an understanding of his medications and how to cope with side effects, and notes how they can help him meet his goals. He knows that marijuana and cocaine make his symptoms worse and explains that when he feels down, he now knows three constructive ways to help himself feel better.

Note: Additional nursing interventions for patients with schizophrenia can be found in Table 12.3.

TABLE 12.3 Additional Nursing Interventions for the Person Experiencing Psychosis

Problem	Considerations	Nursing Care
Poor hygiene	Contributing factors include: Apathy, avolition, negativism, disorganized thinking, impaired memory, distractibility, reduced awareness of social expectations, reduced recognition of own appearance/odor (due to altered sensory perception/processing, internal preoccupation)	1. Concisely and explicitly identify expected hygiene. Have patient try out each hygiene action while observing, assisting when needed, and providing positive reinforcement for each success. 2. Break tasks into smaller, easier to manage steps. 3. Use visual cues to prompt attention to hygiene tasks, such as putting a toothbrush and towels in the bathroom and clean clothes on bed. 4. Suggest ways that improved hygiene will benefit the patient, perhaps greater acceptance by peers, increased privileges. 5. Guide patient to use napkin or towel around neck when eating or if experiencing drooling. 6. Periodically remind patient and refocus to hygiene tasks as needed.
Resistance to treatment, nonadherence	Anosognosia causes treatment to seem illogical (why accept medication for an illness one does not have?). Side effects, stigma, inconvenience, a belief that the treatment will not help, expense, impaired memory, and mistrust of the prescriber also discourage adherence.	1. Do not be judgmental—treat patient with respect. 2. Establish trust and involve the patient collaboratively in planning treatment. 3. Explore concerns about treatment and suggest solutions. Perhaps medications that cause fatigue can be taken at bedtime. 4. Convey in a clear, concrete, and confident manner your belief that the patient will benefit from the treatment. 5. Tie the treatment to the patient's own goals. For example, the patient may not agree to take the medication for an *illness*, but if he believes it will quiet the voices or help him keep his job (his goals), then he will see more value to treatment.
Cheeking or palming medications	See "Resistance to Treatment"	1. Address underlying reasons for wanting to avoid medications. 2. Seek to switch medication to a more difficult to conceal form such as a liquid or fast-dissolving tablet. 3. Long-acting injectable forms need only be addressed every 2-4 weeks or every 3 months.

Continued

TABLE 12.3 Additional Nursing Interventions for the Person Experiencing Psychosis—cont'd

Problem	Considerations	Nursing Care
Anosognosia	Anosognosia occurs in most people with severe mental illness. It is not denial and it is not resistance—the patient quite literally is unable to see the illness.	1. Establish a trusting relationship. Even a simple act such as offering the patient gum each day can increase patient comfort with staff. 2. Seek areas of commonality: What can both the patient and others agree upon? 3. Agree to disagree about whether these issues do or don't indicate an illness, but seek agreement that they are a problem. 4. The patient may be aware of illness in others. If so, suggest that, just as another patient cannot see his own illness, something similar might be happening in him or her as well. 5. Involve the patient in activities where he will encounter peers who have gained insight despite once having had anosognosia. A patient may find the reports of the peer to be more valid than similar information originating with staff.
Avoids interaction with peers	Contributing factors include: asociality, impaired social skills, preoccupation with hallucinatory or other internal experiences, actual or potential rejection by peers, fear of embarrassment.	1. Actively convey acceptance and *meet the patient where he is now* and build from there. 2. Regularly engage with the patient. Connect at intervals and interact briefly about low-anxiety topics like the weather. Gradually increase the duration and/or frequency as interaction becomes more comfortable. 3. Offer encouragement to participate in unit activities, without pressure, such as "We would love to see you at the morning meeting." 4. Assure the patient he has control over his choices when possible. For example if he becomes uncomfortable in a group, he can leave and try another day. 5. Reinforce each step toward greater interaction. "It was nice to see you in the morning meeting today." 6. Pet therapy may help patients increase comfort with people.
Depression, hopelessness, and despair	Depression is common with schizophrenia. It can also be a reaction to living with a serious mental illness. In schizophrenia, the person may be dealing with loss and recognize that the illness has affected her life, and she may grieve for the dreams that have been taken from her.	1. Engage in connecting regularly with the patient. 2. Actively convey empathy. "Sometimes having a mental illness can feel very discouraging…I wonder how you are feeling?" 3. If he cannot identify his feelings, suggest those that may apply. "Sometimes it's hard to say what you're feeling. Do you feel sad, frustrated, or lost?" 4. Validate the feeling is understandable and that he is not alone. Identify options for coping with those feelings such as keeping a journal. 5. Teach activities that reduce depression: physical activity, self-nurturing (such as taking a relaxing bath or listening to uplifting music), seeking support from others, and spending more time in outside if possible.
Poor self-esteem	Contributing factors include: inability to achieve personal goals due to illness, stigma, isolation, depression.	1. Actively convey unconditional acceptance. 2. Engage regularly and supportively with the patient, guiding him to identify and express feelings. 3. Help the patient to recognize positive traits or accomplishments. 4. Educate the patient about how the illness may distort a person's self-view. Guide the patient to question distorted beliefs, and to replace these with a more realistic self-appraisal. 5. Arrange for interaction with individuals who also once experienced poor self-esteem but who have since improved.
Fall risk	Contributing factors include: impaired balance, bradykinesia, orthostatic hypotension that causes an alteration in one's ability to accurately perceive spatial relationships.	1. Walk with all patients to assess their gait, providing physical support as needed. 2. Assess for orthostatic hypotension with lying and standing blood pressure checks. 3. With orthostatic hypotension, ensure that the patient is well hydrated and teach him to slowly change position from lying to sitting to standing. 4. Encourage the use of handrails or seek assistance when unsteady. 5. People who fear falling tend to look at their feet when they walk. Guide the patient to look ahead instead of down. 6. Locate the patient's room close to the nurses' station so that help is readily available.
Choking risk	Contributing factors include: difficulty swallowing (dysphagia) due to muscle stiffness or dry mouth, failing to chew food thoroughly, taking bites which are too large (all of these routine functions can be disrupted in schizophrenia).	1. Assess all patients for difficulty swallowing and identify causes if possible. 2. Address causes that can be corrected. With dry mouth, taking a sip of a beverage with each bite can make swallowing much easier. 3. Encourage smaller bites that are then thoroughly chewed. 4. Ensure that patients are not rushed to complete their meals, and encourage fast eaters to eat more slowly. 5. Be available at mealtime to assist if needed. This can give patients greater confidence, reducing anxiety and improving swallowing.

TABLE 12.3 Additional Nursing Interventions for the Person Experiencing Psychosis—cont'd

Problem	Considerations	Nursing Care
Restlessness, agitation	Contributing factors include: akathisia, interpersonal conflict, sensory overload, paranoia, hallucinations, anxiety, unrealistic expectations by others, concerns about the future.	1. Reduce excess stimulation—dim the lights, lower TV volume, redirect patient to less-stimulating areas or activities. 2. Assess for and treat akathisia with anti-EPS medications and anxiety reduction interventions. 3. Explore patient's feelings and perceptions that may be contributing and address these as indicated. 4. Promote verbal expression of negative emotions to reduce desperation or negative emotions. 5. Provide safe outlets for physical energy (e.g., walk with patient, allow pacing, provide access to safe exercise equipment). 6. Administer as needed calming medications if agitation is unresponsive to non-pharmacological interventions.
Risk for other-directed violence	Aggression may stem from paranoia (assault may be self-defense in the patient's mind), command hallucinations, conflicts with staff about treatment or limit setting, conflicts with peers (who may be frustrated by intrusive or other patient behaviors, or may tease, speak disparagingly of, or even intentionally provoke distress in the patient).	1. Assess for paranoid thoughts, command hallucinations, interpersonal conflict, irritability, impaired impulse control, increasing tension and desperation, and other factors that may increase the risk of violence. 2. Engaging regularly with the patient increases the opportunity for assessment and communication about concerns that may contribute to risk. 3. Provide increased supervision when risk is present. Placing the patient in a room near the nurses' station facilitates monitoring. 4. Ensure that patient is taking ordered medications (see "Cheeking or Palming Medications" section). 5. Monitor for and promptly de-escalate increasing tension. 6. Take action to help the patient feel safe and secure (e.g., if patient fears harm from outside the unit, note the locked doors and constant presence of staff). 7. Promote communication and venting in a safe manner to reduce desperation levels. 8. Teach and guide patient to practice coping skills to reduce stress and desperation. 9. Provide constructive diversion and outlets for physical energy. 10. If the patient, due to paranoia or other factors, targets specific peers, it may be necessary to relocate the patient or the targeted peer. Similar action may be needed if identifiable staff are targeted. 11. Only when truly necessary: use seclusion and/or chemical (medication) or physical restraint. 12. Search thoroughly on admission and repeat the search any time circumstances suggest the patient may have had an opportunity to make or acquire a weapon. 13. Refer to Chapter 27 for a more information on caring for an aggressive patient.
Risk for self-directed violence		1. Assess for risk to self. Warning signs include a sudden brightening or worsening of mood, termination activities (e.g., saying goodbye or giving away possessions), increased suicidal ideation, or taking action to acquire a means of suicide. Assessment should be repeated regularly, particularly if the patient's situation changes. 2. Provide increased supervision when risk is present. Placing the patient in a room near the nurses' station can facilitate monitoring. 3. Make rounds or checks at predictable intervals such as every 15 minutes provide the patient with a window of opportunity. Preferably rounds should be at unpredictable intervals and adjusted based on risk. 4. Ensure that patient is receiving ordered medications (see "Cheeking or Palming Medications" section). Some medication may help reduce suicidality in schizophrenia (e.g., clozapine). 5. Extra precautions should be taken to assure that the patient has not acquired a weapon. See intervention #8 in the "Risk for Self-Directed Violence" section. 6. Implement interventions from the Depression, Hopelessness/ despair, and Poor Self-Esteem sections.

Teamwork and Safety

A therapeutic milieu provides structure (a planned consistent routine) and external limits that create a sense of security. It is a physical and social environment that maximizes safety, opportunities for learning and practicing skills (such as conflict resolution, stress reduction, and symptom management techniques), and therapeutic activities (e.g., games that promote socialization, therapy groups that help develop insight or coping abilities) while minimizing undue stress and stimulation. Hospital alternatives (e.g., crisis centers, partial hospital programs) also provide a therapeutic milieu in a less-restrictive setting.

Activities and Groups

Participation in activities and groups appropriate to the patient's needs and abilities may decrease withdrawal, enhance motivation, modify unacceptable behaviors, improve understanding of the illness, facilitate support and feedback from staff and peers, and increase social competence and other skills. Drawing, poetry, journaling, and listening to music promote the recognition and expression of feelings. Self-esteem is enhanced via task completion and participation in activities for which there is a high likelihood of success.

Recreational activities such as picnics and outings to stores or restaurants are not simply diversions; they teach and provide practice opportunities that improve constructive leisure skills (the ability to make meaningful and rewarding use of free time), increase social comfort, build interactional skills, promote independence, and improve boundaries. Outpatient programs can provide structure after discharge.

Counseling and Communication Techniques

Therapeutic communication techniques for patients with schizophrenia aim to build trust and reduce anxiety. Staff should remember that patients with schizophrenia may have memory and attentional impairment and require repetition and visual and verbal reminders to promote learning and task completion. People who think concretely also benefit from concrete examples during education (e.g., counting out the equivalent number of sugar cubes found in a bottle of cola to show its sugar content). Shorter (less than 30 minutes) but more frequent interactions may be less stimulating and better tolerated than fewer longer interactions.

Intervening with Hallucinations

When a patient is hallucinating, the nurse focuses on understanding the patient's experiences and responses. Suicidal or homicidal themes or commands necessitate appropriate safety measures. For example, if internal voices tell a patient that a peer plans to do harm, it may lead the patient to act aggressively against that person. In this case, close monitoring, helping the patient feel safe, and maintaining separation of the patient and potential victim would be indicated.

Hallucinations are real to the person who is experiencing them and may be distracting during interactions. They can be supportive or terrifying, faint or loud, episodic or constant. They can be sounds or voices, and are sometimes attributed to specific sources (e.g., a parent or God). Nursing care includes calling the patient by name, speaking simply and loudly enough to be understood during auditory hallucinations, presenting in a supportive manner, maintaining eye contact, and redirecting the patient's focus to your conversation as needed (see Box 12.3 regarding helping patients experiencing hallucinations).

Intervening with Delusions

Impaired reality testing prevents self-correction of irrational thoughts that normally would be disregarded. When the nurse attempts to see the world through the patient's eyes, it becomes easier to understand the patient's delusion. For example:

Patient: You people are all alike...all part of the FBI plot to destroy me.

Nurse: It seems to you like people want to hurt you. That must be very frightening. I will not hurt you, and we can work together to help you feel safer.

Here the nurse acknowledges the patient's experience and feelings, conveys empathy about the patient's fearfulness, provides reassurance about her intentions, avoids questioning the delusion itself, and focuses on helping the patient feel safer (addressing the underlying theme of fear). Focus on the delusion itself, the beliefs about the FBI, is not helpful. Focusing on fear, its causes, and what can help the patient feel more secure is therapeutic.

Until reality testing improves it is *never* useful to try to prove that the delusion is incorrect. This can instead intensify the delusion and cause the patient to view staff as individuals who cannot be trusted. However, it *is* helpful to clarify misinterpretations of the environment and gently suggest, as tolerated, a more reality-based perspective. For example:

Patient: I see the doctor is here. He wants to kill me.

Nurse: It is true the doctor wants to see you as he talks with all patients about their treatment. Would you feel more comfortable if I stayed with you during your meeting?

Focusing on activities and events occurring in the present keeps the focus on reality and provides opportunities to distinguish what is real. Work with the patient to find and promote helpful coping strategies. Box 12.4 provides strategies for working with patients experiencing delusions.

Intervening with Associative Looseness

Associative looseness is a reflection of idiosyncratic and disorganized thinking. Increased anxiety or overstimulation worsens cognitive disorganization. Guidelines for helping those with disorganized thinking include:

- Do *not* pretend (or allow the patient to think) that you understand when you don't.
- Place the difficulty in understanding on yourself, *not* on the patient. Example: "I'm having trouble following what you are saying," *not* "You're not making any sense."
- Tell the patient what you *do* understand, and reinforce clear communication of needs, feelings, and thoughts when it occurs.
- Look for recurring issues and *themes* in the patient's communications, and *tie these to possible triggers.* Example: "You've mentioned trouble with your brother several times, usually after your family has visited. Tell me about your brother and your visits with him."
- Summarize or paraphrase the patient's communications to role model clearer communication and to give the patient a chance to correct anything you may have misunderstood.
- Speak concisely, clearly, and concretely in sentences rather than paragraphs.

Health Teaching and Health Promotion

Ideally patients and family members or caregivers are included in teaching. Often home lives have been stressed by the illness. Significant others may have become critical, controlling, or

BOX 12.3 Helping Patients Who Are Experiencing Hallucinations

Nursing Care

1. Watch the patient for hallucinating cues such as eyes tracking an unheard speaker, muttering or talking to self, appearing distracted, suddenly stopping conversing as if interrupted, or intently watching a vacant area of the room.
2. Ask about the content of the hallucinations and how he is reacting to them. Assess for command hallucinations and if the hallucinations are causing fear or distress.
3. Avoid referring to hallucinations as if they are real. Do not ask, "What are the voices saying to you?" Ask, "What are you hearing?"
4. Be alert to signs of anxiety, which may indicate that hallucinations are intensifying, or that they are of a command type.
5. Do not negate the patient's experience, but offer your own perceptions and convey empathy. "I don't hear angry voices that you hear, but that must be very frightening for you."
6. Focus on reality-based "here-and-now" activities such as conversations or simple projects. Tell the patient, "The voice you hear is part of your illness, and it cannot hurt you. Try to listen to me and the others you can see around you."
7. Address any underlying emotion, need, or theme that seems to be indicated by the hallucination such as fear with menacing voices or guilt with accusing voices.
8. Promote and guide reality testing. If the patient has frightening hallucinations, guide him to scan the area to see if others appear frightened, and if they are not, encourage the patient to consider that these might be hallucinations.
9. As the patient begins to develop insight, guide him to interpret the hallucinations as a symptom of his illness.

Teach the Patient to:

1. Manage stress and stimulation
   - Avoid overly loud or stressful places or activities.
   - Avoid negative or critical people and seek out supportive people.
   - Learn assertive communication skills so you can tell others "no" if they pressure or upset you.
   - When stressed, slow and deepen your breathing. Count slowly from one to four as you inhale, hold the breath, and exhale.
   - Gently tense and then relax your muscles, one area of the body at a time, starting at your head (e.g., closing your eyes then opening them, clenching your teeth then relaxing your jaw) and working your way down to your hands and feet.
   - Discover other ways that help you manage stress (e.g., going for a walk, meditation, taking a hot bath, reading or listening to music, imagining yourself in a less-stressful situation [sometimes called a *mental vacation*]).
2. Use other sounds that compete with the hallucinations (sometimes called *competing auditory stimuli*)
   - Talk with others
   - Listen to music or television (but not too loud)
   - Read aloud
   - Sing, whistle, or hum
3. Find out what is and isn't real (called *promoting reality testing*)
   - Look at others; do they seem to be hearing/seeing what you are?
   - Ask trusted others if they are experiencing what you are.
   - If the answers to these questions are "no" then although it seems very real to you, it is most likely not real and you can safely ignore the voices/images.
4. Engage in activity that can take your mind off what you hear
   - Walk
   - Clean
   - Take a relaxing bath or shower
   - Play music or an instrument or sing
   - Go to the any place you enjoy being, where others will be present: a coffee shop, a mall, a library
5. Talk (quietly if others are nearby)
   - Tell the voices or thoughts to go away.
   - Tell yourself that the voices and thoughts are a symptom and aren't real.
   - Tell yourself that no matter what you hear, you will be safe and you can ignore what you hear.
6. Make contact with others
   - Talk with a trusted friend, relative or staff member.
   - Call a help line or go to a drop-in center.
   - Visit a public place where you are comfortable.
7. Develop a plan for how to cope with hallucinations; options include:
   - Any of the above activities that work for you
   - Taking extra medication when ordered (call your prescriber)
   - Using breathing exercises and other relaxation methods

From Buccheri, R., Trygstad, L., Buffum, M., Birmingham, P., & Dowling, G. (2013). Self-management of unpleasant auditory hallucinations: A tested practice model. *Journal of Psychosocial Nursing and Mental Health Services, 51*(11), 26–34; Herzog, E. (2014). Caring for the hallucinating patient: Non-pharmacological interventions. Presentation at the American Psychiatric Nurses Association 28th Annual Conference, October 22, 2014.

BOX 12.4 Helping Patients Who Are Experiencing Delusions

- Build trust by being open, honest, genuine, and reliable.
- Respond to suspicion in a matter-of-fact, empathic, supportive, and calm manner.
- Ask the patient to describe his beliefs. "Tell me more about someone trying to hurt you."
- Never debate the delusional content. Supportively convey doubt where appropriate. "Although it is frightening for you, it seems as if it would be hard for a girl that small to hurt you."
- Validate if part of the delusion is real. "Yes, there was a man at the nurse's station, but I did not hear him talk about you."
- Focus on the feelings or themes of delusion. If a patient believes he is a famous leader, comment: "You seem to wish you could be more powerful." If the patient believes others intend to hurt him, comment: "It must feel frightening to believe others want to hurt you."
- Use reality-based interventions that help meet underlying needs. If the patient believes he is powerful it may represent a sense of powerlessness. Increase the patient's control such as asking the patient when he would like to take his medications.
- Acknowledge that while the belief seems very real to the patient illnesses can make things seem true even though they aren't. Introducing this indirectly can make it less confrontational: "I wonder if that might be what is happening here, because what seems true to you does not seem true to others."
- Do not dwell excessively on the delusion. Instead, refocus onto reality-based topics. If the patient obsesses about delusions, set limits on the amount of time you will talk about them, and explain your reason.
- Help the patient to identify triggers for delusions and find ways to avoid such triggers or reduce associated anxiety.
- Promote reality testing by questioning beliefs: "I wonder if there might be any other explanation why others might be avoiding you? Instead of hating you, might they simply be busy?"

From Farhall, J., Greenwood, K. M., & Jackson, H. J. (2007). Coping with hallucinated voices in schizophrenia: A review of self-initiated strategies and therapeutic interventions. *Clinical Psychology Review, 27*, 476–493.

BOX 12.5 Patient and Family Teaching: Schizophrenia

1. Have regular contact with supportive individuals.
2. Keep healthy and stay in balance.
3. Taking care of one's diet, health, and hygiene helps prevent medical illnesses.
4. Minimize the use of tobacco and caffeine as they may make your medicines less effective and hurt your health.
5. Maintain a stable weight and work to lose weight if you are overweight (staff can help you with information about how to do this).
6. Maintain a regular sleep pattern.
7. Keep active (hobbies, friends, groups, sports, job, special interests).
8. Nurture yourself and practice stress-reduction activities daily.
9. Join support groups such as the National Alliance on Mental Illness (NAMI.org), which provides support, educational resources, and advocacy for those with severe mental illness. NAMI works actively to help those who live with severe mental illness and those who care about them with national, state, and local branches.
10. Learn all you can about the illness (e.g., through NAMI's Family-to-Family program).
11. Read books about severe mental illness such as:
    - *Surviving Schizophrenia (6th Edition): A Family Manual* by E. Fuller Torrey (2014, New York: HarperCollins. ISBN-13: 978-0062268853)
    - *I Am Not Sick, I Don't Need Help! How to Help Someone with Mental Illness Accept Treatment (10th anniversary edition)* by Xavier Amador (2012, Peconic, NY: Vida Press. ISBN-13: 2940014075459).
12. Access trusted websites and online videos including:
    - *Living with Schizophrenia* (X. Amador and others, LEAP Institute). Provides basic information and hope for recovery via interviews with people living with schizophrenia, as well as mental healthcare professionals.
    - *I Am Not Sick, I Don't Need Help.* X. Amador discusses the lived experience of schizophrenia, anosognosia, and helping those who cannot recognize the need for help.
    - *National Alliance on Mental Illness*: about schizophrenia.
    - *Schizophrenia.com*, a source of online support and information about schizophrenia.
    - *National Institute of Mental Health*: Provides information about schizophrenia and other mental health disorders, including research and treatment.
    - *Fred Frese, PhD*, is a psychologist who lives with schizophrenia. He is an advocate for others with the disorder and offers helpful suggestions for coping with the illness.
    - *Minds on the Edge*, a panel discussion on issues often experienced by those seeking to obtain help for a mental illness.
    - *Out of the Shadow* captures the issues that can occur when children are raised by a parent with severe mental illness. It also documents the obstacles to treatment created by an underfunded mental health system.
    - *Schizophrenia and Related Disorders Alliance of America*, a support and advocacy organization for those who live with mental illness and those who care about them.

Further information can be found in the Substance Abuse and Mental Health Services Administration (SAMHSA) pamphlet, *Developing a recovery and wellness lifestyle: A self-help guide*, available at http://store.samhsa.gov/shin/content//SMA-3718/SMA-3718.pdf.

intrusive. Lack of understanding of the disease and its symptoms can lead others to mistake symptoms such as apathy and poor hygiene as intentionally bad behavior. A warm, concerned, and supportive environment free of conflict and chaos promotes recovery. Teaching significant others how to recognize and respond helpfully to symptoms, and how to negotiate to achieve needed changes, is very important.

Education should include the causes and nature of the illness, what to expect, how it is treated, ways to cope and control the illness, medications and side effects, helpful resources, and relapse prevention. This knowledge and skill helps the patient and family to become actively involved in managing symptoms and the illness. Including family members reduces family anxiety and distress and helps them reinforce the patient's and staff's efforts. Box 12.5 identifies patient and family teaching about schizophrenia.

Additional nursing interventions for patients with schizophrenia are listed in Table 12.3.

Psychobiological Interventions

Antipsychotic medications, those used to treat psychotic disorders such as schizophrenia, first became available in the 1950s. Previously available medications provided sedation but did not reduce psychosis. Until the late 1960s, patients with schizophrenia usually spent months or years in state or private hospitals, resulting in great emotional and financial costs to patients, families, and society. Antipsychotic drugs at last provided symptom control and allowed most patients to live and be treated in the community.

Drugs used to treat psychotic disorders include:

1. **First-generation antipsychotics** (FGAs)—traditional dopamine (D_2 receptor) antagonists, also known as *typical antipsychotics* or *neuroleptics (e.g., haloperidol [Haldol])*.
2. **Second-generation antipsychotics** (SGAs)—serotonin ($5\text{-}HT_{2A}$ receptor) and dopamine (D_2 receptor) antagonists (e.g., clozapine [Clozaril]); other drugs are antagonist in areas of high dopamine activity, but agonists in areas of low dopamine activity (e.g., aripiprazole [Abilify]).

The FGAs primarily affect positive symptoms (e.g., hallucinations and delusions) but have little effect on negative symptoms. Second-generation antipsychotics treat positive symptoms and can also help negative symptoms (e.g., asociality, blunted affect) though improvement in negative and cognitive symptoms is usually less. Second-generation drugs are generally an improvement on earlier drugs while reducing the overall burden of side effects.

All antipsychotic agents usually take 2 to 6 weeks to achieve the desired effects. Patient-specific dosage adjustment is required to obtain an optimal balance between effectiveness and side effects. Treatment guidelines recommend monotherapy or the use of a single medication. After the failure of two monotherapy trials, a clozapine (Clozaril) monotherapy trial is warranted. Polypharmacy is avoided if at all possible. However, if clozapine results in failure or intolerance, an adjunctive antipsychotic may be used to improve the response of another.

Antipsychotics are not addictive. However, they should be discontinued gradually to minimize a discontinuation syndrome that can include dizziness, nausea, tremors, insomnia, electric shock-like pains, and anxiety. Antipsychotics are unlikely to be lethal in overdose situations. A lesser-known risk of all antipsychotic medications, due to dopamine blockade or sedation, is impaired swallowing. This may cause drooling and risk of choking (Chen et al., 2015). Also, patients taking antipsychotics are at increased fall risk due to orthostatic (postural) hypotension, sedation, and gait impairment (Wynaden et al., 2015).

Liquid or fast-dissolving forms, available for selected antipsychotics, can make it difficult for a person to cheek or palm his medicine (hide it in his cheek or palm and later dispose of it). See Table 12.3 for interventions to prevent cheeking and palming.

Injectable Antipsychotics

Some antipsychotics are available in short-acting injectable form, used primarily for treatment of agitation, behavioral emergencies such as assaultiveness, or when a patient refuses court-mandated oral antipsychotics. Side effects can be intensified and less easily managed when medication is administered directly into the system intramuscularly (IM).

Some are available in **long-acting injectable (LAI)** formulations that only need to be administered every 2 to 4 weeks and in one case, every 3 months. Some require special administration protocols (Table 12.4). By requiring less frequent medication administration, adherence is improved and conflict about taking medications is reduced. The downside is lack of dosing flexibility and patients may feel like they have less control and are coerced.

Additional information on antipsychotic medications can be found in Table 12.5.

TABLE 12.4 Long-Acting Injectable Antipsychotics

Generic (Trade)	Usual Frequency	Nursing Considerations
First-Generation Antipsychotics		
Haloperidol decanoate (Haldol Decanoate)	Every 4 weeks	Viscous, deltoid or gluteal site Z-track method
Fluphenazine decanoate (generic only)	Every 2 weeks	Viscous, deltoid or gluteal site Z-track method
Second-Generation Antipsychotics		
Olanzapine pamoate (Zyprexa Relprevv)	Every 2-4 weeks	Must monitor patient for excess sedation for three hours post injection Gluteal site only Shake vigorously just before administering
Paliperidone palmitate (Invega Sustenna)	Every 4 weeks	When initiating, the first two injections must be given deltoid. Deltoid or gluteal site afterward. Shake vigorously just before administering
Paliperidone palmitate (Invega Trinza)	Every 3 months	Deltoid or gluteal site Shake vigorously just before administering
Risperidone microspheres (Risperidal Consta)	Every 2 weeks	Deltoid or gluteal site Shake vigorously just before administering
Aripiprazole (Abilify Maintena)	Every 4 weeks	Deltoid or gluteal site Shake vigorously just before administering
Aripiprazole (Aristada)	Every 4 weeks; highest strength every 6 weeks	Deltoid for lowest strength or gluteal site Shake vigorously just before administering

From US Food and Drug Administration. (2016). FDA online label repository. Retrieved from http://labels.fda.gov/; Burchum, J., & Rosenthal, L. (2016) *Lehne's pharmacology for nursing care* (9th ed.). St. Louis, MO: Elsevier.

First-Generation Antipsychotics

FGAs are used less in schizophrenia because of their minimal impact on negative symptoms and their generally higher level of side effects. However, they are as effective against positive symptoms as newer antipsychotics and are much less expensive than some SGAs. For patients untroubled by their side effects, FGAs remain an appropriate choice, especially when cost or metabolic syndrome (more common in SGA drugs and described later in this chapter) is a concern.

First-generation antipsychotics are dopamine (D_2) antagonists in both limbic and motor centers. Blockage of D_2 receptors in motor areas causes **extrapyramidal side effects (EPS)** including:

1. **Acute dystonia**—Sudden, sustained contraction of one or several muscle groups, usually of the head and neck. Acute dystonias can be frightening and painful, but unless they involve muscles affecting the airway, which is rare, they are not dangerous. However, they cause significant anxiety and should be treated promptly.
2. **Akathisia**—A motor restlessness that causes pacing, repetitive movements, or an inability to stay still or remain in one place. It can be severe and distressing to patients. It can be mistaken for anxiety or agitation. Sometimes more of the drug that caused the akathisia is mistakenly given, which makes the side effect worse. A tardive form can persist despite treatment.
3. **Pseudoparkinsonism**—A temporary group of symptoms that looks like Parkinson's disease: tremor, reduced accessory movements (e.g., arms swinging when walking), gait impairment, reduced facial expressiveness (mask facies), and slowing of motor behavior (bradykinesia).

Lowering dosages can minimize EPS, and EPS can be treated or prevented by using antipsychotics less prone to causing EPS. These unusual side effects may diminish with time. Oral **antiparkinsonian drugs** are also useful. However, these drugs have their own side effects because most are anticholinergic. Abuse of antiparkinsonian drugs is also a problem because they can cause an enjoyable altered sensorium. Trihexyphenidyl (Artane) is the most common drug in this category, but other anticholinergics drugs such as benztropine (Cogentin) are also used to get a high.

Tardive dyskinesia is a persistent EPS side effect involving involuntary rhythmic movements. Tardive dyskinesia develops in 10% or more of patients, usually after prolonged

TABLE 12.5 Antipsychotic Drugs: Classification and Relative Side-Effect Profile

			INCIDENCE OF SIDE EFFECTS							
Drug	Trade Name	Equivalent Oral Dose (mg)*	Extrapyramidal Effects†	Sedation	Orthostatic Hypotension	Anticholinergic Effects	Metabolic Effects: Weight Gain, Diabetes Risk, Dyslipidemia	Significant QT Prolongation	Prolactin Elevation	Metabolized by CYP3A4
First-Generation (Conventional) Antipsychotics										
Low Potency										
Chlorpromazine	generic only	100	Moderate	High	High	Moderate	Moderate	Yes	Low	—
Thioridazine	generic only	100	Low	High	High	High	Moderate	Yes	Low	—
Medium Potency										
Loxapine	Loxitane	13	Moderate	Moderate	Low	Low	Low	No	Moderate	—
Perphenazine	generic only	8	Moderate	Moderate	Low	Low	—	No	Low	—
High Potency										
Fluphenazine	generic only	1	Very high	Low	Low	Low	—	No	Moderate	—
Haloperidol	Haldol	2	Very high	Low	Low	Low	Moderate	Yes	Moderate	—
Pimozide	Orap	1	High	Moderate	Low	Moderate	—	Yes	Moderate	—
Thiothixene	Navane	2	High	Low	Moderate	Low	Moderate	No	Moderate	—
Trifluoperazine	generic only	1	High	Low	Low	Low	—	No	Moderate	—
Second-Generation (Atypical) Antipsychotics										
Aripiprazole	Abilify	2	Very low	Low	Low	None	None/low	No	Low	Yes
Asenapine	Saphris	4	Moderate	Moderate	Moderate	Low	Low	Yes	Low	Slightly
Clozapine	Clozaril, FazaClo, Versacloz	75	Very low	High	Moderate	High	High	No	Low	Yes
Iloperidone	Fanapt	4	Very low	Moderate	Moderate	Moderate	Moderate	Yes	Low	Yes
Lurasidone	Latuda	10	Moderate	Moderate	Low	None	None/low	No	Low	Yes
Olanzapine	Zyprexa	3	Low	Moderate	Moderate	Moderate	High	No	Low	No
Paliperidone	Invega	2	Moderate	Low	Low	None	Moderate	Yes	High	Slightly
Quetiapine	Seroquel	95	Very low	Moderate	Moderate	None	Moderate/high	Yes	Low	Yes
Risperidone	Risperdal	1	Moderate	Low	Low	None	Moderate	No	High	No
Ziprasidone	Geodon, Zeldox	20	Low	Moderate	Moderate	None	None/low	Yes	Low	Yes

*Doses listed are the therapeutic equivalent of 100 mg of oral chlorpromazine.

†Incidence here refers to *early* extrapyramidal reactions (acute dystonia, parkinsonism, akathisia). The incidence of *late* reactions (tardive dyskinesia) is the same for all traditional antipsychotics.

Data from Burchum, J., & Rosenthal, L. (2016). *Lehne's pharmacology for nursing care* (9th ed.). St. Louis, MO: Elsevier.

treatment, and often persists even after the medication has been discontinued. This side effect usually begins in oral and facial muscles and progresses to include the fingers, toes, neck, trunk, or pelvis. More common in women, tardive dyskinesia varies from mild to severe and can be disfiguring or incapacitating.

The National Institute of Mental Health (NIMH) developed the Abnormal Involuntary Movement Scale (AIMS, Fig. 12.2), to identify and track involuntary movements. Using the AIMS is a key nursing role in treating this population.

The FDA recently approved valbenazine capsules (Ingrezza) for the treatment of tardive dyskinesia in adults (FDA, 2017). Valbenazine is a selective vesicular monoamine transporter inhibitor that reduces the severity of abnormal involuntary movements in tardive dyskinesia. Adverse effects include sleepiness and QT prolongation. It is contraindicated with congenital long QT syndrome or with abnormal heartbeats associated with a prolonged QT interval. It should be used with caution for people who drive or operate heavy machinery or do other dangerous activities until it is known how the drug affects them.

ABNORMAL INVOLUNTARY MOVEMENT SCALE (AIMS)

Public Health Service
Alcohol, Drug Abuse, and Mental Health Administration
National Institute of Mental Health

Name: ____________
Date: ____________
Prescribing Practitioner: ____________

Code: 0 = None
1 = Minimal, may be extreme normal
2 = Mild
3 = Moderate
4 = Severe

Instructions: Complete Examination Procedure before making ratings.

	Movement ratings: Rate highest severity observed. Rate movements that occur upon activation one *less* than those observed spontaneously. Circle movement as well as code number that applies.	Rater Date	Rater Date	Rater Date	Rater Date
Facial and Oral Movements	**1. Muscles of facial expression** (e.g., movements of forehead, eyebrows, periorbital area, cheeks, including frowning, blinking, smiling, grimacing)	0 1 2 3 4	0 1 2 3 4	0 1 2 3 4	0 1 2 3 4
	2. Lips and perioral area (e.g., puckering, pouting, smacking)	0 1 2 3 4	0 1 2 3 4	0 1 2 3 4	0 1 2 3 4
	3. Jaw (e.g., biting, clenching, chewing, mouth opening, lateral movement)	0 1 2 3 4	0 1 2 3 4	0 1 2 3 4	0 1 2 3 4
	4. Tongue: Rate only increases in movement both in and out of mouth — *not* inability to sustain movement. Darting in and out of mouth.	0 1 2 3 4	0 1 2 3 4	0 1 2 3 4	0 1 2 3 4
Extremity Movements	**5. Upper (arms, wrists, hands, fingers):** Include choreic movements (i.e., rapid, objectively purposeless, irregular, spontaneous) and athetoid movements (i.e., slow, irregular, complex, serpentine). *Do not include tremor* (i.e., repetitive, regular, rhythmic).	0 1 2 3 4	0 1 2 3 4	0 1 2 3 4	0 1 2 3 4
	6. Lower (legs, knees, ankles, toes) (e.g., lateral knee movement, foot tapping, heel dropping, foot squirming, inversion and eversion of foot)	0 1 2 3 4	0 1 2 3 4	0 1 2 3 4	0 1 2 3 4
Trunk Movements	**7. Neck, shoulder, hips** (e.g., rocking, twisting, squirming, pelvic gyrations)	0 1 2 3 4	0 1 2 3 4	0 1 2 3 4	0 1 2 3 4
Global Judgments	**8. Severity of abnormal movements overall**	0 1 2 3 4	0 1 2 3 4	0 1 2 3 4	0 1 2 3 4
	9. Incapacitation due to abnormal movements	0 1 2 3 4	0 1 2 3 4	0 1 2 3 4	0 1 2 3 4
	10. Patient's awareness of abnormal movements: Rate only patient's report. No awareness 0 Aware, no distress 1 Aware, mild distress 2 Aware, moderate distress 3 Aware, severe distress 4	0 1 2 3 4	0 1 2 3 4	0 1 2 3 4	0 1 2 3 4
Dental Status	**11. Current problems with teeth and/or dentures**	No Yes	No Yes	No Yes	No Yes
	12. Are dentures usually worn?	No Yes	No Yes	No Yes	No Yes
	13. Edentia	No Yes	No Yes	No Yes	No Yes
	14. Do movements disappear in sleep?	No Yes	No Yes	No Yes	No Yes

FIG. 12.2 Abnormal Involuntary Movement Scale (AIMS).

Continued

AIMS Examination Procedure
Either before or after completing the Examination Procedure, observe the patient unobtrusively, at rest (e.g., in waiting room).

The chair to be used in this examination should be a hard, firm one without arms.

1. Ask patient to remove shoes and socks.
2. Ask patient whether there is anything in his or her mouth (e.g., gum, candy) and, if there is, to remove it.
3. Ask patient about the *current* condition of his or her teeth. Ask patient if he or she wears dentures. Do teeth or dentures bother the patient *now?*
4. Ask patient whether he or she notices any movements in mouth, face, hands, or feet. If yes, ask to describe and to what extent they *currently* bother patient or interfere with his or her activities.
5. Have patient sit in chair with hands on knees, legs slightly apart, and feet flat on floor. Look at entire body movements while in this position.
6. Ask patient to sit with hands hanging unsupported: if male, between legs; if female and wearing a dress, hanging over knees. Observe hands and other body areas.
7. Ask patient to open mouth. Observe tongue at rest within mouth. Do this twice.
8. Ask patient to protrude tongue. Observe abnormalities of tongue movement. Do this twice.
9. Ask patient to tap thumb, with each finger, as rapidly as possible for 10 to 15 seconds, separately with right hand, then with left hand. Observe each facial and leg movement.
10. Flex and extend patient's left and right arms (one at a time). Note any rigidity.
11. Ask patient to stand up. Observe in profile. Observe all body areas again, hips included.
12. Ask patient to extend both arms outstretched in front with palms down. Observe trunk, legs, and mouth.
13. Have patient walk a few paces, turn, and walk back to chair. Observe hands and gait. Do this twice.

FIG. 12.2, Cont'd

The first-generation antipsychotics cause anticholinergic (ACh) side effects by blocking muscarinic cholinergic receptors. Anticholinergic side effects include urinary retention, dilated pupils, constipation, reduced visual accommodation (blurred near vision), tachycardia, dry mucous membranes, reduced peristalsis (rarely, leading to paralytic ileus and risk of bowel obstruction), and cognitive impairment. Taking multiple medications with ACh side effects increases the risk of anticholinergic toxicity, covered later in this chapter. In general, FGAs have strong EPS potential or strong anticholinergic potential. That is, when one side effect is prominent, the other is not.

Other Side Effects of FGAs

Other side effects of FGAs include sedation, orthostatic (postural) hypotension, lowered seizure threshold (leading to seizures), photosensitivity, cataracts or other visual changes (with chlorpromazine [Thorazine] and thioridazine [Mellaril]), and increased release of prolactin (hyperprolactinemia), which can result in sexual dysfunction (impotence, anorgasmia, impaired ejaculation), galactorrhea (flow of fluid from the breasts), amenorrhea, and gynecomastia. Weight gain can be more than 50 pounds per year, causing significant psychological distress and increasing the risk of cardiovascular disorders and diabetes.

Some side effects such as sedation occur initially but improve thereafter. Potentially dangerous side effects are infrequent but include anticholinergic toxicity, neuroleptic malignant syndrome, and prolongation of the QT interval, all discussed later in this section. Note that side effects that are not addressed increase the risk of nonadherence to treatment. Some have noted possible neurotoxicity in haloperidol and perhaps other FGAs as well, and haloperidol may cause a form of encephalopathy if combined with lithium carbonate (Nasrallah, 2013). Nursing care for common or potentially dangerous side effects is located in Table 12.6.

Second-Generation Antipsychotics

SGAs include drugs such as clozapine (Clozaril), risperidone (Risperdal), olanzapine (Zyprexa), quetiapine (Seroquel), and ziprasidone (Geodon). They antagonize D_2 receptors as do FGAs but also bind to serotonin receptors as well. They are often chosen as first-line antipsychotics because they are equally effective for positive symptoms and also help negative symptoms.

Side Effects of Second-Generation Antipsychotics

Like FGAs, SGAs can cause sedation, sexual dysfunction, seizures, and increased mortality in elderly individuals with dementia. However, most SGAs are less likely to cause tardive dyskinesia or significant EPS. Although they have the same potential side effects as the FGAs, SGA side effects are usually fewer, milder, and better tolerated.

When the first SGA, clozapine (Clozaril), was approved in 1989, it produced dramatic improvement in some patients whose disorder had been resistant to FGAs and helped improve negative symptoms as well. Unfortunately, clozapine causes agranulocytosis in 0.5% to 1% of those who take it. As a result, patients taking clozapine must have neutrophil monitoring (discussed later).

Clozaril can also cause myocarditis and life-threatening bowel emergencies. Due to these serious problems, clozapine use declined in the United States and many clinicians reserve its use for patients who do not respond adequately to other antipsychotics. However, it is one of the few drugs that have Food and Drug Administration (FDA) approval for the treatment of suicidality in schizophrenias.

TABLE 12.6 **Side Effects of Antipsychotic Medication**

Side Effect	Nursing Care and Considerations
Dry mouth	Encourage ice chips or frequent sips of water. Sugarless candy or gum stimulates salivation. Xylitol-containing moisture supplements or other saliva substitutes can be helpful.
Urinary retention and hesitancy	Check for distended bladder. Try running water and a warm moist towel on abdomen. Consider catheterization if no results.
Constipation	Ensure adequate fluid and fiber intake. Promote physical activity. Consider stool softeners, laxatives, or dietary laxatives (e.g., prune juice).
Blurred vision	May improve in 1-2 weeks. Use reading or magnifying glasses. If intolerable, consult prescriber regarding medication change.
Dry eyes	Use artificial tears. Minimize wind exposure. Humidifier may help at home.
Sexual dysfunction	Consult prescriber—patient may need alternative medication. Artificial lubricants for vaginal dryness.
Anticholinergic toxicity Reduced or absent peristalsis (can lead to bowel obstruction); urinary retention; mydriasis; hyperpyrexia without diaphoresis (hot dry skin); delirium with tachycardia, unstable vital signs, agitation, disorientation, hallucinations, reduced responsiveness; worsening of psychotic symptoms; seizure; repetitive motor movements	***Potentially life-threatening medical emergency*** Hold all medications. Consult prescriber immediately. Implement emergency cooling measures as ordered (cooling blanket, alcohol, or ice bath). Urinary catheterization as needed. Administer a benzodiazepine or other sedation as ordered. Physostigmine, an antidote to reverse the toxicity of anticholinergic effects, may be ordered. Evaluate for anticholinergic toxicity any time psychosis appears to be worsening.
Pseudoparkinsonism Masklike face, stiff and stooped posture, shuffling gait, drooling, tremor, "pill-rolling" finger movements, dysphagia or reduction in spontaneous swallowing	Administer antiparkinsonian agent such as trihexyphenidyl (Artane) or benztropine (Cogentin). If intolerable, consult prescriber regarding dose reduction or medication change. Provide towel or handkerchief to wipe excess saliva. Teach how to reduce fall risk.
Acute dystonic reactions Acute painful contractions of tongue, face, neck, and back (usually tongue and jaw first) Spasm of the muscles causing backward arching of the head, neck (torticollis), and spine Eyes roll back (oculogyric crisis) Laryngeal dystonia: could threaten airway (rare)	Monitor and assure open airway. Administer antiparkinsonian agent as above (IM for faster response). Relief usually occurs in 5-15 minutes. Also consider diphenhydramine hydrochloride (Benadryl) 25-50 mg IM/IV. Prevent further dystonias with antiparkinsonian agent. Reassure patient that although frightening, dystonias are not dangerous except for rare airway complications. Stay with the patient to provide comfort and support. Assist patient to understand the event and avert mistrust of medications.
Akathisia Motor restlessness (e.g., pacing, unable to stand still or stay in one location, rocking while seated or shifting from one foot to other while standing)	Consult prescriber regarding possible medication change. Give antiparkinsonian agent or lorazepam (Ativan) as ordered. Propranolol (Inderal), lorazepam (Ativan), or diazepam (Valium) may be used. Relaxation exercises may be helpful. Take care to distinguish akathisia (inability to sit still, generalized muscle restlessness) from simple anxious repetitive movement (which usually involve only the extremities). In severe cases, may cause great distress and contribute to suicidality. Usually subsides when antipsychotic is discontinued (exception: tardive form of akathisia).
Tardive dyskinesia *Face:* protruding or writhing tongue; blowing, smacking, licking; facial distortion Limbs: Chorea: rapid, purposeless, and irregular movements Athetoid: slow, complex, and serpentine movements *Trunk:* neck and shoulder movements, hip jerks and rocking, or twisting pelvic thrusts	Possibly 20% of patients taking these drugs for >2 years may develop tardive dyskinesia. No FDA approved treatment in the United States, but tetrabenazine sometimes used off-label. Screening for abnormal movements at least every 3 months. Purposeful muscle contraction overrides and masks involuntary tardive movements. Discontinuing the drug rarely relieves symptoms but onset may merit reconsideration of medication. Movements associated with tardive dyskinesia may contribute to stigmatizing response by others. Provide support. Teach patient ways to conceal involuntary movements such as holding one hand with the other.
Hypotension and orthostatic (postural) hypotension Upon standing, systolic rises, diastolic decreases, and pulse increases	Monitor lying or sitting and standing blood pressure. Hold dose and consult prescriber if systolic pressure is <80 mm Hg when standing. Advise patient to arise slowly to prevent dizziness and to hold onto railings/furniture while arising to reduce falls. If lying down, patient should first move slowly to sitting position and pause until he any dizziness passes before standing. Effect usually subsides in 1-2 weeks. Ensure adequate hydration.

Continued

TABLE 12.6 Side Effects of Antipsychotic Medication—cont'd

Side Effect	Nursing Care and Considerations
Tachycardia, irregular pulse	Patients, especially those with existing cardiac problems, should always be evaluated before antipsychotic drugs are administered. Monitor pulse for tachycardia and irregularities. Abnormal Q-T interval can be a contraindication for certain antipsychotics.
Agranulocytosis Symptoms include reduced neutrophil counts and increased frequency and severity of infections. Any symptoms suggesting infection (e.g., sore throat, fever, malaise, body aches) should be carefully evaluated	***Potentially fatal blood dyscrasia*** Monitor for neutropenia weekly for 6 months, then twice monthly for 6 more months, then monthly. If neutropenia develops, hold drug and consult prescriber. Moderate neutropenia (ANC 500-999 μL) and severe neutropenia (ANC <500 μL) should result in treatment interruption (Clozapine REMS, 2015). In some cases clozapine may be reinstituted once the ANC returns to normal. Reverse isolation may be initiated temporarily. Teach patient to observe for signs of infection and to report these promptly to prescriber.
Cholestatic jaundice Rare, reversible, and usually benign if caught in time; early symptoms are fever, malaise, nausea, and abdominal pain; jaundice appears 1 week later.	Consult prescriber regarding possible medication change. Bed rest and high-protein, high-carbohydrate diet if ordered. Liver function tests should be performed every 6 months.
Neuroleptic malignant syndrome (NMS) Rare but dangerous. Severe muscle rigidity, dysphasia, flexor-extensor posturing, reduced or absent speech and movement, decreased responsiveness. *Hyperpyrexia is the main feature:* temperature over 103°F Autonomic dysfunction: hypertension, tachycardia, diaphoresis, incontinence Delirium, stupor, coma	***Acute, life-threatening medical emergency*** Early detection increases patient's chance of survival. Hold all antipsychotics. Transfer to a critical care unit (if in community, 911 transport to ER; notify ER of referral and reason). Bromocriptine (Parlodel) and dantrolene (Dantrium) can relieve muscle rigidity and reduce the heat (fever) generated by muscle contractions. Cool body to reduce fever (cooling blankets; alcohol, cool water, or ice bath as ordered). Maintain hydration with oral or IV fluids; correct electrolyte imbalance. Treat dysrhythmias. Small doses of heparin may decrease possibility of pulmonary emboli.
Metabolic syndrome Weight gain, dyslipidemia (abnormal lipid levels), increased insulin resistance, leading to increased risk of cardiovascular disease, diabetes, and other serious medical conditions	Teach patient how to minimize weight gain through proper nutrition and physical activity, e.g. help the patient to identify low-calorie snacks that he enjoys, engage the patient in regular physical activity, and help the patient to identify and pursue enjoyable physical activities such as walking or cycling. Teach the patient and family about the importance of regular medical evaluation and care to identify and correct possible changes that could lead to this syndrome and increase the risk of premature illness and death.

Data from Burchum, J., & Rosenthal, L. (2016) *Lehne's pharmacology for nursing care* (9th ed.). St. Louis, MO: Elsevier.

All SGAs carry a risk of **metabolic syndrome**, which includes weight gain (especially in the abdominal area), dyslipidemia, increased blood glucose, and insulin resistance. This metabolic syndrome is a significant concern and increases the risk of diabetes, certain cancers, hypertension, and cardiovascular disease, making its prevention an important role for nurses (see Table 12.6).

Some SGAs also have antidepressant properties and are FDA approved for adjunctive use in the treatment of major depressive disorder. As with all antidepressants, they carry a theoretical risk of increased suicidality, particularly in adolescents. Other potentially dangerous SGA side effects include anticholinergic toxicity, neuroleptic malignant syndrome, and prolongation of the QT interval, all discussed later in this section.

A subset of the SGAs is sometimes referred to as third-generation antipsychotics. These drugs are aripiprazole (Abilify), brexpiprazole (Rexulti), and cariprazine (Vraylar). They can be described as dopamine system stabilizers that act by reducing dopamine activity in some brain regions while increasing it in others. Aripiprazole and brexpiprazole act as D_2 partial agonists (meaning they attach to the D_2 receptor without fully activating it, reducing the effective level of dopamine activity). Cariprazine acts as a partial agonist more on D_3 than D_2 receptors, which may help improve cognitive symptoms.

Additional information about antipsychotics can be found in Tables 12.4 and 12.5. Table 12.6 describes common antipsychotic side effects and related nursing care.

Dangerous Antipsychotic Side Effects

Nurses need to know about some rare, but serious and potentially fatal, effects of antipsychotic drugs including anticholinergic toxicity, neuroleptic malignant syndrome, and agranulocytosis. Nurses in psychiatry, primary care, and emergency services need to be aware of and monitor for the early signs and symptoms of these side effects. Patients and their families should be taught how to recognize and respond to dangerous side effects. More information and nursing care for these side effects is included in Table 12.6.

Anticholinergic toxicity is a potentially life-threatening medical emergency caused by antipsychotics or other medications with anticholinergic effects including many antiparkinsonian drugs. Older adults and those on multiple anticholinergic drugs are at greatest risk. Symptoms include autonomic nervous system instability and delirium with altered mental status.

Mental status changes can include hallucinations and may be mistaken for a worsening of the patient's psychosis, so people whose psychosis is inexplicably worsening should be immediately evaluated for possible anticholinergic toxicity.

Neuroleptic malignant syndrome (NMS) occurs in about 0.2% to 1% of patients who have taken first-generation antipsychotics and is characterized by reduced consciousness and responsiveness, increased muscle tone (generalized muscular rigidity), and autonomic dysfunction. Although less likely, NMS can also occur with second-generation antipsychotics. Caused by excessive dopamine receptor blockade, NMS is a life-threatening medical emergency that is fatal in up to 10% of cases. It usually occurs early in therapy but has also occurred 20 years into treatment.

Early detection, discontinuation of the antipsychotic, management of fluid balance, temperature reduction, and monitoring for complications such as deep vein thrombosis and rhabdomyolysis (protein in the blood from muscle breakdown, which can cause organ failure) are essential.

Agranulocytosis, while most associated with clozapine (Clozaril), is possible with most other antipsychotics as well. Neutropenia can also develop and can be fatal. Monitoring for neutropenia is done as part of the complete blood count through an absolute neutrophil count (ANC). Symptoms of agranulocytosis include signs of infection (e.g., fever, chills, sore throats) or increased susceptibility to infection.

Some individuals have lower normal levels of ANC. It is referred to as benign ethnic neutropenia (BEN). Among these people are those from African descent (about 25% to 50%), some Middle Eastern groups, and other non-Caucasians with darker skin. They are not at greater risk for developing agranulocytosis but should have a baseline ANC before starting clozapine.

Prolongation of the QT interval may contribute to sudden death of unknown origin that occasionally occurs in individuals with schizophrenia. SGAs quetiapine (Seroquel), risperidone (Risperdal), and ziprasidone (Geodon) can prolong the QT interval. FGAs chlorpromazine (Thorazine), haloperidol (Haldol), and thioridazine (Mellaril) have also been implicated in this cardiac emergency. Electrocardiograms should evaluate all people for existing QT prolongation (which magnifies the risk from medication-related prolongation) before being started on any antipsychotic.

Liver impairment may also occur during antipsychotic therapy, particularly with FGAs. SGAs also lead to serum enzyme elevations but rarely with injury or jaundice. Liver impairment usually occurs in the first weeks of therapy. This makes monitoring of liver function values essential. Signs of liver problems include yellowish skin and eyes, abdominal pain, ascites, vomiting, swelling in lower extremities, dark urine, pale or tar-colored stool, and easy bruising. The patient may complain of itchy skin, chronic fatigue, nausea, and a loss of appetite.

Disorders co-occurring with schizophrenia should be actively treated. Depression is common in schizophrenia and is typically treated with **antidepressants and other interventions** (see Chapter 14). **Antidepressants and mood-stabilizing agents** may be needed for mood symptoms in schizoaffective disorder. **Benzodiazepines** (e.g., lorazepam [Ativan]) can reduce agitation and anxiety (which can worsen other symptoms and is quite common in schizophrenia) and can help lessen positive and negative symptoms.

Advanced Practice Interventions

Services that may be provided by advanced practice registered nurses include individual and group psychotherapy (e.g., cognitive-behavioral therapy [CBT]), psychoeducation, medication prescription and monitoring, health assessment, and family therapy. Cognitive deficits can be addressed with cognitive remediation therapy, which teaches recall, attentional, and other skills to increase the patient's ability to function and maximize ultimate quality of life. While these are advance practice roles, components of some, such as helping patients identify and correct distortions in thinking, can also be implemented by any nurse.

Family therapy is an important advanced practice role. Families often endure considerable distress related to living with individuals who have acute and residual symptoms of schizophrenia, particularly if they are the direct caregivers or the patient becomes abusive. They may not know how to help their loved ones with schizophrenia. Families can become isolated from their peers, communities, and support systems due to the stigma of mental illness and shame they may feel. In family therapy sessions, fears, faulty communication patterns, and distortions are identified; communication and problem-solving skills are taught; healthier alternatives to conflict are explored; and guilt and anxiety can be lessened.

Family therapy and groups such as NAMI and the Schizophrenia and Related Disorders Alliance of America provide support, education, and opportunities to vent one's frustrations. This helps make families full partners in the treatment process, helps them find better ways to solve problems and reduce conflict, and improves the quality of life for the patient and family. This combined approach of family therapy and support groups recognizes that families are secondary victims of a biological illness (hence the name *secondary consumers* for significant others) and carry a heavy burden as caregivers.

This example shows how one family came to understand schizophrenia and learn how to help their loved one:

> *I went to the group therapy session. We all shared what it was like for us, dealing with the illness. Then my daughter and others there with schizophrenia talked about what it was like for them, how it made it hard for them to take a shower or to listen and focus when you are hearing voices or having upsetting thoughts. I really didn't understand it before—I used to think my daughter was just being lazy…I didn't know it was her illness. I thought she could make the symptoms stop if she tried hard enough…I felt so bad for those times I yelled at her or pressured her to get a job before she was ready. We all had a good cry and everyone agreed to talk more and to try harder to understand the other person.*

EVALUATION

Patients' progress should be reevaluated regularly and treatment adjusted when needed. Staff, patents, and families should remember that progress may occur erratically or slowly, and that gains may be small and difficult to see. Even after the person's symptoms seem to have improved considerably to others, inside the patient may still be recovering. As with other serious illnesses, full recovery can take months. Setting small goals makes it easier to identify progress that may occur in small increments.

Active staff involvement and interest in the patient's progress communicates concern and caring helps the patient to maximize progress, promotes treatment adherence, and reduces feelings of helplessness. Involving the patient collaboratively as a true partner in his or her care is consistent with the Recovery Model that increases patient trust, motivation, and "buy-in." Staff must remain objective, actively engage with the patient, and stay abreast of developing treatments to ensure that care is evidence-based and of the highest quality.

QUALITY IMPROVEMENT

Incorporating evidence-based treatment, creatively developing and incorporating treatment innovations, and examining outcomes data can improve patient care and outcomes. Professional organizations have developed standards of care and guidelines for the treatment of schizophrenia, incorporating evidence-based practices that include:

- Effective affordable medications titrated to effective dosages
- Using second-generation antipsychotics for individuals with first-episode psychosis or prominent negative symptoms
- Monitoring and treatment for risk of suicide
- Monitoring and treatment for concurrent substance use disorders
- Preventing metabolic side effects
- Assessment and management of concurrent medical disorders
- Monitoring for and promptly managing dangerous medication side effects
- Monitoring for and promptly managing other medication side effects
- Monitoring for and promptly managing fall and choking risk
- Involving the patient in active case management services to ensure coordination of care and prevent "falling through the cracks"
- Involving the patient in cognitive remediation programs and other activities that build cognitive skills
- Promoting involvement in self-help and support groups (e.g., NAMI.org) and in other activities and resources consistent with the Recovery Model

EVIDENCE-BASED PRACTICE

Improving Attention with Nicotine?

Problem

People with schizophrenia smoke at much higher rates than the general population: 70% versus 22%. Individuals with schizophrenia also smoke more cigarettes and obtain higher amounts of nicotine from each cigarette. Smoking is a significant risk factor for cancers, respiratory disorders, and cardiovascular disease, adding significantly to the already high mortality rates associated with this disorder.

Purpose of Study

One hypothesis to explain these much higher rates of nicotine consumption is that the nicotine has neurological benefits. Nicotine is a form of self-medication for the cognitive deficits seen in schizophrenia. This study sought to test this hypothesis by evaluating the effect of nicotine on the ability to maintain attention.

Methods

A sample of 17 patients with schizophrenia and 20 controls who did not have a serious mental illness took part in this study. They were randomly assigned to receive either nicotine through nicotine patches or no nicotine through a placebo. At the same time their ability to attend to a task despite a distracting recording of urban environment noises was assessed. Functional magnetic resonance imaging scans were used to determine areas of the brain that were affected by the nicotine.

Key Findings

- Without nicotine, people with schizophrenia evidenced hyperactivity in thinking and diminished capacity to focus.
- Nicotine appeared to enhance the ability of individuals with schizophrenia to maintain their attention despite the distracting sounds.

Implications for Nursing Practice

Due to smoking's physical consequences, nurses cannot support smoking as a means to address impaired concentration or distractibility. However, agents with a safer delivery system such as patches, lozenges, and gums may be useful adjuncts for treatment of cognitive impairment. However, nicotine also interferes with the effectiveness of some antipsychotic medications (e.g., clozapine), requiring a dosage adjustment if nicotinic drugs or smoking are initiated or discontinued while patients are on those medications.

Smucny, J., Olincy, A., Rojas, D., & Tregellas, J. (2016). Neuronal effects of nicotine during auditory selective attention in schizophrenia. *Human Brain Mapping. 37*, 410–421.

KEY POINTS TO REMEMBER

- Schizophrenia spectrum disorders are biological disorders of the brain.
- Schizophrenia is a group of related disorders with overlapping symptoms and treatments but varying etiologies.
- Neurochemical, genetic, and neuroanatomical findings help explain the symptoms of schizophrenia. No one theory accounts fully for the complexities of schizophrenia.
- Schizophrenia varies from person to person in terms of which symptoms dominate, their severity, the impairment in affect and cognition, and their impact on functioning.
- Psychotic symptoms are often more pronounced and obvious than symptoms of other disorders, making schizophrenia more apparent to others and increasing stigmatization.
- *Positive symptoms* of schizophrenia (e.g., hallucinations, delusions, associative looseness) are easier to recognize and respond the best to antipsychotic drug therapy.
- *Negative symptoms* of schizophrenia (e.g., reduction in affect, social withdrawal and dysfunction, lack of motivation, inability to experience pleasure) respond less well to antipsychotic therapy and can be more debilitating. Psychosocial

interventions such as support groups improve negative symptoms.

- Comorbid anxiety and depression must be identified and treated to reduce the potential for suicide, substance abuse, nonadherence, and relapse. Helping the patient to learn to regulate emotions (e.g., via stress management techniques, self-nurturance, instilling hope, and participating in rewarding activities) is very important.
- Substance use disorders affect the majority of people with schizophrenia and can intensify symptoms and cause relapse. Prevention, screening, and treatment of substance use disorders is very important.
- Outcomes are chosen based on the phase of the disorder and the patient's individual symptoms, needs, strengths, values, and level of functioning. Short-term and intermediate indicators are also developed to better track the incremental progress typical of schizophrenia.
- It is important for nurses to assess and support functions such as hygiene, self-care, nutrition, and rest, and to ensure a therapeutic milieu (e.g., reducing undue stimuli on the unit).
- Antipsychotic medications are essential in treating patients with schizophrenia. Nurses must understand the properties, desired and undesired effects, and dosages of first- and second-generation antipsychotics and other medications used.
- Side effects can be distressing to patients and are the source of nonadherence to the medication regime.
- Some side effects such as neuroleptic malignant syndrome, agranulocytosis, paralytic ileus, bowel obstruction, and anticholinergic toxicity are potentially fatal.

CRITICAL THINKING

1. Andrea, 24, diagnosed with schizophrenia, was hospitalized after accusing colleagues of trying to poison her. Andrea is being discharged to her mother's care. Andrea's mother is overwhelmed and asks how she is going to cope: "I can hardly talk to Andrea without upsetting her. She is still mad at me because I had her admitted. She says there is nothing wrong with her, and I'm worried she'll stop her medication once she is home. What am I going to do?"
   - **a.** Explain Andrea's behavior and symptoms to a classmate as you would to Andrea's mother.
   - **b.** How would you respond to the mother's immediate concerns?
   - **c.** What priority concerns should the nurse address before discharge?
   - **d.** What community resources could help support this family and how?
   - **e.** How might this situation affect Andrea's prognosis?

CHAPTER REVIEW

Questions

1. Which characteristic in an adolescent female is sometimes associated with the prodromal phase of schizophrenia?
   - **a.** Always afraid another student will steal her belongings.
   - **b.** An unusual interest in numbers and specific topics.
   - **c.** Demonstrates no interest in athletics or organized sports.
   - **d.** Appears more comfortable among males.
2. Which nursing intervention is particularly well chosen for addressing a population at high risk for developing schizophrenia?
   - **a.** Screening a group of males between the ages of 15 and 25 for early symptoms.
   - **b.** Forming a support group for females aged 25 to 35 who are diagnosed with substance use issues.
   - **c.** Providing a group for patients between the ages of 45 and 55 with information on coping skills that have proven to be effective.
   - **d.** Educating the parents of a group of developmentally delayed 5- to 6-year-olds on the importance of early intervention.
3. To provide effective care for the patient diagnosed with schizophrenia, the nurse should frequently assess for which associated condition? *Select all that apply.*
   - **a.** Alcohol use disorder
   - **b.** Major depressive disorder
   - **c.** Stomach cancer
   - **d.** Polydipsia
   - **e.** Metabolic syndrome
4. A female patient diagnosed with schizophrenia has been prescribed a first-generation antipsychotic medication. What information should the nurse provide to the patient regarding her signs and symptoms?
   - **a.** Her memory problems will likely decrease.
   - **b.** Depressive episodes should be less severe.
   - **c.** She will probably enjoy social interactions more.
   - **d.** She should experience a reduction in hallucinations.
5. Which characteristic presents the greatest risk for injury to others by the patient diagnosed with schizophrenia?
   - **a.** Depersonalization
   - **b.** Pressured speech
   - **c.** Negative symptoms
   - **d.** Paranoia
6. Gilbert, age 19, is described by his parents as a "moody child" with an onset of odd behavior about at age 14, which caused Gilbert to suffer academically and socially. Gilbert has lost the ability to complete household chores, is reluctant to leave the house, and is obsessed with the locks on the windows and doors. Due to Gilbert's early and slow onset of what is now recognized as schizophrenia, his prognosis is considered:
   - **a.** Favorable with medication
   - **b.** In the relapse stage
   - **c.** Improvable with psychosocial interventions
   - **d.** To have a less positive outcome

7. Which therapeutic communication statement might a psychiatric-mental health registered nurse use when a patient's nursing diagnosis is altered thought processes?
   a. "I know you say you hear voices, but I cannot hear them."
   b. "Stop listening to the voices, they are NOT real."
   c. "You say you hear voices, what are they telling you?"
   d. "Please tell the voices to leave you alone for now."
8. When patients diagnosed with schizophrenia suffer from anosognosia, they often refuse medication, believing that:
   a. Medications provided are ineffective.
   b. Nurses are trying to control their minds.
   c. The medications will make them sick.
   d. They are not actually ill.
9. Kyle, a patient with schizophrenia, began to take the first-generation antipsychotic haloperidol (Haldol) last week. One day you find him sitting very stiffly and not moving. He is diaphoretic, and when you ask if he is okay he seems unable to respond verbally. His vital signs are: BP 170/100, P 110, T 104.2°F. What is the priority nursing intervention? *Select all that apply.*
   a. Hold his medication and contact his prescriber.
   b. Wipe him with a washcloth wet with cold water or alcohol.
   c. Administer a medication such as benztropine IM to correct this dystonic reaction.
   d. Reassure him that although there is no treatment for his tardive dyskinesia, it will pass.
   e. Hold his medication for now and consult his prescriber when he comes to the unit later today.
10. Tomas is a 21-year-old male with a recent diagnosis of schizophrenia. Tomas's nurse recognizes that self-medicating with excessive alcohol is common in this disease and can co-occur along with:
   a. Generally good health despite the mental illness.
   b. An aversion to drinking fluids.
   c. Anxiety and depression.
   d. The ability to express his needs.

Answers

1. **a;** 2. **a;** 3. **a, b, d, e;** 4. **d;** 5. **d;** 6. **d;** 7. **c;** 8. **d;** 9. **a, b;** 10. **c**

Ⓔ Visit the Evolve website for a posttest on the content in this chapter: http://evolve.elsevier.com/Varcarolis

Post-Test interactive review

REFERENCES

Akbarian, S., & Kundakovic, M. (2015). CHRNA7 and CHRFAM7A: psychosis and smoking? Blame the neighbors! *American Journal of Psychiatry, 172*(11), 1054–1066.

American Psychiatric Association. (2013). *Diagnostic and statistical manual of mental disorders* (5th ed.). Washington, DC: Author.

Andreou, D., Söderman, E., Axelsson, T., Sedvall, G., Terenius, L., Agartz, I., & Jönsson, E. (2015). Cerebrospinal fluid monoamine metabolite concentrations as intermediate phenotypes between glutamate-related genes and psychosis. *Psychiatry Research, 229*(1-2), 497–504.

Aschengrau, A., Weinberg, J., Janulewicz, P., Romano, M., Gallagher, L., Winter, M., Martin, B., Vieira, V., Webster, T., White, R., & Ozonoff, D. (2012). Occurrence of mental illness following prenatal and early childhood exposure to tetrachloroethylene (PCE)-contaminated drinking water: a retrospective cohort study. *Environmental Health: A Global Access Science Source, 11*(1), 1–12.

Berry, A., & Cirulli, F. (2016). Toward a diathesis-stress model of schizophrenia in a neurodevelopmental perspective. In V. Mikhail, & J. L. Waddington (Eds.), *Handbook of behavioral neuroscience* (pp. 209–224). St. Louis, MO: Elsevier.

Blomström, A., Karlsson, H., Gardner, R., Jörgensen, L., Magnusson, C., & Dalman, C. (2016). Associations between maternal infection during pregnancy, childhood infections, and the risk of subsequent psychotic disorder—a Swedish cohort study of nearly 2 million individuals. *Schizophrenia Bulletin, 42*(1), 125–133.

Castellani, C., Melka, M., Gui, J., O'Reilly, R., & Singh, S. (2015). Integration of DNA sequence and DNA methylation changes in monozygotic twin pairs discordant for schizophrenia. *Schizophrenia Research, 169*(1-3), 433–440.

Chen, C.-F., Chen, Y.-F., Chan, C.-H., Lan, T.-H., & Loh, E.-W. (2015). Common factors associated with choking in psychiatric patients. *Journal of Nursing Research, 23*(2), 94–99.

Clozapine REMS. (2015). *Clozapine and the risk of neutropenia: A guide for healthcare providers.* Retrieved from https://www.clozapinerems.com/CpmgClozapineUI/rems/pdf/resources/Clozapine_REMS_HCP_Guide.pdf.

Dean, D., Orr, J., Bernard, J., Gupta, T., Pelletier-Baldelli, A., Carol, E., & Mittal, V. (2016). Hippocampal shape abnormalities predict symptom progression in neuroleptic-free youth at ultrahigh risk for psychosis. *Schizophrenia Bulletin, 42*(1), 161–169.

Evans, G.J., Reid, G., Preston, P., Palmier-Claus, J., & Sellwood, W. (2015). Trauma and psychosis: The mediating role of self-concept clarity and dissociation. *Psychiatry Research, 228*(3), 626–632.

Frankle, W., Cho, R., Prasad, K., Mason, N., Paris, J., Himes, M., Walker, C., & Narendran, R. (2015). In vivo measurement of GABA transmission in healthy subjects and schizophrenia patients. *American Journal of Psychiatry, 172*, 1148–1159.

Goldman, M. B. (2009). The mechanism of life-threatening water imbalance in schizophrenia and its relationship to underlying illness. *Brain Research Reviews, 61*, 210–220.

Haddad, L., Schäfer, A., Streit, F., Lederbogen, F., Grimm, O., Wüst, S., & Meyer-Lindenberg, A. (2015). Brain structure correlates of urban upbringing, an environmental risk factor. *Schizophrenia Bulletin, 41*(1), 115–122.

Marquez-Arrico, J., Benaiges, I., & Adan, A. (2015). Strategies to cope with treatment in substance use disorder male patients with and without schizophrenia. *Psychiatry Research, 228*(3), 752–759.

Miller, B. (2016). Neuroinflammation marker may foretell psychosis. *Psychiatric Times.* Retrieved from http://www.psychiatrictimes.com/schizophrenia/neuroinflammation-marker-may-foretell-psychosis.

Moorhead, S., Johnson, M., Maas, M. L., & Swanson, E. (2013). *Nursing outcomes classification (NOC)* (5th ed.). St. Louis, MO: Mosby.

Morgan, C., Freeman, T., Powell, J., & Curran, H. (2016). AKT1 genotype moderates the acute psychotomimetic effects of naturalistically smoked cannabis in young cannabis smokers. *Translational Psychiatry, 6*(e738).

Nasrallah, H. (2013). Haloperidol clearly is neurotoxic. Should it be banned? Why use an old and harmful antipsychotic when safer alternatives are available? *Current Psychiatry*, *12*(7), 7–8.

Rao, S., Raney, L., & Xiong, G. (2015). Reducing medical comorbidity and mortality in severe mental illness: collaboration with primary and preventive care could improve outcomes. *Current Psychiatry*, *14*(7), 14–20.

Sekar, A., Bialas, A., de Rivera, H., Davis, A., Hammond, T., Kamitaki, N., Tooley, K., & McCarroll, M. C. (2016). Schizophrenia risk from complex variation of complement component 4. *Nature*, *530*(7589), 177–183.

U.S. Food and Drug Administration. (2017, April 11). FDA approves first drug to treat tardive dyskinesia. Retrieved from https://www.fda.gov/NewsEvents/Newsroom/PressAnnouncements/ucm552418.htm.

Waters, F. (2014). Auditory hallucinations in adult populations. *Psychiatric Times*, December 30, 2014. Retrieved from http://www.psychiatrictimes.com/schizophrenia/auditory-hallucinations-adult-populations.

Wynaden, D., Tohotoa, J., Heslop, K., & Omari, O. (2015). Recognizing falls (sic) risk in older adult mental health patients and acknowledging the difference from the general older adult population. *Collegian*, *23*(1), 97–102.

13

Bipolar and Related Disorders

Margaret Jordan Halter

Visit the Evolve website for a pretest on the content in this chapter: http://evolve.elsevier.com/Varcarolis Pre-Test interactive review

OBJECTIVES

1. Describe the signs and symptoms of bipolar I, bipolar II, and cyclothymic disorder.
2. Distinguish between mania and hypomania.
3. Formulate three nursing diagnoses appropriate for a patient with mania.
4. Explain the rationale behind five methods of communication that may be used with a patient experiencing mania.
5. Describe common medications used for bipolar disorders.
6. Distinguish between signs of early and severe lithium toxicity.
7. Write a medication care plan specifying five areas of patient and family teaching regarding lithium carbonate.
8. Evaluate specific indications for the use of seclusion for a patient experiencing mania.
9. Discuss the use of electroconvulsive therapy for a patient in specific situations.

OUTLINE

KEY TERMS AND CONCEPTS

anticonvulsant drugs
bipolar I disorder
bipolar II disorder
circumstantial speech
clang association
cyclothymic disorder
delusions
electroconvulsive therapy (ECT)
flight of ideas
hypomania
lithium
loose associations
mania
mood stabilizers
pressured speech
rapid cycling
tangential speech

Commonly known as *manic-depression*, the bipolar disorders are chronic recurrent illnesses that must be carefully managed throughout a person's life. Bipolar disorder frequently goes unrecognized, and people suffer for years before receiving a proper diagnosis and treatment.

CLINICAL PICTURE

The three types of bipolar and related disorders that we will discuss in this chapter are bipolar I, bipolar II, and cyclothymic disorder.

Bipolar I Disorder

Bipolar I disorder is the most severe bipolar disorder. It is marked by shifts in mood, energy, and ability to function. Periods of normal functioning may alternate with periods of illness (highs, lows, or a combination of both). Many individuals continue to experience chronic interpersonal or occupational difficulties even during remission. The mortality rate for bipolar disorder is severe. Suicide accounts for 5% of deaths among women and 10% of deaths among men with bipolar disorder compared with 1% and 2% in the general population (Crump et al., 2013).

Individuals with bipolar I disorder have experienced at least one manic episode. **Mania** is a period of intense mood disturbance with persistent elevation, expansiveness, irritability, and extreme goal-directed activity or energy. These periods last at least 1 week for most of the day, every day. Symptoms of mania are so severe that this state is a psychiatric emergency. Manic episodes usually alternate with depression or a mixed state of anxiety and depression (refer to Chapter 14 for a full discussion of depression).

Initially, individuals experiencing a manic episode are the happiest, most excited, and most optimistic people you could meet. They feel euphoric and energized, they don't sleep or eat, and are in perpetual motion. Because they feel so important and powerful, they take horrific chances and engage in hazardous activities. Unfortunately, the person with mania does not recognize the behaviors as being problematic and resists treatment.

As the mania intensifies, individuals may become psychotic and experience hallucinations, delusions, and dramatically disturbed thoughts. Hallucinations tend to be auditory and individuals may begin to hear voices, sometimes the voice of God.

The initial euphoria of mania gives way to agitation and irritability. Utter exhaustion eventually happens and many people ultimately collapse into depression. Depression and the agitated state of mania is a dangerous combination that can lead to extreme behaviors such as violence or attempted suicide.

People may be at equal risk for developing anxiety as depression after an episode of mania (Olfson et al., 2016). They may even experience a major depressive disorder and generalized anxiety disorder simultaneously after a manic event. If clinicians adopted a broader definition of bipolar disorder that includes anxiety as an alternating symptom, we may identify bipolar disorder earlier and develop different treatment approaches. Individuals whose main symptom is anxiety should be assessed for a history of mania before being treated for anxiety (see *DSM-5* box).

Bipolar II Disorder

Individuals with **bipolar II disorder** have experienced at least one hypomanic episode and at least one major depressive episode. **Hypomania** refers to a low-level and less dramatic mania.

DSM-5 CRITERIA FOR BIPOLAR I DISORDER

For a diagnosis of bipolar I disorder, it is necessary to meet the following criteria for a manic episode. The manic episode may have been preceded by and may be followed by hypomanic or major depressive episodes.

Manic Episode

A. A distinct period of abnormally and persistently elevated, expansive, or irritable mood and abnormally and persistently increased goal-directed activity or energy, lasting at least 1 week and present most of the day, nearly every day (or any duration if hospitalization is necessary).

B. During the period of mood disturbance and increased energy or activity, three (or more) of the following symptoms (four if the mood is only irritable) are present to a significant degree and represent a noticeable change from usual behavior:
   1. Inflated self-esteem or grandiosity.
   2. Decreased need for sleep (e.g., feels rested after only 3 hours of sleep).
   3. More talkative than usual or pressure to keep talking.
   4. Flight of ideas or subjective experience that thoughts are racing.
   5. Distractibility (i.e., attention too easily drawn to unimportant or irrelevant external stimuli), as reported or observed.
   6. Increase in goal-directed activity (either socially, at work or school, or sexually) or psychomotor agitation (i.e., purposeless non–goal-directed activity).
   7. Excessive involvement in activities that have a high potential for painful consequences (e.g., engaging in unrestrained buying sprees, sexual indiscretions, or foolish business investments).

C. The mood disturbance is sufficiently severe to cause marked impairment in social or occupational functioning or to necessitate hospitalization to prevent harm to self or others, or there are psychotic features.

D. The episode is not attributable to the physiological effects of a substance (e.g, a drug of abuse, a medication, other treatment) or to another medical condition.

Continued

DSM-5 CRITERIA FOR BIPOLAR I DISORDER—cont'd

Note: A full manic episode that emerges during antidepressant treatment (e.g., medication, electroconvulsive therapy) but persists at a fully syndromal level beyond the physiological effect of that treatment is sufficient evidence for a manic episode and, therefore, a bipolar I diagnosis.

Note: Criteria A through D constitute a manic episode. At least one lifetime manic episode is required for the diagnosis of bipolar I disorder.

From American Psychiatric Association. (2013). *Diagnostic and statistical manual of mental disorders* (5th ed.). Washington, DC: Author.

The hypomania of bipolar II disorder tends to be euphoric and often increases functioning. Like mania, hypomania is accompanied by excessive activity and energy for at least 4 days and involves at least three of the behaviors listed under Criterion B in the *DSM-5*. Unlike mania, psychosis is never present with hypomania. Psychotic symptoms may, however, accompany the depressive side of the disorder.

Hypomania is not usually severe enough to cause serious impairment in occupational or social functioning. Hospitalization is rare. However, the depressive symptoms can be quite profound and may put those who suffer from it at particular risk for suicide.

Among adults, bipolar II disorder is believed to be underdiagnosed and is often mistaken for major depression or personality disorders, when it actually may be the most common form of bipolar disorder. Clinicians may downplay bipolar II and consider it to simply be the milder version of bipolar disorders. However, it is a source of significant morbidity and mortality, particularly due to the occurrence of severe depression. Anyone with major depression should be assessed for symptoms of hypomania because these symptoms are frequently associated with a progression to bipolar disorder.

Cyclothymic Disorder

In cyclothymic disorder symptoms of hypomania alternate with symptoms of mild to moderate depression for at least 2 years in adults and 1 year in children. Hypomanic and depressive symptoms do not meet the criteria for either bipolar II or major depression, yet the symptoms are disturbing enough to cause social and occupational impairment.

As part of the spectrum of bipolar disorders (Fig. 13.1), cyclothymic disorder may be difficult to distinguish from bipolar II disorder. Individuals with cyclothymic disorder tend to have irritable hypomanic episodes. Children with cyclothymic disorder experience irritability and sleep disturbance.

Some people experience **rapid cycling** and may have at least four mood episodes in a 12-month period. The cycling can also occur within the course of a month or even a 24-hour period. Rapid cycling is associated with more severe symptoms, such as poorer global functioning, high recurrence risk, and resistance to conventional somatic treatments.

Other Bipolar Disorders

Several other bipolar and related disorders are included in the *DSM-5*. They include:

- Substance/Medication-Induced Bipolar and Related Disorder
- Bipolar and Related Disorder Due to Another Medical Condition
- Other Specified Bipolar and Related Disorder
- Unspecified Bipolar and Related Disorder

EPIDEMIOLOGY

Bipolar I and Bipolar II Disorders

The lifetime risk, or the percentage of the population that will ever have a bipolar I or bipolar II disorder, is nearly 4% (Merikangas et al., 2012). Table 13.1 provides a snapshot of statistics regarding the bipolar disorders in adults and adolescents ages 13 to 18.

Men and women have nearly equal rates of bipolar disorders, yet they respond somewhat differently to their condition. Men with a bipolar disorder are more likely to have legal problems and commit acts of violence. Women with a bipolar disorder are more likely to abuse alcohol, commit suicide, and develop thyroid disease.

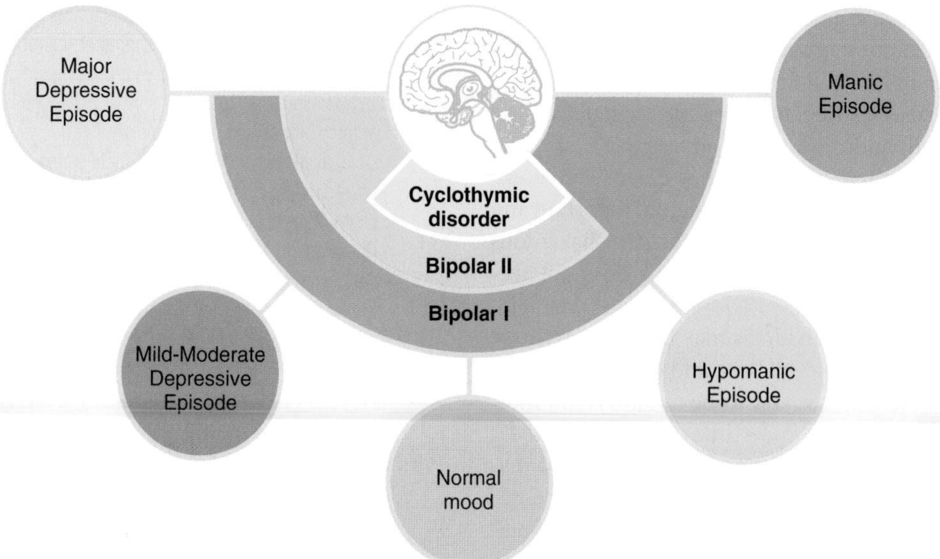

FIG. 13.1 Continuum of bipolar symptoms.

Women who experience a severe postpartum psychosis within 2 weeks of giving birth have a four times greater chance of subsequent conversion to bipolar disorder (Munk-Olsen et al., 2011). Giving birth may act as a trigger for the first symptoms of bipolar disorder. The precipitant may be hormonal changes and sleep deprivation.

Children and Adolescents

The existence of bipolar disorder in nonadults has been the subject of controversy. At the beginning of the 21st century, there was an alarming increase in the number of children and adolescents being diagnosed with bipolar disorder. This diagnosis was given to young people who had chronic irritability and anger along with frequent verbal or behavioral outbursts that were an overreaction to the situation. A bipolar diagnosis for this troubled population provided for financial reimbursement from insurance companies, an answer for bewildered parents, and an established treatment pathway.

However, clinicians and parents alike had concerns over the bipolar disorder in children trend. The most fundamental issue was that these children and adolescents did not usually go on to have bipolar disorder as adults. More commonly, they would eventually be diagnosed with major depression. Unfortunately, a bipolar diagnosis is a lifelong label, one that is stigmatized more than depression. This diagnosis also results in exposure to powerful medications during crucial growth periods. In 2013 a new diagnosis—disruptive mood dysregulation disorder—was developed to reverse this troubling diagnostic problem. Chapter 14 discusses the new disorder in more detail.

Bipolar disorder in adolescence, particularly late adolescence, is a serious problem. Prevalence rates in this age group mirrors that of adults (Merikangas et al., 2012). Researchers estimate that one in five young people with mania plus depression will attempt suicide. Also, these young people experience nearly 2 months per year of role impairment. This impairment has significant implications for individuals who are positioning themselves for a lifetime and a career, as well as developing relationship patterns.

Cyclothymic Disorder

Cyclothymic disorder usually begins in adolescence or early adulthood. There is a 15% to 50% risk that an individual with this disorder will subsequently develop bipolar I or bipolar II disorder. A major risk factor for developing cyclothymic disorder is having a first degree relative—parent, sibling, or child—with bipolar I.

TABLE 13.1 Statistics Related to Bipolar I and II Disorders in Adults and Adolescents

	Bipolar I	Bipolar II
Lifetime prevalence: adult	1.0%	1.1%
Lifetime prevalence: adolescent	2.5%	
12-month prevalence: adult	0.6%	0.8%
12-month prevalence: adolescent	2.2%	
Mean age of onset	18 years	20 years

From American Psychiatric Association. (2013). *Diagnostic and statistical manual of mental disorders* (5th ed.). Washington, DC: Author.

COMORBIDITY

Bipolar I Disorder

Nearly all the anxiety disorders are associated with bipolar I, affecting about 75% of people with this disorder. Individuals may experience panic attacks, social anxiety disorder, and specific phobias.

Other challenging disorders may complicate the clinical presentation and management of the often dramatic bipolar I. They include attention-deficit/hyperactivity disorder and all the disruptive, impulse-control, or conduct disorders. A substance use disorder is present in more than half of individuals with bipolar I, perhaps in an attempt to self-medicate. More than 50% of individuals have an alcohol use disorder, a problem associated with an increased risk for suicide.

Further complicating the picture is a higher than normal rate of serious medical conditions. Migraines are more common. Metabolic syndrome, a cluster of problems such as high blood pressure, high blood glucose, excess body fat around the waist, and abnormal cholesterol levels, may lead to premature death due to heart disease, stroke, and diabetes.

Bipolar II Disorder

As with bipolar I, about 75% of individuals with bipolar II disorder have comorbid anxiety disorders. Typically, the anxiety disorders come about before the hypomania and depressive symptoms. Eating disorders, particularly binge-eating disorder, affects about 14% of this population. Substance use disorders are also common and impact about 37% of people with bipolar I. Anxiety and eating disorders seem to be associated with the depressive side of bipolar II, while substance use disorder symptoms arise along with hypomanic symptoms.

Cyclothymic Disorder

As with the bipolar disorders, substance use disorders are common with cyclothymic disorder. This may be due to efforts to self-medicate and subdue the bipolar symptoms. Sleep disorders where people have difficulty going to sleep and staying asleep are often present in this disorder. Attention-deficit/hyperactivity disorder is more common among children with cyclothymic disorder than with other mental health conditions.

RISK FACTORS

Biological Factors

Genetics

The lifetime prevalence for bipolar disorder is 3.9% (Kessler et al., 2005). However, the illness tends to run in families, and the lifetime risk for individuals with an affected parent is 15% to 30% greater (Fusar-Poli et al., 2012). The concordance rate among identical twins is around 70%. This means that if one twin has the disorder, 70% of the time the other one will too.

Despite the high concordance rate in identical twins, it is uncommon for clinicians to find a positive family history for bipolar disorder (Kerner, 2014). This finding probably means that the disease is polygenic or that a number of genes contribute to its expression. Recent research suggests there may be an overlap between rare genetic variations linked to bipolar disorder and those implicated in schizophrenia and autism (Goes et al., 2016).

Some evidence suggests that bipolar disorders are more prevalent in adults who had high intelligence quotients (IQs), particularly verbally, as children (Smith et al., 2015). People with bipolar disorders appear to achieve higher levels of education and higher occupational status than individuals with unipolar depression. Also, the proportion of patients with bipolar disorders among creative writers, artists, highly educated men and women, and professionals is higher than in the general population.

Neurotransmitters

Neurotransmitters such as norepinephrine, dopamine, and serotonin were the early focus for researchers who studied mania and depression. A simple explanation is that too few of these chemical messengers will result in depression, and an overabundance will bring about mania. However, proportions of neurotransmitters in relation to one another may be more important. Receptor site insensitivity could also be at the root of the problem; even if there is enough of a certain neurotransmitter, it is not getting to where it needs to go.

Brain Structure and Function

Structural neuroimaging techniques (e.g., computed tomography [CT] and magnetic resonance imaging [MRI]) provide still pictures of the scalp, skull, and brain. Structural imaging is useful in viewing bones, tissues, blood vessels, tumors, infection, damage, or bleeding. *Functional* neuroimaging techniques (e.g., positron emission tomography [PET], functional MRI [fMRI], and magnetoencephalography [MEG]) provide measures related to brain activity. Functional imaging reveals activity and chemistry by measuring the rate of blood flow, chemical activity, and electrical impulses in the brain during specific tasks.

With bipolar disorder, functional imaging techniques reveal dysfunction in the prefrontal cortical region, the region associated with executive decision making, personality expression, and social behavior (Phillips & Schwartz, 2014). Dysfunction is also evident in the hippocampus, which is primarily associated with memory, and the amygdala, which is associated with memory, decision making, and emotion. Dysregulation in these areas results in the characteristic emotional lability, heightened reward sensitivity, and emotional dysregulation of bipolar disorder. These abnormalities may be due to gray matter loss in these areas.

Neuroendocrine

The hypothalamic-pituitary-thyroid-adrenal (HPTA) axis has been the object of significant research in bipolar disorder. In fact, hypothyroidism is one of the most common physical abnormalities associated with bipolar disorder. Typically, the thyroid dysfunction is not dramatic and the problem is often undetected.

In both manic and depressive states peripheral inflammation is increased. This inflammation tends to decrease in between episodes (Maletic & Raison, 2014). These findings are consistent with changes in the HPTA axis, which are known to drive inflammatory activation.

Environmental Factors

Children who have a genetic and biological risk of developing bipolar disorder are most vulnerable in bad environments. Stressful family life and adverse life events may result in a more severe course of illness in these individuals. Stress is also a common trigger for mania and depression in adults.

Psychological Factors

With the advent of improved neuroimaging techniques and treatment advances, psychological theories are largely dismissed. Mania was once thought to be a defense against underlying anxiety and depression. Mania was also thought to help individuals tolerate loss or tragedy, such as the death of a loved one. Psychodynamic theorists believed that a faulty ego uses mania when it is overwhelmed by pleasurable impulses such as sex or feared impulses such as aggression. An overactive and critical superego is replaced with the euphoria of mania and has also been suggested as the cause.

APPLICATION OF THE NURSING PROCESS

ASSESSMENT

Individuals with bipolar disorder are often misdiagnosed or underdiagnosed. Early diagnosis and proper treatment can help people avoid:

- Suicide attempts
- Alcohol or substance abuse
- Marital or work problems
- Development of medical comorbidity

Fig. 13.2 presents Altman's Self-Rating Mania Scale. The items in this scale are useful in capturing a picture of the patient's placement on the depression to mania continuum. Scores of 6 or higher suggest mania or hypomania and the need for further assessment and/or treatment.

General Assessment

Individuals with bipolar disorder tend to spend more time in a depressed state than in a manic state. For a complete discussion of nursing care for the depressive aspects of bipolar, refer to Chapter 14. In this chapter we will focus on nursing care for individuals experiencing mania. The characteristics of mania discussed in the following sections are (1) mood, (2) behavior, (3) thought processes and speech patterns, thought content, and (4) cognitive function.

Mood

People with mania are often described as having an expansive mood, which is defined as having an elevated and unrestrained emotional expressiveness. During this euphoria period, the

Level 2—Mania—Adult
Altman Self-Rating Mania Scale (ASRM)

1. Please read each group of statements/question carefully.
2. Choose the one statement in each group that best describes the way you have been feeling for the past week.
3. Check the box next to the number/statement selected.
4. Please note: The word "occasionally" when used here means once or twice, "often" means several times or more, and "frequently" means most of the time.

Question 1		Score
1	I do not feel happier or more cheerful than usual.	
2	I occasionally feel happier or more cheerful than usual.	
3	I often feel happier or more cheerful than usual.	
4	I feel happier or more cheerful than usual most of the time.	
5	I feel happier or more cheerful than usual all of the time.	
Question 2		
1	I do not feel more self-confident than usual.	
2	I occasionally feel more self-confident than usual.	
3	I often feel more self-confident than usual.	
4	I frequently feel more self-confident than usual.	
5	I feel extremely self-confident all of the time.	
Question 3		
1	I do not need less sleep than usual.	
2	I occasionally need less sleep than usual.	
3	I often need less sleep than usual.	
4	I frequently need less sleep than usual.	
5	I can go all day and all night without any sleep and still not feel tired.	
Question 4		
1	I do not talk more than usual.	
2	I occasionally talk more than usual.	
3	I often talk more than usual.	
4	I frequently talk more than usual.	
5	I talk constantly and cannot be interrupted.	
Question 5		
1	I have not been more active (either socially, sexually, at work, home, or school) than usual.	
2	I have occasionally been more active than usual.	
3	I have often been more active than usual.	
4	I have frequently been more active than usual.	
5	I am constantly more active or on the go all the time.	
	TOTAL SCORE:	

FIG. 13.2 Altman Self-Rating Mania Scale (ASRM). Reprinted from Altman, E.G., Hedeker, D., Peterson, J.L., Davis, J.M. (1997). The Altman Self-Rating Mania Scale. *Biological Psychiatry 42*, 948–955, with permission from Elsevier.

patient may experience intense feelings of well-being, being "cheerful in a beautiful world," or is becoming "one with God." The overly joyous mood may seem out of proportion to what is going on, and cheerfulness may be inappropriate for the circumstances.

People experiencing a manic state may laugh, joke, and talk in a continuous stream with uninhibited familiarity. They often demonstrate boundless enthusiasm, treat others with confidential friendliness, and incorporate everyone into their plans and activities. They know no strangers, and energy and self-confidence seem boundless.

The euphoric mood associated with mania is unstable because this mood may change quickly to irritation and anger when the person is thwarted. The irritability and belligerence may be short-lived, or it may become the prominent feature of the manic phase of bipolar disorder.

The following is a patient's description of the painful transition from hypomania to mania (Jamison, 1995):

> *At first when I'm high, it's tremendous…ideas are fast…like shooting stars you follow until brighter ones appear…all shyness disappears, the right words and gestures are suddenly*

there...uninteresting people, things become intensely interesting. Sensuality is pervasive; the desire to seduce and be seduced is irresistible. Your marrow is infused with unbelievable feelings of ease, power, well-being, omnipotence, euphoria...you can do anything...but somewhere this changes...

The fast ideas become too fast and there are far too many...overwhelming confusion replaces clarity...you stop keeping up with it—memory goes. Infectious humor ceases to amuse—your friends become frightened...everything now is against the grain...you are irritable, angry, frightened, uncontrollable, and trapped in the blackest caves of the mind—caves you never knew were there. It will never end. Madness carves its own reality.

Behavior

When people experience hypomania, they have voracious appetites for social engagement, spending, and activity, even indiscriminate sex. Constant activity and a reduced need for sleep prevent proper rest. Although short periods of sleep are possible, some patients may not sleep for several days in a row. This nonstop physical activity and the lack of sleep and food can lead to physical exhaustion and worsening of mania.

The individuals may pursue elaborate schemes to get rich, famous, and powerful despite objections and realistic constraints. Sometimes the person will make excessive phone calls and e-mails, often to well-known and influential people. Being manic means being busy during all hours of the day and night, furthering grandiose plans and wild schemes. To the person experiencing mania, no aspirations are too high and no distances are too far.

In the manic state, a person often gives away money, prized possessions, and expensive gifts. The person experiencing mania may throw lavish parties and visit expensive nightclubs and restaurants. While out, they may spend money freely on friends and strangers alike—"I'll buy the next round for everyone!" This excessive spending, use of credit cards, and high living continue even in the face of seriously depleted resources. The individual often needs intervention to prevent financial ruin.

EVIDENCE-BASED PRACTICE

Fuzzy Thinking in Bipolar Disorder

Problem

We know that bipolar disorder causes significant problems with thought processing. This happens during mind racing manic phases and also with sluggish depressive phases. In between episodes people with bipolar disorder often say that they are not thinking as well as they used to and that their brains feel "fuzzy."

Purpose of Study

Researchers wanted to know if there are actual measurable deficits in thinking in between acute episodes of mania and/or depression.

Methods

To take gender considerations out of the mix, the researchers focused on women.

Part I: More than 600 women participated in the first part of the study. About one-third were healthy controls and two-thirds had experienced either mania or depression. As they looked at a screen with a random sequence of letters, they were asked to react rapidly when specific letters flashed on a screen

Part II: Researchers also used a representative subsample (N=52) of the group and ran detailed brain scans while the women took tests.

Findings

- Compared with the group with no mental health conditions, groups of women with histories of bipolar disorder or depression performed equally poorly on the test.
- Individually, some of the women with psychiatric histories performed as well as their disorder-free counterparts.
- Nearly all of the bottom 5% scores had one of the two mood disorders.
- Brain scans demonstrated some differences in the executive functioning area of the brain—the right posterior parietal cortex. Subjects with depression showed increased activity in this area, while subjects with bipolar histories showed decreased activity in this area.

Why Should Nurses be Interested in This Study?

This study supports the idea that bipolar disorders may impact individuals in between acute episodes of mania and depression. Nurses can be instrumental in validating and understanding a patient's concern about not feeling quite right in between episodes.

Ryan, K.A., Dawson, E.L., Kassel, M.T., Weldon, A.L., Marshall, D.F., Meyers, K.K...Langenecker, S.A. (2015). Shared dimensions of performance and activation dysfunction in cognitive control in females with mood disorders. *Brain, 138*(5), 1424–1434.

Distractibility is a hallmark symptom of mania. People with mania lose their focus and go from one activity or place to another. Many projects are started, but few, if any, are completed. Inactivity is impossible, even for the shortest period of time. Hyperactivity may range from mild constant motion to frenetic wild activity.

Individuals experiencing mania may be manipulative, profane, faultfinding, and skilled at detecting and then exploiting others' vulnerabilities. They constantly push limits. These behaviors often alienate family, friends, employers, healthcare providers, and others.

Choices of clothing often reflect the person's grandiose yet tenuous grasp of reality. Dress may be outlandish, bizarre, colorful, and noticeably inappropriate. Makeup may be gaudy and overdone.

People often emerge from a manic state startled and confused by the shambles of their lives. The following description conveys one patient's experience (Jamison, 1995):

Now there are only others' recollections of your behavior—your bizarre, frenetic, aimless behavior—at least mania has the grace to dim memories of itself...now it's over, but is it?... Incredible feelings to sort through... Who is being too polite? Who knows what? What did I do? Why? And most hauntingly, will it, when will it, happen again? Medication to take, to resist, to resent, to forget...but always to take. Credit cards revoked...explanations at work...bad checks and apologies overdue...memory flashes of vague men (what did I do?)...friendships gone, a marriage ruined.

Thought Processes and Speech Patterns

If a person is thinking clearly, he or she is able to communicate clearly and get to the point. Mania causes a person to experience disorganized thoughts and speech patterns. This disorganization is clearly evident in several specific ways.

- **Pressured speech** is fast, ranging from rapid to frenetic that conveys an inappropriate sense of urgency. As the name implies, the speech is pressured—if normal speech is analogous to the flow of a garden hose, pressured speech is like the stream from a fire hose. This type of speech tends to be loud, rapid, and incoherent. Individuals may talk nonstop and usually have no interest in feedback or conversation.
- **Circumstantial speech** is adding unnecessary details when communicating with others. Unlike some of the other verbal derailments, the person eventually gets to the point.

  I planned to have my oil changed today. When I got in my car, I noticed that the leather on the seat was dirty. The dog. We got a brown and white beagle because Jim insisted upon it. He's a barker. That's how things have gone since we got married in 1986 at a lovely church. I'll never forget the minister wore a green suit and dirty shoes… After I cleaned the seat I drove to the garage and four guys swarmed around the car and changed the oil.

- **Tangential speech** is similar to circumstantial speech with one key difference. When people think tangentially, they lose the point that they were trying to make and never find it again. Awareness of losing the point is an indicator of severity of thought disturbance. "Sorry I'm so scattered, I've got a lot on my mind," indicates insight. The degree of tangentiality also helps identify how serious the thought disturbance is. Often, a common word connects sentences.

  I did the laundry that day because it was Saturday. On Saturday I always watched Ninja Turtles on television. Have you seen those 60-inch televisions? Giants. I used to think of giants as I fell asleep and I thought that sleep activated them.

- **Loose associations** represent the disordered way that a person is processing information. Thoughts are only loosely connected to each other in the person's conversation. For example, a patient may say, "The sky's the limit now that I have money, I took a flight you know from Kennedy, drinking beer is a belly full of bags."
- **Flight of ideas** is a continuous flow of *accelerated* speech with abrupt changes from topic to topic. The speech is usually based on understandable associations or plays on words. At times, the attentive listener can keep up with the flow of words, even though direction changes from moment to moment. Speech is rapid, verbose, and circumstantial. When the condition is severe, speech may be disorganized and incoherent. The incessant talking often includes joking, puns, and teasing:

  How are you doing, kid, no kidding around, I'm going home…home sweet home…home is where the heart is, the heart of the matter is I want out and that ain't hay…hey, Doc…get me out of this place.

Speech is not only profuse but also loud, bellowing, or even screaming. One can hear the force and energy behind the rapid words. As mania escalates, the flight of ideas may give way to clang associations. **Clang associations** are the stringing together of words because of their rhyming sounds, without regard to their meaning:

Cinema I and II, last row. Row, row, row your boat. Don't be a cutthroat. Cut your throat. Get your goat. Go out and vote. And so I wrote.

Thought Content

The content of speech is often sexually explicit and ranges from grossly inappropriate to vulgar. Themes in the communication of the individual with mania may revolve around extraordinary sexual skill, brilliant business ability, or unparalleled artistic talents (e.g., writing, painting, and dancing). The person may actually have only average ability in these areas.

Mania brings about disturbing ways of viewing others and the world. These distorted and generally false thoughts are called **delusions**.

- **Grandiose delusions** are manifested by a highly inflated self-regard. It is apparent in both the ideas expressed and the person's behavior. People with mania may exaggerate their achievements or importance, state that they know famous people, or believe they have great powers. Religious ("I am the Messiah"), science fiction ("I was abducted"), and supernatural ("I am possessed by my dead father") themes are common in grandiose delusions. Sometimes it is difficult to distinguish fact from fiction ("I made an absolute fortune during the real estate crash of 2008").
- **Persecutory delusions** are also disturbingly common. For example, people may think that God is punishing them, that the FBI is spying on them, or that the mayor is harassing them. Sensory perceptions may become altered as the mania escalates, and hallucinations may occur. Rarely, patients may resort to violence in retaliation for this imagined persecution.

Cognitive Function

The onset of bipolar disorder is often preceded by comparatively high cognitive function. However, there is growing evidence that about one-third of patients with bipolar disorder display significant and persistent cognitive problems and difficulties in psychosocial areas. Cognitive deficits in bipolar disorder are milder but similar to those in patients with schizophrenia. Cognitive impairments are greater in bipolar I but are also present in bipolar II.

The potential cognitive dysfunction among many people with bipolar disorder has specific clinical implications:

- Cognitive function affects overall function.
- Cognitive deficits correlate with a greater number of manic episodes, history of psychosis, chronicity of illness, and poor functional outcome.
- Early diagnosis and treatment are crucial to prevent illness progression, cognitive deficits, and poor outcome.

- Medication selection should consider not only the efficacy of the drug in reducing mood symptoms but also the cognitive impact of the drug on the patient.

Self-Assessment

If you are around someone experiencing mania, you will probably feel uncomfortable. This discomfort may be brought on, in part, by the patient's decreased personal space and intrusive comments. You may find yourself feeling afraid, inadequate, or even angry. Understanding, acknowledging, and sharing these responses will enhance your professional ability to care for the patient. Collaborating with staff, your nursing faculty member, and sharing your experience with peers in post conference may be helpful.

ASSESSMENT GUIDELINES

Bipolar Disorder

1. Assess whether the patient is a danger to self and others:
   - Patients may not eat or sleep, often for days at a time.
   - Poor impulse control may result in harm to others or self.
2. Assess the need for protection from uninhibited behaviors. External control may be needed to protect the patient from such consequences as bankruptcy.
3. Assess the need for hospitalization to safeguard and stabilize the patient.
4. Assess medical status. A thorough medical examination helps determine whether mania is primary (a mood disorder—bipolar disorder or cyclothymic disorder) or secondary to another condition.
   - Mania may be secondary to a general medical condition.
   - Mania may be substance-induced (caused by use or abuse of a drug or substance or by toxin exposure).
5. Assess the patient's and family's understanding of bipolar disorder, knowledge of medications, and knowledge of support groups and organizations that provide information on bipolar disorder.

DIAGNOSIS

A primary consideration for a patient in acute mania is the prevention of exhaustion. Because of the patient's poor judgment, excessive and constant motor activity, probable dehydration, and difficulty evaluating reality, *risk for injury* is a likely and appropriate diagnosis. Table 13.2 lists signs, symptoms, potential nursing diagnoses, and outcomes for bipolar disorders.

OUTCOMES IDENTIFICATION

The primary outcome for an acute manic phase is injury prevention. For example, the patient will:

- Be well hydrated.
- Maintain stable cardiac status.
- Maintain/obtain tissue integrity.
- Get sufficient sleep and rest.
- Demonstrate thought self-control with aid of staff or medication.
- Make no attempt at self-harm.

PLANNING

During an acute manic phase, planning focuses on medically stabilizing the patient while maintaining safety, and the hospital is usually the safest environment for accomplishing this (see the Case Study and Nursing Care Plan). Nursing care is geared toward managing medications, decreasing physical activity, increasing food and fluid intake, ensuring at least 4 to 6 hours of sleep per night, and intervening so that self-care needs are met. Seclusion, restraint, or electroconvulsive therapy (ECT) may be considered during the acute phase.

TABLE 13.2 Signs and Symptoms, Nursing Diagnoses, and Outcomes for Mania

Signs and Symptoms	Nursing Diagnoses	Outcomes
Alteration in cognitive functioning, compromised nutrition, alteration in affective orientation	*Risk for injury*	Remains in secure area when unaccompanied, can be redirected from unsafe activities, free from injury
Alteration in cognitive functioning, impulsiveness, sexual advances, threatening violence, psychotic disorder	*Risk for other-directed violence*	Refrains from harming others, controls impulses, avoids violating others' space
Agitation, anxiety, confusion, perceptual disorders, restlessness	*Sleep deprivation*	Sleeps 4-6 hours a night, reports feeling rejuvenated after sleep
Grandiosity, difficulty organizing and attending to information, poor concentration, agitation, hallucinations	*Altered thought processes**	Demonstrates increase in concentration, improved memory, and hallucinations are absent
Minimal calorie intake, poor hygiene, clothing unclean	*Self-care deficit (feeding, bathing, dressing)*	Completes meals, tends to hygiene, dresses in clean clothing
Dysfunctional interaction with others, pressured speech, flight of ideas, annoyance or taunting of others, loud and crass speech	*Impaired social interaction*	Initiates and maintains goal-directed and mutually satisfying verbal exchanges

*Non-NANDA diagnosis

Herdman, T.H., & Kamitsuru, S. (Eds.). (2014). *NANDA International nursing diagnoses: Definitions and classification, 2015-2017*. Oxford, UK: Wiley-Blackwell; Moorhead, S., Johnson, M., Maas, M. L., & Swanson, E. (2013). *Nursing outcomes classification (NOC)* (5th ed.). St. Louis, MO: Mosby.

IMPLEMENTATION

Patients with bipolar disorders are often ambivalent about treatment. Only 39% of people experiencing symptoms of bipolar disorder seek treatment within the first year, and the median delay of treatment is 6 years (Wang, 2005). Self-medicating through alcohol or substances complicates the clinical picture and contributes to treatment delay. Patients may minimize the destructive consequences of their behaviors or deny the seriousness of the disease, and some are reluctant to give up the increased energy, euphoria, and heightened sense of self-esteem of hypomania.

Unfortunately, lack of adherence to mood-stabilizing medication is a major cause of relapse. Establishing a therapeutic alliance with the individual with bipolar disorder is crucial to support continued treatment.

Depressive Episodes

Depressive episodes of bipolar disorder have the same symptoms and risks as major depression (refer to Chapter 14) although they are often more intense. Hospitalization may be required if suicidal ideation, psychosis, or catatonia is present. Pharmacological treatment is impacted by concerns of bringing on a manic phase. A discussion of medication therapy is included in this chapter.

Manic Episodes

Hospitalization provides safety for a patient experiencing acute mania (bipolar I disorder), imposes external controls on destructive behaviors, and provides for medication stabilization. Staff members continuously set limits in a firm, nonthreatening, and neutral manner to prevent further escalation of mania and provide safe boundaries for the patient and others.

There are unique approaches to communicating with and maintaining the safety of the patient during the hospitalization period. Table 13.3 lists interventions for individual experiencing mania.

TABLE 13.3 Interventions for Mania

Intervention	Rationale
Communication	
Use firm and calm approach: "John, come with me. Eat this sandwich."	Structure and control are provided for a patient who is out of control. Believing that someone is in control may improve feelings of security.
Use short and concise explanations or statements.	Short attention span limits comprehension to small bits of information.
Be consistent in approach and expectations.	Consistent limits and expectations minimize potential for patient's manipulation of staff.
Identify expectations in simple, concrete terms with consequences. Example: "John, do not yell at or hit Peter. If you cannot control yourself, we will help you." Or "The seclusion room will help you feel less out of control and prevent harm to yourself and others."	Clear expectations help the patient experience outside controls, as well as understand reasons for medication, seclusion, or restraints (if he or she is not able to control behaviors).
Hear and act on legitimate complaints.	Underlying feelings of helplessness are reduced, and acting-out behaviors are minimized.
Firmly redirect energy into more appropriate and constructive channels.	Distractibility is the most effective tool with the patient experiencing mania.
Structure in a Safe Milieu	
Maintain low level of stimuli in patient's environment (e.g., away from bright lights, loud noises, and people).	Escalation of anxiety can be decreased.
Provide structured solitary activities with nurse or aide.	Structure provides security and focus.
Provide frequent high-calorie fluids.	Serious nutritional deficiencies and dehydration are addressed.
Encourage frequent rest periods.	Exhaustion is prevented.
Redirect aggressive behavior.	Physical exercise can decrease tension and provide focus.
In acute mania use as needed medication seclusion, and/or restraint to minimize physical harm.	Exhaustion can result from dehydration, lack of sleep, and constant physical activity.
Observe for signs of lithium toxicity.	There is a small margin of safety between therapeutic and toxic doses.
Store valuables in hospital safe until rational judgment returns.	Patient is protected from giving away money and possessions.
Physiological Safety: Self-Care Needs	
Nutrition	
Monitor intake, output, and vital signs.	Adequate fluid and calorie intake are ensured; development of dehydration and cardiac collapse is minimized.
Offer frequent, high-calorie protein drinks and finger foods (e.g., sandwiches, fruit, milkshakes).	Fluid and calorie replacement are needed. Finger foods allow for "eating on the run."
Frequently remind patient to eat. "Tom, finish your milkshake." "Taylor, eat this banana."	The patient experiencing mania is unaware of bodily needs and is easily distracted. Needs supervision to eat.

Continued

TABLE 13.3 Interventions for Mania—cont'd

Intervention	Rationale
Sleep	
Encourage frequent rest periods during the day.	Lack of sleep can lead to exhaustion and increase mania.
Keep patient in areas of low stimulation.	Relaxation is promoted, and manic behavior is minimized.
At night, provide warm baths, soothing music, and medication when indicated. Avoid caffeine.	Relaxation, rest, and sleep are promoted.
Hygiene	
Encourage appropriate clothing choices.	The potential is decreased for ridicule, which lowers self-esteem and increases the need for manic defense. The patient is helped to maintain dignity.
Give step-by-step reminders for hygiene and dress. "Here is your razor. Shave the left side…now the right side. Here is your toothbrush. Put the toothpaste on the brush."	Distractibility and poor concentration are countered through simple, concrete instructions.
Elimination	
Offer fluids and foods that are high in fiber. Evaluate need for laxative. Encourage patient to go to the bathroom.	Fecal impaction resulting from dehydration and decreased peristalsis is prevented.

CASE STUDY AND NURSING CARE PLAN

Mania

The police report that when they pulled over Jasmine's weaving car, she told them she was "driving to fame and fortune." She had an open bottle of bourbon on the seat next to her. She proceeded to talk rapidly and make light of the situation. Dressed provocatively, she flirted with the police officers, while chanting, "Boys in blue are fun to do..."

When the police explained that they wanted to take her to the hospital for evaluation, her mood turned to anger and rage. Minutes after getting into the police car, she was singing "Rolling in the Deep."

In the emergency department a psychiatric nurse practitioner saw Jasmine who loudly says, "I'm here because I was driving to fame and fortune." Jasmine then begins to pace.

Her sister arrived and reported that Jasmine stopped taking her lithium about 5 weeks ago. Her behavior had deteriorated rapidly. Apparently, Jasmine had not eaten in days, stayed up all night calling friends and strangers, and finally fled the house when the sister called an ambulance to take her to the hospital. The nurse practitioner receives her old charts with history and medical management. Jasmine is hospitalized, and lithium therapy is restarted.

Self-Assessment

Jeff has worked as a registered nurse on the psychiatric unit for 3 years. He has learned to deal with many of the challenging behaviors associated with mania.

Yet Jeff is uncomfortable with Jasmine's sexual comments such as "Let me be…set me free, lover." He discusses his concerns with the unit coordinator. They decide that two nurses should care for Jasmine. A female nurse will spend time with her in her room, and Jeff will provide care for her on the unit. They agree that neither Jeff nor any male staff member should be alone with Jasmine in her room.

Assessment

Subjective Data

- "I'm here because I was driving myself to fame and fortune."
- "Let me be…set me free, lover."
- Told the police, "Boys in blue are fun to do..."
- Quit lithium 5 weeks ago
- Behavior deteriorated rapidly
- Limited nutritional intake for days
- Limited sleep for days

Objective Data

- Impaired concentration
- Poor judgment
- Constant physical activity
- Loud voice
- Flight of ideas
- Seductive clothing
- Comments suggest grandiose thinking

Priority Diagnosis

Risk for injury as evidenced by inability to meet own physiological needs and set limits on own behavior.

Outcomes Identification

Physical status will remain stable during manic phase.

Planning

The nurse plans interventions that will help de-escalate Jasmine's activity to minimize potential physical injury (e.g., dehydration, cardiac instability) through the use of medication and providing a nonstimulating environment.

Implementation

Jeff makes the following nursing care plan.

CASE STUDY AND NURSING CARE PLAN—cont'd

Mania

Short-Term Goal	Intervention	Rationale	Evaluation
1. Patient will be well hydrated, as evidenced by good skin turgor and normal urinary output and specific gravity, within 24 hours.	1a. Offer high-calorie, high-protein drink (8 oz) every hour in quiet area. 1b. Frequently remind patient to drink: "Take two more sips." 1c. Offer finger food frequently in quiet area. 1d. Maintain record of intake and output. 1e. Weigh patient daily.	1a. Proper hydration is mandatory for maintenance of cardiac status. 1b. Patient is easily distracted; reminders and small goals are useful 1c. Patient is unable to sit and snacks can be eaten while pacing 1d. A record allows staff to make accurate nutritional assessment for patient's safety. 1e. Monitoring of nutritional status is necessary.	**GOAL MET** After 3 hours, patient takes small amounts of fluid (2-4 oz per hour). After 5 hours, patient starts taking 8 oz per hour with encouragement. After 24 hours, urine specific gravity is within normal limits.
2. Patient will sleep or rest 3 hours during the first night in the hospital with aid of medication and nursing interventions.	2a. Give programmed and prn medication as ordered. 2b. Direct patient to unit areas with minimal activity. 2c. Encourage short rest periods throughout the day (e.g., 3-5 minutes every hour) when possible. 2d. Patient should drink decaffeinated drinks only—decaffeinated coffee, tea, or colas. 2e. Provide nursing measures at bedtime that promote sleep: warm milk, soft music.	2a. Antipsychotic and mood stabilizers will reduce physical activity. 2b. Lower levels of stimulation can decrease excitability. 2c. Patient may be unaware of feelings of fatigue. Can collapse from exhaustion if hyperactivity continues without periods of rest. 2d. Caffeine is a central nervous system stimulant that inhibits needed rest or sleep. 2e. Such measures promote nonstimulating and relaxing mood.	**GOAL NOT MET** Patient is awake most of the first night. Slept for 2 hours from 4-6 a.m. Patient is able to rest on the second day for short periods and engage in quiet activities for short periods (5-10 minutes).
3. Patient's blood pressure (BP) and pulse (P) will be within normal limits within 24 hours with the aid of medication and nursing interventions.	3a. Monitor BP and P frequently throughout the day (every 30 minutes). 3b. Keep staff informed by verbal and written reports of baseline vital signs and patient progress.	3a. Overactivity is a great strain on the patient's heart. 3b. Alerting staff regarding patient's status can increase medical intervention if a change in status occurs.	**GOAL MET** Medical records indicate that baseline BP is 130/90 mm Hg and baseline P is 88 beats per minute. BP at end of 24 hours is 130/70 mm Hg; P is 80 beats per minute.

Evaluation

After 2 days Jasmine's vital signs are within normal limits, she is consuming sufficient fluids, and her urinary output is normal. She slept 4 hours during the second night.

As the effect of the medications progresses, Jasmine's activity level decreases. Eventually she sleeps 6 hours. By discharge, she is able to discuss concerns with Jeff and make some decisions about her future. Follow-up care will be provided at the community center. She and her sister will attend a family psychoeducational group for patients with bipolar disorder.

PSYCHOPHARMACOLOGICAL INTERVENTIONS

Agitation

Individuals with bipolar disorder may be on multiple medications. For severe agitation, lithium (Eskalith, Lithobid) or valproate (Depakote) and a second-generation antipsychotic such as olanzapine (Zyprexa) or risperidone (Risperdal) are recommended. Individuals experiencing less severe symptoms may be given only one of these.

There may be times when a benzodiazepine antianxiety agent can help reduce agitation or anxiety. Due to concern of dependency, use of benzodiazepines is usually short term until the mania subsides. The high-potency antianxiety benzodiazepines clonazepam (Klonopin) and lorazepam (Ativan) are useful in the treatment of acute mania. They may calm agitation and reduce insomnia, aggression, and panic.

Mood Stabilization

Mood stabilizers refer to classes of drugs used to treat symptoms associated with bipolar disorder. The original intent of the term "mood stabilizers" was to indicate that these drugs were effective in the treatment of both mania and depression. This is not precisely true. While all of the medications in this category are effective in treating mania, not all of them do as well in treating depression.

Lithium

The chemical name for **lithium** carbonate is $LiCO_3$, although you may see it abbreviated as Li^+. Lithium (Eskalith, Lithobid)

TABLE 13.4 Lithium Side Effects and Signs of Lithium Toxicity

Plasma Level	Signs	Interventions
Expected Side Effects		
<1.5 mEq/L	Nausea, vomiting, diarrhea, thirst, polyuria (producing too much urine), lethargy, sedation, and fine hand tremor	Symptoms often subside during treatment
		Doses should be kept low
	Renal toxicity may occur with long-term use	Kidney function and thyroid levels should be assessed before treatment and then on an annual basis
	Goiter and hypothyroidism	
Early Signs of Toxicity		
1.5-2.0 mEq/L	Gastrointestinal upset, coarse hand tremor, confusion, hyperirritability of muscles, electroencephalographic changes, sedation, incoordination	Medication should be withheld, blood lithium levels measured, and dosage reevaluated.
Advanced Signs of Toxicity		
2.0-2.5 mEq/L	Ataxia, giddiness, serious electroencephalographic changes, blurred vision, clonic movements, large output of dilute urine, seizures, stupor, severe hypotension, coma. Death is usually secondary to pulmonary complications.	Hospitalization is indicated. The drug is stopped, and excretion is hastened. Whole bowel irrigation may be done to prevent further absorption of lithium.
Severe Toxicity		
>2.5 mEq/L	Convulsions, oliguria (producing none or small amounts of urine), and death can occur.	In addition to the interventions above, hemodialysis may be used in severe cases.

Data from Burchum, J.R., & Rosenthal, L.D. (2016). *Lehne's pharmacology for nursing care* (9th ed.). St. Louis, MO: Elsevier Saunders.

has Food and Drug Administration (FDA) approval for both acute mania and maintenance treatment. Onset of action is usually within 10 to 21 days. Because the onset of action is so slow, it is usually supplemented in the early phases of treatment by atypical antipsychotics, anticonvulsants, or antianxiety medications.

The clinical benefits of lithium can be incredible. However, newer drugs have been introduced and approved that carry lower toxicity, have more favorable side effects, and require less frequent laboratory testing. The use of these newer drugs has resulted in a decline in lithium use.

Lithium is particularly effective in reducing the following:

- Elation, grandiosity, and expansiveness
- Flight of ideas
- Irritability and manipulation
- Anxiety
- Self-injurious behavior

To a lesser extent, lithium controls the following:

- Insomnia
- Psychomotor agitation
- Threatening or assaultive behavior
- Distractibility
- Hypersexuality
- Paranoia

Actress Patty Duke describes her response to lithium after years of alternating depression, elation, and bad choices (Moore, 2008):

Lithium saved my life. After just a few weeks on the drug, death-based thoughts were no longer the first I had when I got up and last when I went to bed. The nightmare that had spanned 30 years was over. I'm not a Stepford wife; I still feel the exultation and sadness that any person feels. I'm just not required to feel them 10 times as long or as intensively as I used to.

Therapeutic and toxic levels. In the acute manic phase lithium is usually started at 600 to 1200 mg a day in two or three divided doses. It is then increased every few days by 300 mg a day with a maximum dose of 1800 mg a day. Many patients respond well to lower dosages during maintenance or prophylactic lithium therapy.

There is a small window between the therapeutic and toxic levels of lithium. Lithium must reach therapeutic blood levels to be effective. This usually takes 7 to 14 days, or longer for some patients. Blood serum should reach a level of 0.6 to 1.2 mEq/L (Sadock et al., 2015). Lithium levels should not exceed 1.5 mEq/L to avoid serious toxicity. Table 13.4 details expected side effects of lithium, signs of lithium toxicity, and interventions for both.

Lithium levels should be measured at least 5 days after beginning lithium therapy and after any dosage change, until the therapeutic level has been reached. Blood levels are determined every month. After 6 months to a year of stability, it is common to measure blood levels every 3 months. Blood should be drawn in the morning, 10 to 12 hours after the last dose of lithium is taken. For older adult patients, the principle of **start low and go slow** still applies.

Box 13.1 outlines patient and family teaching regarding lithium therapy.

Contraindications. Before administering lithium, complete a baseline assessment of renal function and thyroid status, including levels of thyroxine and thyroid-stimulating hormone. Perform other clinical and laboratory assessments, including an electrocardiogram as needed, depending on the individual's physical condition.

BOX 13.1 Patient and Family Teaching: Lithium Therapy

The patient and the patient's family should receive the following information, be encouraged to ask questions, and be given the material in written form as well.

- Lithium is a mood stabilizer and helps prevent relapse. It is important to continue taking the drug even after the current episode subsides.
- Lithium is not addictive.
- It is important to monitor lithium blood levels closely until a therapeutic level is reached. After this level is reached continued monitoring will be required to prevent toxicity. You will need more frequent blood level monitoring at first, then once every several months after that.
- It is important to maintain a consistent fluid intake (1500-3000 mL/day or six 12-oz glasses of fluid).
- Sodium intake can affect lithium levels. High sodium intake leads to lower levels of lithium and less therapeutic effect. Low sodium intake leads to higher lithium levels, which could produce toxicity. Aim for consistency in sodium intake.
- You should stop taking lithium if you have excessive diarrhea, vomiting, or sweating. All of these symptoms can lead to dehydration and increase blood lithium to toxic levels. Inform your care provider if you have any of these problems.
- Let your prescriber know if you take diuretics (water pills).
- Talk to your prescriber about having your thyroid, parathyroid, and renal function checked periodically due to risk for hypothyroidism, hyperthyroidism, hyperparathyroidism, and decreased kidney function.
- Don't take over-the-counter medicines without checking with your prescriber. Even non-steroidal anti-inflammatory drugs (e.g., ibuprofen, naproxen) may influence lithium levels.
- Take lithium with meals to avoid stomach irritation.
- In the first week you may gain up to 5 pounds of water weight. Additional weight gain may occur, particularly with females. Discuss how much weight gain is acceptable with your prescriber.
- Groups are available to provide support for people with bipolar disorder and their families. A local self-help group is [give name and telephone number].
- You can find out more information by calling [give name and telephone number].
- Keep a list of side effects and toxic effects handy, along with the name and number of a contact person (see Table 13.4).
- If lithium is to be discontinued, the dosage will be tapered gradually to minimize the risk of relapse.

Lithium therapy is generally contraindicated in patients with cardiovascular disease, brain damage, renal disease, thyroid disease, or myasthenia gravis. Whenever possible, lithium is not given to women who are pregnant because it may harm the fetus. Lithium use is also contraindicated in mothers who are breast-feeding and in children younger than 12 years of age.

Anticonvulsant Drugs

Anticonvulsant drugs were developed to treat convulsions associated with epilepsy. They are commonly used to treat acute mania and bipolar maintenance. They are generally:

- Superior for continuously cycling patients
- More effective when there is no family history of bipolar disease
- Effective at diminishing impulsive and aggressive behavior in some nonpsychotic patients
- Helpful in cases of alcohol and benzodiazepine withdrawal
- Beneficial in controlling mania (within 2 weeks) and depression (within 3 weeks or longer)

Valproate. Valproate (available as divalproex sodium [Depakote] and valproic acid [Depakene]) has surpassed lithium in treating acute mania. Valproate is also helpful in preventing future manic episodes. Although serious complications are rare, it is important to monitor liver function and platelet count periodically.

Carbamazepine. Carbamazepine (Tegretol, Equetro) is an alternative to lithium, valproate, or a second-generation antipsychotic. It seems to work better in patients with rapid cycling and in severely paranoid angry patients experiencing manias rather than in euphoric, overactive, overfriendly patients experiencing mania. It is also thought to be more effective in dysphoric patients experiencing manias.

Liver enzymes should be monitored at least weekly for the first 8 weeks of treatment because the drug can increase levels of liver enzymes that can speed its own metabolism. In some instances, this can cause bone-marrow suppression and liver inflammation. Complete blood counts should also be drawn periodically since carbamazepine is known to cause leukopenia and aplastic anemia.

Lamotrigine. Lamotrigine (Lamictal) is an FDA-approved maintenance therapy medication. Patients usually tolerate lamotrigine well, but there is one serious but rare dermatological reaction: a potentially life-threatening rash. Instruct patients to seek immediate medical attention if a rash appears although most are likely benign.

Second-Generation Antipsychotics

Many of the second-generation antipsychotics are approved for acute mania. In addition to showing sedative properties during the early phase of treatment (help with insomnia, anxiety, agitation), the second-generation antipsychotics seem to have mood-stabilizing properties. Most evidence supports the use of olanzapine (Zyprexa) or risperidone (Risperdal).

This classification of drugs may bring about serious side effects. These serious side effects stem from a tendency toward weight gain that may lead to insulin resistance, diabetes, dyslipidemia, and cardiovascular impairment.

Bipolar Depression

Treatment of bipolar with a common antidepressant alone increases the risk of bringing on a manic episode (Viktorin et al., 2014). This risk vanishes when combining the antidepressant with a mood stabilizer.

Specific medications are indicated for bipolar depression. The second-generation antipsychotics lurasidone (Latuda) and quetiapine (Seroquel) have FDA approval for the treatment of bipolar depression. Symbyax is another drug with approval for this type of depression. It is made up of the second-generation olanzapine (Zyprexa) and the selective serotonin reuptake inhibitor fluoxetine (Prozac).

Table 13.5 identifies drugs with FDA approval for bipolar disorder. You may notice that your patient is taking a drug without specific FDA approval. This is called using the medication *off-label* meaning that they are not officially approved, but practitioners often prescribe them.

Integrative Therapy

A few generations ago, children resisted a nightly dose of cod liver oil that mothers swore by as constipation prevention. While the foul-tasting evil-smelling liquid undoubtedly helped win that particular battle, it may have had other benefits as well.

TABLE 13.5 FDA Approved Drugs for Bipolar Disorder

Generic (Trade) Name	Bipolar Depression	Acute Mania	Bipolar Maintenance
Mood Stabilizer			
Lithium (Eskalith, Eskalith CR, Lithobid)	—	FDA approved	FDA approved
Anticonvulsant Mood Stabilizers			
Divalproex sodium delayed release (Depakote), divalproex sodium extended release (Depakote ER)	—	FDA approved	—
Valproic acid delayed release (Stavzor)	—	FDA approved	—
Carbamazepine (Equetro)	—	FDA approved	—
Lamotrigine (Lamictal)	—	—	FDA approved
First-Generation Antipsychotics			
Chlorpromazine (Thorazine)	—	FDA approved	—
Loxapine (Adasuve) inhaled	—	FDA approved bipolar I agitation	—
Second-Generation Antipsychotics			
Aripiprazole (Abilify)	—	FDA approved	FDA approved
Asenapine (Saphris)	—	FDA approved	—
Cariprazine (Vraylar)	—	FDA approved	—
Lurasidone (Latuda)	FDA approved	—	—
Olanzapine (Zyprexa)	—	FDA approved	FDA approved
Quetiapine (Seroquel, Seroquel XR)	FDA approved	FDA approved	FDA approved
Risperidone (Risperdal)	—	FDA approved	—
(Risperdal Consta)	—	—	FDA approved
Ziprasidone (Geodon)	—	FDA approved	FDA approved
Combination Second-Generation Antipsychotic and Antidepressant			
Olanzapine (Zyprexa) + fluoxetine (Prozac) = Symbyax	FDA approved	—	—

Food and Drug Administration. (2016). FDA online label repository. Retrieved from http://labels.fda.gov/; Howland, R.H. (2015). Drugs to treat bipolar disorder. *Journal of Psychosocial Nursing, 53*(6), 17–18.

Cod liver oil is rich in omega-3 fatty acids, which have drawn increasing attention as being important in mood regulation. Fish oil is the target of this attention. It contains two omega-3 fatty acids, eicosapentaenoic acid (EPA) and docosahexaenoic acid (DHA), which are important in CNS functioning.

The interest in these particular fatty acids developed as research began to suggest that people who live in areas with low seafood consumption, especially cold water seafood, exhibited higher rates of depression and bipolar disorder. This led researchers to explore the influence of omega-3 fatty acids as protective for bipolar disorder.

In 2012 Sarris and colleagues reviewed published research about omega-3 and its influence on mania and depression. They concluded that there is no evidence to support the use of omega-3 in treating mania. However, they found strong evidence that increasing the use of this fatty acid may improve bipolar depressive symptoms.

CONSIDERING CULTURE

Racial Influence on the Diagnosis and Treatment of Bipolar Disorder

Jason, a 28-year-old Caucasian male, arrives at a community mental health center complaining of an inability to sleep. His speech is rapid, he paces, and he talks about the inability of the mayor to cleanse the sewers of chlorine gas. He jumps from topic to topic but seems to always return to his family being Russian rulers in exile. The nurse practitioner tentatively diagnoses him as having bipolar disorder, manic phase, and prescribes a mood stabilizer, lithium, and an antipsychotic, Zyprexa.

Shortly after that, George, a 32-year-old African American male, arrives at the center. He is irritated that his wife threw him out for running up their credit card debt and being involved with another woman. George says that he is superhuman and no longer needs to eat or sleep. He wrings his hands, jumps up from his chair, and looks nervously around the room as if he is afraid or is hearing something. The nurse practitioner diagnoses him with a psychotic disorder (with a need to rule out schizophrenia) and prescribes Zyprexa.

What's the difference between the patients? It is quite likely their races. African Americans frequently receive a diagnosis of schizophrenia rather than bipolar disorder. Implications of this study and many others are that bipolar disorder is not being treated uniformly among different races. As a result, patients are suffering needlessly when cost-effective pharmacotherapy is available. Lithium is far less expensive than either second-generation antipsychotic agents or mood stabilizers.

From Haeri, S., Williams, J., Kopeykina, I., Johnson, J., Newmark, A., Cohen, L., & Galynker, I. (2011). Disparities in diagnosis of bipolar disorder in individuals of African and European descent. *Journal of Psychiatric Practice, 17*(6), 394–403.

Electroconvulsive Therapy

Electroconvulsive therapy (ECT) is used to subdue severe manic behavior, especially in patients with treatment-resistant mania and patients with rapid cycling (i.e., those who experience four or more episodes of illness per year).

ECT seems to be far more effective than drug-based therapy for treatment-resistant bipolar depression (Schoeyen et al., 2015). Depressive episodes—particularly those with severe, catatonic, or treatment-resistant depression—are an indication for this treatment.

Teamwork and Safety

Interprofessional staff work together to create a climate of teamwork and safety. This is essential for patients who are at risk of self-harm during a depressive phase or at risk for self-harm or other harm during the acute phase. The whole treatment team is trained to recognize changes that may lead to unsafe behavior.

Frequent team meetings to plan strategies for dealing with challenging patient behaviors are essential. These meetings help to minimize staff splitting and may reduce feelings of anger, fear, and isolation. Limit setting (e.g., lights out after 11 p.m.) is the main theme in treating a person in a manic state.

Seclusion and Restraint

Control of hyperactivity during the acute phase almost always includes immediate treatment with an antipsychotic drug. When a patient is dangerously out of control, however, use of the seclusion room or restraints may be necessary. The use of seclusion or restraints is associated with complex therapeutic, ethical, and legal issues. Most state laws prohibit the use of unnecessary physical restraint or isolation. Unless it is an emergency, the use of seclusion and restraints requires the patient's consent.

Seclusion and restraint may be warranted when documented data collected by the nursing and medical staff reflect the following points:

- Substantial risk of harm to others or self is clear.
- The patient is unable to control actions.
- Other measures have failed (e.g., setting limits beginning with verbal de-escalation or using chemical restraints).

Most facilities have well-defined practices for treatment with seclusion and restraint, including a proper reporting procedure through the chain of command when a patient is to be secluded. For example, the use of seclusion and restraint is permitted only on the written order of an authorized care provider (e.g., physician, advanced practice nurse, or a physician assistant), which must be reviewed and rewritten every 24 hours. The order must include the type of restraint to be used. Only in an emergency may the charge nurse place a patient in seclusion or restraint; under these circumstances, a written order must be obtained within a specified period of time (15 to 30 minutes).

Protocols identify specific nursing responsibilities such as how often to observe and document the patient's behavior (e.g., every 15 minutes), how often to offer the patient food and fluids (e.g., every 30 to 60 minutes), and how often the patient can use the restroom (e.g., every 1 to 2 hours). Caregivers should measure vital signs frequently (e.g., every 1 to 2 hours).

Communication with a patient in seclusion is concrete, direct, and empathetic. Patients need reassurance that seclusion is only a temporary measure and that they will be returned to the unit when they demonstrate the ability to safely be around others.

Restraints and seclusion are never for punishment or for the convenience of the staff. Refer to Chapter 6 for a more detailed discussion of the legal implications of seclusion and restraints.

Support Groups

Patients with bipolar disorder, as well as their friends and families, benefit from support groups such as those sponsored by the Depression and Bipolar Support Alliance (DBSA), the National Alliance for the Mentally Ill (NAMI), the National Mental Health Association, and the Manic-Depressive Association.

Health Teaching and Health Promotion

Patients and families need information about bipolar illness, with particular emphasis on its chronic and highly recurrent nature. In addition, patients and families need to learn the warning signs and symptoms of impending episodes. For example, changes in sleep patterns are especially important because they usually precede, accompany, or precipitate mania. Even a single night of unexplainable sleep loss can be taken as an early warning of impending mania. Health teaching stresses the importance of establishing regularity in sleep patterns, meals, exercise, and other activities. Box 13.2 lists health-teaching guidelines for patients with bipolar disorder and their families.

Most of the medications used to treat bipolar disorder may cause weight gain and other metabolic disturbances such as altered metabolism of lipids and glucose. These alterations increase the risk for diabetes, high blood pressure, dyslipidemia, cardiac problems, or all of these in combination (metabolic syndrome). Not only do these disturbances impair quality of life and life span, but they are also a major reason for nonadherence. Teaching aimed at weight reduction and management is essential to keeping patients physically healthy and emotionally stable.

Recovery concepts are particularly important for patients with bipolar disorder who often have issues with adherence to treatment. The best method of addressing this problem is to follow a collaborative-care model in which responsibilities for treatment adherence are shared. In this model, patients are responsible for making it to appointments and openly communicating information, and the healthcare provider is responsible for keeping current on treatment methods and listening

BOX 13.2 Patient and Family Teaching: Bipolar Disorder

1. Patients with bipolar disorder and their families need to know:
   - The chronic and episodic nature of bipolar disorder
   - The fact that bipolar disorder is long term. Treatment will require that one or more mood-stabilizing agents be taken for a long time
   - The expected side effects and toxic effects of the prescribed medication, as well as whom to call and where to go in case of an adverse reaction
   - The signs and symptoms of relapse that may "come out of the blue"
   - The role of family members and others in preventing a full relapse
   - The phone numbers of emergency contact people, which should be kept in an easily accessed place
2. The use of alcohol, drugs of abuse, caffeine (particularly in energy drinks), and over-the-counter medications can cause a relapse.
3. Good sleep hygiene is critical to stability. Frequently, the early symptom of a manic episode is lack of sleep. In some cases, mania may be averted by the use of sleep medications.
4. Coping strategies are important for dealing with work, interpersonal, and family problems for lowering stress; for enhancing a sense of personal control; and for increasing community functioning.
5. Group and individual therapy are valuable for gaining insight and skills in relapse prevention, providing social support, increasing coping skills in interpersonal relations, improving adherence to the medication regimen, reducing functional morbidity, and decreasing need for hospitalization.

carefully as the patient shares perceptions. Through this sharing, treatment adherence becomes a self-managed responsibility.

The National Institute of Mental Health (2015) provides two colorful, downloadable brochures about bipolar disorder in adults and children and adolescents. They are available in both English and Spanish that you can provide to your patient. The link is: http://www.nimh.nih.gov/health/publications/bipolar-disorder-listing.shtml.

Advanced Practice Interventions

Many psychiatric-mental health advanced practice registered nurses (PMH-APRNs) are able to diagnose and prescribe medications for treating bipolar disorder. In addition, they may use psychotherapy to help the patient cope more adaptively to stresses in the environment and decrease the risk of relapse. Specific approaches to psychotherapy include cognitive-behavioral therapy, interpersonal and social rhythm therapy, and family-focused therapy.

Many patients have strained interpersonal relationships, marriage and family problems, academic and occupational problems, and legal or other social difficulties. Psychotherapy can help them work through these difficulties, decrease some of the psychic distress, and increase self-esteem. Psychotherapeutic treatments can also help patients improve their functioning between episodes and attempt to decrease the frequency of future episodes.

Cognitive-Behavioral Therapy

Cognitive-behavioral therapy (CBT) is typically used as an adjunct to pharmacotherapy in many psychiatric disorders. It involves identifying maladaptive thoughts ("I am always going to be a loser") and behaviors ("I might as well drink") that may be barriers to a person's recovery and ongoing mood stability.

CBT focuses on adherence to the medication regimen, early detection and intervention for manic or depressive episodes, stress and lifestyle management, and the treatment of depression and comorbid conditions. Some research demonstrates that patients treated with cognitive therapy are more likely to take their medications as prescribed than are patients who do not participate in therapy, and psychotherapy results in greater adherence to the lithium regimen.

Interpersonal and Social Rhythm Therapy

Depression and manic-type states impair a person's ability to interact with others. Even in between episodes, relationships have been so damaged it may seem impossible to correct the problems. The APRN can use a specialized approach, interpersonal and social rhythm therapy. This approach aims to regulate social routines and stabilize interpersonal relationships to improve depression and prevent relapse. Psychoeducation is a major component of this therapy and includes symptom recognition, adherence with medication and sleep routines, stress management, and maintenance of social supports.

Family-Focused Therapy

Family-focused therapy helps improve communication among family members. During depressive and manic episodes, family life can become a challenge or even intolerable. Negative patterns of communicating develop and become part of the fabric of the family. APRNs can help people recognize and reduce negative expressed emotion and stressors that provoke episodes.

EVALUATION

Outcome criteria often dictate the frequency of evaluation of short-term and intermediate indicators. Are the patient's vital signs stable? Is he or she well hydrated? Is the patient able to control personal behavior or respond to external controls? Is the patient able to sleep for 4 or 5 hours a night or take frequent short rest periods during the day? Does the family have a clear understanding of the patient's disease and need for medication? Do the patient and family know which community agencies may help them?

After reassessing the outcomes and care plan, the plan is revised, if indicated. Longer-term outcomes include:

- Adherence to the medication regimen
- Resumption of functioning in the community
- Achievement of stability in family, work, and social relationships and in mood
- Improved coping skills for reducing stress.

QUALITY IMPROVEMENT

Nurses are increasingly involved in finding methods to improve care by examining outcomes data to improve the quality and safety of our care. The Standards for Bipolar Excellence Project is a comprehensive project that addresses the quality of care for bipolar disorders (Centers for Quality Assessment and Improvement in Mental Health Care, 2007). This project provides 15 evidence-based performance measures regarding screening, assessment, treatment, and monitoring bipolar disorder and its care. Many valuable tools for research, teaching, and quality improvement are readily available:

- Screening for bipolar mania/hypomania
- Assessment for risk of suicide
- Assessment for substance use
- Use of antimanic agent in bipolar I disorder: manic phase
- Use of mood-stabilizing or antimanic agent in bipolar I disorder: depressed phase
- Avoidance of antidepressant monotherapy in bipolar I disorder
- Monitoring weight
- Monitoring for extrapyramidal symptoms
- Monitoring lithium serum levels
- Screening for hyperglycemia and hyperlipidemia when a second-generation antipsychotic is prescribed
- Providing condition-specific education/information
- Monitoring change in symptom complex
- Recommending adjunctive psychosocial interventions
- Monitoring change in level of functioning

The assessment forms used for monitoring care given to patients with bipolar disorder are available and quite interesting. You are encouraged to review some of the assessment forms listed previously and consider how your patient might respond or try them out for yourself. They are available at http://www.cqaimh.org/stable.html.

KEY POINTS TO REMEMBER

- Bipolar I disorder is characterized by the presence of history of at least one manic episode, whereas bipolar II is characterized by the presence or history of at least one hypomanic episode.
- Cyclothymia is a bipolar-related disorder with symptoms of hypomania and symptoms of mild-moderate depression.
- Genetics play a strong role in the risk for the bipolar disorders.
- Early detection of bipolar disorder can help diminish comorbid substance abuse, suicide, and decline in social and personal relationships and may help promote more positive outcomes.
- Nurses assess the patient's mood (i.e., mania, hypomania, and depression), behavior, and thought processes and are alert to cognitive dysfunction.
- During the acute phase of mania, physical needs often take priority and demand nursing interventions.
- Support groups, psychoeducation, and guidance for the family can greatly affect the patient's adherence to the medication regimen.
- Patients experiencing mania can be demanding and manipulative. Nurses set limits in a firm, neutral manner and tailor communication techniques and interventions to maintain the patient's safety.
- Healthcare workers, family, and friends often feel angry and frustrated by the patient's disruptive behaviors. When these feelings are not examined and shared with others, the therapeutic potential of the staff is reduced, and feelings of confusion and helplessness remain.
- Mood stabilizers are usually the first line of defense for bipolar disorder and include lithium and several anticonvulsants.
- Lithium is approved for treating acute mania and maintenance. Blood levels, kidney function, and thyroid function should be assessed regularly.
- Most anticonvulsant drugs are approved for acute mania. Lamotrigine (Lamictal) is approved for maintenance.
- Antipsychotic agents, particularly the second-generation antipsychotics, are used for their sedating and mood-stabilizing properties. Screening for metabolic problems (e.g., diabetes) is essential in this population.
- For some patients, ECT may be an appropriate medical treatment.
- Patient and family teaching takes many forms and is most important in encouraging adherence to the medication regimen and reducing the risk of relapse.
- Evaluation includes examining the effectiveness of the nursing interventions, changing the outcomes as needed, and reassessing the nursing diagnoses. Evaluation is an ongoing process and is part of each of the other steps in the nursing process.

CRITICAL THINKING

1. Donald has a history of bipolar disorder and has been taking lithium for 4 months. During his clinic visit, he tells you that he does not think he will be taking his lithium anymore because he feels great and is able to function well at his job and at home with his family. He tells you his wife agrees that he "has this thing licked."
   a. What are Donald's needs in terms of teaching?
   b. What are the needs of the family?
   c. Write a teaching plan or use an already constructed plan. Include the following issues with sound rationales for these teaching topics:
   - Use of alcohol, drugs, caffeine, over-the-counter medications
   - Need for sleep, hygiene
   - Types of community resources available
   - Signs and symptoms of relapse

   d. Role-play with a classmate how you can teach this family about bipolar illness and approach effective medication teaching, stressing the need for adherence and emphasizing those things that may threaten adherence.
   e. What referral information (websites, associations) can you give Donald and his family if they ask where they can access further information regarding this disease?

CHAPTER REVIEW

Questions

1. Which nursing response demonstrates accurate information that should be discussed with the female patient diagnosed with bipolar and her support system? *Select all that apply.*
   a. "Remember that alcohol and caffeine can trigger a relapse of your symptoms."
   b. "Due to the risk of a manic episode, antidepressant therapy is never used with bipolar disorder.
   c. "It's critical to let your healthcare provider know immediately if you aren't sleeping well."
   d. "Is your family prepared to be actively involved in helping manage this disorder?"
   e. "The symptoms tend to come and go and so you need to be able to recognize the early signs."
2. Which statement made by the patient demonstrates an understanding of the effective use of newly prescribed lithium to manage bipolar mania? *Select all that apply.*
   a. "I have to keep reminding myself to consistently drink six 12-ounce glasses of fluid every day."
   b. "I discussed the diuretic my cardiologist prescribed with my psychiatric care provider."

c. "Lithium may help me lose the few extra pounds I tend to carry around."
d. "I take my lithium on an empty stomach to help with absorption."
e. "I've already made arrangements for my monthly lab work."

3. The nurse is providing medication education to a patient who has been prescribed lithium to stabilize mood. Which early signs and symptoms of toxicity should the nurse stress to the patient? *Select all that apply.*
   a. Increased attentiveness
   b. Getting up at night to urinate
   c. Improved vision
   d. An upset stomach for no apparent reason
   e. Shaky hands that make holding a cup difficult
4. A male patient calls to tell the nurse that his monthly lithium level is 1.7 mEq/L. Which nursing intervention will the nurse implement initially?
   a. Reinforce that the level is considered therapeutic.
   b. Instruct the patient to hold the next dose of medication and contact the prescriber.
   c. Have the patient go to the hospital emergency room immediately.
   d. Alert the patient to the possibility of seizures and appropriate precautions.
5. Which intervention should the nurse implement when caring for a patient demonstrating manic behavior? *Select all that apply.*
   a. Monitor the patient's vital signs frequently.
   b. Keep the patient distracted with group-oriented activities.
   c. Provide the patient with frequent milkshakes and protein drinks.
   d. Reduce the volume on the television and dim bright lights in the environment.
   e. Use a firm but calm voice to give specific concise directions to the patient.
6. Substance abuse is often present in people diagnosed with bipolar disorder. Laura, a 28-year-old with a diagnosis of bipolar disorder, drinks alcohol instead of taking her prescribed medications. The nurse caring for this patient recognizes that:
   a. Anxiety may be present.
   b. Alcohol ingestion is a form of self-medication.
   c. The patient is lacking a sufficient number of neurotransmitters.
   d. The patient is using alcohol because she is depressed.
7. Ted, a former executive, is now unemployed due to manic episodes at work. He was diagnosed with bipolar I 8 years ago. Ted has a history of IV drug abuse, which resulted in hepatitis C. He is taking his lithium exactly as scheduled, a fact that both Ted's wife and his blood tests confirm. To reduce Ted's mania the psychiatric nurse practitioner recommends:
   a. Clonazepam (Klonopin)
   b. Fluoxetine (Prozac)
   c. Electroconvulsive therapy (ECT)
   d. Lurasidone (Latuda)
8. A 33-year-old female diagnosed with bipolar I disorder has been functioning well on lithium for 11 months. At her most recent checkup, the psychiatric nurse practitioner states, "You are ready to enter the maintenance therapy stage, so at this time I am going to adjust your dosage by prescribing":
   a. A higher dosage
   b. Once a week dosing
   c. A lower dosage
   d. A different drug
9. Tatiana has been hospitalized for an acute manic episode. On admission the nurse suspects lithium toxicity. What assessment findings would indicate the nurse's suspicion as correct?
   a. Shortness of breath, gastrointestinal distress, chronic cough
   b. Ataxia, severe hypotension, large volume of dilute urine
   c. Gastrointestinal distress, thirst, nystagmus
   d. Electroencephalographic changes, chest pain, dizziness
10. Luc's family comes home one evening to find him extremely agitated and they suspect in a full manic episode. The family calls emergency medical services. While one medic is talking with Luc and his family, the other medic is counting something on his desk. What is the medic most likely counting?
   a. Hypodermic needles
   b. Fast food wrappers
   c. Empty soda cans
   d. Energy drink containers

Answers

1. **a, c, d, e**; 2. **a, b, e**; 3. **d, e**; 4. **b**; 5. **a, c, d, e**; 6. **b**; 7. **c**; 8. **c**; 9. **b**; 10. **d**

Visit the Evolve website for a posttest on the content in this chapter: http://evolve.elsevier.com/Varcarolis

Post-Test interactive review

REFERENCES

Crump, C., Sundquist, K., Winkleby, M. A., & Sundquist, J. (2013). Comorbidities and mortality in bipolar disorder: A Swedish national cohort study. *JAMA Psychiatry*, *70*(9), 931–939.

Fusar-Poli, P., Howes, O., Bechdolf, A., & Borgwardt, S. (2012). Mapping vulnerability to bipolar disorder: A systematic review and meta-analysis of neuroimaging studies. *Journal of Psychiatry Neuroscience*, *37*(3), 170–184.

Goes, F. S., Pierooznia, M., Parla, J. S., Kramer, M., Ghiban, E., Mavruk, S., & Potash, J. B. (2016). Exome sequencing of familial bipolar disorder. *Journal of the American Medical Association Psychiatry*.

Jamison, K. R. (1995). *An unquiet mind*. New York, NY: Knopf.

Kerner, B. (2014). The genetics of bipolar disorder. *Application of Clinical Genetics*, *7*, 33–42.

Kessler, R. C., Berglund, P. A., Demler, O., Jin, R., & Walters, E. E. (2005). Lifetime prevalence and age-of-onset distributions of DSM-IV disorders in the National Comorbidity Survey Replication. *Archives of General Psychiatry*, *62*(6), 593–602.

Maletic, V., & Raison, C. (2014). Integrated neurobiology of bipolar disorder. *Frontiers in Psychiatry*, *5*, 98. Retrieved from http://www.ncbi.nlm.nih.gov/pmc/articles/PMC4142322/.

Merikangas, K., Cui, L., Kattan, G., Carlson, G., Youngstrom, E., & Angst, J. (2012). Mania with and without depression in a community sample of U.S. adolescents. *Archives of General Psychiatry*, *69*(9), 943–951.

Moore, M. (2008). *Patty Duke puts celebrity face on bipolar disorder. Missoulian*. Retrieved from http://missoulian.com/articles/2008/10/11/news/local/news05.txt.

Munk-Olsen, T., Lauresen, T. M., Meltzer-Brody, S., Mortensen, P. B., & Jones, I. (2012). Psychiatric disorders with postpartum onset: Possible early manifestations of bipolar affective disorders. *Archives of General Psychiatry*, *69*(4), 428–434.

National Institute of Mental Health. (2015). Publications about bipolar disorder. Retrieved from https://www.nimh.nih.gov/health/publications/bipolar-disorder-listing.shtml.

Olfson, M., Mojtabai, R., Merikangas, K. R., Compton, W. M., Wang, S., Grant, B. F., & Blanco, C. (2017). Reexamining associations between mania, depression, anxiety and substance use disorders: Results from a prospective national cohort. *Molecular Psychiatry*, *22*, 235–241.

Phillips, M. L., & Swartz, H. A. (2014). A critical appraisal of neuroimaging studies of bipolar disorder: Toward a new conceptualization of underlying neural circuitry and roadmap for future research. *American Journal of Psychiatry*, *171*(8), 829–843.

Sadock, B. J., Sadock, V. A., & Ruiz, P. (2015). *Synopsis of psychiatry* (11th ed.). Philadelphia: Wolters Kluwer.

Sarris, J., Mischoulon, D., & Schweitzer, I. (2012). Omega-3 for bipolar disorder: Meta-analyses of use in mania and bipolar depression. *Journal of Clinical Psychiatry*, *73*(1), 81–86.

Schoeyen, H. K., Kessler, U., Andreassen, O. A., Auestad, B. H., Bergsholm, P., Malt, U. F., & Vaaler, A. (2015). Treatment resistant bipolar depression: A randomized controlled trial of ECT therapy versus algorithm-based pharmacological treatment. *American Journal of Psychiatry*, *172*(1), 41–51.

Smith, D. J., Anderson, J., Zammit, S., Meyeter, T. D., Pell, J. P., & Mackay, D. (2015). Childhood IQ and risk of bipolar disorder in adulthood: Prospective birth cohort study. *British Journal of Psychiatry Open*, *1*, 74–80.

Viktorin, A., Lichtenstein, P., Thase, M. E., Larson, H., Lundholm, C., Magnusson, P. K. E., & Landen, M. (2014). The risk of switch to mania in patients with bipolar disorder during treatment with an antidepressant alone and in combination with a mood stabilizer. *American Journal of Psychiatry*, *171*(10), 1067–1073.

Wang, P. S., Berglund, P., Olfson, M., Pincus, H. A., Wells, K. B., & Kessler, R. C. (2005). Failure and delay in initial treatment contact after first onset of mental disorders in the National Comorbidity Survey Replication. *Archives of General Psychiatry*, *62*, 603–613.

14

Depressive Disorders

Margaret Jordan Halter, Mallie Kozy

Visit the Evolve website for a pretest on the content in this chapter:
http://evolve.elsevier.com/Varcarolis Pre-Test interactive review

OBJECTIVES

1. Identify symptoms of disruptive mood dysregulation disorder, persistent depressive disorder (dysthymia), and premenstrual dysphoric disorder.
2. Discuss the origins of major depressive disorder.
3. Assess behaviors in a patient with depression in regard to each of the following areas: (a) affect, (b) thought processes, (c) mood, (d) feelings, and (e) physical behavior.
4. Formulate five nursing diagnoses for a patient with depression and include outcome criteria.
5. Name unrealistic expectations a nurse may have while working with a patient with depression and compare them to your own personal thoughts.
6. Role-play six principles of communication that are useful in working with patients with depression.
7. Identify the major classifications of antidepressants and general advantages and disadvantages of each.
8. Discuss non-pharmaceutical interventions for major depressive disorder such as electroconvulsive therapy (ECT).

OUTLINE

KEY TERMS AND CONCEPTS

affect
anergia
anhedonia
bereavement exclusion
deep brain stimulation
electroconvulsive therapy (ECT)
light therapy
major depressive disorder
persistent depressive disorder
premenstrual dysphoric disorder
serotonin syndrome
suicidal ideation
transcranial magnetic stimulation
vagus nerve stimulation
vegetative signs of depression

One of the most important aspects of studying psychiatric nursing is to learn about the depressive disorders. In this chapter we will focus on disorders that share symptoms of sadness, emptiness, irritability, somatic (body) concerns, and impairment of thinking. All of the disorders impact a person's ability to function adequately. While the focus in this chapter will be on the classic condition of major depressive disorder, we will begin with a discussion of the other depressive disorders:

- Disruptive mood dysregulation disorder
- Persistent depressive disorder (formerly called dysthymia)
- Premenstrual dysphoric disorder
- Substance/medication-induced depressive disorder
- Depressive disorder due to another medical condition

Disruptive Mood Dysregulation Disorder

Disruptive mood dysregulation disorder was introduced in 2013 in response to an alarming number of children and adolescents being diagnosed with bipolar disorder. A bipolar diagnosis resulted in exposure to powerful medications that probably were not helping and a lifelong label of serious mental illness. Perhaps the most compelling reason to change this diagnostic practice was that most of the young people who received a diagnosis of bipolar did not go on to exhibit classic bipolar symptoms as adults. In fact, most children and adolescents once diagnosed with bipolar disorder actually converted to major depressive disorder or an anxiety disorder in adulthood.

The basic symptoms of disruptive mood dysregulation disorder are constant and severe irritability and anger in individuals between the ages of 6 and 18. Onset is before age 10. Temper tantrums with verbal or behavioral outbursts out of proportion to the situation occur at least three times a week. Sometimes children and adolescents with this problem can maintain control in certain settings such as school. To be diagnosed with disruptive mood dysregulation disorder, individuals need to exhibit the irritability, anger, and temper tantrums in at least two of these settings: home, school, and with peers.

Disruptive mood dysregulation disorder prevalence rate is believed to fall in the range of 2% to 5%. It is more common in males than females, and it is more common in children than adolescents.

There is little information available on the treatment of disruptive mood dysregulation disorder. Sadock and colleagues (2015) suggest a symptom-based approach. If the disorder resembles major depression, antidepressants may be considered. If the disorder is accompanied by attention-deficit/hyperactivity disorder (ADHD), medications for that condition could be tried. Antidepressants may be used to address irritability. The second-generation antipsychotics risperidone (Risperdal) and aripiprazole (Abilify) have FDA approval for irritability in autism and are sometimes used for disruptive mood dysregulation disorder.

Psychosocial interventions such as cognitive behavioral therapy (CBT) are essential considering the degree of turmoil this disorder brings about. Parent training helps parents to interact with a child in such a way to predict and reduce aggression and irritability through consistency and rewarding appropriate behavior. There is some evidence that these young people may be misperceiving others' facial expressions as angry. Computer-based training can help them become more aware of the meaning of facial expressions.

Persistent Depressive Disorder

Persistent depressive disorder, formerly known as dysthymia, is diagnosed when feelings of depression occur most of the day, for the majority of days. These low-level depressive feelings last at least 2 years in adults and 1 year in children and adolescents. In addition to depressed mood individuals with this disorder have at least two of the following: decreased appetite or overeating, insomnia or hypersomnia, low energy, poor self-esteem, difficulty thinking, and hopelessness.

The symptoms are difficult for the patient to live with and bring about social and occupational distress, but they are usually not severe enough to require hospitalization. Because the onset of persistent depressive disorder is usually in the teenage years, patients will frequently express that they have "always felt this way" and that being depressed seems like a normal way of functioning. It is not uncommon for people with this low-level depression to also have periods of full-blown major depressive episodes.

The prevalence of persistent depressive disorder ranges from 0.5% to 1.5%. The problem tends to have an early onset and, as the name suggests, it is a chronic illness.

Treatment for this disorder is similar to that of major depressive disorder, which we will discuss in more depth later in this chapter. Psychotherapy, particularly CBT, is quite useful in managing the symptoms. Antidepressants such as selective serotonin reuptake inhibitors (SSRIs), serotonin and norepinephrine reuptake inhibitors (SNRIs), and tricyclics are the other main treatments.

Premenstrual Dysphoric Disorder

Premenstrual dysphoric disorder is a relatively new addition to the diagnostic system for psychiatry. It refers to a cluster of symptoms that occur in the last week before the onset of a woman's period. Premenstrual dysphoric disorder causes problems severe enough to interfere with the ability of a woman to work or interact with others. Symptoms include mood swings, irritability, depression, anxiety, feeling overwhelmed, and difficulty concentrating. Other physical manifestations include lack of energy, overeating, hypersomnia or insomnia, breast tenderness, aching, bloating, and weight gain. Symptoms decrease significantly or disappear with the onset of menstruation.

The prevalence of premenstrual dysphoric disorder is about 2% to 6% of menstruating women. Symptoms cease after menopause, although they may return with hormone replacement therapy.

Treatment for this disorder includes regular exercise, particularly aerobic exercise. Other recommendations include eating food rich in complex carbohydrates and getting sufficient sleep. Acupuncture, light therapy, and relaxation therapy have also been used to reduce symptoms.

Several drugs have FDA approval for treatment of this disorder. A drosperinone and ethinyl estradiol combination (Yaz) is a contraceptive that improves symptoms. SSRIs have been used successfully and three have FDA approval. They are fluoxetine (Prozac, Serafem), sertraline (Zoloft), and controlled release paroxetine (Paxil CR). Diuretics may be useful in reducing bloating and weigh gain brought on by water retention.

Substance/Medication-Induced Depressive Disorder

Substance/medication-induced depressive disorder is a depressive disorder, such as major depressive disorder, that is a result of prolonged use of or withdrawal from drugs and alcohol. The depressive symptoms last longer than the expected length of physiological effects, intoxication, or withdrawal of the substance. The person with this diagnosis would not experience depressive symptoms in the absence of drug or alcohol use or withdrawal. Symptoms appear within 1 month of use. Once the substance is removed, depressive symptoms usually remit within a few days to several weeks.

The lifetime prevalence rate is fairly low—about 0.25%. Medications associated with depressive symptoms include antiviral agents, cardiovascular drugs, retinoic acid derivatives, antidepressants, anticonvulsants, antimigraine agents, antipsychotics, hormonal agents, smoking cessation agents, and immunological agents.

Depressive Disorder Due to Another Medical Condition

Depressive disorder due to another medical condition may be caused by disorders that affect the body's systems or from long-term illnesses that cause ongoing pain. The depressive symptoms are the same as the diagnostic criteria for the depressive disorders. It is important to review medications being used for the medical condition to rule them out as being the causative agents.

There are clear associations, along with neuroanatomical changes, with some disease states. The prevalence rate of depression in people who have suffered a cerebrovascular accident (stroke) is high—30-50% in the first year (Flaster et al., 2013). Parkinson's disease, Huntington's disease, Alzheimer's disease, and traumatic brain injury are also clearly associated with depressive disorders. Neuroendocrine conditions such as Cushing's disease and hypothyroidism are also commonly accompanied by depression. Arthritis, back pain, metabolic conditions (e.g., vitamin B_{12} deficiency), HIV, diabetes, infection, cancer, and autoimmune problems may also contribute to depression.

Table 14.1 summarizes the medical problems and substances that are associated with major depression.

TABLE 14.1 Medical Conditions and Substances/Medications Associated with Major Depressive Disorder

Substances/Medication	
Central nervous system depressants	Alcohol, barbiturates, benzodiazepines, clonidine
Central nervous system medications	Amantadine, bromocriptine, levodopa, phenothiazines, phenytoin
Psychostimulants	Amphetamines
Systemic medications	Corticosteroids, digoxin, diltiazem, enalapril, ethionamide, isotretinoin, mefloquine, methyldopa, metoclopramide, quinolones, reserpine, statins, thiazides, vincristine
Medical Conditions	
Neurological	Epilepsy, Parkinson's disease, multiple sclerosis, Alzheimer's disease, Huntington's disease, traumatic brain injury, cerebrovascular accident
Infectious or inflammatory	Neurosyphilis, HIV
Cardiac disorders	Ischemic heart disease, cardiac failure, cardiomyopathies
Endocrine	Hypothyroidism, diabetes mellitus, vitamin deficiencies, parathyroid disorders
Inflammatory disorders	Collagen-vascular diseases, irritable bowel syndrome, chronic liver disorders
Neoplastic disorders	Central nervous system tumors, paraneoplastic syndromes

MAJOR DEPRESSIVE DISORDER

Clinical Picture

Major depressive disorder is one of the most common psychiatric disorders. In 2014 it affected approximately 16 million adults in the United States or nearly 7% of the population (Center for Behavioral Health Statistics and Quality, 2015). Major depressive disorder, or major depression, is characterized by a persistently depressed mood lasting for a minimum of 2 weeks.

The length of a depressive episode may be 5 to 6 months (McInnis et al., 2014). About 20% of cases become chronic (i.e., lasting more than 2 years). While depression begins with a single occurrence, most people experience recurrent episodes. People experience a recurrence within the first year about 50% of the time and within a lifetime up to 85% of the time. The full criteria for major depressive disorder are listed in the *DSM-5* box.

DSM-5 CRITERIA FOR MAJOR DEPRESSIVE DISORDER

A. Five (or more) of the following symptoms have been present during the same 2-week period and represent a change from previous functioning; at least one of the symptoms is either (1) depressed mood or (2) loss of interest of pleasure.

Note: Do not include symptoms that are clearly attributable to another medical condition.

1. Depressed mood most of the day, nearly every day, as indicated by either subjective report (e.g., feels sad, empty, hopeless) or observation made by others (e.g., appears tearful). (**Note:** In children and adolescents, it can be irritable mood.)
2. Markedly diminished interest or pleasure in all, or almost all, activities most of the day, nearly every day (as indicated by either subjective account or observation).
3. Significant weight loss when not dieting or weight gain (e.g., a change of more than 5% of body weight in a month) or decrease or increase in appetite nearly every day. (**Note:** In children, consider failure to make expected weight gain.)
4. Insomnia or hypersomnia nearly every day.
5. Psychomotor agitation or retardation nearly every day (observable by others, not merely subjective feelings of restlessness or being slowed down).
6. Fatigue or loss of energy nearly every day.
7. Feelings of worthlessness or excessive or inappropriate guilt (which may be delusional) nearly every day (not merely self-reproach or guilt about being sick).
8. Diminished ability to think or concentrate or indecisiveness nearly every day (either by subjective account or as observed by others).
9. Recurrent thoughts of death (not just fear of dying), recurrent suicidal ideation without a specific plan, or a suicide attempt or a specific plan for committing suicide.

B. The symptoms cause clinically significant distress or impairment in social, occupational, or other important areas of functioning.

C. The episode is not attributable to the physiological effects of a substance or to another medical condition.

Note: Criteria A through C represent a major depressive episode.

Note: Responses to a significant loss (bereavement, financial ruin, losses from a natural disaster, a serious medical illness or disability) may include the feelings of intense sadness, rumination about the loss, insomnia, poor appetite, and weight loss as noted in Criterion A, which may resemble a depressive episode. Although such symptoms may be understandable or considered appropriate to the loss, the presence of a major depressive episode in addition to the normal response to a significant loss should also be carefully considered. This decision inevitably requires the exercise of clinical judgment based on the individual's history and the cultural norms for the expression of distress in the context of loss.

D. The occurrence of the major depressive episode is not better explained by schizoaffective disorder, schizophrenia, schizophreniform disorder, delusional disorder, or other specified and unspecified schizophrenia spectrum and other psychotic disorders.

E. There has never been a manic or a hypomanic episode.

Note: This exclusion does not apply to all of the manic-like or hypomanic-like episodes that are substance-induced or are attributable to the physiological effects of another medical condition.

American Psychiatric Association. (2013). *Diagnostic and statistical manual of mental disorders* (5th ed.). Washington, DC: Author.

Depression and Grieving

People who experience a significant loss can exhibit feelings and behaviors similar to depression. They may cry, feel hopeless about the future, have disruptions in eating and sleeping, and lose pleasure in everyday activities. They may even experience a lack interest in caring for themselves and neglect normal hygiene. At what point does grief become pathological? This is a controversial question and one that is not easily answered.

Until recently, clinicians were advised against diagnosing a person with depression in the first 2 months following a significant loss. This was called the **bereavement exclusion**. The rationale for avoiding a psychiatric diagnosis follows:

1. Normal mourning could be labeled pathological.
2. A psychiatric diagnosis could result in a life-long label.
3. Unnecessary medications might be prescribed.

Although controversial, a diagnosis of depression can now be given in the first 2 months following death of a loved one or other loss. The reason for the change is that grief, like other stressors, can result in depression. For some people, waiting 2 months for an official diagnosis of major depression may delay treatment and adversely affect prognosis. Further research about grief may clarify diagnostic categories and prevent overdiagnosis of depression in the presence of grief.

EPIDEMIOLOGY

Major depressive disorder is the leading cause of disability in the United States. As previously stated, in 2014 it affected approximately 16 million adults in the United States or nearly 7% of the population (Center for Behavioral Health Statistics and Quality, 2015). This results in a significant loss of productivity in addition to the more personal individual and family distress. Beginning in early adolescence, females are more likely than males to be affected by depression at a rate of 1:2.

Children and Adolescents

Because symptoms vary by age and circumstance, depression in children, until recently, has been underrecognized. We now know that even infants can display symptoms of depression. With this understanding, we are just beginning to get a realistic view of the epidemiology of depression in children. We have more information about adolescents. Nearly 3 million (about

11%) individuals between 13 and 18 years of age experienced depression in 2014 (Center for Behavioral Health Statistics and Quality, 2015). This prevalence rate is higher than for adults, which is especially troubling since a youth onset carries a high recurrence rate, setting the stage for lifelong periods of depression.

Older Adults

Although depression in older adults is common, it is not a normal result of aging. The risk of depression increases as health deteriorates. About 1% to 5% of older adults who live in the community have depression. This statistic rises to 11.5% of hospitalized older adults and 13.5% for those requiring home care (National Institute of Mental Health [NIMH], 2012). A disproportionate number of older adults with depression are likely to die by suicide.

Many older adults suffer from *subsyndromal depression* in which they experience many, but not all, of the symptoms of a major depressive episode. These individuals have an increased risk of eventually developing major depression. Sometimes the psychomotor slowing and cognitive effects of depression lead others to believe that the older adult is developing a neurocognitive disorder such as Alzheimer's disease. This condition is referred to as pseudodementia, a problem that can be reversed when the underlying depression is treated and eliminated.

COMORBIDITY

A depressive syndrome frequently accompanies other psychiatric problems such as schizophrenia, substance abuse, eating disorders, schizoaffective disorder, and borderline personality disorder. The combination of anxiety and depression is perhaps one of the most common psychiatric presentations. Symptoms of anxiety occur in an average of 70% of cases of major depression. Some clinicians believe that mixed anxiety and depression should be a stand-alone diagnosis and be treated as a distinct entity.

RISK FACTORS

Although many theories attempt to explain the cause of depression, the combination of psychological, biological, and cultural variables make identification of any one cause difficult. Furthermore, it is unlikely there is a single cause for depression. The high variability in symptom manifestation, response to treatment, and course of the illness supports the supposition that depression may result from a complex interaction of causes. For example, genetic predisposition to the illness combined with childhood stress may lead to significant changes in the central nervous system (CNS) that result in depression. However, there seem to be several common risk factors for depression, as listed in Box 14.1.

BOX 14.1 Primary Risk Factors for Depression

- Female gender
- Adverse childhood experiences
- Stressful life events
- First-degree family members with major depressive disorder
- Neuroticism (a negative personality trait characterized by anxiety, fear, moodiness, worry, envy, frustration, jealousy, and loneliness)
- Other disorders such as substance use, anxiety, and personality disorders
- Chronic or disabling medical conditions

From American Psychiatric Association. (2013). *Diagnostic and statistical manual of mental disorders* (5th ed.). Washington, DC: Author.

Biological Factors

Genetic

Twin studies consistently show that genetic factors play a role in the development of depressive disorders. The concordance rate for major depressive disorder among monozygotic (identical) twins is nearly 50%. That is, if one twin is affected, the second has about a 50% chance of being affected as well. It is likely that multiple genes are involved, each one having a small but substantial role in the development and severity of depression. For instance, certain genetic markers seem to be related to depression when accompanied by early childhood maltreatment or a history of stressful life events. In this case, there is no gene directly related to the development of the mood disorder. There is a genetic marker associated with depression in the context of stressful life events.

EVIDENCE-BASED PRACTICE

Completed Suicide Often Happens on the First Attempt

Problem

The top 10 leading causes of death have gradually declined or held steady except for one: suicide. Suicide rates have been steadily rising despite the fact that this cause of death is largely preventable.

Purpose of Study

The purpose of this study was to determine the relationship between previous attempts at suicide and eventual completion of the act.

Methods

Researchers reviewed records of completed suicides in a California County during a 3-year period. There were 205 people in the sample.

Key Findings

- 86% of the sample had never made a previous suicide attempt.
- 65% had no previous psychiatric diagnosis.
- Previous attempts were associated with borderline personality disorder and substance use disorders.
- Females were more likely than males to have a history of previous attempts (28% versus 9%).

Implications for Nursing Practice

This study supports better detection of mental illness and suicidal ideation in general medical settings, as well as in psychiatric care settings especially in at-risk populations. It also highlights the fact that previous attempts are serious indicators for eventual completed suicide.

Ramsinghani, N., & Leigh, H. (2015). Suicide: Epidemiology, risk, competency, and history of prevention techniques. Scientific and clinical report presented at the 168th Meeting of the American Psychiatric Association (APA), May 16, 2015.

One of the more important aspects of understanding the role of genetics in relation to mental illness such as major depression may be in pharmacological treatments. Understanding genetic

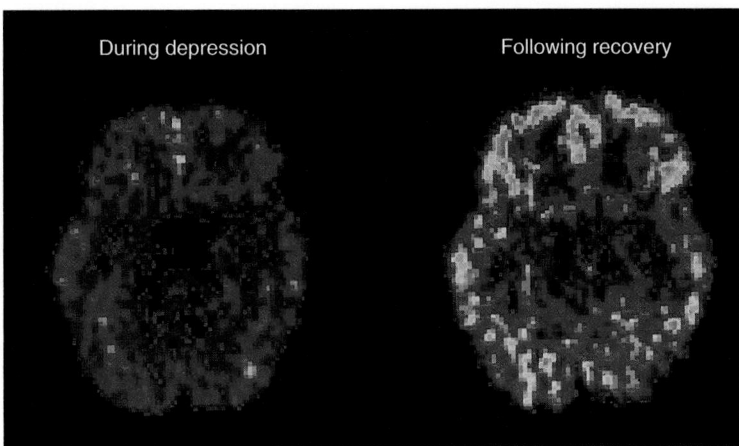

FIG. 14.1 Positron emission tomographic (PET) scans of a 45-year-old woman with recurrent depression. The scan on the left was taken when the patient was on no medication and very depressed. The scan on the right was taken several months later when the patient was well after she had been treated with an antidepressant. Note that her entire brain, particularly the left prefrontal cortex, is more active when she is well. (Courtesy Mark George, MD, Biological Psychiatry Branch, National Institute of Mental Health.)

influences on the role of the transport of certain neurotransmitters, such as serotonin, across synapses will make it much easier to prescribe effective medical treatment of depression based on individual genetic patterns.

Biochemical

The brain is a highly complex organ that contains billions of neurons. There is much evidence to support the concept that many CNS neurotransmitter abnormalities may cause clinical depression. These neurotransmitter abnormalities may be the result of genetic or environmental factors or other medical conditions, such as cerebral infarction, Parkinson's disease, hypothyroidism, acquired immunodeficiency syndrome (AIDS), or drug use.

Two of the main neurotransmitters involved in mood are serotonin (5-hydroxytryptamine [5-HT]) and norepinephrine. Serotonin is an important regulator of sleep, appetite, and libido. Therefore, serotonin-circuit dysfunction can result in sleep disturbances, decreased appetite, low sex drive, poor impulse control, and irritability. Norepinephrine modulates attention and behavior. It is stimulated by stressful situations, which may result in overuse and a deficiency of norepinephrine. A deficiency, an imbalance as compared with other neurotransmitters, or an impaired ability to use available norepinephrine can result in apathy, reduced responsiveness, or slowed psychomotor activity.

Research suggests that depression results from the dysregulation of a number of neurotransmitter systems beyond serotonin and norepinephrine. For example, glutamate is a common neurotransmitter that increases the ability of a nerve fiber to transmit information. A deficit in glutamate can interfere with normal neuron transmission in the areas of the brain that affect mood, attention, and cognition.

Stressful life events, especially losses, seem to be a significant factor in the development of depression. Norepinephrine, serotonin, and acetylcholine play a role in stress regulation. When these neurotransmitters become overtaxed through stressful events, neurotransmitter depletion may occur. Research indicates that stress is associated with a reduction in neurogenesis, which is the ability of the brain to produce new brain cells.

At this time, no single mechanism of depressant action has been found. The relationships among the serotonin, norepinephrine, dopamine, acetylcholine, gamma-aminobutyric acid (GABA), and glutamate systems are complex and need further assessment and study. However, treatment with medication that helps regulate these neurotransmitters has proved empirically successful in the treatment of many patients. Fig. 14.1 shows a positron emission tomographic (PET) scan of the brain of a woman with depression before and after taking medication. Refer to Chapter 3 for further discussion of brain imaging and depression.

Hormonal

The neuroendocrine characteristic most widely studied in relation to depression has been hyperactivity of the hypothalamic-pituitary-adrenal cortical axis. People with major depression have increased urine cortisol levels and elevated corticotrophin-releasing hormone. Dexamethasone, an exogenous steroid that suppresses cortisol, is used in the dexamethasone suppression test (DST) for depression. Results of this test are abnormal in about 50% of people with depression, which indicates hyperactivity of the hypothalamic-pituitary-adrenal cortical axis.

Depression rates are almost equal for males and females in the years preceding puberty and in older adults. This has led to more research into the effect of hormones on depression in women (Ryan et al., 2012). Recent studies have found that estradiol, a form of estrogen, affects receptors sensitive to serotonin in the areas of the brain responsible for mood in rats. As the relationships between sex hormones such as estrogen in women and testosterone in males are better understood, more effective therapies may be developed.

Inflammation

Inflammation is the body's natural defense to physical injury. There is growing evidence that inflammation may be the result of psychological injury as well. Researchers have focused in on two important blood components related to inflammation, C-reactive protein and interleukin-6. In young females with a history of adversity, depression is accompanied by elevations in these blood components but not in children without a history of adversity (Miller & Cole, 2012). Adversity in life may compromise resilience and place children at risk for depression and other disorders.

While we do not believe that inflammation causes depression, research indicates that it does play a role (Krishnadas & Cavanagh, 2012). Support for this belief includes that about a third of people with major depression have elevated inflammatory biomarkers in the absence of a physical illness. Also, people who have inflammatory diseases have an increased risk of major depression. Finally, people treated with cytokines to enhance immunity during cancer treatment develop major depression at a high rate.

Diathesis-Stress Model

The diathesis-stress model of depression takes into account the interplay between genetic and biological predisposition toward depression and life events. The physiological vulnerabilities such as genetic predispositions, biochemical makeup, and personality structure are referred to as a diathesis. The stress part of this model refers to the life events that impact individual vulnerabilities. This explains why two persons exposed to relatively similar events may respond differently. One person may demonstrate resilience and another may develop depression.

Biochemically, the diathesis-stress model of depression is believed to work this way. Psychosocial stressors and interpersonal events trigger neurophysical and neurochemical changes in the brain. Early life trauma may result in long-term hyperactivity of the CNS corticotropin-releasing factor (CRF) and norepinephrine systems with a consequent neurotoxic effect on the hippocampus, which leads to overall neuronal loss. These changes could cause sensitization of the CRF circuits to even mild stress in adulthood, leading to an exaggerated stress response (Gillespie & Nemeroff, 2005).

Psychological Factors

Cognitive Theory

In cognitive theory, the underlying assumption is that a person's thoughts will result in emotions. If a person looks at life in a positive way, the person will experience positive emotions, but negative interpretation of life events can result in sorrow, anger, and hopelessness. Cognitive theorists believe that people may acquire a psychological predisposition to depression due to early life experiences. These experiences contribute to negative, illogical, and irrational thought processes that may remain dormant until they are activated during times of stress (Beck & Rush, 1995).

Beck found that people with depression process information in negative ways, and tend to ignore positive aspects of their lives. He believed that automatic, negative, repetitive, unintended, and not-readily-controllable thoughts perpetuate depression. Three assumptions constitute Beck's cognitive triad:

1. A negative, self-deprecating view of self
2. A pessimistic view of the world
3. The belief that negative reinforcement (or no validation for the self) will continue in the future

APPLICATION OF THE NURSING PROCESS

ASSESSMENT

Major depressive disorder often goes unrecognized and underdiagnosed, yet early treatment can result in improved outcomes. Nurses at both the generalist and advanced practice levels are frequently in the position to screen and assess for signs of depression, thereby facilitating early and appropriate treatment.

General Assessment

Assessment Tools

Numerous standardized depression-screening tools that help assess the type and severity of depression are available. Common screening tools are the Beck Depression Inventory, the Hamilton Depression Scale, and the Geriatric Depression Scale. The Patient Health Questionnaire-9 (PHQ-9) is a short inventory that highlights predominant symptoms seen in depression. It is presented here because of its ease of use (Fig. 14.2) in primary care and community settings. Administering these tools at baseline and then again periodically allows clinicians to follow changes in the patient's symptoms and depression severity over time.

Assessment of Suicide Potential

The most dangerous aspect of major depressive disorder is a preoccupation with death. A patient may fantasize about her funeral or experience recurring dreams about death. Beyond these passive fantasies are thoughts of wanting to die. As a whole, all these nihilistic thoughts are referred to as **suicidal ideation**. These thoughts may be relatively mild and fleeting, or persistent and involve a plan. Suicidal ideation, especially those in which the patient has a plan and the means to carry the plan out, represents an emergency requiring immediate intervention (refer to Chapter 25). Suicidal thoughts are a major reason for hospitalization for patients with major depression.

Patients diagnosed with major depressive disorder should always be evaluated for suicidal ideation. Risk for suicide is increased when depression is accompanied by hopelessness, substance use problems, a recent loss or separation, a history of past suicide attempts, and acute suicidal ideation. The following statements and questions help set the stage for assessing suicide potential:

- "You said you are depressed. Tell me what that is like for you."
- "When you feel depressed, what thoughts go through your mind?"
- "Have you gone so far as to think about taking your own life? Do you have a plan?"
- "Do you have the means to carry out your plan?"
- "Is there anything that would prevent you from carrying out your plan?"

Refer to Chapter 25 for a detailed discussion of suicide, critical risk factors, warning signs, and strategies for suicide prevention. Also see the Case Study and Nursing Care Plan.

PATIENT HEALTH QUESTIONNAIRE-9 (PHQ-9)

Over the last 2 weeks, how often have you been bothered by any of the following problems?	**Not at all**	**Several days**	**More than half the days**	**Nearly every day**
1. Little interest or pleasure in doing things	0	1	2	3
2. Feeling down, depressed, or hopeless	0	1	2	3
3. Trouble falling or staying asleep, or sleeping too much	0	1	2	3
4. Feeling tired or having little energy	0	1	2	3
5. Poor appetite or overeating	0	1	2	3
6. Feeling bad about yourself — or that you are a failure or have let yourself or your family down	0	1	2	3
7. Trouble concentrating on things, such as reading the newspaper or watching television	0	1	2	3
8. Moving or speaking so slowly that other people could have noticed? Or the opposite — being so fidgety or restless that you have been moving around a lot more than usual	0	1	2	3
9. Thoughts that you would be better off dead or of hurting yourself in some way	0	1	2	3
	0 +	______ +	______ +	______
			=Total score:	______

If you checked off any problems, how difficult have these problems made it for you to do your work, take care of things at home, or get along with other people?

Not difficult at all	**Somewhat difficult**	**Very difficult**	**Extremely difficult**
☐	☐	☐	☐

I confirm this information is accurate.	Patient's/Subject's initials:	Date:

A

PHQ-9 SCORING CARD FOR SEVERITY DETERMINATION

for health care professional use only

Scoring—add up all checked boxes on PHQ-9

Total Score	**Depression Severity**
0-4	None
5-9	Mild
10-14	Moderate
15-19	Moderately severe
20-27	Severe

B

FIG. 14.2 A, Patient Health Questionnaire-9 (PHQ-9). B, Scoring the PHQ-9. (Copyright 2005 by Pfizer, Inc. Developed by Drs. Robert L. Spitzer, Janet B. Williams, Kurt Kroenke, and colleagues.)

CASE STUDY AND NURSING CARE PLAN

Depression

Ms. Glessner is a 35-year-old licensed practical nurse who is brought into the emergency department by her neighbor. Ms. Glessner reports that she has been depressed for as long as she can remember, yet she has become hopeless since her boyfriend left her. She has superficial cuts on her wrists. Her affect is blunted, she has poor eye contact, and is slumped down in her chair.

Ms. Glessner is about 20 pounds overweight. Her neighbor states that Ms. Glessner often stays awake late into the night, drinking alone and watching television. She sleeps through most of the day on the weekends.

After receiving treatment in the ED, Ms. Glessner is seen by a psychiatrist. The initial diagnosis is persistent depressive disorder with suicidal ideation and an order is written to hospitalize her.

The nurse, Carrie, admits Ms. Glessner to the unit from the emergency department.

Nurse: Hello, Ms. Glessner, I'm Carrie Wolfe. I'll be your primary nurse.

Ms. Glessner: Yeah…I don't need a nurse, a doctor, or anyone else. I just want to get away from this pain.

Nurse: You want to get away from your pain?

Ms. Glessner: Look at me. I'm fat…ugly…and I'm not good enough. No one wants me.

Nurse: Who doesn't want you?

Ms. Glessner: My husband didn't want me…and now Jerry left me to go back to his wife.

Nurse: You think because Jerry went back to his wife that no one else could care for you?

Ms. Glessner: Well…he doesn't anyway.

Nurse: Who is in your life that supports you?

Ms. Glessner: No one…except my sons…I do love my sons, even though I don't often show it.

Nurse: Tell me more about your sons.

Carrie continues to speak with Ms. Glessner. Ms. Glessner talks about her sons with some affect and apparent affection. However, she continues to state that she does not think of herself as worthwhile.

Self-Assessment

Carrie, a registered nurse, is aware that when patients have depression, they can be negative, think life is hopeless, and be hostile toward those who want to help. When Carrie was new to the unit, she was uncomfortable with depressed patients. After working with this population for 2 years, she now looks forward to the improvement that can be made in people's lives.

Assessment

Subjective Data

- Recently broke off with boyfriend
- Stays awake late at night, drinking by herself
- Poor self-image of herself for 3 years since divorce
- Cares about her two sons
- "I just want to get away from this pain."
- "I'm fat and ugly…no good to anyone."

Objective Data

- Cuts on wrist
- 20 pounds overweight
- Blunted affect
- Poor eye contact
- Slumped in the chair

Priority Diagnosis

Risk for suicide as evidenced by an actual suicide attempt, cuts on her wrists, loss of a relationship, and drinking alone at night.

Outcomes Identification

Patient refrains from attempting suicide.

Planning

Because Ms. Glessner is discharged after 48 hours, the issue of disturbance in self-esteem will be addressed in therapy after discharge. Carrie later reviews the goals for her work with Ms. Glessner in the community.

Implementation

Ms. Glessner's plan of care is personalized as follows:

Short-Term Goal	Intervention	Rationale	Evaluation
1. Patient will remain safe while in the hospital.	1a. Observe patient every 15 minutes while she is suicidal. 1b. Remove all dangerous objects from patient.	1a. Patient safety is ensured. 1b. Impulsive self-harmful behavior is minimized.	**GOAL MET** Ms. Glessner experienced no suicide gestures or acts during the hospitalization.
2. Patient expresses at least one reason to live, and this is apparent by the second day of hospitalization.	2a. Spend regularly scheduled periods of time with patient throughout the day.	2a. This interaction reinforces that patient is worthwhile and builds up experience to begin to relate better to nurse on one-to-one basis.	**GOAL MET** By the end of the second day, she states that her sons are a reason to live and that she would never want to hurt them.
	2b. Assist patient in evaluating both positive and negative aspects of her life.	2b. A depressed person is often unable to acknowledge any positive aspects of life unless others point them out.	

CASE STUDY AND NURSING CARE PLAN—cont'd

Depression

Short-Term Goal	Intervention	Rationale	Evaluation
	2c. Encourage appropriate expression of angry feelings.	2c. Providing for expression of pent-up hostility in a safe environment can reinforce more adaptive methods of releasing tension and may minimize need to act out self-directed anger.	
	2d. Accept patient's negativism.	2d. Acceptance enhances feelings of self-worth.	
3. Patient will identify two outside supports she can call upon if she feels suicidal in the future.	3a. Assist patient in identifying members of her support system.	3a. Strengths and weaknesses in support available can be evaluated.	**GOAL MET** By discharge, Ms. Glessner states that she will contact her oldest son or best friend if she becomes hopeless again. She also discussed joining a women's support group that meets once a week in a neighboring town.
	3b. Suggest community-based support groups she might wish to attend.	3b. Patient needs to be aware of community supports to use them.	

Evaluation

During the course of her work with Carrie, Ms. Glessner decides to go to some meetings of Parents Without Partners. She states that she is looking forward to getting back to work and feels more hopeful about life. She has also lost 3 pounds while attending Weight Watchers. She states, "I need to get back into the world."

Key Assessment Findings

A depressed mood and anhedonia are the key symptoms in depression.

Anxiety is also a common symptom in depression. When people experience a depressive episode, their thinking is slow, and their memory and concentration are usually negatively affected. They also dwell on and exaggerate their perceived faults and failures and are unable to focus on their strengths and successes. A person with major depression may experience delusions of being punished for committing bad deeds or being a terrible person. Feelings of worthlessness, hopelessness, guilt, anger, and helplessness are common.

Depression and chronic pain are commonly seen together in primary care. Neurotransmitters for both problems are shared, as are nerve pathways, which can interact in a vicious cycle. Then there is the two-way interaction between pain and depression. Being in constant pain creates negative thinking overall and dampens brain chemistry, resulting in depression. On the other hand, depression magnifies pain and may also create a vulnerability to other physical problems.

Areas to Assess

Affect

Affect is the outward representation of a person's internal state of being and is an objective finding based on the nurse's assessment. A person who has depression sees the world through gray-colored glasses. Posture is poor, and the patient may look older than the stated age. Facial expressions convey sadness and dejection, and the patient may have frequent bouts of weeping. Conversely, the patient may say that he or she feels numb or is unable to cry. Feelings of **hopelessness** and **despair** are readily reflected in the person's affect. For example, the patient may not make eye contact, may speak in a monotone, may show little or no facial expression (flat affect), and may make only yes or no responses. Frequent sighing is common.

Thought Processes

During a depressive episode, the person's ability to solve problems and think clearly is negatively affected. Judgment, or the ability to make reasonable decisions, is poor. This poor judgment leads to indecisiveness, which makes it difficult to make simple decisions such as what to wear or what to eat. The individual may claim that his mind is slowing down. Memory and concentration are poor. Patients might complain of intrusive negative thoughts. In extreme depression, a person may become mute.

In cases of severe and profound depression, evidence of delusions (false thoughts) may also be present. An example of a delusional thought is, "I am responsible for Elvis Presley's death.

I worked in a factory that made pill molds. Elvis died from an overdose. I deserve to die."

Mood

Mood is the patient's subjective experience of sustained emotions or feelings. Asking a person how he feels can assess a person's mood. **Anhedonia** (*an* "without" + *hedone* "pleasure" = inability to feel happy) refers to the absence of happiness or pleasure in aspects of life that once made them happy.

Feelings

Feelings frequently reported by those with depression include worthlessness, guilt, helplessness, hopelessness, and anger. Feelings of worthlessness range from feeling inadequate to having an unrealistically negative evaluation of self-worth. These feelings reflect the low self-esteem that is a painful partner to depression. Statements such as "I am no good" or "I'll never amount to anything" are common.

Guilt is a nearly universal accompaniment to depression. A person may ruminate over present or past failings,"I was never a good parent," or "It's my fault that project at work failed." These thoughts tend to occur over and over again and are difficult for the patient to stop. These negative ruminations fill in the hours of lost sleep.

Cognitive Changes

Helplessness is demonstrated by a person's inability to solve problems in response to common concerns. In severe situations helplessness may be evidenced by the inability to carry out the simplest tasks (e.g., grooming, doing housework, working, caring for children) because they seem too difficult to accomplish. With feelings of helplessness come feelings of hopelessness, which are particularly correlated with suicidality. Even though most depressive episodes are time limited, people experiencing them believe things will never change. This feeling of utter hopelessness can lead people to view suicide as a way out of constant mental pain. Hopelessness includes the following attributes:

- Negative expectations for the future
- Loss of control over future outcomes
- Passive acceptance of the futility of planning to achieve goals
- Emotional negativism, as expressed in despair, despondency, or depression

Anger and irritability are natural outcomes of profound feelings of helplessness. Anger in depression is often expressed inappropriately through hurtful verbal attacks, physical aggression toward others, or destruction of property, and anger may be directed toward the self in the form of suicidal or otherwise self-destructive behaviors (e.g., alcohol abuse, substance abuse, overeating, smoking). These behaviors often reinforce feelings of low self-esteem and worthlessness.

Physical Behavior

Most people with depression experience **anergia**, which refers to an abnormal lack of energy. Anergia may result in psychomotor retardation, in which movements are extremely slow, facial expressions are decreased, and gaze is fixed. The continuum of psychomotor retardation may range from slowed and difficult movements to complete inactivity and incontinence. Conversely, some patients experience psychomotor agitation, manifested in pacing, nail biting, finger tapping, or engaging in some other tension-relieving activity. Subjectively, patients commonly feel fidgety and unable to relax.

Vegetative signs of depression refer to alterations in those activities necessary to support physical life and growth (e.g., eating, sleeping, elimination, and sex). Appetite changes vary in individuals experiencing depression. Appetite loss is common, and sometimes patients can lose up to 5% of their body weight in less than a month. Other patients find they eat more often and complain of weight gain.

Change in sleep pattern is a cardinal sign of depression. Often, people experience insomnia, wake frequently, and have a total reduction in sleep, especially deep-stage sleep. Waking at 3 or 4 a.m. and then staying awake is common as is sleeping for short periods only. The light sleep of a person with depression tends to prolong the agony of depression over a 24-hour period. For some, sleep is increased (hypersomnia) and provides an escape from painful feelings. In any event, sleep is rarely restful or refreshing.

Changes in bowel habits are common. Constipation is seen most frequently in patients with psychomotor retardation. Diarrhea occurs less frequently, often in conjunction with psychomotor agitation or anxiety.

Sexual interest declines (loss of libido) during depression. Some men experience impotence, and a declining interest in sex often occurs among both men and women, which can further complicate marital and social relationships.

Grooming, dressing, and personal hygiene may be markedly neglected. People who usually take pride in their appearance and dress may allow themselves to look shabby and unkempt. They may neglect to bathe, change clothes, or engage in other basic self-care activities.

Age Considerations

Assessment in Children and Adolescents

As children grow and develop, they may display a wide range of moods and behavior, making it easy to overlook signs of depression. The core symptoms of depression in children and adolescents are the same as for adults, which are sadness and loss of pleasure. What differs is how these symptoms are displayed. For example, a very young child may cry, a school-age child might withdraw, and a teenager may become irritable in response to feeling sad or hopeless. Younger children may suddenly refuse to go to school while adolescents may engage in substance abuse or sexual promiscuity and be preoccupied with death or suicide.

Assessment of Older Adults

Because they are more likely to complain of physical illness than emotional concerns, depression might be overlooked. Older patients actually do have comorbid physical problems, and it is difficult to determine whether fatigue, pain, and weakness are the result of an illness or depression. The Geriatric Depression Scale is a 30-item tool that is both valid and reliable in screening for depression in the older adult (Sheikh & Yesavage, 1986). Its "yes" or "no" format makes this scale easier to administer with patients with cognitive deficits. It can be helpful in determining suicidality in this population.

Self-Assessment

Patients with depression often reject the advice, encouragement, and understanding of the nurse and others, and they often appear unresponsive to nursing interventions and resistant to change. When this occurs, the nurse may experience feelings of frustration, hopelessness, and annoyance. These problematic responses can be altered in the following ways:

- Recognizing unrealistic expectations for yourself or the patient
- Identifying feelings that the patient may be experiencing
- Understanding the roles biology and genetics play in the precipitation and maintenance of a depressed mood

As a student, your personal feelings should be recognized, named, and examined. You can discuss feelings with peers, staff, and faculty to separate personal feelings from those originating with the patient. Ultimately, supervision or peer support can increase your therapeutic potential and self-esteem while caring for individuals with depression.

ASSESSMENT GUIDELINES

Depression

1. Always evaluate the patient's risk of harm to self or others. Overt hostility is highly correlated with suicide
2. Depression is a mood disorder that can be secondary to a host of medical or other psychiatric disorders and medications. A thorough medical and neurological examination helps determine if the depression is primary or secondary to another disorder. Evaluate whether:
   - The patient is psychotic.
   - The patient has taken drugs or alcohol.
   - Medical conditions are present.
   - The patient has a history of a comorbid psychiatric syndrome (eating disorder, borderline or anxiety disorder).
3. Assess the patient's history of depression and suicidality. Determine what strategies helped alleviate depressive symptoms in the past.
4. Assess support systems, family, significant others, and the need for information and referrals.

DIAGNOSIS

Major depressive disorder is a complex disorder, and patients have a variety of needs. Therefore, there are many applicable diagnoses. A high priority for the nurse is determining the risk of suicide, and the nursing diagnosis of *risk for suicide* is always considered. Refer to Chapter 25 for assessment guidelines and interventions for suicidal individuals.

OUTCOMES IDENTIFICATION

The recovery model emphasizes that healing is possible and attainable for individuals with psychiatric disorders, including depression. Recovery is attained through partnerships between patients and healthcare providers who focus on the patient's strengths. Treatment goals are mutually developed based on the patient's personal needs and values, and interventions are evidenced-based. The recovery model is consistent with the focus on patient-centered care and is a key component of safe quality healthcare.

Major depressive disorder can be a recurrent and chronic illness. Care should be directed not only at resolution of the acute phase but also at long-term management. The nurse and the patient identify realistic outcome criteria and formulate concrete, measurable, short-term and long-term goals.

Table 14.2 identifies signs and symptoms commonly experienced in depression, offers potential nursing diagnoses, and suggests outcomes.

PLANNING

The planning of care for patients with depression is geared toward the patient's phase of depression, particular symptoms, and personal goals. At all times students, nurses, and members of the healthcare team must be aware of the potential for suicide. Assessment of risk for self-harm (or harm to others) is ongoing. A combination of therapy (cognitive, behavioral, or interpersonal) and psychopharmacology is an effective approach to the treatment of depression across all age groups. Safety is always the highest priority.

IMPLEMENTATION

There are three phases in treatment and recovery from major depression:

1. The acute phase (6 to 12 weeks) is directed at reduction of depressive symptoms and restoration of psychosocial and work function. Hospitalization may be required, and medication or other biological treatments may be initiated.
2. The continuation phase (4 to 9 months) is directed at prevention of relapse through pharmacotherapy, education, and depression-specific psychotherapy.
3. The maintenance phase (1 year or more) of treatment is directed at prevention of further episodes of depression. Depending on the risk factors for relapse, medication may be phased out or continued.

It is important to keep in mind that both the continuation and maintenance phases are geared toward maintaining the patient as a functional and contributing member of the community after recovery from the acute phase.

Counseling and Communication Techniques

Nurses often have difficulty communicating with patients without talking. However, some patients with depression are so

TABLE 14.2 Signs and Symptoms, Nursing Diagnoses, and Outcomes for Depression

Signs and Symptoms	Nursing Diagnoses	Outcomes
Previous suicidal attempts, putting affairs in order, giving away prized possessions, suicidal ideation (has plan, ability to carry it out), overt or covert statements regarding killing self, feelings of worthlessness, hopelessness, helplessness	*Risk for self-directed violence* *Risk for suicide*	Expresses feelings, verbalizes suicidal ideas, refrains from suicide attempts, plans for the future
Difficulty with simple tasks, inability to function at previous level, poor problem solving, poor cognitive functioning, verbalizations of inability to cope	*Ineffective coping*	Identifies ineffective and effective coping, uses support system, uses new coping strategies, engages in personal actions to manage stressors effectively
Dull/sad affect, no eye contact, preoccupation with own thoughts, seeks to be alone, uncommunicative, withdrawn, feels rejected and not good enough	*Social isolation*	Attends group meetings, interacts spontaneously with others, talks with the nurse in 1:1, demonstrates interest in engaging with family and others
Feelings of helplessness, hopelessness, powerlessness	*Hopelessness* *Powerlessness*	Expresses hope for a positive future, believes that personal actions impact outcomes, demonstrates optimism and describes plans for the future
Questioning meaning of life and existence, anger toward greater power, feeling abandoned, perceived suffering	*Spiritual distress*	Shares feelings of connectedness with self, others, and a higher power, identifies meaning and purpose in life
Exaggerates negative feedback about self, excessive seeking of reassurance, guilt, indecisive and nonassertive behavior, poor eye contact, shame	*Chronic low self-esteem*	Identifies strengths, verbalizes self-acceptance, participates in groups, expresses a personal judgment of self-worth
Vegetative signs of depression: grooming and hygiene deficiencies, significantly reduced appetite, changes in sleeping, eating, elimination, sexual patterns	*Self-care deficit (bathing, dressing)* *Insomnia* *Imbalanced nutrition: less than body requirements* *Constipation* *Sexual dysfunction*	Increases baseline personal care each day, reports adequate sleep, eating and elimination normalize, returns to a normal level of physiologic activity

Herdman, T. H., & Kamitsuru, S. (Eds.). (2014). *NANDA International nursing diagnoses: Definitions and classification, 2015-2017.* Oxford, UK: Wiley-Blackwell.; Moorhead, S., Johnson, M., Maas, M. L., & Swanson, E. (2013). *Nursing outcomes classification (NOC)* (5th ed.). St. Louis, MO: Mosby.

TABLE 14.3 Guidelines for Communication with Severely Withdrawn Persons

Intervention	Rationale
When a patient is silent, use the technique of making observations: "There are many new pictures on the wall." "You are wearing your new shoes."	When a patient is not ready to talk, direct questions can raise the patient's anxiety level and frustrate the nurse. Pointing to commonalities in the environment draws the patient into and reinforces reality.
Use simple, concrete words.	Slowed thinking and difficulty concentrating impair comprehension.
Allow time for the patient to respond.	Slowed thinking necessitates time to formulate a response.
Listen for covert messages, and ask about suicide plans.	People often experience relief and decrease in feelings of isolation when they share thoughts of suicide.
Avoid platitudes such as "Things will look up" or "Everyone gets down once in a while."	Platitudes tend to minimize the patient's feelings and can increase feelings of guilt and worthlessness, because the patient cannot "look up" or "snap out of it."

withdrawn that they are unwilling or unable to speak and just sitting with them in silence may seem like a waste of time or be noticeably uncomfortable. As your anxiety increases, you may start daydreaming, feel bored, and believe that you should be doing something. It is important to be aware that this time can be meaningful, especially if you have a genuine interest in learning about and supporting the patient with depression.

It is difficult to say when a withdrawn patient will be able to respond, but certain techniques are known to be useful in guiding effective nursing interventions. Some communication techniques to use with a severely withdrawn patient are listed in Table 14.3. Counseling guidelines for use with patients with depression are offered in Table 14.4.

TABLE 14.4 Guidelines for Counseling People with Depression

Intervention	Rationale
Help the patient question underlying assumptions and beliefs and consider alternate explanations to problems.	Reconstructing a healthier and more hopeful attitude about the future can alter depressed mood.
Work with the patient to identify cognitive distortions that result in a negative self-perception. For example:	Cognitive distortions reinforce a negative inaccurate perception of self and world.
a. Overgeneralizations	a. Taking one fact or event and making a general rule out of it ("He always…"; "I never…").
b. Self-blame	b. Consistently blaming self.
c. Mind reading	c. Despite a lack of evidence, assumes that others don't like him or her.
d. Discounting of positive attributes	d. Focusing on the negative.
Help the patient identify current coping skills and explore alternate coping skills.	Many depressed people use ineffective coping skills. Exploring and adopting alternate effective coping skills will improve the patient's outlook.
Encourage exercise, such as running and/or weight lifting.	Exercise can improve self-concept and improve the brain's neurochemistry.
Encourage formation of supportive relationships, such as individual therapy, support groups, and peer support.	Such relationships reduce social isolation and enable the patient to work on personal goals and relationship needs.
Provide information referrals, when needed, for religious or spiritual support (e.g., pastoral visits, readings, programs, tapes, community resources).	Spiritual and existential issues may be heightened during depressive episodes; many people find strength, support, and comfort in spirituality or religion.

CONSIDERING CULTURE

Access to Quality Mental Health Treatment for Racial and Ethnic Minorities

Is it really more difficult to access the mental healthcare system and get quality care if you come from a racial or ethnic minority in the United States? Based on the work of Alegria and colleagues (2015), the answer is yes.

In this study data were used from 8762 people to evaluate access to and quality of depression treatment. Adequate treatment in a year's time was considered: four or more healthcare visits with antidepressants prescribed and used for 30 days *or* eight or more specialty care visits lasting at least 30 minutes without antidepressants prescribed.

Researchers found that 32% of Latinos, 31% of Asians, and 41% of African Americans successfully accessed psychiatric care for depression in the past year. Comparatively, about 60% of non-Latino whites successfully accessed mental healthcare. The researchers concluded that minorities correctly anticipated limited quality care available for them in healthcare facility.

Minorities were reluctant to leave work to seek care, were more concerned about being stigmatized, and were mistrustful of healthcare providers. For minorities who did access the mental healthcare system, they were still less likely to be treated. This may be due to clinicians' inexperience in diagnosing minority populations. For example, in Latinos depressive symptoms tend to be expressed somatically rather than emotionally.

What's the solution? One possible intervention is the use of nurse-run quality improvement programs to increase quality of care for minority groups. Home visits were suggested as another way to engage patients. The researchers believe that future studies focus on developing and evaluating these and other strategies for engaging minority populations in essential care for depression.

From Alegria, M., Chatterji, P., Wells, K., Cao, Z., Chen, C., Takeuchi, D., Jackson, J., & Meng, X. (2015). Disparity in depression treatment among racial and ethnic minority populations in the United States. *Psychiatric Services, 59*(11), 1264–1272.

Health Teaching and Health Promotion

A basic premise of the recovery model of mental illness is that individuals exercise personal control of treatment based on individual goals. Within this model, health teaching is paramount because it allows patients to make informed choices. Health teaching points include:

- Depression is an illness beyond a person's voluntary control.
- Although it is beyond voluntary control, depression can be managed through medication and lifestyle.
- Chronic illness management depends in large part on understanding personal signs and symptoms of relapse.
- Illness management depends on understanding the role of medication and possible medication side effects.
- Long-term management works best if the patient receives psychotherapy along with medication.
- Identifying and coping with the stress of interpersonal relationships—whether they are familial, social, or occupational—are key to stable illness management.

Including the family in discharge planning is also important. It helps the patient by:

- Increasing the family's understanding and acceptance of the family member with depression during the aftercare period
- Increasing the patient's use of aftercare facilities in the community
- Contributing to higher overall adjustment in the patient after discharge

Promotion of Self-Care Activities

Nursing measures for improving physical well-being and promoting adequate self-care are essential. Some effective interventions targeting physical needs in depression are listed in Table 14.5. Nurses in the community can work with family members to encourage a family member with depression to perform and maintain self-care activities.

Teamwork and Safety

Safe quality inpatient care requires the skills of a well-coordinated team. Treating a patient with depression require the skills of nurses and prescribers. Other members of the team include

TABLE 14.5 Interventions Targeting the Vegetative Signs of Depression

Intervention	Rationale
Nutrition (Anorexia)	
Offer small, high-calorie, and high-protein snacks frequently throughout the day and evening.	Low weight and poor nutrition render the patient susceptible to illness. Small, frequent snacks are more easily tolerated than large plates of food when the patient is anorexic.
Offer high-protein and high-calorie fluids frequently throughout the day and evening.	These fluids prevent dehydration and can minimize constipation.
When possible, encourage family or friends to join the patient during meals.	Eating is a social event. This strategy reinforces the idea that someone cares, can raise the patient's self-esteem, and can serve as an incentive to eat.
Include the patient in choosing foods and drinks. Involve a dietitian if necessary.	The patient is more likely to eat the foods provided.
Weigh the patient weekly, and observe the patient's eating patterns.	Monitoring the patient's status gives the information needed for revision of the intervention.
Sleep (Insomnia)	
Provide periods of rest after activities.	Fatigue can intensify feelings of depression.
Encourage the patient to get up and dress and to stay out of bed during the day.	Minimizing sleep during the day increases the likelihood of sleep at night and the establishment of healthy routines.
Encourage the use of relaxation measures in the evening (e.g., a warm bath, warm milk, soothing music or sounds).	These measures induce relaxation and sleep.
Provide decaffeinated coffee and soda.	Decreasing caffeine increases the possibility of sleep.
Self-Care Deficits	
Encourage the use of toothbrush, washcloth, soap, makeup, and shaving supplies.	Being clean and well-groomed can improve self-esteem.
When appropriate, give step-by-step reminders, such as, "Wash the right side of your face, now the left."	Slowed thinking and difficulty concentrating make organizing simple tasks difficult.
Elimination (Constipation)	
Monitor intake and output, especially bowel movements.	Many depressed patients are constipated. If the condition is not addressed, fecal impaction can occur.
Offer foods high in fiber, and provide periods of exercise.	Roughage and exercise stimulate peristalsis.
Encourage the intake of fluids.	Fluids help prevent constipation.
Evaluate the need for laxatives and enemas.	These measures prevent constipation.

mental health technicians, pharmacists, dietitians, social workers, and the patient's significant others.

Safety becomes the most important issue facing a team that cares for people with depression who may be at high risk for suicide. Suicide precautions are usually instituted and include the removal of all harmful objects such as "sharps" (e.g., razors, scissors, and nail files), strangulation risks (e.g., belts), and medication that can be used to overdose. Some patients with severe depression may need to have someone check on them frequently, perhaps every 15 minutes, or even have 1:1 observation. A full discussion of inpatient safety measures is provided in Chapter 4.

PSYCHOBIOLOCIAL INTERVENTIONS

Pharmacological Interventions

At the cellular level mood disorders are caused by problems with neurotransmitters. It follows that medications that alter brain chemistry are an important component in their treatment. Antidepressant therapy is an effective strategy for most cases of major depressive disorder, particularly in severe cases. A combination of psychotherapies and antidepressant therapy is superior to either psychotherapy or psychopharmacological treatment alone (Institute for Clinical Systems Improvement, 2016).

Neurobiology of Depression and the Effect of Antidepressants

Imbalance of certain neurotransmitters (serotonin and norepinephrine) contribute to depression in certain parts of the brain.
Prefrontal cortex: regulates role in executive functions and emotional control and memory.

Limbic system: regulates activities such as emotions, physical and sexual drives, and the stress response, as well as processing, learning, and memory (amygdala, hypothalamus, hippocampus).

Anterior cingulate cortex: regulates heart rate and blood pressure. Other functions include decision making, emotional regulation, error detection, preparation for tasks, and executive functions.

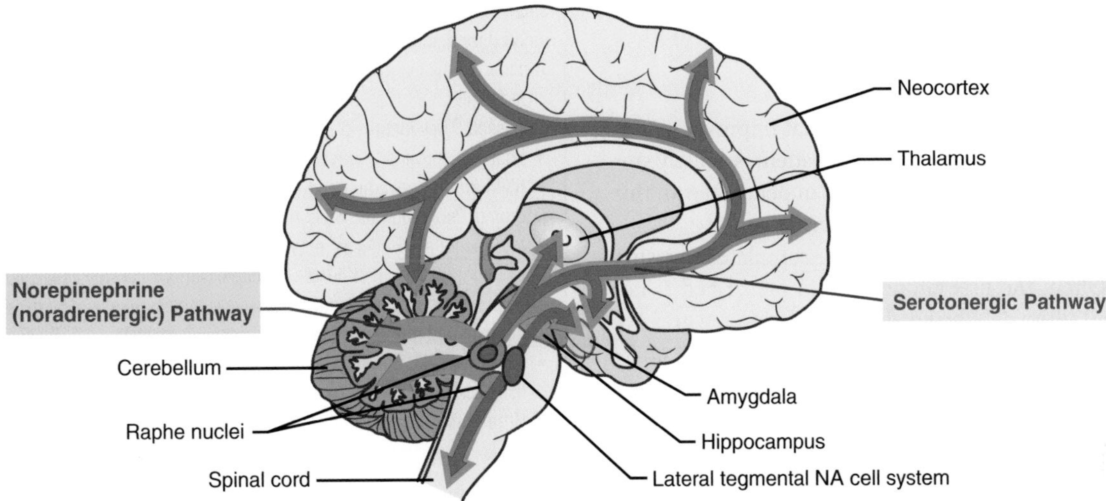

Various Parts of the Brain Along the Noradrenergic Pathway
The axons of these neurons project upward through the forebrain to the cerebral cortex, the limbic system, the thalamus, and the hippocampus.

Norepinephrine (NE) and the Noradrenergic System: plays a major role in mood and emotional behavior as well as energy, drive, anxiety, focus, and metabolism.

Various Parts of the Brain Along the Serotonergic Pathway
The axons of serotonergic neurons originate in the raphe nuclei of the brainstem and project to the cerebral cortex, the limbic system, cerebellum, and spinal cord.

Serotonin (5-HT) and the Serotonergic System: involved in the regulation of pain, depression, pleasure, anxiety, panic arousal, sleep cycle, carbohydrate craving, and premenstrual syndrome.

Medications for Depression
Medications for depression include the selective serotonin reuptake inhibitors (**SSRIs**), serotonin norepinephrine reuptake inhibitors (**SNRIs**), serotonin antagonists and reuptake inhibitors (**SARIs**), norepinephrine dopamine reuptake inhibitor (**NDRI**), noradrenergic and specific serotonergic antidepressants (**NaSSAs**), tricyclic antidepressants (**TCAs**), and monoamine oxidase inhibitors (**MAOIs**).
They all work equally well and are chosen by their safety profile and side effects.* All have a delayed response, a discontinuation syndrome, and a Black Box Warning for suicide.

Patient's Problem*	Side-Effect Profile*	Example of Drug*
Fatigue	Stimulates the CNS	Fluoxetine (SSRI)
Insomnia	Substantial sedation	Mirtazapine (NaSSAs)
Sexual dysfunction	Enhances libido	Bupropion (NDRI)
Chronic pain	Relieves pain	TCAs or duloxetine (SNRI)

*Adapted from Burchum, J.R., & Rosenthal, L.D. (2016). *Lehne's pharmacology for nursing care* (9th ed.). St. Louis, MO: Elsevier.

Antidepressant Drugs

Antidepressant drugs can positively impact poor self-concept, social withdrawal, vegetative signs of depression, and activity level. Target symptoms include the following:

- Sleep disturbance
- Appetite disturbance (decreased or increased)
- Fatigue
- Decreased sex drive
- Psychomotor retardation or agitation
- Diurnal variations in mood (often worse in the morning)
- Impaired concentration or forgetfulness
- Anhedonia

A drawback of antidepressant drugs is that improvement in mood may take 1 to 3 weeks or longer. If a patient is acutely suicidal, electroconvulsive therapy (discussed in detail later in this chapter) may be a reliable and effective alternative.

The goal of antidepressant therapy is the complete remission of symptoms. Often, the first antidepressant prescribed is not the one that will ultimately bring about remission. Aggressive treatment helps in finding the proper treatment. An adequate trial for the treatment of depression is 3 months. Individuals experiencing their first depressive episode are maintained on antidepressants for 6 to 9 months after symptoms of depression remit. Some people may have multiple episodes of depression or may have a chronic form and benefit from indefinite antidepressant therapy. Genetic testing holds some promise in individualizing antidepressant therapy (Box 14.2).

Antidepressants may precipitate a psychotic episode in a person with schizophrenia or a manic episode in a patient with bipolar disorder. Patients with bipolar disorder often receive a mood-stabilizing drug along with an antidepressant.

Choosing an antidepressant. All antidepressants work to increase the availability of one or more of the neurotransmitters, serotonin, norepinephrine, and dopamine. All antidepressants have demonstrated similar efficacy in pharmaceutical trials. Each of the antidepressants has different adverse effects, costs, safety issues, and maintenance considerations. Selection of the appropriate antidepressant is based on the following considerations:

- Symptom profile of the patient
- Side-effect profile (e.g., sexual dysfunction, weight gain)
- Ease of administration
- History of past response
- Safety and medical considerations
- Genotyping (when available)

Table 14.6 provides an overview of antidepressants used in the United States.

Selective serotonin reuptake inhibitors. The selective serotonin reuptake inhibitors (SSRIs) selectively block the neuronal uptake of serotonin (e.g., 5-HT, 5-HT_1 receptors). This blockage increases the availability of serotonin in the synaptic cleft. Refer to Chapter 3 for a more detailed discussion of how the SSRIs work.

SSRI antidepressant drugs have a relatively low side-effect profile compared with the older antidepressants (tricyclics—discussed later in this chapter). They do not create anticholinergic effects, dry mouth, blurred vision, or urinary retention, making it easier for patients to take these medications as prescribed.

BOX 14.2 Genetic Testing for More Precise Antidepressant Selection?

Anyone who has ever been given or prescribed medication for depression can tell you that choosing the best drug is somewhat hit or miss. Some medications work, some do not. Some medications cause intolerable side effects. Why?

Of all the clinical factors that can alter a person's response to drugs—age, sex, weight, general health, and liver function—genetic factors account for about 42% of the variation (Perlis, 2014). One aspect of genetics is the way we metabolize medications. The way you metabolize is largely based on a genetic variation in the cytochrome P450 (CYP450) enzymes.

Genotyping tests can help to identify medications that are more likely to be processed. They identify four types of metabolizers:

- Poor—A missing enzyme causes slow metabolism that may result in a build up of medication and significant side effects such as serotonin syndrome. People in this category should avoid antidepressants.
- Intermediate—Reduced enzyme function in processing drugs causes a slower metabolism of drugs. Antidepressants will likely cause side effects and toxicity is a risk. Some depressive symptom relief can be expected, but not substantially.
- Extensive—People in this category have an expected range for metabolism. Medications will be effective and there will be few side effects.
- Ultrarapid—Medication is processed too quickly, before it has a chance to work. Antidepressants will either not work or will have to be used at higher doses.

The specific CYP450 enzyme with the most variation is the CYP2D6. This enzyme processes common antidepressants including: fluoxetine (Prozac), paroxetine (Paxil, Pexeva), and venlafaxine (Effexor). The CYP2C19 enzyme is involved with metabolizing citalopram (Celexa) and escitalopram (Lexapro).

Despite the fact that several companies market this service, the jury is still out on whether clinicians should routinely use this testing in selecting medications. Large-scale studies are needed to clarify the usefulness of such tests.

From Perlis, R. H. (2014). Pharmacogenomic testing and personalized treatment of depression. *Clinical Chemistry, 60*(1), 53–59.

The SSRIs are effective in depression with anxiety features and depression with psychomotor agitation.

Indications. SSRIs are frequently the first-line treatment in depression. In addition to their use in treating depressive disorders, the SSRIs have been prescribed with success to treat some of the anxiety disorders—in particular obsessive-compulsive disorder and panic disorder. Fluoxetine has been found to be effective in treating some women who suffer from late-luteal-phase dysphoric disorder and bulimia nervosa.

Common adverse reactions. Agents that selectively enhance synaptic serotonin within the CNS may induce agitation, anxiety, sleep disturbance, tremor, sexual dysfunction (primarily anorgasmia), or tension headache. Autonomic reactions (e.g., dry mouth, sweating, weight change, mild nausea, and loose bowel movements) may also be experienced with the SSRIs.

Potential toxic effects. One rare and life-threatening event associated with SSRIs is **serotonin syndrome**. This syndrome is thought to be related to over-activation of the central serotonin receptors caused by either too high a dose or interaction with other drugs. The symptoms are many: abdominal pain, diarrhea, sweating, fever, tachycardia, elevated blood pressure, altered mental state (delirium), myoclonus (muscle spasms),

TABLE 14.6 FDA Approved Drugs for Major Depressive Disorder

Generic (Trade)	Action	Notes	Side Effects	Warnings
Selective Serotonin Reuptake Inhibitors (SSRIs)				
Citalopram (Celexa) Escitalopram (Lexapro) Fluoxetine (Prozac, Prozac Weekly) Paroxetine (Paxil, Paxil CR, Pexeva) Sertraline (Zoloft)	Blocks the synaptic reuptake of serotonin	First line of treatment for major depression Some SSRIs activate and others sedate; choice depends on patient symptoms Risk of lethal overdose minimized with SSRIs	Agitation, insomnia, headache, nausea and vomiting, sexual dysfunction, and hyponatremia	Discontinuation syndrome—dizziness, insomnia, nervousness, irritability, nausea, and agitation—may occur with abrupt withdrawal (depending on half-life); taper slowly
Serotonin Norepinephrine Reuptake Inhibitors (SNRIs)				
Desvenlafaxine (Pristiq, Khedezla)	Blocks the synaptic reuptake of serotonin and norepinephrine	A metabolite of venlafaxine	Nausea, headache, dizziness, insomnia, diarrhea, dry mouth, sweating, constipation	Neonates with in utero exposure have required respiratory support and tube feeding
Duloxetine (Cymbalta)	Blocks the synaptic reuptake of serotonin and norepinephrine	Cymbalta may be more effective than SSRIs in the treatment of severe depression	Nausea, dry mouth, insomnia, somnolence, constipation, reduced appetite, fatigue, sweating, blurred vision	May reduce pain associated with depression and is approved for fibromyalgia and pain of diabetic peripheral neuropathy
Levomilnacipran (Fetzima)	Blocks the synaptic reuptake of serotonin and norepinephrine	Unlike other SNRIs, inhibits reuptake of norepinephrine more than serotonin	Nausea, orthostatic hypotension, constipation, sweating, increased heart rate, palpitations, difficulty urinating, decreased appetite, sexual dysfunction	May increase the effects of anticoagulants
Venlafaxine (Effexor, Effexor XR)	Blocks the synaptic reuptake of serotonin and norepinephrine	Effexor is a popular next-step strategy after trying SSRIs	Hypertension, nausea, insomnia, dry mouth, sedation, sweating, agitation, headache, sexual dysfunction	Monitor blood pressure, especially at higher doses and with a history of hypertension Discontinuation syndrome (see SSRIs discussed previously)
Serotonin Antagonists and Reuptake Inhibitors (SARIs)				
Nefazodone (generic only)	Selective blockade of serotonin-2 receptors and α1-adrenergic receptors	Lower risk of long-term weight gain than SSRIs or TCAs Lower risk of sexual side effects than SSRIs	Sedation, hepatotoxicity, dizziness, hypotension, paresthesias	Life-threatening liver failure is possible but rare; priapism of penis and clitoris is a rare but serious side effect
Trazodone (generic only) Trazodone ER (Oleptro)	Moderate blockade of 5-HT synaptic reuptake	Significant sedative effect. Helps with antidepressant-induced insomnia	Severe sedation, hypotension, nausea	Priapism has been reported
Vilazodone (Viibryd)	Blocks reuptake of serotonin and serotonergic (5-HT_{1A}) receptor partial agonist activity	Take this medication with food to reduce GI disturbances	Diarrhea, nausea, vomiting, dry mouth, dizziness, insomnia	Palpitations, ventricular premature beats, serotonin syndrome
Vortioxetine (Trintellix)	Agonist of serotonin receptors	May improve memory and cognition	Constipation, nausea, vomiting	Hyponatremia, rare induction of manic states, serotonin syndrome
Norepinephrine Dopamine Reuptake Inhibitor (NDRI)				
Bupropion (Wellbutrin, Aplenzin, Forfivo XL, Zyban for smoking cessation)	Blocks the synaptic reuptake of norepinephrine and dopamine	Stimulant action may reduce appetite May increase sexual desire Used as an aid to quit smoking	Agitation, insomnia, headache, nausea and vomiting, seizures (0.4%)	High doses increase seizure risk, especially in people who are predisposed to them
Noradrenergic and Specific Serotonergic Antidepressant (NaSSA)				
Mirtazapine (Remeron)	Enhances the release of norepinephrine and serotonin by blocking α1-adrenergic receptors that normally inhibit norepinephrine and serotonin	Antidepressant effects equal SSRIs and may occur faster	Weight gain/appetite stimulation, sedation, dizziness, headache; sexual dysfunction is rare	Drug-induced somnolence exaggerated by alcohol, benzodiazepines, and other CNS depressants

Continued

TABLE 14.6 FDA Approved Drugs for Major Depressive Disorder—cont'd

Generic (Trade)	Action	Notes	Side Effects	Warnings
Tricyclic Antidepressants (TCAs)				
Amitriptyline (generic only) Amoxapine (generic only) Desipramine (Norpramin) Doxepin (Sinequan) Imipramine (Tofranil) Maprotiline (generic only) Nortriptyline (Aventyl, Pamelor) Protriptyline (Vivactil) Trimipramine (Surmontil)	Inhibits the synaptic reuptake of serotonin and norepinephrine. Antagonizes adrenergic, histaminergic, muscarinic, and dopaminergic receptors	Therapeutic effects similar to SSRIs, but side effects are more prominent May work better in melancholic depression and in people with comorbid medical conditions Some therapeutic serum levels may be monitored	Dry mouth, constipation, urinary retention, blurred vision, hypotension, cardiac toxicity, sedation	Lethal in overdose; use cautiously in older adults with cardiac disorders, elevated intraocular pressure, urinary retention, hyperthyroidism, seizure disorders, and liver or kidney dysfunction
Monoamine Oxidase Inhibitors (MAOIs)				
Isocarboxazid (Marplan) Phenelzine (Nardil, Nardelzine) Selegiline (Eldeprul, EMSAM Transdermal System Patch) Tranylcypromine (Parnate)	Inhibits the enzyme monoamine oxidase, which normally breaks down neurotransmitters, including serotonin and norepinephrine	Efficacy similar to other antidepressants, but strict dietary (tyramine) restrictions and potential drug interactions make this drug class less desirable	Insomnia, nausea, agitation, and confusion; hypertensive crisis	Contraindicated in people taking SSRIs, used cautiously in people taking TCAs; tyramine-rich food could bring about a hypertensive crisis Many other strong drug and dietary interactions

US Food and Drug Administration. (2016). FDA online label repository. Retrieved from http://labels.fda.gov/; Burchum, J. R., & Rosenthal, L. D. (2016). *Lehne's pharmacology for nursing care* (9th ed.). St. Louis, MO: Elsevier.

BOX 14.3 Serotonin Syndrome: Signs and Interventions

Symptoms

- Hyperactivity or restlessness
- Tachycardia → cardiovascular shock
- Fever → hyperpyrexia
- Elevated blood pressure
- Altered mental states (delirium)
- Irrationality, mood swings, hostility
- Seizures → status epilepticus
- Myoclonus, incoordination, tonic rigidity
- Abdominal pain, diarrhea, bloating
- Apnea → death

Interventions

- Remove offending agent(s)
- Initiate symptomatic treatment:
  - Serotonin-receptor blockade with cyproheptadine, methysergide, propranolol
  - Cooling blankets, chlorpromazine for hyperthermia
  - Dantrolene, diazepam for muscle rigidity or rigors
  - Anticonvulsants
  - Artificial ventilation
  - Induction of paralysis

increased motor activity, irritability, hostility, and mood change. Severe manifestations can induce hyperpyrexia (excessively high fever), cardiovascular shock, or death.

The risk of this syndrome seems to be greatest when an SSRI is administered in combination with a second serotonin-enhancing agent, such as a monoamine oxidase inhibitor (MAOI). A patient should discontinue all SSRIs for 2 to 5 weeks before starting an MAOI. Box 14.3 lists the signs of serotonin syndrome and gives emergency treatment guidelines. Box 14.4 is a useful tool for patient and family teaching about the SSRIs.

Serotonin norepinephrine reuptake inhibitors. The serotonin norepinephrine reuptake inhibitors (SNRIs) inhibit the reuptake of both serotonin and norepinephrine. Pharmacological side effects are similar to the SSRIs, although the SSRIs may be tolerated better. The SNRIs are indicated for major depressive disorder.

Other newer antidepressants. Several other classifications of antidepressants have been introduced and have provided people with depression and prescribers with more options. The name of the classification describes the action of the antidepressants. They are the serotonin antagonists and reuptake inhibitors (SARIs), a norepinephrine dopamine reuptake inhibitor (NDRI), and a noradrenergic and specific serotonergic antidepressant (NaSSA). Chapter 3 provides more detail about these drug classifications.

Tricyclic antidepressants. The tricyclic antidepressants (TCAs) inhibit the reuptake of norepinephrine and serotonin by the presynaptic neurons in the CNS, increasing the amount of time norepinephrine and serotonin are available to the postsynaptic receptors. This increase in norepinephrine and serotonin in the brain is believed to be responsible for mood elevations.

Indications. The sedative effects of the TCAs are attributed to the blockade of histamine receptors. Patients must take therapeutic doses of TCAs for 10 to 14 days or longer before they begin to work. Full effects may not be seen for 4 to 8 weeks. An effect on some symptoms of depression, such as insomnia and anorexia, may be noted earlier. Choosing a TCA for a patient is based on what has worked for the patient or a family member in the past and the drug's adverse effects.

BOX 14.4 Patient and Family Teaching: Selective Serotonin Reuptake Inhibitors (SSRIs)

- May cause sexual dysfunction or lack of sex drive. Inform nurse or primary care provider if this occurs.
- May cause insomnia, anxiety, and nervousness. Inform nurse or primary care provider if this occurs.
- May interact with other medications. Tell primary care provider about other medications patient is taking (e.g., digoxin, warfarin). SSRIs should not be taken within 14 days of the last dose of a monoamine oxidase inhibitor.
- No over-the-counter drug should be taken without first notifying primary care provider.
- Common side effects include fatigue, nausea, diarrhea, dry mouth, dizziness, tremor, and sexual dysfunction or lack of sex drive.
- Because of the potential for drowsiness and dizziness, patient should not drive or operate machinery until these side effects are ruled out.
- Alcohol should be avoided.
- Liver and renal function tests should be performed and blood counts checked periodically.
- Medication should not be discontinued abruptly. If side effects become bothersome, patient should ask primary care provider about changing to a different drug. Abrupt cessation can lead to serotonin withdrawal.
- Any of the following symptoms should be reported to the primary care provider immediately:
  - Increase in depression or suicidal thoughts
  - Rash or hives
  - Rapid heartbeat
  - Sore throat
  - Difficulty urinating
  - Fever, malaise
  - Anorexia and weight loss
  - Unusual bleeding
  - Initiation of hyperactive behavior
  - Severe headache

BOX 14.5 Patient and Family Teaching: Tricyclic Antidepressants (TCAs)

- The patient and family should be told that mood elevation may take from 7 to 28 days. Up to 6 to 8 weeks may be required for the full effect to be reached and for major depressive symptoms to subside.
- The family should reinforce this frequently to the depressed family member because depressed people have trouble remembering and respond to ongoing reassurance.
- The patient should be reassured that drowsiness, dizziness, and hypotension usually subside after the first few weeks.
- When the patient starts taking TCAs, the patient should be cautioned to be careful working around machines, driving cars, and crossing streets because of possible altered reflexes, drowsiness, or dizziness.
- Alcohol can block the effects of antidepressants. The patient should be told to refrain from drinking.
- If possible, the patient should take the full dose at bedtime to reduce the experience of side effects during the day.
- If the patient forgets the bedtime dose (or the once-a-day dose), the patient should take the dose within 3 hours; otherwise, the patient should wait until the usual medication time the next day. The patient should not double the dose.
- Suddenly stopping TCAs can cause nausea, altered heartbeat, nightmares, and cold sweats in 2 to 4 days. The patient should call the primary care provider or take one dose of TCA until the primary care provider can be contacted.

A stimulating TCA, such as desipramine (Norpramin) or protriptyline (Vivactil), may be best for a patient who is lethargic and fatigued. If a more sedating effect is needed for agitation or restlessness, drugs such as amitriptyline and doxepin (Sinequan) may be more appropriate choices. Regardless of which TCA is given, the initial dose should always be low and increased gradually.

Common adverse reactions. The chemical structure of the TCAs closely resembles that of antipsychotic medications, and the **anticholinergic** actions are similar (e.g., dry mouth, blurred vision, tachycardia, constipation, urinary retention, and esophageal reflux). These side effects are more common and more severe in patients taking antidepressants. They usually are not serious and are often transitory, but **urinary retention** and **severe constipation** warrant immediate medical attention. Weight gain is also a common complaint among people taking TCAs.

The α-adrenergic blockade of the TCAs can produce postural-orthostatic hypotension and tachycardia. Postural hypotension can lead to dizziness and increase the risk of falls. For this reason older patients on TCAs must be monitored carefully for dizziness and falls.

Administering the total daily dose of TCA at night is beneficial for two reasons. First, most TCAs have sedative effects and thereby aid sleep. Second, the minor side effects occur while the individual is sleeping, which increases compliance with drug therapy.

Potential toxic effects. The most serious effects of the TCAs are cardiovascular: dysrhythmias, tachycardia, myocardial infarction, and heart block. Because the cardiac side effects are so serious, TCA use is considered a risk in older adults and patients with cardiac disease. Patients should have a thorough cardiac workup before beginning TCA therapy.

Adverse drug interactions. A few of the more common medications usually *not* given while TCAs are being used are MAOIs, phenothiazines, barbiturates, disulfiram (Antabuse), oral contraceptives (or other estrogen preparations), anticoagulants, some antihypertensives (clonidine, guanethidine, reserpine), benzodiazepines, and alcohol. A patient who is taking any of these medications along with a TCA should have medical clearance because some of the reactions can be fatal.

Contraindications. People who have recently had a myocardial infarction (or other cardiovascular problems), those with narrow-angle glaucoma or a history of seizures, and women who are pregnant should not be treated with TCAs except with extreme caution and careful monitoring.

Patient and family teaching. Areas for the nurse to discuss when teaching patients and their families about TCA therapy are presented in Box 14.5.

Monoamine oxidase inhibitors. The enzyme monoamine oxidase is responsible for inactivating, or breaking down, monoamine neurotransmitters in the brain such as norepinephrine, serotonin, dopamine, and tyramine. When a person takes an MAOI, fewer amines get inactivated, resulting in an increase of the mood-elevating neurotransmitters.

TABLE 14.7 **Foods that Can Interact with Monoamine Oxidase Inhibitors**

FOODS THAT CONTAIN TYRAMINE

Category	Unsafe Foods (High Tyramine Content)	Safe Foods (Little or No Tyramine)
Vegetables	Avocados, especially if overripe; fermented bean curd; fermented soybean; soybean paste	Most vegetables
Fruits	Figs, especially if overripe; bananas, in large amounts	Most fruits
Meats	Meats that are fermented, smoked, or otherwise aged; spoiled meats; liver, unless very fresh	Meats that are known to be fresh (exercise caution in restaurants; meats may not be fresh)
Sausages	Fermented varieties; bologna, pepperoni, salami, others	Nonfermented varieties
Fish	Dried or cured fish; fish that is fermented, smoked, or otherwise aged; spoiled fish	Fish that is known to be fresh; vacuum-packed fish, if eaten promptly or refrigerated only briefly after opening
Milk, milk products	Practically all cheeses	Milk, yogurt, cottage cheese, cream cheese
Foods with yeast	Yeast extract (e.g., Marmite, Bovril)	Baked goods that contain yeast
Beer, wine	Some imported beers, Chianti wines	Major domestic brands of beer; most wines
Other foods	Protein dietary supplements; soups (may contain protein extract); shrimp paste; soy sauce	

FOODS THAT CONTAIN OTHER NONTYRAMINE VASOPRESSORS

Food	Comments
Chocolate	Contains phenylethylamine, a pressor agent; large amounts can cause a reaction.
Fava beans	Contain dopamine, a pressor agent; reactions are most likely with overripe beans.
Ginseng	Headache, tremulousness, and mania-like reactions have occurred.
Caffeinated beverages	Caffeine is a weak pressor agent; large amounts may cause a reaction.

From Burchum, J.R., & Rosenthal, L.D. (2016). *Lehne's pharmacology for nursing care* (9th ed.). St. Louis, MO: Elsevier.

The inability to break down tyramine sufficiently can result in a serious problem. Certain foods are quite rich in tyramine. Individuals who take MAOIs and eat these foods are at risk for a hypertensive crisis, which is severe high blood pressure that can lead to a cerebrovascular accident. People taking these drugs must reduce or eliminate their intake of foods and drugs that contain high amounts of tyramine (Table 14.7 and Box 14.6).

Indications. MAOIs are particularly effective for people with unconventional depression (characterized by mood reactivity, oversleeping, and overeating), as well as panic disorder, social phobia, generalized anxiety disorder, obsessive-compulsive disorder, posttraumatic stress disorder, and bulimia. MAOIs with FDA approval are phenelzine (Nardil), tranylcypromine (Parnate), and isocarboxazid (Marplan). A transdermal patch, selegiline (EMSAM), does not require strict dietary restrictions.

Common adverse reactions. Some common and troublesome long-term side effects of the MAOIs are orthostatic hypotension, weight gain, edema, change in cardiac rate and rhythm, constipation, urinary hesitancy, sexual dysfunction, vertigo, overactivity, muscle twitching, hypomanic and manic behavior, insomnia, weakness, and fatigue.

Potential toxic effects. The most serious reaction to the MAOIs is an increase in blood pressure with the possible development of intracranial hemorrhage, hyperpyrexia, convulsions, coma, and death. Therefore routine monitoring of blood pressure, especially during the first 6 weeks of treatment, is necessary.

Because many drugs, foods, and beverages can cause an increase in blood pressure in patients taking MAOIs, hypertensive crisis is a constant concern. The hypertensive crisis usually occurs within 15 to 90 minutes of ingestion of the contraindicated substance. Early symptoms include irritability, anxiety, flushing, sweating, and a severe headache. The patient then becomes anxious, restless, and develops a fever. Eventually the fever becomes severe, seizures ensue, and coma or death is possible.

When a hypertensive crisis is suspected, immediate medical attention is crucial. If ingestion is recent, gastric lavage and charcoal may be helpful. Pyrexia is treated with hypothermic blankets or ice packs. Fluid therapy is essential, particularly with hyperthermia. A short-acting antihypertensive agent such as nitroprusside, nitroglycerine, or phentolamine may be used. Intravenous benzodiazepines are useful for agitation and seizure control.

BOX 14.6 **Drugs that Can Interact with Monoamine Oxidase Inhibitors (MAOIs)**

- Over-the-counter medications for colds, allergies, or congestion (any product containing ephedrine, phenylephrine hydrochloride, or phenylpropanolamine)
- Tricyclic antidepressants (imipramine, amitriptyline)
- Narcotics
- Antihypertensives (methyldopa, guanethidine, reserpine)
- Amine precursors (levodopa, L-tryptophan)
- Sedatives (alcohol, barbiturates, benzodiazepines)
- General anesthetics
- Stimulants (amphetamines, cocaine)

TABLE 14.8 **Adverse Reactions to and Toxic Effects of Monoamine Oxidase Inhibitors**

Adverse Reactions	Comments
Hypotension Sedation, weakness, fatigue Insomnia Changes in cardiac rhythm Muscle cramps Anorgasmia or sexual impotence Urinary hesitancy or constipation Weight gain	Hypotension is an expected side effect of MAOIs. Orthostatic blood pressures should be taken—first lying down, then sitting or standing after 1-2 minutes. This may be a dangerous side effect, especially in older adults who may fall and sustain injuries as a result of dizziness from the blood pressure drop.
Toxic Effects	**Comments**
Hypertensive crisis Severe headache Tachycardia, palpitations Hypertension Nausea and vomiting	Patient should go to local emergency department immediately—blood pressure should be checked. One of the following may be given to lower blood pressure: 5 mg intravenous phentolamine (Regitine) or sublingual nifedipine to promote vasodilation. Patients may be prescribed a 10-mg nifedipine capsule to carry in case of emergency.

Table 14.8 identifies common side effects and toxic effects of the MAOIs, and Box 14.7 can be used as an MAOI teaching guide for patients and their families.

Contraindications. The use of MAOIs may be contraindicated with each of the following:

- Cerebrovascular disease
- Hypertension and congestive heart failure
- Liver disease
- Consumption of foods containing tyramine, L-tryptophan, and dopamine (see Table 14.7)
- Use of certain medications (see Box 14.6)
- Recurrent or severe headaches
- Surgery in the previous 10 to 14 days
- Age younger than 16 years

Use of antidepressants by pregnant women. The risk of depression in pregnant women may be as high as 20% (Olivier et al., 2015). There is evidence that depression has a negative effect on birth outcomes. Preeclampsia, diabetes, and hypertension have all been associated with maternal depression. Low birth weight, preterm birth, and small size for gestational age have been noted effects in infants born to depressed mothers. We know that antidepressants cross the placenta. Treatment of severe depression, particularly with suicidal ideation, must weigh out the risks versus the benefits.

Use of antidepressants by children and adolescents. In 2004 FDA issued a black-box warning for all antidepressants. It alerted the public to an increased risk of suicidal thinking or attempts in children or adolescents taking antidepressants. Following the black-box warning, the number of prescriptions written for SSRIs for children, adolescents, and adults decreased (Friedman, 2014).

Unfortunately, suicide attempts increased after the black-box warning was instituted. The risk for suicide is greater in children and adolescents with depression who do not take antidepressants. To minimize the risk of suicide in persons taking antidepressants, close monitoring by healthcare professionals and patient/caregiver education are essential. Chapter 25 has a more detailed discussion of suicide risk factors and warning signs.

BOX 14.7 **Patient and Family Teaching: Monoamine Oxidase Inhibitors (MAOIs)**

- Tell the patient and family to avoid certain foods (especially those that are aged, cured, or ripened) and all medications (especially cold remedies) unless prescribed by and discussed with the patient's primary care provider.
- Give the patient a wallet card describing the MAOI regimen.
- Instruct the patient to avoid Asian restaurants (sherry, brewer's yeast, and other contraindicated products may be used).
- Tell the patient to go to the emergency department immediately if he or she has a severe headache.
- Ideally, blood pressure should be monitored during the first 6 weeks of treatment (for both hypotensive and hypertensive effects).
- After the MAOI is stopped, instruct the patient that dietary and drug restrictions should be maintained for 14 days.

Use of antidepressants by older adults. Polypharmacy and the normal metabolic processes of aging contribute to concerns about prescribing antidepressants for older adults. SSRIs are a first-line treatment for older adults, but this population has the potential for aggravated side effects. Starting doses are recommended to be half the lowest adult dose, with dose adjustments occurring no more frequently than every 7 days ("start low and go slow").

TCAs and MAOIs have side-effect profiles that are more dangerous for older adults, specifically cardiotoxicity with TCAs and hypotension with both classes. Any medication with a side effect of hypotension or sedation in older adults increases the risk of falls. Older adults should be cautioned against abrupt discontinuation of antidepressants because of the possibility of discontinuation syndrome, which causes anxiety, dysphoria, flulike symptoms, dizziness, excessive sweating, and insomnia.

BIOLOGICAL INTERVENTIONS

Electroconvulsive Therapy

Despite being a highly effective somatic (physical) treatment for psychiatric disorders, electroconvulsive therapy (ECT) has a bad reputation. This may be due, in part, to past practices of restraining a conscious individual while having a full-blown seizure induced. In fact, before paralytic drugs, more than 30% of ECT patients experienced compression fractures of the spine (Welch, 2016). Given the current sophistication of anesthetic and paralytic agents, ECT is actually not dramatic at all.

Indications

ECT is the most effective acute treatment for depression (Welch, 2016). Psychotic illnesses are the second most common indication for ECT. For drug-resistant patients with psychosis, a combination of ECT and antipsychotic medication has resulted in sustained improvement about 80% of the time. Depression associated with bipolar disorder remits in about 50% of the cases after ECT.

While medication is generally the first line of treatment for ease of use, ECT may be a primary treatment in the following cases:

- Severely malnourished, exhausted, and dehydrated due to lengthy depression (after rehydration)
- ECT is often more safe than medications with certain medical conditions
- Delusional depression
- Previous medication trials have failed
- Schizophrenia with catatonia

Risk Factors

Using ECT requires clinicians to weigh the risk of using this method versus the risk of suicide and diminished quality of life. Several conditions pose risks and require careful workup and management. Because the heart can be stressed at the onset of the seizure and for up to 10 minutes after, careful assessment and management in hypertension, congestive heart failure, cardiac arrhythmias, and other cardiac conditions is warranted (Welch, 2016). ECT also stresses the brain as a result of increased cerebral oxygen, blood flow, and intracranial pressure. Conditions such as brain tumors and subdural hematomas may increase the risk of using ECT.

Procedure

The procedure is explained to the patient, and informed consent is obtained if the patient is being treated voluntarily. For a patient treated involuntarily, permission may be obtained from the next of kin although in some states treatment must be court-ordered. The patient is usually given a general anesthetic to induce sleep and a muscle-paralyzing agent to prevent muscle distress and fractures. These medications have revolutionized the comfort and safety of ECT.

Patients should have a pre-ECT workup including a chest x-ray, electrocardiogram, urinalysis, complete blood count, blood urea nitrogen, and an electrolyte panel. Benzodiazepines should be discontinued as they will interfere with the seizure process.

An electroencephalogram (EEG) monitors brain waves, and an electrocardiogram (ECG) monitors cardiac responses. Brief seizures (30 to 60+ seconds) are deliberately induced by an electrical current (as brief as 1 second) transmitted through electrodes attached to one or both sides of the head (Fig. 14.3).

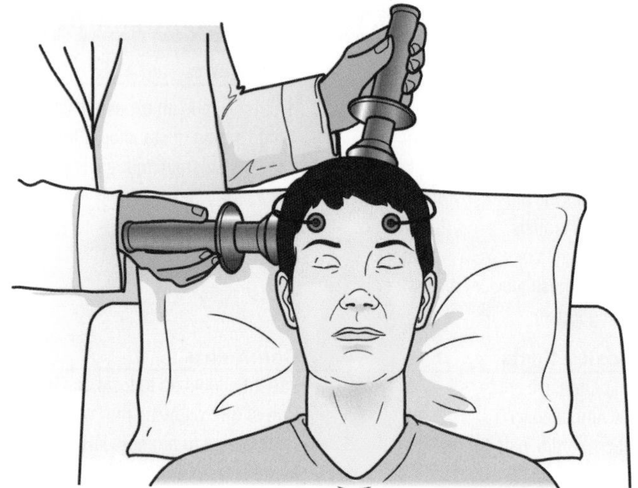

FIG. 14.3 Electroconvulsive therapy. (Photo from National Institute of Mental Health.)

To ensure that patients experience a seizure over the entire brain, a blood pressure cuff may be inflated on the lower arm or leg before administration of the paralytic agent. In that way, the convulsion can be visualized in the unparalyzed extremity.

The usual course of ECT for a patient with depression is two or three treatments per week to a total of 6 to 12 treatments. Continuation ECT along with medication may help to decrease relapse rates.

Adverse Reactions

Patients wake about 15 minutes after the procedure. The patient is often confused and disoriented for several hours. The nurse and family may need to orient the patient frequently during the course of treatment. Most people experience what is called retrograde amnesia, which is a loss of memory of events leading up to and including the treatment itself.

Transcranial Magnetic Stimulation

Transcranial magnetic stimulation (TMS) is a noninvasive treatment modality. It uses MRI-strength magnetic pulses to stimulate focal areas of the cerebral cortex.

Indications

In 2008 the FDA approved the use of TMS for patients who have been unresponsive to other methods of treatment for depression. Some researchers suggest that TMS be used to enhance cognitive function in healthy, non-depressed individuals (Clark et al., 2013).

Risk Factors

The only absolute contraindication to this procedure is the presence of metal in the area of stimulation. Cochlear implants, brain stimulators, or medication pumps are examples of metals that could interfere with the procedures (Camprodon et al., 2016).

Procedure

Outpatient treatment with TMS takes about 30 minutes and is typically ordered for 5 days a week for 4 to 6 weeks. Patients

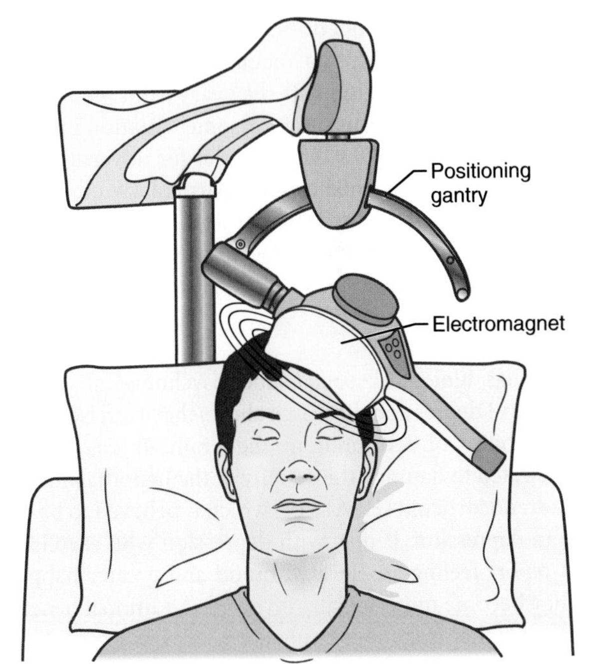

FIG. 14.4 Transcranial magnetic stimulation. (Photo from National Institute of Mental Health.)

are awake and alert during the procedure. An electromagnet is placed on the patient's scalp, and short, magnetic pulses pass into the prefrontal cortex of the brain (Fig. 14.4). These pulses are similar to those used by MRI scanners but are more focused. The pulses cause electrical charges to flow and induce neurons to fire or become active. During TMS, patients feel a slight tapping or knocking in the head, contraction of the scalp, and tightening of the jaws.

Potential Adverse Reactions

After the procedure, patients may experience a headache and lightheadedness. No neurological deficits or memory problems have been noted. Seizures are a rare complication of TMS. Most of the common side effects of TMS are mild and include scalp tingling and discomfort at the administration site.

Vagus Nerve Stimulation

The use of vagus nerve stimulation (VNS) originated as a treatment for epilepsy. Clinicians noted that in addition to decreasing seizures, VNS also seemed to improve mood in a population that normally experiences higher rates of depression. The theory behind VNS relates to the action of the vagus nerve, the longest cranial nerve, which extends from the brainstem to organs in the neck, chest, and abdomen. Electrical stimulation of the vagus nerve results in boosting the level of neurotransmitters, thereby improving mood and also enhancing the action of antidepressants.

Indications

Nearly a decade after VNS was approved for use in Europe, the FDA granted approval for VNS use in the United States for treatment-resistant depression. The efficacy of VNS in treating depression is still being established. Other potential applications of VNS include anxiety, obesity, and pain.

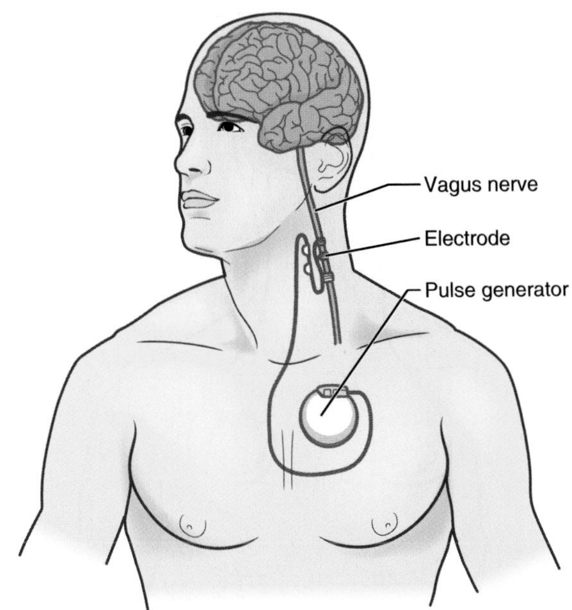

FIG. 14.5 Vagus nerve stimulation. (Photo from National Institute of Mental Health.)

Initiating Vagus Nerve Stimulation

The surgery to implant VNS is typically an outpatient procedure. A pacemaker-like device is implanted surgically into the left chest wall. The device is connected to a thin flexible wire that is threaded up and wrapped around the vagus nerve on the left side of the neck (Fig. 14.5). After surgery, an infrared magnetic wand is held against the chest while a personal computer or personal digital assistant is used to program the frequency of pulses. Pulses are usually delivered for 30 seconds, every 5 minutes, for 24 hours a day. Antidepressant action usually occurs in several weeks.

Potential Adverse Reactions

The implantation of VNS (see Fig. 14.5) is a surgical procedure, carrying with it the risks inherent in any surgical procedure (e.g., pain, infection, sensitivity to anesthesia). Side effects of active VNS therapy are due to the proximity of the lead on the vagus nerve, which is close to the laryngeal and pharyngeal branches of the left vagus nerve. Voice alteration and hoarseness are common side effects. Other side effects include neck pain, cough, paresthesia, and dyspnea, which tend to decrease with time. The device can be temporarily turned off at any time by placing a special magnet over the implant. This may be especially helpful when engaging in public speaking or heavy exercise.

Deep Brain Stimulation

Deep brain stimulation (DBS) is a treatment whereby electrodes are surgically implanted into specific areas of the brain to stimulate those regions identified to be underactive in depression. DBS is a long-approved surgical treatment for Parkinson's disease but is just now being investigated as an effective treatment in depression. As in VNS, a device is implanted in the chest wall designed to provide electrical stimulation. It differs from VNS in that electrodes are implanted directly into the brain to modify brain activity. DBS is also more invasive and as such poses more of a risk, which includes the potential of intracranial

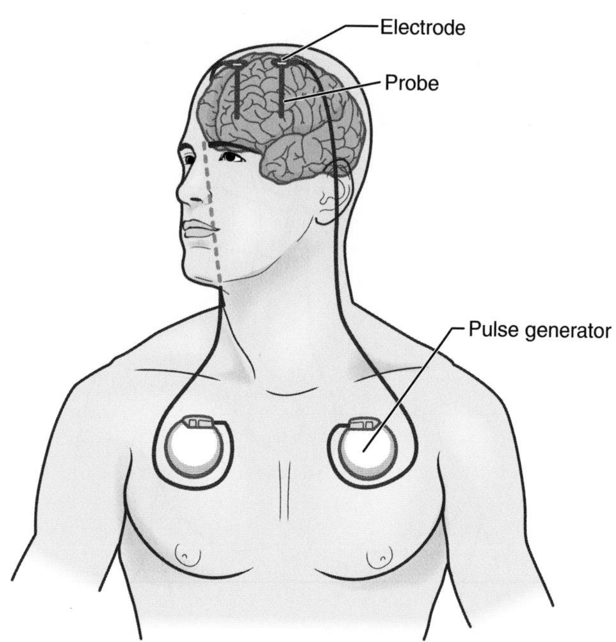

FIG. 14.6 Deep brain stimulation. (Photo from National Institute of Mental Health.)

hemorrhage. DBS is being evaluated primarily in regard to treatment-resistant major depression. Fig. 14.6 illustrates DBS.

Light Therapy

Light therapy has been researched for nearly 20 years and is accepted as a first-line treatment for seasonal affective disorder (SAD). In the *DSM-5* (2013), SAD is considered a subtype of major depressive disorder and listed as "with seasonal pattern." People with SAD often live in regions in which there are marked seasonal differences in the amount of daylight.

Light therapy's effectiveness is thought to be the influence of light on melatonin. Melatonin is secreted by the pineal gland and is necessary for maintaining and shifting biological rhythms. Exposure to light suppresses the nocturnal secretion of melatonin, which seems to have a therapeutic effect on people with SAD.

Ideal treatment consists of 30 to 45 minutes of exposure daily to a 10,000-lux light source. Morning exposure is best. However, success has been reported when exposure occurs at other times of the day or in divided doses. Anecdotal reports suggest that increasing the available light by adding additional light sources may also help to elevate mood. For those affected by SAD, light therapy has been found to be as effective in reducing depressive symptoms as medications. Negative side effects include headache and jitteriness.

St. John's Wort

St. John's wort *(Hypericum perforatum)* is a flower that can be processed into tea or tablets. This herb may increase the amount of serotonin, norepinephrine, and dopamine in the brain, resulting in antidepressant effects. Studies of St. John's wort used in the treatment of depression provide mixed evaluations. It has generally been found to be as effective as antidepressants in the treatment of mild to moderate depression, but usefulness in severe depression has not been established (Carpenter, 2011). Because St. John's wort is not regulated by the FDA, concentrations of the active ingredients may vary from preparation to preparation, which may account for some variation in research results. St. John's wort has the potential for adverse reactions when taken with other medications, particularly other antidepressants. Neither safety nor standardization of dose has been established. Therefore it should be used with caution during pregnancy or in children.

Exercise

Exercise has biological, social, and psychological effects on symptoms of depression. Research shows that exercise increases the availability of serotonin in the brain. It has also been demonstrated to dampen the activity of the hypothalamic-pituitary-adrenocorticoid (HPA) axis, which is believed to be overly active in depression. People with depression who exercise regularly report feeling an elevated mood and greater happiness, and they become more socially involved. Additional benefits of exercise are that it is more easily accessed, less expensive, and results in fewer side effects than taking antidepressants.

Advanced Practice Interventions

Psychiatric-mental health advanced practice registered nurses are qualified to provide individual therapy and group therapy (American Nurses Association et al., 2014). In some states, nurses who have met appropriate educational standards may be certified to prescribe medication to treat depression.

Individual Therapy

CBT, interpersonal therapy (IPT), time-limited focused psychotherapy, and behavioral therapy all are especially effective in the treatment of depression. However, only CBT and IPT demonstrate superiority in the maintenance phase. CBT helps people reconstruct their negative thought patterns and behaviors, leading to lasting mood improvements, whereas IPT focuses on working through personal relationships that may contribute to depression.

Group Therapy

Group therapy is a widespread modality for the treatment of depression. It increases the number of people who can receive treatment at a decreased cost per individual. Another advantage is that groups offer patients an opportunity to socialize and share common feelings and concerns, which decreases feelings of isolation, hopelessness, helplessness, and alienation. Therapy groups also provide a controlled environment in which patients can explore their patterns of interaction and response to others, which may contribute to or exacerbate their depression.

EVALUATION

Because each patient presents differently, outcome evaluation will be tailored to each patient's unique presentation. Based on your evaluation, modification of nursing diagnoses, goals, and interventions is made.

When suicidal ideation is present the following questions should be addressed: Are these thoughts still present? How frequently do they occur? Does the patient have a plan? Is the patient able to stop suicidal thoughts and formulate alternatives to suicidal thoughts? If the depression is severe and the patient has demonstrated psychotic features, the nurse will ask about auditory hallucinations and evaluate for signs of delusions.

Basic self-care issues should be addressed. Is the patient taking in a sufficient number of calories and liquids? In an inpatient setting the nurse will also evaluate the patient's sleep pattern. Is the patient able to fall asleep? Stay asleep? Has the number of hours of sleep increased since admission? What about personal hygiene and grooming?

Thought processes, self-esteem, and social interactions are evaluated because these areas are often problematic in people with depression. The nurse should assess self-esteem. How do you feel about yourself now as compared with when you were admitted? The nurse will evaluate negativity and if the patient is able to identify positive aspects of individual functioning.

QUALITY IMPROVEMENT

National objectives for outcomes improvement related to major depressive disorder have been set by the US Department of Health and Human Services in *Healthy People 2020* (Mental Health and Mental Objectives, 2012). National goals include increasing the percentage of individuals with major depressive disorder who receive treatment to 75% (an increase from 68% in 2008). Other goals involve increasing the number of physicians' offices who routinely screen for depression.

For quality improvement to be successful, nurses and other members of the healthcare team must try new approaches to improve various aspects of care. The Center for Quality Assessment and Improvement in Mental Health (CQAIMH, n.d.) has links to reliable outcome measures for patients with major depression, covering a variety of aspects of care that include treatment and screening. These tools are available at http://www.cqaimh.org/quality.html.

KEY POINTS TO REMEMBER

- Children and adolescents with disruptive mood dysregulation disorder had previously been diagnosed with bipolar disorder. Usually children with this disorder grow up and are diagnosed with major depressive disorder or an anxiety disorder.
- Persistent depressive disorder is a low-level depression that tends to be chronic. Treatment for this disorder is similar to major depressive disorder.
- Premenstrual dysphoric disorder is diagnosed for women with physical discomfort and emotional symptoms similar to major depression. These symptoms disappear at the onset of menstruation.
- The symptoms of major depressive disorder are usually severe enough to interfere with a person's social or occupational functioning. A person with depression may or may not have psychotic symptoms. The most severe consequence of major depressive disorder is suicide.
- Many theories exist about the cause of depression. Biochemical abnormalities are strongly supported in the scientific community. The diathesis-stress theory suggests a dynamic interaction between psychosocial stressors and interpersonal events with neurochemical changes in the brain.
- Nursing assessment includes the evaluation of affect, thought processes (especially suicidal thoughts), mood, feelings, and physical behavior. The nurse also must be aware of the symptoms that may mask depression.
- Nursing diagnoses are numerous. Risk for suicide is always the priority diagnosis when suicidal ideation is present. Other common nursing diagnoses are *chronic low self-esteem, imbalanced nutrition, constipation, disturbed sleep pattern, ineffective coping,* and *disabled family coping.*
- Interventions include using specific principles of communication, planning activities of daily living, administering or participating in psychopharmacological therapy, maintaining a therapeutic environment, and teaching patients about the biochemical aspects of depression.
- Depression is often overlooked in children, adolescents, and older adults.
- Planning and interventions for patients with depression are based on the recovery model, which involves a therapeutic alliance with healthcare professionals to achieve outcomes based on individual patient's needs and values.
- Evaluation is ongoing throughout the nursing process, and patients' outcomes are compared with the stated outcome criteria and short-term and intermediate indicators. The care plan is revised when indicators are not being met.

CRITICAL THINKING

1. You are spending time with Mr. Plotsky, who is undergoing a workup for depression. He hardly makes eye contact, slouches in his seat, and wears a blank but sad expression. Mr. Plotsky has had numerous bouts of major depression in the past and says to you, "This will be my last depression. I will never go through this again."
   - Because safety is the first concern, what are the appropriate questions to ask Mr. Plotsky at this time?
   - In terms of behaviors, thought processes, activities of daily living, and ability to function at work and home, give examples of the kinds of signs and symptoms you might find when assessing a patient with depression.
   - Mr. Plotsky tells you that he has been on every medication there is, but none has worked. He asks you about the herb St. John's wort. What should you tell him about its effectiveness for severe depression, interactions with other antidepressants, and regulatory status?
   - What might be some somatic options for a person resistant to antidepressant medications?

- Mr. Plotsky asks what causes depression. In simple terms, how might you respond to his query?
- Mr. Plotsky tells you that he has never tried therapy because he thinks it is for weaklings. What information could you give him about various therapeutic modalities that have proven effective for other patients with depression?

2. You are working with Ms. Folk, a 28-year-old with major depression on long-term antidepressant therapy. She asks you about the possibility of pregnancy while taking her SSRIs.
   - What are some of the things Ms. Folk might want to consider about taking antidepressants if she plans to get pregnant?
   - If she decides to stop taking her antidepressants, what are some things she might do to help manage her depression?

CHAPTER REVIEW

Questions

1. Which response by a 15-year-old demonstrates a common symptom observed in patients diagnosed with major depressive disorder?
   a. "I'm so restless. I can't seem to sit still."
   b. "I spend most of my time studying. I have to get into a good college."
   c. "I'm not trying to diet, but I've lost about 5 pounds in the past 5 months."
   d. "I go to sleep around 11 p.m. but I'm always up by 3 a.m. and can't go back to sleep."
2. Which assessment question asked by the nurse demonstrates an understanding of comorbid mental health conditions associated with major depressive disorder? *Select all that apply.*
   a. "Do rules apply to you?"
   b. "What do you do to manage anxiety?"
   c. "Do you have a history of disordered eating?"
   d. "Do you think that you drink too much?"
   e. "Have you ever been arrested for committing a crime?"
3. Which nursing intervention focuses on managing a common characteristic of major depressive disorder associated with the older population?
   a. Conducting routine suicide screenings at a senior center.
   b. Identifying depression as a natural, but treatable result of aging.
   c. Identifying males as being at a greater risk for developing depression.
   d. Stressing that most individuals experience just a single episode of major depression in a lifetime.
4. Which characteristic identified during an assessment serves to support a diagnosis of disruptive mood dysregulation disorder? *Select all that apply.*
   a. Female
   b. 7 years old
   c. Comorbid autism diagnosis
   d. Outbursts occur at least once a week
   e. Temper tantrums occur at home and in school
5. Which chronic medical condition is a common trigger for major depressive disorder?
   a. Pain
   b. Hypertension
   c. Hypothyroidism
   d. Crohn's disease
6. Tammy, a 28-year-old with major depressive disorder and bulimia nervosa, is ready for discharge from the county hospital after 2 weeks of inpatient therapy. Tammy is taking citalopram (Celexa) and reports that it has made her feel more hopeful. With a secondary diagnosis of bulimia nervosa, what is an alternative antidepressant to consider?
   a. Fluoxetine (Prozac)
   b. Isocarboxazid (Marplan)
   c. Amitriptyline
   d. Duloxetine (Cymbalta)
7. Cabot has multiple symptoms of depression including mood reactivity, social phobia, anxiety, and overeating. With a history of mild hypertension, which classification of antidepressants dispensed as a transdermal patch would be a safe medication?
   a. Tricyclic antidepressants
   b. Selective serotonin reuptake inhibitors
   c. Serotonin and norepinephrine reuptake inhibitors
   d. Monoamine oxidase inhibitor
8. When a nurse uses therapeutic communication with a withdrawn patient who has major depression, an effective method of managing the silence is to:
   a. Meditate in the quiet environment
   b. Ask simple questions even if the patient will not answer
   c. Use the technique of making observations
   d. Simply sit quietly and leave when the patient falls asleep
9. The biological approach to treating depression with electrodes surgically implanted into specific areas of the brain to stimulate the regions identified to be underactive in depression is:
   a. Transcranial magnetic stimulation
   b. Deep brain stimulation
   c. Vagus nerve stimulation
   d. Electroconvulsive therapy
10. Two months ago, Natasha's husband died suddenly and she has been overwhelmed with grief. When Natasha is subsequently diagnosed with major depressive disorder, her daughter, Nadia, makes which true statement?
    a. "Depression often begins after a major loss. Losing dad was a major loss."
    b. "Bereavement and depression are the same problem."
    c. "Mourning is pathological and not normal behavior."
    d. "Antidepressant medications will not help this type of depression."

Answers

1. **d;** 2. **b, c, d;** 3. **a;** 4. **b, c, e;** 5. **a;** 6. **a;** 7. **d;** 8. **c;** 9. **b;** 10. **a**

Visit the Evolve website for a posttest on the content in this chapter: http://evolve.elsevier.com/Varcarolis

Post-Test interactive review

REFERENCES

American Nurses Association, American Psychiatric Nurses Association, & International Society of Psychiatric-Mental Health Nurses (2014). *Psychiatric-mental health nursing*. Silver Spring, MD: nursesbooks.org.

American Psychiatric Association. (2013). *Diagnostic and statistical manual of mental disorders* (5th ed.). Washington, D.C. Author.

Beck, A. T., & Rush, A. J. (1995). Cognitive therapy. In H. I. Kaplan & B. J. Sadock (Eds.), *Comprehensive textbook of psychiatry/VI* (Vol. 2) (pp. 1847–1856). Baltimore, MD: Williams & Wilkins.

Camprodon, J. A., Kaur, N., Rauch, S. L., & Dougherty, D. D. (2016). Neurotherapeutics. In T. Stern, M. Fava, T. E. Wilens, & J. F. Rosenbaum (Eds.), *Massachusetts General Hospital handbook of general hospital psychiatry* (2nd ed.). Philadelphia, PA: Elsevier.

Carpenter, D. (2011). St. John's wort and S-adenosyl methionine as "natural" alternatives to conventional antidepressants in the era of the suicidality boxed warning: What is the evidence for clinically relevant benefit? *Alternative Medicine Health Review, 16*(1), 17–39.

Center for Behavioral Health Statistics and Quality. (2015). Behavioral health trends in the United States: Results from the 2014 National Survey on Drug Use and Health (HHS Publication No. SMA 15–4927, NSDUH Series H-50). Retrieved from http://www.samhsa.gov/data/.

Center for Quality Assessment and Improvement in Mental Health. (n.d.). National inventory of mental health quality measures. Retrieved from https://www.cqaimh.org/quality.html.

Clark, V. P., & Parasuraman, R. (2013). Neuroenhancement: Enhancing brain and mind in health and disease. *NeuroImage, 85*, 889–894.

Flaster, M., Sharma, A., & Rao, M. (2013). Poststroke depression. *Topics in Stroke Rehabilitation, 20*(2), 139–150.

Friedman, R. A. (2014). Antidepressants' black-box warning 10 years later. *New England Journal of Medicine, 371*, 1666–1668.

Institute for Clinical Systems Improvement. (2016). Depression in primary care. Retrieved from https://www.icsi.org/_asset/xm2nqq/DeprPC0216.pdf.

Krishnadas, R., & Cavanagh, J. (2012). Depression: An inflammatory illness? *Journal of Neurology, Neurosurgery, and Psychiatry, 83*(5), 495–502.

McInnis, M. G., Riba, M., & Greden, J. F. (2014). Depressive disorders. In R. E. Hales, S. C. Yudofsky, & L. W. Roberts (Eds.), *Textbook of psychiatry*. Washington, DC: American Psychiatric Publishing.

Mental Health and Mental Objectives. (2012). *Healthy people 2020*. Washington, DC: US Department of Health and Human Services.

Miller, G. E., & Cole, S. W. (2012). Clustering of depression and inflammation in adolescents previously exposed to childhood adversity. *Biological Psychiatry, 72*(1), 34–40.

National Institute of Mental Health. (2012). Older adults: Depression and suicide facts (fact sheet). Retrieved from http://www.nimh.nih.gov/health/publications/older-adults-and-depression/older-adults-and-depression_141998.pdf.

Olivier, J. D. A., Akerud, H., & Promomaa, I. S. (2015). Antenatal depression and antidepressants during pregnancy. *European Journal of Pharmacology, 753*, 257–262.

Ryan, J., & Ancelin, M. (2012). Polymorphisms of estrogen receptors and risk of depression. *Drugs, 72*(13), 1725–1738.

Sadock, B. J., Sadock, V. A., & Ruiz, P. (2015). *Kaplan and Sadock's synopsis of psychiatry* (11th ed.). Philadelphia, PA: Wolters Kluwer.

Sheikh, J., & Yesavage, J. (1986). Geriatric depression scale (GDS): Recent evidence and development of a shorter version. *Clinical Gerontologist, 5*(1–2), 165–173.

US Department of Health and Human Services. (2012). Mental health and mental disorders. Retrieved from http://www.healthypeople.gov/2020/topicsobjectives2020/objectiveslist.aspx?topicId=28.

Welch, C. A. (2016). Electroconvulsive therapy. In T. A. Stern, M. Fava, T. E. Wilens, & J. F. Rosenbaum (Eds.), *Comprehensive clinical psychiatry* (2nd ed.). St. Louis, MO: Elsevier.

15

Anxiety and Obsessive-Compulsive Disorders

Margaret Jordan Halter

Visit the Evolve website for a pretest on the content in this chapter: http://evolve.elsevier.com/Varcarolis Pre-Test interactive review

OBJECTIVES

1. Compare and contrast the four levels of anxiety in relation to perceptual field, ability to problem solve, and other defining characteristics.
2. Identify defense mechanisms and consider one adaptive and one maladaptive (if any) use of each.
3. Describe clinical manifestations of each anxiety and obsessive-compulsive disorder.
4. Identify genetic, biological, psychological, and cultural factors that may contribute to anxiety and obsessive-compulsive disorders.
5. Describe feelings that may be experienced by nurses caring for patients with anxiety and obsessive-compulsive disorders.
6. Formulate four priority nursing diagnoses that can be used in treating a person with anxiety and obsessive-compulsive disorders.
7. Propose realistic outcome criteria for a patient with (a) generalized anxiety disorder, (b) panic disorder, and (c) obsessive-compulsive disorder.
8. Describe five basic nursing interventions used for patients with anxiety and obsessive-compulsive disorders.
9. Discuss the classes of medications used to treat anxiety and obsessive-compulsive disorders.
10. Describe basic-level and advanced-practice interventions for anxiety and obsessive-compulsive disorders.

OUTLINE

KEY TERMS AND CONCEPTS

agoraphobia
antianxiety drugs
anxiety
body dysmorphic disorder
defense mechanisms
excoriation (skin picking) disorder
generalized anxiety disorder
hoarding disorder
mild anxiety
moderate anxiety
obsessive-compulsive disorder
panic
panic disorder
separation anxiety disorder
severe anxiety
social anxiety disorder
specific phobia
trichotillomania (hair pulling) disorder

For most people, anxiety is a part of everyday life. "I felt really nervous when I couldn't find a parking space right before my final exam. I know I would have done better if that hadn't happened." For some people, however, anxiety-related symptoms become severely debilitating and interfere with normal functioning. "Today I got so worried I wouldn't find a parking space before the final exam, I stayed home." In this chapter, we will examine the concept of anxiety, defenses against anxiety, and an overview of anxiety and obsessive-compulsive disorders and their treatment.

ANXIETY

Anxiety is a universal human experience and is among the most basic of emotions. It can be defined as a feeling of apprehension, uneasiness, uncertainty, or dread resulting from a real or perceived threat. Fear is a reaction to a specific danger, whereas anxiety is a vague sense of dread related to an unspecified or unknown danger. However, the body reacts physiologically in similar ways to both anxiety and fear. Another important distinction between anxiety and fear is that anxiety affects us at a deeper level. It invades the central core of the personality and erodes feelings of self-esteem and personal worth.

Normal anxiety is a healthy reaction necessary for survival. Without anxiety our ancestors would have had little motivation to run from the saber tooth tiger or hunt the mastodon. Anxiety provides the energy needed to carry out the tasks involved in living and striving toward goals. Anxiety motivates people to make and survive change. It prompts constructive behaviors, such as studying for an examination, being on time for a job interview, preparing for a presentation, and working toward a promotion.

An understanding of the levels and defensive patterns used in response to anxiety is basic to psychiatric-mental health nursing care. This understanding is essential for assessing and planning interventions to lower a patient's level of anxiety (as well as one's own) effectively. With practice, you will become skilled at identifying levels of anxiety, understanding the defenses used to alleviate anxiety, and evaluating the possible stressors that contribute to increased levels of anxiety.

LEVELS OF ANXIETY

As discussed in Chapter 2, Hildegard Peplau had a profound role in shaping the specialty of psychiatric-mental health nursing. She identified anxiety as a key element in her theory of interpersonal relationships. Peplau (1968) developed a useful anxiety model that consists of four levels: mild, moderate, severe, and panic. The boundaries between these levels are not distinct, and the behaviors and characteristics of individuals experiencing anxiety can and often do overlap. Identification of a general level of anxiety is helpful in selecting interventions based on the *degree* of the patient's anxiety.

Mild Anxiety

Mild anxiety occurs in the normal experience of everyday living and allows an individual to perceive reality in sharp focus. A person experiencing a mild level of anxiety sees, hears, and grasps more information, and problem solving becomes more effective. Physical symptoms may include slight discomfort, restlessness, irritability, or mild tension-relieving behaviors (e.g., nail biting, foot or finger tapping, fidgeting).

Moderate Anxiety

As anxiety increases, the perceptual field narrows, and some details are excluded from observation. The person experiencing moderate anxiety sees, hears, and grasps less information and may demonstrate **selective inattention** in which only certain things in the environment are seen or heard unless they are pointed out. The ability to think clearly is hampered, but learning and problem solving can still take place although not at an optimal level.

TABLE 15.1 **Levels of Anxiety**

Mild	Moderate	Severe	Panic
Perceptual Field			
Heightened perceptual field Focus is flexible and is aware of the anxiety	Narrowed perceptual field Grasps less of what is going on Focuses on the source of the anxiety Less able to pay attention.	Greatly reduced and distorted perceptual field Focuses on details or one specific detail Attention is scattered	Unable to attend to the environment Focus is lost; may feel unreal (depersonalization) or that the world is unreal (derealization)
Ability to Problem Solve			
Able to work effectively toward a goal and examine alternatives	Able to solve problems but not at optimal ability	Problem solving feels impossible. Unable to see connections between events or details	Completely unable to process what is happening Disorganized or irrational reasoning
Mild and moderate levels of anxiety can alert the person that something is wrong and can stimulate appropriate action.		Severe and panic levels of anxiety prevent problem solving. Unproductive relief behaviors perpetuate a vicious cycle.	
Physical or Other Characteristics			
Slight discomfort Attention-seeking behavior Restlessness Easily startled Irritability or impatience Mild tension-relieving behavior (foot or finger tapping, lip chewing, fidgeting)	Voice tremors Change in voice pitch Poor concentration Shakiness Somatic complaints (urinary frequency, headache, backache, insomnia) Increased respiration, pulse, and muscle tension More tension-relieving behavior (pacing, banging of hands on table)	Feelings of dread Confusion Purposeless activity Sense of impending doom More intense somatic complaints (chest discomfort, dizziness, nausea, sleeplessness) Diaphoresis (sweating) Withdrawal Loud and rapid speech Threats and demands	Experience of terror Immobility or severe hyperactivity or flight Unintelligible communication or inability to speak Somatic complaints increase (numbness or tingling, shortness of breath, dizziness, chest pain, nausea, trembling, chills, overheating, palpitations) Severe withdrawal Hallucinations or delusions Likely out of touch with reality

Sympathetic nervous system symptoms begin to kick in at this level. The individual may experience tension, pounding heart, increased pulse and respiratory rate, perspiration, and mild somatic symptoms (e.g., gastric discomfort, headache, urinary urgency). Voice tremors and shaking may be noticed. Mild or moderate anxiety levels can be constructive because anxiety may be a signal that something in the person's life needs attention or is dangerous.

Severe Anxiety

The perceptual field of a person experiencing severe anxiety is greatly reduced. A person with **severe anxiety** may focus on one particular detail or many scattered details and have difficulty noticing what is going on in the environment, even when another points it out. Learning and problem solving are not possible at this level, and the person may be dazed and confused. Behavior is automatic and aimed at reducing or relieving anxiety. Somatic symptoms (e.g., headache, nausea, dizziness, insomnia) often increase. Trembling and a pounding heart are common, and the person may experience hyperventilation and a sense of impending doom or dread.

Panic

Panic is the most extreme level of anxiety and results in markedly dysregulated behavior. Someone in a state of panic is unable to process what is going on in the environment and may lose touch with reality. The behavior that results may be manifested as pacing, running, shouting, screaming, or withdrawal. Hallucinations, or false sensory perceptions (e.g., seeing people or objects not really there) may be experienced. Physical behavior may become erratic, uncoordinated, and impulsive. Automatic behaviors are used to reduce and relieve anxiety, although such efforts may be ineffective. Acute panic may lead to exhaustion. See the Case Study and Nursing Care Plan for panic level anxiety on the Evolve website.

Review Table 15.1, which distinguishes among the levels of anxiety in regard to their (1) effects on perceptual field, (2) effects on problem solving, and (3) physical and other defining characteristics.

DEFENSES AGAINST ANXIETY

Sigmund Freud and his daughter, Anna Freud, outlined most of the defense mechanisms we recognize today. **Defense mechanisms** are automatic coping styles that protect people from anxiety and maintain self-image by blocking feelings, conflicts, and memories. Although they operate all the time, defense mechanisms are not always apparent to the individual using them.

Adaptive use of defense mechanisms helps people lower anxiety to achieve goals in acceptable ways. Maladaptive use of defense mechanisms occurs when one or several are used in excess, particularly in the overuse of immature defenses. Fig. 15.1 operationally defines anxiety and shows how defenses come into play.

With the exception of sublimation and altruism, which are always healthy coping mechanisms, most defense mechanisms can be used in both healthy and unhealthy ways. Most people use a variety of defense mechanisms but not always at the same

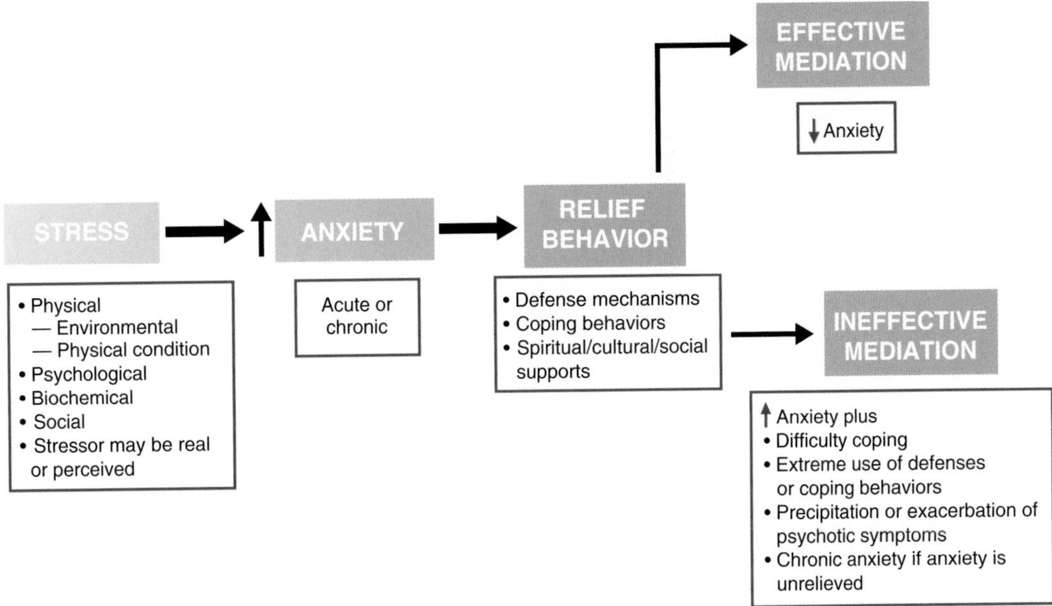

FIG. 15.1 Anxiety operationally defined.

level. Keep in mind that evaluating whether the use of defense mechanisms is adaptive or maladaptive is determined for the most part by their *frequency*, *intensity*, and *duration* of use. Table 15.2 describes defense mechanisms and their adaptive and maladaptive uses.

ANXIETY DISORDERS

Individuals with anxiety disorders use rigid, repetitive, and ineffective behaviors to try to control their anxiety. The common element of such disorders is that those affected experience a degree of anxiety that interferes with personal, occupational, or social functioning. The presence of chronic anxiety disorders may increase the rate of cardiovascular system–related deaths. Anxiety disorders tend to be persistent and often disabling.

CLINICAL PICTURE

According to the American Psychiatric Association (2013), the term *anxiety disorder* refers to a number of disorders including:

- Separation anxiety disorder
- Specific phobia
- Social anxiety disorder (social phobia)
- Panic disorder
- Agoraphobia
- Generalized anxiety disorder

A closely related set of disorders anxiety results in abnormal selective overattention or obsessions. These obsessive-compulsive and related disorders include the following:

- Obsessive-compulsive disorder
- Body dysmorphic disorder
- Hoarding disorder
- Trichotrillomania (hair pulling) disorder
- Excoriation (skin picking) disorder

Separation Anxiety Disorder

Separation anxiety is a normal part of infant development that begins around 8 months of age, peaks about 18 months, and begins to decline after that. People with **separation anxiety disorder** exhibit *developmentally inappropriate* levels of concern over being away from a significant other. There may also be fear that something horrible will happen to the other person and that it will result in permanent separation. The anxiety is so intense that it distracts sufferers from their normal activities and causes sleep disruptions and nightmares. The separation anxiety is often manifested in physical symptoms such as gastrointestinal disturbances and headaches.

Recently, clinicians have begun to recognize an adult form of separation anxiety disorder that may begin either in childhood or in adulthood. Those who are the subject of the attachment—a parent, a spouse, a child, or a friend—may become alienated due to the constant neediness and clinginess. In fact, adults with this disorder often have extreme difficulties in romantic relationships and are more likely to be unmarried. Characteristics of adult separation anxiety disorder include harm avoidance, worry, shyness, uncertainty, fatigability, and a lack of self-direction (Mertol & Alkin, 2012). It is accompanied by a significant level of discomfort and disability that impairs social and occupational functioning and does not respond well to the most popular type of psychotherapy, cognitive-behavioral therapy.

This problem is typically diagnosed before the age of 18 after about a month of symptoms. The 12-month prevalence rates of separation anxiety disorder in children, adolescents, and adults is 4%, 1.9%, and 0.9% to 1.9%, respectively. It is the most common anxiety disorder in children. Females are more likely to be affected.

Environmental stresses such as a significant loss through death of a relative or pet, separation from significant others, or a change in environment by moving or immigration can bring about symptoms of this disorder. A physical or sexual assault

TABLE 15.2 Adaptive and Maladaptive Uses of Defense Mechanisms

Defense Mechanism	Adaptive Use	Maladaptive Use
Compensation is used to counterbalance perceived deficiencies by emphasizing strengths.	A shorter-than-average man becomes assertively verbal and excels in business.	An individual drinks alcohol when self-esteem is low to temporarily diffuse discomfort.
Conversion is the unconscious transformation of anxiety into a physical symptom with no organic cause.	No example. Almost always a pathological defense.	A man becomes blind after seeing his wife flirt with other men.
Denial involves escaping unpleasant, anxiety-causing thoughts, feelings, wishes, or needs by ignoring their existence.	A man reacts to the death of a loved one by saying "No, I don't believe you" to initially protect himself from the overwhelming news.	A woman whose husband died 3 years earlier still keeps his clothes in the closet and talks about him in the present tense.
Displacement is the transference of emotions associated with a particular person, object, or situation to another nonthreatening person, object, or situation.	A child yells at his teddy bear after being picked on by the school bully.	A child who is unable to acknowledge fear of his father becomes fearful of animals.
Dissociation is a disruption in consciousness, memory, identity, or perception of the environment that results in compartmentalizing uncomfortable or unpleasant aspects of oneself.	An art student is able to mentally separate herself from the noisy environment as she becomes absorbed in her work.	As the result of an abusive childhood and the need to separate from its realities, a woman finds herself perpetually disconnected from reality.
Identification is attributing to oneself the characteristics of another person or group. This may be done consciously or unconsciously.	An 8-year-old girl dresses up like her teacher and puts together a pretend classroom for her friends.	A young boy thinks a neighborhood pimp with money and drugs is someone to look up to.
Intellectualization is a process in which events are analyzed based on remote, cold facts and without passion, rather than incorporating feeling and emotion into the processing.	Despite the fact that a man has lost his farm to a tornado, he analyzes his options and leads his child to safety.	A man responds to the death of his wife by focusing on the details of day care and operating the household, rather than processing the grief with his children.
Projection refers to the unconscious rejection of emotionally unacceptable features and attributing them to others.	No example. This is considered an immature defense mechanism.	A woman who has repressed an attraction toward other women refuses to socialize. She fears another woman will make homosexual advances toward her.
Rationalization consists of justifying illogical or unreasonable ideas, actions, or feelings by developing acceptable explanations that satisfy the teller and the listener.	An employee says, "I didn't get the raise because the boss doesn't like me."	A man who thinks his son was fathered by another man excuses his malicious treatment of the boy by saying, "He is lazy and disobedient," when that is not the case.
Reaction formation is when unacceptable feelings or behaviors are controlled and kept out of awareness by developing the opposite behavior or emotion.	A recovering alcoholic constantly talks about the evils of drinking.	A woman who has an unconscious hostility toward her daughter is overprotective and hovers over her to protect her from harm, interfering with her normal growth and development.
Regression is reverting to an earlier, more primitive and childlike pattern of behavior that may or may not have been previously exhibited.	A 4-year-old boy with a new baby brother temporarily starts sucking his thumb and wanting a bottle.	A man who loses a promotion starts complaining to others, hands in sloppy work, misses appointments, and comes in late for meetings.
Repression is an unconscious exclusion of unpleasant or unwanted experiences, emotions, or ideas from conscious awareness.	A man forgets his wife's birthday after a marital fight.	A woman is unable to enjoy sex after having pushed out of awareness a traumatic sexual incident from childhood.
Splitting is the inability to integrate the positive and negative qualities of oneself or others into a cohesive image.	No example. Almost always a pathological defense.	A 26-year-old woman initially values her acquaintances yet invariably becomes disillusioned when they turn out to have flaws.
Sublimation is an unconscious process of substituting mature and socially acceptable activity for immature and unacceptable impulses.	A woman who is angry with her boss writes a short story about a heroic woman.	The use of sublimation is always constructive.
Suppression is the conscious denial of a disturbing situation or feeling. For example, Jessica has been studying for the state board examination for a week solid. She says, "I won't worry about paying my rent until after my exam tomorrow."	A businessman who is preparing to make an important speech is told by his wife that morning that she wants a divorce. Although visibly upset, he puts the incident aside until after his speech, when he can give the matter his total concentration.	A woman who feels a lump in her breast shortly before leaving for a 3-week vacation puts the information in the back of her mind until after returning from her vacation.
Undoing is most commonly seen in children. It is when a person makes up for an act or communication.	After flirting with her male secretary, a woman brings her husband tickets to a concert he wants to see.	A man with rigid, moralistic beliefs and repressed sexuality is driven to wash his hands to gain composure when around attractive women.

may also precede symptoms. There is also strong evidence that this illness is inherited genetically (Mervis et al., 2012).

In children, this severe form of separation anxiety is often seen with generalized anxiety disorder and specific phobias. In adults, a range of disorders commonly coexists. They are depressive disorders, bipolar disorders, anxiety disorders, posttraumatic stress disorder, obsessive-compulsive disorder, and personality disorders.

TABLE 15.3 Clinical Names for Common Phobias

Clinical Name	Feared Object or Situation
Acrophobia	Heights
Agoraphobia	Open spaces
Astraphobia	Electrical storms
Claustrophobia	Closed spaces
Glossophobia	Talking
Hematophobia	Blood
Hydrophobia	Water
Monophobia	Being alone
Mysophobia	Germs or dirt
Nyctophobia	Darkness
Pyrophobia	Fire
Xenophobia	Strangers
Zoophobia	Animals

Specific Phobias

A **specific phobia** is a persistent irrational fear of a specific object, activity, or situation that leads to a desire for avoidance or actual avoidance of the object, activity, or situation. Specific phobias are characterized by the experience of high levels of anxiety or fear in response to specific objects or situations such as dogs, spiders, heights, storms, water, blood, closed spaces, tunnels, and bridges.

Characteristically, phobic individuals experience overwhelming and crippling anxiety when faced with the object or situation provoking the phobic response. Daily functioning is compromised, and phobic people go to great lengths to avoid the feared object or situation. A phobic person may not be able to think about or visualize the object or situation without becoming severely anxious. The life of a phobic person becomes more restricted as activities are given up so that the phobic object can be avoided. All too frequently, complications ensue when sufferers try to decrease anxiety through self-medication with alcohol or drugs.

Consider the case of Daniel, who developed a profound fear of elevators after being trapped in one for 3 hours during a power outage. As his fear and anxiety intensified, it became necessary for him to use only stairs or escalators. He obsesses about the possibility that he will be forced to use an elevator in social situations and avoids attending events where this may occur. It has reached a point where even going inside closets or small storage rooms is unbearable. This fear of enclosed spaces is called *claustrophobia*. Other common phobias are listed in Table 15.3.

Twelve-month prevalence rates for specific phobias in children, adolescents, and adults are 5%, 16%, and 8%, respectively. Females are affected twice as often as males.

Negative and traumatic experiences with the feared objects or situations lead to the fear. Phobic reactions tend to run in families. Having a first-degree relative with a specific phobia puts one at greater risk for having the same specific phobia.

Few people are seen in healthcare settings for treatment of phobias. In general, they seek help for comorbid conditions including major depression, anxiety, substance use, somatic symptom disorders, and dependent personality disorder.

Social Anxiety Disorder

Social anxiety disorder, also called *social phobia*, is characterized by severe anxiety or fear provoked by exposure to a social or a performance situation that could be evaluated negatively by others. Situations that trigger this distress include fear of saying something that sounds foolish in public, not being able to answer questions in a classroom, looking awkward while eating or drinking in public, and performing badly on stage. Whenever possible, people with social anxiety disorder avoid these social situations. If they are unable to avoid them, they endure the situation with intense anxiety and emotional distress.

Small children with this disorder may be mute, nervous, and hide behind their parents. Older children and adolescents may be paralyzed by fear of speaking in class or interacting with other children. The worry over saying the wrong thing or being criticized immobilizes them. Conversely, younger people may act out to compensate for this fear, making an accurate diagnosis more difficult. This anxiety often results in physical complaints to avoid social situations, particularly school.

Fear of public speaking is the most common manifestation of social anxiety disorder. Interestingly, this disorder has afflicted famous singers and actors such as Barbra Streisand and Sir Laurence Olivier, both of whom were terrified that they might forget the words to songs and scripts.

The 12-month prevalence of social anxiety disorder is the same for children, adolescents, and adults—about 7%. As with many of the anxiety disorders, females are more likely to be affected.

Risk factors for social anxiety disorder include childhood mistreatment and adverse childhood events. The trait of shyness is also strongly heritable. Having parents who are shy carries a double risk of genetic transmission and parental modeling.

Chronic social isolation may increase the risk for major depression. Substance use disorders are common and may be related to the social isolation and inhibition of this illness. Bipolar disorder and body dysmorphic disorder are also comorbid. In children, comorbidities include high-functioning autism and selective mutism.

Panic Disorder

Panic attacks are the key feature of **panic disorder**. A **panic attack** is the sudden onset of extreme apprehension or fear, usually associated with feelings of impending doom. The feelings of terror present during a panic attack are so severe that normal functioning is suspended, the perceptual field is severely limited, and misinterpretation of reality may occur. People experiencing panic attacks may believe they are losing their minds or having a heart attack. Typically, panic attacks come "out of the blue" (i.e., suddenly and not necessarily in response to stress), are extremely intense, last a matter of minutes, and then subside.

Unpredictability is a key aspect of panic disorder in children and adolescents. The attacks of panic seem to come out of nowhere, last about 10 minutes, and then subside. During the

TABLE 15.4 Generic Care Plan for Panic Disorder

Priority diagnosis: Severe anxiety as evidenced by sudden onset of fear of impending doom or dying, increased pulse and respirations, shortness of breath, possible chest pain, dizziness, and abdominal distress.

Outcome criteria: Panic attacks will become less intense and time between episodes will lengthen so that patient can function at the usual level.

Short-Term Goal	Intervention	Rationale
1. Patient's anxiety will decrease to moderate by (date).	1a. If hyperventilation occurs, instruct patient to take slow, deep breaths. Breathing with the patient may be helpful. 1b. Keep expectations minimal and simple.	1a. Focus is shifted away from distressing symptoms. 1b. Anxiety limits ability to attend to complex tasks.
2. Patient will gain mastery over panic episodes by (date).	2a. Help patient connect feelings before attack with onset of attack: "What were you thinking about just before the attack?" "Can you identify what you were feeling just before the attack?" 2b. Help patient recognize symptoms as resulting from anxiety, not from a catastrophic physical problem. Examples: Explain physical symptoms of anxiety. Discuss the fact that anxiety causes sensations similar to those of physical events, such as a heart attack. 2c. Identify effective therapies for panic episodes. 2d. Teach patient abdominal breathing to be immediately used when anxiety is detected. 2e. Teach patient to use positive self-talk, such as "I can control my anxiety." 2f. Teach patient and family about any medication ordered for patient's panic attacks.	2a. Physiological symptoms of anxiety usually appear first as the result of a stressor. They are immediately followed by automatic thoughts, such as "I'm dying" or "I'm going crazy," which are distorted assessments. 2b. Factual information and alternative interpretations can help patient recognize distortions in thought. 2c. Cognitive-behavioral treatment is highly effective. Anti-anxiety medication is appropriate. 2d. Breathing exercises break the cycle of escalating symptoms of anxiety. 2e. Cognitive restructuring is an effective way to replace negative self-talk. 2f. Patient and family need to know what the medication can do, what the side effects and toxic effects are, and whom to call if untoward reactions occur.

attack the young person is less able to articulate the psychological aspects such as fear. They may become avoidant of situations where help is not available, may develop feelings of hopelessness in controlling these attacks, and may become depressed. Alcohol or substance abuse is not uncommon in adolescents with this disorder.

People who experience these attacks begin to "fear the fear." They become so preoccupied about future episodes of panic that they avoid what could be pleasurable and adaptive activities, experiences, and obligations.

Major depression may occur before the onset of panic disorder or may occur at the same time. Substance use disorder frequently accompanies panic disorder, probably as attempts to self-medicate. Nonpsychiatric disorders are also comorbid. They include hyperthyroidism, dizziness, cardiac arrhythmias, asthma, chronic obstructive pulmonary disease (COPD), and irritable bowel syndrome.

Table 15.4 outlines a generic nursing care plan for panic disorder. The *DSM-5* box contains diagnostic criteria for panic disorder.

DSM-5 CRITERIA FOR PANIC DISORDER

A. Recurrent unexpected panic attacks. A panic attack is an abrupt surge of intense fear or intense discomfort that reaches a peak within minutes and during which time four (or more) of the following symptoms occur:

Note: The abrupt surge can occur from a calm state or an anxious state.

1. Palpitations, pounding heart, or accelerated heart rate.
2. Sweating.
3. Trembling or shaking.
4. Sensations of shortness of breath or smothering.
5. Feelings of choking.
6. Chest pain or discomfort.
7. Nausea or abdominal distress.
8. Feeling dizzy, unsteady, light-headed, or faint.
9. Chills or heat sensations.
10. Paresthesias (numbness or tingling sensations).
11. Derealization (feelings of unreality) or depersonalization (being detached from oneself).
12. Fear of losing control or "going crazy."
13. Fear of dying.

Note: Culture-specific symptoms (e.g., tinnitus, neck soreness, headache, uncontrollable screaming or crying) may be seen. Such symptoms should not count as one of the four required symptoms.

B. At least one of the attacks has been followed by 1 month (or more) of one or both of the following:

1. Persistent concern or worry about additional panic attacks or their consequences (e.g., losing control, having a heart attack, "going crazy").
2. A significant maladaptive change in behavior related to the attacks (e.g., behaviors designed to avoid having panic attacks such as avoidance of exercise or unfamiliar situations).

C. The disturbance is not attributable to the physiological effects of a substance (e.g., a drug of abuse, a medication) or another medical condition (e.g., hyperthyroidism, cardiopulmonary disorders).

D. The disturbance is not better explained by another mental disorder (e.g., the panic attacks do not occur only in response to feared social situations, as in social anxiety disorder; in response to circumscribed phobic objects or situations, as in specific phobia; in response to obsessions, as in obsessive-compulsive disorder; in response to reminders of traumatic events, as in posttraumatic stress disorder; or in response to separation from attachment figures, as in separation anxiety disorder).

Agoraphobia

The term agoraphobia is derived from the Greek *agora* ("open space") and phobia ("fear"). It refers to intense excessive anxiety or fear about being in places or situations from which escape might be difficult or embarrassing, or in which help might not be available. The feared places are avoided in an effort to control anxiety. Situations that are commonly avoided are being alone outside, being alone at home, traveling in a car, bus, or airplane, being on a bridge, and riding in an elevator. These situations may be made more tolerable in the company of another.

Avoidance behaviors can be debilitating and life constricting. Consider the effect on a father whose agoraphobia renders him unable to leave home and prevents him from seeing his child's high school graduation.

Nearly 2% of adolescents and adults experience agoraphobia in a given year. Some children may develop the disorder, but it typically begins in late adolescence or early adulthood. The ratio of females to males with agoraphobia is 2:1.

Adverse childhood events and stressful life events are associated with the development of agoraphobia. Families of origin are often described as emotionally cool and overprotective. Genetics are also implicated in this disorder. Agoraphobia has a strong heritability factor of 61%.

Before the onset of this fear-based disorder, many individuals will experience other anxiety disorders such as phobias, panic, and social anxiety. After the onset of agoraphobia individuals often experience depressive disorders and alcohol use disorder.

EVIDENCE-BASED PRACTICE

Using Simulation to Prepare for Psychiatric Nursing Clinical Experiences

Problem

Students frequently report feelings of anxiety, fear, and negative attitudes before going to psychiatric nursing clinical experiences. The anxiety may be moderate to severe as students anticipate working with patients who are experiencing suicidal ideation, psychosis, mania, or aggressiveness.

Purpose of Study

The purpose of the study was to investigate the impact of clinical simulation on nursing student anxiety before the psychiatric nursing clinical experience.

Methods

Three groups of undergraduate nursing students (N = 44) were given a pretest set of questionnaires that included two anxiety measures (i.e., the State-Trait Anxiety Inventory and the visual analogue scale). Afterward they (1) participated in a 2-hour lecture on therapeutic communication techniques and (2) interacted individually with the simulator (SimMan), which alternated between two scenarios—anxiety accompanied by alcohol use or depression. A posttest using the same anxiety measures followed the simulation experience.

Key Findings

- Before the simulation experience students' state traits were "somewhat" anxious. After the simulation experience students' scores were between "not at all" and "somewhat."
- The visual analogue scale scores also demonstrated a decrease in anxiety.

Implications for Nursing Practice

The authors of this study concluded that clinical simulation improves anxiety levels and support the development of a subsequent therapeutic relationship in the actual clinical area. Improving the quality of the clinical experience may increase students' interest in eventually choosing a career in this area.

Szpak, J.L., & Kameg, K.M. (2013). Simulation decreases nursing student anxiety prior to communication with mentally ill patients. *Clinical Simulation in Nursing, 9*(1), e13-e19.

Generalized Anxiety Disorder

The key pathological feature of generalized anxiety disorder is excessive worry. Children, teens, and adults may experience this worry, which is out of proportion to the true impact of events or situations.

Common worries in generalized anxiety disorder are inadequacy in interpersonal relationships, job responsibilities, finances, and health of family members. Because of this worry, huge amounts of time are spent in preparing for activities. Putting things off and avoidance are key symptoms and may result in lateness or absence from school or employment and overall social isolation. Family members and friends are overtaxed as the person with this disorder seeks continual reassurance and perseverates about meaningless details.

Sleep disturbance is common because the individual worries about the day's events and real or imagined mistakes, reviews past problems, and anticipates future difficulties. Fatigue is a noticeable side effect of this sleep deprivation.

The 12-month prevalence rate of generalized anxiety disorder is nearly 1% in adolescents and nearly 3% in adults. Over a lifetime, the risk of this disorder is 9%. The ratio of affected females to males is 2:1.

Parental overprotection and adverse experiences are associated with anxiety disorders. Genetics account for one-third of the risk for developing generalized anxiety disorder.

This anxiety problem is often comorbid with major depressive disorder. Other anxiety disorders frequently accompany generalized anxiety disorder.

Refer to Table 15.5 for a generic care plan for generalized anxiety disorder. The *DSM-5* box contains diagnostic criteria for generalized anxiety disorder.

DSM-5 CRITERIA FOR GENERALIZED ANXIETY DISORDER

A. Excessive anxiety and worry (apprehensive expectation), occurring more days than not for at least 6 months, about a number of events or activities (such as work or school performance).

B. The individual finds it difficult to control the worry.

C. The anxiety and worry are associated with three (or more) of the following six symptoms (with at least some symptoms having been present for more days than not for the past 6 months):

Note: Only one item is required for children.

1. Restlessness or feeling keyed up or on edge.
2. Being easily fatigued.
3. Difficulty concentrating or mind going blank.

Continued

DSM-5 CRITERIA FOR GENERALIZED ANXIETY DISORDER—cont'd

4. Irritability.
5. Muscle tension.
6. Sleep disturbance (difficulty falling or staying asleep, or restless, unsatisfying sleep).

D. The anxiety, worry, or physical symptoms cause clinically significant distress or impairment in social, occupational, or other important areas of functioning.

E. The disturbance is not attributable to the physiological effects of a substance (e.g., a drug of abuse, a medication) or another medical condition (e.g., hyperthyroidism).

F. The disturbance is not better explained by another mental disorder (e.g., anxiety or worry about having panic attacks in panic disorder, negative evaluation in social anxiety disorder, contamination or other obsessions in obsessive-compulsive disorder, separation from attachment figures in separation anxiety disorder, reminders of traumatic events in posttraumatic stress disorder, gaining weight in anorexia nervosa, physical complaints in somatic symptom disorder, perceived appearance flaws in body dysmorphic disorder, having a serious illness in illness anxiety disorder, or the content of delusional beliefs in schizophrenia or delusional disorder.

Other Anxiety Disorders

Selective mutism is a condition where children do not speak due to fears of negative responses or evaluation. They tend to speak at home around immediate family members. When engaged in activities that do not require speech, these children seem comfortable.

Substance-induced anxiety disorder is characterized by symptoms of anxiety, panic attacks, obsessions, and compulsions that develop with the use of a substance (e.g., alcohol, cocaine, heroin, hallucinogens).

In **anxiety due to a medical condition**, the individual's symptoms of anxiety are a direct physiological result of a medical condition, such as hyperthyroidism, pulmonary embolism, or cardiac dysrhythmias. To determine whether the anxiety symptoms are due to a medical condition, a careful and comprehensive assessment of multiple factors is necessary. Refer to Table 15.6 for a list of medical disorders that may contribute to anxiety symptoms.

OBSESSIVE-COMPULSIVE DISORDERS

Obsessive-compulsive disorders are a group of related disorders that all have obsessive-compulsive characteristics. **Obsessions** are defined as thoughts, impulses, or images that persist and recur so that they cannot be dismissed from the mind even though the individual attempts to do so. Obsessions often seem senseless to the individual who experiences them (ego-dystonic), and their presence causes severe anxiety.

Compulsions are ritualistic behaviors an individual feels driven to perform in an attempt to reduce anxiety or prevent an imagined calamity. Performing the compulsive act temporarily reduces anxiety, but because the relief is only temporary, the compulsive act must be repeated again and again.

Although obsessions and compulsions can exist independently of each other, they most often occur together. Examples of common obsessions and compulsions are given in Table 15.7.

TABLE 15.5 Generic Care Plan for Generalized Anxiety Disorder

Priority diagnosis: Ineffective coping related to persistent anxiety, fatigue, difficulty concentrating.
Outcome criteria: Patient will maintain role performance.

Short-Term Goal	Intervention	Rationale
1. Patient will state that immediate distress is relieved by end of session.	1a. Stay with patient. 1b. Speak slowly and calmly. 1c. Use short simple sentences. 1d. Assure patient that you are in control and can assist him or her. 1e. Give brief directions. 1f. Decrease excessive stimuli; provide quiet environment. 1g. After assessing level of anxiety, administer appropriate dose of antianxiety drug as needed.	1a. Conveys acceptance and ability to give help. 1b. Conveys calm and promotes security. 1c. Promotes comprehension. 1d. Counters feeling of loss of control that accompanies severe anxiety. 1e. Reduces indecision. Conveys belief that patient can respond in a healthy manner. 1f. Reduces need to focus on diverse stimuli. Promotes ability to concentrate. 1g. Reduces anxiety and allows patient to use coping skills.
2. Patient will be able to identify precipitants of anxiety by (date).	2a. Encourage patient to discuss preceding events. 2b. Link patient's behavior to feelings. 2c. Teach a cognitive therapy principle: Anxiety is the result of automatic thinking with a dysfunctional appraisal of a situation. 2d. Ask questions that clarify and dispute illogical thinking: "What evidence do you have?" "Are you basing that conclusion on fact or feeling?" "What's the worst thing that could happen?" 2e. Encourage patient to provide an alternative interpretation.	2a. Promotes future change through identification of stressors. 2b. Promotes self-awareness. 2c. Provides a basis for behavioral change. 2d. Helps promote accurate cognition. 2e. Broadens perspective. Helps patient think in a new way about problem or symptom.
3. Patient will identify strengths and coping skills by (date).	3a. Identify what has provided relief in the past. 3b. Have patient write assessment of strengths. 3c. Reframe situation in ways that are positive.	3a. Provides awareness of self as individual with some ability to cope. 3b. Increases self-acceptance. 3c. Provides a new perspective and converts distorted thinking.

Obsessive-Compulsive Disorder

Obsessive-compulsive behavior exists along a continuum. Most sufferers may experience mildly obsessive-compulsive behavior such as nagging doubts as to whether a door is locked or the stove is turned off. These doubts require the person to go back to check the door or stove. Mild compulsions about timeliness, orderliness, and reliability are valued traits in US society.

At the pathological end of the continuum is **obsessive-compulsive disorder (OCD)** with symptoms that occur on a daily basis and may involve issues of sexuality, violence, contamination, illness, or death. Pathological obsessions or compulsions cause marked distress to individuals who often feel humiliation and shame regarding these behaviors.

The rituals are time-consuming and interfere with normal routines, social activities, and relationships with others. Severe OCD occupies so much of the individual's mental processes that the performance of cognitive tasks is impaired. English soccer player David Beckham has shared his struggle with OCD. He has a compulsion to count his clothes and line his magazines up in a straight line.

The 12-month prevalence of OCD is 1.2%. Females are slightly more affected, but males have an earlier age of onset (about 25% before age 10). Onset after age 35 is rare.

Sexual and physical abuse in childhood or trauma increases the risk of this disorder. Some children develop OCD along with a postinfectious autoimmune syndrome. Genetics are strongly associated with this disorder. First-degree relatives have twice the risk. Early onset OCD results in a 10 times greater risk in first-degree relatives.

OCD tends to occur along with anxiety disorders 76% of the time. Other comorbid conditions for OCD include major depressive disorder, bipolar disorder, and eating disorders. About 30% of individuals with this problem also have a tic disorder.

See the *DSM-5* box for diagnostic criteria.

TABLE 15.6 Common Medical Causes of Anxiety

System	Disorders
Respiratory	Chronic obstructive pulmonary disease
	Pulmonary embolism
	Asthma
	Hypoxia
	Pulmonary edema
Cardiovascular	Angina pectoris
	Arrhythmias
	Congestive heart failure
	Hypertension
	Hypotension
	Mitral valve prolapse
Endocrine	Hyperthyroidism
	Hypoglycemia
	Pheochromocytoma
	Carcinoid syndrome
	Hypercortisolism
Neurological	Delirium
	Essential tremor
	Complex partial seizures
	Parkinson's disease
	Akathisia
	Otoneurological disorders
	Postconcussion syndrome
Metabolic	Hypercalcemia
	Hyperkalemia
	Hyponatremia
	Porphyria

DSM-5 CRITERIA FOR OBSESSIVE-COMPULSIVE DISORDER

A. Presence of obsessions, compulsions, or both.

Obsessions are defined by (1) and (2):

1. Recurrent and persistent thoughts, urges, or images that are experienced, at some time during the disturbance, as intrusive and unwanted, and that in most individuals cause marked anxiety or distress.
2. The individual attempts to ignore or suppress such thoughts, urges, or images or to neutralize them with some other thought or action (i.e., by performing a compulsion).

Compulsions are defined by (1) and (2):

1. Repetitive behaviors (e.g., hand washing, ordering, checking) or mental acts (e.g., praying, counting, repeating words silently) that the individual feels driven to perform in response to an obsession or according to rules that must be applied rigidly.

Continued

TABLE 15.7 Common Obsessions and Compulsions

Type of Obsession	Example	Accompanying Compulsion
Losing control and religious concerns	A middle-age man worries, "If I go to church, what will stop me from blurting out obscenities?"	Despite his desire to attend services, has not gone to church in 2 years.
Harm	"If I don't turn the light switch off, the room will catch on fire, and my mom will die while I am at school," worries a 9-year-old girl.	Returns to her room four times before school, checks that the light is turned off, and taps the four sides of the light switch.
Unwanted sexual thoughts	A young man has a recurrent thought: "What if I get a sexually transmitted disease from a prostitute during sleepwalking?"	Ritualistically locks the doors of the house with a key each night and hides his wallet.
Perfectionism	"My work is never second best," proclaims an administrative assistant.	Gets to work early, leaves work late, never has a messy desk, always completes tasks.
Violence	A man repeatedly has the thought "I should kill her" when he sees a blonde woman.	Abruptly turns head away from women and squints eyes to try to avoid seeing blondes.
Contamination	A woman ruminates, "Everything is covered in germs."	Avoids touching all objects; scrubs hands if forced to touch any object.
Superstitions	"All lists need to end in an even number," thinks a college professor.	Adds or deletes items from tests, agendas, and other numbered items.

DSM-5 CRITERIA FOR OBSESSIVE-COMPULSIVE DISORDER—cont'd

2. The behaviors or mental acts are aimed at preventing or reducing anxiety or distress or preventing some dreaded event or situation; however, these behaviors or mental acts are not connected in a realistic way with what they are designed to neutralize or prevent or are clearly excessive.

Note: Young children may not be able to articulate the aims of these behaviors or mental acts.

B. The obsessions or compulsions are time-consuming (e.g., take more than 1 hour per day) or cause clinically significant distress or impairment in social, occupational, or other important areas of functioning.

C. The obsessive-compulsive symptoms are not attributable to the physiological effects of a substance (e.g., a drug of abuse, a medication) or another medical condition.

D. The disturbance is not better explained by the symptoms of another mental disorder (e.g., excessive worries, as in generalized anxiety disorder; preoccupation with appearance, as in body dysmorphic disorder; difficulty discarding or parting with possessions, as in hoarding disorder; hair pulling, as in trichotillomania, skin picking, as in excoriation disorder; stereotypes, as in stereotypic movement disorder; ritualized eating behavior, as in eating disorders; preoccupation with substances or gambling, as in substance-related and addictive disorder; preoccupation with having an illness, as in illness anxiety disorder; sexual urges or fantasies, as in paraphilic disorders; impulses, as in disruptive, impulse-control, and conduct disorders; guilty ruminations, as in major depressive disorder; thought insertion or delusional preoccupations, as in schizophrenia spectrum and other psychotic disorders; or repetitive patterns of behavior, as in autism spectrum disorder.

Reprinted with permission from American Psychiatric Association. (2013). *Diagnostic and statistical manual* (5th ed.). Washington, D.C: Author.

Body Dysmorphic Disorder

Body dysmorphic disorder was first described over a century ago and continues to be a challenge to treat. Patients with body dysmorphic disorder are commonly seen in community, psychiatric, cosmetic surgery, and dermatological settings. Although patients tend to have a normal appearance, their preoccupation with an imagined defective body part results in obsessional thinking and compulsive behavior such as mirror checking and camouflaging. In body dysmorphic disorder levels of insight vary. People may be well aware that their thoughts are distorted, or they may be completely sure about existence of the defect.

False assumptions about the importance of appearance, fear of rejection by others, perfectionism, and conviction of being disfigured lead to overwhelming emotions of disgust, shame, and depression. Patients are frequently concerned with their skin, hair, nose, stomach, teeth, weight, and breasts/chest. Men tend to be concerned with body build and the appearance of their genitals and body build. Women focus on the appearance of their skin, stomach, weight, breasts, buttocks, thighs, legs, hips, and toes.

Often the patient keeps the disorder secret for many years. The disorder is chronic and response to treatment is limited. Suicide risk is high in this population.

The prevalence of body dysmorphic disorder is slightly higher in females (2.5%) than males (2.2%). The rate of this problem is higher among patients seeking cosmetic surgery, dermatology treatment, adult orthodontia, and oral/maxillofacial surgery.

Individuals with this disorder often come from homes with abuse and neglect. Body dysmorphic disorder seems to be related to OCD because first-degree relatives often share those conditions.

The most common comorbid disorder is major depressive disorder, which usually comes on after body dysmorphic disorder. Social anxiety disorder, OCD, and substance use disorders are also seen along with this disorder.

Hoarding Disorder

Have you ever reached the point where there is just too much clutter in your closet and you proceed to sort through it and make stacks of keep, give away, and donate? You probably have, and for most of us this is neither a pleasant nor painful experience. For individuals with **hoarding disorder**, this purging would have been extremely distressing. In fact, the accumulation of belongings that may have little nor no value prevents some people from leading normal lives. Belongings literally fill every available surface and area in their residences, and guests can (or will) no longer visit. The problem may progress to the point where the home is nearly uninhabitable due to unsafe and unsanitary conditions. Individuals who hoard may or may not be aware of the problem and how the quest to collect has consumed their lives and alienated others.

It is difficult to determine the age of onset for this disorder as children do not have the means to add to their collections as adults do. Symptoms usually emerge in adolescence, begin to interfere with functioning in the 20s, and significantly impair functioning in the 30s. The condition worsens with each decade of life. While more women are treated for hoarding disorder, it is likely that men are affected at much the same rate but do not seek treatment for this problem. Estimates of prevalence from the United Kingdom are about 1.5% (Nordsletten et al., 2013).

Indecisiveness is associated with hoarding. Stressful life events seem to precede the onset of symptoms. The disorder is strongly heritable with a twin concordance rate (percentage of time one twin will be affected when the other one is) of 50%.

Nearly all hoarders (75%) also experience major depressive and/or anxiety disorders. Not surprisingly, about 20% of this population also has obsessive-compulsive disorder. It is the presence of these other disorders that may cause these individuals to get treatment because they resist seeing hoarding as a problem.

Trichotillomania and Excoriation Disorder

Trichotillomania, or **hair pulling disorder**, and **excoriation disorder**, or **skin picking disorder**, are two distressing problems that may result in varying degrees of disability, social stigma, and altered appearance. Both of the activities are irresistible to the individual who typically tries to hide the activity. These disorders have been linked to symptoms of OCD. It occurs more often in children than adults and may begin as early as 1 year of age.

Trichotillomania (tricho·til·lo·ma·nia) may be one of the oldest recorded psychiatric problems. The phrase "I was so annoyed that I wanted to pull my hair out" attests to the anxiety-related component of the disorder. Typically, it is the hair of the head, but it may come from anywhere on the body including eyebrows, eyelashes, pubic areas, axilla, and limbs. The amount of hair removed ranges from small patches to complete baldness. For some, the pain brought on by hair pulling results in anxiety reduction, similar to those who engage in cutting. Most individuals may be unaware of the behavior until they notice a wad of hair close by.

Trichophagia, or secretly swallowing the pulled hair, is common in this disorder. This ingestion may lead to hair masses, or trichobezoar, in the gastrointestinal system. The masses can be fatal if they progress to abdominal obstruction or perforation. You may be interested to know that the masses of digested hair are also referred to as the Rapunzel syndrome.

The disorder may begin in childhood, adolescence, or even adulthood and may last weeks to decades. The 12-month prevalence in adolescents and adults is about 2%. Females are affected more frequently than males, with a ratio around 10:1. There is no gender difference in children.

The disorder seems to run in families. Individuals with relatives who have OCD tend to have higher rates of trichotillomania. People who obsessively pull their hair also often have major depressive disorder. Trichotillomania is often accompanied by excoriation disorder.

The skin picking of **excoriation** (ex·co·ri·ay·shun) **disorder** is typically confined to the face, although other areas of the body may be targeted. As with hair pulling, the individual may engage in skin picking as a means to deal with stress and relieve anxiety, while others may engage in this activity without thinking about it. Most people occasionally pick at their skin, nails, and scabs; however people with skin picking disorder damage their skin. Fingers and fingernails are the usual implements, but biting, nail cutters, and tweezers are also used. The most common areas of focus are the face, head, cuticles, back, arms and legs, and hands and feet. Complications include pain, sores, scars, and infections.

The lifetime prevalence of this problem is 1.4%. Seventy-five percent of those affected are females. The onset is in adolescence and frequently begins with conditions such as acne.

A risk factor for this disorder is having relatives with obsessive-compulsive disorder. Excoriation disorder is often accompanied by obsessive-compulsive disorders and trichotillomania.

Other Compulsive Disorders

Substance-induced obsessive-compulsive and related disorders are characterized by obsessions and compulsions that develop with the use of a substance or within a month of stopping use of the substance. Drugs used to treat the movement disorders in Parkinson's disease have been reported to cause obsessions with gambling, irresistible urges for sex, and out-of-control spending. This diagnosis is based on a thorough history, physical examination, and laboratory findings.

In **obsessive-compulsive or related disorders due to a medical condition**, the individual's symptoms of obsessions and compulsions are a direct physiological result of a medical condition such as a postencephalatic syndrome, postanoxic event, traumatic brain injury, Huntington's disease, seizures, and cerebral infarctions. To determine whether the symptoms are due to a medical condition, a careful and comprehensive assessment of multiple factors is necessary. Evidence must be present in the history, physical examination, or laboratory findings for this diagnosis.

RISK FACTORS

There is no longer any doubt that biological factors predispose some individuals to pathological anxiety states (e.g., phobias, panic attacks). By the same token, traumatic life events, psychosocial factors, and sociocultural factors are also etiologically significant.

Biological Factors

Genetic

Numerous studies substantiate that anxiety disorders tend to cluster in families. Genetic variants have been identified that are associated with increased risk for anxiety and obsessive-compulsive disorders. Twin studies demonstrate the existence of a genetic component to both panic disorder and OCD. First-degree biological relatives of those with OCD or phobias have a higher frequency of these disorders than exists in the general population.

Neurobiological

The amygdala plays a role in anxiety and obsessive-compulsive disorders. The amygdala alerts the brain to the presence of danger and brings about fear or anxiety to preserve the system. Memories with emotional significance are stored in the brain and have been implicated in phobic responses such as fear of snakes, heights, or open spaces.

Certain anatomic pathways (e.g., the limbic system) provide the transmission structure for the electrical impulses that occur when anxiety-related responses are sent or received. Neurons release chemicals (i.e., neurotransmitters) that convey these messages. The neurochemicals that regulate anxiety include epinephrine, norepinephrine, dopamine, serotonin, and gamma-aminobutyric acid (GABA).

The jury is still out on the role of serotonin in anxiety disorders. Because selective serotonin reuptake inhibitors (SSRIs) increase neural serotonin, researchers have assumed that low levels of serotonin are at least partially to blame for anxiety symptoms. Recently, Frick and colleagues (2015) discovered that serotonin in one anxiety problem, social anxiety disorder, was actually elevated in the amygdala. This finding calls into question the role of the SSRIs in improving anxiety symptoms.

GABA, an inhibitory neurotransmitter that puts a brake on excitatory neurotransmitters, is commonly the focus of pharmacological therapy for anxiety symptoms. GABA slows neuron activity, which plays a role in lowering anxiety. It is believed that people with too little GABA may suffer from anxiety disorders.

Psychological Factors

Psychodynamic theories suggest that unconscious childhood conflicts are the basis for future symptom development. Sigmund Freud posited that anxiety results when threatening repressed ideas or emotions are close to breaking through from the unconscious mind into the aware and conscious mind. Freud also suggested that ego-defense mechanisms are used to keep anxiety at manageable levels (refer to Chapter 2). The use of defense mechanisms may result in overuse of behavior that is not wholly adaptive because of its rigidity and repetitive nature.

Harry Stack Sullivan (1953) believed that anxiety is linked to the emotional distress caused when early needs go unmet or disapproval is experienced (**interpersonal theory**). He also suggested that anxiety is "contagious," being transmitted to the infant from the mother or caregiver. Thus the anxiety felt early in life becomes the prototype for anxiety responses when unpleasant events occur later in life.

Behavioral theories suggest that anxiety is a learned response to specific environmental stimuli (classical conditioning). An example of classical conditioning is a boy who is anxious in the presence of his abusive mother. He then generalizes this anxiety as a response to all women. Conditioning can be reversed through the influence of safe and loving female friends and significant others.

The social learning model suggests that anxiety is learned through the modeling of parents or peers. For example, a mother who is fearful of thunder and lightning and hides in closets during storms may transmit her anxiety to her children. These children continue to immitate this fearful behavior into adult life. Such individuals can unlearn this behavior by observing others who react normally to a storm by lighting candles and telling stories.

Cognitive theorists believe that anxiety disorders are caused by distortions in an individual's thoughts and perceptions. Because individuals with such distortions exaggerate any mistake and believe that they will have catastrophic results, they experience acute anxiety. People who tend to perceive events and situations as being potentially dangerous may be overly responsive and become anxious or even experience panic attacks.

Cultural Considerations

Sociocultural variation in symptoms of anxiety disorders has been noted. In some cultures, individuals express anxiety through somatic symptoms, whereas in other cultures, cognitive symptoms predominate. Panic attacks in Latin Americans and Northern Europeans often involve sensations of choking, smothering, numbness, or tingling, as well as fear of dying. In other cultural groups, panic attacks involve fear of magic or witchcraft. Social anxiety in Japanese and Korean cultures may relate to beliefs that the individual's blushing, eye contact, or body odor is offensive to others.

The Considering Culture box discusses factors relevant to one anxiety disorder (ataque de nervios) primarily experienced by people from Hispanic cultures. Refer to Chapter 5 for more discussion of cultural issues.

CONSIDERING CULTURE

Attack of the Nerves in Hispanic People

Technology and the commonplace of travel have resulted in a "smaller" world. Psychiatric-mental health nurses in the United States will be exposed to culture-bound syndromes with which they may be unfamiliar.

One example of a culture-bound syndrome is ataque de nervios, or in English, "attack of the nerves." This is a disorder found primarily among Hispanic populations in response to stressful events such as a death, acute family discord, or witnessing an accident. Symptoms are dramatic: sudden trembling, faintness, palpitations, out-of-control shouting, heat that moves from the chest to head, and seizure-like activities. After the episode, the affected individual often has little memory of it. This disorder is more common in socially disadvantaged females with less than a high school education.

What do these symptoms sound like to you? Some clinicians and researchers believe that it is closely related to an anxiety disorder and could even be a form of panic attack. Unlike people who have panic attacks individuals with this disorder are responding to a precipitating event, and they do not typically experience fear or apprehension before the attack.

Henderson, D. C., Vincenzi, B., Yeung, A. S., & Fricchione, G. L. (2016). Culture and psychiatry. In T. A. Stern, M. Fava, T. E. Wilens, & J. F. Rosenbaum (Eds.), *Massachusetts General Hospital comprehensive clinical psychiatry* (2nd ed.). Philadelphia, PA: Elsevier.

APPLICATION OF THE NURSING PROCESS

ASSESSMENT

General Assessment

People with anxiety and obsessive-compulsive disorders rarely need hospitalization unless they are suicidal or have compulsions that cause injury (e.g., cutting self, infected sores from picking). Most of these individuals are encountered incidentally in a variety of community settings. A common example is someone taken to an emergency department to rule out a heart attack when in fact the individual is experiencing a panic attack. It is essential to determine whether the anxiety is the primary problem, as in an anxiety disorder, or secondary to another source (medical condition or substance).

Your assessment should be *patient-centered* to be helpful or meaningful. First and foremost is the recognition that the patient is the expert when it comes to his or her own illness. Elicit information about what has helped in the past. Identify expectations for the patient's personal participation in care and for the family or significant other's participation in care. Assess for specific cultural, ethnic, and social backgrounds that may impact the care that you and the patient plan.

Objectively, there are a variety of scales available to measure anxiety and anxiety-related symptoms, and most are available online. The Yale-Brown Obsessive Compulsive Scale measures severity of compulsive behavior. The Hoarding Scale Self-Report measures hoarding; phobias are measured on the Fear Questionnaire; and panic symptoms are measured on the Panic Disorder Severity Scale. The Severity Measure for Generalized Anxiety Disorder in Adults is a popular tool for measuring anxiety (Fig. 15.2). High scores may indicate generalized anxiety disorder or panic disorder, although it is important to note that high anxiety scores may also be a symptom of major depressive disorder.

Self-Assessment

As a nurse working with an individual with an anxiety or obsessive-compulsive disorder, you may have feelings of frustration, especially if it seems that his or her symptoms are a matter of choice or under personal control. The rituals of the patient with obsessive-compulsive disorder may seriously slow your ability to complete certain nursing tasks within the usual time. How do you respond to a person with a phobia who acknowledges that the fear is exaggerated and unrealistic yet continues to engage in avoidant behavior?

Behavioral change is often accomplished slowly. The recovery process is very different from what is seen in physical disorders such as an infection. After being given antibiotics, improvement may be seen in as little as 24 hours. Planning outcomes in small attainable steps can help prevent you from feeling overwhelmed by the patient's slow progress and help the patient gain a sense of control.

DIAGNOSIS

The North American Nursing Diagnosis Association International (Herdman & Kamitsuru, 2014) provides many nursing diagnoses that can be considered for patients with anxiety and obsessive-compulsive disorders. The related-to component will vary with the individual patient.

Severity Measure for Generalized Anxiety Disorder—Adult

Name: ____________ Age: ____ Sex: Male ☐ Female ☐ Date: ____________

Instructions: The following questions ask about thoughts, feelings, and behaviors, often tied to concerns about family, health, finances, school, and work. **Please respond to each item by marking (✓ or x) one box per row.**

During the PAST 7 DAYS, I have...	Never	Occasionally	Half of the time	Most of the time	All of the time	Clinician use: Item Score
1 felt moments of sudden terror, fear, or fright	☐ 0	☐ 1	☐ 2	☐ 3	☐ 4	
2 felt anxious, worried, or nervous	☐ 0	☐ 1	☐ 2	☐ 3	☐ 4	
3 had thoughts of bad things happening, such as family tragedy, ill health, loss of a job, or accidents	☐ 0	☐ 1	☐ 2	☐ 3	☐ 4	
4 felt a racing heart, sweaty, trouble breathing, faint, or shaky	☐ 0	☐ 1	☐ 2	☐ 3	☐ 4	
5 felt tense muscles, felt on edge or restless, or had trouble relaxing or trouble sleeping	☐ 0	☐ 1	☐ 2	☐ 3	☐ 4	
6 avoided, or did not approach or enter, situations about which I worry	☐ 0	☐ 1	☐ 2	☐ 3	☐ 4	
7 left situations early or participated only minimally due to worries	☐ 0	☐ 1	☐ 2	☐ 3	☐ 4	
8 spent lots of time making decisions, putting off making decisions, or preparing for situations, due to worries	☐ 0	☐ 1	☐ 2	☐ 3	☐ 4	
9 sought reassurance from others due to worries	☐ 0	☐ 1	☐ 2	☐ 3	☐ 4	
10 needed help to cope with anxiety (e.g., alcohol or medication, superstitious objects, or other people)	☐ 0	☐ 1	☐ 2	☐ 3	☐ 4	
Total/partial raw score:						
Prorated total raw score: (if 1–2 items left unanswered)						
Average total score:						

FIG. 15.2 Severity Measure for Generalized Anxiety Disorder in Adults.

ASSESSMENT GUIDELINES

Anxiety and Obsessive-Compulsive Disorders

1. Ensure that a sound physical and neurological examination is performed to help determine whether the anxiety is primary or secondary to another psychiatric disorder, medical condition, or substance use.
2. Determine current level of anxiety (mild, moderate, severe, or panic).
3. Assess for the potential for self-harm and suicidal ideation. People suffering from high levels of intractable anxiety may become desperate and attempt suicide.
4. Perform a psychosocial assessment. Always ask the person, "What is going on in your life that may be contributing to your anxiety?" The patient may identify a problem (stressful marriage, recent loss, stressful job, or school situation) that should be addressed by counseling.

OUTCOMES IDENTIFICATION

The *Nursing Outcomes Classification (NOC)* identifies desired outcomes for patients with anxiety-related or obsessive-compulsive disorders (Moorhead et al., 2013). Outcomes are linked with signs and symptoms and nursing diagnoses in Table 15.8.

PLANNING

Whenever possible, the patient should be encouraged to participate actively in planning. By sharing decision making with the patient, you can increase the likelihood that the treatment regimen will be successful. Owning responsibility for health outcomes improves adherence. Shared planning is especially appropriate for someone with mild or moderate anxiety. When experiencing severe levels of anxiety, a patient may be unable to participate in planning, and the nurse may be required to take a more directive role.

IMPLEMENTATION

When working with patients with anxiety and obsessive-compulsive disorders, you must first determine what level of anxiety they are experiencing. A general framework for anxiety interventions can then be built on a solid foundation.

Mild to Moderate Levels of Anxiety

A person experiencing a mild to moderate level of anxiety is still able to solve problems; however, the ability to concentrate decreases as anxiety increases. A patient can be helped to focus and solve problems when you use specific nursing communication techniques such as asking open-ended questions, giving broad openings, and exploring and seeking clarification. Closing off topics of communication and bringing up irrelevant topics can increase a person's anxiety, making the *nurse*, not the *patient*, feel better.

Reducing the patient's anxiety level and preventing escalation to more distressing levels can be aided by providing a calm presence, recognizing the anxious person's distress, and being willing to listen. Evaluation of effective past coping mechanisms is also useful. Often you can help the patient consider alternatives to problem situations and offer activities that may temporarily relieve feelings of inner tension. Table 15.9 identifies interventions useful in assisting people experiencing mild to moderate levels of anxiety.

Severe to Panic Levels of Anxiety

A person experiencing a severe to panic level of anxiety is unable to solve problems and may have a poor grasp of what is happening in the environment. Unproductive relief behaviors may take over, and the person may not be in control.

Priority nursing interventions are to provide for the safety of the patient and others and to meet physical needs (e.g., fluids, rest) to prevent exhaustion. Anxiety-reduction measures may take the form of guiding the person to a quiet environment. The use of medications and restraints/seclusion may have to be considered. As always, both medications and restraints should be used only after other less-restrictive interventions have failed to decrease anxiety to safer levels.

Because individuals experiencing severe to panic levels of anxiety are unable to solve problems, the techniques suggested for communicating with people with mild to moderate levels of anxiety are not as effective at more severe levels. Patients experiencing severe to panic anxiety levels are out of control, so

TABLE 15.8 Signs and Symptoms, Nursing Diagnoses, and Outcomes for Anxiety-Related Disorders

Signs and Symptoms	Nursing Diagnoses	Outcomes
Separation from significant other, concern that a panic attack will occur, exposure to phobic object or situation, presence of obsessive thoughts, fear of panic attacks, preoccupation with perceived physical flaws, apprehension about losing prized possessions, pulling hair or picking skin	*Anxiety (moderate, severe, panic)*	Monitors intensity of anxiety, uses relaxation techniques, decreases environmental stimuli as needed, controls anxiety response, maintains role performance
Unable to attend social functions or take employment, anxiety interferes with the ability to work, avoidance behaviors (phobia, agoraphobia), inordinate time taken for obsession and compulsions	*Ineffective coping*	Identifies ineffective coping patterns, asks for assistance, seeks information about illness and treatment, identifies multiple coping strategies, modifies lifestyle as needed
Exaggerated negative perception of physical appearance, ashamed of the appearance of the house due to hoarding activity, believes that others are disgusted with his appearance, embarrassment about the hair or skin condition	*Chronic low self-esteem*	Verbalizes self-acceptance, communicates openly, increases confidence, describes a positive sense of self-worth
Skin excoriation related to rituals of excessive washing, excessive picking at the skin, or pulling hair out	*Self-mutilation*	Identifies feelings that lead to impulsive actions, practices self-restraint of compulsive behaviors

From Herdman, T. H., & Kamitsuru, S. (Eds.). (2014). *Nursing diagnoses—Definitions and classification 2015-2017*. Oxford, UK: Wiley Blackwell. Copyright © 2014, 1994-2012 by NANDA International. Used by arrangement with John Wiley & Sons Limited; Moorhead, S., Johnson, M., Maas, M. L., & Swanson, E. (2013). *Nursing outcomes classification (NOC)* (5th ed.). St. Louis, MO: Mosby.

TABLE 15.9 Interventions for Mild to Moderate Levels of Anxiety

Priority diagnosis: Anxiety (moderate) related to situational event or psychological stress, as evidenced by increase in vital signs, moderate discomfort, narrowing of perceptual field, and selective inattention.

Intervention	Rationale
Help the patient identify anxiety. "Are you comfortable right now?"	It is important to validate observations with the patient, name the anxiety, and start to work with the patient to lower anxiety.
Anticipate anxiety-provoking situations.	Escalation of anxiety to a more disorganizing level is prevented.
Use nonverbal language to demonstrate interest (e.g., lean forward, maintain eye contact, nod your head).	Verbal and nonverbal messages should be consistent. The presence of an interested person provides a stabilizing focus.
Encourage the patient to talk about his or her feelings and concerns.	When concerns are stated aloud, problems can be discussed and feelings of isolation decreased.
Avoid closing off avenues of communication that are important for the patient. Focus on the patient's concerns.	When staff anxiety increases, changing the topic or offering advice is common but leaves the person isolated.
Ask questions to clarify what is being said. "I'm not sure what you mean. Give me an example."	Increased anxiety results in scattering of thoughts. Clarifying helps the patient identify thoughts and feelings.
Help the patient identify thoughts or feelings before the onset of anxiety. "What were you thinking right before you started to feel anxious?"	The patient is assisted in identifying thoughts and feelings, and problem solving is facilitated.
Encourage problem solving with the patient.*	Encouraging patients to explore alternatives increases sense of control and decreases anxiety.
Assist in developing alternative solutions to a problem through role play or modeling behaviors.	The patient is encouraged to try out alternative behaviors and solutions.
Explore behaviors that have worked to relieve anxiety in the past.	The patient is encouraged to mobilize successful coping mechanisms and strengths.
Provide outlets for working off excess energy (e.g., walking, playing ping-pong, dancing, exercising).	Physical activity can provide relief of built-up tension, increase muscle tone, and increase endorphin levels.

*Patients experiencing mild to moderate anxiety levels can problem solve.

they need to know they are safe from their own impulses. Firm, short, and simple statements are useful. Reinforcing commonalities in the environment and pointing out reality when there are distortions can also be useful interventions for severely anxious people. Table 15.10 suggests some basic nursing interventions for patients with severe to panic levels of anxiety.

Anxiety management and reduction are primary concerns when working with patients who have anxiety and obsessive-compulsive disorders, but they may have a variety of other needs. When developing a plan of care, the psychiatric-mental health registered nurse can utilize the *Psychiatric-Mental Health Nursing: Scope and Standards of Practice* (American Nurses Association [ANA] et al., 2014). The *Nursing Interventions Classification (NIC)* offers pertinent interventions in the behavioral and safety domains (Bulechek et al., 2013). Refer to Box 15.1 for potential nursing interventions for patients experiencing anxiety.

Guidelines for basic nursing interventions are:

1. Use counseling, milieu therapy, promotion of self-care activities, and psychobiological and health teaching interventions as appropriate.
2. Guide patients through slow, deep breathing exercises along with progressive muscle relaxation.
3. Identify community resources that can offer the patient specialized treatment proven to be highly effective for people with a variety of anxiety disorders.
4. Identify community support groups for people with specific anxiety disorders and their families.

Counseling

Basic-level psychiatric-mental health registered nurses use counseling to reduce anxiety, enhance coping and communication skills, and intervene in crises. When patients request or prefer to use integrative therapies, the nurse performs assessment and teaching as appropriate.

Teamwork and Safety

As mentioned earlier, most patients who demonstrate anxiety disorders and obsessive-compulsive disorders can be treated successfully as outpatients. Hospital admission is necessary only if severe anxiety or compulsive symptoms interfere with the individual's health or if the individual is suicidal. When hospitalization is necessary, the healthcare team can be especially effective by:

- Collaborating to develop a multidisciplinary treatment plan to address goals, interventions, and outcomes that includes the patient's input.
- Evaluating and refining the plan of care at regular intervals.
- Documenting the plan and other essential communication electronically through an interactive and secure system.
- Identifying specific members of the treatment team to be responsible for carrying out specific actions of the plan.
- Maximizing safety through the provision of calm and consistent care.
- Stressing the value of unconditional positive regard.
- Maintaining a safe environment with an atmosphere of low-level stimulation.
- Providing ongoing education and training for the team to recognize escalating or problematic behaviors.

Promotion of Self-Care Activities

Respecting the patients' preferences for how involved they are in self-care, while recognizing that they may require more or

TABLE 15.10 Interventions for Severe to Panic Levels of Anxiety

Priority diagnosis: Anxiety (severe, panic) related to perception of a severe threat as evidenced by verbal or physical acting out, extreme immobility, sense of impending doom, and inability to problem solve.

Intervention	Rationale
Maintain a calm manner.	Anxiety is communicated interpersonally. The quiet calm of the nurse can serve to calm the patient. The presence of anxiety can escalate anxiety in the patient.
Always remain with the person experiencing an acute severe to panic level of anxiety.	Alone with immense anxiety, a person feels abandoned. A caring face may be the patient's only contact with reality when confusion becomes overwhelming.
Minimize environmental stimuli. Move to a quieter setting, and stay with the patient.	Helps minimize further escalation of patient's anxiety.
Use clear and simple statements and repetition.	A person experiencing a severe to panic level of anxiety has difficulty concentrating and processing information.
Use a low-pitched voice; speak slowly.	A high-pitched voice can convey anxiety. Low pitch can decrease anxiety.
Reinforce reality if distortions occur (e.g., seeing objects that are not there or hearing voices when no one is present).	Anxiety can be reduced by focusing on and validating what is going on in the environment.
Listen for themes in communication.	In severe to panic levels of anxiety, verbal communication themes may be the only indication of the patient's thoughts or feelings.
Attend to physical and safety needs when necessary (e.g., need for warmth, fluids, elimination, pain relief, family contact).	High levels of anxiety may obscure the patient's awareness of physical needs.
Because safety is an overall goal, physical limits may need to be set. Speak in a firm, authoritative voice: "You may not hit anyone here. If you can't control yourself, we will help you."	A person who is out of control is often terrorized. Staff must offer the patient and others protection from destructive and self-destructive impulses.
Provide opportunities for exercise (e.g., walk with nurse, punching bag, ping-pong game).	Physical activity helps channel and dissipate tension and may temporarily lower anxiety.
When a person is constantly moving or pacing, offer high-calorie fluids.	Dehydration and exhaustion must be prevented.
Assess need for medication or seclusion after other interventions have been tried and have been unsuccessful.	Exhaustion and physical harm to self and others must be prevented.

BOX 15.1 Select NIC Interventions for Anxiety Disorders

Coping Enhancement

Definition: Facilitation of cognitive and behavioral efforts to manage perceived stressors, changes, or threats that interfere with meeting life demands and roles.

Activities:

- Provide an atmosphere of acceptance.
- Encourage verbalization of feelings, perceptions, and fears.
- Acknowledge the patient's spiritual/cultural background.
- Discourage decision making when the patient is under severe stress.

Hope Inspiration

Definition: Enhancing the belief in one's capacity to initiate and sustain actions.

Activities:

- Assist the patient to identify areas of hope in life.
- Demonstrate hope by recognizing the patient's intrinsic worth and viewing the patient's illness as only one facet of the individual.
- Avoid masking the truth.
- Help the patient expand spiritual self.

Self-Esteem Enhancement

Definition: Assisting a patient to increase his or her personal judgment of self-worth.

Activities:

- Make positive statements about the patient.
- Monitor frequency of self-negating verbalizations.
- Explore previous achievements.
- Explore reasons for self-criticism or guilt.

Relaxation Therapy

Definition: Use of techniques to encourage and elicit relaxation for the purpose of decreasing undesirable signs and symptoms such as pain, muscle tension, or anxiety.

Activities:

- Demonstrate and practice the relaxation technique with the patient.
- Provide written information about preparing and engaging in relaxation techniques.
- Anticipate the need for the use of relaxation.
- Evaluate and document the response to relaxation therapy.

From Bulechek, G. M., Butcher, H. K., Dochterman, J. M., & Wagner, C. (2013). *Nursing interventions classification (NIC)* (6th ed.). St. Louis, MO: Mosby.

less guidance depending on their level of ability, is a fine balance. Including the patient in care decisions is essential whenever possible. Patients with anxiety and obsessive-compulsive disorders are usually able to meet their own basic physical needs. Self-care activities that are most likely to be affected are discussed in the following sections.

Nutrition and Fluid Intake

Patients with high levels of anxiety are not focused on eating and drinking. Some phobic patients may be so afraid of germs that they cannot eat. In home settings, individuals who hoard may have created an environment that is so dysfunctional that normal intake may be impossible. Likewise, people who engage in ritualistic

TABLE 15.11 **FDA Approved Drugs for Anxiety Disorders**

Anxiety Disorder	Selective Serotonin Reuptake Inhibitors	Serotonin Norepinephrine Reuptake Inhibitors	Benzodiazepines	Other
Generalized anxiety disorder	Escitalopram (Lexapro) Paroxetine (Paxil)	Venlafaxine (Effexor) Duloxetine (Cymbalta)	Alprazolam (Xanax) Chlordiazepoxide (Librium) Clorazepate (Tranxene) Diazepam (Valium) Lorazepam (Ativan) Oxazepam (Serax)	Buspirone (BuSpar)
Panic disorder	Fluoxetine (Prozac) Paroxetine (Paxil) Sertraline (Zoloft)	Venlafaxine (Effexor)	Alprazolam (Xanax) Clonazepam (Klonopin)	
Social anxiety disorder	Paroxetine (Paxil) Sertraline (Zoloft)	Venlafaxine (Effexor)		
Obsessive-compulsive disorder	Fluoxetine (Prozac) Fluvoxamine (Luvox) Paroxetine (Paxil) Sertraline (Zoloft)			Clomipramine (Anafranil)

Food and Drug Administration. (2016). *FDA label repository*. Retrieved from labels.fda.gov; Burchum, J., & Rosenthal, L. (2016). *Lehne's pharmacology for nursing care* (9th ed.). St Louis, MO: Elsevier.

behaviors may be too involved with their rituals to take time to eat and drink. In general, nutritious diets with snacks should be provided. Adequate intake should be firmly encouraged, but power struggles should be avoided. Weighing patients frequently (e.g., three times a week) is useful in assessing nutrition.

Personal Hygiene and Grooming

Some patients with anxiety and obsessive-compulsive disorders are indecisive about bathing or about what clothing should be worn. For the latter, limiting choices to two outfits is helpful. In the event of severe indecisiveness, simply presenting the patient with the clothing to be worn may be necessary. You may also need to remain with the patient to give simple directions: "Put on your shirt. Now put on your slacks." Matter-of-fact support is effective in assisting patients to independently perform as much of a task as possible. Encourage patients to express thoughts and feelings about self-care. This communication can provide a basis for future health teaching or for ongoing dialogue about the patient's abilities.

Some patients, especially those with obsessive-compulsive disorder and phobias, may be excessively neat and engage in time-consuming rituals associated with bathing and dressing. Hygiene, dressing, and grooming may take several hours. Maintenance of skin integrity may become a problem when the rituals involve excessive washing and skin becomes excoriated and infected. Assessment of skin integrity is also a concern for individuals who pull their hair or pick at their skin.

Elimination

Patients with severe obsessive-compulsive disorder may be so involved with the performance of rituals that they may suppress the urge to void and defecate. Urinary tract infections and constipation may result. Interventions may include creating a regular schedule for taking the patient to the bathroom.

Sleep

Patients experiencing anxiety and obsessive-compulsive disorders frequently have difficulty sleeping, particularly in falling asleep. Patients with generalized anxiety disorder often experience sleep disturbance from nightmares. Separation anxiety disorder may have such profound fears that sleep seems impossible. Patients may perform rituals to the exclusion of resting and sleeping, and physical exhaustion may occur. Teaching patients how to discover ways to promote sleep (e.g., warm bath, warm milk, and relaxing music) and monitoring sleep through a sleep record are useful interventions. Chapter 19 offers an in-depth discussion of sleep disturbances.

Pharmacological Interventions

Several classes of medications have been found to be effective in the treatment of anxiety disorders. Table 15.11 identifies medications approved by the US Food and Drug Administration (FDA) for the treatment of anxiety disorders. Refer to Chapter 3 for a more detailed explanation of the actions of psychotropic medications.

Antidepressants

SSRIs are considered the first line of defense in most anxiety and obsessive-compulsive–related disorders. These SSRIs include paroxetine (Paxil), fluoxetine (Prozac), escitalopram (Lexapro), fluvoxamine (Luvox), and sertraline (Zoloft). Some of these antidepressants exert more of an activating effect than others and may actually increase anxiety initially. Fluoxetine and sertraline tend to be the most activating. Paroxetine seems to have a more calming effect than the other SSRIs. Antidepressants have the secondary benefit of treating comorbid depressive disorders.

Venlafaxine (Effexor) is a serotonin norepinephrine reuptake inhibitor (SNRI) that is quite successful in the treatment of several anxiety disorders. Another SNRI, duloxetine (Cymbalta), is effective in the treatment of generalized anxiety disorder.

Monoamine oxidase inhibitors (MAOIs) are reserved for treatment-resistant conditions because of the risk of life-threatening hypertensive crisis if the patient does not follow dietary restrictions (patients cannot eat foods containing tyramine and must be given specific dietary instructions). The risk of hypertensive crisis also makes the use of MAOIs contraindicated in patients with comorbid substance use disorders. See Chapter 14 for a full discussion of antidepressants.

Antianxiety Drugs

Antianxiety drugs are often used to treat the somatic and psychological symptoms of anxiety disorders. When moderate or severe anxiety is reduced, patients are better able to participate in treatment of their underlying problems. Benzodiazepines are most commonly used because they have a quick onset of action. However, due to the potential for dependence, these medications should be used for short periods, only until other medications or treatments reduce symptoms.

An important nursing intervention is to monitor for side effects of the benzodiazepines including sedation, ataxia, and decreased cognitive function. Paradoxical reactions—reactions that are the exact opposite of intended responses—sometimes occur. Symptoms such as anxiety, agitation, talkativeness, and loss of impulse control may occur when using this classification of medications. Benzodiazepines are not recommended for patients with a substance use disorder. They are not recommended for elderly patients due to risk of delirium, falls, and fractures.

The decision to use benzodiazepines during pregnancy should be made by weighing the risk of fetal exposure versus the risk of untreated anxiety disorders (US Department of Health and Human Services, 2012). Benzodiazepine use shortly before delivery can result in a dystonia and muscle weakness in the newborn known as floppy infant syndrome. Withdrawal symptoms in the neonate have been known to occur. Prenatal benzodiazepine exposure increases the risk of oral cleft lip and palate, although the absolute risk increases by only 0.01%. The FDA warns against breastfeeding while taking these drugs since they pass into breast milk.

Box 15.2 summarizes important information for patient teaching.

BOX 15.2 Patient and Family Teaching: Antianxiety Drugs

1. Caution the patient:
   Not to change dose or frequency of medication without consultation with the prescriber.
   These medications may make it unsafe to handle mechanical equipment (e.g., cars, saws, and machinery).
   Avoid alcoholic beverages and other antianxiety drugs, due to unsafe depressant effects when combined.
   Avoid drinking beverages containing caffeine because they decrease the desired effects of the drug.
   Review prescription medications and doses that may cause or increase anxiety (e.g., thyroid hormones, steroids, decongestants).
2. Discuss the risks to the fetus and the risk of untreated anxiety disorders with prescriber should pregnancy occur or be considered.
3. Advise the patient to discuss breastfeeding with prescriber because these drugs are excreted in the milk and could have adverse effects on the infant.
4. Teach a patient who is taking monoamine oxidase inhibitors about the details of a tyramine-restricted diet (refer to Chapter 3).
5. Teach the patient that:
   Cessation of benzodiazepine use after 3 to 4 months of daily use may cause withdrawal symptoms such as insomnia, irritability, nervousness, dry mouth, tremors, convulsions, and confusion.
   Medications should be taken with or shortly after meals or snacks to reduce gastrointestinal discomfort.
   Drug interactions can occur: Antacids may delay absorption; cimetidine interferes with metabolism of benzodiazepines, causing increased sedation; central nervous system depressants, such as alcohol and barbiturates, cause increased sedation.

Buspirone (BuSpar) is an alternative antianxiety medication that does not cause dependence, but 2 to 4 weeks are required for it to reach full effects. The drug may be used for long-term treatment and should be taken regularly. Side effects include dizziness, nausea, headache, nervousness, lightheadedness, and excitement.

Buspirone is not recommended for individuals with impaired hepatic or renal function since in increased plasma levels and lengthened half-life may result. There is no direct evidence that this medication poses a danger to the developing infant. The FDA recommends using the drug during pregnancy and breastfeeding only if clearly necessary.

Other Classes of Medications

Other classes of medications sometimes used to treat anxiety disorders include beta-blockers, antihistamines, anticonvulsants, and antipsychotics. These agents are often added if the first course of treatment is ineffective. Beta-blockers block the receptors that, when stimulated, cause the heart to beat faster. The beta-blockers reduce physical manifestations of anxiety by slowing the heart rate and reducing blushing and have been used to treat social anxiety disorder.

Anticonvulsants have shown some benefit in the management of generalized anxiety disorder and social anxiety disorder. Gabapentin (Neurontin) and pregabalin (Lyrica), for example, are commonly prescribed.

Antihistamines are a safe nonaddictive alternative to benzodiazepines to lower anxiety levels and again are helpful in treating patients with substance use problems. Antipsychotic medications are useful in treating more severe symptoms of anxiety disorders.

There are no FDA-approved drugs for the treatment of the following disorders: separation anxiety, specific phobia, body dysmorphic, hoarding, trichotillomania, and excoriation. Despite the lack of approval, these conditions are often treated with antidepressants, antianxiety agents, and the other classes of medications previously described.

Pharmacological Interventions in Children and Adolescents

A few drugs are approved specifically for anxiety and obsessive-compulsive disorders in children and adolescents. The FDA approved the SNRI duloxetine (Cymbalta) in 2014 for children aged 7 to 17 years for generalized anxiety disorder. The FDA has approved four medications for use in children with obsessive-compulsive disorder. They are clomipramine (Anafranil), fluoxetine (Prozac), fluvoxamine (Luvox), and sertraline (Zoloft).

However, medications approved for other age groups are still prescribed off label. SSRIs are being used for generalized anxiety disorder, panic disorder, and social anxiety disorder with good results. For children with obsessive-compulsive and related disorders, SSRIs are also often used.

Neurobiology of Anxiety Disorders and the Effects of Antianxiety Medications

An imbalance of certain neurotransmitters are thought to disrupt specific brain regions that contribute to various anxiety disorders.
Frontal cortex: cognitive interpretations (e.g., potential threat)
Hypothalamus: activation of the stress response (fight-or-flight response)
Hippocampus: associated with memory related to fear responses
Amygdala: fear, especially related to phobic and panic disorders

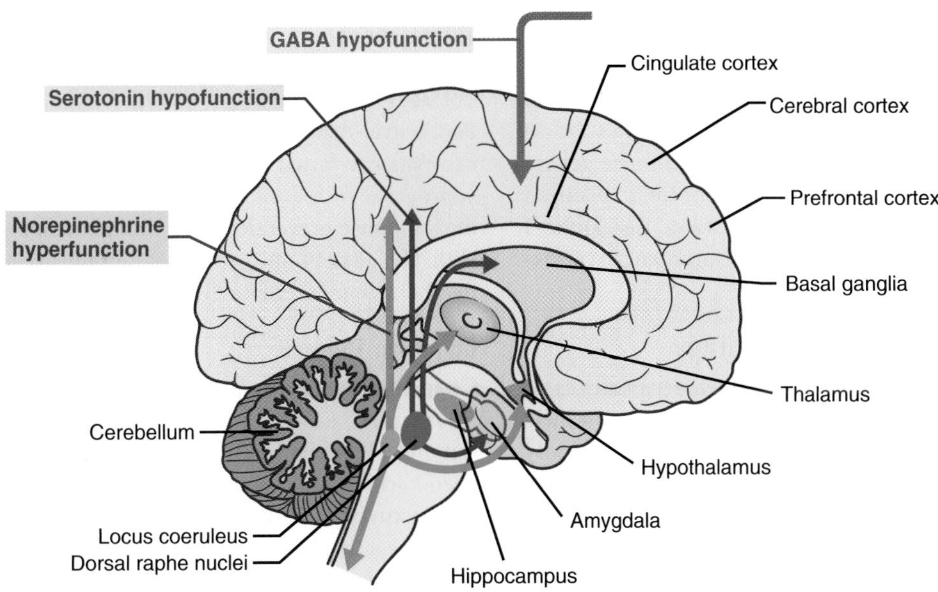

Serotonin: midbrain, ventral tegmental area (VTA), cerebral cortex, and hypothalamus. Helps regulate mood, sleep, sexual desire, appetite, and inhibits pain. In anxiety disorders it is believed that there are reduced levels of serotonin transmission. Low levels of serotonin are believed to play a role in anxiety disorders as well as depression.

Gamma-aminobutyric acid (GABA): neurotransmitters are widely distributed in the brain. GABA slows neuron activity which plays a role in lowering anxiety and also effects memory. There appears to be strong support that problems with the GABA neurotransmitter system in the brain is related to anxiety disorders.

Norepinephrine: midbrain, VTA, cerebral cortex, and hypothalamus. Plays a role in sensitization, fear conditioning, stress response (increases blood pressure and heart rate). Excessive and unregulated norepinephrine thought to be related to anxiety disorders

Antianxiety Agent	How It Works	Examples of Use
SSRIs–first-line treatment	Blocks reuptake of serotonin-increasing levels in the brain	Paroxetine (Paxil)—helpful in GAD
SNRI–first-line treatment	Blocks both serotonin and norepinephrine in the brain	Venlafaxine (Effexor)—mixed anxiety/depression, anxiety, and nerve pain
Noradrenergic drugs	Propranolol—blocks adrenergic receptor activity Clonidine—stimulates adrenergic receptors	Propranolol—short-term relief of social anxiety and performance anxiety Clonidine—anxiety disorders, panic attacks
Benzodiazepines	Binds to benzodiazepine receptors, facilitates action of GABA, slowing neural transmission thus lowering anxiety	Alprazolam—may be used short term to treat panic disorder and agoraphobia
Buspirone (BuSpar)	Functions as a serotonin 5-HT_{1A} receptor partial agonist resulting in anxiolytic and antidepressant effects	Can treat the worry associated with GAD rather than the muscle tension

Psychobiological Interventions

Besides medication, there are few biological interventions available to disrupt the course of the anxiety and anxiety-related disorders. Surgery has been used in obsessive-compulsive disorder for those most severely affected. A Gamma Knife® creates irreversible damage known as *lesions* to certain areas of the brain, resulting in a disconnect of overactive circuits or regions.

A relatively new reversible surgical treatment being used for obsessive-compulsive disorder is deep brain stimulation. This technique is considered a valid treatment (Alonso et al., 2015). Electrodes are surgically placed in the subthalamic nucleus of the brain. Then an implanted pulse generator in the chest activates a low-dose current for a specified period of time (several months in some cases). Researchers have reported a decrease of 35% on a measurement of obsessive-compulsive symptoms.

Complementary and Integrative Therapy

Chapter 35 identifies a number of complementary practices or integrative therapies that people use to cope with stress in their lives. Herbal therapy and dietary supplements are commonly used, yet they are not subject to the same rigorous testing as prescription medications. Also, herbs and dietary supplements may not be uniformly prepared or dosed, and there is no guarantee of bioequivalence of the active compound among preparations. Problems that can occur with the use of psychotropic herbs include toxic side effects and herb-drug interactions. Nurses and other healthcare providers should stay current regarding these popular products in order to assist their patients in making informed decisions.

One example is kava, which is derived from the roots of *Piper methysticum,* a South American plant. Kava is used as a sedative with antianxiety effects. As an alternative to seeking professional care, people with anxiety disorders may try kava in the belief that herbs are safer than medications, but it has a dark side. In 2010 the FDA issued a warning regarding its risk of liver damage. Kava is known to dramatically inhibit the P450 liver enzyme necessary for the metabolism of many medications. This inhibition could result in liver failure, especially when taken along with alcohol or other medications such as central nervous system depressants (antianxiety agents fall into this category).

Health Teaching

Health teaching is a significant nursing intervention for patients with anxiety disorders. Patients may conceal symptoms for years before seeking treatment and often come to the attention of healthcare providers during a co-occurring problem. People with panic disorder and generalized anxiety disorder seem more motivated than those with other anxiety disorders to get treatment; most seek help during the first year of symptoms (Wang et al., 2005).

Teaching about the specific disorder and available effective treatments is a major step toward improving the quality of life for those with anxiety disorders. Whether in a community or hospital setting, nurses can teach patients about signs and symptoms of anxiety disorders, presumed causes or risk factors (especially substance abuse), medications, the use of relaxation techniques, and the benefits of psychotherapy.

Relaxation exercises for breathing or muscle groups are extremely useful in initiating a relaxation response. The relaxation response is the opposite of the stress response and results in a reduced heart rate and breathing and relaxed muscles. Refer to Chapter 10 for a description of different approaches to relaxation training.

Advanced Practice Interventions

Psychiatric-mental health advanced practice registered nurses use evidence-based cognitive treatment approaches. Behavioral approaches such as modeling, systematic desensitization, flooding, response prevention, and thought stopping are also useful with the anxiety and obsessive-compulsive disorders. Cognitive-behavioral therapies link both of these approaches.

Cognitive Therapy

Cognitive therapy is based on the belief that patients make errors in thinking that lead to mistaken negative beliefs about self and others. For example, "I have to be perfect or my boyfriend will not love me." Through a process called **cognitive restructuring**, the therapist helps the patient (1) identify automatic negative beliefs that cause anxiety, (2) explore the basis for these thoughts, (3) reevaluate the situation realistically, and (4) replace negative self-talk with supportive ideas.

Behavioral Therapy

There are currently several forms of **behavioral therapy**, which involve teaching and physical practice of activities to decrease anxious or avoidant behavior:

- **Modeling:** The therapist or significant other acts as a role model to demonstrate appropriate behavior in a feared situation, and then the patient imitates it. For example, the role model rides in an elevator with a claustrophobic patient.
- **Systematic desensitization:** The patient is gradually introduced to a feared object or experience through a series of steps, from the least frightening to the most frightening (graduated exposure). The patient is taught to use a relaxation technique at each step when anxiety becomes overwhelming. For example, a patient with agoraphobia would start with opening the door to the house to go out on the steps and advance to attending a movie in a theater. The therapist may start with imagined situations in the office before moving on to in vivo (live) exposures.
- **Flooding:** Unlike systematic desensitization, this method exposes the patient to a large amount of an undesirable stimulus in an effort to extinguish the anxiety response. The patient learns through prolonged exposure that survival is possible and that anxiety diminishes spontaneously. For example, an obsessive patient who usually touches objects with a paper towel may be forced to touch objects with a bare hand for 1 hour. By the end of that period, the anxiety level is lower.
- **Response prevention:** This method is used for compulsive behavior. The therapist does not allow the patient to perform

the compulsive ritual (e.g., hand washing), and the patient learns that anxiety does subside even when the ritual is not completed. After trying this in the office, the patient learns to set time limits at home to gradually lengthen the time between rituals until the urge fades away.

- **Thought stopping:** Through this technique a negative thought or obsession is interrupted. The patient may be instructed to say "Stop!" out loud when the idea comes to mind or to snap a rubber band worn on the wrist. This distraction briefly blocks the automatic undesirable thought and cues the patient to select an alternative, more positive idea. (After learning the exercise, the patient gives the command silently.)

Cognitive-Behavioral Therapy

Cognitive-behavioral therapy combines cognitive therapy with specific behavioral therapies to reduce the anxiety response. Cognitive-behavioral therapy includes cognitive restructuring, psychoeducation, breath restraining and muscle relaxation, teaching of self-monitoring for panic and other symptoms, and in vivo (real life) exposure to feared objects or situations.

EVALUATION

Identified outcomes serve as the basis for evaluation. In general, evaluation of outcomes for patients with anxiety and obsessive-compulsive disorders deals with questions such as the following:

- Is the patient experiencing a reduced level of anxiety?
- Does the patient recognize symptoms as anxiety related?
- Does the patient continue to display signs and symptoms such as obsessions, compulsions, phobias, worrying, or other symptoms of anxiety disorders? If still present, are they more or less frequent? More or less intense?
- Is the patient able to use new behaviors to manage anxiety?
- Does the patient adequately perform self-care activities?
- Can the patient maintain satisfying interpersonal relations?
- Is the patient able to assume usual roles?

QUALITY IMPROVEMENT

Quality improvement attempts to quantitatively measure severity of disorders, develop outcomes and guidelines for care, and monitor patients' progress. In primary care (where most people seek mental healthcare), evidence-based practice guidelines result in practitioners being more confident in their skills and more likely to treat anxiety. Evidence-based treatment includes using cognitive-behavioral therapy, prescribing appropriate medication, and following up with patients. Primary care providers may need expert support to provide this care (Roy-Byrne et al., 2010).

A variety of instruments are used in quality improvement initiatives for psychiatric disorders. A simple tool for measuring quality improvement for anxiety care is the Clinical Global Impression-Severity (CGI-S) scale for inpatient, outpatient, or primary care. It asks the clinician to rate the severity of illness on a seven-point continuum from normal-not ill to among the most extremely ill. Versteeg and colleagues (2012) developed the following outcomes for use with the tool:

- At least 80% of patients with anxiety disorders are monitored every 6 weeks with the CGI-S scale.
- After 6 months of treatment, 50% of patients with severe anxiety disorders will score less than three on the CGI-S.

Nurses are at the forefront in gathering information to improve the quality of care in all settings. Understanding anxiety disorders and their treatment is more fully accomplished when we consider the seriousness and importance of continuous quality improvement in providing care.

KEY POINTS TO REMEMBER

- Anxiety has an unknown or unrecognized source, whereas fear is a reaction to a specific threat.
- Peplau operationally defined four levels of anxiety (mild, moderate, severe, and panic). The patient's perceptual field, ability to learn, and other characteristics are different at each level.
- Defenses against anxiety can be adaptive or maladaptive and viewed in a hierarchy from healthy to intermediate to immature.
- Anxiety disorders are the most common psychiatric disorders in the United States and frequently co-occur with depression or substance abuse.
- Another closely related set of disorders is obsessive-compulsive disorders in which anxiety results in abnormal selective overattention.
- Research has identified biological, psychological, and environmental factors in the etiology of anxiety and obsessive-compulsive disorders.
- Patients with anxiety and obsessive-compulsive disorders suffer from debilitating anxiety, panic attacks, irrational fears, excessive worrying, uncontrollable rituals, or severe reactions to stress.
- Embarrassment and shame often prevent people from seeking psychiatric help. Instead, they may go to primary care providers with multiple somatic complaints.
- Psychiatric treatment is effective for anxiety and obsessive-compulsive disorders.
- Understanding the levels of anxiety will help in planning basic care including how much direction your patient will need, what precautions should be taken to prevent harm, and how able your patient is to learn.
- Basic-level nursing interventions include counseling, milieu therapy, promotion of self-care activities, psychobiological intervention, and health teaching.
- Advanced practice nursing interventions include behavioral and cognitive-behavioral therapies.
- Quality improvement initiatives help to measure severity of symptoms and to establish interventions that are evidence based rather than tradition based.

CRITICAL THINKING

1. Corey is a senior in college and is taking his final examinations for an engineering course. The professor catches him copying from the examination of his willing partner, Katie, and takes his exam away. Corey's heart immediately begins to pound, his pulse and respiration rates increase, and he has to wipe perspiration from his hands and face several times. He feels like he may vomit and has a throbbing in his head.

   After the examination, he approaches the professor, but has difficulty focusing; when he starts to speak, his voice trembles. Corey says that Katie suggested that cheating is no big deal, that he needed to do it to be competitive, and that it was done all the time. Corey goes on to say that this "silly exam" doesn't mean anything anyway and that he already passed the important courses. He tells the professor, "I thought you were the greatest, and now I see that you're a fool."

   The professor remains calm and explains that regardless of Corey's thoughts on this matter, he was, in fact, caught cheating, and he will have to take responsibility for his actions. The professor will refer Corey to the disciplinary board. When Corey realizes how serious this incident is, he flips out and yells at the professor and calls him offensive names. Another professor walking past the classroom witnesses this encounter.
   a. Identify the level of anxiety Corey was experiencing once he was caught cheating, and describe the signs and symptoms that helped you determine this level.
   b. Identify and define five defense mechanisms Corey used to lessen his anxiety.

   Given the circumstances once Corey was caught, how could he have reacted using healthier coping defenses in a manner that would have reflected more self-responsibility?
2. Tiffany, a teenager with obsessive-compulsive disorder, washes her hands until they are cracked and bleeding. Your nursing goal is to promote healing of her hands. What interventions will you plan?
3. This is Logan's third emergency department visit in a week. He is experiencing severe anxiety accompanied by many physical symptoms. He clings to you, desperately crying, "Help me! Help me! Don't let me die!" Diagnostic tests have ruled out a physical disorder. The patient outcome has been identified as "Patient's anxiety level will be reduced to moderate/mild within 1 hour."
   a. What interventions should you use? Be comprehensive in your approach.
   b. Logan is given an appointment at the anxiety disorders clinic. How will you explain the importance of keeping the clinic appointment? Are there any factors you would have to consider while providing patient education?
4. Liz is a patient with generalized anxiety disorder. She has a history of substance abuse and is now a recovering alcoholic. During a clinic visit, she tells you she plans to ask the psychiatrist to prescribe diazepam (Valium) to use when she feels anxious. She asks whether you think this is a good idea. How would you respond? What action could you take?

CHAPTER REVIEW

Questions

1. The nurse is providing care for a patient demonstrating behaviors associated with moderate levels of anxiety. What question should the nurse ask initially when attempting to help the patient deescalate their anxiety?
   a. "Do you know what will help you manage your anxiety?"
   b. "Do you need help to manage your anxiety?"
   c. "Can you identify what was happening when your anxiety began to increase?"
   d. "Are you feeling anxious right now?"
2. Which patient has an increased risk for the development of anxiety and will require frequent assessment by the nurse? *Select all that apply.*
   a. Exacerbation of asthma signs and symptoms
   b. History of peanut and strawberry allergies
   c. History of chronic obstructive pulmonary disease
   d. Current treatment for unstable angina pectoris
   e. History of a traumatic brain injury
3. Which medication should the nurse be prepared to educate patients on when they are prescribed a selective serotonin reuptake inhibitor (SSRI) for panic attacks?
   a. Alprazolam (Xanax)
   b. Fluoxetine (Prozac)
   c. Clonazepam (Klonopin)
   d. Venlafaxine (Effexor)
4. Which statement(s) made by the nurse demonstrates an understanding of the effective use of relaxation therapy for anxiety management? *Select all that apply.*
   a. "Relaxation therapy's main goal is to prevent exhaustion by removing muscle tension."
   b. "Muscle relaxation promotes the relaxation response."
   c. "Show me how you learned to deep breathe in yesterday's therapy session."
   d. "You've said that going to group makes you nervous so let's start relaxing now."
   e. "I've given you written descriptions of the various relaxation exercises for you to review."
5. To maximize the therapeutic effect, which lifestyle practice should the nurse discourage for a patient who has been recently prescribed an antianxiety medication?
   a. Eating high protein foods.
   b. Using acetaminophen without first discussing it with a healthcare provider
   c. Taking medications after eating dinner or while having a bedtime snack
   d. Buying a large coffee with sugar and extra cream each morning on the way to work

6. In a parent teacher conference, the school nurse meets with the parents of a profoundly shy 8-year-old girl. The parents hold hands, speak softly, respond briefly, and have poor eye contact. The nurse recognizes that the child is most likely exposed to parental modeling and:
   a. The inherited shyness trait
   b. A lack of affection in the home
   c. Severe punishment by the parents
   d. Is afraid to say something foolish
7. Isabel is a straight-A student, yet she suffers from severe test anxiety and seeks medical attention. The nurse interviews Isabel and develops a plan of care. The nurse recognizes effective teaching about mild anxiety when Isabel states:
   a. "I would like to try a benzodiazepine for my anxiety."
   b. "If I study harder, my anxiety level will go down."
   c. "Mild anxiety is okay because it helps me to focus."
   d. "I have fear that I will fail at college."
8. The activity of gamma-aminobutyric acid (GABA) contributes to a slowing of neural activity. Which of the following drugs facilitates the action of GABA?
   a. Benzodiazepines
   b. Antihistamines
   c. Anticonvulsants
   d. Noradrenergic
9. Samantha is a new patient to the mental health clinic and is seeking assistance for what she describes as "severe anxiety." In addition to daily self-medicating with alcohol, Samantha describes long-term use of herbal kava. The nurse knows that kava is associated with inhibiting P450 and orders which of the following tests?
   a. Electrocardiogram
   b. Liver enzymes
   c. Glomerular filtration rate
   d. Complete blood count
10. A homebound patient diagnosed with agoraphobia has been receiving therapy in the home. The nurse evaluates patient teaching is effective when the patient states:
   a. "I may never leave the house again."
   b. "Having groceries delivered is very convenient."
   c. "My risk for agoraphobia is increased by my family history."
   d. "I will go out again, someday, just not today."

Answers

1. **c**; 2. **a, c, d, e**; 3. **b**; 4. **b, c, d, e**; 5. **d**; 6. **a**; 7. **c**; 8. **a**; 9. **b**; 10. **c**

Visit the Evolve website for a posttest on the content in this chapter: http://evolve.elsevier.com/Varcarolis

Post-Test interactive review

REFERENCES

Alonso, P., Cuadras, D., Gabriels, L., Denys, D., Goodman, W., Greenberg, B. D., & Menchon, J. M. (2015). Deep brain stimulation for obsessive-compulsive disorder: A meta-analysis of treatment outcome and predictors of response. *PLOS [online]*. Retrieved from http://journals.plos.org/plosone/article?id=10.1371/journal.pone.0133591.

American Nurses Association, American Psychiatric Nurses Association, & International Society of Psychiatric-Mental Health Nurses. (2014). *Psychiatric-mental health nursing: Scope and standards of practice* (2nd ed.). Silver Spring, MD: NurseBooks.org.

American Psychiatric Association. (2013). *Diagnostic and statistical manual of mental disorders* (5th ed.). Washington, D.C.: Author.

Bulechek, G. M., Butcher, H. K., Dochterman, J. M., & Wagner, C. (2013). *Nursing interventions classification (NIC)* (6th ed.). St. Louis, MO: Mosby.

Frick, A., Ahs, F., Engman, J., Jonasson, M., Alaie, I., Bjorkstrand, J., Furmark, T. (2015). Serotonin synthesis and reuptake in social anxiety disorder. *JAMA Psychiatry*, *72*(8), 794–802.

Herdman, T. H., & Kamitsuru, S. (Eds.). (2014). *NANDA International nursing diagnoses: Definitions and classification*. Oxford, UK: Wiley Blackwell, 2015–2017.

Mertol, S., & Alkin, T. (2012). Temperament and character dimensions of patients with adult separation anxiety disorder. *Journal of Affective Disorders*, *139*(2), 199–203.

Mervis, C. B., Dida, J., Lam, E., Crawford-Zelli, N. A., Young, E. J., Henderson, D. R., & Osborne, L. R. (2012). Duplication of GTF21 results in separation anxiety in mice and humans. *American Journal of Human Genetics*, *90*(6), 1064–1070.

Moorhead, S., Johnson, M., Maas, M., & Swanson, E. (2013). *Nursing outcomes classification (NOC)* (5th ed.). St. Louis, MO: Mosby.

Nordsletten, A. E., Reichenberg, A., Hatch, S. L., Fernandez de la Cruz, L., Pertusa, A., Hotopf, M., & Mataix-Cols, D. (2013). Epidemiology of hoarding disorder. *British Journal of Psychiatry [online]*. Retrieved from http://bjp.rcpsych.org/content/early/2013/10/17/bjp.bp.113.130195.short.

Peplau, H. E. (1968). A working definition of anxiety. In S. F. Burd & M. A. Marshall (Eds.), *Some clinical approaches to psychiatric nursing* (pp. 323–327). New York, NY: Macmillan.

Roy-Byrne, P., Craske, M. G., Sullivan, G., Rose, R. D., Edlund, M. J., Lang, A. J., et al. (2010). Delivery of evidence-based treatment for multiple anxiety disorders in primary care: A randomized controlled trial. *Journal of the American Medical Association*, *303*(19), 1921–1928.

Sullivan, H. S. (1953). *The interpersonal theory of psychiatry*. New York, NY: W. W. Norton.

Versteeg, M. H., Laurant, M. G. H., Franx, G. C., Jacobs, A. J., & Wensing, M. J. P. (2012). Factors associated with the quality improvement collaboratives in mental healthcare: An exploratory study. *Implementation Science*, *7*(1). Retrieved from http://www.implementationscience.com/content/7/1/1.

US Department of Health and Human Services. (2012). Use of psychiatric medications in pregnancy and lactation. Retrieved from https://www.guideline.gov/summaries/summary/12490.

Wang, P. S., Berglund, P., Olfson, M., Pincus, H. A., Wells, K. B., & Kessler, R. C. (2005). Failure and delay in initial treatment contact after first onset of mental disorders in the national comorbidity survey replication. *Archives of General Psychiatry*, *62*, 603–613.

16

Trauma, Stressor-Related, and Dissociative Disorders

Kathleen Wheeler

Visit the Evolve website for a pretest on the content in this chapter: http://evolve.elsevier.com/Varcarolis Pre-Test interactive review

OBJECTIVES

1. Describe clinical manifestations of each disorder covered under the general umbrella of trauma-related and dissociative disorders.
2. Describe the symptoms, epidemiology, comorbidity, and risk factors of trauma-related disorders in children.
3. Discuss at least five of the neurobiological changes that occur as the result of trauma.
4. Apply the nursing process to the care of children who are experiencing trauma-related disorders.
5. Differentiate between the symptoms of posttraumatic stress, acute stress, and adjustment disorders in adults.
6. Describe the symptoms, epidemiology, comorbidity, and risk factors of trauma-related disorders in adults.
7. Discuss how to deal with common reactions the nurse may experience while working with a patient who has suffered trauma.
8. Apply the nursing process to trauma-related disorders in adults.
9. Develop a teaching plan for a patient with posttraumatic stress disorder.
10. Identify dissociative disorders including depersonalization/derealization disorder, dissociative amnesia, and dissociative identity disorder.
11. Create a nursing care plan incorporating evidence-based interventions for symptoms of dissociation, including flashbacks, amnesia, and impaired self-care.
12. Role-play intervening with a patient experiencing a flashback.

OUTLINE

OUTLINE—cont'd

KEY TERMS AND CONCEPTS

acute stress disorder
adjustment disorder
alternate personality (alter)
debriefing
depersonalization
derealization
disinhibited social engagement disorder
dissociation
dissociative amnesia
dissociative fugue
dissociative identity disorder
eye movement desensitization and reprocessing
flashbacks
neuroplasticity
posttraumatic stress disorder (PTSD)
reactive attachment disorder
resilience
trauma-informed care
window of tolerance

Traumatic life events are associated with a wide range of psychiatric and other medical disorders. Traumatic events are not always as extraordinary as war and may be as common as interpersonal trauma, sexual abuse, physical abuse, severe neglect, emotional abuse, repeated abandonment, or sudden and traumatic loss in childhood, adolescence, or adulthood.

Our understanding of the long-term physiological and psychological effects of trauma has expanded, and effective treatments are available. However, people who need these treatments do not always get the care that they need. Integrating trauma-informed care into all health care settings, both behavioral and medical, can reduce the effects of trauma and help to prevent the pervasive and damaging psychological and physical consequences of trauma.

Trauma often precedes many psychiatric disorders. According to the American Psychiatric Association (APA, 2013), disorders included under the trauma umbrella include:

- Posttraumatic stress disorder
- Attachment disorders
  1. Reactive attachment disorder
  2. Disinhibited social engagement disorder
- Acute stress disorder
- Adjustment disorders

Because trauma impacts children in related, but different ways, the two populations will be addressed separately. This chapter begins with trauma-related disorders in children and then discusses adult trauma-related disorders.

The last part of the chapter addresses dissociative disorders. Dissociative disorders are also related to trauma, specifically early interpersonal trauma. These disorders include:

- Depersonalization/derealization disorder
- Dissociative amnesia
- Dissociative identity disorder

TRAUMA-RELATED DISORDERS IN CHILDREN

POSTTRAUMATIC STRESS DISORDER

Tragically, children are exposed to many traumatic events without the strength or coping skills to adequately defend themselves. Abuse, interpersonal violence, automobile accidents, natural disasters, war, medical procedures, and illnesses are all traumatizing incidents. Children who have been abused and neglected by their caretakers and other adults are at great risk for developing physical illnesses and psychological problems as a result of their traumatic experiences.

According to the National Child Abuse and Neglect Data System (2015), nearly 679,000 children were victims of abuse and neglect in 2013. Neglect is the most prevalent form of child abuse in the United States. Of those children who died from abuse and neglect, about 74% were younger than 3 years old. One or both parents are responsible for nearly 80% of child fatalities, and boys suffer a higher child fatality rate than girls. These statistics only reflect known cases of abuse. There is little doubt that far more children suffer abuse and neglect than are reported to child protective services agencies.

Sexual abuse of a child is a particularly reprehensible act. Sexual abuse ranges from forcing a child to observe lewd acts, to fondling, and all the way to sexual intercourse. All instances of sexual abuse are devastating to a child who lacks the mental capacity or emotional maturation to consent to this type of a relationship. Children who are starved for affection may be particularly vulnerable and confused by this attention.

Witnessing violence is traumatizing and a well-documented risk factor for many mental health problems, including depression, anxiety, **posttraumatic stress disorder (PTSD)**, aggressive and delinquent behavior, drug use, academic failure, and low self-esteem (Weiland, 2015). Children who have been abused are at risk for abusing others and developing dysfunctional patterns in close interpersonal relationships.

CLINICAL PICTURE

PTSD in preschool children may manifest as a reduction in play, repetitive play that includes aspects of the traumatic event, social withdrawal, and negative emotions such as fear, guilt, anger, horror, sadness, shame, or confusion. Children may blame themselves for the traumatic event and manifest persistent negative thoughts about themselves such as "I am a bad person." In addition there may be a feeling of detachment or estrangement from others and diminished interest or participation in significant activities. Often there is irritability, aggressive or self-destructive behavior, sleep disturbances, problems concentrating, and hypervigilance.

The *DSM-5* box provides criteria for PTSD in adolescents and adults followed by criteria for children under the age of 7.

DSM-5 CRITERIA FOR POSTTRAUMATIC STRESS DISORDER

I. Posttraumatic Stress Disorder for Adults, Adolescents, and Children Older than 6 Years

A. Exposure to actual or threatened death, serious injury, or sexual violence in one (or more) of the following ways:
1. Directly experiencing the traumatic event(s).
2. Witnessing, in person, the event(s) as it occurred to others.
3. Learning that the traumatic event(s) occurred to a close family member or close friend. In cases of actual or threatened death of a family member or friend, the event(s) must have been violent or accidental.
4. Experiencing repeated or extreme exposure to aversive details of the traumatic event(s) (e.g., first responders collecting human remains; police officers repeatedly exposed to details of child abuse).

Note: Criterion A4 does not apply to exposure through electronic media, television, movies, or pictures, unless this exposure is work related.

B. Presence of one (or more) of the following intrusion symptoms associated with traumatic event(s), beginning after the traumatic event(s) occurred:
1. Recurrent, involuntary, and intrusive distressing memories of the traumatic event(s).

Note: In children older than 6 years, repetitive play may occur in which themes or aspects of the traumatic event(s) are expressed.

2. Recurrent distressing dreams in which the content and/or affect of the dream are related to the traumatic event(s).
3. Note: In children, there may be frightening dreams without recognizable content.
4. Dissociative reactions (e.g., **flashbacks**) in which the individual feels or acts as if the traumatic event(s) were recurring. (Such reactions may occur on a continuum, with the most extreme expression being a complete loss of awareness of present surroundings.)

Note: In children, trauma-specific reenactment may occur in play.

5. Intense or prolonged psychological distress at exposure to internal or external cues that symbolize or resemble an aspect of the traumatic event(s).
6. Marked physiological reactions to internal or external cues that symbolize or resemble an aspect of the traumatic event(s).

C. Persistent avoidance of stimuli associated with the traumatic event(s), beginning or worsening after the traumatic event(s) occurred, as evidenced by two (or more) of the following:
1. Avoidance of or efforts to avoid distressing memories, thoughts, or feelings about or closely associated with the traumatic event(s).
2. Avoidance of or efforts to avoid external reminders (people, places, conversations, activities, objects, situations) that arouse distressing memories, thoughts, feelings about or closely associated with the traumatic event(s).

D. Negative alterations in cognitions and mood associated with the traumatic event(s), beginning or worsening after the traumatic event(s) occurred, as evidenced by two (or more) of the following:
1. Inability to remember an important aspect of the traumatic event(s) (typically due to dissociative amnesia and not to other factors such as head injury, alcohol, or drugs).
2. Persistent and exaggerated negative beliefs or expectations about oneself, others, or the world (e.g., "I am bad," "No one can be trusted," "The world is completely dangerous," "My whole nervous system is permanently ruined").
3. Persistent distorted cognitions about the cause of consequences of the traumatic event(s) that lead the individual to blame himself/herself or others.
4. Persistent negative motional state (e.g., fear, horror, anger, guilt, or shame).
5. Markedly diminished interest or participation in significant activities.
6. Feelings of detachment or estrangement from others.
7. Persistent inability to experience positive emotions (e.g., inability to experience happiness, satisfaction, or loving feelings).

E. Marked alterations in arousal and reactivity associated with the traumatic event(s), beginning or worsening after the traumatic event(s) occurred, as evidenced by two (or more) of the following:
1. Irritable behavior and angry outburst (with little or no provocation) typically expressed as verbal or physical aggression toward people or objects.
2. Reckless or self-destructive behavior.
3. Hypervigilance.
4. Exaggerated startle response.
5. Problems with concentration.
6. Sleep disturbance (e.g., difficulty falling or staying asleep or restless sleep).

F. Duration of the disturbance (Criteria B, C, D, and E) is more than 1 month.

G. The disturbance causes clinically significant distress or impairment in social, occupational, or other important areas of functioning.

H. The disturbance is not attributable to the physiological effects of a substance (e.g., medication, alcohol) or another medical condition.

Specify whether:

With dissociative symptoms: The individual's symptoms meet the criteria for posttraumatic stress disorder and in addition, in response to the stressor, the individual experiences persistent or recurrent symptoms of either of the following:
1. **Depersonalization:** Persistent or recurrent experiences of feeling detached from, and as if one were an outside observer of, one's mental processes or body (e.g., feeling as though one were in a dream; feeling a sense of unreality of self or body or of time moving slowly).

DSM-5 BOX DIAGNOSTIC CRITERIA FOR POSTTRAUMATIC STRESS DISORDER—cont'd

2. **Derealization:** Persistent or recurrent experiences of unreality of surroundings (e.g., the world around the individual is experienced as unreal, dreamlike, distant, or distorted).

Note: To use this subtype, the dissociative symptoms must not be attributable to the physiological effects of a substance (e.g., blackouts, behavior during alcohol intoxication) or another medical condition (e.g., complex partial seizures).

Specify if:

With delayed expression: If the full diagnostic criteria are not met until at least 6 months after the event (although the onset and expression of some symptoms may be immediate).

II. Posttraumatic Stress Disorder for Children 6 Years and Younger

A. In children 6 years and younger, exposure to actual or threatened death, serious injury, or sexual violence in one (or more) of the following ways:
   1. Directly experiencing the traumatic event(s).
   2. Witnessing, in person, the event(s) as it occurred to others, especially primary caregivers.

Note: Witnessing does not include events witnessed only in electronic media, television, movies, or pictures.

   3. Learning that the traumatic event(s) occurred to a parent or caregiving figure.

B. Presence of one (or more) of the following intrusion symptoms associated with the traumatic event(s), beginning after the traumatic event(s) occurred:
   4. Recurrent, involuntary, and intrusive distressing memories of the traumatic event(s).

Note: Spontaneous and intrusive memories may not necessarily appear distressing and may be expressed as play reenactment.

   5. Recurrent distressing dreams in which the content and/or affect of the dream are related to the traumatic event(s).

Note: It may not be possible to ascertain that the frightening content is related to the traumatic event.

   6. Dissociative reactions (e.g., flashbacks) in which the child feels or acts as if the traumatic event(s) were recurring. (Such reactions may occur on a continuum, with the most extreme expression being a complete loss of awareness of present surroundings.) Such trauma-specific reenactment may occur in play.
   7. Intense or prolonged psychological distress at exposure to internal or external cues that symbolize or resemble an aspect of the traumatic event(s).
   8. Marked physiological reactions to reminders of the traumatic event(s).

C. One (or more) of the following symptoms, representing either persistent avoidance of stimuli associated with the traumatic event(s) or negative alterations in cognitions and mood associated with the traumatic event(s), must be present, beginning after the event(s) or worsening after the event(s).

Persistent Avoidance of Stimuli

1. Avoidance of or efforts to avoid activities, places, or physical reminders that arouse recollections of the traumatic event(s).
2. Avoidance of or efforts to avoid people, conversations, or interpersonal situations that arouse recollections of the traumatic event(s).

Negative Alterations in Cognitions

1. Substantially increased frequency of negative emotional states (e.g., fear, guilt, sadness, shame, confusion).
2. Markedly diminished interest or participation in significant activities, including constriction of play.
3. Socially withdrawn behavior.
4. Persistent reduction in expression of positive emotions.

D. Alterations in arousal and reactivity associated with the traumatic event(s), beginning or worsening after the traumatic event(s) occurred, as evidenced by two (or more) of the following:
   1. Irritable behavior and angry outbursts (with little or no provocation) typically expressed as verbal or physical aggression toward people or objects (including extreme temper tantrums).
   2. Hypervigilance.
   3. Exaggerated startle response.
   4. Problems with concentration.
   5. Sleep disturbance (e.g., difficulty falling or staying asleep or restless sleep).

E. The duration of the disturbance is more than 1 month.

F. The disturbance cases clinically significant distress or impairment in relationships with parents, siblings, peers, or other caregivers or with school behavior.

G. The disturbance is not attributable to the physiological effects of a substance (e.g., medication or alcohol) or another medical condition.

Specify whether:

With dissociative symptoms: The individual's symptoms meet the criteria for posttraumatic stress disorder and the individual experiences persistent or recurrent symptoms of either of the following:

1. **Depersonalization:** Persistent or recurrent experiences of feeling detached from, and as if one were an outside observer of, one's mental processes or body (e.g., feeling as though one were in a dream; feeling a sense of unreality of self or body or of time moving slowly).
2. **Derealization:** Persistent or recurrent experiences of unreality of surroundings (e.g., the world around the individual is experienced as unreal, dreamlike, distant, or distorted).

Note: To use this subtype, the dissociative symptoms must not be attributable to the physiological effects of a substance (e.g., blackouts) or another medical condition (e.g., complex partial seizures).

Specify if:

With delayed expression: If the full diagnostic criteria are not met until at least 6 months after the event (although the onset and expression of some symptoms may be immediate).

American Psychiatric Association. (2013). *Diagnostic and statistical manual of mental disorders* (5th ed.). Washington, D.C.: Author.

EPIDEMIOLOGY

Prevalence rates for PTSD in children under 13 years of age are not available. Research on adolescents indicates a rate of 5% (US Department of Veterans Affairs, 2015). The prevalence for girls is higher than for boys—8% and 2.3%, respectively. Virtually 100% of children who witness their parent's murder or sexual assault will develop PTSD. Other alarming statistical relationships with PTSD are for children who are sexually abused (90%), exposed to a shooting at school (77%), and who see community violence (39%).

COMORBIDITY

Comorbidities increase the child's vulnerability to developing or exacerbating (making worse) PTSD symptoms. Children and adolescents who have suffered toxic stress and trauma often meet the criteria for more than one diagnostic category. Even if a child does not have sufficient symptoms for a diagnosis of PTSD, he or she can still suffer from overwhelming nightmares or difficulties with trust, phobias, somatic problems, impulse control, and identity issues. Learning and attention problems, behavioral problems, sleep disorders, depression, suicide attempts, dissociation, and substance-abuse problems are all significant comorbidities (Weiland, 2015). These comorbidities cause children to be subjected to an endless cycle of medications, punishments, and inadequate responses that revictimize and stigmatize the child.

RISK FACTORS

Biological Factors

Genetic

Genetic variability might play a role in how individuals react to stress. Environmental factors also influence the expression of genotype. Research on animals and humans has found that prenatal exposure to maternal stress can influence later responses to stress and behavioral outcomes in the offspring (Monk et al., 2012).

Also, early adversity has been found to alter the DNA in the brain through a process called methylation (Bick et al., 2012). Methyl groups are attached to genes that govern the production of stress hormone receptors in the brain. This in turn prevents the brain from regulating its response to stress. Parental nurturing may mediate this response. In the absence of nurturing, children have difficulties with attention and following directions. They are more likely to engage in high-risk behavior as teenagers and show increased aggression, impulsivity, weakened cognition, and an inability to discriminate between real and imagined threats as adults.

Neurobiological

The most rapid phase of brain development occurs during the first 5 years of life, which makes a child particularly vulnerable to adverse events. The right hemisphere develops first. It is involved in processing social-emotional information, promoting attachment functions, regulating body functions, and supporting the individual in coping with stress. Because the right brain develops first and is involved with developing templates for relationships and regulation of emotion and bodily function, early attachments are particularly important for healthy development.

It is in the context of attachments that regulatory functions develop in the child. Through day-to-day interactions with a caring person, the child develops adaptive coping strategies that support healthy physical and emotional regulation. Neural connections between the limbic system and prefrontal cortex are established between 10 and 18 months of age, and these neural pathways play a crucial role in modulating arousal and emotional regulation.

Normally, we take in information from the environment through our senses, match it against previous experiences, and process it adaptively. Experiences are integrated into memory in a way that allows for connection with other memories. In a normal stress response, the hyperarousal in the sympathetic system is balanced by the parasympathetic system. Neuronal circuits connect the amygdala, our emotional brain, to the prefrontal lobe, our logical brain. The prefrontal lobe serves as the translator of the emotion so that amygdala activation can be modulated. The prefrontal area also keeps track of where information has been stored in long-term memory. It is responsible for retrieving memories and then integrating them with sensory input for decision making.

Trauma causes a disruption of the integration of these neural networks. The more intense the arousal, the less likely it is that the experience will be processed (Bergmann, 2012). The more helpless and less in control of the situation the person feels, the more vulnerable to pathophysiological changes a person is.

In response to trauma, the parasympathetic response triggers a hypoaroused state with dysregulation of the hypothalamic-pituitary-adrenal axis resulting in **dissociation**. Dissociation is a disconnection of thoughts, emotions, sensations, and behaviors connected with a memory. This dissociation is different from the normal experience of spacing out and losing time during a movie or when driving. Severe dissociation occurs for those who have suffered significant trauma (Boon, et al., 2012). When dissociation fails, intrusive symptoms such as flashbacks occur.

Polyvagal theory posits that the autonomic nervous system is not limited to a fight-or-flight response to a threat and actually consists of three different responses (Porges, 2011). The sympathetic and parasympathetic systems are controlled by the tenth cranial nerve or vagus nerve. The vagus nerve sends and receives information between the body and the brain through two major vagus nerves: ventral and dorsal. Responses are as follows:

1. Myelinated ventral vagal responses are activated during social or intellectual engagement when the individual is "on," in a state of pleasant, not overwhelming, arousal. This state serves as a gentle brake by inhibiting sympathetic responses of the autonomic system.
2. Unmyelinated ventral vagus responses are activated when we perceive a threat. The attending sympathetic arousal symptoms of rapid heart rate and rapid respiration prepare the person for fight-or-flight responses. After many hours, days, or months the body cannot sustain this state.
3. The third response is the dorsal vagal response that occurs to dampen down the sympathetic nervous system. This is a parasympathetic response with the heart rate and respiration slowing down and a decrease in blood pressure. Animals in the wild illustrate the ultimate dorsal vagal shutdown by playing dead when extremely threatened.

Subjectively, the person may just want to sleep or escape through mind-numbing activities and stay in this hypoarousal or depression. This hypoarousal may alternate with hyperarousal and anxiety. This theory provides an explanation of why many people with PTSD also suffer from depression.

Psychological Factors

Attachment Theory

A psychological theory with implications for trauma-related disorders is attachment theory based on the work of Bowlby (1988). This theory describes the importance and dynamics of the early relationship between the infant and the caretaker. Attachment patterns or schemas are formed early in life through interaction and experiences with caregivers, and this relationship is embedded in memories. Research has demonstrated that these patterns of attachment persist into adulthood.

Environmental Factors

Neuroplasticity of the brain describes how experiences reorganize neural pathways. This reorganization is particularly intense in children. It is this neuroplasticity along with a dependency on others that can increase vulnerability to adverse childhood experiences (ACEs). External factors in the environment can either support or put stress on children and adolescents and shape development. Young people are vulnerable in an environment in which systems (e.g., schools, court systems) and adults (e.g., parents, counselors) have power and control.

Parents model behavior and provide the child with a view of the world. If parents are abusive, rejecting, or overly controlling, the child may suffer negative effects during the period of development when the trauma occurs. Most children, however, who suffer traumatic and stressful events, do develop normally.

Poverty, parental substance abuse, and exposure to violence have received increasing attention and place minority children at greater risk for trauma and stress. Differences in cultural expectations, presence of stresses, and lack of support by the dominant culture may have profound effects and increase the risk of mental, emotional, and academic problems. Family stability may provide cushioning effects in the face of poverty and adversity.

Children brought up in a chaotic or non-nurturing environment suffer neurological consequences that are long lasting and difficult to remediate (Shonkoff & Garner, 2012). Toxic stress and ACEs often result in lifelong consequences for both psychological and physical health. Trauma in early childhood also plays a role in the intergenerational transmission of disparities in health outcomes.

Intriguingly, some children who live with severe or chronic ACEs respond with strength and overcome circumstances that would leave most adults terribly shaken. The term resilience refers to positive adaptation, or the ability to maintain or regain mental health despite adversity. Studies have shown that factors that enhance resilience are the presence of social support and protective factors that include positive emotions and self-efficacy (Lee et al., 2013).

EVIDENCE-BASED PRACTICE

Can We Help Children Become Resilient?

Problem

Adverse childhood experiences (ACEs) are correlated with risk behaviors of smoking, disordered eating, and alcohol and substance abuse. Such behaviors can lead to significant public health problems of chronic obstructive pulmonary disease, obesity, liver disease, and hypertension. We know that some people with ACEs do not appear to suffer negative consequences but instead bounce back.

Purpose of Study

The purpose of this pilot study was to explore the benefits of a program called the Empower Resilience Intervention (ERI). The ERI was developed to help increase resilience and health behaviors with young adults who have high ACE scores.

Methods

All 28 participants had an ACE score of 4, which is significant for ACEs. A 4-week psychoeducation ERI program was provided for 17 undergraduate students. A control group of 11 students did not receive this intervention. Components of ERI included mindful meditation, building personal strength, improving cognitive flexibility, and increasing social support. Both the experimental group and the control group completed a pretest and posttest that compared symptoms, health behaviors, resilience, and asked for personal impressions of themselves.

Key Findings

- There was no significant change in risk behaviors or resilience score by cohort.
- Young adults in the intervention group reported building strengths, reframing resilience, and creating support connections.

Implications for Nursing Practice

An increase in health behavior should be possible with a strength-based intervention such as this. The sample may have been too small. Evaluating this intervention with a larger sample is important in determining its effects. This short-term intervention holds promise as an opportunity to build on strengths to positively impact the future.

Chandler, G. E., Roberts, S. J., & Chiodo, L. (2015). Resilience intervention for young adults with adverse childhood experiences. *Journal of the American Psychiatric Nurses Association, 21*(6), 406–416.

APPLICATION OF THE NURSING PROCESS

ASSESSMENT

A child or adolescent with a trauma or stressor-related disorder is one whose development may be delayed if adequate assessment, diagnosis, and treatment are not available. It is important for nurses working in school, community settings, and juvenile detention to assess for PTSD and the safety of the environment for young people who have been traumatized or experienced abuse and a history of violence.

The type of data collected to assess the child depends on the setting, the severity of the presenting problem, and the availability of resources. However, assessment is an ongoing process throughout treatment. Methods of collecting data include interviewing, screening, testing (neurological, psychological, intelligence), observing, and interacting with the child or adolescent. Ideally, histories are taken from multiple sources including parents, other caregivers, the child or adolescent, and other adults such as teachers. A genogram, which is a drawing of the family tree with descriptions of individuals and relationships, can provide a clearer illustration of the family (refer to Chapter 35).

Assessment of the mental status of children is similar to that of adults. It identifies problems with thinking, feeling, and behaving. Broad categories to assess include safety, general appearance, socialization, activity level, speech, coordination and motor function, affect, manner of relating, intellectual function, thought processes and content, and characteristics of play.

The observation-interaction part of a mental health assessment begins with a semi-structured interview in which the nurse asks the young person to describe the home environment, parents, and siblings. Information about the school environment, teachers, and peers is also collected.

Play activities, such as games, drawings, and puppets, are used for younger children who cannot respond to a direct approach. The initial interview is key to observing interactions among the child, caregiver, and siblings (if available) and to building trust and rapport.

Essential assessment data include posttraumatic symptoms such as:

- Nightmares
- Night terrors
- Hallucinations
- Intrusive traumatic thoughts and memories
- Reexperiencing or flashbacks of trauma
- Traumatic reenactments in play
- Self-injurious behaviors

Traumatized children may have dramatic mood swings and exhibit uncontrollable rage and negative symptoms such as numbing and avoidance. Somatic symptoms may manifest as headaches, stomachaches, or pain. Memory problems include amnesia, forgetfulness, difficulty concentrating, or trance states.

Specific assessment tools include the Child Dissociative Checklist (Putnam et al., 1993), Trauma Symptoms Checklist for Children (Briere, 1996), and the Child Sexual Behavior Inventory (Friedrich et al., 2001).

Developmental Assessment

The developmental assessment provides information about the child's or adolescent's maturational level. Is he behaving and functioning at his chronological age or are there areas where he lags behind the norms and peers? The Denver II Developmental Screening Test for infants and children up to 6 years of age is a popular assessment tool (Frankenburg et al., 1992). For adolescents, tools may be tailored to specific areas of assessment such as neuropsychological, physical, hormonal, and biochemical. Computer-based screening tools for children and adolescents are used in primary care settings to gather sensitive information.

Abnormal findings in the developmental and mental status assessments may be temporary. Parents are understandably relieved to learn that behaviors are stress related. However, intervening early to replace maladaptive coping behaviors with adaptive coping is important to reduce the risk of developing psychiatric disorders.

DIAGNOSIS

After a comprehensive trauma assessment, two priority nursing diagnoses are applicable (Herdman & Kamitsuru, 2014). The first is *risk for impaired attachment*, which is defined as being "vulnerable to disruption of the interactive process between parent/significant other and child that fosters the development of a protective and nurturing reciprocal relationship" (p. 289). Risk factors include:

- Anxiety associated with the parent role
- Ill infant/child who is unable to effectively initiate parental contact due to altered behavioral organization
- Inability of parents to meet personal needs
- Parental conflict due to altered behavior
- Substance use
- Separation

Another nursing diagnosis is *risk of delayed development*. This is "being vulnerable to delay of 25% or more in one or more of the areas of social or self-regulatory behavior, or in cognitive, language, gross or fine motor skills" (p. 452). Risk factors include:

- Substance use
- Failure to thrive
- Unstable home
- Unwanted pregnancy
- Poverty

OUTCOMES IDENTIFICATION

A child with a trauma-related disorder is at risk for developmental and regulatory disorders. A number of outcomes have been identified related to the nursing diagnoses listed previously (Moorhead et al., 2013). An overall attachment outcome would be for the parent and infant/child to demonstrate an enduring affectionate bond. With regard to development, general outcomes would pertain to meeting age-appropriate milestones.

IMPLEMENTATION

The overall treatment plan for trauma includes psychobiological, psychological, and family goals within a staged treatment protocol. The model of treatment for trauma includes the following stages:

Stage 1: Providing safety and stabilization by creating a safe predictable environment; stopping self-destructive behaviors; providing education about trauma and its effects.

Stage 2: Reducing arousal and regulating emotion through symptom reduction and memory work; finding comfort from others; integrating suppressed emotions and accepting ambivalence; overcoming avoidance; improving attention and decreasing dissociation; working with memories; and transforming memories.

Stage 3: Developmental skills catch up through enhancing problem-solving skills; nurturing self-awareness; social skills training; and developing a value system. Interventions in this phase should focus on teaching coping skills to deal with trauma, supporting efforts to achieve socially appropriate goals, and facilitating use of healthy social support systems.

Treatment strategies for the traumatized child are designed to modulate arousal so that the child is helped to stay within a window of tolerance. The **window of tolerance** is a term that means a balance between sympathetic and parasympathetic arousal (Porges, 2011). See the earlier neurobiological discussion and Fig. 16.1.

Traumatized children have difficulty shifting their emotional and physiological states to adapt to different environments. They alternate between hyperarousal (anxiety, fear, hyperactivity, aggression) and hypoarousal (withdrawal, isolation, numbness). You can help increase the child's ability to self-regulate using the interventions described in this chapter. These interventions will help to widen the window of tolerance.

Interventions

The traumatized child has suffered significant fragmentation of relationships with others. An essential healing ingredient is improving relationships and connection to others. The nurse-patient relationship provides a foundation of connection and caring. Box 16.1 identifies interventions appropriate for a child who has suffered a specific trauma.

Interventions for the traumatized child are used in a variety of settings such as inpatient, residential, outpatient, day

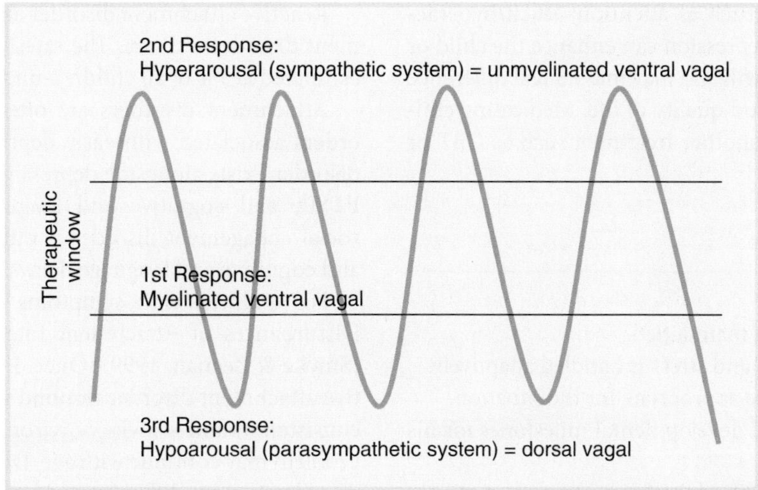

FIG. 16.1 Therapeutic window of arousal (Porges). Redrawn from Wheeler, K. (2014). *Psychotherapy for the advanced practice psychiatric nurse: A how-to guide for evidence-based practice.* New York, NY: Springer.

BOX 16.1 Trauma Interventions for a Child with PTSD

Establish trust and safety in the therapeutic relationship.
Use developmentally appropriate language to explore feelings.
Teach relaxation techniques before trauma exploration to restore a sense of control over thoughts and feelings.
Help the child to identify and cope with feelings through the use of art and play to promote expression.
Involve the parents or appropriate caretakers in 1:1s unless they are the cause of the trauma.
Educate the child and parents about the grief process and response to the trauma.
Assist parents in resolving their own emotional distress about the trauma.
Coordinate with social work for protections as indicated.

Bulechek, G. M., Butcher, H. K., Dochterman, J. M., & Wagner, C. (2013). *Nursing interventions classification (NIC)* (6th ed.). St. Louis, MO: Mosby.

treatment, outreach programs in schools, and home visits. Many of the modalities can encompass activities of daily living, learning activities, multiple forms of play and recreational activities, and interactions with adults and peers. Other therapies include family therapy, group therapy, play therapy, mutual storytelling, therapeutic games, bibliotherapy, therapeutic drawing, and mindfulness exercises.

If possible, the family is critical in helping a child recover from trauma. Family counseling and education are key components of treatment. Teaching the family how to set limits without being punitive helps the child to feel in control.

Often traumatized children need help in dealing with flashbacks, amnesia, or hallucinations. You may, for example, work with a child who developed an imaginary friend as a coping mechanism. She may even think that the friend is really a part of her and not a separate person. In such a case, you can offer reassurance and education. "Sometimes when really bad things happen, our brain helps us by forgetting and creating special parts of ourselves that we may think of as friends."

Traumatized children need to learn strategies to regulate emotion and arousal levels. Teaching deep breathing techniques and mindfulness techniques helps decrease arousal levels and restore natural rhythms. Soothing strategies that redirect behavior might also include warm baths, singing, distraction, listening to music, and guided imagery. These strategies help the child to manage feelings. Talking about feelings and helping the child to identify emotions are essential.

Advanced Practice Interventions

International guidelines recommend the use of two therapies with this population: cognitive-behavioral therapy (CBT) and **eye movement desensitization and reprocessing** (EMDR) therapy. These are first-line treatments for traumatized children (World Health Organization, 2013). CBT uses a range of strategies such as psychoeducation, behavior modification, cognitive therapy, exposure therapy, and stress management to help the child manage behavior and change maladaptive beliefs and thoughts.

EMDR therapy is an innovative evidence-based therapy used to treat children and adults by professionals with advanced training (Wheeler, 2014). EMDR therapy processes traumatic memories though a specific eight-phase protocol. The advanced practice nurse asks the patient to think about the traumatic event. At the same time the patient attends to other stimulation such as eye movements, audio tones, or tapping. The combination of thinking and other stimuli bring about neurological and physiological changes that help people process and integrate traumatic memories. Specific protocols have been developed for the treatment of children. Even if the child does not remember what happened, EMDR therapy can be helpful.

Psychopharmacology

Currently there are no FDA approved medications for children with PTSD. Selective serotonin reuptake inhibitors (SSRIs) may improve social and school functioning and decrease avoidance, numbing, and dissociation. Medications that target specific symptoms or comorbidities such as attention-deficit/hyperactivity disorder (ADHD) or depression can enhance the child or adolescent's potential for growth and may make a real difference in a family's ability to cope and quality of life. Medicating children works best along with another treatment such as CBT or EMDR.

EVALUATION

Treatment is effective when:

1. The child's safety has been maintained.
2. Anxiety has been reduced and stress is handled adaptively.
3. Emotions and behavior are appropriate for the situation.
4. The child achieves normal developmental milestones for his or her chronological age.
5. The child is able to seek out adults for nurturance and help when needed.

ATTACHMENT DISORDERS

Attachment at its most basic level ensures survival of the species. Lack of attachment is counter to such a basic drive. Tizard (1977) conducted one of the best known, but tragic studies related to attachment disorders. Children in this study were abandoned by their parents and lived in an institution. They were provided with play areas, books, and basic needs. They were not provided with an adequate number of caregivers, and caregivers were instructed not to form attachments with the children. After 4 years, 8 of the 26 children managed to somehow form an attachment with caregivers, 8 of the children became emotionally unresponsive, and 10 of the children became indiscriminately social and attention seeking.

Children may suffer relationship trauma from a grossly inadequate caregiving environment. Disordered responses to these environments may be one of the two extremes described above: severe emotional inhibition or indiscriminately social behaviors. Children with **reactive attachment disorder** have a consistent pattern of inhibited and emotionally withdrawn behavior. The child rarely directs attachment behaviors toward any adult caregivers and does not seek comfort from them when distressed. This problem is caused by a lack of bonding experiences with a primary caregiver by the age of 8 months. This lack of bonding may be due to severe neglect, repeated changes of primary caregivers, or care in an institutional setting

A seemingly opposite response to inadequate parenting is manifested in **disinhibited social engagement disorder**. These children come across as being remarkably friendly and confident. They demonstrate no normal fear of strangers and are usually willing to go off with people who are unknown to them. Their words (e.g., "I really like you") and physical behavior (e.g., attempts to sit on a stranger's lap) are overly familiar and inconsistent with culturally sanctioned and age-appropriate social boundaries. Children with disinhibited social engagement disorder rarely check back with adult caregivers and seemed unfazed by separation from them. By attaching to everyone they are really not attaching to anyone.

Reactive attachment disorder and disinhibited social engagement disorder are rare. The rates of these problems have been estimated at 1% of all children under the age of 5.

Attachment disorders are often comorbid with other disorders associated with early deprivation. Reactive attachment disorder exists alongside depressive disorders, social problems, PTSD, and cognitive and language problems. Disinhibited social engagement disorder is often seen with ADHD, PTSD, and cognitive and language delays.

For children with symptoms of attachment disorder, the Disturbances of Attachment Interview may be administered (Smyke & Zeanah, 1999). Once diagnosed, children with reactive attachment disorder respond surprisingly well to structure, consistency, and a loving environment. Some evidence of the problem may continue with age. Disinhibited social engagement disorder is more difficult to address. The indiscriminate behavior and attention seeking persists into adolescence, but becomes less pronounced with adults and more focused on peers.

Attachment therapies involve improving the interaction between caregiver and child and are quite effective. Some other attachment therapies are controversial. The most common is holding therapy in which a child is forcibly held or even lain upon by therapists or parents. Through a combination of restraint and confrontation the goal is to produce a certain amount of rage that results in a catharsis or release. At that point the child may become infantile and then re-parented by cradling, rocking, and even bottle-feeding.

TRAUMA-RELATED DISORDERS IN ADULTS

POSTTRAUMATIC STRESS DISORDER

As in children, PTSD in adults is characterized by persistent reexperiencing of a highly traumatic event that involves actual or threatened death or serious injury to self or others, to which the individual responded with intense fear, helplessness, or horror. PTSD may occur after any traumatic event that is outside the range of usual experience. Examples are military trauma, natural disasters, human disasters (e.g., airplane crashes), crime-related events, or a diagnosis of a life-threatening illness.

PTSD may be brought about by indirect exposure to trauma, such as learning that a loved one or friend has experienced violence or accidentally died. First responders who are subjected to repeated or extreme exposure to gruesome scenes or details are also at risk. PTSD symptoms can begin after a month from exposure, but a delay of months or years is not uncommon. See the *DSM-5* box with the criteria for PTSD.

The flashbacks and hypervigilance of PTSD can be terrifying. When the person recalls a traumatic memory, physiological reactions (e.g., sensation of terror in the stomach, heart palpitations, muscles tensing) occur. The person often does not know where these sensations are coming from and attributes them to present circumstances, and the past becomes the present. Because of the changes in the brain, the individual can fluctuate radically from moments of overstimulation and anxiety to moments of complete shutdown and depression. Just when the person feels at rest, as while asleep, intrusive flashbacks may occur. Victims who suffer from PTSD begin to feel permanently damaged and often hate themselves for feeling so needy and helpless.

EPIDEMIOLOGY

Epidemiological studies confirm that most (55% to 90%) people have experienced at least one traumatic event in their lifetimes with an average of five traumatic events reported per person (Centers for Disease Control and Prevention, 2010). An individual's response and the long-term sequelae of a disturbing event are highly variable. Responses depend on a multitude of factors such as the person's age, developmental stage, coping skills, support system, cognitive deficits, preexisting neural physiology, and the nature of the trauma.

Following a traumatic event, nearly 8% of people will develop PTSD (Kessler et al., 1995) with some populations particularly vulnerable. The lifetime prevalence for PTSD is 3.5% of the adult population in the United States with more than a third of these cases classified as severe (National Institute of Mental Health, 2015). The average age of onset is 23 years old with women more than twice as likely as men (10% versus 4%) to develop PTSD. This may be due to the greater incidence of sexual assault on women and also the higher likelihood for women to have a past mental health problem such as anxiety and depression, which may make them more vulnerable to response to a traumatic event (Gradus, 2016).

COMORBIDITY

Comorbidities for adults with PTSD include major depressive disorder, anxiety disorders, sleep disorders, and dissociative disorders. Often substances are used to try to manage the feelings and symptoms. Individuals with PTSD are sad, anhedonic, aggressive, angry, guilty, dissociative, and abuse substances. Difficulty with interpersonal, social, or occupational relationships nearly always accompanies PTSD, and trust is frequently an issue of concern. Presenting symptoms include chronic pain, migraines, and vague somatic complaints. Anxiety or depression, irritability, avoidance, anger or nonadherence, self-risk behavior, threatening or aggressive behavior, dissociative symptoms, or a change in functioning are also common. Some individuals who are victims of spousal abuse may be hypervigilant and irritable. Sometimes people with PTSD use substances in an attempt to self-medicate to relieve anxiety.

RISK FACTORS

See earlier discussion on biological factors in trauma-related disorders for children.

APPLICATION OF THE NURSING PROCESS

ASSESSMENT

Screening tools for PTSD in adults include the Primary Care PTSD Screen (PC-PTSD; Prins et al., 2003) and the PTSD Checklist (PCL-5; Weathers et al., 2013). A more comprehensive assessment is indicated for those who initially screen positive. The Severity of Posttraumatic Stress Scale (Kilpatrick et al., 2013) is provided in Fig. 16.2.

Additional history about the time of onset, frequency, course, severity, level of distress, and degree of functional impairment is important. Further assessment for suicidal or violent ideation, family and social supports, insomnia, social withdrawal, functional impairment, current life stressors, medication, past medical and psychiatric history, and a mental status exam are indicated (refer to Chapter 7). The diagnosis of PTSD involves a comprehensive clinical interview that assesses all symptoms collectively.

DIAGNOSIS

After a comprehensive assessment, a priority nursing diagnosis is applicable (Herdman & Kamitsuru, 2014). *Posttrauma syndrome* is defined as having a "sustained maladaptive response to a traumatic overwhelming event" (p. 315).

Based on this definition, a diagnostic statement would be posttrauma syndrome with a related factor of a distressing event that is considered to be outside the range of usual human experience.

OUTCOMES IDENTIFICATION

Outcomes for trauma-related disorders for an adult are to:

1. Manage anxiety as demonstrated by use of relaxation techniques, adequate sleep, and ability to maintain role or work requirements.
2. Increase self-esteem as demonstrated by maintenance of grooming/hygiene, maintenance of eye contact, positive statements about self, and acceptance of self-limitations.
3. Improve ability to cope as demonstrated by a decrease in physical symptoms, an ability to ask for help, and in seeking information about treatment.

IMPLEMENTATION

A stage model of treatment as previously described for children is the standard for trauma treatment for adults as well. A primary consideration for caring for the person with PTSD is establishing a therapeutic relationship through nonjudgmental acceptance and empathy. In this context, the nurse assists the person in managing his or her arousal level. The latter can be accomplished through providing a safe predictable environment.

Teaching strategies to manage anxiety such as deep breathing, imagery, and mindfulness exercises is a fairly simple intervention. You can also help the patient to connect with support groups, family, and friends. The person often feels guilty and responsible for the event, and the nurse, as a witness through listening and reflecting back to the person his or her concerns, can gently suggest that the person was not responsible for what happened. By sharing the experience, the patient can begin to heal and integrate what happened into his or her life.

Severity of Posttraumatic Stress Symptoms—Adult
National Stressful Events Survey PTSD Short Scale (NSESSS)

Name: ______________________ Age:______ Sex: Male ☐ Female ☐ Date: ____________

Please list the traumatic event that you experienced: ______________________

Date of the traumatic event: ______________________

Instructions: People sometimes have problems after extremely stressful events or experiences. How much have you been bothered during the PAST SEVEN (7) DAYS by each of the following problems that occurred or became worse after an extremely stressful event/experience? **Please respond to each item by marking (✓ or x) one box per row.**

	Not at all	A little bit	Moderately	Quite a bit	Extremely	Clinician use: Item Score
1 Having "flashbacks," that is, you suddenly acted or felt as if a stressful experience from the past was happening all over again (for example, you re-experienced parts of a stressful experience by seeing, hearing, smelling, or physically feeling parts of the experience)?	☐ 0	☐ 1	☐ 2	☐ 3	☐ 4	
2 Feeling very emotionally upset when something reminded you of a stressful experience?	☐ 0	☐ 1	☐ 2	☐ 3	☐ 4	
3 Trying to avoid thoughts, feelings, or physical sensation that reminded you of a stressful experience?	☐ 0	☐ 1	☐ 2	☐ 3	☐ 4	
4 Thinking that a stressful event happened because you or someone else (who didn't directly harm you) did something wrong or didn't do everything possible to prevent it, or because of something about you?	☐ 0	☐ 1	☐ 2	☐ 3	☐ 4	
5 Having a very negative emotional state (for example, you were experiencing lots of fear, anger, guilt, shame, or horror) after a stressful experience?	☐ 0	☐ 1	☐ 2	☐ 3	☐ 4	
6 Losing interest in activities you used to enjoy before having a stressful experience?	☐ 0	☐ 1	☐ 2	☐ 3	☐ 4	
7 Being "super alert," on guard, or constantly on the lookout for danger?	☐ 0	☐ 1	☐ 2	☐ 3	☐ 4	
8 Feeling jumpy or easily startled when you hear an unexpected noise?	☐ 0	☐ 1	☐ 2	☐ 3	☐ 4	
9 Being extremely irritable or angry to the point where you yelled at other people, got into fights, or destroyed things?	☐ 0	☐ 1	☐ 2	☐ 3	☐ 4	
Total/partial raw score:						
Prorated total raw score: (if 1–2 items left unanswered)						
Average total score:						

FIG. 16.2 Severity of posttraumatic stress symptoms scale.

Psychoeducation

Initial education should include reassurance that reactions to trauma are common and that these reactions do not indicate personal failure or weakness. The nurse should inform the patient and significant others of the many ways that trauma can be manifested. Interpersonal problems with family and friends, occupational problems, and/or substance-use disorders and problems with alcohol use are common symptoms. Strategies to improve coping, enhance self-care, and facilitate recognition of problems are essential. Patients experiencing such severe stress will benefit from relaxation techniques and in the avoidance of caffeine and alcohol.

Psychopharmacology

The best evidence supports the use of selective serotonin reuptake inhibitors (SSRIs) for PTSD symptoms. Currently, the FDA has approved two drugs: sertraline (Zoloft) and paroxetine (Paxil). From the perspective of the FDA, all other medications are used off label.

Phenelzine (Nardil) is a monoamine oxidase inhibitor that has been used with some success in PTSD. A serotonin norepinephrine reuptake inhibitor (SNRI) such as venlafaxine (Effexor) may be used to decrease anxiety and depressive symptoms. Tricyclic antidepressants (TCAs) or mirtazapine (Remeron) may be prescribed if SSRIs or SNRIs are not tolerated or do not work.

Clonidine (Catapres) is a centrally acting alpha-2 receptor agonist used to address hyperarousal and intrusive symptoms. Prazosin (Minipress) is an alpha-receptor antagonist used for nightmares and sleep disturbances. Propranolol (Inderal), a beta-blocker, is used for hyperarousal and panic. The most difficult to tolerate side effect of these medications is hypotension.

The FDA recently agreed to new trials for MDMA, the illegal party drug known as Ecstasy, as a relief for PTSD patients (Phillips, 2016). Phase III clinical trials of the drug are under way as a final step for approval of Ecstasy as a prescription drug. After three doses of MDMA, patients reported a 56% decrease in symptom severity on average. Follow-up examinations found that improvements lasted more than a year after therapy. The drug reduces painful memories and helped patients to stop substance use.

CASE STUDY AND NURSING CARE PLAN

Posttraumatic Stress Disorder

A distraught wife brings Mr. Blake, 46, to the emergency department after she finds him writing a suicide note and planning to shoot himself in the woods with a handgun. Mr. Blake is subdued, shows minimal affect, and his breath smells of alcohol. He states that he is worthless and that his family would be better off if he were dead. He is hospitalized to protect him from danger to himself.

Mr. Blake's wife states that her husband is a contractor who served during the Iraq War. He lost half his squad from a roadside bombing and narrowly escaped with his life. Upon returning home he told his wife, "I don't deserve to live. I should have died with the others." Over the next 6 months, Mrs. Blake noticed that he was having trouble sleeping, his mood was irritable or withdrawn, and he started to drink daily. He complained of nightmares but wouldn't talk about them. He agreed to go to his primary care nurse practitioner for sleep medication.

On the psychiatric unit, Mr. Blake is assigned to Ms. Dawson, a registered nurse. She observes that Mr. Blake is quiet as he is oriented to the unit but that he looks around vigilantly and is easily startled by sounds.

Self-Assessment

Ms. Dawson is a registered nurse with an associate degree and 3 years of experience on this unit. Initially she feels sympathy for Mr. Blake, and he reminds her of her Uncle James who served in Vietnam. She is concerned because his suicide plan was lethal and he is not sharing his thoughts or feelings. Ms. Dawson implements suicide precautions while demonstrating an attitude of hope and acceptance to develop trust.

Assessment

Mr. Blake was administered the PCL-5, which is a 20-item self-report scale of symptoms of PTSD. He scored significant for PTSD with this measure. The nurse obtained the following subjective and objective data:

Subjective Data

"I don't deserve to live; I should have died with the others."
Sleep difficulty, nightmares
Feels estranged from wife and children
Refusal of treatment and safety contract
Plan for suicide

Objective Data

Hypervigilant
Alcohol on breath
Irritability
Withdrawn mood
Constricted/reduced range of affect

Priority Diagnosis

Risk for suicide as evidenced by suicide plan and verbalization of intent.

Outcomes Identification

Patient will remain safe while in the hospital.

Planning

The initial plan is to maintain safety for Mr. Blake while encouraging him to express feelings and recognize that his situation is not hopeless.

Implementation

Mr. Blake's plan of care is personalized as follows:

Short-Term Goal	Intervention	Rationale	Evaluation
1. Patient will speak to staff whenever experiencing self-destructive thoughts.	1a. Administer medications with mouth checks.	1a. Addresses risk of hiding medications for future overdose.	**GOAL MET** After 8 hours, patient contracts for safety every shift and starts to discuss feelings of self-harm.
	1b. Provide ongoing surveillance of patient and environment.	1b. Provides one-to-one monitoring for safety.	
	1c. Use direct, nonjudgmental approach in discussing suicide.	1c. Shows acceptance of patient's situation with respect.	
2. Patient will express feelings by the third day of hospitalization.	2a. Interact with patient at regular intervals to convey caring and openness and to provide an opportunity to talk.	2a. Encourages development of trust.	**GOAL MET** By second day, patient occasionally answers questions about feelings and admits to anger and grief.
	2b. Use silence and listening to encourage expression of feelings.	2b. Shows positive expectation that patient will respond.	
	2c. Be open to expressions of loneliness and powerlessness.	2c. Allows patient to voice these uncomfortable feelings.	
	2d. Share observations or thoughts about patient's behavior or response.	2d. Directs attention to here-and-now treatment situation.	

Continued

CASE STUDY AND NURSING CARE PLAN—cont'd

Posttraumatic Stress Disorder

Short-Term Goal	Intervention	Rationale	Evaluation
3. Patient will express desire to live by discharge from unit.	3a. Listen to expressions of grief. 3b. Encourage identification of strengths and abilities. 3c. Explore with patient previous methods of dealing with life problems. 3d. Assist in identifying available support systems. 3e. Refer to spiritual advisor of individual's choice.	3a. Supports patient, communicating that such feelings are natural. 3b. Affirms patient's worth and potential to survive. 3c. Reinforces patient's past coping skills and ability to problem solve now. 3d. May have pushed others away. Support systems can also be community groups. 3e. Allows opportunity to explore spiritual values and self-worth.	**GOAL MET** By third day, patient becomes tearful and states that he does not want to hurt his wife and daughter.

Evaluation

See individual outcomes and evaluation within the care plan.

Advanced Practice Interventions

Evidence-based treatments for PTSD include trauma-focused psychotherapy that may include components of exposure and/or cognitive restructuring and EMDR therapy. These modalities are often combined with anxiety management/stress reduction that focuses on alleviation of symptoms. Other helpful strategies include brief psychodynamic psychotherapy, imagery, relaxation techniques, hypnosis, and group therapy.

EVALUATION

Treatment is effective when:

1. The patient recognizes symptoms as related to the trauma.
2. The patient is able to use new strategies to manage anxiety.
3. The patient experiences no flashbacks or intrusive thoughts about the traumatic event.
4. The patient is able to sleep adequately without nightmares.
5. The patient can assume usual roles and maintains satisfying interpersonal relationships.

(See the Case Study and Nursing Care Plan.)

ACUTE STRESS DISORDER

Acute stress disorder (ASD) may develop after exposure to a highly traumatic event such as those listed in the section on PTSD. Symptoms develop immediately after the event, but a diagnosis is not made until they have persisted for 3 days. The diagnosis must be made within a month of the trauma. After a period of a month the stress response will begin to resolve or go on to become PTSD.

VIGNETTE: At a party, a male sexually assaults John, a 22-year-old college student. After John is brought to the emergency department by a friend, he describes feeling detached from his body. He can't remember his surroundings during the assault, "It feels like it took place in a vacuum." He is agitated, irritable, and tells his friend to leave. John has difficulty concentrating on the examiner's questions. After a week, John still feels as though his mind is detached from his body. He reports having difficulty sleeping, nightmares, headaches, not being able to concentrate, and startling whenever anyone touches him.

DIAGNOSIS

As with PTSD, an appropriate nursing diagnosis for a patient with ASD (NANDA, 2012) is *posttrauma syndrome related to victimization* as manifested by:

- Alterations in concentration
- Anger
- Dissociative amnesia
- Headache
- Irritability
- Nightmares

OUTCOMES IDENTIFICATION

Outcomes will focus on attaining mood equilibrium and well-being. For anxiety, a general outcome may be that the patient's anxiety level be maintained at mild to moderate.

IMPLEMENTATION

The nurse's role in caring for a patient with ASD begins with establishing a therapeutic relationship with the person. Based on this relationship the nurse can help keep the person safe and monitor response to treatment. Promoting problem solving, connecting the person to supports such as family and friends, and providing education about ASD are also important interventions. Other responsibilities include coordination of care through collaboration with others and providing referrals for continued treatment.

There are few studies that evaluate the efficacy of treatments for ASD. Historically, critical incident stress debriefing (CISD) has been used for those who had suffered from acute trauma. Typically **debriefing** occurs within 12 to 48 hours after the traumatic event and is often offered as a group intervention. Group members receive information on the facts of the event and psychological consequences of trauma and the possible ways of coping, and they exchange the details of the incident. Research on CISD has not supported its efficacy as an intervention after a traumatic event.

In fact several studies have found a higher incidence of PTSD for those who received CISD (Bisson & Andrew, 2007).

Advanced Practice Interventions

CBT is effective in reducing the subsequent development of PTSD for people with ASD. Other promising new therapies for ASD include specialized protocols for EMDR: the EMDR Protocol for Recent Critical Incidents (EMDR-PRECI), the Recent Event Protocol, and the Recent Traumatic Episode Protocol (R-TEP; Luber, 2014).

EVALUATION

See the Evaluation section for PTSD previously discussed in this chapter.

ADJUSTMENT DISORDER

What may be considered to be a milder less specific version of ASD and PTSD is **adjustment disorder**. Like ASD and PTSD, it is precipitated by a stressful event. However, the event—including retirement, chronic illness, or a breakup—may not be as severe and may not be considered a traumatic event. This problem may be diagnosed immediately or within 3 months of exposure. The hallmarks of adjustment disorder are cognitive, emotional, and behavioral symptoms that negatively impact functioning. Responses to the stressful event may include combinations of depression, anxiety, and conduct disturbances.

Symptoms of adjustment disorder run the gamut of all forms of distress including guilt, depression, anxiety, and anger. These feelings may be combined with other manifestations of distress, including physical complaints, social withdrawal, or work or academic inhibition. Quality of life scores are higher with adjustment disorder than for major depression but lower than for people without any disorder (Fernández et al., 2012).

There is a type of adjustment disorder that addresses the needs of those who have lost a loved one within the past 12 months—a sort of complicated grief. This type of adjustment disorder is manifested by intense yearning/longing for the deceased and intense sorrow and emotional pain or preoccupation with the deceased or the circumstances of the death. In addition, the person may feel anger, a diminished sense of self, emptiness, and/or difficulty in relationships or in planning future activities. This may be in accordance with cultural norms.

The reported prevalence of adjustment disorder varies widely depending on the setting studied. For example, in those hospitalized, adjustment disorder was found to occur in 50% of the population (APA, 2013), whereas in a primary care setting, it is estimated at 3% of the population (Fernández et al., 2012). Thus treatment of adjustment disorder is not uniform due to the lack of specificity of the problem, and practitioners do not usually recognize this disorder. Symptoms are generally treated with antidepressants.

DISSOCIATIVE DISORDERS

Dissociative disorders occur after significant adverse experiences/traumas, and individuals respond to stress with a severe interruption of consciousness. Dissociation is an unconscious defense mechanism that protects the individual against overwhelming anxiety through an emotional separation. However, this separation results in disturbances in memory, consciousness, self-identity, and perception.

Patients with dissociative disorders have intact reality testing. This means that although the person may have flashbacks or images, these are triggered by current events, relate to the past trauma, and are not delusions or hallucinations. Mild fleeting dissociative experiences are relatively common to all of us. For example, we say we are on "auto pilot" when we drive home from work and cannot recall the last 15 minutes before reaching the house.

These common experiences are distinctly different from the processes of pathological dissociation. Dissociation is involuntary and results in failure of the normal control over a person's mental processes and normal integration of conscious awareness. Dimensions of a memory that should be linked are not and are fragmented. For example, a person may be aware of a sound or smell, but these sensations would not be linked to the actual event itself, leaving the person fearful and/or confused. In addition, the person may reenact, as well as re-experience, trauma without consciously knowing why.

Symptoms of dissociation may be either positive or negative. Positive symptoms refer to unwanted additions to mental activity such as flashbacks. Negative symptoms refer to deficits such as memory problems or the ability to sense or control different parts of the body. Dissociation decreases the immediate subjective distress of the trauma and also continues to protect the individual from full awareness of the disturbing event.

Dissociation can also be somewhat protective for a child to maintain an attachment with abusive or neglectful caregivers. This highlights the importance of attachments and relationships in allowing the child to grow socially, intellectually, and cognitively. If abuse or neglect has occurred, these memories become compartmentalized and often do not intrude into awareness until later in life when the person is in a stressful situation. Dissociative disorders include (1) depersonalization/derealization disorder, (2) dissociative amnesia, and (3) dissociative identity disorder.

DEPERSONALIZATION/DEREALIZATION DISORDER

Depersonalization/derealization is found in both adolescents and adults often in response to acute stress. In **depersonalization** the focus is on oneself. It is an extremely uncomfortable feeling of being an observer of one's own body or mental processes. In **derealization** the focus is on the outside world. It is the recurring feeling that one's surroundings are unreal or distant. The person may feel mechanical, dreamy, or detached from the body. Some people suffer episodes of these problems that come and go while others have episodes that begin with stressors and eventually become constant. Patients describe these experiences as very distressing.

VIGNETTE: Elizabeth, a 42-year-old executive, gasps as she looks in the mirror. She can't believe the changes in her appearance. She thinks that her body looks wavy and out of focus. She says that it feels as though she is floating in a fog and her feet are not actually touching the ground. "I wonder if I am really awake or if my life is a dream." As she is admitted to the stress-management unit, Elizabeth confides to the nurse that her son has recently been charged with insider trading in the stock market and that he may be facing a lengthy jail sentence.

DISSOCIATIVE AMNESIA

Dissociative amnesia may occur in any age group from children to adults. The amnesia is often related to trauma, and memory usually returns spontaneously after the individual is removed from the stressful situation (ISSTD, 2012). **Dissociative amnesia** is marked by the inability to recall important personal information often of a traumatic or stressful nature. The amnesia may also be localized (the patient is unable to remember all events in a certain period) or selective (the patient is able to recall some but not all events in a certain period).

A subtype of dissociative amnesia is **dissociative fugue**. It is characterized by sudden unexpected travel and an inability to recall one's identity and information about some or all of the past. In rare cases, an individual with dissociative fugue assumes a whole new identity. In fugue states, individuals often function adequately in their new identities by choosing simple undemanding occupations and having few intimate social interactions. After a few weeks to a few months, they may remember their former identities and then become amnesic for the time spent in the fugue state. Usually a traumatic event precedes a dissociative fugue.

VIGNETTE: A young woman found wandering in a Florida park is partly dressed and poorly nourished. She has no knowledge of who she is. Her parents identify her 2 weeks later when she appears in an interview on a national television show. Her boyfriend of 3 years had committed suicide before the fugue state.

DISSOCIATIVE IDENTITY DISORDER

The essential feature of **dissociative identity disorder** is the presence of two or more distinct personality states that recurrently take control of behavior. Each **alternate personality (alter)** has its own pattern of perceiving, relating to, and thinking about the self and the environment. It is believed that severe sexual, physical, or psychological trauma in childhood predisposes an individual to the development of dissociative identity disorder.

Dissociative identity disorder is associated with at least two dissociative identity states: one is a state or personality that functions on a daily basis and blocks access and responses to traumatic memories, and another state (also referred to as an *alter state*) is fixated on traumatic memories. Each alter is a complex unit with its own memories, behavioral patterns, and social relationships that dictate how the person acts when that personality is dominant. Often the original or primary personality is religious and moralistic, and the alters are pleasure-seeking and nonconforming. The alter personalities may behave as individuals of a different sex, race, or religion. The dominant hand and the voice may also be different; intelligence and electroencephalographic findings may also be altered.

The primary personality or host is usually not aware of the alters and is perplexed by lost time and unexplained events. Experiences such as finding unfamiliar clothing in the closet, being called a different name by a stranger, or not having childhood memories are characteristic of dissociative identity disorder. Alters may be aware of the existence of each other to some degree. Transition from one personality to another (switching) occurs during times of stress and may range from a dramatic to a barely noticeable event. Some patients experience the transition when awakening. Shifts may last from minutes to months, although shorter periods are more common.

Several movies and TV shows that explore case studies of individuals diagnosed with dissociative identity disorder have been produced. They include *Sybil* (1976), *The Three Faces of Eve* (1957), *Fight Club* (1999), *Me, Myself and Irene* (2000), and the television series *The United States of Tara.*

EPIDEMIOLOGY

The lifetime prevalence of dissociative disorders ranges from 2% to 10% (International Society for the Study of Trauma and Dissociation [ISSTD], 2012). Depersonalization/derealization disorder is about 2%. Females and males are equally affected by this problem. Dissociative amnesia is also fairly common with a prevalence of about 2% to 7%. Females are affected at more than twice the rate of men. Dissociative identity disorder has a 12-month prevalence of 1.5%. Males and females are equally represented in this disorder.

COMORBIDITY

Comorbidity is common with dissociative disorders. Major depressive disorder, panic attacks, eating disorders, PTSD, somatoform symptoms, eating disorders, obsessive-compulsive disorder (OCD), reactive attachment disorder, and attention-deficit disorder commonly co-occur with the dissociative disorders. Personality disorders such as borderline personality disorder, substance-use disorders, and sexual and sleep disorders, are also comorbid with dissociative disorders (ISSTD, 2012).

Dissociative amnesia may be comorbid with conversion disorder or a personality disorder. Dissociative fugue may co-occur with PTSD. Depersonalization and derealization also occur in hypochondriasis, mood and anxiety disorders, obsessive-compulsive disorder, and schizophrenia.

RISK FACTORS

Childhood physical, sexual, or emotional abuse and other traumatic life events are associated with adults experiencing dissociative symptoms. Dissociative symptoms, or "mindflight," actually reduce disturbing feelings and protect the person from full awareness of the trauma.

Biological Factors

Genetic

Although genetic variability is thought to play a role in stress reactivity, dissociation is largely due to extreme stress or environmental factors.

Neurobiological

The limbic system is involved in the development of dissociative disorders. Animal studies show that early and prolonged detachment from the caretaker negatively affects the development of the limbic system. Traumatic memories are processed in the limbic system, and the hippocampus stores this information. Individuals with dissociative disorders have altered communication between higher and lower brain structures due to the massive release of endogenous opioids at the time of severe threat. This inhibits the thalamus from connecting with the limbic area with the neocortex and integration across the hemispheres through the corpus callosum (Lanius et al., 2014).

People with temporal lobe epilepsy experience depersonalization, derealization, anxiety, and dissociation. This overlap of symptoms results in people without epilepsy being treated with anticonvulsants. Conversely, but less likely, people with epilepsy may be treated for a psychiatric disorder

Psychological Factors

One of the most primitive ego defense mechanisms is dissociation. The theory of structural dissociation of the personality proposes that patients with complex trauma have different parts of their personality—the apparently normal part and the emotional part—that are not fully integrated with each other (Steele et al., 2005). Each part has its own responses, feelings, thoughts, perceptions, physical sensations, and behaviors. These different parts may not be aware of one another with only one dominant personality operating depending on the situation and circumstance of the moment.

Environmental Factors

Dissociative disorders are responses to acute overwhelming trauma and as such are due to environmental factors. These may include any experience that is overwhelming to the person such as a motor vehicle accident, combat, emotional/verbal abuse, incest, neglectful or abusive caregivers, imprisonment, and many other types of traumatic events.

Cultural Considerations

Certain culture-bound disorders exist that are similar to dissociative fugue. They are characterized by a high level of activity, a trancelike state, and running or fleeing, followed by exhaustion, sleep, and amnesia regarding the episode. These syndromes include *piblokto* seen in native people of the Arctic, *frenzy* witchcraft among the Navajo, and *amok* among Western Pacific natives. These syndromes, if observed in individuals native to the corresponding geographical areas, are different from dissociative disorders and the nurse should take this into account.

CONSIDERING CULTURE

Are Culture Bound Syndromes Always Culture Bound?

The *DSM-5* identifies syndromes specific to certain cultures. Some syndromes have predominantly dissociative syndromes. For example ataque de nervios occurs among individuals of Latino descent. It is characterized by acute anxiety, anger, grief, shouting, crying, trembling, and heat in the upper part of the body. The person may become verbally and physically aggressive. Dissociative episodes such as depersonalization, derealization, amnesia, seizures, and fainting also can occur.

An interesting study included 100 mainly white inpatients in the United States with a history of childhood and/or sexual abuse (87%) and dissociative disorders (73%). Researchers found that many symptoms that tend to be considered culture-bound occurred with surprising frequency in these patients. Participants reported that they were possessed and were involved with various exorcism procedures. Among the procedures were having a healer enter a trance state during a ritual, animal sacrifice, or ritual dancing. The most common exorcism practice involved prayer, which is consistent with mainstream Christian beliefs.

The authors conclude that not all classical culture-bound syndromes are really culture bound. Dissociative symptoms are similar no matter the culture. Referring to dissociative symptoms as a unique cultural syndrome may be an epidemiological error and one based on American and DSM ethnocentricity.

Ross, C., Schroeder, B. A., & Ness, L. (2013). Dissociation and symptoms of culture-bound syndromes in North America: A preliminary study. *Journal of Trauma and Dissociation, 14*, 224–235.

APPLICATION OF THE NURSING PROCESS

ASSESSMENT

Many patients with dissociative disorders seek help for depressive and anxiety disorders. Living with symptoms such as feeling unreal, perceiving the world as unreal, forgetting significant events, and losing track of time are obviously disturbing and depressing. Specific information about life events, memory, suicide risk, and the impact of the disorder on the patient and the family are important dimensions to assess.

Life Events

The nurse gathers information about events in the person's life. Has the patient sustained a recent injury such as a concussion? Does the patient have a history of epilepsy, especially temporal lobe epilepsy? Does the patient have a history of early trauma such as physical, mental, or sexual abuse? If you suspect dissociative identity disorder, ask the following questions:

1. Have you ever found yourself wearing clothes you cannot remember buying?
2. Have you ever had strange persons greet and talk to you as though they were old friends?
3. Does your ability to engage in things such as athletics, artistic activities, or mechanical tasks seem to change?
4. Do you have differing sets of memories about childhood?

Memory

The nurse should consider the following when assessing memory:

1. Can the patient remember recent and past events?
2. Is the patient's memory clear and complete or partial and fuzzy?

3. Is the patient aware of gaps in memory such as lack of memory for events such as a graduation or a wedding?
4. Do the patient's memories place the self with a family, in school, or in an occupation?
5. Is the patient oriented to time, place, person, and situation?
6. Does the patient ever lose time or have blackouts?
7. Does the patient ever find herself or himself in places with no idea how she or he got there?

Suicide Risk

Whenever a patient's life has been substantially disrupted, the patient may have thoughts of suicide. Nurses should be alert for expressions of hopelessness, helplessness, or worthlessness. Directly addressing the possibility of suicidal ideation, intent, and plans are always important interventions when working with this population. Asking questions for self-mutilating compulsions and behaviors is important, as is directly assessing for physical harm since dissociative patients may be unaware of injury.

Impact on Patient and Family

Dissociative disorders impair an individual's ability to relate to the world, which results in significant impairment of interpersonal relationships. Feelings of being unreal or the world being unreal negatively impact normal communication patterns and satisfaction in relationships. Patients with depersonalization/derealization disorder are often fearful that others may perceive their appearance as distorted and may avoid being seen in public.

Patients with dissociative amnesia and identity disorder often have employment and family problems. Memory loss often renders them unable to work and impairs normal relationships. Employers dislike the lost time that may occur due to dissociative symptoms. Families often direct considerable attention toward the patient but may express concern over having to assume roles that were once assigned to the patient. Families find it difficult to accept the seemingly erratic behaviors of the patient. The high anxiety that accompanies dissociative disorders makes it difficult to keep relationships stable.

Assessment Tools

Reviewing assessment tools can help you remember the symptoms of dissociation and to understand what your patient is experiencing. Scales have been developed to assess dissociation. The Cambridge Depersonalization Scale (Sierra & Berrios, 2000) measures both depersonalization and derealization. General dissociation is assessed with the Dissociative Experience Scale (DES; Bernstein & Putnam, 1986) and the Somatoform Dissociation Questionnaire (SDQ; Nijenhuis et al., 2012). Both are available online.

General Guidelines for Assessment

General guidelines for assessment of a patient with a dissociative disorder include:

1. Assess for a history of self-harm.
2. Evaluate level of anxiety and signs of dissociation.
3. Identify support systems through a psychosocial assessment.
4. Refer patient to therapist.

Self-Assessment

It is natural to experience feelings of discomfort when working with people who lose self-awareness. You may simply be skeptical that someone could forget who they are and believe that they are being manipulative and want to leave their responsibilities behind. On the other hand, some nurses experience feelings of fascination and are caught up in the intrigue of caring for a patient with these dramatic disorders. Self-awareness, managing overly negative or positive responses, and recognizing professional boundaries are essential skills when working with this population.

DIAGNOSIS

See Table 16.1 for potential nursing diagnoses.

OUTCOMES IDENTIFICATION

The overall goal for dissociative disorder is to develop an integrated and complete perception of self. See Table 16.1 for possible short-term outcomes for dissociative disorders.

TABLE 16.1 Signs and Symptoms, Diagnoses, and Outcomes for Dissociative Disorders

Signs and Symptoms	Nursing Diagnoses	Outcomes
Amnesia or fugue related to a traumatic event, symptoms of depersonalization, feelings of unreality and/or body image distortions	*Disturbed personal identity*	Verbalizes clear sense of personal identity, perceives environment accurately, performs social roles well
Alterations in consciousness, memory, or identity, abuse of substances, disorganization or dysfunction in usual patterns of behavior (absence from work, withdrawal from relationships, changes in role function)	*Ineffective role performance*	Performs family, parental, intimate, community, and work roles adequately; reports comfort with role expectations; recovers deficits in memory
Feeling of being out of control of memory, behaviors, and awareness, inability to explain actions or behaviors when in altered state	*Anxiety self-control*	Monitors intensity of anxiety, identifies triggers that lead to switching; uses effective coping strategies to manage anxiety

From Herdman, T. H., & Kamitsuru, S. (Eds.). (2014). *Nursing diagnoses—Definitions and classification 2015-2017.* Oxford, UK: Wiley Blackwell. Copyright © 2014, 1994-2012 by NANDA International. Used by arrangement with John Wiley & Sons Limited; Moorhead, S., Johnson, M., Maas, M. L., & Swanson, E. (2013). *Nursing outcomes classification (NOC)* (5th ed.). St. Louis, MO: Mosby.

PLANNING

The setting and presenting problem influence the planning of nursing care for the patient with a dissociative disorder. However, a phase-oriented treatment model is recommended and includes the following:

Phase 1: Establishing safety, stabilization, and symptom reduction.

Phase 2: Confronting, working through, and integrating traumatic memories.

Phase 3: Identity integration and rehabilitation.

The nurse will most often encounter the patient in times of crisis (i.e., when the patient is admitted to the hospital for suicidal or homicidal behavior). The care plan will focus on Phase 1 strategies to ensure safety and crisis intervention. The patient may also come for treatment of a comorbid depression or anxiety disorder in the community setting. Planning will address the presenting complaint with appropriate referrals for treatment of the dissociative disorder.

IMPLEMENTATION

Healing trauma can be thought of as a process of integration and linking neural networks that have become disconnected during an overwhelming event. You should offer an emotional presence during the recall of painful experiences, provide a sense of safety, and encourage an optimal level of functioning. *NIC* topics that offer relevant interventions include *anxiety reduction, coping enhancement, self-awareness enhancement, self-esteem enhancement,* and *emotional support.* Refer to Table 16.2 for examples of basic-level interventions.

Psychoeducation

Patients with dissociative disorders need to learn about their illness and be given ongoing instruction about coping skills and stress management. Normalizing experiences by explaining symptoms as adaptive responses to overwhelming events is important. Often the victim of childhood trauma grows up with the false negative belief that the abuse was deserved punishment.

Grounding techniques promote the individual's ability to be "in the moment" and help counter dissociative episodes. For example, dissociation can be disrupted by: stomping feet, taking a shower, holding an ice cube, exercising, deep breathing, or touching the upholstery on a chair. Patients can learn to keep a daily journal to increase awareness of feelings and to identify triggers to dissociation. If a patient has never written a journal, the nurse should suggest beginning with a 5- to 10-minute daily writing exercise.

Pharmacological Interventions

There are no specific medications for patients with dissociative disorders, but appropriate medications are often prescribed for the hyperarousal and intrusive symptoms that accompany PTSD and dissociation (ISSTD, 2012). These might include antidepressant medication, antianxiety agents, and antipsychotics. Substance-use disorders and suicidal risk, which are common, must be assessed carefully in selecting safe and appropriate pharmacotherapy. In the acute setting, the nurse may witness dramatic memory retrieval in patients with dissociative amnesia or fugue after treatment with intravenous benzodiazepines.

Advanced Practice Interventions

Advanced practice psychiatric-mental health registered nurses use therapies discussed previously: CBT and (modified) EMDR. Other therapies that may be useful with dissociative conditions

TABLE 16.2 Basic-Level Nursing Interventions for Dissociative Disorders

Intervention	Rationale
Provide undemanding, simple routine.	Reduces anxiety.
Ensure patient safety by providing safe, protected environment and frequent observation.	Sense of bewilderment may lead to inattention to safety needs; some alters may be thrill-seeking, violent, or careless.
Confirm identity of patient and orientation to time and place.	Supports reality and promotes ego integrity.
Encourage patient to do things for self and make decisions about routine tasks.	Enhances self-esteem by reducing sense of powerlessness and reduces secondary gain associated with dependence.
Assist with major decision making until memory returns.	Lowers stress and prevents patient from having to live with the consequences of unwise decisions.
Support patient during exploration of feelings surrounding the stressful event.	Helps lower the defense of dissociation used by patient to block awareness of the stressful event.
Do not flood patient with data regarding past events.	Memory loss serves the purpose of preventing severe to panic levels of anxiety from overtaking and disorganizing the individual.
Allow patient to progress at own pace as memory is recovered.	Prevents undue anxiety and resistance.
Provide support through empathetic listening during disclosure of painful experiences.	Can be healing, while minimizing feelings of isolation.
Teach patient grounding techniques such as taking a shower, deep breathing, touching fabric on chair, exercising or stomping feet.	Helps keep the person in the present and decrease dissociation.
Accept patient's expression of negative feelings.	Conveys permission to have negative or unacceptable feelings.
Teach stress-reduction methods.	Provides alternatives for anxiety relief.
If patient does not remember significant others, work with involved parties to reestablish relationships.	Helps patient experience satisfaction and relieves sense of isolation.

include psychodynamic psychotherapy, exposure therapy, hypnotherapy, neurofeedback, ego state therapies, and somatic therapies.

Somatic Therapy

Dissociation causes people to experience a distressing fragmentation of consciousness and a sense of separation from themselves. Disturbances of perception, sensation, autonomic regulation, and movement are common for those who have suffered significant trauma because trauma is often stored physically in the body. Verbal and bodily psychotherapies are seen as complementary by the discipline of Dance Movement Therapists in working with traumatized dissociative patients in emotional recovery (Koch & Harvey, 2012).

Sensorimotor psychotherapy combines talk therapy with body-centered interventions and movement to address dissociative symptoms (Ogden et al., 2006). This therapy is based on the premise that the body, mind, emotions, and spirit are interrelated, and a change at one level results in changes in the others. Awareness, focusing on the present, and recognizing touch as a means of communicating are some of the principles of this therapy. During psychotherapy sessions, the patient describes current physical sensations. The goal is to safely disarm the pathological defense mechanism of dissociation and replace it with other resources, especially body awareness and mindfulness.

EVALUATION

Overall, treatment effectiveness for dissociative disorders is evaluated by integration. In general, treatment for dissociative disorders is considered successful when outcomes are met. In the final analysis, the evaluation is positive when:

1. Patient safety has been maintained.
2. Anxiety has been reduced, and the patient has returned to a functional state.
3. Integration of the fragmented memories has occurred.
4. New coping strategies have permitted the patient to function at a better level.
5. Stress is handled adaptively, without the use of dissociation.

KEY POINTS TO REMEMBER

- Childhood trauma changes the brain and can cause medical and psychological problems in adulthood.
- A phase model of treatment is most effective with safety and stabilization first.
- Evidenced-based treatments for trauma are eye movement desensitization and reprocessing (EMDR) therapy and cognitive-behavioral therapy (CBT).
- Understanding patients as traumatized changes the conversation from "What is wrong with this person?" to "What happened to this person?"
- Trauma is stored in the body and often manifests as physical symptoms. Healing involves connection and integration.
- Dissociative disorders involve a disruption in consciousness with significant impairments in memory, identity, and perception of self.
- Assessment is especially important in clarifying the history of symptoms and obtaining a complete picture of the current physical, psychological, and safety status.
- Psychotherapy is the treatment of choice for trauma, with medication prescribed only to ameliorate symptoms.
- Patients with trauma-related disorders are often treated on an outpatient basis except during a period of crisis such as suicidal risk.
- Crisis intervention is important for stabilization. Referral for psychotherapy to attain sustained improvement in level of functioning is typically necessary.

CRITICAL THINKING EXERCISES

1. Jeanne is a 48-year-old with dissociative identity disorder who was admitted to the crisis unit for a short-term stay after a suicide threat. On the unit, she has repeated the statement that she will kill herself to get rid of "all the others," meaning her alters.
   a. How do you think that staff reacts to working with patients such as Jeanne?
   b. What do you believe needs to be done to protect Jeanne?
2. Steven is an 8-year-old who was in a devastating earthquake and came to the outpatient clinic with his parents because he was having nightmares and trouble sleeping. How would you explain what is happening to Steven?
3. John, a 24-year-old, returned from the Iraq War last month. Since then he has become increasingly irritable, isolated, and depressed. His wife says he does not want to go anywhere and won't leave his home for days at a time. In the interview with the nurse at the clinic, he indicates that he feels helpless and anxious and jumpy.
   a. Identify priorities in providing care for this patient.
   b. What type of medication would you anticipate being ordered for John?

CHAPTER REVIEW

Questions

1. Which statement made by the patient demonstrates an understanding of the treatment of choice for patients managing the effects of traumatic events?
   a. "I attend my therapy sessions regularly."
   b. "Those intrusive memories are hidden for a reason and should stay hidden."
   c. "Keeping busy is the key to getting mentally healthy."
   d. "I've agreed to move in with my parents so I'll get the support I need."

2. Which goal should be addressed initially when providing care for 10-year-old Harper who is diagnosed with posttraumatic stress disorder (PTSD)?
   a. Harper will be able to identify feelings through the use of play therapy.
   b. Harper and her parents will have access to protective resources available through social services.
   c. Harper will demonstrate the effective use of relaxation techniques to restore a sense of control over disturbing thoughts.
   d. Harper and her parents will demonstrate an understanding of the personal human response to traumatic events.
3. The care plan of a male patient diagnosed with a dissociative disorder includes the nursing diagnosis *ineffective coping*. Which behavior demonstrated by the patient supports this nursing diagnosis?
   a. Has no memory of the physical abuse he endured.
   b. Using both alcohol and marijuana.
   c. Often reports being unaware of surroundings.
   d. Reports feelings of "not really being here."
4. Which statement accurately describes the effects of emotional trauma on the individual physically?
   a. Emotional trauma is a distinct category and unrelated to physical problems
   b. The physical manifestations of emotional trauma are usually temporary
   c. Emotional trauma is often manifested as physical symptoms
   d. Patients are more aware of the physical problems caused by trauma
5. The school nurse has been alerted to the fact that an 8-year-old boy routinely playacts as a police officer "locking up" other children on the playground to the point where the children get scared. The nurse recognizes that this behavior is most likely an indication of:
   a. The need to dominate others
   b. Inventing traumatic events
   c. A need to develop close relationships
   d. A potential symptom of traumatization
6. A pregnant woman is in a relationship with a male who routinely abuses her. Her unborn child may engage in high-risk behavior as a teen as a result of:
   a. Maternal stress
   b. Parental nurturing
   c. Appropriate stress responses in the brain
   d. Memories of the abuse
7. Maggie, a child in protective custody, is found to have an imaginary friend, Holly. Her foster family shares this information with the nurse. The nurse teaches the family members about children who have suffered trauma and knows her teaching was effective when the foster mother states:
   a. "I understand that imaginary friends are abnormal."
   b. "I understand that imaginary friends are a maladaptive behavior."
   c. "I understand that imaginary friends are a coping mechanism."
   d. "I understand that we should tell the child that imaginary friends are unacceptable."
8. An incest survivor undergoing treatment at the mental health clinic is relieved when she learns that her anxiety and depression are:
   a. Going to be eradicated with treatment
   b. Normal and will soon pass
   c. Abnormal but will pass
   d. A normal reaction to posttraumatic events
9. During a routine health screening, a grieving widow whose husband died 15 months ago reports emptiness, a loss of self, difficulty thinking of the future, and anger at her dead husband. The nurse suggests bereavement counseling. The widow is most likely suffering from:
   a. Major depression
   b. Normal grieving
   c. Adjustment disorder
   d. Posttraumatic stress disorder
10. A young child is found wandering alone at a mall. A male store employee approaches and asks where her parents are. She responds, "I don't know. Maybe you will take me home with you?" This sort of response in children may be due to:
   a. A lack of bonding as an infant
   b. A healthy confidence in the child
   c. Adequate parental bonding
   d. Normal parenting

Answers

1. **a**; 2. **c**; 3. **b**; 4. **c**; 5. **d**; 6. **a**; 7. **c**; 8. **d**; 9. **c**; 10. **a**

Visit the Evolve website for a posttest on the content in this chapter: http://evolve.elsevier.com/Varcarolis

Post-Test interactive review

REFERENCES

American Psychiatric Association (APA). (2013). *Diagnostic and statistical manual of mental disorders* (5th ed.). Washington, DC: American Psychiatric Publishing.

Bergmann, U. (2012). *Neurobiological foundations for EMDR practice.* New York, NY: Springer.

Bernstein, E. M., & Putnam, F. W. (1986). Development, reliability, and validity of a dissociation scale. *Journal of Nervous and Mental Disease, 174*(12), 727–735.

Bick, J., Naumova, O., Hunter, S., Barbot, B., Lee, M., Luthar, S., Raefsi, A., & Grigorenko, E. (2012). Childhood adversity and DNA methylation of genes involved in the hypothalamus–pituitary–adrenal axis and immune system: Whole-genome and candidate-gene associations. *Developmental Psychopathology, 24*(4), 1417–1425.

Bisson, J., & Andrew, M. (2007). Psychological treatment of post-traumatic stress disorder (PTSD). *Cochrane Database of Systematic Reviews, 3*, CD003388.

Boon, S., Steele, K., & van der Hart, O. (2011). *Coping with trauma-related dissociation: Skills training for patients and therapists*. New York, NY: Norton.

Bowlby, J. (1988). *A secure base: clinical applications of attachment theory*. London, UK: Routledge.

Briere, J. (1996). *The trauma symptom checklist for children*. Retrieved from http://www4.parinc.com/Products/Product.aspx?ProductID5TSCC .

Centers for Disease Control and Prevention. (2010). Adverse childhood experiences reported by adult—Five states, 2009. *Morbidity and Mortality Weekly Report, 59*(49), 1609–1613.

Fernández, A., Mendive, J. M., Salvador-Carulla, L., Rubio-Valera, M., Luciano, J. V., Pinto-Meza, A., et al. (2012). Adjustment disorders in primary care: Prevalence, recognition, and use of services. *British Journal of Psychiatry, 201*, 137–142.

Frankenburg, W. K., Dodds, J., Archer, P., Shapiro, H., & Bresnick, B. (1992). The Denver II: A major revision and restandardization of the Denver Developmental Screening test. *Pediatrics, 89*(1), 91–97.

Friedrich, W., Gerber, P., Koplin, B., Davis, M., Giese, J., Mykelebust, C., & Franckowiak, D. (2001). Multimodal assessment of dissociation in adolescents: inpatients and juvenile sex offenders. *Sexual Abuse: Journal of Research and Treatment, 13*, 167–177.

Gradus, J. L. (2016). Epidemiology of PTSD. Retrieved from http://www.ptsd.va.gov/professional/PTSD-overview/epidemiological-facts-ptsd.asp.

Herdman, T. H., & Kamitsuru, S. (Eds.). (2014). *NANDA International nursing diagnoses: Definitions and classifications, 2015-2017*. Oxford, UK: Wiley-Blackwell.

International Society for the Study of Trauma and Dissociation. (2012). Guidelines for treating dissociative identity disorder in adults, 3rd rev. *Journal of Trauma and Dissociation, 12*(2), 115–187.

Kessler, R. C., Sonnega, A., Bromet, E., Hughes, M., & Nelson, C. (1995). Posttraumatic stress in the national comorbidity survey. *Archives of General Psychiatry, 52*, 1048–1060.

Kilpatrick, D. G., Resnick, H. S., & Friedman, M. J. (2013). Severity of posttraumatic stress symptoms – adult. Retrieved from http://www.psychiatry.org/practice/dsm/dsm5/online-assessment-measures.

Koch, S. C., & Harvey, S. (2012). Dance/movement therapy with traumatized dissociative patients. In S. C. Koch, T. Fuchs, M. Summa, & C. Muller (Eds.), *Body memory, methaphor and movement* (pp. 369–386). Philadelphia, PA: John Benjamins.

Lanius, U. F., Paulson, S. L., & Corrigan, F. M. (2014). Dissociation: cortical deafferentation and the loss of self. In U. F. Lanius, S. L. Paulsen, & F. M. Corrigan (Eds.), *Neurobiology and treatment of traumatic dissociation: Toward an embodied self* (pp. 5–28). New York, NY: Springer.

Lee, J. H., Nam, S. K., Kim, A., Kim, B., Lee, M. Y., & Lee, S. M. (2013). Resilience: A meta-analytic approach. *Journal of Counseling & Development, 91*(3), 269–279.

Luber, M. (2014). *EMDR early mental health interventions*. New York, NY: Springer.

Monk, C., Spicer, J., & Champagne, F. (2012). Linking prenatal maternal adversity to developmental outcomes in infants: The role of epigenetic pathways. *Developmental Psychopathology, 24*(4), 1361–1376.

Moorhead, S., Johnson, M., Maas, M. L., & Swanson, E. (Eds.). (2013). *Nursing outcome classification (NOC)* (5th ed.). St. Louis, MO: Mosby.

National Child Abuse and Neglect Data System. (2015). *Child abuse and neglect statistics*. Retrieved from https://www.childwelfare.gov/topics/systemwide/statistics/can/.

National Institute of Mental Health. (2015). *Posttraumatic stress disorder among children*. Retrieved from http://www.nimh.nih.gov/health/statistics/prevalence/post-traumatic-stress-disorder-among-children.shtml.

Nijenhuis, E. R. S., Spinhoven, P., Van Dyck, R., Van der Hart, O., & Vanderlinden, J. (1996). The development and the psychometric characteristics of the somatoform dissociation questionnaire (SDQ-20). *Journal of Mental and Nervous Disease, 184*, 688–694.

Ogden, P., Minton, K., & Pain, C. (2006). *Trauma and the body: A sensorimotor approach to psychotherapy*. New York, NY: Norton.

Phillips, D. (2016, November 29). F.D.A. agrees to new trials for Ecstasy as relief for PTSD patients. *New York Times*. Retrieved from http://nyti.ms/2gGt6kS.

Porges, S. W. (2011). *The polyvagal theory*. New York, NY: W.W. Norton.

Prins, A., Ouimette, P., Kimerling, R., Cameron, R. P., Hugelshofer, D. S., Shaw-Hegwer, J., & Sheikh, J. I. (2003). The primary care PTSD screen (PC-PTSD): Development and operating characteristics. *Primary Care Psychiatry, 9*, 9–14.

Putnam, F. W., Helmers, K., & Trickett, P. K. (1993). Development, reliability, and validity of a child dissociation scale. *Child Abuse & Neglect, 17*, 731–742.

Shonkoff, J. P., & Garner, A. S. (2012). The lifelong effects of early childhood adversity and toxic stress. *Pediatrics, 129*(1). Retrieved from http://pediatrics.aappublications.org/content/129/1/e232.

Sierra, M., & Berrios, G. E. (2000). The Cambridge Depersonalization Scale: A new instrument for the measurement of depersonalization. *Psychiatry Research, 93*(2), 153–164.

Smyke, A., & Zeanah, C. H. (1999). *Disturbances of attachment interview*. Unpublished manuscript.

Steele, K., van der Hart, O., & Nijenjuis, E. (2005). Phase-oriented treatment of structural dissociation in complex traumatization: Overcoming trauma-related phobias. *Journal of Trauma and Dissociation, 6*(3), 11–53.

Tizard, B. (1977). *Adoption: a second chance*. London, UK: Open Books.

United States Department of Veterans Affairs. (2015). *PTSD in children and adolescents*. Retrieved from http://www.ptsd.va.gov/professional/pages/ptsd_in_children_and_adolescents_overview_for_professionals.asp .

Weathers, F. W., Litz, B. T., Keane, T. M., Palmieri, P. A., Marx, B. P., & Schnurr, P. P. (2013). The PTSD checklist for DSM-5 (PCL-5). Scale available from the National Center for PTSD at www.ptsd.va.gov .

Weiland, S. (2015). *Dissociation in traumatized children and adolescents: Theory and clinical interventions*. New York, NY: Routledge.

Wheeler, K. (2014). *Psychotherapy for the advanced practice psychiatric nurse: A how-to guide for evidence-based practice* (2nd ed.). New York, NY: Springer.

World Health Organization. (2013). *Guidelines for the management of conditions specifically related to stress*. Geneva, Switzerland: Author.

17

Somatic Symptom Disorders

Lois Angelo

Visit the Evolve website for a pretest on the content in this chapter: http://evolve.elsevier.com/Varcarolis Pre-Test interactive review

OBJECTIVES

1. Describe clinical manifestations of each of the somatic symptom disorders.
2. Discuss biological, psychological, behavioral, cognitive, environmental, and cultural factors influencing the onset and course of the somatic symptom disorders.
3. Analyze the impact of childhood trauma on adult somatic preoccupation.
4. Describe how anxiety, depression, and trauma can result in physical distress.
5. Apply the nursing process to individuals with somatic symptom disorders.
6. Evaluate the importance of assessing the patient's coping skills and strengths.
7. Describe five psychosocial interventions for the care of the patient who has a somatic symptom disorder.
8. Identify the role of the advanced practice psychiatric-mental health registered nurse in managing somatic symptom disorders in the primary care setting.
9. Define factitious disorder as a distinct, but related problem about which registered nurses need to know.

OUTLINE

KEY TERMS AND CONCEPTS

conversion disorder
factitious disorder
holistic approach
illness anxiety disorder
la belle indifference
malingering
psychological factors affecting medical condition
secondary gain
somatic symptom disorder
somatization

Soma is the Greek word for "body." **Somatization** is the expression of stress through physical symptoms. These symptoms may be manifestations of psychological and emotional distress. Instead of feeling anxiety, depression, or irritability, some individuals experience pain, paralysis, unexplained skin rashes, and other symptoms. Somatic symptoms disorders have been around for centuries and have disrupted countless lives. These complex disorders confuse both patients and healthcare providers. Many factors, including biological, cognitive, psychological, and social factors, play a role in the development of somatic symptoms.

When psychiatric disorders occur along with general medical conditions, they may increase the likelihood of increased healthcare costs and length of stay. They also can negatively impact outcomes and increase morbidity and mortality. Anxiety, depression, and trauma exert a powerful influence on the mind and may lead to a variety of clinical conditions—both mental and physical.

This chapter helps prepare nurses to utilize a **holistic approach** in nursing care for individuals with somatic symptom disorder. This approach emphasizes the multidimensional interplay of biological, psychological, and sociocultural needs and its effects on the somatization process. The material in this chapter is important for psychiatric nurses who care for patients with physical illnesses. It is also important for nurses who work outside of psychiatric settings to be aware of the influence of environment, stress, individual lifestyle, a support network, and coping skills of each patient.

DSM-5 CRITERIA FOR SOMATIC SYMPTOM DISORDER

A. One or more somatic symptoms that are distressing or result in significant disruption of daily life.
B. Excessive thoughts, feelings, or behaviors related to the somatic symptoms or associated health concerns as manifested by at least one of the following:
   1. Disproportionate and persistent thoughts about the seriousness of one's symptoms.
   2. Persistently high level of anxiety about health or symptoms.
   3. Excessive time and energy devoted to these symptoms or health concerns.
C. Although any one somatic symptom may not be continuously present, the state of being symptomatic is persistent (typically more than 6 months).

Specify if:
With predominant pain (previously pain disorder): This specifier is for individuals whose somatic symptoms predominantly involve pain.
Specify if:
Persistent: A persistent course is characterized by severe symptoms, marked impairment, and long duration (more than 6 months).
Specify current severity:
Mild: Only of the symptoms specified in Criterion B is fulfilled.
Moderate: Two or more of the symptoms specified in Criterion B are fulfilled.
Severe: Two or more of the symptoms specified in Criterion B are fulfilled plus there are multiple somatic complaints (or one very severe somatic symptoms).

From the American Psychiatric Association. (2013). *Diagnostic and statistical manual of mental disorders* (5th ed.). Washington, DC: Author.

CLINICAL PICTURE

According to the American Psychiatric Association (APA; 2013), the somatic symptom and related disorders include the following:

- Somatic symptom disorder
- Illness anxiety disorder
- Conversion disorder
- **Psychological factors affecting medical condition**
- Factitious disorder

Somatic Symptom Disorder

Somatic symptom disorder is characterized by a focus on somatic (physical) symptoms, such as pain or fatigue, to the point of excessive concern, preoccupation, and fear. Patients' suffering is authentic and they typically experience a high level of functional impairment. Criteria for somatic symptom disorder are listed in the *DSM-5* box.

In somatic symptom disorder there tends to be a high level of help seeking, which rarely alleviates the patient's concerns. Among common symptoms for primary care visits are chest pain, fatigue, dizziness, headache, swelling, back pain, shortness of breath, insomnia, abdominal pain, and numbness. While these symptoms account for 40% of all visits to primary care providers, a biological cause for these symptoms is identified in only 26% of patients (Edwards et al., 2010). Health-related quality of life is frequently severely impaired, and patients see their bodily symptoms as unduly threatening, harmful, or troublesome, often fearing the worst about their health.

When the care provider is unable to make a clear diagnosis explaining the discomfort, patients feel discounted and misunderstood. There is, in fact, some basis for these feelings. Providers tend to use less patient-centered communication in this population as compared with patients with more straightforward symptoms, even though their visits are longer. A "difficult" patient may receive a somatic diagnosis more readily than a "pleasant" patient, which could contribute to an inadequate workup. The strongest predictor of misdiagnosing somatic disorders is the primary care provider's dissatisfaction with the clinical encounter (Huang & McCarron, 2011).

Illness Anxiety Disorder

You have probably heard the term *hypochondriasis* and are probably somewhat familiar with the symptoms. This term was retired in 2013 and replaced with the descriptive diagnosis of illness anxiety disorder. **Illness anxiety disorder** is characterized by extreme worry and fear about the possibility of having a disease. This worry leads to frequent scanning of the body for signs of illness. Actual symptoms and complaints of symptoms are either mild or absent. Illness anxiety is quite obsessive as thoughts about illness may be intrusive and hard to dismiss even when the patients realize their fears are unrealistic. Constantly talking about health and possible illness is common. Some individuals with this disorder are care seekers and some are care avoiders. The *DSM-5* box provides criteria for illness anxiety disorder.

DSM-5 CRITERIA FOR ILLNESS ANXIETY DISORDER

A. Preoccupation with having or acquiring a serious illness.

B. Somatic symptoms are not present or, if present, are only mild in intensity. If another medical condition is present or there is a high risk for developing a medical condition (e.g., strong family history is present), the preoccupation is clearly excessive or disproportionate.

C. There is a high level of anxiety about health, and the individual is easily alarmed about personal health status.

D. The individual performs excessive health-related behaviors (e.g., repeatedly checks his or her body for signs of illness) or exhibits maladaptive avoidance (e.g., avoids doctor appointments and hospitals).

E. Illness preoccupation has been present for at least 6 months, but the specific illness that is feared may change over that period of time.

F. The illness-related preoccupation is not better explained by another mental disorder such as somatic symptom disorder, panic disorder, generalized anxiety disorder, body dysmorphic disorder, obsessive-compulsive disorder, or delusional disorder, somatic type.

Specify whether:

Care-seeking type: Medical care, including physician visits or undergoing tests and procedures, is frequently used.

Care-avoidant type: Medical care is rarely used.

From the American Psychiatric Association. (2013). *Diagnostic and statistical manual of mental disorders* (5th ed.). Washington, DC: APA.

Care providers may suggest a consultation with a mental health professional, but the patient typically refuses it. The course of the illness is chronic and relapsing with symptoms becoming amplified during times of increased stress. Depression may play a role in increasing concerns. Consider the case of a 72-year-old woman with illness anxiety who was treated with electroconvulsive therapy (ECT), a treatment most often used for depression. After one session her somatic complaints stopped abruptly. This patient's success with ECT may indicate that depressive symptoms were the catalyst for her symptoms, leading to the diagnosis of illness anxiety (Dols et al., 2012).

Overall, the illness anxiety patient uses about 41% to 78% more healthcare services per year than patients with well-defined medical conditions (Fink, 2010). It is important that clinicians possess basic skills in identifying and treating this disorder. If patient health concerns are addressed at an early stage, repeated consultations, multiple trials of medications, and medical examinations can be prevented (Fink, 2010).

Exposure to media that urge us to use certain health screens or suggest we talk to our doctor about specific medications may also contribute to fears about health. Social media in particular seems to increase fears. For example, following a large-scale trauma or disaster, use of Twitter and YouTube are significantly associated with higher stress responses (Goodwin et al., 2015).

Conversion Disorder

Conversion disorder (also known as **functional neurological disorder**) manifests itself as neurological symptoms in the absence of a neurological diagnosis. Conversion disorder is marked by the presence of deficits in voluntary motor or sensory functions including paralysis, blindness, movement disorder, gait disorder, numbness, paresthesia (tingling or burning sensations), loss of vision or hearing, or episodes resembling epilepsy.

In conversion disorder, emotional conflicts or stressors are transferred to physical symptoms. This transfer may have a physical basis. Some MRI studies suggest that patients with conversion disorder have an abnormal pattern of cerebral activation (Feinstein, 2011).

One of the most striking aspects of conversion disorder is that many patients show a lack of emotional concern about often dramatic symptoms. This response is called **la belle indifference**, or "the grand" indifference. Imagine someone casually discussing sudden blindness. Despite the calm response of the afflicted, care providers should assume there is an organic cause to the symptoms until physical pathology has been ruled out.

Comorbid psychiatric conditions include depression, anxiety, posttraumatic stress disorder, other somatic disorders, and personality disorders. There are also cases in which a comorbid medical or neurological condition exists, and the conversion disorder is an exaggeration of the original problem.

Lifetime prevalence of conversion disorder ranges from 2 to 5 per 100,000 people (APA, 2013). In neurology clinics, the rate climbs to 5%. This disorder is up to three times more common in females. Risk factors include low socioeconomic and educational status, low psychological sophistication, and rural settings. Childhood physical or sexual abuse is common in patients with conversion disorder.

Psychological Factors Affecting Medical Condition

Both medical and mental health professionals recognize the interrelationships between medical and psychiatric comorbidities. Psychological factors may increase a risk for medical disease or they may magnify and adversely affect a medical condition. For example, there is a growing body of evidence that links between psychiatric disorders with cardiovascular disease. Major depressive disorder is a risk factor in the occurrence of coronary heart disease (Marwijk et al., 2015). A link between depression and cancer incidence has been suggested since the time of the ancient Greeks. Depression is such a powerful condition that it is associated with increased risk of death from nearly all major medical causes (Zivin et al., 2015).

Stress is certainly a psychological factor that can affect the disease process. Hans Selye (1956) was the first to introduce the concept of stress into the fields of medicine and physiology. Cannon (1914) identified the fight-or-flight response and Selye described the general adaptation syndrome. Both theories provide insight into the biological and molecular reactions to stressors. Extensive studies have left little doubt that psychosocial stress can affect the course and severity of illness (Table 17.1).

VIGNETTE: Gerald is a 63-year-old real estate agent who was recently hospitalized for increased symptoms of congestive heart failure, particularly high blood pressure and shortness of breath. Because of insomnia, lack of appetite, and chronic anger toward his wife, his primary care provider refers him for a mental health consultation.

He tells the psychiatric-mental health registered nurse practitioner, "I'm very scared. I worry about my health and my retirement. I don't know where I would get the money to live or to pay for medical insurance if I get sick again. I am too old to start another career."

After a thorough assessment and medical workup, Gerald is diagnosed with major depressive disorder with anxious distress. The nurse practitioner suggests that these problems may have increased the symptoms of congestive heart failure. Gerald has responded well to couples therapy and a men's support group. His blood pressure has decreased, his breathing has become less strained, and his mood is improved.

TABLE 17.1 Common Medical Conditions Negatively Affected by Stress

Medical Condition	Incidence	Genetic and Biological Correlates	Common Precipitating Factors	Holistic Therapies in Addition to Medical Management
Cardiovascular disease (e.g., coronary heart disease)	Rates higher in males until age 60 years Rates higher in white population than in African American population	Family history of cardiac disease a risk factor Other risk factors include hypertension, increased serum lipid levels, obesity, sedentary lifestyle, and cigarette smoking Psychosocial risk factors (stress, depression, loneliness) High anxiety risk in patient with prior cardiac events	Often, myocardial infarction occurs after sudden stress preceded by a period of losses, frustration, and disappointments	Relaxation training, stress management, group social support, and psychosocial intervention Support groups for type A personalities and type A modification helpful Anxiolytics (benzodiazepines) and antidepressants when indicated
Peptic ulcer (caused by *Helicobacter pylori* infection)	Occurs in 12% of men, 6% of women (more prevalent in industrialized societies)	Infection with *H. pylori* is associated with 95%-99% of peptic ulcers Both peptic and duodenal ulcers cluster in families, but separately from each other	Periods of social tension and increased life stress After losses; often after menopause	Biofeedback can alter gastric acidity; cognitive-behavioral approaches are used to reduce stress (stress management)
Cancer	Men: most common in lung, prostate, colon, and rectum Women: most common in breast, uterus, colon, and rectum Death rate higher in men (especially African American men) than in women	Genetic evidence suggests dysfunction of cellular proliferation Familial patterns for breast cancer, colorectal cancer, stomach cancer, melanoma	Prolonged and intensive stress Stressful life events (e.g., separation from or loss of significant other 2 years before diagnosis) Feelings of hopelessness, helplessness, and despair (depression) may precede the diagnosis of cancer	Relaxation (e.g., meditation, autogenic training, self-hypnosis) Visualization Psychological counseling Support groups Massage therapy Stress management
Tension headache	Occurs in 80% of population when under stress Begins at end of workday or early evening		Associated with anxiety and depression	Psychotherapy usually prescribed for chronic tension headaches Learning to cope or avoiding tension-creating situations or people Relaxation techniques, stress management techniques, cognitive restructuring techniques
Essential hypertension	Rates higher in males until age 60 years	Family history of cardiac disease and hypertension a risk factor	Life changes and traumatic life events Stressful job (e.g., air traffic controller) Hypothesized to be found more in areas of social stress and conflict	Behavioral feedback, stress reduction techniques, meditation, yoga, hypnosis Note: pharmacological treatment considered primary for treatment of hypertension

EPIDEMIOLOGY

It is significant that women report more somatization. It may be that women are more aware of their bodily sensations, have different health-seeking behaviors, and use more healthcare services than men. In particular young women ages 16 to 25 are more likely to receive a somatic diagnosis than men or older individuals (Huang & McCarron, 2011).

Somatic symptoms are common, especially among children and adolescents. Approximately 20% to 25% of children suffer from abdominal pain, headaches, and musculoskeletal pains (van Gils et al., 2014). Recurrent somatic complaints in childhood are associated with adult emotional disorders (Shanahan et al., 2015). Childhood maltreatment has been associated with elevated levels of C-reactive protein, a biomarker of inflammation that may play a role in autoimmune diseases in adults 20 years later (Dube et al., 2009).

Depression is linked with physical illness in several ways. It is associated with a significantly increased risk of autoimmune disease compared with those without a history of depression (Andersson et al., 2015). Also depression later in life may have a more physical presentation compared with depression earlier in life (Hegeman et al., 2015). People over the age of 55 with major depressive disorder may be up to three times more likely to have cardiovascular disease than nondepressed patients (Marwijk et al., 2015).

RISK FACTORS

Somatization is a complex biopsychosocial phenomenon with many factors influencing the onset and course of the illness. Studies have shown that patients with somatic symptom disorders are more sensitive to negativity, less resilient in response to stress, and more prone to catastrophic thinking and negative interpretation to life events (Miller, 2009). In early development, stress has been implicated as a triggering factor, most often stemming from parents and the pressure to perform. Somatization is often the "tip of the iceberg" that calls for attention to a psychiatric disorder necessitating mental health treatment. Unfortunately, many untreated children risk continuous somatization as adults.

Biological Factors

People with somatic symptom disorder may have low thresholds for and low tolerance of physical discomfort (Sadock et al., 2015). For example, what most people would consider abdominal pressure, people with somatic symptom disorder would describe as abdominal pain.

Conversion disorder may have a biological basis. Hypometabolism in the dominant hemisphere and hypermetabolism in the non-dominant hemisphere may lead to impaired hemispheric communication (Sadock et al., 2015). Excess cortisol may set off negative feedback loops between the cerebral cortex and the brainstem. This cortical output may inhibit the patient's awareness of bodily sensations, thereby resulting in sensory deficits.

Psychological Factors

Psychoanalytic Theory

Psychoanalytic theory originally dominated medical thinking about somatization, which Sigmund Freud considered a "mysterious leap from mind to body" (Stone et al., 2010). Psychoanalytic theorists viewed the psychogenic complaints of pain, illness, or loss of physical function as a cover-up for conflicted feelings and/or unwelcome experiences. Transforming anxiety into a physical symptom is symbolically related to the conflict.

For example, in conversion disorder, conversion symptoms allow a forbidden wish or urge to be partly expressed but sufficiently disguised so that the individual does not have to face the unacceptable wish. The symptoms also permit the individual to communicate a need for special treatment or consideration from others.

Anger, aggression, or hostility that had its source in past losses or a disappointment may be expressed as a need for help and concern from others. Illness anxiety may also be a defense against guilt or low self-esteem. In the patient's view, the somatic symptoms often serve as deserved punishment.

Behavioral Theory

Behaviorists suggest that people with somatic symptoms learn methods of communicating helplessness and that these methods help the individuals gain care from others. The symptoms become more intense when they are reinforced by attention from others. Seeking formal care may also reinforce this behavior because care providers are attentive and responsive to a patient's reports of pain. Other reinforcers include avoiding activities the individual considers distasteful, obtaining financial benefit, or gaining some advantage in interpersonal relationships.

Cognitive Theory

Cognitive theorists believe that the somatic disorders are the result of negative, distorted, and catastrophic thoughts and reinforcement of these thoughts. Patients focus on body sensations, misinterprets their meaning, and respond with excessive alarm.

EVIDENCE-BASED PRACTICE

Twitter Predicts Heart Disease Mortality

Problem

Hostility and chronic stress are known risk factors for heart disease. Language patterns reflecting negativity have emerged as risk factors. Positive emotions and psychological engagement have emerged as protective factors.

Purpose of Study

Researchers wanted to determine if negative language is associated with increased risk for atherosclerotic heart disease (AHD).

Methods

An analysis of the social media forum, Twitter, was done to identify psychological characteristics associated with mortality. Data were collected from 1347 United States counties from about 50,000 tweets. Language measures were correlated with AHD mortality rates in the counties.

Findings

- Greater use of anger, negative relationship, negative emotion, and disengagement words was significantly correlated with greater AHD mortality.
- Greater use of optimism, positive emotion, and engagement words was associated with lower AHS mortality.

Continued

EVIDENCE-BASED PRACTICE—cont'd

Twitter Predicts Heart Disease Mortality

Why Should Nurses Be Interested in This Study?

The typical Twitter user has a median age of 31. The people tweeting are not the people dying. However, the tweets of younger adults may disclose characteristics of their county reflecting a shared economic, physical, and psychological environment. Nurses are in a unique position to teach patients about the power of positive thinking and actions.

Eichstaedt, J., Schwartz, H. A., Kern, M. L., Park, G., Labarthe, D. L., Merchant, R. M. ... Seligman, M. E. P. (2015). Psychological language on twitter predicts county-level heart disease mortality, *Psychological Science, 26*(2), 159–169.

Cultural Considerations

The type and frequency of somatic symptoms vary across cultures. Burning hands and feet or the sensation of worms in the head or ants under the skin is more common in Africa and southern Asia than in North America. Alteration of consciousness with falling is a symptom commonly associated with culture-specific religious and healing rituals. Somatic symptom disorder, which is rarely seen in men in the United States, is often reported in Greek and Puerto Rican men. This suggests that cultural customs may permit these men to use somatization as an acceptable approach to dealing with life stress. Somatization related to posttraumatic stress and depression was the most prevalent psychiatric symptom in North Korean defectors to South Korea (Kim et al., 2011)

West Indians (Caribbean) attribute somatic symptoms to chronic overwork and the irregularity of daily living, citing symptoms such as dizziness, fatigue, joint pain, and muscle tension. Patients from Korea may explain some distress as *hwa-byung*, a syndrome of both somatic and depressive symptoms, commonly attributed to suppressed anger or rage (Edwards et al., 2010).

In some cultures, certain physical symptoms are believed to be the result of spells being cast. Spellbound individuals often seek the help of traditional healers in addition to modern medical staff. The medical provider may diagnose a non–life-threatening somatic symptom disorder, whereas the traditional healer may offer an entirely different explanation and prognosis. The individual may not show improvement until the traditional healer removes the spell.

In contemporary Western culture, there has been unprecedented growth and comfort in the past few decades. However, levels of health have not increased. Core values such as materialism, consumerism, and individualism may be damaging to individuals' sense of well-being and health including a high incidence of somatization.

Abraham Maslow's hierarchy of needs indicates that humans shift attention to higher-level needs (social, intellectual, spiritual) once basic lower-level needs (food, shelter, clothing) are satisfied. However, Western culture has become fixated upon materialism and resisting movement to higher-level needs such as love, belonging, and respect for others. Acting to enhance belonging through inclusion results in more adaptive physiological and psychological outcomes and increased social self-esteem (Begen & Turner-Cobb, 2015).

In addition, somatization among the immigrant population in the United States in primary care is significantly related to traumatic events. Immigrants frequently experience multiple traumatic events, both intentional and unintentional, in premigration and postmigration life. A study of asylum seekers reported 79% had experienced a traumatic event such as witnessing killings, being assaulted, or suffering torture and captivity. It is important for primary care providers evaluating immigrants to be aware of the possible link between somatization symptoms reported by the patient and undisclosed traumatic experiences.

CONSIDERING CULTURE

Culture, Trauma, and Somatization in Primary Care

Immigrants and refugees, as well as patients from ethnic and racial minorities, frequently seek care for a spectrum of physical and psychological symptoms. These symptoms are best understood within the context of their cultural background and experiences.

Carlos is a 27-year-old from El Salvador. He fled his native country after finding out that his name was on a death squad list for execution. Nine months after his arrival in the United States, he learned his wife was killed during an attempt to extract information about Carlos's whereabouts.

Carlos visited a primary care provider at a community clinic. He described multiple symptoms, including weakness, which caused him to be terminated from his temporary job. He also complained of abdominal pain, chest pain, insomnia, and weight loss. After extensive diagnostic studies, Carlos's primary care provider could find no physical cause for his symptoms.

He was then referred to a psychiatric nurse practitioner (NP). The NP diagnosed somatization and prescribed a low-dose antidepressant along with individual therapy.

Carlos grew more aware of the emotional factors that exacerbated his symptoms and developed new coping strategies. He joined a group of local Central American refugees, where he was encouraged to write and to recite poetry as a therapeutic tool. During the following months, his somatic symptoms gradually decreased.

Patients across cultures with somatic symptoms often offer clues about their underlying concerns and want more emotional support from their healthcare provider in comparison to other patients. They are most satisfied with their care when their healthcare provider shares their understanding of the presenting problems and treatment options (Edwards et al., 2010).

APPLICATION OF THE NURSING PROCESS

ASSESSMENT

Assessment of patients with somatic symptom disorders is a complex process that requires careful and complete documentation. This section outlines several areas that are important in the assessment of a patient with a suspected somatic symptom disorder.

ASSESSMENT GUIDELINES

Somatic Symptom Disorders

1. Assess for nature, location, onset, characteristics, and duration of the symptom(s).
2. Explore past history of adverse childhood events.
3. Identify symptoms of anxiety, depression, and past trauma that may be contributing to somatic symptoms and ability to meet basic physical, and safety/security needs.
4. Determine current quality of life, social support, and coping skills including spirituality.
5. Identify any secondary gain that the patient is experiencing from symptom(s).
6. Explore the patient's cognitive style and ability to communicate feelings and needs.
7. Assess current psychosocial and biological needs.
8. Screen for misuse of prescribed medication and substance use.

Assessment should begin with collection of data about the nature, location, onset, character, and duration of the symptom or symptoms. A thorough medical and psychosocial history is also essential. Assessment of nutrition, fluid balance, and elimination needs should be a high priority as patients with somatic symptom disorders often complain of gastrointestinal distress, diarrhea, constipation, and anorexia.

Fig. 17.1 provides a tool to quantify somatic symptoms. This measure was adapted from the Patient Health Questionnaire Physical Symptoms.

In addition, nurses should gather information about patients' ability to meet their own basic needs. Rest, comfort, activity, and hygiene needs may be altered as a result of patient problems such as fatigue, weakness, insomnia, muscle tension, pain, and avoidance of diversional activity. Safety and security needs may be threatened by patient experiences of blindness, deafness, loss of balance and falling, and anesthesia of various parts of the body.

During assessment, it is important to determine whether symptoms are under the patient's voluntary control. Somatic symptoms *are not under the individual's voluntary control.* Although the relationship between symptoms and interpersonal conflicts may be obvious to others, the patient cannot see it.

Symptom reporting will vary depending upon the disorder. Patients with conversion disorder may matter-of-factly report having a sudden loss in function of a body part: "I woke up this morning and couldn't move my arm." In contrast, patients with somatic symptom disorder and illness anxiety disorder usually discuss their symptoms in dramatic terms. They may use colorful metaphors and exaggerations: "The pain was searing, like a hot sword drawn across my forehead." "My symptoms are so rare that I've stumped hundreds of doctors."

Table 17.2 provides an outline for a psychosocial assessment of a patient with a medical condition. You perform a psychosocial assessment in tandem with a thorough physical workup and mental status examination.

Coping Skills

Assessing how a patient has dealt with adversity in the past provides information about coping skills available for use now and in the future. Healthcare workers can also support the patient in gaining additional coping skills that may help an individual better manage a healthier lifestyle.

Spirituality and Religion

Spirituality or religion may play an important role in many patients' lives. Support from a priest, pastor, rabbi, or other religious leader may be indicated, especially in a case of spiritual distress. Beliefs and practices are forces that promote resilience; the practice of healthy coping depends upon the capacity to create meaning from life experiences.

Communication

Patients with somatic disorders have difficulty communicating their emotional needs. Although they are able to describe their physical symptoms, they frequently do not verbalize feelings, especially those related to anger, guilt, and dependence. The somatic symptom may be the patient's chief means of communicating emotional needs. Psychogenic blindness or hearing loss may represent the symbolic statement "I can't face this knowledge." For example, after a woman overheard friends discussing her husband's sexual infidelity, she developed total deafness.

Dependence on Medication

Individuals experiencing somatic complaints often become dependent on medication to relieve pain or anxiety or to induce sleep. Primary care providers prescribe antianxiety drugs for patients who seem highly anxious and concerned about their symptoms. Patients often return to the primary care provider for prescription renewal or seek treatment from numerous primary care providers. It is important that the nurse assess the type and amount of medications being used.

Secondary Gains

The nurse tries to identify secondary gains the patient may be receiving from the symptoms. **Secondary gains** are those benefits derived from the symptoms alone; for example, in the sick role, the patient is not able to perform the usual family, work, and social functions and receives extra attention from loved ones. If a patient derives personal benefit from the symptoms, giving up the symptoms is more difficult. The clinician works with the patient to achieve the same benefits through healthier avenues such as learning to communicate more adaptively and connect with others. One approach to identifying the presence of secondary gains is to ask the patient questions such as:

- What are you unable to do now that you used to be able to do?
- How has this problem affected your life?

Self-Assessment

Working with patients with somatic symptom disorders can be frustrating and unsatisfying. When a physiological basis for the patient's symptoms is absent, you may wonder why this patient is taking up valuable time that might better be spent on a "sick"

Level 2—Somatic Symptom—Adult Patient
Adapted from the Patient Health Questionnaire Physical Symptoms (PHQ-15)

Instructions: On the DSM-5 Level 1 cross-cutting questionnaire that you just completed, you indicated that *during the past 2 weeks* you (the individual receiving care) have been bothered by "unexplained aches and pains," and/or "feeling that your illnesses are not being taken seriously enough" at a mild or greater level of severity. The questions below ask about these feelings in more detail and especially how often you (the individual receiving care) have been bothered by a list of symptoms **during the past 7 days. Please respond to each item by marking (✓ or x) one box per row.**

During the past 7 days, how much have you been bothered by any of the following problems?	**Not bothered at all (0)**	**Bothered a little (1)**	**Bothered a lot (2)**
1 Stomach pain	☐	☐	☐
2 Back pain	☐	☐	☐
3 Pain in your arms, legs, or joints (knees, hips, etc.)	☐	☐	☐
4 Menstrual cramps or other problems with your periods *WOMEN ONLY*	☐	☐	☐
5 Headaches	☐	☐	☐
6 Chest pain	☐	☐	☐
7 Dizziness	☐	☐	☐
8 Fainting spells	☐	☐	☐
9 Feeling your heart pound or race	☐	☐	☐
10 Shortness of breath	☐	☐	☐
11 Pain or problems during sexual intercourse	☐	☐	☐
12 Constipation, loose bowels, or diarrhea	☐	☐	☐
13 Nausea, gas, or indigestion	☐	☐	☐
14 Feeling tired or having low energy	☐	☐	☐
15 Trouble sleeping	☐	☐	☐

FIG. 17.1 Somatic symptom—adult patient.

patient. You may feel resentment or anger toward such a patient. Negative feelings occur whether the patient is being cared for in a medical setting or in a psychiatric setting.

It is helpful to remember that the symptom the patient is experiencing feels *real* to him or her, even though the objective data may not support a physiological basis. It is important for clinicians not to convey by word or body language their own frustration about the difficult and time-consuming task they are facing with somatic symptom disorders. Clinicians should also avoid the temptation to perform unnecessary, repetitive, or extensive testing in an attempt to demonstrate to the patient and/or family that the presenting complaint is of somatic origin.

Anger may also arise when staff members find themselves dealing with a patient who uses somatic symptoms to manipulate the environment and the people within it. Being unable to make a patient realize that symptoms have no organic basis can be a source of frustration. Patients who use somatization exhibit remarkable resistance to change. As you plan the care of this patient, a useful strategy is to set goals with staged outcomes (i.e., small attainable steps) to offset feelings of helplessness or ineffectuality.

It is helpful for you, no matter the setting, to discuss responses to these patients in postconference with other students, faculty, or staff. Ultimately, your increased self-awareness and increased

TABLE 17.2 Psychosocial Assessment of Patients with Medical Conditions

Areas to Assess	Specific Questions to Ask
Social Supports and Cultural Issues	
Family	What were the effects of the patient's illness, treatments, and recovery on the family in the past?
Friends	Who can the patient share painful feelings with?
	Does the patient have friends to joke and laugh with?
	Are there people the patient believes would stand by him or her?
Religious or spiritual beliefs	Does the patient find comfort and support in spiritual practices?
	Is the patient a member of a spiritual or religious group in the community (church, temple, other place of worship)?
	Does the patient find inner peace and strength in religious or spiritual practices?
	The following statements may be used in performing a spiritual assessment of a patient:
	I [often/sometimes/seldom] believe that life has value, meaning, and direction.
	I [often/sometimes/seldom] feel a connection with the universe.
	I [often/sometimes/seldom] believe in a power greater than myself.
	I [often/sometimes/seldom] believe that my actions make a difference.
	I [often/sometimes/seldom] believe that my actions express my true self.
Cultural beliefs	Does the patient use specific culture-oriented treatments or remedies for his or her condition?
	Do the patient's cultural beliefs allow for adequate treatment by Western medical standards?
Work	Are there colleagues at work the patient can count on for support?
Concurrent Physical Conditions Affecting Psychosocial Well-Being	
Physical pain	Is the patient in pain?
	How does the patient cope with it?
	Is the pain disabling?
	Are there pain-reducing techniques that might help?
Major illness	Does the patient have a co-occurring major illness that will negatively affect his or her current condition?
	Is the patient undergoing treatments that are affecting daily life more than expected?
	Are there interventions that would help the patient better cope with the sequelae of the illness and treatments?
	Has the patient been hospitalized in the past?
	How many times?
	For what?
	How did the patient cope?
Addictions and mental health	Does the patient have a co-occurring mental health problem (depression, anxiety, compulsions)?
	Has the patient suffered a mental disease in the past?
	Does the patient participate in any compulsive behavior (e.g., smoking, overworking, excessive spending, gambling, cybersex)?
	Does the patient abuse substances (alcohol, drugs [illicit, over the counter, prescription])?

skill will help you to provide strong and consistent care for this population.

NURSING DIAGNOSIS

Patients with somatic disorders present various nursing problems. *Ineffective coping* is a priority in this population. Other potential nursing diagnoses include *anxiety, risk for loneliness, powerlessness, hopelessness, social isolation, pain, altered family processes,* and *risk for suicide.*

OUTCOMES IDENTIFICATION

Because shared decision making promotes goal attainment, the patient should participate in identifying desired outcomes. Outcome criteria must be realistic and attainable. Structuring outcomes in small steps helps the patient see concrete evidence of progress. Table 17.3 describes signs and symptoms, potential nursing diagnoses, and outcomes for somatic symptom disorders.

IMPLEMENTATION

Because patients are seldom admitted to psychiatric care settings specifically for treatment of somatic disorders, long-term interventions usually take place on an outpatient basis. The nurse may initiate short-term planning if the patient is admitted to a medical-surgical unit. Such a stay is usually brief, and discharge will occur after the results of diagnostic tests are negative.

Patients who somatize often do not mention psychological symptoms and attribute their symptoms to physical problems when consulting healthcare providers. Somatization is common in primary care, but providers are not confident in managing it and often prescribe unnecessary treatments. Because comorbidities between somatic disorders and major depression and anxiety are common in primary care, it is essential that an integrated model of care exist between psychiatric care providers and medical clinicians (Steinbrecher et al., 2011).

Initially, nursing interventions should focus on establishing a helping relationship with the patient. The therapeutic relationship is vital to the success of the care plan given (1) the patient's

TABLE 17.3 Signs and Symptoms, Nursing Diagnoses, and Outcomes for Somatic Symptom Disorders

Signs and Symptoms	Nursing Diagnoses	Outcomes
Ineffective coping strategies, insufficient access of social support, insufficient problem-solving skills, inability to meet role expectations	*Ineffective coping*	Identifies ineffective coping patterns, identifies alternate coping strategies, uses support system
Presence of secondary gains by adoption of sick role	*Pain, acute or chronic*	Recognizes associated symptoms of pain, reports pain control
Absence of support system, disabling condition, preoccupation with own thoughts, friends and family alienated by physical obsessions	*Social isolation*	Identifies support system, willing to call on others for assistance, identifies a support group
Nonassertive behavior, exaggerates negative feedback about self, excessive seeking of reassurance, repeatedly unsuccessful in life events	*Chronic low self-esteem*	Verbalizes positive regard for self, describes self as successful, strong beliefs that decisions and actions control health outcomes

From Herdman, T. H., & Kamitsuru, S. (Eds.). (2014). *Nursing diagnoses—Definitions and classification 2015-2017*. Oxford, UK: Wiley Blackwell. Copyright © 2014, 1994-2012 by NANDA International. Used by arrangement with John Wiley & Sons Limited; Moorhead, S., Johnson, M., Maas, M. L., & Swanson, E. (2013). *Nursing outcomes classification (NOC)* (5th ed.). St. Louis, MO: Mosby.

BOX 17.1 Reattribution Treatment to Link Physical Complaints and Psychological Distress

Reattribution treatment is a structured intervention designed to provide a simple explanation of somatic symptoms to patients. Reattribution skills from the healthcare provider help the patient feel understood and help the patient make the link between physical complaints and psychological distress.

The four stages of reattribution are:

Stage 1: Feeling Understood

Empathetic listening skills are used in taking the history of physical, emotional, and psychosocial factors of the presenting symptoms including patient beliefs and perceptions of the causality of illness, when is it worse, and what helps. This stage includes a brief focused physical examination.

Stage 2: Broadening the Agenda

The care provider gives feedback and implications of assessment findings, and acknowledges the patient's distress.

Stage 3: Making the Link

The care provider uses patient cues to give an empowering explanation of the symptoms. For example, "You may have a heightened sensitivity to particular stressors that is affected by genetics, your personal experiences, and the environment" is a patient-centered comment that removes any sense of blame from the patient (Fuller-Thomson et al., 2011).

Stage 4: Negotiating Further Treatment

The provider and the patient create a treatment plan that includes regular follow-up visits.

Walters, P., Tylee, A., Fisher, J., & Goldberg, D. (2007). Teaching junior doctors to manage patients who somatise: Is it possible in an afternoon? *Medical Education, 41*, 995–1001; Fuller-Thomson, E., Sulman, J., Brennenstuhl, S., & Merchant, M. (2011). Functional somatic syndromes and childhood physical abuse in women: Data from a representative community-based sample. *Journal of Aggression, Maltreatment and Trauma, 20*, 445–469.

resistance to the concept that no physical cause for the symptom exists and (2) the patient's tendency to go from caregiver to caregiver.

To be successful, therapeutic interventions address ways to help the patient get needs met without resorting to somatization. The secondary gains derived from illness behaviors become less important to the patient when underlying needs can be met directly. A specific treatment approach for somatization is provided in Box 17.1.

Given that multiple healthcare providers are often involved in the management of this disorder, good communication among treating clinicians is required to maintain a consistent approach. In an ideal situation, a multidisciplinary team of caretakers, including an advanced practice psychiatric-mental health registered nurse who provides consultation to nurses outside of psychiatry, would be involved in the treatment of patients with somatic symptom disorders. Using the data from the holistic assessment, nurse clinicians, along with a physician, are in a position to provide useful and effective interventions.

People who have distressing symptoms are vulnerable to a variety of psychosocial stresses. How they cope with these stresses may make the difference between living with an acceptable quality of life and giving in to despair, withdrawal, helplessness, or hopelessness. Nurses are in a position to assess and understand patients' psychosocial stressors, identify needed coping skills, and teach stress-management techniques. Nurses can play an important role not only in managing patients' immediate care but also in helping patients to improve their ability to cope and increase the quality of life during the course of somatic disorders.

Patients can learn various effective **coping skills** such as assertiveness training, cognitive reframing, problem-solving skills, and social supports. Nurses are in key positions to assess, educate, or provide referrals to a patient to enable healthier ways of looking at and dealing with illness. Teaching relaxation techniques, such as progressive muscle relaxation, meditation, guided imagery, and breathing exercises, promotes self-care and provides a distraction from obsessive somatic thoughts.

HEALTH POLICY

Primary Care and Mental Health Services: A Call for Integration

For many symptoms seen in primary healthcare, there is no evidence of physical disease. The high prevalence of behavioral health problems and the interrelated nature of mental and physical treatment have led the Institutes of Medicine (IOM) to call for integration of behavioral and physical care.

One of the advantages for integrating mental health services into primary healthcare includes less stigmatization. Because primary healthcare services are not associated with any specific health conditions, individuals reduce the stigma when seeking mental healthcare from a primary healthcare provider.

In the Netherlands, several models have been developed to integrate behavioral health and primary care. They launched the Depression Initiative Primary Mental Health Collaborative Care Model. This model consists of a primary care provider prescribing an antidepressant, a psychiatrist available for consult, and a nurse case manager who monitors patient progress and provides behavioral healthcare. The Netherlands expects that 80% of mental disorders will be treated in the primary care setting.

Psychiatric-mental health nurses can bring a strong perspective in assessing and managing both physical and mental health needs in such integrated care settings. Advocating for models such as the one used in the Netherlands is an important aspect of leadership in nursing.

Pincus, H. A., Jun, M., Franx, G., van der Feltz-Cornelis, C., Ito, H., & Mossialos, E. (2015). How can we link general medical and behavioral healthcare? International models for practice and policy. *Psychiatric Services, 66*(8), 775–777.

The following interventions have all been shown to positively affect a patient's recovery:

- Educating the patient regarding specific treatments
- Referring the patient to community support groups (or systems)
- Teaching patients more effective coping skills that take into consideration patients' values, preferences, and lifestyle
- Focusing on a patient's strengths and reinforcing coping skills that work (e.g., prayerfulness, participation in hobbies, relaxation techniques)

General recommendations for healthcare providers in working with patients with somatic symptoms include six key elements for effective relationships and treatment:

1. Provide continuity of care.
2. Avoid unnecessary tests and procedures.
3. Provide frequent, brief, and regular office visits.
4. Always conduct a physical examination.
5. Avoid making disparaging comments such as, "Your symptoms are all in your head."
6. Set reasonable therapeutic goals such as maintaining function despite ongoing pain.

Psychosocial Interventions

Nursing interventions for patients with somatic symptom disorders generally take place in the home or clinic setting and entail helping the patient improve overall functioning through the development of effective coping strategies. The *Nursing Interventions Classification (NIC)* offers several categories pertinent to caring for patients with somatic symptom disorders: *assertiveness training, family involvement promotion, limit setting, self-awareness enhancement,* and *self-esteem enhancement* (Bulechek et al., 2013).

Promotion of Self-Care Activities

When somatization is present, the patient's ability to perform self-care activities may be impaired, and nursing intervention is necessary. In general, interventions involve the use of a matter-of-fact approach to support the highest level of self-care of which the patient is capable.

For patients manifesting paralysis, blindness, or severe fatigue, an effective nursing approach is to support patients while expecting them to support themselves. For example, the patient who demonstrates paralysis of an arm can be expected to eat using the other arm. To encourage the patient experiencing blindness to feed himself, he can be told at what numbers on an imaginary clock the food is located on the plate. These strategies are effective in reducing secondary gain.

Assertiveness training is often identified as appropriate teaching for patients with somatic symptom disorders. Use of assertiveness techniques gives patients a direct means of getting needs met, thereby decreasing the need for somatic symptoms. Teaching an exercise regimen, such as doing range-of-motion exercises for 15 to 20 minutes daily and taking regular walks if possible, can help the patient feel in control, increase endorphin levels, and help decrease anxiety.

Table 17.4 provides basic-level interventions for somatic symptom disorders.

Pharmacological Interventions

It is unclear whether medications are useful for treatment of the somatic symptom disorders. Certainly if there are underlying psychiatric diagnoses, appropriate utilization of medication is indicated and may result in a decrease of somatic symptoms. The decision to medicate patients with a somatic symptom disorder should weigh the benefits against the possibility that these patients may misuse their medication or take it irregularly.

While there are no medications that have received FDA approval specifically for somatic disorders, some medications are used off-label. Tricyclic antidepressants (TCAs) and selective serotonin reuptake inhibitors (SSRIs) may be helpful in somatic disorders directly by reducing depressive symptoms and subsequent somatic responses. They may also help by affecting nerve circuits that affect not only mood but fatigue, pain perception, gastrointestinal distress, and other somatic symptoms.

Medication trials with other antidepressants including serotonin norepinephrine reuptake inhibitors (SNRIs)—venlafaxine (Effexor) and duloxetine (Cymbalta)—and a noradrenergic specific serotonergic antidepressant—mirtazapine (Remeron)—have been effective with somatic disorders, but further controlled trials are necessary (Garcia-Martin et al., 2012).

Patients may also benefit from short-term use of benzodiazepine antianxiety medication, which must be monitored carefully because of the risk of dependence. The nurse may administer these medications in certain settings, but teaching patients and families about the medication is helpful in all settings.

Health Teaching and Health Promotion

Patients who use somatization as a way of coping with anxiety tend to be less educated than average. Teaching these patients

TABLE 17.4 Basic-Level Interventions for Somatic Symptom Disorders

Intervention	Rationale
Offer explanations and support during diagnostic testing.	Reduces anxiety while ruling out organic illness
After physical complaints have been investigated, avoid further reinforcement (e.g., do not take vital signs each time patient complains of palpitations).	Directs focus away from physical symptoms
Spend time with patient at times other than when patient summons nurse to voice physical complaint.	Rewards non–illness-related behaviors and encourages repetition of desired behavior
Observe and record frequency and intensity of somatic symptoms. (Patient or family can give information.)	Establishes a baseline and later enables evaluation of effectiveness of interventions
Do not imply that symptoms are not real.	Acknowledges that psychogenic symptoms are real to the patient
Shift focus from somatic complaints to feelings or to neutral topics.	Conveys interest in patient as a person rather than in patient's symptoms; reduces need to gain attention via symptoms
Assess secondary gains "physical illness" provides for patient (e.g., attention, increased dependency, and distraction from another problem).	Allows these needs to be met in healthier ways and thus minimizes secondary gains
Use matter-of-fact approach to patient exhibiting resistance or covert anger.	Avoids power struggles; demonstrates acceptance of anger and permits discussion of angry feelings
Have patient direct all requests to case manager.	Reduces manipulation
Help patient look at effect of illness behavior on others.	Encourages insight; can help improve intrafamily relationships
Show concern for patient while avoiding fostering dependency needs.	Shows respect for patient's feelings while minimizing secondary gains from "illness"
Reinforce patient's strengths and problem-solving abilities.	Contributes to positive self-esteem; helps patient realize that needs can be met without resorting to somatic symptoms
Teach assertive communication.	Provides patient with a positive means of getting needs met; reduces feelings of helplessness and need for manipulation
Teach patient stress-reduction techniques, such as meditation, relaxation, and mild physical exercise.	Provides alternate coping strategies; reduces need for medication

basic information about bodily functions is often necessary. Pictures and charts can be helpful, and it is useful to review the same information with the family because their knowledge may also be faulty.

Case Management

"Doctor shopping" is common among patients with somatic symptom disorders. They go from provider to provider, clinic to clinic, or hospital to hospital, hoping to establish a physical basis for their distress. Repeated computed tomographic scans, magnetic resonance images, and other diagnostic tests are often documented in the medical record.

Case management can help limit healthcare costs associated with such visits. The case manager can recommend to the primary care provider that the patient be scheduled for brief appointments every 4 to 6 weeks at set times, rather than on demand, and that laboratory tests be avoided unless they are absolutely necessary. The patient who establishes a relationship with the case manager often feels less anxiety because the patient has someone to contact and knows that a healthcare expert is a partner.

Advanced Practice Interventions

Psychiatric-mental health advanced practice registered nurses may use various types of psychotherapy or consultation with the primary care provider in the treatment of somatic symptom disorders. As nursing is a profession with a major focus on viewing the patient in a holistic way, the advanced practice nurse can lead the healthcare team in assessing each patient's unique biological, environmental, psychological, spiritual, and sociocultural needs to develop the most comprehensive, individualized plan of care to alleviate the distress of somatic symptoms.

Advanced practice nurses use cognitive behavioral therapy (CBT), the most evidence-based approach for the treatment of somatic disorders. CBT helps patients to find ways to reframe their thoughts and gain control of their situation and break what can become a self-fulfilling cycle of pain, despair, and health-seeking behaviors. Refer to Chapter 2 for a more complete explanation of CBT. Table 17.5 provides a summary of advanced practice interventions.

Managing psychiatric symptoms and physical symptoms can be a challenge for general medical nurses. Advanced practice psychiatric nurses can bridge that gap as liaisons. The first meeting is with the nurse who initiated the consultation. The advanced practice nurse reviews the medical records, discusses the case with the admitting care provider, and interviews the patient. Afterward, the liaison nurse discusses the assessment and suggestions with the referring nurse. If a psychiatric consultation is necessary, the psychiatric liaison nurse initiates the consultation by contacting the patient's physician. A case conference is sometimes needed to enhance communication and consistency in the care of a particular patient.

EVALUATION

Evaluation of patients with somatic symptom disorders is a straightforward process when you have written measurable behavioral outcomes clearly and realistically. For these patients,

TABLE 17.5 Advanced Practice Interventions for Somatic Symptom Disorders

Disorder	Course	Interventions
Somatic symptom disorder	Chronic and relapsing	Consistent primary care provider with regular patient visits, limited tests Group therapy Cognitive-behavioral therapy
Illness anxiety disorder	Chronic and relapsing, but 50% of patients improve	Cognitive-behavioral therapy Insight-oriented therapy Group therapy Psychopharmacological management for comorbid conditions Stress management
Conversion disorder	Usually acute onset; resolves quickly	Suggest that the conversion symptom will gradually improve Behavioral therapy Insight-oriented therapy Hypnosis Antianxiety drugs
Psychological factors affecting medical condition	Acute and chronic; variable resolution	Treat psychiatric symptoms Tailor treatment to address both the psychological symptom and the medical condition
Factitious disorder	Highly treatment-resistant	Confrontation is counterproductive Emphasis on management over cure Legal interventions may be necessary in the case of factitious disorder imposed on another

you might often find that goals and outcomes are only partially met. Patients are likely to report the continuing presence of somatic symptoms, but they often say they are less concerned about the symptoms. Families frequently report relatively high satisfaction with outcomes even without total eradication of the patient's symptoms.

FACTITIOUS DISORDER

Whereas other somatic disorders are not under conscious control, people with a **factitious disorder** consciously pretend to be ill to get emotional needs met and attain the status of patient. The term *factitious* comes from the Latin word meaning "artificial or contrived." Patients with this disorder artificially, deliberately, and dramatically fabricate symptoms or self-inflict injury with the goal of assuming the sick role. Similar to substance use disorders, this problem is compulsive and individuals consciously conceal the true nature of the illness through deception. Factitious disorder results in disability and immeasurable costs to the healthcare system.

The contrived illness may be physical or psychiatric. Examples of manufactured illnesses include bleeding, fever, hypoglycemia, seizures, hallucinations, and even cancer. Individuals with factitious disorder may report depression and suicidality after the death of a spouse despite the fact that the death is not true or that he was not even married (APA, 2013).

An older term for factitious disorder is **Munchausen syndrome,** which was named for Baron Karl Friedrich Hieronymus von Münchausen (1720–1797). He was an 18th-century German officer with a reputation for fabricating outrageous tales such as traveling to the moon, riding a cannonball, or fighting a 40-foot crocodile.

CLINICAL PICTURE

Factitious Disorder Imposed on Self

Admission to the hospital often begins in the emergency room with a dramatic description of an illness using unusually proper medical terminology. The patient is often reluctant for professionals to speak with family members, friends, or previous healthcare providers. Once admitted, the patient is frequently demanding and requests specific treatments and interventions. Negative test results are often followed by new or additional symptoms. If the healthcare team sets limits and does not follow through with requests, the patient may become angry and accuse the staff of incompetence and maltreatment.

Patients go from one primary care provider or hospital to another. Serious complications and sepsis may result from self-injections of toxins such as *E. coli.* Patients may have "crisscrossed" or "railroad-track" abdomens due to scars from numerous exploratory surgeries to investigate unexplained symptoms. In the extreme, amputations may even result from this disorder.

Factitious Disorder Imposed on Another

The most insidious form of factitious disorder is **factitious disorder imposed on another** (also known as *Munchausen syndrome by proxy*) in which a caregiver deliberately falsifies illness in a vulnerable dependent. The diagnosis is imposed on the perpetrator and not the victim. People with this disorder do not do it to receive awards such as insurance money or other compensation. They do it for the purpose of the attention and excitement and to perpetuate the relationship with healthcare providers of that dependent. The parent or guardian is frequently a healthcare worker or someone with extensive knowledge of the healthcare system.

The disorder results in unnecessary medical visits and sometimes-harmful medical procedures. Examples of this falsified problem include inducing premature delivery by rupturing the amniotic sac with a fingernail, infant apnea and sudden infant death, and introducing microorganisms into a child's wound. Falsification of illnesses results in extreme pain, surgical procedures, and even the death of dependents.

EPIDEMIOLOGY

Epidemiological studies estimate an incidence rate of 0.8% to 1.3%. Explanation for the low incidence rate includes the belief that a large number of cases are missed due to frequent denial of factitious disorder behaviors, the challenge to differentiate between real and feigned illness, and the fact that many patients often flee the healthcare setting. Factitious disorder, however, is more prevalent than previously recognized with suggestions that up to 6% of healthcare provider contacts may involve factitious disorder. Nurses should consider this diagnosis in complicated patients, especially those with a history of emotional or physical distress, excessive dependence, and resistance to discharge.

COMORBIDITY

People with factitious disorders tend to complain of physical problems although some patients may also try to convince clinicians that they have a psychiatric disorder. Patients may describe symptoms of depression, dissociation, conversion, and psychoses and seek treatment for these problems. According to some reports, substance use, borderline personality disorders, and sexual disorders are frequently present along with a normal to high intelligence quotient (IQ) and an intimate knowledge of the healthcare system.

RISK FACTORS

Biological Factors

Research points to brain dysfunction as a possible source of the symptoms of factitious disorders (Sadock et al., 2015). Specifically, impaired information processing is a potential cause. There does not seem to be a genetic pattern, and there are no abnormalities in electroencephalographic studies among people with factitious disorder.

Psychological Factors

It is difficult to determine or understand the psychological basis of these disorders because of the patients' intention to skew the facts. There is some evidence that persons with these disorders suffered abuse and neglect as children and may have been hospitalized more frequently than is typical (Sadock et al., 2015). These hospitalizations may have been perceived as a refuge from a chaotic home life. Patients with factitious disorders may have a masochistic side and feel a need to be punished through painful procedures.

APPLICATION OF THE NURSING PROCESS

ASSESSMENT AND DIAGNOSIS

Many of the principles of care for somatic symptom disorders apply to factitious disorders. Often, determining if a patient's signs and symptoms are conscious or unconscious (i.e., whether they are a somatic disorder or a factitious disorder) is a challenge for clinicians, particularly those in the position to diagnose psychiatric disorders. Your role as a nurse, whether you work in psychiatry or any other setting, is to carefully assess the patient and document your care. A general principle in treating people with a factitious disorder is to avoid confrontation, which may result in the patient's defensiveness, elusiveness, or departure from the treatment facility.

Self-Assessment

Nurses who work with patients with factitious disorders—patients who intentionally and consciously fake illnesses—are often angry and resentful. After all, there are patients who really need care and have no control over how sick they are, and then there are patients with factitious disorders who are probably causing their own problems. If this happens to you, it helps to acknowledge and address these reactions through discussions with other members of the treatment team.

PLANNING AND IMPLEMENTATION

In cases of self-directed factitious disorder and particularly other-directed factitious disorder, the nurse must consider safety. Nurses must carefully monitor patients who may purposefully inflict damage to themselves, and report suspicious activities to the healthcare team for discussion. It is essential that the nurse share any information that may prevent a person or a vulnerable and unsuspecting child from undergoing unnecessary surgery or treatments.

EVALUATION

Evaluation with factitious disorders is positive when you maintain patient safety and explore conflicts. New coping strategies should permit the patient to function at a higher level, and the patient should handle stress adaptively without the desire or need of the pretense of a physiological disorder.

Malingering

While not a specific mental disorder, **malingering** is mentioned here as a condition related to the factitious disorders. Malingering is a consciously motivated act of fabricating an illness or exaggerating symptoms. This is done for secondary gain to become eligible for such things as disability compensation, committing fraud against insurance companies, obtaining prescription medications, evading military service, or receiving a reduced prison sentence. Reported pains are vague and hard for clinicians to prove or disprove (e.g., back pain, stomach ailments, headache, or toothache).

Malingering is likely more common in men than in women. It is nearly impossible to determine the prevalence of malingering due to the concealment of its origins. Childhood neglect and abuse are possible causes. A childhood history of frequent illnesses, especially those that result in hospitalization, may also be present in people who develop this disorder. Malingering is associated with antisocial, narcissistic, and borderline personality disorders.

CASE STUDY AND NURSING CARE PLAN

Somatic Symptom Disorder

Cara, age 49, a recently divorced mother of twin teenage daughters, works as a copy editor for a local newspaper. She has been trying to sell her house to downsize after her daughters graduate from high school next year. Cara feels "nervous most of the time" and that she only leaves the house for work or to do grocery shopping. She reports no social life and states, "I don't have any friends."

She reports being been referred to a variety of specialists who found no evidence of organic origins of her pathophysiology. Today, she went to the emergency room with tachycardia in normal sinus rhythm, shortness of breath, and fatigue. All diagnostic tests were normal.

Cara agreed to attend an intensive outpatient program (IOP) three mornings each week. After two days in the IOP she has not engaged in treatment. She is worried about losing her job if she does not return to work soon. She is frustrated that her fatigue and physical symptoms are continuing. "My mood is fine, but my body is the major problem."

Self-Assessment

Heather is a registered nurse with 3 years of experience in the IOP. She recognizes her own feelings of frustration toward Cara for refusing to identify emotional concerns and wanting to leave the program and return to work.

Heather realizes she has to monitor her emotional reactions to Cara and adopt a persistent matter-of-fact approach to encourage the patient to be more assertive, self-aware, and independent. Heather plans to actively support Cara in creating her discharge plan.

Assessment

Subjective Data

- Reports no history of diagnosed physical illness or psychiatric disorders.
- Reports shortness of breath and a rapid heart rate.
- "I don't have any friends."
- Reports feeling "nervous most of the time" and only leaving the house for work or to do grocery shopping.
- "My mood is fine, but my body is the major problem."

Objective Data

- Vital signs are within normal limits
- Diagnostic tests are negative.
- Onset of symptoms coincides with a divorce and impending graduation of her daughters.

Nursing Diagnoses

1. *Complicated grieving* related to loss of significant other and anticipatory losses of children and home as evidenced by multiple somatic symptoms, anxiety, and depressed mood.
2. *Social isolation* related to fatigue/pain as evidenced by decreased contact and interaction with family and friends.

Outcomes Identification

Long-term goal: Patient will identify and express emotions without physical symptoms.

Planning

The initial plan is to encourage Cara to explore feelings related to recent and impending losses and to develop a support system.

Implementation

The plan of care for Cara is personalized as follows:

Short-Term Goal	Intervention	Rationale	Evaluation
1. Patient will identify levels of anxiety in at least three situations and encounters with IOP patients and staff.	1. Teach the patient techniques to identify and manage anxiety.	1. Identifying anxiety and anxiety reduction techniques helps manage distress and provides patient with self-care behaviors, thereby enhancing self-esteem.	**GOAL MET**
2. Patient will develop a contract in conjunction with staff to plan for behavior change.	2. Develop a relationship with the patient that includes a mutually agreed upon contract that details expected changes in behaviors.	2. A concrete means to keep track of patient actions will enhance self-direction and independent actions.	**GOAL MET**
3. Patient will seek support from staff and patients when feelings of anxiety become difficult to handle or physical symptoms increase.	3. Educate the patient about sharing feelings of loss with staff, friends, and family members.	3. Communication and expression of feelings with family and friends helps alleviate stress and often provides a more supportive environment.	**GOAL MET**
4. Patient will make a list with contacts and phone numbers of community resources of interest to her.	4. Assist in the identification of available support systems.	4. Patients are more successful with stressful life events if there is adequate support.	**GOAL MET**
5. Patient will utilize the therapeutic milieu to increase her ability to express feelings.	5. Support expression of feelings via the arts such as writing, music, and role-playing.	5. Various forms of artistic expression encourage promotion of feelings	**GOAL MET**

Continued

CASE STUDY AND NURSING CARE PLAN—cont'd

Somatic Symptom Disorder

Short-Term Goal	Intervention	Rationale	Evaluation
6. Patient will be active in unit activities.	6. Assist the patient in identification of appropriate diversional activities.	6. Diversional activities assist the patient to be less attentive to inner turmoil. The patient is more likely to use activities that are of specific interest.	**GOAL MET**
7. Patient will challenge negative and self-defeating thoughts and replace them with positive thoughts.	7. Encourage the patient to use positive self-talk such as, "I can do this one step at a time," "Right now I need to stretch and breathe," and "I don't need to be perfect."	7. Cognitive techniques focus on changing behaviors and feelings by changing thoughts. Replacing negative thoughts with positive ones helps to decreased anxiety.	**GOAL MET**

Evaluation

Short-term goals met: After spending 3 weeks in the IOP, Cara developed a trusting relationship with one staff person and two patients. Heather arranged a family meeting with Cara and her daughters where Cara was able to express her feelings. Her daughters expressed their concerns and emotions about leaving home as well. Cara also became more active expressing her grief, particularly in the assertiveness and anger-management classes. Cara felt the music group amazingly improved her mood. Following discharge from the IOP, Cara decided to take piano lessons and also enrolled in some of her town's adult education classes. She is meeting more people in the community.

Long-term goal, partially met: Many of Cara's symptoms have decreased. In particular, there have been no further episodes of tachycardia. Cara will continue to see her nurse therapist weekly, work on assertiveness skills, identification and expression of feelings, and a healthier lifestyle.

KEY POINTS TO REMEMBER

- There is irrefutable evidence that emotional conditions may precipitate and often increase the severity of physical symptoms. Likewise, physical illnesses are often accompanied by a spectrum of emotional responses.
- Somatic symptom disorders are characterized by the presence of multiple real physical symptoms with or without an identifiable medical illness.
- Somatic symptom disorders are responses to psychosocial stress although the patient often shows no insight in the potential stressors.
- The course of somatic symptom disorders may be brief, with acute onset and spontaneous remission, or chronic, with a gradual onset and prolonged impairment.
- The nursing assessment is especially important to identify symptoms of adverse childhood events, depression, anxiety, posttraumatic stress disorder, and substance use that are contributing to the somatic symptom disorder.
- Integrated holistic interventions target both the psychological and medical problems to increase adherence to the care regimen, maximize quality of life, promote healing, and minimize healthcare costs.
- The advanced practice psychiatric-mental health registered nurse is in a key position to assist other healthcare personnel to view patients in an integrated, holistic approach in both inpatient and outpatient settings.
- Factitious disorders, in contrast to other somatic disorders, are under conscious control. Nurses are challenged to provide care for persons who are pretending to have disorders when there are others with real illnesses who need their time.

CRITICAL THINKING

1. A patient with suspected somatic symptom disorder has been admitted to the medical-surgical unit after an episode of chest pain with possible electrocardiographic changes. While on the unit, she frequently complains of palpitations, asks the nurse to check her vital signs, and begs staff to stay with her. Some nurses take her pulse and blood pressure when she asks. Others evade her requests. Most of the staff tries to avoid spending time with her.
   a. Consider why staff wish to avoid her. How would you feel as a nurse in this situation?
   b. Design interventions to cope with the patient's behaviors. Give rationales for your interventions.
2. Maria Valdez is a 45-year-old who has learned that she is HIV-positive. She is asymptomatic, has a normal physical examination, and all routine laboratory tests are normal. Her CD4 cell count is 325 cells per cubic millimeter, and her plasma HIV-1 RNA level is 60,000 copies per milliliter (both confirmed on repeated testing). She and her ex-husband have been divorced for years but maintain a good relationship. Maria has a supportive extended family, church community, and neighbors. She has a full-time job and several committed friends that she grew up with. Maria has been seeing her current boyfriend for 2 years; however, she was not aware that he was engaging in unprotected sex outside of their relationship. Maria is distraught. "How can I live with myself? I am a disgrace to my children and family." Within several weeks, Maria returns to work and starts to assume more daily household responsibilities. When she is encouraged to talk about her feelings and see a therapist, Maria states, "I will be able to do everything I did before.

I feel healthy." The nurse has several concerns including Maria's focus on self-care, acceptance and understanding of her HIV-positive status, and her willingness to disclose her status to sexual/intimate partners.

a. How would you evaluate Maria's social support system?
b. What other information would you like to know about her situation that might help your assessment?
c. What do you need to know about her cultural beliefs about illness?
d. What recommendations or referrals could you make for her? How would you approach these recommendations?
e. From what you know about Maria, identify the strengths she has that you would support and encourage.

CHAPTER REVIEW

Questions

1. The care plan of a patient diagnosed with a somatic disorder includes the nursing diagnosis *ineffective coping*. Which patient behavior demonstrates a successful outcome for that nursing diagnosis?
   a. Showers and dresses in clean clothes daily
   b. Calls a friend to talk when feeling lonely
   c. Spends more time talking about pain in her abdomen
   d. Maintains focus and concentration
2. Which patient is at greatest risk for developing a stress-induced myocardial infarction?
   a. A patient who lost a child in an accidental shooting 24 hours ago
   b. A woman who has begun experiencing early signs of menopause
   c. A patient who has spent years trying to sustain a successful business
   d. A patient who was diagnosed with chronic depression 10 years ago
3. What precipitating emotional factor has been associated with an increased incidence of cancers? *Select all that apply.*
   a. Anxiety
   b. Job-related stress
   c. Acute grief
   d. Feelings of hopelessness and despair from depression
   e. Prolonged, intense stress
4. You are caring for Aaron, a 38-year-old patient diagnosed with somatic symptom disorder. When interacting with you, Aaron continues to focus on his severe headaches. In planning care for Aaron, which of the following interventions would be appropriate?
   a. Call for a family meeting with Aaron in attendance to confront Aaron regarding his diagnosis.
   b. Educate Aaron on alternative therapies to deal with pain.
   c. Improve reality testing by telling Aaron that you do not believe that the headaches are real.
   d. After a limited discussion of physical concerns, shift focus to feelings and effective coping skills.
5. Living comfortable and materialistic lives in Western societies seems to have altered the original hierarchy proposed by Maslow in that:
   a. Once lower level needs are satisfied, no further growth feels necessary
   b. Self-actualization is easier to achieve with financial stability
   c. Esteem is more highly valued than safety
   d. Focusing on materialism reduces interests in love, belonging, and family
6. Diane, a 63-year-old mother of three, was brought to the community psychiatric clinic. Diane and her son had a bitter fight over finances. Ever since Diane has been complaining of "a severe pain in my neck." She has seen several doctors who cannot find a physical basis for the pain. The nurse knows that:
   a. Showing concern for Diane's pain will increase her obsessional thinking.
   b. Diane's symptoms are manipulative and under conscious control.
   c. Diane believes there is a physical cause for the pain and will resist a psychological explanation.
   d. Diane is trying to make her son feel bad about the argument.
7. Conversion disorder is described as an absence of a neurological diagnosis that manifests in neurological symptoms. Channeling of emotions, conflicts, and stressors into physical symptoms is thought to be the cause in conversion disorder. Which statement is true?
   a. People with conversion disorder are extremely upset about often dramatic symptoms.
   b. Abnormal patterns of cerebral activation have been found in individuals with conversion disorder.
   c. An organic cause is usually found in most cases of conversion disorder.
   d. Symptoms can be turned off and on depending on the patient's choice.
8. Melanie is a 38-year-old female admitted to the hospital to rule out a neurological disorder. The testing was negative, yet she is reluctant to be discharged. Today she has added lower back pain and a stabbing sensation in her abdomen. The nurse suspects a factitious disorder in which Melanie may:
   a. Consciously be trying to maintain her role of a sick patient
   b. Not recognize her unmet needs to be cared for
   c. Protect her child from illness
   d. Recognize physical symptoms as a coping mechanism
9. You are caring for Yolanda, a 67-year-old patient who has been receiving hemodialysis for 3 months. Yolanda reports that she feels angry whenever it is time for her dialysis treatment. You attribute this to:
   a. Organic changes in Yolanda's brain
   b. A flaw in Yolanda's personality
   c. A normal response to grief and loss
   d. Denial of the reality of a poor prognosis

10. Lucas is a nurse on a medical floor caring for Kelly, a 48-year-old patient with newly diagnosed type 2 diabetes. He realizes that depression is a complicating factor in the patient's adjustment to her new diagnosis. What problem has the most potential to arise?
   a. Development of agoraphobia
   b. Treatment nonadherence
   c. Frequent hypoglycemic reactions
   d. Sleeping rather than checking blood sugar

Answers

1. **b**; 2. **d**; 3. **d, e**; 4. **d**; 5. **d**; 6. **c**; 7. **b**; 8. **a**; 9. **c**; 10. **b**

Ⓔ Visit the Evolve website for a posttest on the content in this chapter: http://evolve.elsevier.com/Varcarolis

Post-Test interactive review

REFERENCES

American Psychiatric Association. (2013). *Diagnostic and statistical manual of mental disorders* (5th ed.). Washington, DC: Author.

Andersson, N. W., Gustafsson, L. N., Okkels, N., Taha, F., Cole, S. W., Munk-Jorgensen, P., & Goodwin, R. D. (2015). Depression and the risk of autoimmune disease: A nationally representative, prospective longitudinal study. *Psychological Medicine, 45*(16), 3559–3569.

Begen, F., & Turner-Cobb, J. M. (2015). Benefits of belonging: Experimental manipulation of social inclusion to enhance psychological and physiological health parameters. *Psychology and Health, 30*(5), 568–582.

Bulechek, G. M., Butcher, H. K., Dochterman, J. M., & Wagner, C. (2013). *Nursing interventions classification (NIC)* (6th ed.). St. Louis, MO: Mosby.

Cannon, W. B. (1914). The emergency function of the adrenal medulla in pain and the major emotions. *American Journal of Physiology, 33*, 356–372.

Dols, A., Rhebergen, D., Eikelenboom, P., & Stek, M. L. (2012). Hypochondriacal delusion in an elderly woman recovers quickly with electroconvulsive therapy. *Clinical and Practice, 2*(11), 21–22.

Dube, S., Fairweather, D., Pearson, W. S., Felitti, V. J., Anda, R. F., & Croft, J. B. (2009). Cumulative childhood stress and autoimmune diseases in adults. *Psychosomatic Medicine, 71*(2), 243–250.

Edwards, T., Stern, A., Clarke, D. D., Ivbijaro, G., & Kasney, L. M. (2010). The treatment of the patient with medically unexplained symptoms in primary care: A review of the literature. *Mental Health in Family Medicine, 7*, 209–221.

Feinstein, A. (2011). Conversion disorder: Advances in our understanding. *Canadian Medical Association Journal, 183*(8), 915–920.

Fink, P. (2010). The outcome of health anxiety in primary care: A two-year follow up study on healthcare costs and self-rated health. *PloS ONE, 5*(3), e9873.

Garcia-Martin, M. I., Miranda, V. E. M., & Soutullo, C. A. (2012). Duloxetine in the treatment of adolescents with somatoform disorders: A report of two cases. *Actas Espanolas de Psiquiatra, 20*(3), 165–168.

Goodwin, R., Palgi, Y., Lavenda, O., Hamama-Raz, Y., & Ben-Ezra, M. (2015). Association between media use, acute stress disorder, and psychological distress. *Psychotherapy and Psychosomatics, 84*, 253–254.

Hegeman, J. M., de Waal, M. W. M., Comijs, H. C., Kok, R. M., & van der Mast, R. C. (2015). Depression in later life: A more somatic presentation? *Journal of Affective Disorders, 170*, 196–202.

Huang, H., & McCarron, R. M. (2011). Medically unexplained symptoms: Evidence-based interventions. *Current Psychiatry, 10*(7), 17–31.

Kim, H. H., Lee, Y. J., Kim, H. K., Kim, J. E., Kim, S. J., Bae, S., et al. (2011). Prevalence and correlates of psychiatric symptoms in North Korean defectors. *Psychiatry Investigation, 8*(3), 179–185.

Marwijk, H. W. J., Kooy, K. G., Stehouwer, C. D., Beekman, A. T., & van Hout, H. P. (2015). Depression increases the onset of cardiovascular disease over and above other determinants in older primary care patients, a cohort study. *BioMed Central Cardiovascular Disorders, 15*(40).

Miller, M. (2009). Treating somatoform disorders. *Harvard Mental Health Letter*. Retrieved from http://www.health.harvard.edu/newsletters/harvard_mental_health_letter/2009/November.

Sadock, B. J., Sadock, V. A., & Ruiz, P. (2015). *Synopsis of psychiatry* (11th ed.). Philadelphia, PA: Wolters.

Selye, H. (1956). *The stress of life*. New York, NY: McGraw-Hill.

Shanahan, L., Zucker, N., Copeland, W. E., Bondy, C. L., Egger, H. L., & Costello, E. J. (2015). Childhood somatic complaints predict generalized anxiety and depressive disorders during young adulthood in a community sample. *Psychological Medicine, 45*(8), 1721–1730.

Steinbrecher, N., Koerber, S., Frieser, D., & Hiller, W. (2011). The prevalence of medically unexplained symptoms in primary care. *Psychosomatics, 52*, 263–271.

Stone, J., Vuilleumier, P., & Friedman, J. H. (2010). Conversion disorder: separating "how" from "why." *Neurology, 74*, 190–191.

van Gils, A., Janssens, K. A., & Rosmalen, J. G. (2014). Family disruption increases functional somatic symptoms in late adolescence: The TRAILS study. *Health Psychology, 33*(11), 1354–1361.

Zivin, K., Yosef, M., Miller, E. M., Valenstein, M., Duffy, S., Kales, H. C., & Kim, H. M. (2015). Association between depression and cause specific death: A retrospective cohort study in the Veterans Health Administration. *Journal of Psychosomatic Research, 78*(4), 324–331.

18

Eating and Feeding Disorders

Carissa R. Enright

Visit the Evolve website for a pretest on the content in this chapter: http://evolve.elsevier.com/Varcarolis Pre-Test interactive review

OBJECTIVES

1. Compare and contrast the signs and symptoms of anorexia nervosa, bulimia nervosa, and binge-eating disorder.
2. Describe the biological, psychological, and environmental factors associated with eating disorders.
3. Apply the nursing process to patients with anorexia nervosa, bulimia nervosa, and binge-eating disorders.
4. Identify three life-threatening conditions, stated in terms of nursing diagnoses, for a patient with an eating disorder.
5. Identify two realistic outcome criteria for a patient with anorexia nervosa, bulimia nervosa, and binge-eating disorder.
6. Describe three feeding disorders: pica, rumination disorder, and avoidant/restrictive food intake disorder.

OUTLINE

KEY TERMS AND CONCEPTS

- anorexia nervosa
- body mass index
- binge-eating disorder
- bulimia nervosa
- ideal body weight
- lanugo
- pica
- refeeding syndrome
- rumination

Of all the psychiatric disorders, eating disorders may be the most perplexing. Eating and sharing food is usually pleasurable and culturally important. It is difficult for many of us to understand how people could starve themselves or reverse the digestive process through vomiting. While there are many theories of the etiology of these disorders to date, the reasons behind the behaviors are still a mystery.

In this chapter we will focus on the three main eating disorders: anorexia nervosa, bulimia nervosa, and binge-eating disorder (American Psychiatric Association, 2013). A summary of characteristics of these disorders is included in Box 18.1. After discussing the eating disorder, we will briefly review feeding disorders.

ANOREXIA NERVOSA

Individuals with **anorexia nervosa** refuse to maintain a minimally normal weight for height and express intense fear of gaining weight. The term *anorexia* is a misnomer, because loss of appetite is rare. Some people with anorexia nervosa restrict their intake of food while others engage in binge eating and purging.

Anorexia nervosa is a chronic illness that waxes and wanes. The 1-year relapse rate approaches 50%, and long-term studies show that up to 40% of patients continue to meet some criteria for anorexia nervosa after 4 years (Harrington et al., 2015). Recovery is evaluated as a stage in the process rather than a fixed event. Factors that influence the stage of recovery include the percentage of ideal body weight that has been achieved, the extent to which self-worth is defined by shape and weight, and the amount of disruption existing in the patient's personal life.

The patient will require long-term treatment that might include periodic brief stays, outpatient psychotherapy, and pharmacological interventions. The combination of individual, group, couples, and family therapy (especially for the younger patient) provides the patient with the greatest chance for a successful outcome.

The *DSM-5* box contains criteria for anorexia nervosa.

DSM-5 CRITERIA FOR ANOREXIA NERVOSA

A. Restrictions of energy intake relative to requirements, leading to a significantly low body weight in the context of age, sex, developmental trajectory, and physical health. Significantly low weight is defined as a weight less than minimally normal or, for children and adolescents, less than that minimally expected.

B. Intense fear of gaining weight or becoming fat or persistent behavior that interferes with weight gain, even though at a significantly low weight.

C. Disturbance in the way in which one's body weight or shape is experienced, undue influence of body weight or shape on self-evaluation, or persistent lack of recognition of the seriousness of the current low body weight.

Coding note: The ICD-9-CM code for anorexia nervosa is 307.1, which is assigned regardless of the subtype. The ICD-10-CM code depends on the subtype (see the following text).

Specify whether:

(F50.01) Restricting type: During the last 3 months, the individual has not engaged in recurrent episodes of binge-eating or purging behavior (i.e., self-induced vomiting or the misuse of laxatives, diuretics, or enemas). This subtype describes presentations in which weight loss is accomplished primarily through dieting, fasting, and/or excessive exercise.

(F50.02) Binge-eating/purging type: During the last 3 months, the individual has engaged in recurrent episodes of binge-eating or purging behavior (i.e., self-induced vomiting or the misuse of laxatives, diuretics, or enemas).

Specify if:

In partial remission: After full criteria for anorexia nervosa were previously met. Criterion A (low body weight) has not been met for a sustained period, but either Criterion B (intense fear of gaining weight or becoming fat or behavior that interferes with weight gain) or Criterion C (disturbances in self-perception of weight and shape) is still met.

In full remission: After full criteria for anorexia nervosa were previously met, none of the criteria have been met for a sustained period of time.

Specify current severity:

The minimum level of severity is based, for adults, on current **body mass index** (BMI; see the following text) or, for children and adolescents, on BMI percentile. The ranges that follow are derived from World Health Organization categories for thinness in adults; for children and adolescents, corresponding BMI percentiles should be used. The level of severity may be increased to reflect clinical symptoms, the degree of functional disability, and the need for supervision.

Mild: BMI $\geq$ 17 kg/m^2
Moderate: BMI 16 to 16.99 kg/m^2
Severe: BMI 15 to 15.99 kg/m^2
Extreme: BMI $<$ 15 kg/m^2

American Psychiatric Association. (2013). *Diagnostic and statistical manual of disorders* (5th ed.). Washington, DC: Author.

EPIDEMIOLOGY

For women, the lifetime incidence of anorexia nervosa is 0.9% and the lifetime incidence for men is 0.24% (Rosenvinge & Petterson, 2015). It is extremely difficult to determine the specific

BOX 18.1 Characteristics of Eating Problems

Anorexia Nervosa	Bulimia Nervosa	Binge Eating

• Intense fear of weight gain
• Distorted body image
• Restricted calories with significantly low BMI
• Subtypes:
  • Restricting (no consistent bulimic features)
  • Binge/eating/purging type (primarily restriction, some bulimic behaviors)
	• Recurrent episodes of uncontrollable binging
	• Inappropriate compensatory behaviors: vomiting, laxatives, diuretics, or exercise
	• Self-image largely influenced by body image
		• Recurrent episodes of uncontrollable binging without compensatory behaviors
		• Binging episodes induce guilt, depression, embarrassment, or disgust

number of people afflicted with eating disorders as fewer than half seek healthcare for their illness. Anorexia nervosa may start as early as between the ages of 7 and 12.

COMORBIDITY

Bipolar, depressive, and anxiety disorders commonly occur with anorexia nervosa. Obsessive–compulsive disorders occurs in some people with anorexia nervosa, particularly in those with the restricting type. Alcohol and substance use disorders are associated with the binge-eating/purging type.

RISK FACTORS

Biological Factors

Genetic

A review of relevant studies suggests that the heritability of anorexia nervosa is 60% (Bienvenu et al., 2011). A genetic vulnerability may lead to poor affect and impulse control or to an underlying neurotransmitter dysfunction, but researchers have not discovered any single causative gene to date. It is likely that a gene-environmental interaction may be responsible for the prevalence of the eating disorders (Campbell et al., 2011).

Neurobiological

Altered brain serotonin function contributes to dysregulation of appetite, mood, and impulse control in eating disorders. Patients consistently exhibit personality traits of perfectionism, obsessive-compulsiveness, and dysphoric mood, all of which correlate with serotonin pathways in the brain modulate. Because these traits appear to begin in childhood—before the onset of actual eating-disorder symptoms—and persist into recovery, experts believe they contribute to a vulnerability to disordered eating (Kaye et al., 2013).

Tryptophan, an amino acid essential to serotonin synthesis, is only available through diet. A normal diet boosts serotonin in the brain and regulates mood. Temporary drops in dietary tryptophan may actually relieve symptoms of anxiety and dysphoria and provide a reward for caloric restriction. However, continued malnutrition will result in a physiological dysphoria. This cycle of temporary relief, followed by more dysphoria, sets up a positive feedback loop that reinforces the disordered eating behavior. This dietary need for tryptophan may account for the fact that antidepressants that boost serotonin do not improve mood symptoms until after an underweight patient has been restored to 90% of optimal weight.

Newer brain imaging capabilities allow for better understanding of the etiological factors of anorexia nervosa (Frank, 2015). Relative to other psychiatric disorders, there are few brain scanning studies of the eating disorders. However, this is a promising area of research that may add significant insights into the diagnosis and treatment of this difficult disease. Studies so far suggest that there is a difference in the reward and executive function parts of the anorexic brain (Kaye et al., 2013).

Psychological Factors

Because anorexia nervosa was observed primarily in girls approaching puberty, early psychoanalytic theories linked the symptoms to an unconscious aversion to sexuality. Throughout the 20th century many authors examined the family dynamics of these patients and concluded that a failure to separate from parents and a rebellion against the maternal bond explained the disordered eating behaviors. Further work by Bruch in the 1970s explored the symptoms as a defense against an overwhelming feeling of ineffectiveness and powerlessness. Even with these theories of unconscious processes, therapies based on this understanding have not made a major impact.

Currently, cognitive-behavioral theorists suggest that anorexia nervosa is based on learned behavior that has positive reinforcement. For example, a mildly overweight 14-year-old has the flu and loses a little weight. She returns to school, and her friends say, “Wow, you look great.” Now she purposefully strives to lose weight. When people say, “Wow, you look really skinny,” she hears, “Wow, you look great.” These comments reinforce her behavior powerfully despite the fact that her health is at risk.

Family theorists maintain that eating disorders are a problem of the whole family, but research has not been able to determine any definitive family characteristics specific to the eating disorders. In general, family therapies focus on facilitating emotional communication and conflict resolution.

Environmental Factors

Studies have shown that culture influences the development of self-concept and satisfaction with body size. The Western cultural ideal that equates feminine beauty to tall, thin models has received much attention in the media as an etiology for anorexia nervosa. However, research has not proven a direct relationship between social ideals portrayed in the media and the development of an eating disorder (Doris et al., 2015).

The rate of obesity in the United States is at an alarming level. Record numbers of men and women are on diets to reduce body weight, but no study has been able to fully explain why only an estimated 0.3% to 3% of the population develops an eating disorder. At this time the assumption is that the "habit" of losing weight becomes entrenched through a reward cycle significantly present in the eating disorders as compared with other dieters (Walsh, 2013).

APPLICATION OF THE NURSING PROCESS

ASSESSMENT

Fundamental to the care of individuals with eating disorders is establishing and maintaining a therapeutic alliance. Patients with anorexia nervosa need a nurse who is able to provide compassionate care that also respects personal boundaries (Wright, 2015). The nursing care starts with a clear understanding of this disease. Box 18.2 lists several thoughts and behaviors associated with anorexia nervosa, and Table 18.1 identifies clinical signs and symptoms of anorexia nervosa along with their causes.

Anorexia nervosa can lead to death. Table 18.2 identifies a number of medical complications that can occur in individuals with anorexia nervosa and bulimia nervosa (discussed later). As you can see, some of the complications are quite severe and life threatening.

BOX 18.2 Thoughts and Behaviors Associated with Anorexia Nervosa

- Terror of gaining weight
- Preoccupation with thoughts of food
- View of self as fat even when emaciated
- Peculiar handling of food: cutting food into small bits
- Pushing pieces of food around plate
- Possible development of rigorous exercise regimen
- Possible self-induced vomiting, use of laxatives and diuretics
- Cognition so disturbed that individual judges self-worth by his or her weight

General Assessment

The patient with the restricting type of anorexia will be severely underweight and may have growth of fine, downy hair called **lanugo** on the face and back. Although cessation of menstruation, amenorrhea, is common in females, it is no longer a required symptom for this disorder. The patient will also have mottled, cool skin on the extremities and low blood pressure, pulse, and temperature readings consistent with a malnourished, dehydrated state (see Table 18.1). Usually, electrolytes will not deviate far from normal ranges. But individuals with anorexia nervosa who also purge may have severe electrolyte imbalance and enter the healthcare system through admission to an intensive care unit.

As with any comprehensive psychiatric nursing assessment, a complete evaluation of biopsychosocial function is mandatory. The areas to be covered include the patient's:

- Perception of the problem
- Eating habits
- History of dieting
- Methods used to achieve weight control (restricting, purging, exercising)
- Value attached to a specific shape and weight
- Interpersonal and social functioning
- Mental status and physiological parameters

Self-Assessment

When caring for a patient with anorexia, you may find it difficult to appreciate the compelling force of the illness, incorrectly believing that the individual has self-imposed

TABLE 18.1 Possible Signs and Symptoms of Anorexia Nervosa

Clinical Presentation	Cause
Low weight	Caloric restriction, excessive exercising
Amenorrhea	Low weight
Yellow skin	Hypercarotenemia
Lanugo	Starvation
Cold extremities	Starvation
Peripheral edema	Hypoalbuminemia and refeeding
Muscle weakening	Starvation, electrolyte imbalance
Constipation	Starvation
Abnormal laboratory values (low triiodothyronine, thyroxine levels)	Starvation
Abnormal computed tomographic scans, electroencephalographic changes	Starvation
Cardiovascular abnormalities (hypotension, bradycardia, heart failure)	Starvation, dehydration Electrolyte imbalance
Impaired renal function	Dehydration
Hypokalemia (<3.5 mEq/L)	Starvation
Anemic pancytopenia	Starvation
Decreased bone density	Estrogen deficiency, low calcium intake

TABLE 18.2 Medical Complications of Anorexia Nervosa and Bulimia Nervosa

	Anorexia Nervosa	Bulimia Nervosa
General		
Cachexia	X	—
Weakness	X	X
Skin		
Lanugo	X	—
Russell's sign (callus on knuckles from self-induced vomiting)	X	X
Yellowing	X	—
Hair loss	X	X
Petechiae/ecchymosis	X	X
Musculoskeletal		
Muscle wasting	X	—
Myopathy	X	—
Osteopenia	X	X
Osteoporosis	X	—
Fracture risk	X	—
Fluid/Electrolyte		
Dehydration	X	X
Hypokalemia	X	X
Hypochloremia	X	X
Alkalosis/acidosis	X	X
Hypophosphatemia	X	—
Hypomagnesemia	X	—
Cardiovascular		
Hypotension	X	X
Bradycardia	X	—
Tachycardia	X	X
Arrhythmias	X	X
Electrocardiographic changes	X	X
QTc prolongation	X	—
ST-T wave abnormalities	X	—
Cardiomyopathy	X	X
Gastrointestinal		
Parotidomegaly	X	X
Dental enamel erosion	X	X
Gastric dilation, rupture	X	X
Esophageal rupture	X	X
Hematemesis	X	X
Constipation/diarrhea	X	X
Central Nervous System		
Neuropathy	X	—
Mild cerebral atrophy	X	X
Cognitive impairment	X	—
Endocrine		
Hypothyroidism, hypercholesterolemia, hypercortisolemia, amenorrhea, ↓ follicle-stimulating hormone, ↓ luteinizing hormone, ↓ estrogen (females), ↓ testosterone (males), ↓ libido	X	—
Renal		
↓ Glomerular filtration rate, ↓ concentrating ability, renal failure, hypokalemic nephropathy	X	—
Hematological		
↓White blood cell count, relative lymphocytosis, ↓ platelets, bone marrow atrophy	X	—

Mitchell, J. E., & Wonderlich, S. A. (2014). Feeding and eating disorders. In R. E. Hales, S. C. Yudofsky, & L.W. Roberts (Eds.), *Textbook of psychiatry* (6th ed.). (pp. 564-565). Washington, DC: American Psychiatric Publishing.

weight restriction, binge eating, and purging. If we see such self-destructive behaviors as choices, it is only natural to blame the patient for any subsequent health problems. The common personality traits of these patients—perfectionism, obsessive thoughts and actions relating to food, intense feelings of shame, people pleasing, and the need to have complete control over their therapy—pose additional challenges. When patients appear to be resistant to change, it is helpful to acknowledge the constant struggle that so characterizes the treatment.

DIAGNOSIS

Imbalanced nutrition: less than body requirements is usually the priority nursing diagnosis for individuals with anorexia. Other nursing diagnoses include *decreased cardiac output, risk for injury* (electrolyte imbalance), and *risk for imbalanced fluid volume* (which would have first priority when problems are addressed). Other nursing diagnoses include *disturbed body image, ineffective coping, chronic low self-esteem,* and *powerlessness.*

ASSESSMENT GUIDELINES

Anorexia Nervosa

1. Determine the patient's perception of the problem, or chief complaint.
2. Perform a complete nursing assessment including vital signs, review of systems, and general appearance.
3. Gather a psychosocial history.
4. Assess nutritional pattern and fluid intake.
5. Assess daily activities including exercise.
6. Review laboratory testing, including:
   - Electrolyte levels
   - Glucose level
   - Thyroid function tests
   - Complete blood count
   - ECG
6. Elicit the patient's goals for treatment.

OUTCOMES IDENTIFICATION

You should always develop outcomes that are patient-centered, ideally in conjunction with the patient or with someone who

TABLE 18.3 Signs and Symptoms, Nursing Diagnoses, and Outcomes for Anorexia Nervosa

Signs and Symptoms	Nursing Diagnoses	Outcomes
Emaciation, dehydration, arrhythmias, inadequate intake, dry skin, decreased blood pressure, decreased urine output, increased urine concentration, weakness	*Imbalanced nutrition: less than body requirements* *Decreased cardiac output* *Risk for injury (electrolyte imbalance)* *Risk for imbalanced fluid volume*	Nutrients are ingested and absorbed to meet metabolic needs; cardiac pump supports systemic perfusion pressure; electrolytes are in balance; fluids are in balance
Excessive self-monitoring, describes self as fat despite emaciation	*Disturbed body image*	Congruence between body reality, body ideal, and body presentation; satisfaction with body appearance
Destructive behavior toward self, poor concentration, inability to meet role expectations, inadequate problem solving	*Ineffective coping*	Demonstrates effective coping, reports decrease in stress, uses personal support system, uses effective coping strategies, reports increase in psychological comfort
Indecisive behavior, lack of eye contact, passive, reports feelings of shame, rejects positive feedback about self	*Chronic low self-esteem*	Verbalizes a positive level of confidence; makes informed life decisions, expresses independence with decision-making processes

From Herdman, T. H., & Kamitsuru, S. (Eds.). (2014). *Nursing diagnoses—Definitions and classification 2015-2017*. Oxford, UK: Wiley Blackwell. Moorhead, S., Johnson, M., Maas, M. L., & Swanson, E. (2013). *Nursing outcomes classification (NOC)* (5th ed.). St. Louis, MO: Mosby.

can represent the patient. To evaluate the effectiveness of treatment, establish outcome criteria to measure treatment results. The most important outcome is the attainment of a safe weight. Table 18.3 identifies signs and symptoms commonly experienced with anorexia nervosa, offers potential nursing diagnoses, and suggests outcomes.

PLANNING

Planning depends on the acuity of the patient's situation. When a patient with anorexia is experiencing extreme electrolyte imbalance or weighs below 75% of **ideal body weight**, the plan is to provide immediate medical stabilization, most likely on an inpatient unit. Other criteria for hospitalization includes less than 10% body fat, a daytime heart rate of less than 50 beats per minute, a systolic blood pressure of less than 90, a temperature of less than 96, and arrhthymias. If a specialized eating-disorder unit is not available, hospitalization on a cardiac or medical unit is usually brief, providing only limited weight restoration and addressing only the acute complications (e.g., electrolyte imbalance and dysrhythmias) and acute psychiatric symptoms (e.g., significant depression).

With the initiation of therapeutic nutrition, malnourished patients may need treatment on a medical unit. During prolonged starvation the body switches from glucose-based energy to fat- and protein-based energy. When nutrients are restored, insulin stimulates glycogen, fat, and protein synthesis, a process that requires minerals such as phosphate and magnesium. In severely malnourished patients a **refeeding syndrome** may occur. This is a potentially lethal treatment complication that may result in fluid-balance abnormalities, abnormal glucose metabolism, hypophosphatemia, hypomagnesemia, and hypokalemia. Thiamine deficiency can also occur (Myatt, 2014). Reintroduction of nutrients must proceed slowly to avoid this syndrome.

Once a patient is medically stable, the plan addresses the issues underlying the eating disorder. These psychological issues are usually addressed on an outpatient basis. The plan of care will include individual, group, and family therapy, as well as psychopharmacological therapy during different phases of the illness. The nature of the treatment depends on the intensity of the symptoms—which may vary over time—and the experienced disruption in the patient's life.

Discharge planning is a critical component in treatment. Often, family members benefit from counseling. The discharge planning process includes living arrangements, school, work, the feasibility of independent financial status, applications for state and/or federal program assistance (if needed), and follow-up outpatient treatment.

IMPLEMENTATION

Acute Care

Typically, a patient with an eating disorder is admitted to the inpatient psychiatric facility in a crisis state. The initial focus depends on the results of a comprehensive assessment. Address any acute psychiatric symptoms, such as suicidal ideation, immediately. You are challenged to both establish trust while monitoring the eating pattern.

Psychosocial Interventions

After resolving acute symptoms, the patient with anorexia begins a weight restoration program that allows for incremental weight gain. Based on the patient's height, a treatment goal is set at 90% of ideal body weight, the weight at which most women are able to menstruate.

As patients begin to re-feed, they ideally participate in the unit's milieu. In this setting, the patient should feel accepted and safe from judgmental evaluations. The focus should be on the eating behavior and underlying feelings of anxiety, dysphoria, low self-esteem, and lack of control. Approach discussions about physical appearance carefully because the patient could misinterpret comments.

CONSIDERING CULTURE

Does Faith-Based Fasting Have an Impact on Women with Anorexia Nervosa?

Researchers compared the impact of faith and traditional fasting in relation to body image and eating distress. The sample included 205 Caucasian women living in Bulgaria. Part of the group met criteria for anorexia nervosa, and part of the group did not. They found that faith-based fasting had different effects on eating behavior:

- Women without an eating disorder were more likely to use fasting in the way intended by religious scripture that has nothing to do with body image.
- Women with anorexia nervosa used this religious practice as a weight management practice that camouflaged the eating disorder.
- In eating disordered women, religious fasting may spur a punishing behavior to meet the demands of their faith.

Culturally sensitive nursing care requires that nurses seek out and understand the cultural influences that may contribute to the disordered eating. The decision to reinforce or de-emphasize spiritual beliefs in our patients must be made in the context of those cultural differences.

Angelova, R. A., & Utermohlen, V. (2013). Culture-specific influences on body image and eating distress in a sample of urban Bulgarian women: The roles of faith and traditional fasting. *Eating Behaviors, 14*(3), 386–389.

Pharmacological Interventions

There are no drugs approved by the US Food and Drug Administration (FDA) for the treatment of anorexia nervosa, and research does not support the use of pharmacological agents to treat the core symptoms (Harrington et al., 2015). The selective serotonin reuptake inhibitor (SSRI) fluoxetine (Prozac), however, has proven useful in reducing obsessive-compulsive behavior *after* the patient has reached a maintenance weight.

Complementary and Integrative Approaches

Patients with eating disorders may benefit from a number of complementary and integrative approaches (Smith et al., 2014). A comprehensive treatment plan can include the usual medical and nutritional interventions along with the beneficial effects of massage, biofeedback, acupuncture, or yoga to manage mood. It is also important that the nurse ask if patients are taking herbals, such as St. John's wort for depression, valerian for sleep, or chamomile for anxiety. Patients need guidance and education to assist them when they choose to add these therapies to their recovery program.

Health Teaching and Health Promotion

Self-care activities are an important part of the treatment plan. These activities include learning more constructive coping skills, improving social skills, and developing problem-solving and decision-making skills. The skills become the focus of both therapy sessions and supervised food-shopping trips. As the patient approaches the goal weight, encourage him or her to expand the repertoire to include eating out in a restaurant, preparing a meal, and eating forbidden foods.

Teamwork and Safety

Patients admitted to an inpatient unit designed to treat eating disorders participate in a combination of therapeutic modalities provided by a multidisciplinary team. These modalities normalize eating patterns and begin to address the medical, family, and social issues raised by the illness.

The milieu of an eating-disorder unit is purposefully organized to assist the patient in establishing more adaptive behavioral patterns, including normalization of eating. The highly structured environment includes precise meal times, adherence to the selected menu, observation during and after meals, and regularly scheduled weighing.

Close monitoring of patients includes all trips to the bathroom after eating to prevent self-induced vomiting. Patients may also need monitoring on bathroom trips after seeing visitors and after any hospital pass to ensure they have not had access to and ingested any laxatives or diuretics. Often, there is a link between patient privileges and weight gain and treatment-plan adherence. The vignette demonstrates monitoring the bathroom as a therapeutic intervention.

VIGNETTE: A 20-year-old woman who primarily restricts her eating has also resorted to purging when her family forces her to eat. As part of her treatment plan on a general psychiatric unit, the dietitian ordered specific meals for her. She became visibly distressed after eating one of these meals and requested permission to go to the bathroom alone because she had "embarrassing gas." The nurse agreed to stand away from the bathroom door if the patient agreed not to flush the toilet until the nurse was able to inspect the contents. However, the patient flushed the toilet. The treatment team concluded that she broke the contract with the nurse and was not able to adhere to her prescribed treatment without additional structure. The treatment team established a new goal that she gain 2 pounds and an intervention that she wait 30 minutes after every meal before she was allowed supervised bathroom breaks.

Advanced Practice Interventions

Psychotherapy

Psychiatric-mental health advanced practice registered nurses provide individual, group, or family therapy in a variety of settings. The goals of treatment are weight restoration with normalization of eating habits and initiation of the treatment of psychological, interpersonal, and social issues that personally affect each individual patient.

Outpatient partial hospitalization programs designed to treat eating disorders are structured to achieve outcomes comparable to those of inpatient eating-disorders units. The advanced practice nurse, along with other therapists, might contract with patients with anorexia regarding the terms of treatment. For example, outpatient treatment can continue only if the patient maintains a contracted weight. If weight falls below the goal, the nurse must make other treatment arrangements until the patient returns to the goal weight.

This highly structured approach to treating patients whose weight is below 75% of ideal body weight is necessary, even for therapists who approach treatment from a more emotional or cognitive model of therapy. Assisting the patient with a daily meal plan, reviewing a journal of meals and dietary intake maintained by the patient, and providing for weekly weighing (ideally two to three times a week) are essential if the patient is to reach a medically stable weight.

Families frequently report feeling powerless in the face of behavior that is mystifying. For instance, patients are often unable to experience compliments as supportive and therefore are unable to internalize the support. They often seek attention from others but feel shamed when they receive it. Patients express that they want their families to care for and about them but are unable to recognize expressions of care. When others do respond with love and support, patients do not perceive this as positive.

Often, family members and significant others seek ways to communicate clearly with the patient with anorexia but find that they are frequently misunderstood and that overtures of concern are misinterpreted. Consequently, families experience the tension of saying or doing the wrong thing and then feeling responsible if a setback occurs. Advanced practice psychiatric-mental health registered nurses have an important role in assisting families and significant others to develop strategies for improved communication and search for ways to be comfortably supportive to the patient.

EVALUATION

The process of evaluation is built into the outcomes specified by *NOC* (Moorhead et al., 2013). Evaluation is ongoing, and the nurse can revise short-term indicators as necessary to achieve the treatment outcomes established. The indicators provide a daily guide for evaluating success and the nurse must continually reevaluate them for their appropriateness. The Case Study and Nursing Care Plan presents a patient with anorexia nervosa.

CASE STUDY AND NURSING CARE PLAN

Anorexia Nervosa

Cynthia is a 20-year-old woman who is brought to the inpatient eating-disorders unit of a psychiatric research hospital by two older brothers who physically support her on both sides. She is profoundly weak, holding her head up with her hands. During the intake interview, Cynthia denies being underweight and says, "I need treatment because I get fatigued so easily." She is particularly concerned about fat on her thighs. "I check my legs every night. I'm so afraid of getting fat. I hate it if my legs touch each other." A self-described perfectionist, Cynthia comments, "I don't like to start anything until I know I can do it perfectly the first time. I wouldn't want anyone to see me make a mistake."

Self-Assessment

Mindy Jacobs, a registered nurse, is assigned to care for Cynthia. Three years ago when she began working on the unit, she had difficulty with overidentifying with patients. During college, Mindy struggled with bulimia, but after treatment she has done well. She seeks guidance from her nursing supervisor and the multidisciplinary team. This support allows her to maintain appropriate boundaries while creating a therapeutic alliance with patients.

Assessment

Subjective Data

- Denies being underweight: "I need treatment because I get fatigued so easily."
- "I check my legs every night. I'm so afraid of getting fat. I hate it if my legs touch each other."
- "I don't like to start anything until I know I can do it perfectly the first time. I wouldn't want anyone to see me make a mistake."

Objective Data

- Height: 62 inches (5 feet 2 inches)
- Weight: 58 pounds —50% of ideal body weight
- Blood pressure: 74/50 mm Hg
- Pulse: 54 beats per minute
- Anemic—hemoglobin: 9 g/dL
- Cachexia, pale, fine lanugo
- Sad facial expression

Priority Diagnosis

Imbalanced nutrition: less than body requirements related to restriction of caloric intake secondary to extreme fear of weight gain.

Outcomes Identification

Patient will reach 75% of ideal weight (92 lb) by discharge.

Planning

The initial plan is to address Cynthia's unstable physiological state.

Implementation

Cynthia's care plan is personalized as follows:

Short-Term Goal	Intervention	Rationale	Evaluation
1. Patient will gain a minimum of 2 lb and a maximum of 3 lb weekly through inpatient stay.	1a. Acknowledge the emotional and physical difficulty patient is experiencing. Use patient's extreme fatigue to engage cooperation in the treatment plan.	1a. A first priority is to establish a therapeutic relationship.	**WEEK 1:** Patient increases caloric intake with liquid supplement only. Patient unable to eat solid food. Patient does not gain weight. Patient remains hypotensive, bradycardic, anemic (hemoglobin [HGB] = 9 g/dL).
	1b. Weigh daily for the first week, then three times a week. Weigh in bra and panties only. No oral intake, including water, before the morning weigh-in.	1b. These measures ensure that weight is accurate.	
	1c. Do not negotiate weight with patient or reweigh. Patient may choose not to look at the scale or request that she not be told the weight.	1c. Patient may try to control and sabotage treatment.	**WEEK 2:** Patient gains 2 lb drinking liquid supplement—minimal solid food. Patient remains hypotensive, bradycardic (HGB = 10 g/dL).
	1d. Measure vital signs TID until stable, then daily. Repeat ECG and laboratory tests until stable.	1d. As patient begins to increase in weight, cardiovascular status improves to within normal range, and monitoring is less frequent.	

CASE STUDY AND NURSING CARE PLAN—cont'd

Anorexia Nervosa

Short-Term Goal	Intervention	Rationale	Evaluation
	1e. Provide a pleasant, calm atmosphere at mealtimes. Patient should be told the specific times and duration (usually a half hour) of meals.	1e. Mealtimes become episodes of high anxiety, and knowledge of regulations decreases tension, particularly when patient has given up so much control by entering treatment.	**WEEK 3:** Patient gains l lb drinking liquid supplement. Patient selects meal plan but is unable to eat most of solid food. Patient's blood pressure (BP) = 84/60 mm Hg; pulse = 68 beats per minute, regular; HGB = 11 g/dL.
	1f. Administer liquid supplement as ordered.	1f. Patient may be unable to eat solid food at first.	
	1g. Observe patient during meals to prevent hiding or throwing away of food and for at least 1 hour after eating to prevent purging.	1g. The primary goal is to promote nutrition and a healthy weight - external control is required initially. Cognitive and behavioral changes will occur gradually.	**WEEKS 4-6:** Patient gains an average of 2.5 lb/wk. Patient samples more of solid food selected from meal plan. Patient's BP = 90/60 mm Hg; pulse = 68 beats per minute, regular; HGB = 11.5 g/dL.
	1h. Be empathetic with patient's struggle to give up control of eating and weight as she is expected to make minimum weight gain on a regular basis. Permit patient to verbalize feelings at these times.	1h. Patient is expected to gain at least 0.5 lb on a specific schedule, usually three times a week (Monday, Wednesday, Friday).	**WEEK 7:** Patient weighs 71 lb (almost 60% of ideal body weight); calories are mostly from liquid supplement.
	1i. Monitor patient's weight gain. A weight gain of 2-3 lb/wk is medically acceptable.	1i. Weight gain of more than 5 lb in 1 week may result in pulmonary edema.	Patient selects balanced meals, eating more varied solid food: turkey, carrots, lettuce, fruit.
	1j. Provide teaching regarding healthy eating as the basis of a healthy lifestyle.	1j. Healthy aspects of eating (e.g., increased energy, rather than gaining weight) are reinforced.	Patient's HGB = 12.5 g/dL; normal range of BP and pulse are maintained.
	1k. Use a cognitive-behavioral approach to address patient's fears regarding weight gain. Identify and examine distorted thoughts.	1k. Confronting irrational thoughts and beliefs is crucial to changing eating behaviors.	Patient continues to increase participation in social aspects of eating.
	1l. As patient approaches her target weight, there should be encouragement to make her own choices for menu selection.	1l. Patient can assume more control of her meals, which is empowering for the patient with anorexia.	**WEEKS 8-12:** Patient gains an average of 2.5 lb/wk and weighs 82 lb (approx. 68% of ideal body weight).
	1m. Emphasize social nature of eating. Encourage conversation that does not have the theme of food during mealtimes.	1m. Eating as a social activity, shared with others and with participation in conversation, serves as both a distraction from obsessive preoccupations and a pleasurable event.	Patient is eating more varied solid food, but most caloric intake is still from liquid supplement. Patient maintains normal vital signs and HGB levels.
	1n. Focus on the patient's strengths, including her work in normalizing her weight and eating habits.	1n. Patient who is beginning to normalize weight and eating behaviors has achieved a major accomplishment. Noneating activities are explored as a source of gratification.	Patient maintains social interaction during mealtimes and snacks. **WEEKS 13-16:** Patient has reached medically stable weight at the end of 16th week—92 lb (75% of ideal body weight).
	1o. Provide for a planned exercise program when patient reaches target weight.	1o. Patient experiences a strong drive to exercise; this measure accommodates this drive by planning a reasonable amount.	Patient continues to eat more solid food with relatively less liquid supplement.
	1p. Encourage patient to apply all the knowledge, skills, and gains made from the various individual, family, and group therapy sessions.	1p. Patient has been receiving intensive therapy and education, which have provided tools and techniques that are useful in maintaining healthy behaviors.	Patient is not able to participate in planned exercise program until patient reaches 85% of ideal body weight

Evaluation

By the end of the 16th week, Cynthia has achieved a stable weight of 92 lb. Her BMI is 16.8, which is underweight, but is approaching an acceptable level for Cynthia's frame and age. Her vital signs and hemoglobin levels are consistently within normal levels. She is participating in therapy and consistently communicating satisfaction with her body appearance.

BULIMIA NERVOSA

Individuals with **bulimia nervosa** engage in repeated episodes of binge eating followed by inappropriate compensatory behaviors such as self-induced vomiting misuse of laxatives, diuretics, or other medications; fasting; or excessive exercise. This disorder is characterized by a significant disturbance in the perception of body shape and weight. The *DSM-5* box contains criteria for bulimia nervosa.

DSM-5 CRITERIA FOR BULIMIA NERVOSA

A. Recurrent episodes of binge eating. An episode of binge eating is characterized by both of the following:
   1. Eating, in a discrete period of time (e.g., within any 2-hour period), an amount of food that is definitely larger than what most individuals would eat in a similar period of time under similar circumstances.
   2. A sense of lack of control over eating during the episode (e.g., feeling that one cannot stop eating or control what or how much one is eating).

B. Recurrent inappropriate compensatory behavior to prevent weight gain such as self-induced vomiting; misuse of laxatives, diuretics, or other medications; fasting; or excessive exercise.

C. The binge eating and inappropriate compensatory behaviors both occur, on average, at least once a week for 3 months.

D. Self-evaluation is unduly influenced by body shape and weight.

E. The disturbance does not occur exclusively during episodes of anorexia nervosa.

Specify if:

In partial remission: After full criteria for bulimia nervosa were previously met, some, but not all, of the criteria have been met for a sustained period of time.

In full remission: After full criteria for bulimia nervosa were previously met, none of the criteria have been met for a sustained period of time.

Specify current severity:

The minimum level of severity is based on the frequency of inappropriate compensatory behaviors (see later text). The level of severity may be increased to reflect other symptoms and the degree of functional disability.

Mild: An average of 1 to 3 episodes of inappropriate compensatory behaviors per week.

Moderate: An average of 4 to 7 episodes of inappropriate compensatory behaviors per week.

Severe: An average of 8 to 13 episodes of inappropriate compensatory behaviors per week.

Extreme: An average of 14 or more episodes of inappropriate compensatory behaviors per week.

From American Psychiatric Association. (2013). *Diagnostic and statistical manual of disorders* (5th ed.). Washington, DC: Author.

EVIDENCE-BASED PRACTICE

Is Spirituality a Protective Factor in College Students?

Problem

There is no definitive theory for the etiology or prevention of eating disorders among college students. Dysfunctional eating habits impair the overall health in this population and prevention programs should target strategies that use students' strengths to be most effective.

Purpose of Study

The purpose of the study was to examine relationships between eating disorders and spiritual well-being among college students. If spiritual well-being is correlated with fewer dysfunctional eating behaviors, it could be enhanced as a protective factor in prevention programs for this population.

Methods

Nursing students in a public university volunteered to participate. One hundred three women and twelve men ranging in age from 18 to 35 years were recruited. Women's BMIs ranged from 17.7 to 47.6 with a mean of 22.5, and men's BMI ranged from 20.2 to 35.3 with a mean of 26. Each subject provided basic demographic data and took three self-reported measures of eating and spirituality: the Eating Attitudes Test (EAT-26); the Sick, Control, One Stone, Fat, Food (SCOFF) screening tool, and the Spiritual Well-Being Scale (SWBS).

Key Findings

- Approximately 25% of participants screened positive for eating disorder symptoms.
- Forty percent of the students surveyed experienced periods of binging/purging.
- The majority of students identified themselves as spiritual individuals.
- Higher levels of spirituality were related to lower levels of eating disorder symptoms.
- Participants reported a low to moderate sense of spiritual well-being.

Implications for Nursing Practice

Nurses should be aware of the high prevalence of eating disorders, especially among college students. A large number of nursing students in this sample experienced unreported dysfunctional eating habits. Nursing students may find that exploration and enhancement of spiritual beliefs may be a strong personal intervention to help avoid disordered eating behaviors.

Phillips, L., Kemppainen, J., & Mechling, B. (2015). Eating disorders and spirituality in college students. *Journal of Psychosocial Nursing and Mental Health Services, 53*(1), 30–37.

EPIDEMIOLOGY

The 12-month prevalence of bulimia nervosa among young women is 1% to 1.5%. The lifetime incidence of bulimia nervosa for women is 2.3% and the lifetime incidence for men is 0.5% (Rosenvinge & Petterson, 2015). Bulimia commonly begins in later adolescence when the prevalence peaks into young adulthood. Onset of bulimia nervosa is rare in children younger than 12 and adults older than 40.

COMORBIDTY

Most people with bulimia nervosa will experience at least one other psychiatric disorder and many people will experience multiple comorbidities. Mood disorders such as major depressive disorder and bipolar disorder are commonly comorbid, as are anxiety disorders. Bulimia nervosa is associated with borderline or histrionic personality disorders. Alcohol and substance use is problematic in about a third of this population.

RISK FACTORS

Biological Factors

Genetic

Increased frequency of bulimia nervosa is found in first-degree relatives of people with this disorder. Genetic vulnerabilities for its development are believed to exist. Gene variations that are responsible for serotonin have been implicated in bulimia. Even in recovery from this disorder serotonin levels remain abnormal.

Neurobiological

Cycles of binging and purging may have an association with neurotransmitters. Because antidepressants are helpful with bulimia nervosa and because serotonin is linked with satiety, serotonin and norepinephrine have been implicated. Vomiting may increase plasma endorphin levels. The feeling of well-being that some patients feel after vomiting may be due to endorphins.

Individuals with bulimia nervosa may be predisposed to this disorder based on differences in their brains. Research suggests that affected individuals have increased gray matter in the medial orbitofrontal cortex, an area of the brain associated with reward responses. In one intriguing study women with bulimia and women who had recovered from bulimia demonstrated more activity in that area of the brain when tasting sugar compared with healthy controls (Frank et al., 2013).

Individuals with bulimia are more likely to have attention-deficit/hyperactivity disorder and subclinical attention impairments (Seitz et al., 2016). Functional magnetic resonance imaging (fMRI) demonstrates altered neural activity in all three attentional areas of the brain. Inattention, impulsivity, and poor emotional regulation may result from this altered activity.

Psychological Factors

Anxiety disorder or low self-esteem can contribute to the unusual eating behavior of bulimia. Temperamental qualities including impulsivity and sensation seeking are associated with this disorder. Triggers for bingeing may include stress, poor body self-image, food, restrictive dieting, or boredom.

Environmental Factors

Internalization of a thin body ideal increases the risk for weight worries, which in turn increase the risk for bulimia nervosa. There is also some connection between the disorder and childhood sexual or physical abuse. In some cases traumatic events and environmental stress may be contributing factors.

APPLICATION OF THE NURSING PROCESS

ASSESSMENT

General Assessment

Initially, patients with bulimia nervosa do not appear to be physically or emotionally ill. They are often at or close to ideal body weight. However, as the assessment continues and the nurse makes further observations, the physical and emotional problems of the patient become apparent. The patient may have enlargement of the parotid glands, dental erosion, and caries if the patient has been inducing vomiting. The history may reveal great difficulties with both impulsivity and compulsivity. Family relationships are frequently chaotic and reflect a lack of nurturing. Patients' lives reflect instability and troublesome interpersonal relationships as well. Refer to Table 18.2 for medical complications that can occur and the laboratory findings that may result in individuals with bulimia nervosa.

Box 18.3 lists several thoughts and behaviors associated with bulimia nervosa, and Table 18.4 identifies possible signs and symptoms found on assessment and their causes.

BOX 18.3 Thoughts and Behaviors Associated with Bulimia Nervosa

- Binge-eating behaviors
- Often self-induced vomiting (or laxative or diuretic use) after bingeing
- History of anorexia nervosa in one-fourth to one-third of individuals
- Depressive signs and symptoms
- Problems with:
  - Interpersonal relationships
  - Self-concept
  - Impulsive behaviors
- Increased levels of anxiety and compulsivity
- Possible substance use disorders
- Possible impulsive stealing

VIGNETTE: During the initial assessment, the nurse wonders if Brittany is actually in need of hospitalization on the eating-disorders unit. The nurse is struck by how well the patient appears, seeming healthy, well dressed, and articulate.

Brittany tells of restricting her intake until early evening when she buys her food and begins to binge. Once home, she immediately induces vomiting. For the remainder of the evening and into the early morning hours, she "zones out" while watching television and binge eating. Periodically, she goes to the bathroom to vomit. She does this about 15 times during the evening.

The nurse admitting Brittany reminds her of the goals of the hospitalization including interrupting the binge-purge cycle and normalizing eating. The nurse further explains to Brittany that she has the support of the eating-disorder treatment team and the milieu of the unit to assist her toward recovery.

Self-Assessment

Be aware that the patient is sensitive to the perceptions of others regarding this illness and may feel significant shame and totally out of control. In building a therapeutic alliance, try to empathize with the patient's feelings of low self-esteem, unworthiness, and dysphoria. If you believe the patient is not being honest (e.g., active binge eating or purging goes unreported) or is being manipulative, acknowledge such obstacles and the frustration they provoke and construct alternative ways to view the patient's thinking and behavior. An accepting, nonjudgmental approach, along with a comprehensive understanding of the subjective experience of the patient with bulimia, will help to build trust.

ASSESSMENT GUIDELINES

Bulimia Nervosa

1. Determine the patient's perception of the problem, or chief complaint.
2. Perform a complete nursing assessment including vital signs, review of systems, and general appearance.
3. Gather a psychosocial history.
4. Assess nutritional pattern and fluid intake.
5. Assess binging and purging patterns with direct questions.
6. Assess daily activities including exercise.
7. Review laboratory testing, including:
   - Electrolyte levels
   - Glucose level
   - Thyroid function tests
   - Complete blood count
   - ECG
8. Elicit the patient's goals for treatment.

TABLE 18.4 Possible Signs and Symptoms of Bulimia Nervosa

Clinical Presentation	Cause
Normal to slightly low weight	Excessive caloric intake with purging, excessive exercising
Dental caries, tooth erosion	Vomiting (HCl reflux over enamel)
Parotid swelling	Increased serum amylase levels
Gastric dilation, rupture	Binge eating
Calluses, scars on hand (Russell's sign)	Self-induced vomiting
Peripheral edema	Rebound fluid, especially if diuretic used
Muscle weakening	Electrolyte imbalance
Abnormal laboratory values (electrolyte imbalance, hypokalemia, hyponatremia)	Purging: vomiting, laxative and/or diuretic use
Cardiovascular abnormalities (cardiomyopathy, electrocardiographic changes)	Electrolyte imbalance—**can lead to death**
Cardiac failure (cardiomyopathy)	Ipecac intoxication

TABLE 18.5 Signs and Symptoms, Nursing Diagnoses, and Outcomes for Bulimia Nervosa

Signs and Symptoms	Nursing Diagnoses	Outcomes
Electrolyte imbalances, esophageal tears, cardiac problems, excessive vomiting, self-destructive behaviors	*Decreased cardiac output* *Risk for injury (electrolyte imbalance)*	Cardiac pump supports systemic perfusion pressure; electrolytes are in balance
Obsession with body, denial of problems, dissatisfied with appearance	*Disturbed body image*	Congruence between body reality, body ideal, and body presentation; satisfaction with body appearance
Obsessed with food, substance abuse, impulsive responses to problems; inappropriate use of laxatives, diuretics, enemas, fasting, inadequate problem solving	*Ineffective coping*	Demonstrates effective coping, reports decrease in stress, uses personal support system, uses effective coping strategies, reports increase in psychological comfort
Loss of control with the binge-purge cycle, feelings of shame and guilt, views self as unable to deal with events, excessive seeking of reassurance	*Chronic low self-esteem*	Verbalizes a positive level of confidence, makes informed life decisions, expresses independence with decision-making processes
Absence of supportive significant other(s), hides eating behaviors from others, reports feeling alone	*Social isolation*	Willing to call on others for assistance, develops a confidant relationship, feels a sense of belonging

From Herdman, T. H., & Kamitsuru, S. (Eds.). (2014). *Nursing diagnoses—Definitions and classification 2015-2017.* Oxford, UK: Wiley Blackwell. Copyright © 2014, 1994-2012 by NANDA International. Used by arrangement with John Wiley & Sons Limited; Moorhead, S., Johnson, M., Maas, M. L., & Swanson, E. (2013). *Nursing outcomes classification (NOC)* (5th ed.). St. Louis, MO: Mosby.

DIAGNOSIS

The assessment of the patient with bulimia nervosa yields nursing diagnoses that result from the disordered eating and weight-control behaviors. Problems resulting from purging are a first priority because electrolyte and fluid balance and cardiac function are affected. Common nursing diagnoses include *decreased cardiac output, disturbed body image, ineffective coping, powerlessness, chronic low self-esteem,* and *social isolation.*

OUTCOMES IDENTIFICATION

Outcome criteria are linked to the diagnoses listed previously. Table 18.5 provides an overview of signs and symptoms, nursing diagnoses, and associated outcomes for individuals with bulimia nervosa.

PLANNING

Like the patient with anorexia nervosa, the nurse must prioritize care that addresses life-threatening complications. Criteria for inpatient hospitalization include syncope, serum potassium of less than 3.2 mEq/L, serum chloride of less than 88 mEq/L, esophageal tears, arrhythmias, intractable vomiting, and hematemesis (vomiting blood). Suicide risk in this population also requires hospitalization.

VIGNETTE: Iris weighs 85% of her ideal body weight. She has a history of diuretic abuse, and she becomes edematous when she stops their use and enters treatment. The nurse informs Iris that the edema is related to the use of diuretics (and thus is transient) and that it will resolve after Iris begins to eat normally and discontinues the diuretics. Iris cannot tolerate the weight gain and the accompanying edema that occurs when she stops taking diuretics. She restarts the diuretics, perpetuating the cycle of fluid retention and the risk of kidney damage. The nurse empathizes with Iris's inability to tolerate the feelings of anxiety and dread she experiences because of her markedly swollen extremities.

IMPLEMENTATION

Acute Care

A patient who is medically compromised as a result of bulimia nervosa should be referred to an inpatient eating-disorder unit for comprehensive treatment of the illness. The cognitive-behavioral principles of treatment are highly effective and frequently serve as the cornerstone of the therapeutic approach.

Inpatient units designed to treat eating disorders are especially structured to interrupt the cycle of binge eating and purging and to normalize eating habits. The patient begins therapy to examine the underlying conflicts and body dissatisfaction that sustain the illness. Evaluation for treatment of comorbid disorders, such as major depression and substance abuse, is also undertaken. In most cases of substance dependence, the treatment of the eating disorder must occur after treating the substance dependence.

Pharmacological Interventions

Research has shown that antidepressant medication together with cognitive-behavioral therapy brings about improvement in bulimic symptoms. Fluoxetine (Prozac), an SSRI antidepressant, has FDA approval for acute and maintenance treatment of bulimia nervosa in adult patients. When fluoxetine is used for bulimia, it is typically at a higher dose than is used for depression. Although no other drugs have FDA approval for this disorder, medications such as topiramate (Topamax) have been studied for binge suppression. Tricyclic antidepressants help reduce binge eating and vomiting.

Counseling

Compared with the patient with anorexia, the patient with bulimia nervosa often more readily establishes a therapeutic alliance with the nurse because the eating-disordered behaviors are seen as a problem. The therapeutic alliance allows the nurse, along with other members of the multidisciplinary team, to provide counseling that gives useful feedback regarding the patient's distorted beliefs.

Health Teaching and Health Promotion

Health teaching focuses on not only the eating disorder but also meal planning, use of relaxation techniques, maintenance of a healthy diet and exercise, coping skills, the physical and emotional effects of binging and purging, and the impact of cognitive distortions. This preparation lays the foundation for the second phase of treatment in which the nurse carefully plans challenges to the patient's newly developed skills. For instance the patient is expected to have an unsupervised meal at home and share the feelings this event provoked with others in a group therapy setting.

Once a patient reaches therapeutic goals, it is recommended that patients seek long-term care to solidify those goals. Continued therapy can help the individual address the attitudes and perceptions that may perpetuate the disordered eating symptoms.

Teamwork and Safety

The highly structured milieu of an inpatient eating-disorder unit has as its primary goals the interruption of the binge-purge cycle and the prevention of disordered eating behaviors. Observation during and after meals (to prevent purging), normalization of eating patterns, and maintenance of appropriate exercise are integral elements of such a unit. The multidisciplinary team uses a comprehensive treatment approach to address the emotional and behavioral problems that arise when the patient is no longer binge eating or purging. Like the interruption of other obsessive-compulsive behaviors, preventing the binge-purge pattern allows underlying anxiety to come to the surface and be examined.

Advanced Practice Interventions

Psychotherapy

Psychiatric-mental health advanced practice registered nurses are qualified to use cognitive-behavioral therapy, which is the most effective psychotherapy for bulimia nervosa. Restructuring faulty perceptions and helping individuals develop accepting attitudes toward themselves and their bodies are the primary focus of therapy. When patients do not indulge in bulimic behaviors, issues of self-worth and interpersonal functioning become more prominent.

EVALUATION

Evaluation of treatment effectiveness is ongoing and built into the *NOC* categories. Outcomes are revised as necessary to reach the desired outcomes. The Case Study and Nursing Care Plan presents a patient with bulimia nervosa.

CASE STUDY AND NURSING CARE PLAN

Bulimia Nervosa

Kaitlyn is a 30-year-old college graduate who identifies herself an aspiring actress. In the admission interview she expresses concern that her weight will prevent her from attaining her goals and says, "I can't stand to be fat." However, Kaitlyn is motivated to change. "I'm ashamed that I can't control my binge eating and vomiting-I know it's not good." She is being admitted to a partial hospitalization program that specializes in work with eating disorders. Kaitlyn is diagnosed with bulimia nervosa.

Self-Assessment

Matthew, an experienced nurse in the area of eating disorders, is assigned as case manager for Kaitlyn. Matthew enjoys working with patients with bulimia because he believes he can help them manage their condition.

Assessment

Subjective Data

- "I can't stand to be fat."
- "I'm ashamed that I can't control my binge eating and vomiting—I know it's not good."

Objective Data

- Height: 65 inches (5 feet 5 inches)
- Weight: 127 lb—95% of ideal body weight
- Blood pressure: 120/80 mm Hg sitting; 90/60 mm Hg standing
- Pulse: 70 beats/min sitting; 96 beats/min standing
- Potassium level of 2.7 mmol/L (normal range, 3.3 to 5.5 mmol/L)
- ECG: abnormal—consistent with hypokalemia
- Erosion of teeth enamel, enlarged parotid glands

Priority Diagnosis

Risk for injury as evidenced by low potassium and other physical changes secondary to binge eating and purging.

Continued

CASE STUDY AND NURSING CARE PLAN—cont'd

Bulimia Nervosa

Outcomes Identification

Kaitlyn will demonstrate ability to regulate eating patterns, resulting in consistently normal electrolyte balance.

Planning

Kaitlyn is admitted to a partial hospitalization program designed for patients with eating disorders. She attends the program 3 or 4 days a week and participates in individual and group therapy. She will continue to work as a "temp" for a publishing house.

Implementation

Kaitlyn's care plan is personalized as follows:

Short-Term Goal	Intervention	Rationale	Evaluation
1. Patient will identify signs and symptoms of low potassium (K^+) level, and K^+ level will remain within normal limits throughout hospitalization.	1a. Educate patient regarding the ill effects of self-induced vomiting on K^+ level 1b. Educate patient about binge-purge cycle and its self-perpetuating nature. 1c. Teach patient that fasting sets one up to binge eat.	1a. Health teaching is crucial to promoting self-care. 1b, 1c. The compulsive nature of the binge-purge cycle is maintained by the sequence of intake restriction, hunger, bingeing, purging accompanied by feelings of guilt, and then repetition of the cycle over and over.	**WEEK 1:** Patient begins to select balanced meals. Patient demonstrates knowledge of untoward effects of vomiting and K^+ deficiency. Patient begins to demonstrate understanding of repetitive nature of binge-purge cycle.
	1d. Explore thoughts that trigger binge behavior.	1d. If the patient understands thoughts that trigger binge behavior, irrational thoughts can be challenged.	**WEEK 2:** Patient begins to challenge irrational thoughts and beliefs. Patient continues to plan nutritionally balanced meals including dinner at home. Patient begins to sample "forbidden foods" and discuss thoughts and attitudes about same.
	1e. Challenge irrational thoughts and beliefs about "forbidden" foods.	1e. Challenge forces patient to examine own thinking and beliefs.	**WEEK 3:** Patient discusses triggers to binge and resultant behavior. Patient continues to challenge irrational thoughts and beliefs in individual and group sessions. Patient plans meals including "forbidden foods."
	1f. Teach patient to plan and eat regularly scheduled, balanced meals.	1f. This teaching helps ensure success in maintaining abstinence from binge-purge activity.	**WEEK 4:** Patient reports no binge-purge behaviors at day program or outside. Patient demonstrates understanding of repetitive nature of binge-purge cycle. Patient continues to challenge irrational thoughts and beliefs.

Evaluation

At the end of 4 weeks, Kaitlyn reports no binge-purge cycles and her potassium level remains consistently within normal limits. She is beginning to plan meals and challenge irrational thoughts and beliefs.

VIGNETTE: Becky, a 23-year-old patient with a 6-year history of bulimia nervosa, struggles with issues of self-esteem. She expresses much guilt about "letting her father down" in the past by drinking alcohol excessively and binge eating and purging. She is determined that this time she is not going to fail at treatment. After her initial success in stopping the disordered behaviors, she says defiantly, "I'm doing this for *me*." Becky usually experiences her behavior as either pleasing or disappointing to others, but she begins to realize that her feeling of self-worth is very much dependent on how others see her and that she needs to develop a better sense of herself.

BINGE-EATING DISORDER

Individuals with **binge-eating disorder** engage in repeated episodes of binge eating, after which they experience significant distress. These individuals do not regularly use the compensatory behaviors (e.g., vomiting and laxatives) that are seen in patients with bulimia nervosa. Although individuals who start binge eating may be of normal weight, repeated binge eating inevitably causes obesity in this cohort. The *DSM-5* box contains criteria for binge-eating disorder.

DSM-5 CRITERIA FOR BINGE-EATING DISORDER

A. Recurrent episodes of binge eating. An episode of binge eating is characterized by both of the following:
 1. Eating, in a discrete period of time (e.g., within any 2-hour period), an amount of food that is definitely larger than what most people would eat in a similar period of time under similar circumstances.
 2. A sense of lack of control over eating during the episode (e.g., a feeling that one cannot stop eating or control what or how much one is eating).

B. The binge-eating episodes are associated with three (or more) of the following:
 1. Eating much more rapidly than normal.
 2. Eating until feeling uncomfortably full.
 3. Eating large amounts of food when not feeling physically hungry.
 4. Eating alone because of feeling embarrassed by how much one is eating.
 5. Feeling disgusted with oneself, depressed, or very guilty afterward.

C. Marked distress regarding binge eating is present.

D. The binge eating occurs, on average, at least once a week for 3 months.

E. The binge eating is not associated with the recurrent use of inappropriate compensatory behavior as in bulimia nervosa and does not occur exclusively during the course of bulimia nervosa or anorexia nervosa.

Specify if:

In partial remission: After full criteria for binge-eating disorder were previously met, binge eating occurs at an average frequency of less than one episode per week for a sustained period of time.

In full remission: After full criteria for binge-eating disorder were previously met, none of the criteria have been met for a sustained period of time.

Specify current severity:

The minimum level of severity is based on the frequency of episodes of binge eating (see the following text). The level of severity may be increased to reflect other symptoms and the degree of functional disability.

Mild: 1 to 3 binge-eating episodes per week.
Moderate: 4 to 7 binge-eating episodes per week.
Severe: 8 to 13 binge-eating episodes per week.
Extreme: 14 or more binge-eating episodes per week.

American Psychiatric Association. (2013). *Diagnostic and statistical manual of disorders* (5th ed.). Washington, DC: Author.

EPIDEMIOLOGY

Binge-eating disorder is the most common eating disorder. The 12-month prevalence of binge-eating disorder for US adults is 1.6% in females and 0.8% in males. For women, the lifetime incidence of binge-eating disorder is 3.6% and the lifetime incidence for men is 2.1% (Rosenvinge & Petterson, 2015). The presence of binge eating disorder is higher in overweight populations–3%–than in the general population–2%. All racial and ethnic groups seem to be represented fairly equally.

COMORBIDITY

The most common psychiatric disorders associated with binge-eating disorder are bipolar disorder, major depressive disorder, anxiety disorders, and substance-use disorders. The psychiatric comorbidity is linked to the severity of binge eating and not the degree of obesity.

Biological Factors

Binge-eating disorder tends to run in families, which may demonstrate addictive genetic influences. Biological abnormalities, such as hormonal irregularities, may be associated with compulsive eating and food addition.

Psychological Factors

Low self-esteem and body dissatisfaction can contribute to binge-eating disorder. Reduced levels of coping ability are also associated with this disorder.

Environmental Factors

Adverse childhood events such as sexual abuse can increase the risk of binge eating. Social pressures to be thin can trigger emotional eating.

APPLICATION OF THE NURSING PROCESS

ASSESSMENT

Although obesity puts these patients at risk for diabetes, hypertension, and heart disease, hospitalization to treat the binge eating itself is not indicated. Because the stomach must accommodate larger than normal volumes during a binge, there are also gastrointestinal problems associated with this dilation. In addition to reducing binge eating, the nurse will need to help the patient manage the gastric symptoms associated with the disordered eating.

General Assessment

To some extent, all people with obesity have periods when their eating feels out of their control, and to the nurse, the amount of food consumed during meals may look larger than "normal." This presents a major challenge to the accurate discrimination between people who are obese due to metabolic or lifestyle causes and those who have an obsessive binge-eating pattern of eating. A careful history of the quantity of food consumed in discrete binge-eating episodes and how often they occur is essential to the nursing care plan.

Self-Assessment

It is common for people to believe that obesity is a personality flaw in people who fail to control their eating and exercise habits. Culturally, obesity is still the subject of jokes and discrimination. It is important that the nurse be aware of possible negative reactions to obese patients.

ASSESSMENT GUIDELINES

Binge-Eating Disorder

1. Determine the patient's perception of the problem, or chief complaint.
2. Perform a complete nursing assessment including vital signs, review of systems, and general appearance.
3. Gather a psychosocial history.
4. Assess nutritional pattern.
5. Assess history of weight cycling (i.e., gains and loss).
6. Collect a careful history of binge-eating triggers, foods, and frequency.

DIAGNOSIS

Imbalanced nutrition: more than body requirements is usually the most appropriate initial nursing diagnosis for individuals

TABLE 18.6 Signs and Symptoms, Nursing Diagnoses, and Outcomes for Binge-Eating Disorder

Signs and Symptoms	Nursing Diagnoses	Outcomes
Dysfunctional eating pattern, eating in response to internal cues, sedentary lifestyle, weight significantly over ideal for height and frame, intake exceeds metabolic need	*Imbalanced nutrition: More than body requirements*	Nutrient intake meets metabolic needs
Embarrassment due to weight gain, fear of negative reactions by others, attempts to hide weight gain, body dissatisfaction	*Disturbed body image*	Congruence between body reality, body ideal, and body presentation; satisfaction with body appearance
Eats as a coping method, absence of other more effective coping methods, eats even when full	*Ineffective coping*	Demonstrates effective coping, reports decrease in stress, uses personal support system, uses effective coping strategies, reports increase in psychological comfort
Feelings of discomfort or dread, feelings of inadequacy, focused on self, increased wariness, irritability, heart pounding, increased blood pressure and pulse	*Anxiety*	Verbalizes a positive level of confidence; makes informed life decisions, expresses independence with decision-making processes
Loss of control of eating, feelings of shame and guilt, views self as unable to deal with events	*Chronic low self-esteem* *Powerlessness*	Verbalizes a positive level of confidence; makes informed life decisions, expresses independence with decision-making processes
Absence of supportive significant other(s), eats normally in the presence of others, hides eating behaviors, reports feeling alone	*Social isolation*	Willing to call on others for assistance, develops a confidant relationship, feels a sense of belonging

From Herdman, T. H., & Kamitsuru, S. (Eds.). (2014). *Nursing diagnoses—Definitions and classification 2015-2017.* Oxford, UK: Wiley Blackwell. Moorhead, S., Johnson, M., Maas, M. L., & Swanson, E. (2013). *Nursing outcomes classification (NOC)* (5th ed.). St. Louis, MO: Mosby.

with binge-eating disorder. Other nursing diagnoses are similar to bulimia nervosa and include *disturbed body image, ineffective coping, anxiety, chronic low self-esteem, powerlessness,* and *social isolation.*

OUTCOMES IDENTIFICATION

To evaluate the effectiveness of treatment, establish outcome criteria to measure treatment results. You should include patients when developing outcomes. Table 18.6 provides a summary of signs and symptoms, nursing diagnoses, and general outcomes for binge-eating disorder.

PLANNING

Planning care includes the usual diet and exercise elements for all weight loss programs. One major difference in binge eating is the complications that arise due to the larger than normal volume of food consumed during a binge. These episodes of abnormal eating cause gastrointestinal problems associated with the periodic dilation of the stomach. These patients have significant difficulties with heartburn, dysphagia, bloating, and abdominal pain, as well as diarrhea, urgency, constipation, and a feeling of anal blockage. The nurse will need to help patients manage dysregulation of the entire gastrointestinal tract.

IMPLEMENTATION

Although obesity puts patients in this population at risk for diabetes, hypertension, and heart disease, hospitalization to treat the binge eating itself is not indicated. Treatment is usually provided in an outpatient setting.

Pharmacological Interventions

Because of their efficacy with bulimia nervosa, researchers have studied the use of SSRIs at or near the high end of the dosage range to treat binge-eating disorder. While it seems to help in the short term, patients regained significant weight after stopping their medication. Other medications that are under investigation include the tricyclic antidepressants and antiepileptic agents (McKeever & Clauss, 2015).

Lisdexamfetamine dimesylate (Vyvanse), a central nervous stimulant used to treat attention-deficit/hyperactivity disorder, is approved to treat binge-eating disorder in adults. This drug is the only FDA-approved medication to treat moderate to severe binge-eating disorder. Vyvanse is a stimulant and can be misused. Common side effects include dry mouth and insomnia, but more serious side effects can occur. However, while FDA approved, it still may not be a first-line therapy. Antidepressants are probably still a better option to try first due to more tolerable adverse effects and no risk of abuse.

Other medications, such as drugs used to treat overweight and obesity, may be used off label in patients with binge-eating disorder. The two rationales for their use are (1) binge-eating disorder is associated with obesity and these drugs bring about weight loss, and (2) these drugs may suppress appetite (McElroy et al., 2012). Table 18.7 lists prescription weight loss medications.

Surgical Interventions

Bariatric surgery is a controversial option for the treatment of obesity. While all persons who are obese do not suffer from binge-eating disorder, research has linked individuals with eating disorders that undergo this surgery to possible complications (Mitchell et al., 2015). These complications include

TABLE 18.7 **FDA-Approved Drugs for Weight Reduction**

Generic (Trade) Name	Mechanism of Action	Side Effects
Benzphetamine (Didrex)	Anorectic stimulant	Nervousness, insomnia, dry mouth, constipation, hypertension
Diethylpropion (Tenuate)	Anorectic stimulant	Headache, dry mouth, insomnia, nervousness, nausea, hypertension
Liraglutide (Saxenda)	Human glucagon-like peptide-1 (GLP-1) receptor agonist An injectable medication that stimulates insulin secretion and reduces glucagon secretion	Hypoglycemia, nausea, vomiting, diarrhea, pancreatitis
Lorcaserin (Belviq)	Selective serotonin receptor agonist	Headache, nausea, upper respiratory infections
Methamphetamine (Desoxyn)	Central nervous stimulant	Tachycardia, tremors, headache, insomnia, dizziness, nausea, dry mouth
Naltrexone and bupropion extended-release (Contrave)	Combination medication: Naltrexone, an opioid receptor antagonist, blocks the euphoric effects of opioid substances and bupropion is a norepinephrine and dopamine reuptake inhibitor	Nausea, constipation, headache, vomiting, dizziness
Orlistat (Xenical, Alli—over the counter)	Inhibits pancreatic lipases thereby blocking absorption of dietary fat	Steatorrhea (loose, oily stools), intestinal cramps, fecal urgency, fat soluble vitamin deficiency
Phendimetrazine	Anorectic stimulant	Hypertension, nervousness, insomnia, dry mouth, constipation
Phentermine (Adipex-P, Suprenza)	Anorectic stimulant	Hypertension, nervousness, insomnia, dry mouth, constipation
Phentermine and topiramate extended-release (Qsymia)	Combination medication: Phentermine is central nervous system stimulant Topiramate is an anticonvulsant	Paresthesias, insomnia, dry mouth, dizziness, constipation, changes in sense of taste or smell

impaired fasting glucose levels, high triglycerides, and urinary incontinence. If bariatric surgery is undertaken in this population, it should be accompanied with and followed by counseling and/or psychotherapy to improve emotional responses to food.

Health Teaching and Health Promotion

Patients struggling with binge-eating disorder have been using food to regulate their mood and will need to learn new coping strategies for the challenges in their lives. Education centered on healthy eating and exercise will need to be reinforced within a caring nurse-patient relationship. At first, the focus of change will be the binge eating itself. Once abstinence has been established, the focus may change to slow and steady weight loss to improve the person's overall health.

Advanced Practice Interventions

Psychotherapy

Psychiatric-mental health advanced practice registered nurses can be instrumental in providing care to this population. Cognitive-behavioral therapy, behavior therapy, dialectical behavior therapy, and interpersonal therapy have all been associated with binge frequency reduction rates of 67% or more and significant abstinence rates during active treatment (APA, 2006).

The Case Study and Nursing Care Plan presents a patient with binge-eating disorder.

EVALUATION

Box 18.4 presents relevant *Nursing Interventions Classification (NIC)* interventions for the management of eating disorders.

CASE STUDY AND NURSING CARE PLAN

Binge-Eating Disorder

Angela is a 25-year-old schoolteacher who shares a history of overeating since the age of 10 years. She seeks treatment at a community mental health center because she has recently felt more depressed, stating, "I'll eat anything in sight." She also said, "I wish I wouldn't wake up in the morning."

Self-Assessment

The nurse assigned to Angela is Bernice. Bernice is new to the community mental health center, and her experience as a psychiatric nurse is primarily with people with serious mentally illness. During Bernice's initial contact with Angela, she recognizes some negative feelings toward Angela due to her weight. Bernice does some research and learns that binge-eating disorder is an illness just as schizophrenia is.

Assessment

Subjective Data

- Uncontrollable eating pattern
- Recently felt more depressed
- History of overeating since age of 10
- "I'll eat anything in sight."
- "I wish I wouldn't wake up in the morning."

Continued

CASE STUDY AND NURSING CARE PLAN—cont'd

Binge-Eating Disorder

Objective Data

- Height: 61 inches (5 feet 1 inch)
- Weight: 200 lb—180% of ideal weight
- Sad facial expression

Priority Diagnosis

Imbalanced nutrition: more than body requirements related to compulsive overeating including episodes of binging.

Outcomes Identification

Patient will normalize eating pattern and achieve a specific target weight according to a predetermined plan.

Implementation

Angela's care plan is personalized as follows:

Short-Term Goal	Intervention	Rationale	Evaluation
1. Patient will demonstrate at least two coping strategies that result in adhering to a structured meal schedule.	1a. The advanced practice nurse uses cognitive-behavioral therapy to address weight issues and disordered eating. Asks the patient to begin a journal.	1a. Cognitive-behavioral techniques can be useful in addressing automatic behaviors. Recording what, when, and where one eats begins to identify patterns that can be modified.	**WEEK 1:** Patient selects a meal plan with structured times and places; begins journal and maintains it consistently. Begins to share feelings about eating.
	1b. Teach the patient to structure and plan ahead for times and places where she will have her meals and snacks for the day.	1b. Organization and structure can allow for a different choice.	**WEEK 2:** Patient is able to adhere to structured meal schedule approximately 25% of the time. Patient expresses feelings of tension regarding this schedule; some modifications are made to allow the patient to be more successful. Patient shares contents of journal, which she consistently maintains. Weight is unchanged; patient was unable to change pattern of exercise.
	1c. Teach patient to eat small amounts more frequently to avoid rebound binge eating. 1d. Review the nutritional content of dietary intake to ensure consumption of a balanced diet.	1c, 1d. Extended periods of abstinence, restrictive dietary intake, or very low-calorie diet can result in rebound overeating.	**WEEK 3:** Patient is adhering to schedule 50% of the time. Patient shares journal entries and relates thoughts and feelings concerning eating. 1 lb weight loss. Patient is beginning to walk for a half hour as part of her daily routine.
	1e. Review journal with patient to identify areas for improvement in adhering to the treatment plan. 1f. Explore thoughts and feelings she is experiencing about this new regimen. 1g. Identify thoughts, beliefs, and underlying assumptions that reinforce disordered eating patterns. 1h. Establish a once-a-week schedule of weighing.	1e. The journal is an important tool in modifying eating behaviors. 1f, 1g. Nurse must be empathetic and supportive of patient's experience, which is one of struggle accompanied by feelings of tension. 1h. From day to day, there may be minimal or no weight reduction, which can lead to discouragement.	**WEEK 4:** Patient continues to adhere to structured schedule approximately 75% of the time. Patient walks regularly, experiencing a better sense of well-being. Patient thinks she is up to the challenge of continuing the plan to normalize her eating pattern and increase her energy expenditure. Patient's weight is 196 lb (–4 lb); she acknowledges that progress has and will continue to be slow.

Evaluation

At the end of 4 weeks, Angela's weight is 196 pounds. She adheres to a structured meal plan 75% of the time and has increased her exercise by incorporating daily walks into her routine.

BOX 18.4 *NIC* Interventions for Eating Disorders Management

Definition: Prevention and treatment of severe diet restriction and overexercising or bingeing and purging of food and fluids.

Teamwork

- Collaborate with other members of healthcare team to develop treatment plan; involve patient and/or significant others as appropriate.
- Confer with team and patient to set a target weight if patient is not within a recommended weight range for age and body frame.
- Confer with dietitian to determine daily caloric intake necessary to attain and/or maintain target weight. Encourage patient to discuss food preferences with dietitian.
- Confer with the healthcare team on a routine basis about patient's progress.

Monitoring

- Monitor physiological parameters (vital signs, electrolyte levels) as needed.
- Weigh on a routine basis (e.g., at same time of day and after voiding).
- Monitor daily caloric intake and intake and output of fluids, as appropriate.
- Restrict food availability to scheduled, pre-served meals and snacks.
- Encourage self-monitoring of daily food intake and weight gain/maintenance as appropriate.
- Observe patient during and after meals/snacks to ensure that adequate intake is achieved and maintained.
- Accompany patient to bathroom during designated observation times following meals/snacks.
- Limit time spent in bathroom during periods when not under direct supervision.
- Limit physical activity as needed to promote weight gain.

Support

- Use behavioral contracting with patient to elicit desired weight gain or maintenance behaviors.
- Use behavior modification techniques to promote behaviors that contribute to weight gain and limit weight-loss behaviors, as appropriate.
- Provide reinforcement for weight gain and behaviors that promote weight gain.
- Provide support (e.g., relaxation therapy, desensitization exercises, opportunities to talk about feelings) as patient integrates new eating behaviors, changing body image, and lifestyle changes.
- Encourage patient use of daily logs to record feelings and circumstances surrounding urge to purge, vomit, or overexercise.
- Assist patient (and significant others, as appropriate) to examine and resolve personal issues that may contribute to the eating disorder.
- Assist patient to develop a self-esteem that is compatible with a healthy body weight.

Promote Increasing Independence

- Allow opportunity to make limited choices about eating and exercise as weight gain progresses in desirable manner.
- Initiate maintenance phase of treatment when patient has achieved target weight and has consistently shown desired eating behaviors for designated period of time.
- Place responsibility for choices about eating and physical activity with patient, as appropriate.
- Institute a treatment program and follow-up care (medical, counseling) for home management.

From Bulechek, G. M., Butcher, H. K., Dochterman, J. M., & Wagner, C. (2013). *Nursing interventions classification (NIC)* (6th ed.). St. Louis, MO: Mosby.

BOX 18.5 Characteristics of Feeding Problems

PICA	Rumination	Avoidant/Restrictive
• Eating nonfood items after maturing past toddlerhood • Not culturally sanctioned • Not part of any other mental illness	• Regurgitation with rechewing, reswallowing, or spitting • No GI or medical reason • Not part of other mental illness or eating disorder	• Avoiding or restricting foods starting in childhood • Significantly low BMI • Dependent on enteral feeding or experiencing nutritional deficiencies • No distortion of body image • Not medically explained or part of any other mental illness

FEEDING DISORDERS

We have all witnessed children with picky eating habits. However, children with feeding disorders take this problem to an extreme. The three feeding disorders usually seen in infancy and childhood include pica, rumination **disorder,** and **avoidant/restrictive food intake disorder.** Box 18.5 identifies the diagnostic criteria for these disorders.

Pica

Pica is the persistent eating of substances such as dirt or paint that have no nutritional value. In institutionalized children the rate of this disorder may be as high as 26%. Pica usually begins in early childhood and last for a few months. Eating nonfood items may interfere with eating nutritional items. Eating nonfood items can also be dangerous. Paint may contain lead and result in brain damage. Objects that cannot be digested such as stones can result in intestinal blockage. Sharp objects such as paperclips can result in intestinal damage or laceration. Bacteria from dirt or other soiled objects can result in serious infection. Tooth decay may result from stomach acids.

Monitoring the child's eating behavior is obviously an essential aspect of treating this problem. Behavioral interventions such as rewarding appropriate eating are helpful.

Rumination Disorder

Rumination disorder is characterized by undigested food being returned to the mouth. It is then re-chewed, re-swallowed, or spit out. It may be diagnosed after 1 month of symptoms. Rumination symptoms can occur at any age, and the onset in infants is between 3 and 12 months. Intellectual development disorder is association with rumination. Neglect is a predisposing factor to the development of this disorder. The symptoms frequently remit spontaneously, but may become habitual and result in severe malnutrition and even death.

Interventions include repositioning infants and small children during feeding. Improving the interaction between caregiver and child and making mealtimes a pleasant experience often reduce rumination. Distracting the child when the behavior starts is also helpful. Family therapy may be required.

Avoidant/Restrictive Food Intake Disorder

Up to 40% of all toddlers will experience mealtime difficulties that resolve spontaneously with or without caregiver support and education. About 5% to 20% of children without other disorders may have feeding disorders. Prematurity, failure to thrive, autism, and genetic syndromes result in ranges of 40% to 80% with feeding disorders (Romano et al., 2015). There are no unifying etiologies for food refusal. Lack of interest in eating or food may result in weight loss, growth retardation, and nutritional deficiency. It most commonly begins in infancy or early childhood and may continue into adulthood. Anxiety and family anxiety are risk factors.

The primary treatment modality is some form of behavioral modification to increase regular food consumption. Families caring for a child with a feeding disorder often need support and education in specific behavioral techniques, but family therapy is not usually necessary. Treating anxiety and depressive symptoms may be helpful in some cases.

KEY POINTS TO REMEMBER

- A number of theoretical models help explain the origins of eating disorders.
- Neurobiological theories focus on neurotransmitters in the brain that regulate mood and hunger.
- Psychological theories explore issues of control in anorexia and affective instability and poor impulse control in bulimia.
- Genetic theories postulate the existence of vulnerabilities that may predispose people toward eating disorders.
- Sociocultural models look at our present societal ideal of being thin.
- Anorexia nervosa is a potentially life-threatening eating disorder that includes severe underweight; low blood pressure, pulse, and temperature; dehydration; and dysrhythmias.
- Anorexia may be treated in an inpatient treatment setting in which milieu therapy, psychotherapy (cognitive), development of self-care skills, and psychobiological interventions can be implemented.
- Long-term treatment is provided on an outpatient basis and aims to help patients maintain healthy weight. It includes treatment modalities such as individual therapy, family therapy, group therapy, psychopharmacology, and nutrition counseling.
- Patients with bulimia nervosa are typically within the normal weight range, but some may be slightly below or above ideal body weight.
- Assessment of the patient with bulimia nervosa may show enlargement of the parotid glands, dental erosion, and caries if the patient has induced vomiting.
- Acute care may be necessary when life-threatening complications such as gastric rupture (rare), electrolyte imbalance, and cardiac dysrhythmias are present.
- The goal of interventions is to interrupt the binge-purge cycle. Psychotherapy and self-care skill training are included in the treatment plan.
- Therapy is the long-term treatment focus to address coexisting depression, substance abuse, and/or personality disorders that are causing the patient distress and interfering with the quality of life. Self-worth and interpersonal functioning eventually become issues that are useful for the patient to target.
- Effective treatment for obese patients with binge-eating disorder includes binge abstinence, improvement of depressive symptoms, and achievement of an appropriate weight for the individual.
- Patients with binge-eating disorder often have upper and lower GI problems that bring them to medical professionals for management.
- Feeding disorders have multiple etiologies and are often associated with developmental delays of childhood.
- Feeding disorders may result in significant nutritional deficiencies and can be fatal. Behavioral interventions to increase appropriate food consumption are the primary treatments.

CRITICAL THINKING

1. Logan, a 19-year-old male model, has experienced a rapid decrease in weight over the past 4 months after his agent told him he would have to lose some weight or lose a coveted account. Logan is 6 feet 2 inches tall and weighs 132 pounds, down from his usual 176 pounds. He is brought to the emergency department with a pulse of 40 beats per minute and severe arrhythmias. His laboratory workup reveals severe hypokalemia. He has become extremely depressed, saying, "I'm too fat… I don't want anything to eat… If I gain weight, my life will be ruined. There is nothing to live for if I can't model." Logan's parents are startled and confused, and his best friend is worried and feels powerless to help Logan. "I tell Logan he needs to eat or he will die… I tell him he is a skeleton, but he refuses to listen to me. I don't know what to do."
   - **a.** Which physical and psychiatric criteria suggest that Logan should be immediately hospitalized?
   - **b.** What are some of the questions you would eventually ask Logan when evaluating his biopsychosocial functioning?
   - **c.** What are your feelings toward someone with anorexia? Can you make a distinction between your thoughts and feelings toward women with anorexia and toward men with anorexia?
   - **d.** What are some things you could do for Logan's parents and friend in terms of offering them information, support, and referrals? Identify specific referrals.
   - **e.** Identify at least five criteria that, if met, would indicate that Logan was improving.

2. You and Heather have been close friends since nursing school and are now working on the same surgical unit. Heather told you that in the past she has made several suicide attempts. Today, you come upon her bingeing off the unit, and she looks embarrassed and uncomfortable when she sees you. Several times you notice that she spends time in the bathroom, and you hear sounds of retching. In response to your concern, she admits that she has been binge-purging for several years but that now she is getting out of control and feels profoundly depressed.
   - **a.** Although Heather does not show any physical signs of bulimia nervosa, what would you look for when assessing an individual with bulimia?
   - **b.** What kinds of emergencies could result from bingeing and purging?
   - **c.** What would be the most useful type of psychotherapy for Heather initially, and what issues would need to be addressed?
   - **d.** What kinds of new skills does a person with bulimia need to learn to lessen the compulsion to binge and purge?
   - **e.** What would be some signs that Heather is recovering?

CHAPTER REVIEW

Questions

1. Which patient statement acknowledges the characteristic behavior associated with a diagnosis of pica?
   - **a.** "Nothing could make me drink milk."
   - **b.** "I'm ashamed of it, but I eat my hair."
   - **c.** "I haven't eaten a green vegetable since I was 3 years old."
   - **d.** "I regurgitate and re-chew my food after almost every meal."
2. When considering an eating disorder, what is a physical criterion for hospital admission?
   - **a.** A daytime heart rate of less than 50 beats per minute
   - **b.** An oral temperature of 100°F or more
   - **c.** 90% of ideal body weight
   - **d.** Systolic blood pressure greater than 130 mm Hg
3. When considering the need for monitoring, which intervention should the nurse implement for a patient with anorexia nervosa? *Select all that apply.*
   - **a.** Provide scheduled portion-controlled meals and snacks.
   - **b.** Congratulate patients for weight gain and behaviors that promote weight gain.
   - **c.** Limit time spent in bathroom during periods when not under direct supervision.
   - **d.** Promote exercise as a method to increase appetite.
   - **e.** Observe patient during and after meals/snacks to ensure that adequate intake is achieved and maintained.
4. Which intervention will promote independence in a patient being treated for bulimia nervosa?
   - **a.** Have the patient monitor daily caloric intake and intake and output of fluids.
   - **b.** Encourage the patient to use behavior modification techniques to promote weight gain behaviors.
   - **c.** Ask the patient to use a daily log to record feelings and circumstances related to urges to purge.
   - **d.** Allow the patient to make limited choices about eating and exercise as weight gain progresses.
5. Which patient statement supports the diagnosis of anorexia nervosa?
   - **a.** "I'm terrified of gaining weight."
   - **b.** "I wish I had a good friend to talk to."
   - **c.** "I've been told I drink way too much alcohol."
   - **d.** "I don't get much pleasure out of life anymore."
6. Obesity can be the end result of a binge-eating disorder. The nurse understands that the best treatment option in persons with a binge-eating disorder promotes:
   - **a.** Bariatric surgery
   - **b.** Coping strategies
   - **c.** Avoidance of public eating
   - **d.** Appetite suppression medications
7. Taylor, a psychiatric registered nurse, orients Regina, a patient with anorexia nervosa, to the room where she will be assigned during her stay. After getting Regina settled, the nurse informs Regina:
   - **a.** "I need to go through the belongings you have brought with you."
   - **b.** "You can use the scale in the back room when you need to."
   - **c.** "You will be eating five times a day here."
   - **d.** "The daily structure is based around your desire to eat."
8. Safety measures are of concern in eating-disorder treatments. Patients with anorexia nervosa are supervised closely to monitor: *Select all that apply.*
   - **a.** Foods that are eaten
   - **b.** Attempts at self-induced vomiting
   - **c.** Relationships with other patients
   - **d.** Weight
9. Malika has been overweight all of her life. Now an adult, she has health problems related to her excessive weight. Seeking weight loss assistance at a primary care facility Malika is surprised when the nurse practitioner suggests:
   - **a.** A trial of SSRI antidepressant therapy
   - **b.** Mild exercise to start, increasing in intensity over time
   - **c.** Removing snack foods from the home
   - **d.** Medication treatment for hypertension
10. Malika agrees to try losing weight according to the nurse practitioner's outlined plan. Additional teaching is warranted when Malika states:
    - **a.** "I am willing to admit I am depressed."
    - **b.** "Psychotherapy will be a part of my treatment."
    - **c.** "I prefer to have a gastric bypass rather than use this plan."
    - **d.** "My comorbid conditions may improve with weight loss."

Answers

1. **b**; 2. **a**; 3. **a, c, e**; 4. **d**; 5. **a**; 6. **b**; 7. **a**; 8. **a, b, d**; 9. **a**; 10. **c**

ⓔ Visit the Evolve website for a posttest on the content in this chapter: http://evolve.elsevier.com/Varcarolis

Post-Test interactive review

REFERENCES

American Psychiatric Association (APA). (2006). *Practice guideline for the treatment of patients with eating disorders* (3rd ed.). Washington, DC: Author.

American Psychiatric Association (APA). (2013). *Diagnostic and statistical manual of mental disorders* (5th ed.). Washington, DC: Author.

Bienvenu, O. J., Davydow, D. S., & Kendler, K. S. (2011). Psychiatric 'diseases' versus behavioral disorders and degree of genetic influence. *Psychological Medicine, 41*(1), 33–40.

Campbell, I. C., Mill, J., Uher, R., & Schmidt, U. (2011). Eating disorders, gene-environment interactions and epigenetics. *Neuroscience and Biobehavioral Reviews, 35*(3), 784–793.

Doris, E., Shekriladze, I., Javakhishvili, N., Jones, R., Treasure, J., & Tchanturia, K. (2015). Is cultural change associated with eating disorders? A systematic review of the literature. *Eating and Weight Disorders: EWD, 20*(2), 149–160.

Frank, G. K. W. (2015). Advances from neuroimaging studies in eating disorders. *CNS Spectrums, 20*(4), 391–400.

Frank, G. K., Shott, M. E., Hagman, J. O., & Mittal, V. A. (2013). Alterations in brain structures related to taste reward circuitry. *American Journal of Psychiatry, 170*(10).

Harrington, B. C., Jimerson, M., Haxton, C., & Jimerson, D. C. (2015). Initial evaluation, diagnosis, and treatment of anorexia nervosa and bulimia nervosa. *American Family Physician, 91*(1), 46–52. Retrieved from http://ezproxy.twu.edu:2048/login?url=http://search.ebscohost.com/login.aspx?direct=true&db=ccm&AN=109693701&site=ehost-live&scope=site.

Kaye, W. H., Wierenga, C. E., Bailer, U. F., Simmons, A. N., & Bischoff-Grethe, A. (2013). Nothing tastes as good as skinny feels: The neurobiology of anorexia nervosa. *Trends in Neuroscience, 36*(2), 110–120.

McElroy, S. L., Guerdjikova, A., Mori, N., & O'Melia, A. M. (2012). Pharmacological management of binge eating disorder: Current and emerging treatment options. *Therapeutics and Clinical Risk Management, 8*, 219–241.

McKeever, A., & Clauss, L. J. (2015). Practical strategies for the diagnosis and management of binge eating disorder. *Women's Healthcare: A Clinical Journal for NPs, 3*(1), 8–15. Retrieved from http://ezproxy.twu.edu:2048/login?url=http://search.ebscohost.com/login.aspx?direct=true&db=ccm&AN=103776528&site=ehost-live&scope=site.

Mitchell, J. E., King, W. C., Pories, W., Wolfe, B., Flum, D. R., Spaniolas, K., & Yanovski, S. (2015). Binge eating disorder and medical comorbidities in bariatric surgery candidates. *The International Journal of Eating Disorders, 48*(5), 471–476.

Moorhead, S., Johnson, M., Maas, M. L., & Swanson, E. (2013). *Nursing outcomes classification (NOC)* (5th ed.). St. Louis, MO: Mosby.

Myatt, R. (2014). An overview of cardiac risk in patients with chronic eating disorders. *British Journal of Cardiac Nursing, 9*(6), 287–291. Retrieved from http://ezproxy.twu.edu:2048/login?url=http://search.ebscohost.com/login.aspx?direct=true&db=ccm&AN=103955686&site=ehost-live&scope=site.

Romano, C., Hartman, C., Privitera, C., Cardile, S., & Shamir, R. (2015). Current topics in the diagnosis and management of the pediatric non organic feeding disorders (NOFEDs). *Clinical Nutrition, 34*(2), 195–200.

Rosenvinge, J., & Petterson, G. (2015). Epidemiology of eating disorders part II: An update with a special reference to the DSM-5. *Advances in Eating Disorders, 3*(2), 198–220.

Seitz, J., Hueck, M., Dahmen, B., Schulte-Ruther, M., Legenbauer, T., Herpertz-Dahlmann, B., & Konrad, K. (2016). Attention network dysfunction in bulimia nervosa – an fMRI study. *PLoS One, 11*(9). Retrieved from https://www.ncbi.nlm.nih.gov/pubmed/27607439.

Smith, C., Fogarty, S., Touyz, S., Madden, S., Buckett, G., & Hay, P. (2014). Acupuncture and acupressure and massage health outcomes for patients with anorexia nervosa: Findings from a pilot randomized controlled trial and patient interviews. *Journal of Alternative & Complementary Medicine, 20*(2), 103–112.

Walsh, B. T. (2013). The enigmatic persistence of anorexia nervosa. *American Journal of Psychiatry, 170*(5), 477–484.

Wright, K. M. (2015). Maternalism: A healthy alliance for recovery and transition in eating disorder services. *Journal of Psychiatric and Mental Health Nursing, 22*(6), 431–439.

19

Sleep-Wake Disorders

Margaret Jordan Halter,
Margaret Trussler

Visit the Evolve website for a pretest on the content in this chapter: http://evolve.elsevier.com/Varcarolis Pre-Test interactive review

OBJECTIVES

1. Discuss the impact of inadequate sleep on overall physical and mental health.
2. Describe the social and economic impact of sleep disturbance and chronic sleep deprivation.
3. Recognize the risks to personal and community safety imposed by sleep disturbance and chronic sleep deprivation.
4. Describe normal sleep physiology and explain the variations in normal sleep.
5. Identify the major categories and medical diagnoses for sleep disorders.
6. Identify the predisposing, precipitating, and perpetuating factors for patients with insomnia.
7. Apply the nursing process in caring for individuals with sleep disorders.
8. Describe the use of two assessment tools in the evaluation of patients experiencing sleep disturbance.
9. Formulate three nursing diagnoses for patients experiencing a sleep disturbance.
10. Develop a teaching plan for a patient with insomnia disorder incorporating principles of sleep restriction, stimulus control, and cognitive-behavioral therapy.
11. Develop a care plan for the patient experiencing sleep disturbance incorporating basic sleep hygiene principles.

OUTLINE

KEY TERMS AND CONCEPTS

basal sleep requirement
cataplexy
circadian drive
excessive sleepiness
hypersomnolence
narcolepsy
sleep architecture
sleep continuity
sleep deprivation
sleep drive
sleep efficiency
sleep fragmentation
sleep hygiene
sleep latency
sleep restriction
stimulus control

Sleep and sleep disorders are receiving increased attention in the medical, nursing, research, and social science literature. Obtaining sufficient quality sleep is now recognized as a key determinant of health and well-being. The national health promotion and disease prevention initiative, *Healthy People 2020,* included sleep health in the list of current health topics, making sleep a national health priority.

HEALTH POLICY

Healthy People 2020 and Sleep

Healthy People 2020 added sleep health to the national health agenda with the goal of "increasing public knowledge of how adequate sleep and treatment of sleep disorders improve health, productivity, wellness, quality of life, and safety on roads and in the workplace." Four goals were identified:

1. Increase the proportion of persons with symptoms of obstructive sleep apnea who seek medical evaluation.
2. Reduce the rate of vehicular crashes per 100 million miles traveled that are due to drowsy driving.
3. Increase the proportion of students in grades 9 through 12 who get sufficient sleep.
4. Increase the proportion of adults who get sufficient sleep.

Nurses can be instrumental in advancing the sleep goals of *Healthy People 2020.* As 24/7 care providers, nurses can assess for sleep problems, educate patients about sleep requirements, and promote a restful environment in patient care areas. As healthcare advocates, nurses can bring forth or support policy change that brings the problems of inadequate sleep and its consequences into sharp focus.

Healthy People 2020 offers a simple guide to implementing the Healthy People goals using the MAP-IT (**M**obilize, **A**ssess, **P**lan, **I**mplement, **T**rack) framework. Consider adopting one of the sleep goals to implement a policy change in your community using this framework. For more information and ideas on how to get started see the *Healthy People 2020* website at www.healthypeople.gov/2020/default.aspx, and click on *Implementing Healthy People* (USDHHS, 2012).

The National Center on Sleep Disorder Research (NCSDR) was established in 1996 to facilitate research, training, health information dissemination, and other activities with respect to the basic understanding of sleep and sleep disorders. Under the guidance of the NCSDR and other organizations such as the National Sleep Foundation (NSF) and the American Academy of Sleep Medicine (AASM), there has been exponential growth in the scientific understanding of sleep over the past two decades.

SLEEP

For many people, sleep has become an expendable commodity. In a fast-paced society, sleep is often forfeited, and people subject themselves to schedules that disrupt normal sleep physiology. Sleep is often forfeited to meet other social and vocational demands. The amount of time spent working, engaging in academic activities, and traveling to and from work and school are the strongest determinants of total sleep time. The more time devoted to work-related activities, the less time spent sleeping.

The NSF (2016a) recommends that the average adult get 7 to 9 hours of sleep each night. Yet annual surveys conducted by the NSF between 2002 and 2015 have consistently demonstrated that the average adult gets less than 7 hours of sleep on weeknights. The 2015 NSF *Sleep in America Poll* indicates that, while people prefer to sleep 7.3 hours on weeknights, they report sleeping 6.9 hours, which results in a sleep debt of 26 minutes. Weekend sleep is better with an average of 7.6 hours each night (Fig. 19.1).

Consequences of Sleep Loss

The major consequence of acute or chronic sleep curtailment is **excessive sleepiness**. Excessive sleepiness is a subjective self-report of difficulty staying awake. Individuals with this problem believe that it is serious enough to impact social and work functioning and increase the risk for accident or injury. Sleep restriction may be caused by a disruption of the normal sleep cycle (as seen in shift work), underlying sleep disorders, medications, alcohol and substance use, and medical and psychiatric disorders.

We need only to look to our own experiences with acute or total sleep loss to recognize its consequences. After a poor night's sleep, we feel tired, lethargic, and out of synch. The effects of chronic sleep loss may be less obvious but may have a greater overall impact on health and well-being. A discrepancy between hours of sleep obtained and hours of sleep required for optimal functioning is responsible for a state of **sleep deprivation**. This sleep deprivation has widespread implications for quality of life, health, and safety. Because there can be considerable individual variability in total sleep need, the term *sleep deprivation* applies only to impaired functioning due to sleep loss.

Many of the neurocognitive symptoms of chronic sleep deprivation can mimic psychiatric symptoms, highlighting the importance of a comprehensive sleep evaluation for patients

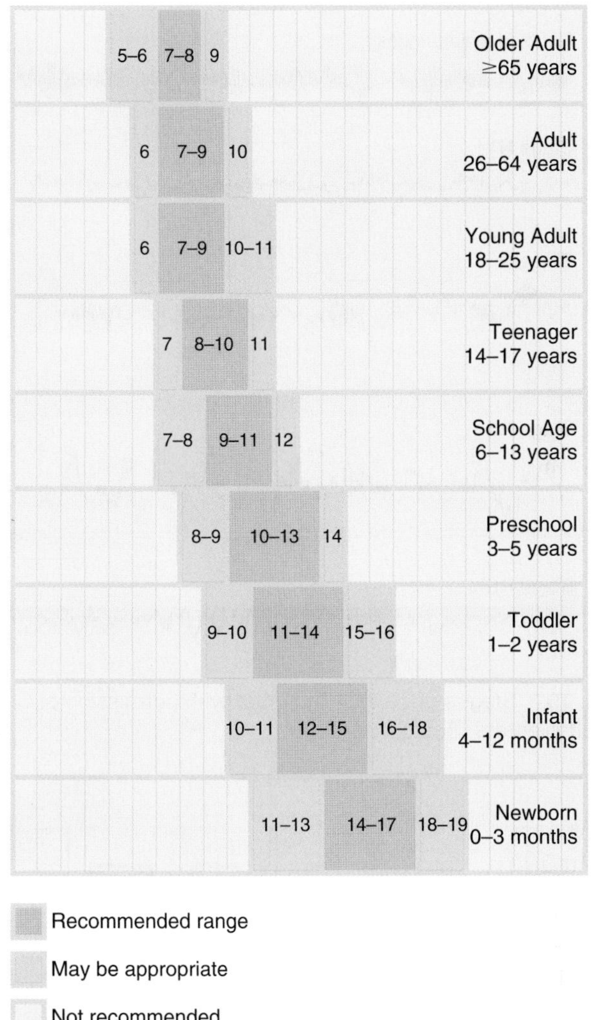

FIG. 19.1 Recommended hours of sleep by age. National Sleep Foundation. (2016). *How much sleep do we really need?* Retrieved from https://sleepfoundation.org/how-sleep-works/how-much-sleep-do-we-really-need.

with mental health disorders. In a multiethnic representative sample of US adults, insufficient sleep/rest was shown to be positively associated with poor self-rated health (Geiger et al., 2012). Adults who sleep less than 6 hours per night are more likely to report fair to poor general health, mood disturbance, increase in pain syndromes/perception, impaired cognitive function and memory disturbance, and reduction in measures of overall quality of life (Grandner et al., 2010).

Short *and* long sleep duration (sleeping less than 6 hours per night or greater than 8 hours per night) are associated with up to a twofold increased risk of obesity, diabetes, hypertension, cardiovascular disease, stroke, depression, substance use, and all-cause mortality in multiple studies (NCSDR, 2011). Less than 6 hours of sleep per night is associated with impaired glucose tolerance, elevated cortisol levels, and alterations in sympathetic nervous system activity. Sleep deprivation may be linked to obesity because it is associated with dysregulation of leptin (a hormone that regulates satiety or feelings of fullness) and ghrelin (a hormone that regulates hunger). Less than 6 hours of sleep per night may also increase proinflammatory markers such as C-reactive protein, tumor necrosis factor, and interleukin (Luyster et al., 2012). All these problems are common pathways to the development of cardiovascular disease and diabetes. Mechanisms linking long sleep time with vascular and metabolic morbidities are unknown but may be related to cofounders such as depression, inactivity, low socioeconomic status, and overall poor general health (Luyster et al., 2012).

Sleep loss diminishes safety and results in the loss of lives and property. Sleep deprivation can produce psychomotor impairments equivalent to those induced by alcohol consumption at or above the legal limit. Daytime wakefulness in excess of 17 to 19 hours can produce psychomotor deficits equivalent to blood alcohol concentrations (BACs) between 0.05% and 0.1% while the legal limit in most states is 0.08% (Insurance Institute for Highway Safety, 2012).

Acute or chronic sleep deprivation can result in episodes of microsleep lasting from 1 second up to 10 seconds when a tired person is trying to stay awake. Many of us have experienced this when sitting in a class or in a meeting. Such lapses can lead to lower capabilities and efficiency of task performance and increased risk for errors (Orzel-Gryglewska, 2010). Some of the most devastating environmental and human tragedies of our time can be linked to human error due to sleep loss and fatigue. The grounding of the Exxon Valdez, the nuclear meltdown at Three Mile Island, and the explosion of the Union Carbide chemical plant in India are prime examples. Sleepiness with driving has become a national epidemic. The 2011 NSF *Sleep in America Poll* indicates that an alarming 52% of respondents admit to driving while sleepy. Another incredible statistic is that one-third of Americans report falling asleep while driving once or twice a month (Centers for Disease Control, 2010).

Although researchers have tried to quantify the financial burden associated with sleep disruption, there are relatively few comprehensive data available on the economic burden of sleep-wake disorders. However, considering the prevalence, impact on overall health and quality of life, and the indirect costs associated with property loss and damage, the economic burden is likely in the billions of dollars. For example, one study estimated that chronic insomnia results in nearly $63.2 billion in direct and indirect expenses annually (Kessler et al., 2011).

Formal training in sleep or sleep disorders within medical and nursing education is limited, and the number of trained clinicians and researchers continues to be insufficient (Institute of Medicine, 2006). Awareness among healthcare providers regarding the prevalence and burden of sleep disruption and the problem of inadequate sleep is underappreciated, and providers do not routinely screen for sleep disturbance or inquire about overall sleep quality. Consequently, sleep disturbances may not be recognized, diagnosed, managed, and treated.

In this chapter, we briefly review the components of normal sleep, sleep regulation, and functions of sleep; give an overview of the most common sleep disturbances encountered in the clinical environment with a focus on their relationship to psychiatric illness; and discuss the nurse's role in the assessment and management of a patient presenting with sleep disturbance.

Normal Sleep Cycle

Sleep is a dynamic neurological process that involves complex interaction between the central nervous system and the environment. Behaviorally, sleep is associated with low or absent motor activity, a reduced response to environmental stimuli, and closed eyes. Neurophysiologically, sleep is categorized according to specific brain wave patterns, eye movements, and general muscle tone. Sleep is measured through an electroencephalogram (EEG) and consists of two distinct physiological states: non-rapid eye movement (NREM) sleep and rapid eye movement (REM) sleep.

Non-rapid eye movement sleep. NREM sleep is divided into three stages (N1, N2, N3) and is characterized by progressive or deeper sleep. Stage 1 (N1) is a brief transition between wakefulness and sleep. It comprises between 2% to 5% of total sleep time. The time it takes to fall asleep is referred to as **sleep latency**. During stage 1 sleep, body temperature declines and muscles relax. Slow rolling eye movements are common. People lose awareness of their environment but are generally easily aroused. Stage 2 (N2) sleep occupies 45% to 55% of total sleep time. During this period, heart rate and respiratory rate decline. Arousal from stage 2 sleep requires more stimuli than stage 1.

Stage 3 (N3) is known as slow wave sleep or delta sleep. Slow wave sleep is relatively short and constitutes only about 13% to 23% of total sleep time. It is characterized by further reduction in heart rate, respiratory rate, blood pressure, and response to external stimuli. The three stages of NREM sleep make up 75% to 80% of total sleep time. Stage 3 sleep is considered to be "restorative sleep," as it is a time of reduced sympathetic activity.

Rapid eye movement sleep. REM sleep comprises 20% to 25% of total sleep time. REM is characterized by reduction and absence of skeletal muscle tone (muscle atonia), bursts of rapid eye movement, myoclonic twitches of the facial and limb muscles, reports of dreaming, and autonomic nervous system variability. The atonia in REM sleep is thought to be a protective mechanism to prevent the acting out of nightmares and dreams. Fig. 19.2 shows the EEG patterns characteristic of these sleep stages.

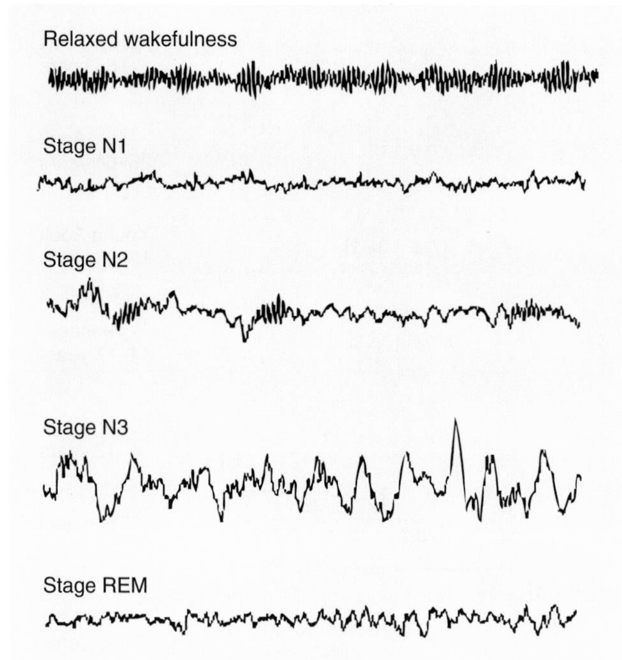
Relaxed wakefulness
Stage N1
Stage N2
Stage N3
Stage REM

FIG. 19.2 Stages of sleep. (Reprinted with permission of Sleep HealthCenters, Boston, MA.)

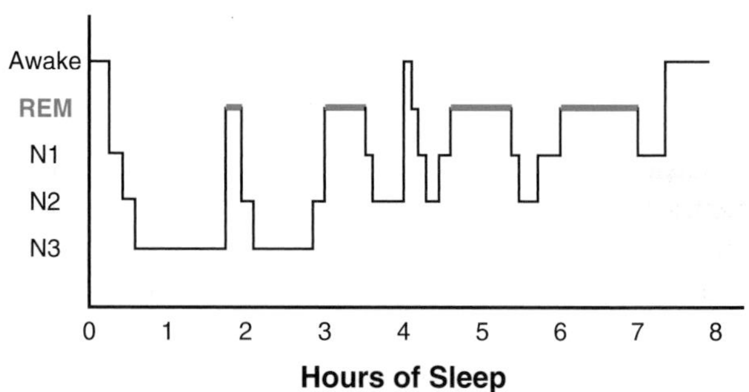
Awake
REM
N1
N2
N3
0
1
2
3
4
5
6
7
8
Hours of Sleep
Normal adult hypnogram: Slow wave sleep (N3) is more prominent during the first portion of the night. REM episodes increase as the night progresses with the longest episode before awakening.

FIG. 19.3 Hypnogram depicting the progression of the sleep stages of an adult. (From David N. Neubauer, MD, Johns Hopkins Sleep Disorders Center, Baltimore, MD *[American Family Physician, 59*(9):2551–2558, May 1, 1999].)

NREM and REM patterns. In the adult, sleep normally begins with NREM sleep. Continuous EEG recordings of sleep demonstrate an alternating cycle between NREM and REM sleep. There are typically four to six cycles of NREM and REM sleep occurring over 90- to 120-minute intervals across the sleep period.

There is also a distinct organization to sleep with NREM predominating the first half of the sleep period and REM sleep predominating during the second half. The shortest REM period occurs 60 to 90 minutes after sleep onset and lasts only for several minutes. The longest REM period occurs at the end of the sleep period and can last up to an hour. This is the reason why many people remember dreaming upon awakening.

The structural organization of NREM and REM sleep is known as **sleep architecture** and is often displayed graphically as a *hypnogram*. Fig. 19.3 is a hypnogram depicting the normal progression of the stages of sleep in an adult. The visual depiction of sleep is helpful in identifying **sleep continuity** (i.e., the distribution of sleep and wakefulness across the sleep period), as well as changes in sleep that may occur as a result of aging, illness, or certain medications.

Disruption of sleep stages as indicated by excessive amounts of stage 1 sleep, multiple brief arousals, and frequent shifts in sleep staging is known as **sleep fragmentation**. Fig. 19.4 is a hypnogram of a patient with a complaint of insomnia, indicating multiple brief arousals.

The function of alternations between NREM and REM sleep is not yet understood. We do know that irregular cycling, absent sleep stages, and sleep fragmentation are associated with many psychiatric disorders, sleep disorders, and medication effects. For example, in patients with depression, the latency period to

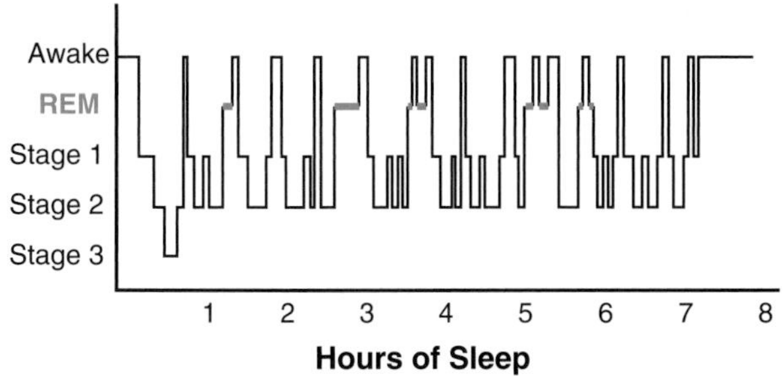

FIG. 19.4 Hypnogram depicting multiple awakenings and sleep fragmentation. (From David N. Neubauer, MD, Johns Hopkins Sleep Disorders Center, Baltimore, MD [*American Family Physician, 59*(9):2551–2558, May 1, 1999].)

REM sleep is frequently reduced, as is the percentage of slow wave sleep. Patients with narcolepsy frequently enter sleep through REM sleep rather than NREM sleep. Benzodiazepines tend to suppress slow wave sleep, whereas serotonergic drugs such as antidepressants suppress REM sleep.

Sleep Patterns

Sleep architecture changes over the lifespan. The percentage in each stage of sleep, as well as the overall **sleep efficiency** or ratio of sleep duration to time spent in bed, varies according to age. For example, infants sleep 16 to 18 hours a day, enter sleep through REM (not NREM) sleep, and spend up to 50% of sleep time in REM sleep. The percentage of REM sleep decreases to 20% to 25% by age 3 and stays relatively constant throughout the lifespan. The amount of slow wave sleep is maximal in young children and declines with age to almost none, particularly in men. This results in a tendency for middle-of-the-night awakenings and reduced sleep efficiency with age (Bliwise, 2011).

Regulation of Sleep

The regulation of sleep and wakefulness is believed to be a complex interaction between two processes, one that promotes sleep—known as the homeostatic process or **sleep drive**—and one that promotes wakefulness, known as the circadian process or **circadian drive**. The homeostatic process is dependent on the number of hours a person is awake. The longer the period of wakefulness, the stronger the sleep drive. During sleep, the sleep drive gradually dissipates.

Circadian drives are near-24-hour cycles of behavior and physiology generated and influenced by endogenous and exogenous factors and are wake-promoting. The exogenous factors are various clues from the environment known as *zeitgebers* (time-givers) that help set our internal clock to a 24-hour cycle. The strongest external cue for wakefulness is light, whereas darkness is the cue for sleep. Other environmental cues include the timing of social events such as meals, work, or exercise.

A *master biological clock* is located in the suprachiasmatic nucleus (SCN) of the hypothalamus. This clock regulates not only sleep but also a host of other biological and physiological functions within the body. Information about the lighting conditions of the external environment is relayed to the SCN from the retina. The SCN also receives information from the thalamus and the midbrain. These two pathways transmit photic and nonphotic information to the circadian clock through an expansive network. In addition to regulating sleep-wake cycles, they also exert control over endocrine regulation, body temperature, metabolism, autonomic regulation, psychomotor and cognitive performance, attention, memory, and emotion (Czeisler et al., 2011).

In addition to the circadian and homeostatic processes, several neurotransmitter systems are responsible for sleep and wakefulness. The wakefulness neurotransmitters are dopamine, norepinephrine, serotonin, acetylcholine, histamine, glutamate, and hypocretin. Sleep-promoting neurotransmitters include adenosine, gamma-aminobutyric acid (GABA), and galanin (Carney et al., 2011). Any medication that crosses the blood-brain barrier may have effects on sleep and wakefulness through modulation of these neurotransmitters.

It is important to appreciate the neurotransmitters involved in sleep and wakefulness. Many of the medications used in psychiatry manipulate these neurotransmitter systems. For example, amphetamines—which promote wakefulness—increase the release of dopamine and norepinephrine. Caffeine (methylxanthine)—which promotes alertness—functions by blocking the sleep-promoting neurotransmitter adenosine. Patients report both difficulty sleeping and drowsiness when beginning treatment with antidepressants classified as selective serotonin reuptake inhibitors (SSRIs).

Functions of Sleep

Despite remarkable advances in the understanding of sleep disorders and the biological and physiological process of sleep, very little is known about the true function of sleep. Most of the information regarding the function of sleep comes to us from animal models of sleep deprivation and human models of partial sleep deprivation. Based on these models, several theories are proposed and include brain tissue restoration, body restoration (NREM sleep), energy conservation, memory reinforcement and consolidation (REM sleep), regulation of immune function, metabolism and regulation of certain hormones, and thermoregulation (Arun et al., 2014).

Sleep Requirements

Sleep architecture and efficiency may change over time, but there is little change in the amount of sleep required once we reach adulthood. Sleep requirements vary from individual to individual and to some degree is probably genetically mediated. While most adults require 7 to 8 hours of sleep for optimal functioning, there is a small percentage of individuals defined as *long sleepers* (requiring 10 or more hours per night) and *short sleepers* (requiring less than 5 hours per night). The amount of sleep necessary to feel fully awake and able to sustain normal levels of performance is known as the **basal sleep requirement**.

How Much Sleep Are You Getting?

Unfortunately, many people allow circumstances to dictate the amount of sleep obtained. However, there is a simple way to determine your basal sleep requirement. The first step is to establish a routine bedtime. Then allow yourself to sleep undisturbed without an alarm for several days. This is usually best accomplished during an extended period of leisure time such as during a vacation. The average of several nights' undisturbed sleep is a good estimate of the basal sleep requirement. Many activity trackers can help you fine-tune your understanding of that mysterious world of sleep. They provide such information as length of time to fall asleep, number of times restless, number of times awake, and the number of steps you take during hours of sleep.

SLEEP DISORDERS

Sleep testing is often indicated for patients complaining of sleep disturbance or excessive sleepiness that impairs social and vocational functioning. There are four common diagnostic procedures used in the evaluation of sleep disorders:

1. **Polysomnography** is the most common sleep test and is used to diagnose and evaluate patients with sleep-related breathing disorders and nocturnal seizure disorders (NSF, 2016b). It usually involves one or two nights of sleep in a lab with electrodes and monitors placed on the head, chest, and legs. Technicians record brain wave activity, eye movement, muscle tone, heart rhythm, and breathing.
2. The **multiple sleep latency test (MSLT)** is a daytime nap test used to objectively measure sleepiness in a sleep-conducive setting. Polysomnography and MSLT performed on the day after polysomnography evaluation are routinely indicated in patients suspected of having narcolepsy.
3. The **maintenance of wakefulness test (MWT)** evaluates a patient's ability to remain awake in a situation conducive to sleep. It is used to document adequate alertness in individuals with careers such as airline pilots for which sleepiness would pose a risk to public safety.
4. **Actigraphy** involves using a wristwatch-type tracker that records body movement over a period of time and is helpful in evaluating sleep patterns and sleep duration. It is used in patients with circadian rhythm disorders and insomnia.

CLINICAL PICTURE

In this chapter, you will review the major categories of sleep disorders. The American Psychiatric Association (2013) identifies the following disorders:

- Insomnia disorder
- Hypersomnolence disorder
- Narcolepsy
- Breathing-related sleep disorders
- Circadian rhythm disorders
- Non-rapid eye movement sleep arousal disorders
- Nightmare disorder
- Rapid eye movement sleep behavior disorder
- Restless legs syndrome
- Substance-induced sleep disorders

Insomnia Disorder

Insomnia is characterized by dissatisfaction with quantity or quality of sleep. It is the most common sleep disorder and may affect up to 45% of adults (Sadock et al., 2015). Females are more frequently affected as are older adults. *DSM-5* criteria for insomnia disorders are listed in the *DSM-5* box.

DSM-5 CRITERIA FOR INSOMNIA DISORDER

Diagnostic Criteria

A. A predominant complaint of dissatisfaction with sleep quantity or quality associated with one (or more) of the following symptoms:
   1. Difficulty initiating sleep. (In children, this may manifest as difficulty initiating sleep without caregiver intervention.)
   2. Difficulty maintaining sleep, characterized by frequent awakenings or problems returning to sleep after awakenings. (In children, this may manifest as difficulty returning to sleep without caregiver intervention.)
   3. Early-morning awakening with inability to return to sleep.

B. The sleep disturbance causes clinically significant distress or impairment in social, occupational, educational, academic, behavioral, or other important areas of functioning.

C. The sleep difficulty occurs at least 3 nights per week.

D. The sleep difficulty is present for at least 3 months.

E. The sleep difficulty occurs despite adequate opportunity for sleep.

F. The insomnia is not better explained by and does not occur exclusively during the course of another sleep-wake disorder (e.g., narcolepsy, a breathing-related sleep disorder, a circadian rhythm sleep-wake disorder, a parasomnia).

G. The insomnia is not attributable to the physiological effects of a substance (e.g., a drug of abuse, a medication).

H. Coexisting mental disorders and medical conditions do not adequately explain the predominant complaint of insomnia.

Specify if:

With nonsleep disorder mental comorbidity, including substance use disorders

With other medical comorbidity

With other sleep disorder

From the American Psychiatric Association. (2013). *Diagnostic and statistical manual of mental disorders* (5th ed.). Washington, DC: Author.

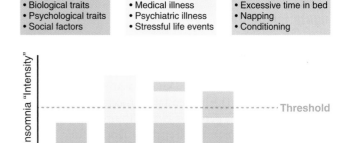

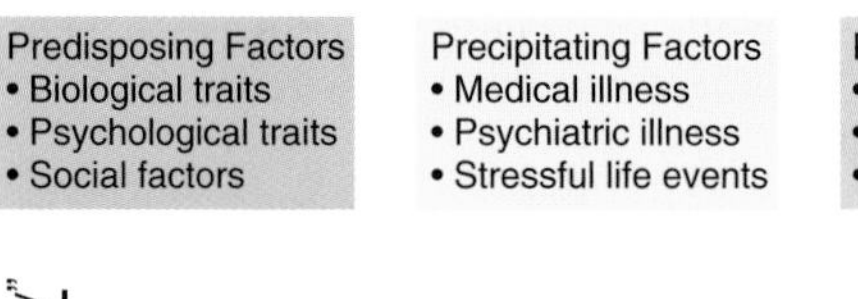

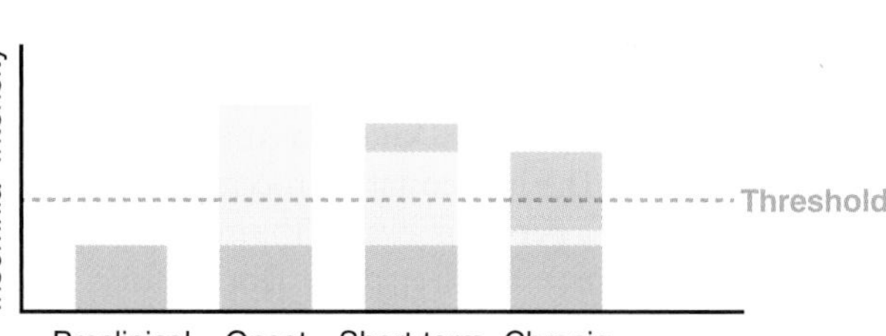

FIG. 19.5 Spielman's 3P model of insomnia. (From Erman, M. K. [2007]. *Primary Psychiatry, 14*[7].)

In addition to a thorough medical, psychiatric, and substance use history, it is helpful to use Spielman's **3P model of insomnia** to comprehensively assess the causes of insomnia, suggest appropriate interventions, and provide rationales for treatment (Spielman & Glovinsky, 2004). This model suggests that there are three factors that contribute to the insomnia complaint: **predisposing, precipitating,** and **perpetuating** factors (Fig. 19.5).

Predisposing factors are individual factors that create a vulnerability to insomnia. These may include a prior history of poor-quality sleep, history of depression and anxiety, or a state of hyperarousal. Patients at risk to develop insomnia may describe themselves as light sleepers and night owls. **Precipitating** factors are external events that trigger insomnia. Personal and vocational difficulties, medical and psychiatric disorders, grief, and changes in role or identity (as seen with retirement) are examples. **Perpetuating** factors are sleep practices and attributes that maintain the sleep complaint such as excessive caffeine or alcohol use, spending excessive amounts of time in bed or napping, and worrying about the consequences of insomnia.

Nursing care for patients experiencing insomnia will be addressed later in the chapter. Medication for its treatment will also be discussed.

Hypersomnolence Disorder

Hypersomnolence disorder is associated with excessive daytime sleepiness and has a prevalence of about 5% to 10% of individuals who seek help in sleep disorder clinics. Hypersomnolence disorder is chronic (3 months or more) and begins in young adulthood. It affects males and females equally.

The patient with hypersomnolence reports recurrent periods of sleep or unintended lapses into sleep, frequent napping, a prolonged main sleep period of greater than 9 hours, nonrefreshing nonrestorative sleep regardless of amount of time slept, and difficulty with full alertness during the wake period. Excessive sleepiness significantly impairs social and vocational functioning by impacting the person's ability to participate in and enjoy relationships and function in the workplace. Cognitive impairment is common as is an increased risk for accident or injury associated with the sleepiness.

Treatment for hypersomnolence disorders focuses on maintaining a regular sleep-wake schedule with an ample sleep opportunity. Some individuals will improve if they allow for an extended sleep opportunity of 10 or more hours. Pharmacotherapy with long-acting amphetamine-based stimulants such as methylphenidate and nonamphetamine-based stimulants such as modafinil (Provigil) are helpful.

Narcolepsy

People with **narcolepsy** have an uncontrollable urge to sleep. It is a relatively rare phenomenon that affects less than 0.05% of the general population. Narcolepsy seems to occur slightly more frequently in men. It usually begins before young adulthood and persists throughout the lifespan.

Narcolepsy may be accompanied by **cataplexy**, which refers to brief episodes of bilateral loss of muscle tone while maintaining consciousness. This is usually triggered by a strong emotion such as anger, frustration, or laughter. This terrifying symptom may last for up to several minutes, and recovery is generally immediate and complete. Cataplexy is probably the occurrence of REM sleep paralysis during wakefulness. Cataplexy occurs in about half of all people with narcolepsy. Some people have one or two episodes in their whole lives, while other people may have up to 20 episodes a day. It can have a major impact on people's social lives, functioning, and even safety.

Two other classic symptoms of narcolepsy are:

- Hypnagogic hallucinations—false auditory, visual, and tactile sensations. They occur at the transition from wakefulness to sleep.
- Sleep paralysis—an inability to move or speak during the transition from sleep to wakefulness.

Additional symptoms of narcolepsy include disturbed nighttime sleep with multiple middle-of-the-night awakenings and automatic behaviors characterized by memory lapses. Patients with narcolepsy generally feel refreshed upon awakening but within 2 or 3 hours begin to feel sleepy again. Individuals with other hypersomnia disorders generally do not feel rested or refreshed regardless of the amount of sleep obtained. Measuring levels of hypocretin, a neuropeptide that regulates arousal and wakefulness, in cerebrospinal fluid can provide an objective basis for diagnosis.

Treatment for narcolepsy includes naps, exercise, and a balanced diet. Medications with US Food and Drug Administration (FDA) approval for excessive daytime sleepiness include the stimulants modafinil (Provigil), armodafinil (Nuvigil), methylphenidate, and amphetamine. Sodium oxybate (Xyrem) is a depressant used to treat daytime sleepiness.

Depending on its severity, cataplexy can be treated with medications and achieve excellent responses. Sodium oxybate has FDA approval for cataplexy. It takes up to 8 weeks to become effective. Some SSRIs and tricyclic antidepressants are used off-label for this condition with good results. They may work by suppressing REM sleep associated with the paralysis.

Breathing-Related Sleep Disorders

The most common disorder of breathing and sleeping is obstructive sleep apnea hypopnea syndrome. It affects about 2% of children and 2% to 20% of adults—rates increase with age. More men than women are affected. This type of apnea is strongly associated with obesity.

This problem is characterized by repeated episodes of upper airway collapse and obstruction that result in sleep fragmentation. Essentially, patients with obstructive sleep apnea are not able to sleep and breathe at the same time. Typical symptoms include loud disruptive snoring, apnea episodes witnessed by others, and excessive daytime sleepiness. Diagnosis is determined by clinical evaluation and polysomnography. Treatment is with continuous positive airway pressure (CPAP) therapy.

Additional breathing-related sleep disorders include central sleep apnea and sleep-related hypoventilation. Central sleep apnea is the cessation of respiration during sleep. This problem is due to instability of the respiratory control system, and there is no compensatory response. Central sleep apnea is seen in older individuals, those with advanced cardiac or pulmonary disease, or those with neurological disorders. Sleep-related hypoventilation is associated with sustained oxygen desaturation during sleep in the absence of apnea or respiratory events. This problem is seen in individuals with morbid obesity, lung parenchymal disease, or pulmonary vascular pathology.

Circadian Rhythm Sleep Disorders

Circadian rhythm sleep disorders occur when there is a misalignment between the timing of the individual's normal circadian rhythm and external factors that affect the timing or duration of sleep. Diagnosis is determined by clinical evaluation, sleep diaries, and actigraphy. Treatment is with aggressive lifestyle management strategies aimed at adapting to or modifying the required sleep schedule. Examples include:

- Delayed sleep phase type—A delay of more than 2 hours between desired time of sleep and actual sleep. Results in delays in waking. Rare in the general population, more common in adolescents (about 7%).
- Advanced sleep phase type—Sleep begins several hours earlier and ends several hours earlier than desired. This problem is thought to affect about 1% of middle age adults and becomes more common with age.
- Irregular sleep-wake type—Sleep is sporadic and fragmented. The longest sleep period lasts about 4 hours and tends to occur between 2:00 a.m. and 6:00 a.m. It is associated with brain disorders such as Alzheimer's and disruptive environments such as hospitals.
- Non-24-hour sleep-wake type—Characterized by a mismatch of the 24-hour environment and the person's internal clock. Sleep tends to occur later and later, eventually resulting in daytime sleeping. This problem is rare in sighted people but is a significant problem for up to 70% of blind individuals. Medication is specifically approved for this problem—tasimelteon (Hetlioz)—which works by increasing melatonin.
- Shift work type—Working outside of the normal work hours (late evening and night) results in excessive sleepiness at work and impaired sleep at home. It is estimated to occur in up to 10% of night shift workers.

VIGNETTE: Sarah had been living with treatment-resistant schizophrenia for many years. Despite multiple medication trials, she was frequently hospitalized. Last year, she was started on clozapine (Clozaril) and within a few months experienced a dramatic reduction in psychotic symptoms.

Despite careful monitoring of her dietary intake and weight by her group home staff, Sarah began to experience weight gain while taking the clozapine. Staff also began to notice a change in her sleeping patterns. She complained of frequently waking in the night and having a morning headache and sore throat. When she returned home from work in the afternoon, it was not unusual for her to have a nap for 60 minutes or longer.

While home on a family visit, her mother noted loud snoring and discussed this with the psychiatrist. A polysomnography was performed, which demonstrated a severe degree of obstructive sleep apnea, most likely related to her recent weight gain. Continuous positive airway pressure (CPAP) therapy was initiated, and she was able to return to her baseline level of functioning.

Non-Rapid Eye Movement Sleep Arousal Disorders

Non-rapid eye movement (NREM) sleep arousal disorders include sleepwalking and sleep terrors. Because individuals in the NREM phase of sleep are not experiencing the loss of muscle tone that characterizes REM sleep, unsafe activities may occur.

Sleepwalking, or somnambulism, consists of a sequence of complex behaviors that begin in the first third of the night during NREM sleep. Individuals leave the bed and walk about without full consciousness or later memory. The individual may dress, go to the bathroom, leave the house, and, in some extreme cases, drive a car.

This problem tends to run in families and is rare in adults (Sadock et al., 2015). It is very common in children between the ages of 4 and 8. Typically, it disappears in adolescence.

Because of the possibility of accident or injury, a sleep specialist should always evaluate somnambulism. Polysomnography is sometimes indicated to rule out the possibility of an underlying disorder of sleep fragmentation. Treatment consists of instructing the patient and family regarding safety measures such as alarms or locks on windows and doors and gating stairways. Attention to sleep hygiene, limiting alcohol before bed, obtaining adequate amounts of sleep, and stress reduction are helpful. Benzodiazepines are frequently prescribed when the risk for accident or injury is likely.

Sleep terrors refer to sudden terrified near-awakenings. Sleep terrors tend to run in families. It is a fairly rare disorder and typically presents between the ages of 4 to 12. Sleep terrors may occur in response to fever or central nervous system depressant withdrawal (Sadock et al., 2015).

Typically, the episodes begin with sitting up in bed followed by a panicked scream. The person is unresponsive to stimuli, is overcome with anxiety, and may vocalize incoherently. There is a tremendous degree of autonomic arousal and intense fear. Sleepwalking may accompany this problem. Sleep terrors generally occur during the first third of the sleep episode arising out of slow wave sleep. Afterward, there is no recollection of dream content.

Sleep terrors are addressed by exploring areas of stress that can be managed. Regular sleep habits (e.g., going to bed at the same time each night) may help reduce their occurrence. Medication is rarely used, but benzodiazepines may be helpful in the short term.

Nightmare Disorder

Nightmare disorder is characterized by long frightening dreams from which people awaken scared. Nightmare disorder begins in preschool. It tends to increase until males reach the age of 13; for females, it tends to increase until the age of 29. About 6% of adults have monthly nightmares.

The nightmares almost always occur during rapid eye movement (REM) sleep and usually after a long REM period late in the night. A nightmare disorder may be diagnosed with repeated occurrences of extremely unsettling dreams that are remembered well upon awakening. Risk factors for nightmares include frequent past adverse events, sleep problems, and a familial disposition for sleep disturbances.

Polysomnography is sometimes necessary to rule out the possibility of an underlying disorder of sleep fragmentation such as obstructive sleep apnea. Treatment for nightmare disorder and night terrors is dependent on the frequency and severity of the symptoms, as well as the underlying cause. Treatment with hypnotic therapy is sometimes indicated. Many patients do well with lifestyle modification measures, attention to sleep hygiene, and stress reduction.

Rapid Eye Movement Sleep Behavior Disorder

REM sleep behavior disorder is characterized by elaborate motor activity associated with dreaming. These patients are actually acting out their dreams. Comedian Mike Birbiglia (2010) shares his experience of dreaming: he was standing on a podium accepting an Olympic medal when he was actually falling off of a tall bookcase in his living room. Another incident occurred while he was on tour and staying in a hotel room. In order to avoid a guided missile headed toward his room, he jumped from a second story window and ended up with 33 stitches.

The prevalence of rapid eye movement behavior disorder is about 0.5% in the general population. It is most frequently seen in elderly men. It may also be the heralding symptom of neurological pathology such as Parkinson's disease. Serotonergic medications such as SSRIs or selective norepinephrine reuptake inhibitors (SNRIs) can induce or exacerbate episodes.

Diagnosis is determined by clinical evaluation and polysomnography with video recording. Treatment focuses on patient and sleep partner safety. Placing the mattress on the floor is sometimes necessary to prevent injury as a result of falling out of bed. The use of an intermediate-acting benzodiazepine can be helpful, especially in cases of severe disruption to the sleep partner and concerns about safety.

VIGNETTE: A primary care provider refers an 80-year-old man with Parkinson's disease to a sleep clinic. The patient's wife became concerned when on several occasions she awoke to find him shouting and thrashing in the bed. It appeared that he was acting out his dreams. The patient reported no memory of these events and had no particular sleep complaint. During one of these episodes, he knocked over the bedside lamp and struck her. When he was awoken, he reported that he was dreaming there was an intruder in the house and he was attempting to save her. A polysomnography examination demonstrated an absence of the muscle atonia normally seen in REM sleep, confirming a diagnosis of REM sleep behavior disorder. He was treated with a low dose of a benzodiazepine and given instructions regarding personal and sleep partner safety.

Restless Legs Syndrome

Restless legs syndrome is a sensory and movement disorder characterized by an uncomfortable sensation in the legs (occasionally the arms and trunk are affected) accompanied by an urge to move. The prevalence rate is about 2% to 7%. Females tend to be affected by this problem more than men. Most of this gender difference is due to the increased risk of restless legs syndrome in pregnancy. Twelve percent of pregnant women are affected, and about half of those affected continue to experience restless legs syndrome postpartum (Hubner et al., 2013) Most people with this disorder had symptoms before adulthood.

Symptoms begin or worsen during periods of inactivity and are relieved or reduced by physical activity such as walking, stretching, or flexing. Symptoms are worse in the evening and at bedtime and can have a significant impact on the individual's ability to fall asleep and stay asleep. SSRIs or SNRIs may precipitate restless legs syndrome.

The cause of restless legs syndrome is unknown. Evidence suggests that it may be related to dysfunction of the brain's basal ganglia circuits that use the neurotransmitter dopamine. There is likely to be a strong genetic component, especially when seen in individuals under 40 years old (National Institute of Neurologic Disorders and Stroke, 2012). Iron deficiency is also associated with restless legs syndrome.

Diagnosis is determined by clinical evaluation. Many patients with restless legs syndrome also have periodic limb movements of sleep that are observed during polysomnography.

Many dopamine receptor agonists are FDA approved for the treatment of restless legs syndrome. Examples are ropinirole (Requip), pramipexole (Mirapex), and rotigotine (Neupro). Unfortunately, long-term use of these drugs can lead to augmentation, or worsening, of symptoms. Another FDA-approved drug is gabapentin enacarbil (Horizant), an anticonvulsant. Iron deficiencies are treated with iron supplements. Levodopa is used off-label for intermittent restless legs syndrome.

The FDA recently approved a nonpharmacological treatment: a pad (Relaxis) that works by providing counterstimulation of the legs in the form of vibration that slowly tapers off through the night. Individuals who have had a deep vein thrombosis within the past 6 months should not use this treatment.

VIGNETTE: Kathy is a 32-year-old woman referred by her primary care provider for a psychiatric evaluation for complaints of anxiety and restlessness. She reported feeling fine during the day, but in the evening, she felt nervous and anxious. The symptoms always started at the same time. As soon as she would settle down for the evening to watch television, she would begin to have a restless sensation in her legs that would make her jump up and pace up and down. She described the sensation as having "soda pop fizzing through my veins." Sometimes she would go out for a walk at night even if it was very late to "calm down." These episodes began to occur almost nightly, and as a result, she was having difficulty getting a good night's sleep. She began to dread the approach of darkness. A full clinical evaluation suggested the diagnosis of restless legs syndrome. A course of the dopamine agonist pramipexole (Mirapex) was initiated in the evening with dramatic improvement in symptoms and total resolution of her sleep complaint.

Substance-Induced Sleep Disorder

A substance-induced sleep disorder can result from the use or recent discontinuance of a substance or medication. While it is quite obvious that many prescriptions and over-the-counter medications may affect sleep, there is less appreciation for the effects of commonly used substances on sleep. Alcohol, nicotine, and caffeine all have an impact on sleep quantity and quality.

- **Alcohol**—despite its great soporific (sleep-inducing) effects—decreases deep sleep (stage 3) and REM sleep and is responsible for middle-of-the-night awakenings with difficulty returning to sleep.
- **Nicotine** is a central nervous system stimulant, increasing heart rate, blood pressure, and respiratory rate. As nicotine levels decline through the night, patients wake in response to mild withdrawal symptoms. Patients should be reminded to remove nicotine delivery patches at bedtime.
- **Caffeine** blocks the neurotransmitter adenosine, promoting wakefulness. It increases sleep latency, reduces slow wave sleep, and acts as a diuretic, causing middle-of-the-night awakening for urination.

CONSIDERING CULTURE

The Role of Sleep in US Culture

Jennifer is a busy 21-year-old college senior. She is working on a degree in social work and has a part-time job working about 20 hours per week as a bartender. She is fully connected with a smartphone, laptop computer, and television. Despite a long and active day, at night before bed, she surfs the internet for several hours and sleeps with the television on. She keeps her cell phone on at night and is sometime awakened when she receives an e-mail or a text message.

The 2011 NSF *Sleep in America Poll* indicated that 90% of respondents aged 19 to 64 reported using some type of technology (laptop/computer, cell phone, television, electronic music device, video game, reader) in their bedrooms in the hour before going to sleep. Individuals under the age of 30 are more likely to do so. Is it possible that our growing cultural attachment to technology is impacting sleep quality by reducing time spent in sleeping and causing sleep fragmentation? The results of the 2011 NSF poll and several recent studies seem to indicate it does.

Individuals who used their cell phone and/or laptop or computer in the hour before bed were *less* likely to report getting a good night's sleep, *more* likely to be categorized as sleepy on the Epworth Sleepiness Scale. They were also *more* likely to drive drowsy.

Communication technology and media are an important part of American culture but may threaten healthy sleep. Media use, particularly of the computer and cell phone, seems to pose particular threats. The use of these devices at bedtime and during the night, coupled with the brightness of the light that they project onto the retina, are believed to trigger changes in sleep patterns, decrease total sleep time, cause sleep fragmentation, and reduce overall sleep quality.

Many Americans prefer more waking hours and fill these hours with technology that they believe keeps them connected to the world at large. Nurses are in key positions to provide anticipatory guidance regarding the impact technology has on sleep quality and to make recommendations to keep it out of the bedroom and limit its use in the hour before bedtime. Recommend all patients to engage in a relaxed quiet activity such as reading, meditating, praying, or crossword puzzles before bed. Encourage them to turn off the television, computer, and cell phone.

National Sleep Foundation (2011). *2011 National Sleep in America Poll: Communication technology in the bedroom*. Retrieved from http://www.sleepfoundation.org/sites/default/files/sleepinamericapoll/ SIAP_2011_Summary_of_Findings.pdf; Mesquita, G., & Reimao, R. (2010). Quality of sleep among university students: Effects of nighttime computer and television use. *Arquivos de Neuropsiquiatria, 68*(5), 720–725.

COMORBIDITY

Multiple studies suggest that sleeping less than 6 hours per night may have a significant impact on cardiovascular, endocrine, immune, and neurological function. Short sleep duration has been associated with obesity, cardiovascular disease and hypertension, impaired glucose tolerance and diabetes, and mood disturbance (Cappuccio et al., 2010).

Many sleep disorders increase the risk for the development of certain medical conditions. For example, obstructive sleep apnea has been associated with hypertension, diabetes, cardiovascular disease, and stroke (Tracova et al., 2008). Individuals with neurological disease, such as Alzheimer's and Parkinson's disease, frequently experience sleep disturbance that worsens with the progression of the illness. Sleep disturbance is a major factor contributing to nursing home placement in patients with dementia.

Virtually all psychiatric disorders are associated with sleep disturbance. Nearly all patients with a major depressive disorder or a bipolar disorder will report some type of a sleep disturbance over the course of the illness. In addition, there is evidence to demonstrate that sleep disruption itself may be a precipitating factor in triggering mood and other psychiatric disorders and increases the risk to relapse, making the identification and management of sleep disturbance in patients with affective disorders critical. Of special concern is that depressed patients with sleep disturbances demonstrate greater degrees of suicidal ideation.

Sleep disturbance is common in patients with alcoholism, and insomnia occurs in most patients in early recovery and persists for months or even years. Sleep disturbance increases the risk for relapse to alcohol abuse. Targeting sleep disturbance during recovery may support continued abstinence.

EVIDENCE-BASED PRACTICE

Impaired Sleep May be a Risk Factor for Adolescents and Young Adults

Problem

Major depressive disorder is a prevalent and serious problem among adolescents and young adults. If we can identify risk factors for depression, we can target interventions to reduce its prevalence. While research demonstrates that a person's chronotype (midpoint of sleep) and social jetlag (sleep loss due to socialization) are associated with depression, research is lacking among adolescents.

Purpose

The objective of this cross-sectional study was to examine the relationship between chronotype and social jetlag with the presence of depression symptoms in young students.

Methods

Researchers assessed 351 students who were between the ages of 12 and 21. Each student provided demographic information (age, sex, and class schedule) and circadian variables for school and free days (sunlight exposure, sleep duration, midpoint of sleep, and social jetlag). They also completed the Munich Chronotype Questionnaire and the Beck Depression Inventory.

Key Findings

- Girls and students who attended school in the evening were more frequently depressed.
- Students whose scores indicated depression had significantly delayed midpoints of sleep during school and free days.
- Two or more hours of social jetlag were not associated with depression.

Implications for Nursing Practice

This study highlights the importance of adequate sleep for everyone, but it seems to be especially true for females. Attending evening classes is a necessity for people who must work during the day. It makes sense that being employed during the day and attending school in the evening would negatively impact sleep due to late evening stress and a full schedule. Psychiatric nurses are often in the position to counsel depressed patients about minimizing stressors. In this case, nurses can help patients to find a balance in their lives, perhaps by reducing hours of employment and/or hours of school.

de Souza, C. M., & Hidalgo, M. P. (2014). Midpoint of sleep on school days is associated with depression among adolescents. *Chronobiology International, 31*(2), 199–205.

APPLICATION OF THE NURSING PROCESS

Regardless of the clinical environment or the presenting complaint, all patients can benefit from an evaluation of their sleep. Assessment of the patient's sleep allows the nurse to identify short- and long-term health risks associated with sleep disorders and sleep deprivation, provide health teaching and counseling regarding sleep needs, and improve clinical outcomes in patients experiencing a sleep disturbance.

The major focus of this section of the chapter is insomnia. However, you will find helpful information for anyone experiencing a sleep-wake disorder

ASSESSMENT

General Assessment

Sleep Patterns

Patients frequently do not report sleep difficulties or discuss their sleep-related concerns with care providers. People tend to minimize or adapt to the consequences of sleep disturbance. Furthermore, there is a lack of appreciation about the impact sleep disturbance and sleep deprivation have on overall functioning and health. Many patients do not complain of sleep disturbance directly but rather complain of associated symptoms such as fatigue, decreased concentration, mood disturbance, or physical ailments.

When assessing an individual who has a sleep complaint, it is important to recognize the 24-hour nature of the sleep disturbance. Sleep disturbance is not confined to the 7 or 8 hours devoted to sleep. Sleep diaries (Fig. 19.6) are helpful in identifying sleep patterns and behaviors that may be contributing to the sleep complaint. Assigning the patient the homework of completing a sleep diary for 2 weeks will help guide the assessment and direct the plan of care. The following questions and comments provide direction for the assessment:

- When did you begin having trouble with sleep? Have you had trouble with sleep in the past?
- Describe your prebedtime routine. What are the activities you customarily engage in before sleep?
- Describe your sleeping environment. Are there things in your sleep environment that are hampering your sleep (such as noise, light, temperature, or overall comfort)?
- Do you use your bedroom for things other than sleep or sexual activity (such as working, eating, or watching television)?

Two-week sleep diary

INSTRUCTIONS:

1 Write the date, day of the week, and type of day: Work, School, Day off, or Vacation.
2 Put the letter "C" in the box when you have coffee, cola or tea. Put "M" when you take any medicine. Put "A" when you drink alcohol. Put "E" when you exercise.
3 Put a line (I) to show when you go to bed. Shade in the box that shows when you think you fell asleep.
4 Shade in all the boxes that show when you are asleep at night or when you take a nap during the day.
5 Leave boxes unshaded to show when you wake up at night and when you are awake during the day.

SAMPLE ENTRY BELOW: On a Monday when I worked, I jogged on my lunch break at 1 PM, had a glass of wine with dinner at 6 PM, fell asleep watching TV from 7 to 8 PM, went to bed at 10:30 PM, fell asleep around midnight, woke up and couldn't get back to sleep at about 4 AM, went back to sleep from 5 to 7 AM, and had coffee and medicine at 7:00 in the morning.

Today's Date	Day of the week	Type of Day Work, School, Off, Vacation	Noon	1 PM	2	3	4	5	6 PM	7	8	9	10	11 PM	Midnight	1 AM	2	3	4	5	6 AM	7	8	9	10	11	
sample	Mon.	Work		E					A				I									C M					
																											Week 1
																											Week 2

FIG. 19.6 Two-week sleep diary. (Modified from the American Academy of Sleep Medicine. (Retrieved from http://www.sleepeducation.com/pdf/sleepdiary.pdf.)

- What time do you go to bed? How long does it take to fall asleep?
- Once asleep, does middle-of-the-night awakening disturb you? If so, what wakes you up? Are you able to return to sleep?
- If you are unable to sleep, what do you do?
- What time do you wake up? What time do you get out of bed?
- How much time do you actually think you sleep?
- Do you sleep longer on weekends or days off?
- Do you nap? If so, for how long? Do you feel refreshed after napping?
- Can you identify any stress or problem that may have initially contributed to your sleep difficulties?
- Tell me about your daily habits, diet, exercise, and medications.
- What changes, if any, have you made to improve your sleep? What were the results?

Identifying Sleep-Wake Disorders

It is helpful to think about sleep-wake disorders according to the predominant symptoms of insomnia, hypersomnia, arousal disorders, and circadian rhythm disorders. Box 19.1 provides pertinent screening questions for each diagnosis. An affirmative answer to any of these questions demands further investigation and evaluation.

BOX 19.1 Sleep Disorders Screening Questions

Insomnia

- Do you have difficulty with falling asleep, staying asleep, or early-morning awakenings?
- Do you feel refreshed and restored in the morning?
- Have you noticed any problems with your energy, mood, concentration, or work quality as a result of your sleep problem?

Hypersomnia

- Obstructive sleep apnea hypopnea syndrome: Have you ever been told that you snore or that it looks as if you stop breathing in your sleep?
- Restless legs syndrome: Do you have an unpleasant or uncomfortable sensation in your legs (or arms) that prevents you from sleeping or wakes you up from sleep and makes you want to move?
- Narcolepsy: Do you have episodes of sleepiness you cannot control? Have you experienced episodes where you were unable to move as you were about to fall asleep or wake up (sleep paralysis)? Unexplained muscle weakness after a strong emotion (cataplexy)? Have you ever seen or heard something that you knew was not real as you were falling asleep or waking up from sleep (hypnogogic hallucination)?
- Primary hypersomnia: Do you ever feel unrested even after an extended sleep period?

Arousal

- Have you ever been told that you have done anything unusual in your sleep, such as walking or talking?
- Have you ever been told that you act out your dreams? (REM sleep behavior disorder)
- Have you been troubled by nightmares or disturbing dreams?

Circadian Rhythm

- Is your desired sleep schedule in conflict with your social and vocational goals?
- What is your preferred sleep schedule?

Functioning and Safety

As previously described, sleep disturbance can result in increased risk for accident and injury and impose serious limitations on quality of life. Several screening tools are available to assist the clinician in evaluating sleep quality and the safety risk associated with excessive sleepiness. The Pittsburgh Sleep Quality Index (PSQI) is a subjective measure of sleep quality. A global sum of 5 or greater indicates poor quality and patterns of sleep (Buysse et al., 1989). The PSQI is available online.

The Epworth Sleepiness Scale (ESS) is a validated psychometric tool used to measure subjective reports of sleepiness and has been validated by objective measures using the MSLT. It is also available online. Scores of less than 10 are considered normal, 10 to 15 is moderately sleepy, and greater than 15 is excessively sleepy (Johns, 1991). In addition to these screening tools, the following questions provide direction for further assessment:

- Have you had an accident or injury as a result of sleepiness?
- Are you sleepy when you drive a car? What do you do if you are sleepy while driving?
- What kind of work do you do? Do you operate heavy equipment or machinery? How many hours a week do you work? How long is your commute?
- How does your sleep disturbance affect your work performance?
- Do you avoid social obligations as a result of your sleep problems?
- Do you feel as if your sleep disturbance is affecting your physical health? How so?

Self-Assessment

Nurses and nursing students are especially vulnerable to the effects of sleep deprivation and sleep disruption. Rotating shifts and night work result in circadian rhythm disruption that can cause problems with insomnia and excessive sleepiness. Long shifts and working overtime may lead to a decrease in total available sleep time. Inadequate sleep time and sleep quality have been shown to impair performance and judgment, both of which may affect patient safety and quality of care. In addition, nurses who work rotating or night shifts may pose an increased risk for accident or injury to themselves and the community as a result of excessive sleepiness while driving.

Nurses need to be able to recognize the effects of chronic partial sleep deprivation on their performance and functioning and take measures to ensure that they are well rested and able to provide safe and competent care. Self-evaluation for a possible sleep disorder and ability to cope with the rigors of shift work is warranted. Consultation with a sleep professional is indicated if there is significant disruption to sleep, physical and mental health, job performance, job satisfaction, and social functioning. Attention to issues of sleep hygiene, limiting overtime, limiting shift work to 8 hours, and obtaining 7 to 8 hours of sleep within a 24-hour period are essential for personal, patient, and community safety.

DIAGNOSIS

There are four specific North American Nursing Diagnosis Association International nursing diagnoses for sleep disturbance (Herdman & Kamitsuru, 2014, pp. 209–213):

1. *Insomnia:* A disruption in amount and quality of sleep that impairs functioning.
2. *Sleep deprivation:* Prolonged periods of time without sleep.
3. *Disturbed sleep pattern:* Changes in sleep routines that cause impairment in social or vocational functioning.
4. *Readiness for enhanced sleep:* A pattern of natural periodic suspension of relative consciousness to provide rest and sustain a desired lifestyle, which can be strengthened.

OUTCOMES IDENTIFICATION

The *Nursing Outcomes Classification* (*NOC*; Moorhead et al., 2013) identifies several appropriate outcomes for the patient experiencing sleep disruption including *sleep, rest, risk control,* and *personal well-being.* Table 19.1 provides signs and symptoms, nursing diagnoses, and short-term and long-term indicators for these categories.

PLANNING

The majority of patients with sleep disorders are treated in the community. The exceptions are cases in which the patient has a primary psychiatric disorder or a medical condition that requires hospitalization. Because longstanding sleep problems are associated with significant occupational, social, interpersonal, psychiatric, and medical conditions, the treatment is multifaceted and frequently requires a team approach under the leadership of a sleep disorder specialist. The role of the nurse is generally to conduct a full assessment, provide support to the patient and family while the appropriate interventions are determined, and teach the patient and family strategies that may improve sleep.

IMPLEMENTATION

Counseling

The nurse's counseling role begins with the assessment of the sleep disorder. The nurse's questions and responses provide support to the patient and family, as well as assurance that the sleep problems are amenable to treatment. The distress caused by chronic sleep difficulties results in hopelessness for many patients. Through the nurse's counseling approach, this hopelessness is identified and countered with encouragement, positive suggestions, and the belief that the patient will be able to manage sleep difficulties.

Health Teaching and Health Promotion

The nurse's role in health teaching cannot be overemphasized. Many people minimize the importance of their sleep and even boast about how little sleep they need to get by. This means that they also do not recognize the importance of a sleep routine or consider factors that influence good sleep. In addition, there are many myths regarding what constitutes "good sleep" and what factors contribute to sleep quality (Box 19.2). The nurse may also be involved in teaching relaxation techniques such as meditation, guided imagery, progressive muscle relaxation, or controlled breathing exercises. Use of these techniques has been linked to sustained benefits for patients with primary insomnia.

Modifying poor sleep habits and establishing a regular sleep-wake schedule can be accomplished using sleep diaries (see Fig. 19.6). As previously mentioned, a period of 2 weeks is helpful in establishing overall sleep patterns and determining overall sleep efficiency ([time in bed divided by total sleep time] × 100). After reviewing sleep diaries, patients are sometimes surprised to discover that their sleep problems are not as bad as previously believed.

BOX 19.2 Sleep Hygiene

- Maintain a regular sleep-wake schedule.
- Develop a presleep routine that signals the end of the day.
- Reserve the bedroom for sleep and a place for intimacy.
- Create an environment that is conducive to sleep (taking into consideration light, temperature, and clothing).
- Avoid clock watching.
- Limit caffeinated beverages to one or two a day and none in the evening.
- Avoid heavy meals before bedtime.
- Use alcohol cautiously and avoid use for several hours before bed.
- Avoid daytime napping.
- Exercise daily, but not right before bed.

TABLE 19.1 Signs and Symptoms, Diagnoses, and Outcomes for Sleep Disorders

Signs and Symptoms	Nursing Diagnoses	Outcomes
Absenteeism, changes in affect and energy; reports changes in mood, quality of life, concentration, and sleep; reports lack of energy, sleep disturbances, early wakening	*Insomnia*	Successful sleep induction, appropriate hours of sleep, consistent sleep pattern, minimal awakening
Acute confusion, agitation, anxiety, apathy, fatigue, poor concentration, irritability, lethargy, malaise, perceptual disorders, slowed reaction	*Sleep deprivation*	Balance between work and sleep, minimal awakening, feeling restored after sleep, sleeping between 7 and 9 hours on average
Changes in normal sleep pattern, decreased ability to function, dissatisfaction with sleep, awakening, no difficulty falling asleep, not feeling well rested	*Disturbed sleep pattern*	Minimal awakening, feeling restored after sleep
Expresses desire to enhance sleep	*Readiness for enhanced sleep*	Reports a satisfactory sleep pattern

From Herdman, T. H., & Kamitsuru, S. (Ed.). (2014). *Nursing diagnoses—Definitions and classification 2015-2017.* Used by arrangement with John Wiley & Sons Limited; Moorhead, S., Johnson, M., Maas, M. L., & Swanson, E. (2013). *Nursing outcomes classification* (*NOC;* 5th ed.). St. Louis, MO: Mosby.

Sleep restriction, or limiting the total sleep time, creates a temporary mild state of sleep deprivation and strengthens the sleep homeostatic drive. This helps decrease sleep latency and improves sleep continuity and quality. If, for example, a patient's sleep diary indicates that he or she is in bed for 8 hours but sleeping only 6 hours, sleep is restricted to 6 hours, and the bedtime and wake time are adjusted accordingly. The sleep time should not be reduced below 5 hours, regardless of sleep efficiency, and patients should be cautioned about the dangers of sleepiness with driving while undergoing a trial of sleep restriction. Once sleep efficiency is improved, total sleep time is gradually increased by 10- to 20-minute increments.

Pharmacological Interventions

Many patients use medication to address their sleep problems. Nurses frequently provide education about the benefits of a particular drug, the side effects, and adverse effects. Nurses explain that medications are usually prescribed for no more than 2 weeks, because tolerance and withdrawal may result. In many settings, the nurse also monitors the effectiveness of the medication. Table 19.2 provides an overview of pharmacological treatment of insomnia.

Generally, long-term sleeping pill use is discouraged because nonpharmacological treatments have shown superior efficacy in reducing insomnia. Other classifications of drugs used for insomnia are antidepressants, anticonvulsants, and antihistamines are also used off-label (without specific approval from the FDA). Second-generation antipsychotics improve sleep in people using them as indicated for other problems such as schizophrenia.

Somatic Interventions

Functional magnetic resonance imaging studies indicate that the prefrontal cortex is overly active with insomnia. Racing thoughts interfere with the individual's ability to sleep. In 2016 the FDA approved a device called the Cerêve Sleep System, which significantly reduced sleep latency from stage 1 to stage 2 in clinical trials. It is a software-controlled bedside device that is placed on the forehead. A fluid-filled pad cools the forehead and reduces activity in the cerebral cortex.

Advanced Practice Interventions

The initial episode of insomnia is frequently associated with a stressful event or crisis that produces anxiety. This anxiety becomes associated with worry about not being able to get to sleep and leads to preoccupation with getting enough sleep. The more the patient tries to sleep, the more elusive sleep becomes and the greater the patient's experienced anxiety.

Successful treatment of insomnia involves an integration of the basic principles of **sleep hygiene** (conditions and practices

TABLE 19.2 FDA-Approved Drugs for Insomnia

			USE IN INSOMNIA		
Generic (Trade) Name	**Onset of Action (Min.)**	**Duration of Action**	**DFA**	**DMS**	**HABIT FORMING**
Benzodiazepines					
Estazolam (ProSom)	15-60	Intermediate	✓	✓	Yes, all drugs in this class are schedule IV
Flurazepam (Dalmane)*	30-60	Long	✓	✓	
Quazepam (Doral)*	20-45	Long	✓	✓	
Temazepam (Restoril)	45-60	Intermediate	-	✓	
Triazolam (Halcion)	15-30	Short	✓	-	
Nonbenzodiazepine Receptor Agonists					
Eszopiclone (Lunesta)	60	Intermediate	✓	✓	Yes, all drugs in this class are schedule IV
Zaleplon (Sonata)	15-30	Ultra Short	✓	-	
Zolpidem	30	Short	✓	-	
Immediate release (Ambien)	30	Short	-	✓	
Immediate release (Intermezzo)**	30	Intermediate	✓	✓	
Extended release (Ambien CR)					
Melatonin Receptor Agonists					
Ramelteon (Rozerem)	30	Short	✓	-	No
Orexin Receptor Antagonist					
Suvorexant (Belsomra)	30	Intermediate	✓	✓	Yes, schedule IV
Tricyclic Antidepressant					
Doxepin (Silenor)	>60	Intermediate	-	✓	No

DFA, Difficulty falling asleep; *DMS,* difficulty maintaining sleep.
*Because of its long duration of action, this drug is generally not recommended.
**A sublingual taken in the middle of the night when there are at least four hours left to sleep.
United States Food and Drug Administration. (2015). *Search FDA*. Retrieved from http://www.fda.gov/Drugs/.

that promote continuous and effective sleep), behavioral therapies, and, in some instances the use of hypnotic medication. Hypnotic medication is always used with caution, and over-the-counter sleeping aids have limited effectiveness. Melatonin, a naturally occurring hormone, is a popular over-the-counter product. To date, there are few data to support its use in the management of insomnia disorder, but new research into prolonged release forms of melatonin are demonstrating some promise.

Advanced practice psychiatric-mental health nurses are qualified to conduct psychotherapy. A specific type of cognitive-behavioral therapy (CBT) has been developed for insomnia (CBT-I). Educational, behavioral, and cognitive components target factors that perpetuate insomnia over time (Morin, 2004). The first objectives are to provide education regarding sleep and sleep needs and to help the patient to set realistic expectations regarding sleep. Patients should be asked what they believe constitutes healthy sleep and have any misconceptions clarified. Determining the total number of hours spent sleeping typically has little value. Many patients are stuck on a set number of sleep hours rather than on the quality of sleep obtained. Focusing on the number of hours slept rather than the quality of sleep and daytime functioning increases the insomnia experience.

Stimulus control is a behavioral intervention that involves some interventions previously discussed with sleep hygiene. Adherence to five basic principles that decrease the negative associations between the bed and bedroom and strengthen the stimulus for sleep is essential. Patients should be instructed to:

1. Go to bed only when sleepy.
2. Use the bed or bedroom only for sleep and intimacy (no television, reading, or other activities in the bedroom).
3. Get out of bed if unable to sleep and engage in a quiet-time activity such as reading or crossword puzzles (no television, work, or computer).
4. Maintain a regular sleep-wake schedule with getting up at the same time each day being the most important factor.
5. Avoid daytime napping. If napping is necessary to avoid accident or injury, it should be limited to 20 to 30 minutes maximum, and a timer should be set.

Other objectives of CBT-I are aimed at identifying and correcting maladaptive attitudes and beliefs about sleep that perpetuate insomnia. For example, patients frequently amplify the consequences of their insomnia and attribute most daytime experiences to their sleep complaint. They may rationalize maladaptive coping behaviors such as excessive time in bed to "catch up" on lost sleep and may exhibit unrealistic expectations about sleep. The nurse offers alternative interpretations regarding the sleep complaint to assist the patient to think about his or her insomnia in a different way, empowering the patient to be in control of sleep. Because CBT-I approaches are not immediately effective and may take several weeks of practice before improvement is seen, success is dependent on both a high degree of motivation in patients and a commitment on the part of the practitioner.

EVALUATION

Evaluation is based on whether or not the patient experiences improved sleep quality as evidenced by decreased sleep latency, fewer nighttime awakenings, a shorter time to get back to sleep after awakening, and improvement in daytime symptoms of sleepiness. This evaluation is accomplished through patient report and patient maintenance of a sleep diary. Just as important as objective changes in the patient's sleep pattern is the patient's perception that there has been an improvement. Objectively, the improvement may be quite modest, but the patient may no longer feel *controlled by* sleep, but instead has *control over* sleep through lifestyle changes and a better sleep routine.

KEY POINTS TO REMEMBER

- Sleep disturbance has major implications for overall health, quality of life, and personal and community safety.
- Research into the physiology of normal sleep, as well as sleep disorders, is expanding.
- Virtually all patients with a mood disorder will report sleep disturbance; recognition and treatment of sleep disturbance in patients with psychiatric disorders improves clinical outcomes.
- Regardless of the clinical environment or the presenting complaint, all patients can benefit from an evaluation of their sleep needs.
- Primary insomnia can be effectively treated with nonpharmacological interventions such as CBT-I, sleep restriction, stimulus control, and attention to issues of sleep hygiene. Long-term pharmacological management is generally not indicated.

CRITICAL THINKING

1. Anthony is a 46-year-old who complains of waking frequently at night. Consequently, he is tired all day and knows that he has not been functioning as well as he should. Whenever he can manage it, he goes out to his car at lunchtime to take a 60-minute nap, because he has fallen asleep at his desk and been given a disciplinary warning. He is drinking 2 to 3 cups of coffee in the afternoon so that he does not feel sleepy while driving home.
   - **a.** What questions would you ask to determine if Anthony might have a sleep disorder?
   - **b.** What recommendations will you make to improve his sleep hygiene?
   - **c.** What instructions and education should you give this patient regarding personal and community safety?
2. Your patient, Vivian, has been using temazepam (Restoril) for several years to treat insomnia. She has been reading that long-term use of hypnotics is not healthy or productive and wants to quit taking them. However, she is focused on needing 9 hours of sleep each night and is extremely worried about what will happen when she discontinues the temazepam.

a. What instructions would you provide to Vivian regarding stimulus control, sleep restriction, and cognitive restructuring of her sleep complaint?
b. Identify alternative pharmacological therapies.

3. Mrs. Levine is a 72-year-old woman with a history of major depression. She takes fluoxetine (Prozac), 10 mg every day, and has experienced significant relief from depression. While reviewing her medications, she tells you she is using a variety of over-the-counter (OTC) sleep aids because she has been having some difficulty sleeping recently. These OTC products include diphenhydramine, melatonin, valerian, and something that her neighbor gave her to try.
   a. In light of the patient's age and history of depression, what are your concerns?
   b. What further assessment is required?
   c. What specific question would you need to ask concerning her use of Prozac?
   d. What instructions and education will you provide?

CHAPTER REVIEW

Questions

1. Which patient statement supports a diagnosis of narcolepsy?
   a. "My wife tells me I snore at night."
   b. "I sleepwalk several nights a week."
   c. "I have no control over when I fall asleep."
   d. "My legs feel funny, and that keeps me awake."
2. Madelyn, a 29-year-old patient recently diagnosed with depression, comes to the mental health clinic complaining of continued difficulty sleeping. One week ago she was started on a selective serotonin reuptake inhibitor (SRRI), fluoxetine (Prozac), for her depressive symptoms. When educating Madelyn your response is guided by the knowledge that:
   a. SSRIs such as fluoxetine more commonly cause hypersomnolence as opposed to difficulty sleeping.
   b. The sleep problem is caused by the depression and is unrelated to the medication.
   c. The neurotransmitters involved in sleep and wakefulness are the same neurotransmitters targeted by many psychiatric medications and the problem may be temporary.
   d. The medication should be discontinued since sleep is the most important element to her recovery.
3. Which behaviors will the nurse encourage a patient diagnosed with insomnia disorder to adopt? *Select all that apply.*
   a. Avoiding exercising at bedtime
   b. Avoiding napping during the day
   c. Eating a hearty snack at bedtime
   d. Getting up at the same time each day
   e. Moving the clock so it is not visible from the bed
4. Which treatment is typically prescribed for primary insomnia? *Select all that apply.*
   a. Cognitive-behavioral therapy-insomnia (CBT-I)
   b. Intravenous medication for sedation
   c. Stimulus control
   d. Sleep restriction
   e. Sleep hygiene measures
5. Light projected into the retina is believed to trigger changes in sleep patterns and quality of sleep. Therefore the nurse should suggest:
   a. Not reading within an hour of bedtime
   b. Exercising before bedtime in a darkened environment
   c. Limiting use of electronic devices in the hour before bedtime
   d. Dimming the screen on cellphones and computers in the evening
6. Sleep disturbances are often overlooked or undiagnosed due to:
   a. A lack of formal nurse and physician training in sleep disturbances
   b. Patients not often accurately describing sleep disturbance patterns
   c. The belief that sleep disturbance is a necessary part of hospitalization
   d. Patients hiding the fact that they have issues with sleep
7. Many people allow life circumstances to dictate their amount of sleep instead of recognizing sleep as a priority. Which statement will the nurse recognize as progress in the patient's sleep hygiene program?
   a. "I go to bed even if I am not sleepy, hoping I will fall asleep."
   b. "I have one glass of red wine at bedtime each night."
   c. "I take a nap each day to 'catch up' on my sleep deficit."
   d. "I have removed the television from my bedroom."
8. Larry is a 50-year-old man who works about 60 hours per week. He arrives at the clinic seeking assistance with a weight gain of 50 pounds over the past year. Larry admits to sleeping 4 to 5 hours a night. The nurse recognizes that the weight gain may be related to:
   a. A new onset of diabetes
   b. Suspected cardiovascular disease
   c. Dysregulation of hormones that influence appetite
   d. Comorbidity of depression with obesity
9. Sleep deprivation is considered a safety issue that results in loss of life and property. Psychomotor impairments of sleep deprivation are similar to symptoms caused by:
   a. Sleeping in excess of 10 hours
   b. Misuse of caffeine products
   c. Alcohol consumption
   d. Working more than 40 hours per week
10. The stage of sleep known as rapid eye movement or REM sleep is characterized by atonia and myoclonic twitches in addition to the actual rapid movement of the eyes. Atonia is thought to be a protective mechanism as it:
   a. Limits physical movements
   b. Prevents nightmares
   c. Enhances the dream state
   d. Regulates the autonomic nervous system

Answers

1. **c**; 2. **c**; 3. **a, b, d, e**; 4. **a, c, d, e**; 5. **c**; 6. **a**; 7. **d**; 8. **c**; 9. **c**; 10. **a**

Visit the Evolve website for a posttest on the content in this chapter: http://evolve.elsevier.com/Varcarolis

Post-Test interactive review

REFERENCES

American Psychiatric Association. (2013). Diagnostic and Statistical Manual of Mental Disorders (5th ed.). Washington, DC: Author.

Arun, S., Sathiamma, S., & Bindu, K. (2014). Current understanding on the neurobiology of sleep and wakefulness. *International Journal of Clinical and Experimental Psychology*, *1*(1), 3–9.

Birbiglia, M. (2010). *Sleepwalk with me*. New York, NY: Simon and Schuster.

Bliwise, D. (2011). Normal aging. In M. Kryger, T. Roth, & W. Dement (Eds.), *Principles and practice of sleep medicine* (5th ed.). Philadelphia, PA: Saunders.

Buysse, D. J., Reynolds, C. F., III, Monk, T. H., Berman, S. R., & Kupfer, D. J. (1989). The Pittsburgh Sleep Quality Index: A new instrument for psychiatric practice and research. *Psychiatry Research*, *28*(2), 193–213.

Cappuccio, E., Miller, M., & Lockley, S. (2010). *Sleep, health, and society: From aetiology to public health*. Oxford, UK; New York, NY: Oxford University Press.

Carney, R., Berry, R., & Geyer, J. (2011). *Clinical sleep disorders* (2nd ed.). Philadelphia, PA: Lippincott, Williams & Wilkins.

Centers for Disease Control. (2010). Youth risk behavior surveillance—United States, 2009. *Morbidity and Mortality Weekly Report*, *59*(SS-5), 1–142.

Czeisler, C., Buxton, O., & Khalsa, S. (2011). The human circadian system and sleep-wake regulation. In M. Kryger, T. Roth, & W. Dement (Eds.), *Principles and practice of sleep medicine* (5th ed.). Philadelphia, PA: Saunders.

Geiger, S. D., Sabanayagam, C., & Shankar, A. (2012). The relationship between insufficient sleep and self-rated health in a nationally representative sample. *Journal of Environmental and Public Health*, *2012*, 518263.

Grandner, M. A., Patel, N. P., Gehrman, P. R., Perlis, M. L., & Pack, A. I. (2010). Problems associated with short sleep: Bridging the gap between laboratory and epidemiological studies. *Sleep Medicine Reviews*, *14*(4), 239–247.

Herdman, T. H., & Kamitsuru, S. (Eds.), (2014). *NANDA International nursing diagnoses: Definitions and classification* (pp. 2015–2017). Oxford, UK: Wiley-Blackwell.

Hubner, A., Krafft, A., Gadient, S., Werth, E., Zimmermann, R., & Bassetti, C. L. (2013). Characteristics and determinants of restless legs syndrome in pregnancy. *Neurology*, *80*(8), 738–742.

Institute of Medicine. (2006). *Sleep disorders and sleep deprivation: An unmet public health problem*. Washington, DC: The National Academies Press.

Insurance Institute for Highway Safety. (2012). *DUI/DWI laws*. Retrieved from http://www.iihs.org/laws/dui.aspx.

Johns, M. W. (1991). A new method for measuring daytime sleepiness: The Epworth Sleepiness Scale. *Sleep*, *14*, 540–545.

Kessler, R. C., Berglund, P. A., Coulouvrat, C., Hajak, G., Roth, T., Shahly, V., et al. (2011). Insomnia and performance of U.S. workers: Results from the American insomnia survey. *Sleep*, *34*(9), 1161–1171.

Luyster, F. S., Strollo, P. J., Zee, P. C., & Walsh, J. K. (2012). Sleep: A health imperative. *Sleep*, *35*(6), 727–734.

Moorhead, S., Johnson, M., Maas, M. L., & Swanson, E. (2013). *Nursing outcomes classification* (NOC; 5th ed.). St. Louis, MO: Mosby.

Morin, C. (2004). Cognitive-behavioral approaches to the treatment of insomnia. *Journal of Clinical Psychiatry*, *65*(Suppl. 16), 33–40.

National Center on Sleep Disorder Research. (2011). *National Institute of Health: Sleep disorders research plan*. Retrieved from http://www.nhlbi.nih.gov/health/prof/sleep/201101011NationalSleepDisordersResearchPlanDHHSPublication11-7820.pdf.

National Institute of Neurologic Disorders and Stroke. (2012). *Restless leg syndrome fact sheet*. Retrieved from http://www.ninds.nih.gov/disorders/restless_legs/detail_restless_legs.htm.

National Sleep Foundation. (2011). *2011 NSF Sleep in America Poll*. Retrieved from https://sleepfoundation.org/sites/default/files/sleepinamericapoll/SIAP_2011_Summary_of_Findings.pdf.

National Sleep Foundation. (2015). *2015 Sleep in America Poll*. Retrieved from https://sleepfoundation.org/sleep-polls-data/2015-sleep-and-pain.

National Sleep Foundation. (2016a). *How much sleep do we really need?* Retrieved from https://sleepfoundation.org/how-sleep-works/how-much-sleep-do-we-really-need.

National Sleep Foundation. (2016b). Sleep studies. Retrieved from https://sleepfoundation.org/sleep-topics/sleep-studies/page/0/1.

Orzel-Gryglewska, J. (2010). Consequences of sleep deprivation. *International Journal of Occupational Medicine and Environmental Health*, *23*(1), 95–114.

Sadock, B. J., Sadock, V. A., & Ruiz, P. (2015). *Kaplan and Sadock's synopsis of psychiatry*. Philadelphia, PA: Wolters Kluwer.

Spielman, A., & Glovinsky, P. (2004). A conceptual framework of insomnia for primary care providers: Predisposing, precipitating, and perpetuating factors. *Sleep Medicine Alert*, *9*(1), 1–6.

Tracova, R., Dorkova, Z., Molcanyiova, A., Radikova, Z., Klimes, I., & Tkac, I. (2008). Cardiovascular risk and insulin resistance in patients with obstructive sleep apnea. *Medical Science Monitor*, *14*(9), CR438–CR444.

U.S. Department of Health and Human Services. (2012). *Healthy People 2020*. Retrieved from http://www.healthypeople.gov/2020/default.aspx.

20

Sexual Dysfunction, Gender Dysphoria, and Paraphilias

Margaret Jordan Halter

Visit the Evolve website for a pretest on the content in this chapter: http://evolve.elsevier.com/Varcarolis Pre-Test interactive review

OBJECTIVES

1. Describe the four phases of the sexual response cycle.
2. Describe clinical manifestations of each major sexual dysfunction.
3. Consider the impact of medical problems and medications on normal sexual functioning.
4. Describe biological, psychological, and environmental factors related to sexual dysfunction.
5. Apply the nursing process to caring for individuals with sexual dysfunction.
6. Discuss the importance of nurses being knowledgeable about and comfortable discussing topics pertaining to sexuality.
7. Describe treatments available for sexual dysfunction.
8. Identify the problem of gender dysphoria in children and adults
9. Identify sexual preoccupations considered to be paraphilic disorders.
10. Discuss personal values and biases regarding sexuality and sexual behaviors.
11. Develop a plan of care for individuals diagnosed with sexual disorders.

OUTLINE

OUTLINE—cont'd

KEY TERMS AND CONCEPTS

delayed ejaculation
erectile disorder
exhibitionistic disorder
female orgasmic disorder
female sexual interest/arousal disorder
fetishistic disorder
frotteuristic disorder
gender dysphoria
gender identity
genito-pelvic pain/penetration disorder
male hypoactive sexual desire disorder
paraphilic disorder
pedophilic disorder
premature ejaculation
sex reassignment surgery
sexual dysfunction
voyeuristic disorder

Practicing professional nursing requires us to engage in matter-of-fact discussions with patients regarding topics generally considered to be extremely private and personal. We perform head-to-toe assessments during which we inquire about everything from headaches and sore throats to difficulties urinating and problems with constipation. The realities of providing physical care necessitate becoming comfortable with a number of skills that concern privacy and modesty such as performing breast examinations, initiating urinary catheters, and inserting rectal medications.

Despite a sort of learned fearlessness when it comes to addressing other intimate issues, the topic of sexuality is often a source of discomfort for not only nurses but also other healthcare providers. Although most of us recognize that addressing sexuality is part of holistic care, many do not routinely include the topic when doing assessments. Nursing curricula typically have a deficiency in training nurses in the fundamentals of sexuality and nursing care. Patients want to know how, for example, medications or treatments will affect their relationships and ability to have satisfying sex lives. Nurses can normalize such issues and foster opportunities to address feelings and fears.

Views regarding sexuality are based on our individual beliefs about ourselves as women and men, mothers and fathers, and generative individuals who create and give to society. Multiple factors, including societal attitudes and traditions, parental views, cultural practices, spiritual and religious teaching, socioeconomic status, and education, affect our sexual beliefs and behaviors and also our attitudes toward the sexual behaviors of others including our patients.

Health promotion and disease prevention are key responsibilities for nurses. Nurses should be educated to assess a patient's sexuality and be prepared to educate, dispel myths, assist with values clarification, refer to appropriate care providers when indicated, and share resources. These actions alleviate or decrease patient illness and suffering and reduce healthcare costs through prevention. As a nursing student, you are introduced to complex aspects of sexual behavior that should help facilitate thoughtful discussion of the topic, make you aware of your personal beliefs, and help you consider the broader perspective of sexual issues as they exist in contemporary society.

This chapter addresses two general categories related to sexuality. In the first half of the chapter we will examine the normal sexual response cycle, clinical disorders related to the disruption or malfunction of this cycle, and guidelines for nursing care. In the second half of the chapter we focus on problems related to sexual preoccupation. These problems may be sources of discomfort and distress to the person experiencing them (e.g., gender dysphoria) and may be a source of pain and trauma for others whose rights are violated (e.g., pedophilia).

SEXUALITY

Phases of the Sexual Response Cycle

Before looking more closely at the dysfunctions of sexual functioning, we will first review normal sexual functioning. According to the early experts in sexuality and sexual functioning, Masters and Johnson (1966), there are four distinct phases:

- Phase 1: Desire
- Phase 2: Excitement
- Phase 3: Orgasm
- Phase 4: Resolution

Desire

Many factors may affect interest in sexual activity, including age, physical and emotional health, availability of a sexual partner, and the context of an individual's life. In fact, for a number of individuals, the lack of sexual desire is not a source of distress either to the person or the partner. In such a situation, decreased or absent sexual desire is not viewed as an illness. Furthermore, desire is not a necessary component of sexual functioning.

CONSIDERING CULTURE

Female Genital Mutilation and Sexual Functioning

Female genital mutilation (FGM) is the surgical altering of female sexual organs for nonmedical reasons. The World Health Organization (2016) condemns this practice as does the United Nations. An estimated 100 to 140 million females currently are living with the consequences of this surgery, which occurs between birth and 15 years of age. It is performed to decrease libido (ensuring chastity and fidelity to spouses), prevent premarital sex, uphold a cultural tradition, or make the girl more feminine and beautiful by removing parts that are considered "male."

The actual practice of FGM varies depending on what structures are removed or altered.

Type 1: *Clitoridectomy.* Partial or total removal of the clitoris.

Type 2: *Excision.* Partial or total removal of the clitoris and the labia minora with or without excision of the labia majora.

Type 3: *Infibulation.* The most extreme form of FGM involves the removal of all external genitalia and stitching the labia together. A small opening allows for urination and menstruation.

Type 4: All other harmful nonmedical procedures to genitalia includes pricking, piercing, incising, scraping, and cauterizing.

The surgery is often done ritualistically and in unsanitary conditions with a razor blade that may be used over and over. The immediate effects are severe pain and infection. Girls and women suffer recurrent urinary tract infections, cysts, infertility, and childbirth complications. Clitoridectomy results in altered sexual responsiveness. Sexual activity is often associated with dyspareunia (painful intercourse).

The procedure occurs mainly in Africa, the Middle East, and Asia. It is increasingly protested and restricted by law resulting in some families taking their daughters abroad for "vacation cutting." Some US doctors suggest that parents should be allowed to have their daughter's genitals ritually nicked to prevent more extreme versions of FGM (Arora & Jacobs, 2016).

Clinicians in the United States also encounter females who have already undergone these procedures. Few healthcare providers are prepared to deal with the mutilation and sexual problems. Developing a trusting relationship with patients who have been subjected to this custom includes understanding the types of mutilation, as well as the culture in which it occurs.

Arora, K. S., & Jacobs, A. J. (2016). Female genital alteration: A compromise solution. *Journal of Medical Ethics, 42(3),* 148–154. World Health Organization. (2016). *Female genital mutilation.* Retrieved from http://www.who.int/(3)mediacentre/factsheets/fs241/en/.

According to Levine (2010), there are three components to desire: drive, motive, and values. He refers to *drive* as the biologically motivated interest based in the cerebral cortex, the limbic, and the endocrine system that prompts a focus on sexually appealing aspects of another, physiological response, and plotting for connection. *Motive* is less physiological and more psychological and is based on choices, aspirations, and motives for interpersonal connection. This is the area that clinicians often target for intervention. *Values* impact sexuality by imparting certain familial, religious, and cultural beliefs and guidelines for our responses and behaviors. It is a significant part of our programming beginning in adolescence. As adults, values are fairly enduring, but they may shift depending on other motivations.

Invariably, there is a difference in sex drive within a relationship, and negotiations are almost always present. Low sexual desire may be a source of frustration, both for the one experiencing it and also for partners. It is sometimes associated with psychiatric or medical conditions. Conversely, excessive sexual desire becomes a problem when it creates difficulties for the individual's partner or when such excessive desire drives the person to demand sexual compliance from or to force it upon unwilling partners.

Testosterone, normally present in the circulation of both males and females but in a much higher level in males, appears to be essential to sexual desire in both men and women. Estrogen does not seem to have a direct effect on sexual desire in women. A secondary effect, however, may be present in the requirement of estrogen for the maintenance of normal vaginal elasticity and lubrication.

Excitement

The excitement phase of the normal human sexual response cycle is that period of time during which sexual tension continues to increase from the preceding level of sexual desire. Traditionally, penile erection and vaginal lubrication have been used as indicators of the presence of sexual excitement. If erection or lubrication does not occur in what, for that individual, is a sexually stimulating and appropriate situation, then there has been an inhibition of sexual excitement, regardless of the causative factors.

Orgasm

The orgasm phase of the human sexual response cycle is attained only at high levels of sexual tension in both women and men. Sexual tension (also described as sexual arousal) is produced by a combination of mental activity—including thoughts, fantasies, and dreams—and erotic stimulation of erogenous areas, which may be more or less specific for each individual. Most men require some penile stimulation and most women some clitoral stimulation, either directly or indirectly, to produce the high levels of sexual tension necessary for orgasm to occur.

Some women who have experienced one orgasm may have repeated orgasms during the continuation of the same sexual activity. The occurrence of multiple orgasms depends on the maintenance of high levels of sexual tension through continued stimulation. On the other hand, once men ejaculate as a part of orgasm, they go through a refractory period. This is the time required to produce another ejaculate, which varies primarily with age. In a young man, this refractory period is measured in minutes whereas in an older man it may last several hours.

Resolution

During the resolution phase, sexual tension developed in prior phases subsides to baseline levels provided sexual stimulation has ceased. The physiological changes that occurred during the earlier phases of the response cycle now tend to dissipate. This is a period of psychological vulnerability and can either be experienced as a period of pleasurable afterglow or described as being uncomfortably emotionally exposed. With the restoration of normal pulse, respiratory rate, and blood pressure, individuals frequently experience increased perspiration.

SEXUAL DYSFUNCTION

Sexual dysfunction is an extremely common problem that involves the disturbance in the desire, excitement, or orgasm phases of the sexual response cycle or pain during sexual intercourse. It may prevent or reduce a person's ability to enjoy sex and can be classified according to the phase of the sexual response cycle in which it occurs. In evaluating a patient with a sexual dysfunction, a physical assessment—including laboratory studies—is performed before exploring psychological factors such as emotional issues, life situation, and experiences. Sexual dysfunctions can be the result of physiological problems, interpersonal conflicts, or a combination of both. Stress of any kind can adversely affect sexual function.

CLINICAL PICTURE

Seven major classes of sexual dysfunction include:

- Male hypoactive sexual desire disorder
- Female sexual interest/arousal disorder
- Erectile disorder
- Female orgasmic disorder
- Delayed ejaculation
- Premature ejaculation
- Genito-pelvic pain/penetration disorder

In addition to these disorders and conditions, there are substance/medication-induced and sexual dysfunction that is not classified (American Psychiatric Association, 2013).

It is important to note that individuals may not have a desire for sexual relations. This is called *asexuality*, which may be a distinct form of sexual orientation. Asexuality is different from celibacy, which is a conscious choice to abstain from sex even though the desire is there. Asexuality is having no sexual attraction. If heterosexuality is attraction to the opposite sex and homosexuality is the attraction to the same sex, then asexuality could legitimize the preference for no sexual attraction. Asexual people may have an interest in cuddling and physical contact but no interest in sex, and asexuals may be married and negotiate for sex or simply do without.

Sexual Desire Disorders

Male Hypoactive Sexual Desire Disorder

The male version of low interest in sex is called male hypoactive sexual desire disorder. This disorder is characterized by a deficiency or absence of sexual fantasies or desire for sexual activity.

Lack of sexual desire in men can be a lifelong problem or may be acute. The acquired version may be situational (the man is not interested in sexual relations with a particular person but continues to have interest in others and/or in masturbation) or generalized (the man has no interest in sexual activity with someone else or solitarily).

The source of this disorder may be physiological, psychological, or a combination of both. Hormonal imbalance, particularly testosterone deficiency, may be an issue. Depression is often implicated in a lack of desire for sexual intimacy in men.

Lack of sexual desire occurs more frequently in older males. About 6% of men ages 18 to 24 compared with 41% of men ages 66 to 74 have this problem.

Female Sexual Interest/Arousal Disorder

The female version of low sexual desire includes the descriptors interest and arousal. This combination places the disorder across both the "desire" category and also the "excitement" category (see the following section). Female sexual interest/arousal disorder is characterized by emotional distress caused by absent or reduced interest in sexual fantasies, sexual activity, pleasure, and arousal. Some women experience these symptoms their whole lives while others may gradually become less interested in sexual activities.

Reasons for the disorder may be clear such as having an abusive mate. In other cases, it is a baffling problem to both the woman and her partner. The cause may be a combination of neurobiological, hormonal, and psychosocial factors. Dopamine, progesterone, estrogen, and testosterone exert an excitatory role while serotonin, prolactin, and opioids inhibit sexual desire.

Sexual desire may decrease with age, particularly after menopause. Female sexual interest/arousal disorder is thought to be fairly common, although exact prevalence rates are unavailable.

Sexual Excitement Disorders

Erectile Disorder

Erectile disorder (also called *erectile dysfunction* and *impotence*) refers to failure to obtain and maintain an erection sufficient for sexual activity. While most men occasionally experience this problem, it is only a disorder if it happens on 75% of sexual occasions and lasts for at least 6 months.

This problem may be a rare lifelong condition in which a man has never been able to obtain an erection sufficient for intercourse. It may also be an acquired condition in which a man has previously been able to have sexual intercourse but has lost the ability.

Aging is associated with erectile disorder. The prevalence in men younger than 40 years old is about 2%. Men older than 60 experience significant erectile problems at a rate of about 40%.

Orgasm Disorders

Female Orgasmic Disorder

Study of the female orgasm is more complicated than the male orgasm, which results in a noticeable ejaculation. Additionally, there is no reproduction associated with the female analog. Comparing female and male responses to orgasm, men are more focused on performance while women tend to be focused on the subjective quality of having sex. Some women are uncertain if orgasm has even occurred.

Female orgasmic disorder is sometimes referred to as *inhibited female orgasm* or *anorgasmia* and is defined as the recurrent or persistent inhibition of female orgasm. It is manifested by the recurrent delay in, or absence of, orgasm after a normal sexual excitement phase achieved by masturbation or coitus. For the recognition of a clinically significant problem, it must happen for at least 6 months and must occur during most sexual encounters.

It may be a lifelong disorder (never having achieved orgasm) or acquired (having had at least one orgasm and then having difficulties). Most cases are lifelong rather than acquired, and once a woman learns how to achieve orgasm it is unusual to lose this capacity. Acquired anorgasmia in women tends to be associated with painful intercourse during or after menopause.

Psychological factors including fears of pregnancy, rejection, or loss of control are associated with anorgasmia. Other factors may include hostility toward or from men and cultural/societal restrictions.

The prevalence of either type of this disorder is estimated between 10% and 42%. There is some evidence to suggest that female orgasmic disorder may be inherited.

Delayed Ejaculation

In **delayed ejaculation**, formerly referred to as *male orgasmic disorder, inhibited orgasm,* or *retarded ejaculation,* a man achieves ejaculation during coitus only with great difficulty. A man with a *lifelong delayed ejaculation* has never been able to ejaculate during coitus. This uncommon condition may result from a rigid background in which sex is believed to be a sin.

Acquired delayed ejaculation develops after previously normal functioning and is fairly common. Interpersonal problems may be the cause. Physical conditions, substance use, and prescribed medication may also cause this problem and should be assessed.

Premature Ejaculation

In **premature ejaculation**, a man persistently or recurrently achieves orgasm and ejaculation before he wishes to. Diagnosis is made when a man regularly ejaculates before or immediately after the penis enters the vagina. Considerations as to age, newness of the relationship, and how often the man has intercourse should be assessed.

Physical factors may be involved. Some men may be more tactilely sensitive and respond more intensely to stimulation. Psychological factors include fear about performance and stressful relationships where the man feels hurried. There is no disorder in women that corresponds to premature ejaculation.

Although this problem is fairly uncommon in the general population (1% to 3%), about 35% to 40% of men who are treated for sexual disorders complain of premature ejaculation.

Genito-Pelvic Pain/Penetration Disorder

The group of disorders previously diagnosed in the psychiatric community included a problem called *dyspareunia,* which referred to pelvic and/or vaginal pain during or after intercourse. It also included vaginismus, which referred to an involuntary constriction response of the muscles of the vagina. Researchers believed that the distinction between the two disorders is too blurry and combined them into a single disorder.

Genito-pelvic pain/penetration disorder interferes with penile insertion during intercourse. It may even be elicited during a normal gynecological examination with a speculum. Individuals experiencing these problems become fearful that pain and spasms will occur during the next encounter. This fear compounds the problem by increasing anxiety and muscle tension.

VIGNETTE: Jessica, a computer programmer, had recently had a baby and was looking forward to renewing her love life with her husband. She said, "My husband would barely begin penetration, and the pain would be awful. The whole area just clenched up." She continued, "I had never had any problems before, and I didn't think I would because I'd had a caesarean, so I didn't think that anything would change. 'Good grief, that hurts,' I thought. 'What is wrong with me?' We were both terribly upset."

Other Sexual Dysfunctions and Problems

Sexual dysfunction due to a general medical condition includes sexual desire disorders, orgasm disorders, and sexual pain disorders. The cause of each is related to a medical condition such as cardiovascular, neurological, or endocrine disease.

The diagnosis *substance-induced sexual dysfunction* is used when evidence of substance intoxication or withdrawal is apparent from the history, physical examination, or laboratory findings. Specified substances include alcohol, amphetamines or related substances, cocaine, opioids, sedatives, hypnotics, antianxiety agents, and other known and unknown substances. Abused recreational substances can have a variety of effects on sexual functioning. In small doses, many substances enhance sexual performance. With continued use, sexual difficulties become the norm.

Sexual dysfunction not elsewhere classified is a category that covers sexual dysfunctions that cannot be classified under one of the other categories. Typically, this is because their presentation is not quite strong enough to meet the criteria for a disorder or because there is not enough information to make a diagnosis.

Box 20.1 provides a discussion regarding the influence of pharmacological treatment for men and psychiatric diagnoses for sexual dysfunction in women.

EPIDEMIOLOGY

Overall, sexual dysfunctions are more common in women than men. There are data that indicate that nearly half of adult women (40% to 45%) and about a third of adult men (20% to 30%) have at least one sexual dysfunction (Lewis et al., 2010).

COMORBIDITY

Sexual functioning may be adversely affected any time there is a disturbance in an individual's ability to develop and maintain stable relationships. This is especially true for patients with schizophrenia who show difficulty coping with stress, a decrease in reality-based orientation to the world, and defense mechanisms that lead to withdrawn behavior. Sexual dysfunction is often associated with depression and personality disorders. A history of sexual trauma is also frequently associated with sexual dysfunction.

Obesity and a sedentary lifestyle contribute to sexual dysfunction from both a psychological and a physiological perspective. Psychologically, an obese person may feel undesirable or may have a partner who is no longer attracted. Physiologically, inactivity results in less vitality overall including sexual ability and responsiveness.

BOX 20.1 Sexual Dysfunction in Women: The Viagra Effect

Experts in psychiatric disorders are expressing concern that women may be overdiagnosed with disorders in sexual function based on criteria in the latest edition of the *Diagnostic and Statistical Manual* (APA, 2013). Normal variation in sexual interest, along with variability within the life cycle, should be taken into consideration when these diagnoses are made (Frances, 2013).

A safeguard in the criteria for female sexual interest/arousal disorder stipulates that emotional distress is necessary. However, the advent of pharmacological innovations such as sildenafil (Viagra) that improve sexual performance in men should be factored into this emotional distress. Expectations on the part of men as treated partners, researchers, and pharmaceutical leaders set the social stage for the overdiagnosis of female sexual dysfunction in women. Only a generation ago, both partners in a couple were aging and experiencing a reduction in sexual interest and appetite. Now, pharmacological innovations may have created a mismatch between treated men and untreated women.

RISK FACTORS

Biological Factors

Aging appears to be a factor in the prevalence of all sexual dysfunction for both men and women. In addition, a variety of physical conditions are related to sexual dysfunction and are presented in Table 20.1.

Psychological Factors

Pioneers in the study of human sexuality include Helen Singer Kaplan (1929–1995). According to Kaplan (1974), sexual dysfunctions are the result of a combination of factors including the following:

- Misinformation or ignorance regarding sexual and social interaction
- Unconscious guilt and anxiety regarding sex
- Anxiety related to performance, especially with erectile and orgasmic dysfunction
- Poor communication between partners about feelings and what they desire sexually

Additional factors have been identified to explain sexual dysfunction. Unacknowledged or unidentified sexual orientation may lead to poor performance with the opposite sex, or the presence of one sexual problem may lead to another. For example, difficulty maintaining an erection may lead to hypoactive sexual desire. Education seems to have a buffering

TABLE 20.1 Medical Conditions and Surgical Procedures that Cause Sexual Dysfunction

System/State	Organic Disorders	Sexual Impairment
Endocrine	Hypothyroidism, adrenal dysfunction, hypogonadism, diabetes mellitus	Low libido, impotence, decreased vaginal lubrication, early impotence
Vascular	Hypertension, atherosclerosis, stroke, venous insufficiency, sickle cell disorder	Impotence, but ejaculation and libido intact
Neurological	Spinal cord damage, diabetic neuropathy, herniated disk, alcoholic neuropathy, multiple sclerosis, temporal lobe epilepsy	Sexual disorder—early signs: low or high libido, impotence, impaired orgasm
Genital	*Male*—Priapism, Peyronie's disease, urethritis, prostatitis, hydrocele	Low libido, impotence
	Female—Imperforate hymen, vaginitis, pelvic inflammatory disease, endometriosis	Genito-pelvic pain, low libido, decreased arousal
Systemic	Renal, pulmonary, hepatic, advanced malignancies, infections	Low libido, impotence, decreased arousal
Psychiatric	Depression	Low libido, erectile dysfunction
	Bipolar disorder (manic phase)	Increased libido
	Generalized anxiety disorder, panic disorder, posttraumatic stress disorder (PTSD), obsessive-compulsive disorder (OCD)	Low libido, erectile dysfunction, reduced vaginal lubrication, anorgasmia
	Schizophrenia	Low desire, bizarre sexual fantasies
	Personality disorders (passive-aggressive, obsessive-compulsive, histrionic)	Low libido, erectile dysfunction, premature ejaculation, anorgasmia
Surgical-postoperative	*Male*—Prostatectomy, abdominal-perineal bowel resection	Impotence, no loss of libido, ejaculatory impairment
	Female—Episiotomy, vaginal prolapse repair, oophorectomy	Genito-pelvic pain, decreased lubrication
	Male and female—Leg amputation, colostomy, ileostomy	Mechanical difficulties in sex, low self- image, fear of odor

Adapted from Shafer, L. C. (2016). Sexual disorders and sexual dysfunction. In T. A. Stern, M. Fava, T. E. Wilens, & J. F. Rosenbaum (Eds.), *Massachusetts General Hospital comprehensive clinical psychiatry* (2nd ed.). (pp. 401–411). Philadelphia, PA: Elsevier.

effect, and people who have more education have fewer sexual problems and are less anxious about issues pertaining to sex (Shafer, 2016).

APPLICATION OF THE NURSING PROCESS

ASSESSMENT

General Assessment

Sexual assessment includes both subjective and objective data. Many psychiatric hospitals use a nursing history tool that is biologically oriented and has few questions on sexual functioning. Health history questions pertaining to the reproductive system may be limited to menstrual history, parity, history of sexually transmitted diseases, method of contraception, and questions regarding safe sex practices. There may be a few vague questions about sexual functioning or sexual concerns.

Patients may cue the nurse into the presence of sexual concerns without explicitly verbalizing them. Box 20.2 presents a discussion of these cues.

The nurse may ask the patient if there is concern in the area of sexual functioning. Generally, it is more comfortable for the patient if the nurse first asks questions in a general manner and then proceeds to the patient's experience. For example, the nurse might say, "Some people who are prescribed this medication find it difficult to achieve an erection. Have you had this problem?" This allows the patient to feel that he is not alone in what he is experiencing. Table 20.2 provides facilitative statements for the interviewer conducting a sexual assessment.

The sexual history includes the patient's perception of physiological functioning and behavioral, emotional, and spiritual aspects of sexuality. It also includes cultural and religious beliefs with regard to sexual behavior and sexual knowledge base. During the assessment, both the nurse and the patient are free to ask questions and clarify information. It is reasonable to defer lengthy sexual health assessment when acute psychiatric symptoms prevent a calm thoughtful discussion. As symptoms subside and rapport is developed, the assessment may be resumed. With experience, the nurse is able to identify those patients who are at greater risk for difficulties in sexual functioning. This includes patients with a history of certain medical problems or surgical procedures (see Table 20.1) and patients taking some drugs (Table 20.3).

Self-Assessment

Discomfort in assessing sexual history may be due to poor training, inexperience, inadequate time, or beliefs that sexual history is not important. Indeed, you may experience discomfort exploring sexual issues with patients, fearing that this discussion will be personally embarrassing and embarrassing to the patient. You may fear that you will not know what questions to ask or why the questions should be asked.

BOX 20.2 Patient Cues that May Indicate Concerns about Sexuality

Nonverbal Behaviors

- Showing discomfort by blushing, looking away, making tight fists, fidgeting, crying
- Openly engaging in overt sexual behaviors (e.g., touching own body parts, masturbating, exposing genitals, placing nurse's hand on genitals, making sexually suggestive sounds)

Verbal Behaviors

- Telling sexually explicit jokes
- Making sexual comments about the nurse
- Asking inappropriate questions about the nurse's sexual activity
- Discussing sexual exploits
- Expressing concern about relationship with partner:
  - "I don't feel the same about my partner."
  - "My partner doesn't feel the same about me."
  - "We're not as close."
  - "Our relationship has changed."
  - "My personal life has changed."
- Expressing concern that sexuality has been diminished (e.g., feeling less of a man, less of a woman):
  - "I've lost my manhood."
  - "I'm not as desirable as I once was."
- Expressing concern over lack of sexual desire:
  - "I'm not interested in sex anymore."
  - "My desire has changed."
  - "I'm not the man/woman I used to be."
  - "We don't click anymore."
- Expressing concern over sexual performance:
  - "I've lost my power."
  - "What will happen to my ability to perform?"
  - "I can't perform like I used to."
- Expressing concern about one's love life:
  - "My love life has changed."
  - "The spark is gone."
- Expressing concern over the sexual impact of drugs, surgery, or some other medical treatment:
  - "Will this drug interfere with my sex life?"
  - "Will I still be able to perform sexually after surgery?"

Concerns related to age and gender differences are understandable. Maybe your patient is approximately your age and of the opposite sex. In this case, you might wonder whether talking about sexuality is inappropriate or whether the patient might decide that you are a little too interested. Discussing issues related to sexuality with people who are your parents' or grandparents' age may also create a level of discomfort, especially if you grew up in a home where such topics were avoided.

Remembering your position as a professional and addressing the topics in a tone and manner appropriate of a professional will increase your comfort, along with the patient's. Also, letting the patient know *why* you are asking such personal questions increases openness and cooperation. For example, "People who are depressed sometimes find that it affects their sexual desire. Because you have been depressed, have you noticed a change in your interest in sex?" Sometimes a more subtle approach that shifts the focus away from the patient is helpful. "Because you

TABLE 20.2 Facilitative Statements for the Interviewer Conducting a Sexual Assessment

Purpose	Facilitative Statement
To provide a rationale for a question	"As a nurse, I'm concerned about all aspects of your health. Many individuals have concern about sexual matters, especially when they are sick or having other health problems."
To give statements of generality or normality	"Most people are hesitant to discuss…" "Many people worry about feeling…" "Many people have concerns about…"
To identify sexual dysfunction	"Most people have difficulties sometime during their sexual relationships. What have yours been?"
To obtain information	"The degree to which unmarried people have sexual outlets varies considerably. Some have sexual partners. Some relieve sexual tension through masturbation. Others need no outlet at all. What has been your pattern?"
To identify sexual myths	"While growing up, most of us have heard some sexual myths or half-truths that continue to puzzle us. Are there any that come to mind?"
To determine whether homosexuality is a source of conflict	"What is your attitude toward your homosexual orientation?"
To identify an older person's concerns about sexual function	"Many people, as they get older, believe or worry that this signals the end of their sex life. Much misinformation continues this myth. What is your understanding about sexuality during the later years? How has the passage of time affected your sexuality (sex life)?"
To obtain and give information (miscellaneous areas)	"Frequently people have questions about…" "What questions do you have about…" "What would you like to know about…"
To close the history	"Is there anything further in the area of sexuality that you would like to bring up now?"

Adapted from Green, R. (1975). *Human sexuality: A health practitioner's text.* Baltimore, MD: Williams & Wilkins.

TABLE 20.3 Drugs that Can Cause Sexual Dysfunction

Category	Drug	Sexual Side Effects
Cardiovascular drugs	Methyldopa	Women: Amenorrhea, galactorrhea, decreased libido Men: Gynecomastia, impotence, decreased libido
	Thiazides	Women: Low libido, decreased lubrication Men: Low libido, impotence
	Clonidine	Men: Impotence, anorgasmia
	Propranolol	Men: Impotence
	Digoxin	Men: Gynecomastia
	Clofibrate	Women: Decreased libido Men: Decreased libido, impotence
	Statins	Men and women: Decreased libido
Gastrointestinal drugs	Cimetidine	Men: Decreased libido, impotence, gynecomastia, reduced sperm count
	Methantheline bromide	Men: Impotence
Sedatives	Alcohol	Women: Increased libido Men: Decreased libido, delayed ejaculation, gynecomastia, testicular atrophy
Antianxiety drugs	Alprazolam Diazepam	Women: Decreased libido, decreased orgasm Men: Impotence, decreased libido, delayed ejaculation
Antipsychotics	First generation antipsychotics	Women: Amenorrhea, galactorrhea Men: Retarded or retrograde ejaculation, impotence, gynecomastia, galactorrhea
	Second generation antipsychotics	Women: Amenorrhea, galactorrhea Men: Abnormal ejaculation, impotence, galactorrhea, gynecomastia
Antidepressants	SSRIs	Women: Lowering of sex drive, delayed or inability to reach orgasm Men: Delayed ejaculation and erectile dysfunction
	SNRIs	Women: Lowering of sex drive, delayed or absent orgasm Men: Erectile dysfunction and abnormal ejaculation
	Atypical (trazodone)	Men: Priapism (sustained erection in the absence of sexual stimuli)
	Tricyclics	Women: Breast enlargement and decreased orgasm Men: Erectile dysfunction and decreased orgasm
	MAOIs	Women: Vaginal dryness, inhibited orgasm Men: Impaired erection, inhibited orgasm
Antimanic drugs	Lithium	Men: Impaired erection

MAOIs, Monoamine oxidase inhibitors; *SSRIs,* selective serotonin reuptake inhibitors; *SNRIs,* serotonin norepinephrine reuptake inhibitors.
Data adapted from Shafer, L. C. (2016). Sexual disorders and sexual dysfunction. In T. A. Stern, M. Fava, T. E. Wilens, & J. F. Rosenbaum (Eds.), *Massachusetts General Hospital comprehensive clinical psychiatry* (2nd ed.). (pp. 401-411). Philadelphia, PA: Elsevier; US Food and Drug Administration. (2016). *Drugs.* Retrieved from http://www.fda.gov/Drugs/default.htm.

have been depressed, has your husband felt as if you are less interested in him?"

Perhaps the most helpful consideration is recognizing that assessing sexuality is part of holistic nursing care. Your role and responsibility is in assisting the patient in dealing with responses to illness and/or the treatment of the illness. Understanding your patient's concerns, acknowledging the patient's discomfort, and providing useful feedback will enhance your professional abilities to care for your patient and perhaps even improve self-understanding.

ASSESSMENT GUIDELINES

Sexual Dysfunction

1. A sexual assessment should be conducted in a setting that allows privacy and eliminates distractions.
2. Although note-taking may be necessary for the beginner, it can be distracting to the patient and interrupt the flow of the interview. When note-taking is necessary, it should be unobtrusive and kept to a minimum.
3. The interviewer should be aware of personal biases and attitudes that could block open discussion of sexual issues.
4. Good eye contact, relaxed posture, and friendly facial expressions facilitate the patient's comfort and communicate openness and receptivity on the part of the nurse.

DIAGNOSIS

A comprehensive sexual assessment can reveal areas of sexual concern and dysfunction for the patient. These data are analyzed to determine the appropriate nursing diagnoses. Priority nursing diagnoses, their definitions, and possible etiology follow (Herdman & Kamitsuru, 2014).

Sexual dysfunction is the state in which an individual experiences a change in sexual function during the sexual response phases of desire, excitation, and/or orgasm. The change is viewed as unsatisfying, unrewarding, or inadequate and may be related to the following:

- Altered body function from medication
- Biopsychosocial alteration of sexuality
- Psychological abuse from significant other

Ineffective sexuality pattern is indicated by expressions of concern regarding one's own sexuality. It may be related to the following:

- Lack of significant other
- Conflicts with sexual orientation
- Impaired relationship with significant other
- Knowledge deficit about alternative responses to illness

OUTCOMES IDENTIFICATION

The diagnosis of *sexual dysfunction* may be paired with *NOC* (Moorhead et al., 2013) outcomes listed under the category of sexual functioning. Each is ranked on a 5-point scale where 1 is "never demonstrated" and 5 is "consistently demonstrated." Examples of outcomes include:

- Attains sexual arousal
- Uses hormone replacement therapy as needed
- Expresses ability to be intimate

The diagnosis of *ineffective sexuality pattern* is linked by *NOC* with the outcome category sexual identity. Useful indicators (ranked the same way as the previous entry) include:

- Exhibits clear sense of sexual orientation
- Reports healthy intimate relationships
- Uses precautions to minimize risks associated with sexual activity

Table 20.4 provides signs and symptoms, nursing diagnoses, and outcomes for sexual disorders.

PLANNING

Planning nursing care for the patient with a sexual dysfunction may occur as part of care for a coexisting disorder. Nurses prepared at the basic level may encounter such patients when they are being treated for a variety of conditions in any setting.

IMPLEMENTATION

An understanding of sexual function and dysfunction is essential for nurses who work in psychiatry and most any specialty area in nursing including oncology, cardiology, and neurology.

TABLE 20.4 Signs and Symptoms, Diagnoses, and Outcomes for Sexual Dysfunction

Signs and Symptoms	Nursing Diagnoses	Outcomes
Alteration in achieving perceived sex role, alteration in relationship with significant other, changes in sexual activities and/or behaviors	*Ineffective sexuality pattern*	Attains sexual arousal, sustains arousal through orgasm, adapts sexual techniques as needed, expresses ability to be intimate, communicates comfortably with partner
Perceived alteration in sexual excitement and/or desire, limitations imposed by disease or therapy, inability to achieve desired satisfaction, verbalization of a problem	*Sexual dysfunction*	Discusses the side effect profile of various antidepressants on sexual functioning, expresses ability to be intimate

All nurses need to be able to facilitate a discussion about sexuality with the patient. To be a facilitator, the nurse must be nonjudgmental, have basic knowledge of sexual functioning, and have the ability to conduct a basic sexual assessment. Once the assessment is completed, the nurse needs to know when and to whom to refer the patient with a sexual complaint. Depending on the nature of the problem, the patient may need a referral to a professional such as a marital counselor, psychiatrist, gynecologist, urologist, clinical nurse specialist, or pastoral counselor.

Box 20.3 provides sample interventions from *Nursing Interventions Classification (NIC;* Bulechek et al., 2013) for sexual counseling.

BOX 20.3 *NIC* Interventions for Sexual Counseling

Definition: Use of an interactive helping process focusing on the need to make adjustments in sexual practice or to enhance coping with a sexual event or disorder.

*Activities**:

- Establish a therapeutic relationship based on trust and respect.
- Provide privacy and ensure confidentiality.
- Discuss the effect of the illness or health situation on sexuality.
- Discuss the effect of medications on sexuality, as appropriate.
- Avoid displaying aversion to an altered body part.
- Provide factual information about sexual myths and misinformation that patients may verbalize.
- Provide reassurance that current and new sexual practices are healthy, as appropriate.
- Include the spouse/sexual partner in the counseling as much as possible, as appropriate.
- Refer patient to a sex therapist, as appropriate.

*Partial list.
Data from Bulechek, G. M., Butcher, H. K., Dochterman, J. M., & Wagner, C. (Eds.). (2013). *Nursing interventions classification (NIC;* 6th ed.). St. Louis, MO: Mosby.

Pharmacological Interventions

Treatments for sexual dysfunction are increasingly becoming the target of pharmaceutical industries. Despite the fact that women with sexual dysfunction greatly outnumber men, most of the available pharmacological treatment for sexual dysfunction is aimed at men. There is one medication approved by the US Food and Drug Administration (FDA) for female sexual disorders. Table 20.5 summarizes treatments for sexual dysfunction.

Pharmacological treatments are available for lifelong premature ejaculation. These treatments include antidepressants in the selective serotonin reuptake inhibitors (SSRIs) category or topical anesthetics. Pharmacotherapy may *cause* erectile dysfunction, and medications may need to be evaluated for change or dose reduction. Erectile dysfunction may also have a biological cause and/or psychogenic etiology. Several strategies for combatting antidepressant-induced sexual dysfunction include the following:

- Waiting to see whether sexual side effects decrease over the course of several weeks.
- Reducing the dose of the antidepressant.

TABLE 20.5 Pharmacological, Psychosocial, and Other Treatments for Sexual Dysfunction

Sexual Disorder	Pharmacological Treatment	Psychosocial Approaches	Other
Male hypoactive sexual desire disorder	Testosterone for males with low levels of this hormone	Individual therapy Couples therapy	
Female sexual interest/arousal disorder	Flibanserin (Addyi)* Testosterone patch for menopausal females Alprostadil cream Lubrication (K-Y Jelly)	Sensate focus exercises Individual therapy Couples therapy	EROS-CTD clitoral suction device* Lubrication (e.g., K-Y Jelly)
Male erectile disorder	Sildenafil (Viagra)* Tadalafil (Cialis)* Vardenafil (Levitra)* Avanafil (Stendra)* Alprostadil (MUSE)* penile self-injection and intraurethral suppository Testosterone (for hypogonadism)	Sensate focus exercises Group therapy Hypnotherapy Systematic desensitization Psychodynamic therapy Couples therapy	Vacuum pump Penile prostheses
Female orgasmic disorder	Sildenafil (Viagra)	Masturbation training Couples therapy Kegel vaginal exercises	
Male orgasmic disorder	Sildenafil (Viagra)	Masturbatory training Systematic desensitization	
Premature ejaculation	(None with FDA approval) SSRIs to delay or retard ejaculation Topical anesthetics	Start-stop technique Squeeze technique Increased sexual frequency	

*FDA approved.
Data adapted from Shafer, L. C. (2016). Sexual disorders and sexual dysfunction. In T. A. Stern, M. Fava, T.E. Wilens, & J. F. Rosenbaum (Eds.), *Massachusetts General Hospital comprehensive clinical psychiatry* (2nd ed.). (pp. 401–411). Philadelphia, PA: Elsevier; US Food and Drug Administration. (2016). *A to Z index.* Retrieved from http://www.fda.gov/Drugs/.

- Planning for sexual activity before taking the antidepressant if the dosing is once a day.
- For men, using phosphodiesterase inhibitors such as Viagra.
- Switching antidepressants to one with a more favorable side effect profile such as mirtazapine (Remeron), bupropion (Wellbutrin), or vilazodone (Viibryd).

EVIDENCE-BASED PRACTICE

How Does Sexting Impact Teenagers?

Problem

Sexting, as most people know, is exchanging sexually suggestive pictures or messages by cell phones or social networking sites. The practice has received tremendous attention. While some people view the activity as mostly harmless, the media are full of warnings about sexting. We have all heard of social devastation when compromising photos or texts are circulated around the school or workplace.

Purpose of Study

Our knowledge of risk factors and outcomes from sexting behaviors has not been established. In this study researchers explored which impulsivity-related traits and expectations influence sexting behaviors. They also examined the prevalence and perceived likelihood of sexting resulting in negative outcomes.

Methods

Researchers used a convenience sample of 611 undergraduate college students. Mean age in the sample was 21.2; about 77% were female and Caucasian. Students completed the following instruments: the Sexting Behaviors Scale, Sexpectancies Measure, the Impulsive Behavior Scale, and a Sexual Hookup Questionnaire.

Key Findings

- Eighty percent of undergraduates report having received sext messages, while 67% report having sent messages.
- Forty-six percent of undergraduates have received picture sexts, while 64% report having sent sexually suggestive images.
- Positive expectations about the outcome (e.g., hooking up) of sexting may drive the behavior, prompting the individual to overlook possible consequences.
- Negative outcomes were rare: Sexts being spread to others was the most common negative sexting experience.

Implications for Nursing Practice

The current generation of undergraduate students may have a more relaxed attitude toward sexting than previous generations. No matter the climate, sexuality and intimacy are sensitive and associated with intense emotions. Nurses should keep themselves current on trends such as sexting and help young people and patients cope with the potential stressors of social media.

Dir, A. L., & Cyders, M. A. (2015). Risks, risk factors, and outcomes associated with phone and internet sexting among university students in the United States. *Archives of Sexual Behavior, 44*(6), 1675–1684.

Health Teaching and Health Promotion

Nurses should help patients weigh the pros and cons of any type of pharmacotherapy. Many drugs cause sexual side effects, and notably psychotropic medications used for psychiatric disorders are common offenders. Nurses tend to ignore or minimize the sexual side effects associated with these medications, perhaps in an attempt to promote adherence. Helping patients to evaluate for themselves the benefits versus the risks of pharmacotherapy empowers them to choose the best course of action that increases their ability to be informed consumers of mental health services.

Advanced Practice Interventions

Advanced practice psychiatric-mental health registered nurses can be qualified to treat sexual dysfunction through advanced training and certification. General therapies include psychoanalytic therapy, couples therapy, group therapy, and hypnotherapy. Some specific therapies available for sexual dysfunction include the following:

- **Sensate focus:** A therapeutic treatment in which patients progress from general touching and cuddling without intercourse to more intimate forms of expression.
- **Behavioral therapy:** Useful for men with premature ejaculation when psychogenic or relationship factors are present and is often best combined with medication in an integrated treatment program.
- **Systematic desensitization:** Involves combining relaxation exercises with sexually anxiety-producing stimuli.
- **Masturbation training:** Especially helpful in women who have never had an orgasm. This approach helps women learn about their bodies and their responses to understand their sexual responsiveness.

VIGNETTE: Maria is a 67-year-old woman, widowed many years, who has recently been approached by a 75-year-old widower with a marriage proposal. Maria is concerned about the sexual implications of a marriage so late in life. She confides in her nurse practitioner, "I really haven't even thought about sex for so many years. I know Joe is just an old goat. He's always after me to take my clothes off." After discussing the possibility of a physiological cause for her lack of interest in sex, Maria's nurse practitioner gives her small doses of testosterone. Within a remarkably short time, Maria stops talking about Joe as "an old goat" and begins talking again about how great life can be with the right partner.

EVALUATION

Evaluation of expected outcomes relates to the level of control and personal satisfaction achieved. Acceptance of sexual dysfunction (e.g., impotence) as being part—but not necessarily the defining characteristic—of sexual behavior can result in greater satisfaction. The degree to which negative attitudes about sex are no longer problematic is also important.

GENDER DYSPHORIA

CLINICAL PICTURE

When we inquire about the birth of an infant, we want to know if it is a boy or a girl. We are asking about the sex of the child (i.e., whether its chromosomes are XX or XY). However, **gender identity**, the sense of maleness or femaleness, is not usually established until a child is about 3 years old.

People tend to be comfortable with the fact that they are male or female. Unfortunately, biological assignment does not necessarily determine whether individuals think of themselves as male or female. When biological sex differs from gender identity, the individual may suffer from **gender dysphoria**, or feelings of unease about their incongruent maleness or femaleness. A man might describe himself as "a woman trapped in a man's body."

It should be noted that gender dysphoria is no longer considered a psychiatric disorder. Until quite recently, this problem was known as *gender identity disorder*, and all transgender people would be considered mentally ill based on the disorder's criteria (Beredjick, 2012).

Symptoms in children include expressions of desire to be the opposite sex. Some children insist that they *are* the opposite sex and ask their families to call them by another name. Only a small percentage of children who display gender dysphoria characteristics will continue to show these characteristics into adolescence or adulthood. More intense childhood symptoms are associated with persistence of the dysphoria into adulthood (Steensma et al., 2013).

Teenagers and adults may also verbalize a desire to be the other sex and to be treated as such. Dressing up and passing for the opposite sex is common. Adolescents may dread the appearance of secondary sexual characteristics and (along with adults) may seek hormones or surgery to alter their masculinity or femininity. These individuals do not usually consider themselves to be homosexual. The biological female who falls in love with a woman believes she is actually a man who loves a woman.

EPIDEMIOLOGY

Gender dysphoria is extremely uncommon. For adult individuals born male, the prevalence is estimated from 0.005% to 0.014%. For adult individuals born female, the prevalence is lower ranging from 0.002 to 0.003%. Research regarding this population is sparse in the United States. However, a Swedish study (Dhejne et al., 2014) tracked sex reassignment by gender over a 50-year period. During that time, 429 male-to-females and 252 female-to-males underwent this procedure.

COMORBIDITY

Children with gender dysphoria may also have anxiety, disruptive and impulse-control problems, and depressive disorders. Autism spectrum disorder has also been associated with gender dysphoria. In adolescents and adults, anxiety disorders are most common followed by mood disorders. Substance use and self-destructive behavior are also common parallels found in people suffering from gender dysphoria.

RISK FACTORS

Biological Factors

While biological factors are not thought to *cause* this problem, they are believed to influence its development. Hormones may play a role as decreased levels of testosterone in males and increased levels in women are associated with gender dysphoria.

There is some evidence to suggest a genetic linkage. Heylens and colleagues (2012) studied concordance rates in monozygotic (identical) and dizygotic (fraternal) twins. Monozygotic twins had a concordance rate for gender dysphoria at 39%. This means that 39% of the time when one twin has the problem, the other does too. No concordance was found for fraternal twins.

Psychosocial Factors

Learning theorists suggest the absence of same-sex role models may contribute to gender dysphoria. In this scenario, caregivers provide either covert or overt approval for cross-gender identification and behaviors.

Psychoanalytic theorists have posited that male children who are deprived of their mothers seek to internally meld or become one with their mothers. This melding prevents them from developing fully as a separate entity.

NURSING CARE FOR GENDER DYSPHORIA

Individuals dealing with gender dysphoria may feel profound social and internal guilt and shame related to their sexual proclivities. "I am disgusted by how hairy my body is" and "I have never wanted to be macho; I have always been sensitive and caring." A nursing diagnosis that goes along with this problem includes *disturbed personal identity* related to incongruence between expressed (beliefs) and assigned (inborn) gender. Outcomes include seeking social support, using healthy coping behaviors to resolve sexual identity issues, and acknowledging and accepting sexual identity.

Advanced Interventions

Psychotherapy

Children. There is lack of consensus as to the best approach in treating children. However, the goal is to optimize the child's psychological adjustment and well-being. One approach is to let the child identify with the opposite gender and provide support for the stresses of familial and peer responses (e.g., bullying). Another is to accept the parents' goal of having the child accept his natal gender and then working on making him comfortable it. In this approach, family dynamics are also examined for their role in perpetuating the cross-gender behavior. Another family-directed approach is to provide supportive therapy while waiting to see whether the dysphoria will continue.

Adolescents and adults. Gender dysphoria in adolescents will likely continue into adulthood. Individual and family therapy is helpful. Adolescents will need help with coping skills to deal with harassment. Long-term psychotherapy is recommended to address gender dysphoria and comorbid conditions (Shafer, 2016). A thorough psychological evaluation is commonly required before sex reassignment.

Pharmacological

Pharmacological interventions in adolescents may be used to delay puberty. Supporters of this reversible approach suggest that this gives adolescents time to explore gender-related issues.

Adults with gender dysphoria may choose to take hormones to alter their chemistry toward their preferred gender. A female who would like to become a male takes testosterone.

This results in more muscle, facial hair, clitoral enlargement, amenorrhea, and increased sex drive. When a male takes estrogen, it results in decreased penis and testicles size, less muscle, more fat on the hips, less facial and body hair, and slight increase in breast size.

Surgical

When gender dysphoria in adults and even adolescents is severe and intractable sex reassignment surgery is an option. If the patient is considered appropriate for sex reassignment, psychotherapy is usually initiated to prepare the patient for the cross-gender role. The patient is then instructed to live in the cross-gender role before surgery—including going to work or attending school—to help the individual determine whether he or she can interact successfully with members of society in the cross-gender mode.

Legal and social arrangements are made such as changing names on legal documents. New employment may be sought if it is necessary to leave a former job because of discrimination. Relationship issues, such as what to tell parents, children, and former spouses, must be addressed. Males are instructed to have electrolysis and to practice female behaviors. Females are instructed to cut their hair, bind or conceal their breasts, and similarly take on the identity of a man.

If these measures have been successful and the patient still wishes reassignment, hormone treatment is begun. After a period of time on hormone therapy, the patient may be considered for surgical reassignment if it is still desired.

In men, surgery may include removal of the penis (penectomy) and testes (orchiectomy) and the addition of a vagina (vaginoplasty). In females, surgical procedures may include the removal of the breasts (mastectomy), optional removal of the uterus (hysterectomy) and ovaries (oophorectomy), and the construction of a penis (phalloplasty) in females. Efforts to create an artificial penis have met with mixed results.

Do people regret having sex reassignment surgery? In a study by Dhejne and colleagues (2014), regret for the surgery was found in only about 2% of people who underwent sex reassignment surgery. Still psychotherapy is indicated after surgery to help the patient adjust to the surgical changes and discuss sexual functioning and satisfaction. Box 20.4 describes a case of sex reassignment gone wrong.

PARAPHILIC DISORDERS

People do not consciously decide what arouses them sexually. Rather, during the maturation process they discover the nature of their own sexual orientation and interests. Individuals differ from one another in terms of the types of partners they find to be erotically appealing and the types of behaviors they find to be erotically stimulating. They also differ in the intensity of the sexual drive, in the degree of difficulty they experience in trying to resist sexual urges, and in their attitudes about whether or not such urges should be resisted.

Sexual disorders include many forms of paraphilic disorders. This term refers to acts or sexual stimuli that are outside of what society considers normal but are required for some individuals to experience desire, arousal, and orgasm. Criteria for being diagnosed with this category of disorders include whether the symptoms occur for at least 6 months. A disorder is characterized by discomfort in the individual or persistent risk or danger to themselves or others.

A small segment of individual with paraphilic disorders actually commit sexual offenses. Many people who meet criteria for paraphilic disorders do not act on their sexual feelings (Sorrentino, 2016).

BOX 20.4 Nature or Nurture? A Case of Sex Reassignment Gone Wrong

Accidents in early infancy may result in sex reassignment. One such fascinating case is that of David Reimer, a Canadian-born identical twin male whose penis was destroyed as the result of a botched circumcision. With the advice of healthcare professionals, the child underwent surgical reassignment and later received hormonal therapy in puberty to induce the development of breasts and secondary female sex characteristics.

While the family psychologist proclaimed the reassignment from male to female a success and concluded that gender identity was primarily based on socialization, David never felt comfortable. He rejected his female designation of Brenda and began living his life as a male at age 14. Shortly after he learned of his biological sex, he had the reassignment surgically reversed, married a woman, and became stepfather to her three children.

However, David always felt uncomfortable and ultimately committed suicide. His case bolstered support for the biological influence of prenatal and early-life exposure to male hormones on gender identity. David Reimer's life is chronicled in the book *As Nature Made Him*, which raises questions about gender reassignment and the modification of an unconsenting minor's genitals.

From Colapinto, J. (2006). *As nature made him: The boy who was raised as a girl.* New York, NY: Harper Collins.

EXHIBITIONISTIC DISORDER

Exhibitionistic disorder involves illegal activity with the intentional display of the genitals in a public place. Almost 100% of cases of **exhibitionism** involve a man exposing himself to a woman or to women. This may occur as a man walks around exposed in a busy shopping mall or exposes himself on a doorstep after ringing the doorbell. Excitement results from the anticipation of the act, and the individual masturbates during or after exposing himself. The exhibitionist becomes aroused by observers' responses of shock and even disgust, and some fantasize that the person will also be aroused by the experience and actually want to be with them sexually.

On the other hand, some people with exhibitionistic disorder may experience deep shame and judge themselves by the same standard that society does and consider themselves perverts. They may cover their actions and live in intense fear that they will be recognized and shame themselves and their families.

Although these behaviors are illegal, it seems to be done more for shock value than as a precursor to sexual assault or rape.

Actual contact is rarely sought. Because few people are arrested for this behavior after age 40, we speculate that it resolves with age (Shafer, 2016).

FETISHISTIC DISORDER

The term fetish is derived from a Portuguese word, *feitico*, which means obsessive fascination. **Fetishistic disorder** is characterized by a sexual focus on objects—such as shoes, gloves, pantyhose, and stockings—that are intimately associated with the human body. Preferred items are shoes, leather or latex items, and underclothing. Basically, it is becoming aroused by something that would not normally arouse other people.

This disorder is far more common in men and is almost unheard of in women. Fetishes may replace sexual partners or the fetish may be a component of sexual activity. Fetishes may become all-consuming and destructive. Many people have fetishes. However, to be diagnosed with a fetishistic disorder, the person needs to experience significant distress or become impaired in his or her overall functioning due to the fetish.

FROTTEURISTIC DISORDER

Rubbing or touching a nonconsenting person characterizes **frotteuristic disorder**. In fact, the word **frotteurism** originates from the French word *frotter*, which means to "rub or scrape." The disorder is usually seen in men. The behavior typically occurs in busy public places, particularly in subways and buses, where the individual can escape after touching his victim. People with this disorder often have no close relationships, and this sort of aggressive contact is their only means of sexual gratification.

PEDOPHILIC DISORDER

Pedophilic disorder is, unfortunately, the most common paraphilic disorder. It involves a predominant or exclusive sexual interest toward prepubescent children (generally 13 years or younger). Sexual fantasies can lead some individuals to seek physical contact with these sexually immature children. A subtype of this disorder refers to pubescents between ages 11 and 14. Termed *hebephilia*, this attraction is unacceptable in most cultures and represents a profound violation of the boundaries of childhood. Critics of pathologizing this attraction to pubescent young people by calling it a mental disorder say that adults have always had sexual interest in this age group and that it is a legal issue and not a disorder.

Because pedophilia is illegal, its exact incidence is unknown. For the definition of pedophilia to be met, the perpetrator must be at least 16 years of age and at least 5 years older than the victim. The nature of the child molestation ranges from undressing and looking at the child, to genital fondling or oral sex, to penetration, and even torture.

HEALTH POLICY

Registered Nurse Advocacy: Eliminating Statutes of Limitations for Reporting Childhood Sexual Abuse

Victims of sexual abuse are reluctant to report the crimes, particularly if someone close abuses them. It may take years or even decades to come to terms with what happened. Unfortunately, statutes of limitations put in place to encourage the timely reporting of crimes reduce the chances that perpetrators will be stopped.

Famous high-profile cases such as those involving comedian Bill Cosby and allegations against the Catholic Church have encouraged activists to challenge these old laws. Forty-three states have statutes of limitations for sex crimes (RAINN, 2016). Of the states with statutes, 27 of them allow for charges to be filed when DNA evidence is involved. Legislation increasing these statues is being considered in California, Illinois, New York, Oklahoma, and Pennsylvania.

Beitsch, R. (2016). *High profile cases spur states to reconsider statutes of limitation for rape. KTOO Public Media.* Retrieved from http://www.ktoo.org/2016/06/02/high-profile-cases-spur-states-reconsider-statutes-limitations-rape/; RAINN. (2016). *About sexual assault.* Retrieved from https://rainn.org/about-sexual-assault.

SEXUAL SADISM DISORDER AND SEXUAL MASOCHISM DISORDER

Sexual sadism is a term derived from the Marquis de Sade (1740–1814), a well-known French writer who was obsessed with sexual violence. This disorder involves the achievement of sexual satisfaction from the physical or psychological suffering (including humiliation) of the victim. The sadist inflicts pain and suffering on (usually) nonconsenting people.

Consenting partners for sadists may be sexual masochists. **Sexual masochism** involves the achievement of sexual satisfaction by being humiliated, beaten, bound, or otherwise made to suffer. Sexual masochistic practices are more common among men than among women. In either case, participants tend to know this is a "game," and actual humiliation or pain is avoided.

TRANSVESTIC DISORDER

In **transvestic disorder,** sexual satisfaction is achieved by dressing in the clothing of the opposite gender. This behavior is related to **fetishism** but often goes beyond the use of one particular object. Generally, this behavior develops early in life and is associated with someone with whom the person is closely associated, whether in a loving relationship or through abuse. Unlike gender dysphoria, there are no sexual orientation issues, and people with transvestic disorder do not desire a sex change. Transvestites are usually heterosexual. Many cross-dress only in specific sexual situations, and they often receive the cooperation and support of their partners. This paraphilia is more common in men than in women. Over time, some men, as well as some women, with transvestic disorder desire to dress and live permanently as the opposite sex.

VOYEURISTIC DISORDER

Voyeurism is another illegal activity that begins in adolescence or early adulthood. It is characterized by seeking sexual arousal through viewing, usually secretly, other people in intimate situations (e.g., naked, in the process of disrobing, or engaging in sexual activity). In the language of the layperson, this behavior is called being a *peeping Tom.* Voyeuristic disorder often begins in adolescence and may become a chronic condition and the only type of sexual activity for the person. Voyeurism may be driven by anger and a need to retaliate. Typically, people who engage in voyeurism also engage in other compulsive sexual behavior and are frequently addicted to pornography and going to strip clubs.

Like an exhibitionist, a person who engages in voyeurism may also be consumed by dissonance. The drive to engage in this activity does not make sense, considering the lengths to which the voyeur goes and the risks taken. "Why am I throwing away 2 or 3 hours staring through these binoculars on the off chance that I will see somebody naked when I can rent a movie, buy a magazine, or even find a real relationship? I must be such a loser." As with all obsessions and compulsions, the shame and anxiety is temporarily relieved by engaging in the very activity that brings it about.

PARAPHILIC DISORDER NOT OTHERWISE SPECIFIED

Other paraphilic disorders include various problems that do not meet the criteria for the other categories. Included in this grouping are:

- **Telephone scatalogia disorder:** Obscene phone calling to an unsuspecting person or sending obscene messages or video images by e-mail
- **Necrophilic disorder:** Obsession with having a sexual encounter with a cadaver
- **Zoophilic disorder:** Incorporation of animals into sexual activity
- **Coprophilic disorder:** Fixation on feces in sexual encounters
- **Klismaphilic disorder:** Sexual activity that incorporates enemas
- **Urophilic disorder:** Sexual activity that involves urinating on one's partner or being urinated on
- **Hypoxyphilia:** Desire to achieve an altered state of consciousness secondary to hypoxia while experiencing orgasm; a drug such as nitrous oxide may be used to produce hypoxia

Many of the people involved in nonstandard sexual practices find no need for therapy because their sexual activities are carried out with a consenting adult partner, and they are neither illegal nor physically or emotionally harmful to either partner. If, however, the person is experiencing relationship difficulties, wishes to change the sexual behaviors, becomes involved in illegal activity, or is physically or emotionally harming others or being harmed, therapy is indicated.

EPIDEMIOLOGY

Although the paraphilic disorders are uncommon, the repetitive and consuming nature of the disorders make the occurrence highly frequent (Sadock et al., 2015). Most people with paraphilic disorders are Caucasian males, and in about 50% of these individuals, the onset of the paraphilic arousal is before age 18 years. The average age of onset is between 8 and 12. The behaviors associated with the disorder tend to peak in the decade between 15 and 25 years of age and then become virtually nonexistent by age 50. Patients with paraphilic disorders often have more than one paraphilia, which can occur simultaneously or at different points in their lives.

COMORBIDITY

Attention-deficit/hyperactivity disorder (ADHD) in childhood, substance abuse, phobic disorders, and major depression/dysthymia are strongly associated with paraphilic disorders (Shafer, 2016). A significant number of pedophiles have previous or current involvement in voyeurism, exhibitionism, or rape. Men with paraphilic disorders may have concurrent sexual arousal disorders related to ambivalence created by an altered sexual focus toward the object of their desire (Ahlers et al., 2009). Researchers believe that substance abuse is strongly associated with sex offenses. In one study (Kraanen & Emmelkamp, 2011), nearly 50% of sex offenders misused alcohol, 20% had a history of drug abuse, and 25% were intoxicated at the time of their offense.

RISK FACTORS

Biological Factors

A variety of theories attempt to identify what predisposes an individual to the development of paraphilic disorders, but these theories are far from conclusive as they have focused primarily on violent offenders. Sexual problems can result from head trauma. Patients who have experienced head trauma with damage to the frontal lobe of the brain may display symptoms of promiscuity, poor judgment, inability to recognize triggers that set off sexual desires, and poor impulse control. Inappropriate sexual arousal has been linked to abnormal levels of androgens.

Psychosocial Factors

Psychoanalytic theories suggest that castration anxiety results in a safer substitution of a symbolic object for the mother, which results in fetishism and transvestism. The need for a safe substitute may result in extreme behaviors such as pedophilia, exhibitionism, and voyeurism.

Learning theorists explain paraphilic disorders in terms of timing and reinforcement. During vulnerable periods, especially puberty, sexual exploration is common. If it is pleasurable and there are no negative consequences, the activity becomes reinforced and is repeated. For example, if an adolescent boy experiments sexually with a 7-year-old boy, does not get caught, and continues to fantasize, he may develop arousal to young boys.

Cognitive theorists identify paraphilic disorders as being based on cognitive distortions. Errors in thought make it seem acceptable for deviant and destructive sexual behaviors to occur. For example, belief that there is agreement on the part of a child makes it okay in the individual's mind to have relations with her; or watching others engage in sexual relations is okay "as long as no one gets hurt." Perhaps the perpetrator of exhibitionistic behavior believes that young girls may get as excited as he does when he exposes himself.

APPLICATION OF THE NURSING PROCESS

ASSESSMENT

General Assessment

Patients with paraphilic disorders rarely are hospitalized as a direct result of their condition. However, people with paraphilic disorders may be overrepresented in psychiatric care settings, due to the frequency of comorbid psychiatric conditions that are undoubtedly exacerbated by the sexual disorder. Nurses who work in forensic settings such as prisons and jails may care for inmates who are imprisoned due to consequences of paraphilic disorders. Depression with suicidal ideation and substance use are common comorbid conditions and should be assessed using principles outlined in Chapters 22 and 25.

During a thorough assessment for any psychiatric disorder (or medical condition as well), you may discover symptoms of one of the paraphilic disorders. For example, you may ask a patient about his family, and he may remark that he and his wife "aren't getting along so great lately." As you explore this area of concern further, he reveals, "My wife wants to do the same old boring things...you know...sexually, all the time." As the assessment continues, you may learn that he is focused on sadistic sorts of activities, is obsessed with pornography, and no longer becomes aroused by his wife.

Self-Assessment

It is reasonable for students to read descriptions of sexual disorders and respond with disgust to objectionable behaviors. It is also common to respond with frustration, anger, and hostility toward people with disorders such as sexual masochism and pedophilia. A major issue is trying to understand human behavior and where to place the blame. Where do we draw the line between considering a person to be a victim of life experiences and considering him to be responsible for his actions?

Providing care for someone who has abused others may be nearly impossible for certain individuals. We may have known someone who was the victim of a voyeur or a pedophile or we may personally have been victimized. Exploring paraphilic disorders, even in an academic context, may evoke significant distress. At this point, talking with a faculty member, a primary care provider, or someone at a mental health clinic can be helpful and important and may even result in better personal understanding and coping.

ASSESSMENT GUIDELINES

Paraphilic Disorders

1. Assess the potential for self-harm because patients with paraphilic disorders may become despondent and be more of a suicide risk.
2. The main focus of the assessment should be on the presenting problem (e.g., depression with suicidal ideation).
3. Elicit the patient's perception of the impact of the sexual disorder upon the current illness.

DIAGNOSIS

Nursing diagnoses for individuals with paraphilic disorder include *risk for suicide, other-directed violence, ineffective impulse control,* and *ineffective sexuality pattern.* Other diagnoses should be considered depending upon the comorbid psychiatric condition that has precipitated the admission.

OUTCOMES IDENTIFICATION

NOC (Moorhead et al., 2013) identifies a number of outcomes for patients with either ineffective sexuality patterns or risk for other-directed violence. Included are *sexual identity* and *impulse self-control.* Table 20.6 provides signs and symptoms, nursing diagnoses, and outcomes for paraphilias.

PLANNING

The setting and presenting problem influence the planning of nursing care for the patient with a paraphilic disorder. The basic-level registered nurse may encounter such a patient during treatment for a comorbid condition especially when the patient is admitted to the hospital for suicidal thoughts and behavior. Sometimes psychiatric care and treatment are mandated such as when a voyeur or exhibitionist gets caught.

The care plan will focus on safety and crisis intervention. The patient may also be treated for comorbid depression or anxiety disorders in the community setting. Planning will address the major complaint along with the sexual disorder.

IMPLEMENTATION

Interventions are aimed at offering a nonjudgmental emotional presence while exploring identity issues, self-esteem, and anxiety and encouraging an optimal level of functioning. Patients with a potential for violating the boundaries of others may require closer observation and firm limit setting. Box 20.5 lists examples of basic-level *NIC* interventions for paraphilic disorders.

Health Teaching and Health Promotion

Education is typically geared toward reducing symptoms from the presenting problem, typically depression and anxiety. Patients with paraphilic disorders can be taught to journal

TABLE 20.6 Signs and Symptoms, Diagnoses, and Outcomes for Sexual Disorders

Signs and Symptoms	Nursing Diagnoses	Outcomes
History of exposing self to others, deep remorse and shame over behavior, wants to control the fantasies, urges, and resultant behaviors	*Ineffective impulse control*	Identifies feelings that lead to impulsive actions, consequences of actions, and alternatives; practices self-restraint of impulsive behaviors
Lacks interest for his spouse, feels an increasing attraction to prepubescent girls, history of arrests	*Risk for other-directed violence (sexual)*	Identifies triggers for maladaptive sexual fantasies and describes techniques to control these fantasies; practices self-restraint of sexual urges and behaviors
Shame when dressing like a woman, fears loss of community respect, wife found a suicide note, increasingly unable to control sexual impulses	*Risk for suicide*	Expresses a determination to live and a sense of control; identifies strategies to manage his urges, refrains from self-destructive urges
Alteration in relationship with significant other, reports difficulties with sexual activities, values conflict	*Ineffective sexuality pattern*	Seeks social support, reports healthy sexual functioning, sets personal sexual boundaries

From Herdman, T. H., & Kamitsuru, S. (Ed.). (2014). *Nursing diagnoses—Definitions and classification 2015–2017.* Copyright © 2014, 1994-2014 by NANDA International. Used by arrangement with John Wiley & Sons Limited; Moorhead, S., Johnson, M., Maas, M. L., & Swanson, E. (2013). *Nursing outcomes classification (NOC*; 5th ed.). St. Louis, MO: Mosby.

BOX 20.5 *NIC* Interventions for Paraphilic Disorders

Behavior Management: Sexual

Definition: Delineation and prevention of socially unacceptable sexual behaviors

*Activities**:

- Discuss consequences of unacceptable behavior.
- Discuss the negative impact that behavior has on others.
- Encourage expression of feelings about past crises.
- Provide opportunities for caregivers to process their feelings about the patient.

Self-Esteem Enhancement

Definition: Assisting a patient to increase his/her personal judgment of self-worth

*Activities**:

- Encourage patient to identify strengths.
- Assist in setting realistic goals to achieve higher self-esteem.
- Assist patient to accept dependence on others, as appropriate.
- Explore previous achievements of success.
- Encourage patient to accept new challenges.

Social Skills Behavior Modification

Definition: Assisting the patient to develop or improve interpersonal social skills

*Activities**:

- Assist in identifying problems resulting from social skill deficits.
- Encourage verbalization of feelings regarding social interaction.
- Identify a specific skill to improve.
- Identify steps to reach skill and role-play the steps.

*Partial list.

Data from Bulechek, G. M., Butcher, H. K., & Dochterman, J. M. (Eds.). (2013). *Nursing interventions classification (NIC*; 6th ed.). St. Louis, MO: Mosby.

their feelings and to begin to identify triggers for pathological behavior.

Teamwork and Safety

When the patient who has a paraphilic disorder is in a crisis that requires hospitalization, providing a safe environment is fundamental. All patients on a psychiatric inpatient unit should be informed on admission about unit rules regarding personal contact between patients and between patients and staff. Limit setting is done consistently when it is needed, and staff work together as a team to this end.

Individuals with paraphilic disorders tend to isolate themselves. The unit environment may be a challenge. Sharing meals with others may result in discomfort, and the patient might wonder what other people are thinking about him or her. A particular challenge may be interacting in formal group settings and the expectation of participation. But the group setting may actually provide patients with the greatest opportunity for growth in that they can experience others as humans with feelings, perhaps learning how much anguish and pain personal violations have caused them. The group milieu can mean having others present who empathize with one's background and current distress.

Pharmacological Interventions

Two classes of pharmacological agents, antiandrogens and serotonergic antidepressants, may be prescribed for paraphilic disorders (Garcia et al., 2013). Medication is not used independently without other interventions. Drugs that reduce levels of testosterone may be used to treat sex offenders. The drugs that are frequently used are progestin derivatives including medroxyprogesterone acetate (MPA; an analog of progesterone) and cyproterone acetate (CPA; an inhibitor of testosterone). Both of these drugs act to decrease libido and reduce compulsive deviant sexual behavior. They work best in patients with paraphilic disorders and a high sexual drive, such as pedophiles and exhibitionists, and less well in those with a low sexual drive or an antisocial personality (Becker et al., 2014).

SSRIs are also used off-label without specific FDA approval in the treatment of sexual disorders. Fluoxetine (Prozac) has been used successfully to treat patients with exhibitionism, voyeurism, and pedophilia and people who have committed rape. These drugs may work to improve mood, reduce impulsivity, decrease sexual obsessions, and cause sexual dysfunction. In addition to fluoxetine, other drugs, such as clomipramine (Anafranil) and fluvoxamine (Luvox), have been used in the treatment of sexual obsessions, addictions, and paraphilic disorders.

Advanced Practice Interventions

Psychotherapy

The usual treatment plan for working with patients with paraphilic disorders is cognitive-behavioral therapy. An attempt is made to help the person learn a new sexual response pattern that will eliminate the need for the activity that is causing the problem. Techniques range from positive reinforcement for appropriate object choices to aversion techniques, in which mild electrical shocks may be applied for inappropriate choices. Other treatment modalities include psychodynamic techniques designed to help the patient understand the origin of the paraphilia.

Advanced practice psychiatric-mental health registered nurses may seek specialized training to enable them to work effectively with patients with gender dysphorias and paraphilic disorders. This preparation allows the nurse to practice sex therapy and conduct sex research. The American Association of Sex Educators, Counselors, and Therapists (AASECT) provides credentialing based on academic preparation, clinical supervision, experience, and skills. Credentialing is a method by which consumers of mental healthcare services can be assured of the professional competency of the therapist treating them.

EVALUATION

Essential evaluative criteria for paraphilic disorders include maintaining the safety of others and self, reducing and/or eliminating behaviors that result in discomfort and shame, and improving interpersonal relationships. Despite progress, people with sexual impulse disorders, especially those that generate victims, may be required to continue treatment, which has been demonstrated to reduce recidivism (relapse into the offending behavior).

KEY POINTS TO REMEMBER

- Sexual dysfunction is an extremely common problem that involves a disturbance in the desire, excitement, or orgasm phases of the sexual response cycle or pain during sexual intercourse.
- There are seven different disorders of sexual dysfunction.
- Sexual problems have the potential to disrupt meaningful relationships.
- Healthcare workers are often uncomfortable asking questions related to sexuality. Providing professional and holistic care requires that nurses include this vital area of assessment.
- Certain medical and surgical conditions and some drugs result in a variety of sexual dysfunctions, including low libido, impotence, erectile dysfunction, anorgasmia, and priapism.
- There are distinctions between biological sex and gender identity. Gender dysphoria is a strong and persistent cross-gender identification accompanied by anxiety, discomfort, and unhappiness.
- Paraphilia is a term used to identify repetitive or preferred sexual fantasies or behaviors that involve preference for use of a nonhuman object, repetitive sexual activity with humans involving real or simulated suffering or humiliation, and repetitive sexual activity with nonconsenting partners.
- Paraphilic disorders include exhibitionistic disorder, fetishistic disorder, frotteuristic disorder, pedophilic disorder, sexual masochism disorder, sexual sadism disorder, transvestic disorder, voyeuristic disorder, and paraphilic disorders not otherwise specified.
- In addition to conducting a sexual assessment, nurses are involved in milieu and behavioral therapy, counseling, education, and medication management.
- Nursing interventions for paraphilic disorders involve administration of medications (e.g., medroxyprogesterone [Depo-Provera] and SSRIs) and therapy.
- Advanced practice nurses may specialize in the area of sexual counseling, treatment, and therapy.

CRITICAL THINKING

1. As a nurse on an adolescent psychiatric-mental health nursing unit, you often encounter teenagers who are misinformed about growth and development, as well as sexuality. What information would you include in a series of teaching sessions that would help these adolescents acquire a greater understanding of the developmental changes they are going through?
2. To understand your own beliefs, answer these questions:
   a. Are you comfortable with your own sexuality? With that of others?
   b. Are you judgmental?
   c. Could you be helpful to someone who has a sexual disorder?
   d. What factors have influenced your beliefs and values regarding sexuality?
   e. What do you think is the impact of sexually explicit television, music videos, and movies on your sexual attitudes, values, and beliefs?
3. During a one-to-one session, Mrs. Chase, a patient who was admitted to your inpatient unit with depression and anxiety, confides concern about her 17-year-old son, Alex. She becomes tearful and says, "I don't know what I've done wrong. Alex was arrested for exposing himself to a girl at school. I'm worried that he may begin doing even worse things."
   a. Provide Mrs. Chase with information regarding Alex's condition and his probable prognosis.
   b. What sort of feelings in yourself about Alex would you need to be aware of in order to be the most helpful to Mrs. Chase?

CHAPTER REVIEW

Questions

1. Which patient statement suggests a concern over one's ability to perform sexually?
   a. "My partner and I aren't as close as we once were."
   b. "I'm not as desirable as I once was."
   c. "My personal life has changed a lot."
   d. "I'm not the partner I used to be."
2. The nurse should plan to educate the male patients prescribed a statin medication on the possible development of which commonly observed side effect?
   a. Impotence
   b. Gynecomastia
   c. Decreased libido
   d. Delayed ejaculation
3. Which medications are currently approved for the treatment of male erectile disorder? *Select all that apply.*
   a. Sildenafil (Viagra)
   b. Flibanserin (Addyi)
   c. Tadalafil (Cialis)
   d. Vardenafil (Levitra)
   e. Avanafil (Stendra)
4. Which statement describes a common sexual side effect of diazepam (Valium)?
   a. "I'm just not interested in sex as much."
   b. "I'm experiencing vaginal dryness."
   c. "I don't have organisms anymore."
   d. "My breasts have gotten larger."
5. Obtaining a sexual history can be embarrassing for the patient and practitioner. Experience with addressing the topic can help, as well as:
   a. Using informal language familiar to the patient's age
   b. Avoiding specifics and keeping the interview on general topics
   c. Avoiding eye contact
   d. Using a professional tone of voice and a relaxed posture
6. Which patient has the greatest risk for suicide?
   a. A patient who expresses the inability to stop searching the internet for child pornography.
   b. A patient who reports having lost interest in having a sexual relationship with his wife.
   c. A patient with a history of exposing himself to female strangers on the bus.
   d. A patient whose attraction to prepubescent girls has increased.
7. When Melissa was a small child, she insisted that she was a boy, refused to wear dresses, and wanted to be called Mitch. As Melissa reached puberty, she no longer displayed a desire to be male. This change in identity is considered:
   a. Gender dysphoria
   b. Reaction formation
   c. Normal
   d. Early transgender syndrome
8. Phillip, a 63-year-old male, has exposed his genitals in public for all of his adult life, but the act has lost some of the former thrill. A rationale for this change in his experience may be:
   a. An increasing sense of shame
   b. Disgust over his lack of control
   c. Desire waning with age
   d. Progression into actual assault
9. A male arrested for inappropriate sexual contact in a subway car denies the allegation. Upon interviewing the man, the nurse suspects frotteuristic disorder due to his:
   a. Lack of relationships
   b. Overall aggressive nature
   c. Criminal history including robbery
   d. Intense hatred of women
10. Pedophilic disorder is the most common paraphilic disorder where adults who have a primary or exclusive sexual preference for prepubescent children. A subset of this disorder is termed hebephilia and is defined as attraction to:
    a. Infants
    b. Pubescent individuals
    c. Teens between the ages of 15 and 19
    d. Males only

Answers

1. **d;** 2. **c;** 3. **a, c, d, e;** 4. **a;** 5. **d;** 6. **a;** 7. **c;** 8. **c;** 9. **a;** 10. **b**

Visit the Evolve website for a posttest on the content in this chapter: http://evolve.elsevier.com/Varcarolis

Post-Test interactive review

REFERENCES

Ahlers, C. J., Schaefer, G. A., Mundt, I. A., Roll, S., Englert, H., Willich, S. N., et al. (2009). How unusual are the contents of paraphilias? Paraphilia-associated sexual arousal patterns in a community based sample of men. *The Journal of Sexual Medicine*, *8*(5), 1362–1370.

American Psychiatric Association. (2013). *DSM-5 table of contents.* Retrieved from http://www.psychiatry.org/dsm5.

Becker, J. V., Johnson, B. R., & Perkins, A. (2014). Paraphilic disorders. In R. E. Hales, S. C. Yudofsky, & L. W. Roberts (Eds.), *Textbook of psychiatry* (pp. 895–925). Washington, DC: American Psychiatric Publishing.

Beredjick, C. (2012). *DSM-V to rename gender identity disorder 'gender dysphoria.' Advocate.com.* Retrieved from http://www.advocate.com/politics/transgender/2012/07/23/dsm-replaces-gender-identity-disorder-gender-dysphoria.

Bulechek, G. M., Butcher, H. K., Dochterman, J. M., & Wagner, C. (2013). *Nursing interventions classification* (*NIC*, 6th ed.). St. Louis, MO: Mosby.

Dhejne, C., Oberg, K., Arver, S., & Landen, M. (2014). An analysis of all applications for sex reassignment surgery in Sweden, 1960–2010: Prevalence, incidence, and regrets. *Archives of Sexual Behavior*, *43*(8), 1535–1545.

Frances, A. (2013). *Essentials of psychiatric diagnosis*. New York, NY: Guilford Press.

Garcia, D. V., Delavenne, H. G., deFatima, A., Assumpcao, A., & Thibaut, F. (2013). Phamacologic treatment of sex offenders with paraphilic disorder. *Current Psychiatry Reports, 15* [online]. Retrieved from http://link.springer.com/article/10.1007/s11920.013-0356-5#/page-1.

Heylens, G., DeCuypere, G., Zucker, K. J., Schelfaut, C., Elaut, E., Vanden Bossche, H., & T'Sjoen, G. (2012). Gender identity disorder in twins: A review of the case report literature. *The Journal of Sexual Medicine*, *9*(3), 751–757.

Herdman, T. H., & Kamitsuru, S. (Eds.). (2014). *NANDA International nursing diagnoses: Definitions and classification* (pp. 2015–2017). Oxford, UK: Wiley-Blackwell.

Kaplan, H. S. (1974). *The new sex therapy: Active treatment of sexual dysfunctions*. New York, NY: Brunner/Mazel.

Kraanen, F. L., & Emmelkamp, P. M. G. (2011). Substance misuse and substance use in sex offenders: a review. *Clinical Psychology Review*, *31*(3), 478–489.

Levine, H. B. (2010). What patients mean by love, intimacy, and sexual desire. In H. B. Levine, C. B. Risen, & S. E. Althof (Eds.), *Handbook of clinical sexuality for mental health professionals* (pp. 41–56). New York, NY: Taylor and Francis.

Lewis, R. W., Fugl-Meyer, K. S., Corona, G., Hayes, R. D., Laumann, E. O., Moreira, E. D., & Segraves, T. (2010). Definitions/epidemiology/risk factors for sexual dysfunction. *The Journal of Sexual Dysfunction*, *7*(4 Pt 2), 1598–1607.

Masters, W. H., & Johnson, V. E. (1966). *Human sexual response*. Boston, MA: Little, Brown.

Moorhead, S., Johnson, M., Maas, M. L., & Swanson, E. (2013). *Nursing outcomes classification* (*NOC*, 5th ed.). St. Louis, MO: Mosby.

Sadock, B. J., Sadock, V. A., & Ruiz, P. (2015). *Kaplan & Sadock's synopsis of psychiatry* (11th ed.). Philadelphia, PA: Wolters Kluwer.

Shafer, L. C. (2016). Sexual disorders and sexual dysfunction. In T. A. Stern, M. Fava, T. E. Wilens, & J. F. Rosenbaum (Eds.), *Massachusetts General Hospital comprehensive clinical psychiatry* (2nd ed.) (pp. 401–411). Philadelphia, PA: Elsevier.

Sorrentino, R. (2016). DSM-5 and paraphilias: What psychiatrists need to know. *Psychiatric Times*. Retrieved from http:/www.psychiatrictimes.com/dsm-5-0/dsm-5-and-paraphilias-what-psychiatrists-need-know/page/0/1.

Steensma, T., McGuire, J. K., Kreukels, B. P. C., Beekman, A. J., & Cohen-Kettinis, P. T. (2013). Factors associated with desistence and persistence of childhood gender dysphoria. *Child and Adolescent Psychiatry*, *52*(6), 582–590.

21

Impulse Control Disorders

Sandra Yaklin, Margaret Jordan Halter

Visit the Evolve website for a pretest on the content in this chapter: http://evolve.elsevier.com/Varcarolis Pre-Test interactive review

OBJECTIVES

1. Describe clinical manifestations of oppositional defiant disorder, intermittent explosive disorder, and conduct disorder.
2. Discuss comorbidities of and risk factors for the impulse control disorders.
3. Describe biological, psychological, and environmental factors related to the development of impulse control disorders.
4. Compare your feelings about working with someone who has an impulse control disorder with someone in your class.
5. Formulate three nursing diagnoses for impulse control disorders, identifying patient outcomes and interventions for each.
6. Identify evidence-based treatments for oppositional defiant disorder, intermittent explosive disorder, and conduct disorder.

OUTLINE

KEY TERMS AND CONCEPTS

cognitive-behavioral therapy (CBT)
conduct disorder
dialectical behavioral therapy (DBT)
expressed emotion
intermittent explosive disorder
kleptomania
oppositional defiant disorder
pyromania

The development of a psychiatric illness can be devastating to people and their significant others. Disorders such as autism and schizophrenia can alter the entire direction of a person's life, yet it is usually evident that there is a psychiatric basis to the disorders. Comparatively, people with impulse control disorders may seem like children whose parents cannot control them or adults who simply do not choose to control their behavior.

Disruptive, impulse control, and conduct disorders are characterized by aggressive behaviors and emotions. Problems relating to others in socially acceptable ways result in a lack of healthy relationships, leaving the individual isolated and the family devastated. The behaviors related to these disorders can have severe criminal consequences and long-lasting negative personal impact.

Recognizing and treating aggressive and impulsive behaviors while a person is young can prevent further problems and avoid interactions with the criminal justice system. Unfortunately, stigma and misconceptions around mental illness may cause individuals and their families to conceal these conditions. Concealment can limit help-seeking and professional care, preventing timely intervention.

According to the American Psychiatric Association (APA; 2013), major disorders considered under this umbrella include:

- Oppositional defiant disorder
- Intermittent explosive disorder
- Conduct disorder

OPPOSITIONAL DEFIANT DISORDER

A certain amount of oppositional behavior and contrariness is normal and developmentally appropriate for children and early adolescents. For instance, 2-year-old children and early adolescents often assert their growing autonomy by saying "No!" There are children and adolescents whose behavior exceeds the boundaries of what is socially acceptable. **Oppositional defiant disorder** impacts both emotions (e.g., anger and irritation) and behaviors (e.g., argumentativeness and defiance).

A child or adolescent with oppositional defiant disorder is not just difficult or defiant. This disorder impairs the child's life and makes it extremely difficult for him or her to attend school, to have friends, or be a functioning member of the family. The behaviors may be confined to only one setting or, in more severe cases, present in multiple settings such as both at home and in school. Children and adults with oppositional defiant disorder show a preference for large rewards and pay little attention to increasing penalties.

Left untreated, most children outgrow this disorder. However, some do not and continue to experience social difficulties, conflicts with authority figures, and academic problems that impact their whole lives. Because impairment may persist into adulthood, some researchers suggest we reconsider this as a problem not limited to childhood (Burke et al., 2013).

The APA (2013) differentiates emotional (e.g., anger), behavioral (e.g., defiance), and spiteful/vindictive (e.g., revenge-seeking) behaviors. This system is important as emotional symptoms tend to be linked to future mood and anxiety disorders, while spiteful and vindictive behaviors are predictive of future conduct disorder and delinquency. Diagnostic criteria for oppositional defiant disorder are listed in the *DSM-5* box.

DSM-5 CRITERIA FOR OPPOSITIONAL DEFIANT DISORDER

A. A pattern of angry/irritable mood, argumentative/defiant behavior, or vindictiveness lasting at least 6 months as evidenced by at least four symptoms from any of the following categories and exhibited during interaction with at least one individual who is not a sibling.

Angry/Irritable Mood

1. Often loses temper.
2. Is often touchy or easily annoyed.
3. Is often angry and resentful.

Argumentative/Defiant Behavior

4. Often argues with authority figures or, for children and adolescents, with adults.
5. Often actively defies or refuses to comply with requests from authority figures or with rules.
6. Often deliberately annoys others.
7. Often blames others for his or her mistakes or misbehavior.

Vindictiveness

8. Has been spiteful or vindictive at least twice within the past 6 months.

Note: The persistence and frequency of these behaviors should be used to distinguish a behavior within normal limits from a behavior that is symptomatic. For children younger than 5 years, the behavior should occur on most days for a period of at least 6 months unless otherwise noted (Criterion A8). For individuals 5 years or older, the behavior should occur at least once per week for at least 6 months unless otherwise noted (Criterion A8). While these frequency criteria provide guidance on a minimal level of frequency to define

Continued

DSM-5 CRITERIA FOR OPPOSITIONAL DEFIANT DISORDER—cont'd

symptoms, other factors should also be considered such as whether the frequency and intensity of the behaviors are outside a range normative for the individual's developmental level, gender, and culture.

B. The disturbance in behavior is associated with distress in the individual or others in his or her immediate social context (e.g., family, peer group, work colleagues) or it impacts negatively on social, educational, occupational, or other important areas of functioning.

C. The behaviors to not occur exclusively during the course of a psychotic, substance use, depressive, or bipolar disorder. Also, the criteria are not met for disruptive mood dysregulation disorder.

Specify current severity:

Mild: Symptoms are confined to only one setting (e.g., at home, at school, at work, with peers).

Moderate: Some symptoms are present in at least two settings.

Severe: Some symptoms are present in three or more settings.

From the American Psychiatric Association. (2013). *Diagnostic and statistical manual of mental disorders* (5th ed.). Washington, DC: Author.

Epidemiology

Oppositional defiant disorder is typically diagnosed around 8 years of age, but it may be seen as early as age 3 and usually not later than early adolescence. The prevalence of oppositional defiant disorder is globally consistent and similar across race and ethnicity. The lifetime prevalence is nearly 13%.

Males are diagnosed three times more often than females (Loeber et al., 2009). Various factors may account for this gender difference. For example, some traits of the disorder are seen more in boys than girls. For example, boys are more likely to annoy and blame others, and girls argue more. Additionally, clinicians may view and judge an individual's display of behavior differently depending on the person's gender. For example, it may be more socially appropriate in many cultures for a boy to express aggression than a girl.

Comorbidity

The most common condition associated with oppositional defiant disorder is attention-deficit/hyperactivity disorder with rates reaching nearly 40% (Speltz et al., 1999). Anxiety and depressive disorders are also commonly present in this population.

Conduct disorder, which we will discuss later, and oppositional defiant disorder are both related to conflict with adults and authority. The difference between the two is that conduct disorder is more severe and includes aggression toward people or animals, destruction of property, stealing, and deceit. Also, the emotional dysregulation (e.g., anger, irritability) in oppositional defiant disorder is not present in conduct disorder.

Oppositional defiant disorder shares criteria with disruptive mood dysregulation disorder, a depressive disorder. Its symptoms include a chronic negative mood and temper outbursts. Since symptoms tend to be more severe in disruptive mood dysregulation disorder, if the individual meets the criteria for this disorder, a diagnosis of oppositional defiant disorder is not given. The World Health Organization, however, does not support two separate diagnoses and suggests that disruptive mood dysregulation disorder is part of the spectrum of oppositional defiant disorder (Mayes et al., 2016).

RISK FACTORS

Biological

Physiological

Researchers have studied resting heart rates in children and adolescents diagnosed with oppositional defiant disorder. A low resting heart rate is positively correlated with increased aggression. The precise reason why a low resting heart rate is a risk factor for impulsive, disruptive, and aggressive behaviors is not known. However, low heart rate may be caused by lower arousability, increased vagal tone, reduced sympathetic nervous response, or reduced right hemispheric functioning. Individuals with low resting heart rates in late adolescence are at increased risk of becoming violent adults (Latvala et al., 2015).

Genetic

Oppositional defiant disorder tends to manifest at a young age, and more than 100 studies have supported that aggressive and antisocial behavior has a 40% to 60% genetic basis (Raine, 2014). Many individuals diagnosed with this disorder have a family history of another mental illness.

Neurobiological

A growing body of research supports the neurobiological basis of aggressive behavior. Gray matter is less dense in the left prefrontal cortex, an area associated with impulse control and self-regulation, in individuals with oppositional defiant disorder (Fahim et al., 2012). Noordermeer and colleagues (2016) analyzed controlled studies that used both structural (sMRI) and functional MRI (fMRI) in individuals diagnosed with oppositional defiant disorder and conduct disorder. Individuals with either disorder had smaller brain structures and lower brain activity in the bilateral amygdala, bilateral insula, right striatum, left medial/superior frontal gyrus, and left precuneus.

People with oppositional defiant disorder have increased gray matter in the left temporal area, which is associated with impulsivity, aggression, and antisocial personality. In boys, the structural abnormalities of the brain are more pronounced. Neurotransmitter and hormonal changes have also been observed in the serotonin, norepinephrine, and dopamine systems in addition to low cortisol and elevated testosterone levels.

Environmental

Factors associated with oppositional defiant disorder include family distress, inadequate parenting, and problems with attachment. Conflict in the marriage is more important than whether or not the parents separate. Children from larger and impoverished families are also at risk for these disorders.

Children with insecure attachment as a result of high levels of maternal criticism are often more aggressive (Cyr et al., 2014). Oppositional defiant disorder is more common in children and adolescents with insecure attachment stemming from chaotic caregiving or harsh neglectful families. Coercive or inconsistent parental behavior and child abuse are also correlated with the development of disruptive behaviors. Other factors, such as socioeconomic status, neighborhood violence, and lack of structure within the home, all contribute some risk toward the development of this disorder.

TREATMENT APPROACHES

Psychosocial Interventions

Treatment approaches for oppositional defiant disorder target the unique needs of both the child and the family (Taylor et al., 2014). Children can be helped to manage anger, improve problem solving, develop techniques to reduce impulsivity, and improve social interactions. Psychosocial interventions include parent training, group therapy, and anger management. Cognitive-behavioral approaches are also helpful. When treating preschool children, parental intervention is an essential component. Home visits and programs such as Head Start can reduce future oppositional behaviors and delinquency (Taylor et al., 2014).

Psychobiological Interventions

Pharmacological Treatment

The US Food and Drug Administration (FDA) has not approved any drugs for the treatment of oppositional defiant disorder. Medications available for oppositional defiant disorder are primarily used for control of anger and aggression rather than the disruptive behaviors. Divalproex sodium (Depakote), an antiseizure medication, has been shown to reduce reactive aggression and irritability.

Oppositional defiant disorder is comorbid with several diagnoses that do have effective pharmacological treatment—attention-deficit/hyperactivity disorder, depression, and anxiety. Medications may be used to address symptoms related to these other diagnoses. Evidence indicates that psychostimulants work best for disruptive and aggressive behaviors in addition to core attention-deficit/hyperactivity symptoms. Some studies support the use of alpha-2 agonists and atomoxetine (Strattera), a nonstimulant used for attention-deficit/hyperactivity disorder as well.

INTERMITTENT EXPLOSIVE DISORDER

Intermittent explosive disorder is a pattern of behavioral outbursts characterized by an inability to control aggressive impulses. The aggression can be verbal or physical and targeted toward other persons, animals, property, or even themselves.

Anything can trigger the aggressive reaction to the situation. A man may be unable to locate his favorite video game and impulsively punches his fist through a pane of glass. He may tear his room apart, break furniture, or damage costly properly. As the rage continues, he may attack anyone who intervenes and often causes injury. The explosive anger may occur during a competitive sport such as lashing out at opposing baseball fans when his team loses.

A pattern that commonly emerges is going from rage to remorse. The first stage is tension and arousal based on some environmental stimuli such as someone driving too slowly in the passing lane on the expressway. This is followed by explosive behavior and aggression. A response to the slow driver may be hitting the gas and dangerously passing the person on the shoulder of the road. Immediately after, the person feels a sense of relief and release, taking satisfaction by looking at the offender in the rearview mirror and delivering a negative hand signal. Delayed consequences include feelings of remorse, regret, and embarrassment over the aggressive behavior. After the event, reality may set in. "Wow, I just risked my life to pass an 80-year-old man to get to a party that will go on for hours. I have to stop doing this."

This disorder can impair a person's functioning by leading to problems with interpersonal relationships and occupational difficulties. It can lead to legal problems as well. Significant problems with physical health, such as hypertension and diabetes, have been linked to this disorder (McCloskey et al., 2010). Being in a heightened state of stress and agitation for a prolonged period of time may be the correlation for these outcomes.

Individuals with intermittent explosive disorder may feel a range of emotions, and not just anger, stronger than other people. The problem is a general form of emotional dysregulation, and explosive anger is just one manifestation (Fettich et al., 2015).

Diagnostic criteria for intermittent explosive disorder are listed in the *DSM-5* box.

DSM-5 CRITERIA FOR INTERMITTENT EXPLOSIVE DISORDER

A. Recurrent behavioral outbursts representing a failure to control aggressive impulses as manifested by either of the following:
   1. Verbal aggression (e.g., temper tantrums, tirades, verbal arguments, or fights) or physical aggression toward property, animals, or other individuals, occurring twice weekly, on average, for a period of 3 months. The physical aggression does not result in damage or destruction of property and does not result in physical injury to animals or other individuals.
   2. Three behavioral outbursts involving damage or destruction of property and/or physical assault involving physical injury against animals or other individuals occurring with a 12-month period.

B. The magnitude of aggressiveness expressed during the recurrent outbursts is grossly out of proportion to the provocation or to any precipitating psychosocial stressors.

C. The recurrent aggressive outbursts are not premeditated (i.e., they are impulsive and/or anger-based) and are not committed to achieve some tangible objective (i.e., money, power, intimidation).

D. The recurrent aggressive outbursts cause either marked distress in the individual or impairment in occupational or interpersonal functioning or are associated with financial or legal consequences.

E. Chronological age is at least 6 years (or equivalent developmental level).

F. The recurrent aggressive outbursts are not better explained by another mental disorder (e.g., major depressive disorder, bipolar disorder, disruptive mood dysregulation disorder, a psychotic disorder, antisocial personality disorder, borderline personality disorder) and are not attributable to another medical condition (e.g., head trauma, Alzheimer's disease) or to the physiological effects of a substance (e.g., a drug of abuse, a medication). For children aged 6 to 18 years, aggressive behavior that occurs as part of an adjustment disorder should not be considered for this diagnosis.

Note: This diagnosis can be made in addition to the diagnosis of attention-deficit/hyperactivity disorder, conduct disorder, oppositional defiant disorder, or autism spectrum disorder when recurrent impulsive aggressive outbursts are in excess of those usually seen in these disorders and warrant independent clinical attention.

From the American Psychiatric Association. (2013). *Diagnostic and statistical manual of mental disorders* (5th ed.). Washington, DC: Author.

Epidemiology

Lifetime prevalence of intermittent explosive disorder is about 7%. It is more common in males than in females (McCloskey et al., 2010). This disorder tends to begin in childhood and is more prevalent in people under the age of 50.

Comorbid Conditions

The most commonly associated comorbid conditions associated with intermittent explosive disorder are depressive disorders, anxiety disorders, and substance use disorders. Antisocial and borderline personality disorder, attention-deficit/hyperactivity disorder, and people with a history of the other disruptive disorders (e.g., conduct disorder, oppositional defiant disorder) are also associated with this disorder.

RISK FACTORS

Biological

Physiological

Individuals with intermittent explosive disorder have been found to have higher than normal levels of inflammatory markers (Coccaro et al., 2014). These inflammatory markers may facilitate aggression by modulating certain neurotransmitters. Research demonstrates a direct correlation between high levels of these markers and actual measures of aggression. Also, higher levels of the hormone testosterone have been associated with intermittent explosive disorder

Neurobiological

Intermittent explosive disorder is associated with the loss of neurons in both the amygdala and hippocampus. These changes may play a role in the pathophysiology of impulsive aggression (Coccaro et al., 2015). Abnormalities in serotonin in the limbic area of the brain have been found in individuals with this diagnosis.

Environmental

Intermittent explosive disorder is associated with conflict and violence in the family of origin. Being exposed to violence at an early age makes it more likely that, as the children mature, the behavior will be repeated. It is common for these families to have a history of addiction and substance abuse.

Impulsivity and aggression are distinctive characteristics of intermittent explosive disorder and are also risk factors for suicide (self-aggression). Childhood maltreatment is a factor strongly associated with impulsive aggression. Physical abuse is a specific risk factor for developing intermittent explosive disorder (Fanning et al., 2014). Sexual abuse is also associated with the development of this disorder (Nickerson et al., 2012).

TREATMENT APPROACHES

Psychosocial Interventions

Similar to oppositional defiant disorder treatment, a combination of therapy and psychopharmacology is most beneficial. Both individual and group cognitive behavioral therapy has been shown to be an effective treatment for intermittent explosive disorder (McCloskey et al., 2008).

Psychobiological Interventions

Pharmacological Treatment

Several medications are used off-label (i.e., not for their intended us). Selective serotonin reuptake inhibitors (SSRIs) such as fluoxetine (Prozac) or paroxetine (Paxil) are used based on the premise that explosive temper is the result of serotonergic dysfunction. Another SSRI, escitalopram (Lexapro), has also been shown to improve social cognition, empathy, and understanding of others (Cremers et al., 2015). Mood stabilizers, such as lithium, or some of the anticonvulsant agents, may be used along with an SSRI to increase its beneficial effects (Ploskin, 2012).

Antipsychotics may also exert a calming effect on the outbursts associated with intermittent explosive disorder. Beta-blocking medications may also help calm individuals with intermittent explosive disorder by slowing the heart rate and reducing blood pressure. Benzodiazepine medications should be avoided, however, as they may further reduce inhibitions and self-control in much the same way as alcohol.

EVIDENCE-BASED PRACTICE

Emotional Intelligence: A Deficit in Intermittent Explosive Disorder?

Problem

The hostility that people with intermittent explosive disorder exhibit comes at a high cost for both the afflicted and those around him or her. Researchers hypothesized that individuals with this disorder may have deficits in emotional intelligence, that is, the ability to recognize and understand emotional information and cues.

Purpose of Study

To determine if people with intermittent explosive disorder had deficits in emotional intelligence.

Methods

Researchers compared 44 people with a diagnosis of intermittent explosive disorder with 44 people without it. A test was used to assess experiential and strategic emotional intelligence.

Findings

- Intermittent explosive disorder subjects had lower scores on strategic emotional intelligence.
- Lower scores were associated and accounted for by greater hostile attribution and hostile automatic thoughts in those subjects with a history of aggression.

Why Should Nurses Be Interested in This Study?

Understanding sources of the problem can give clinicians new targets in the treatment of this disorder. Nurses can help patients to understand the connection between angry thoughts and negative behaviors. Replacing negative views and negative thoughts with positive ones is the basis for cognitive-behavioral therapy and also a simple counseling tool.

Coccaro, E. F., Solis, O., Fanning, J., & Lee, R. (2015). Emotional intelligence and impulsive aggression in intermittent explosive disorder. *Journal of Psychiatric Research, 61*, 135–140.

CONDUCT DISORDER

Conduct disorder is a persistent pattern of behavior in which the rights of others are violated and societal norms or rules are disregarded. The behavior is usually abnormally aggressive and can frequently lead to destruction of property or physical injury. Persons with this disorder initiate physical fights and bully, and they may steal or use a weapon to intimidate or hurt others. Coercion into an activity against another's will, including sexual activity, is characteristic of this disorder. These behaviors are enduring patterns and continue over a period of 6 months and beyond.

People affected by this disorder may have a normal intelligence, but they tend to skip class or disrupt school so much that they fall behind and may fail, be expelled, or drop out. Complications associated with conduct disorder include juvenile delinquency, drug and alcohol abuse and dependency, and juvenile court involvement (Harvard Medical School, 2011). People with conduct disorder crave excitement and do not worry as much about consequences as others do.

Though the literature tends to focus on children and adolescents with conduct disorder, it is quite a problem in adults as well. In adults, conduct disorder has similar characteristics of aggression, destruction of property, stealing, deceitfulness, and criminal behavior.

There are two subtypes of conduct disorder—child-onset and adolescent-onset—both of which can occur in mild, moderate, or severe forms.

Childhood-onset conduct disorder occurs before age 10 and occurs mostly in males. These boys are physically aggressive, have poor peer relationships, show little concern for others, and lack feelings of guilt or remorse. They tend to interpret others' intentions as hostile and believe their aggressive responses are justified.

Violent children also often display antisocial reasoning, such as "he deserved it," when rationalizing aggressive behaviors. Children with childhood-onset conduct disorder attempt to project a strong image, but they actually have a low self-esteem. Limited frustration tolerance, irritability, and temper outbursts are hallmarks of this disorder. Individuals with childhood-onset conduct disorder are more likely to have problems that persist through adolescence, and without intensive treatment they may later develop antisocial personality disorder as adults.

In adolescent-onset conduct disorder, no clinically significant symptoms are present before age 10. Affected adolescents tend to act out in the context of their peer group through sexual behavior, substance use, or risk-taking behaviors. Males are more likely to fight, steal, vandalize, and have school discipline problems. Girls tend to lie, be truant, run away, abuse substances, and engage in promiscuity. The male-to-female ratio is not as high as for the childhood-onset type indicating that more girls become aggressive during this period of development.

A subset of people with conduct disorder is referred to by the especially dangerous terms of callous and unemotional. Callousness is characterized by a lack of empathy and being unconcerned about the feelings of others. Expression of guilt is absent except when facing punishment. School and family obligations are unimportant to affected individuals. Callousness may be a predictor of future antisocial personality disorder in adults (Burke et al., 2010). Unemotional traits include a shallow, unexpressive, and superficial affect.

Diagnostic criteria for conduct disorder are listed in the *DSM-5* box.

DSM-5 CRITERIA FOR CONDUCT DISORDER

A. A repetitive and persistent pattern of behavior in which the basic rights of others or major age-appropriate societal norms or rules are violated as manifested by the presence of at least three of the following 15 criteria in the past 12 months from any of the following categories with at least one criterion present in the past 6 months:

Aggression to People and Animals

1. Often bullies, threatens, or intimidates others.
2. Often initiates physical fights.
3. Has used a weapon that can cause serious physical harm to others (e.g., a bat, brick, broken bottle, knife, gun).
4. Has been physically cruel to people.
5. Has been physically cruel to animals.
6. Has stolen while confronting a victim (e.g., mugging, purse snatching, extortion, armed robbery).
7. Has forced someone into sexual activity.

Destruction of Property

8. Has deliberately engaged in fire setting with the intention of causing serious damage.
9. Has deliberately destroyed others' property (other than by fire setting).

Deceitfulness or Theft

10. Has broken into someone else's house, building, or car.
11. Often lies to obtain goods or favors to avoid obligations (i.e., "cons" others).
12. Has stolen items of nontrivial value without confronting a victim (e.g., shoplifting but without breaking and entering; forgery).

Serious Violations of Rules

13. Often stays out at night despite parental prohibitions, beginning before age 13 years.
14. Has run away from home overnight at least twice while living in the parental or parental surrogate home, or once without returning for a lengthy period.
15. Is often truant from school beginning before age 13 years.

B. The disturbance in behavior causes clinically significant impairment in social, academic, or occupational functioning.

C. If the individual is age 18 years or older, criteria are not met for antisocial personality disorder.

Specify whether:

Childhood-onset type: Individuals show at least one symptom characteristic of conduct disorder before age 10 years.

Adolescent-onset type: Individuals show no symptom characteristic of conduct disorder before age 10 years.

Unspecified onset: Criteria for a diagnosis of conduct disorder are met, but there is not enough information available to determine whether the onset of the first symptom was before or after age 10 years.

Specify if: With limited prosocial emotions

Specify current severity: Mild, Moderate, Severe

From the American Psychiatric Association. (2013). *Diagnostic and statistical manual of mental disorders* (5th ed.). Washington, DC: Author.

Epidemiology

Conduct disorder carries a lifetime prevalence of nearly 7%. Conduct disorder may be higher in urban settings as compared with rural areas. Childhood onset is more common in males than in females; in adolescent onset, the numbers are nearly equal. It is stable across races and ethnicities (Polanczyk et al., 2015). The diagnosis of conduct disorder is four times more common in individuals who have previously been diagnosed with oppositional defiant disorder (Loeber et al., 2009).

Comorbidity

Attention-deficit/hyperactivity disorder and oppositional defiant disorder are both common in people with conduct disorder. The combination of both predicts worse outcomes. Conduct disorders are often comorbid with one or more of the following disorders: specific learning disorder, anxiety disorders, depressive or bipolar disorders, and substance use disorders.

RISK FACTORS

Biological

Physiological

A slower resting heart rate has been associated with people who have conduct disorder. Increased testosterone is also found in males with conduct disorder.

Genetic

Conduct disorder seems to be influenced by genetic factors. The risk is increased in children with a biological parent or a sibling with the disorder. However, it is difficult to tease out the contribution of genetics versus that of the environment. Do people inherit traits associated with antisocial behavior or do they learn to be antisocial by the intergenerational mirroring of characteristics?

Neurobiological

Adolescents with conduct disorder have been found to have significantly reduced gray matter in the anterior insulate cortex and the left amygdala. The insulate cortex is believed to be involved in emotion and empathy, and the amygdala helps process emotional reactions and rewards (Byrd et al., 2013). Individuals with conduct disorder who display limited prosocial emotions, specifically those who are callous and unemotional, have more folds in their cortical insula (Fairchild et al., 2015).

Brain changes in people with conduct disorder are not simply structural, they are also functional. Investigators asked children with conduct disorder who displayed callousness to respond to images of others being harmed. Functional MRIs indicated the children experienced diminished blood flow in the region of the brain associated with empathy and emotional response as compared to healthy controls (Michalska et al., 2015).

Environmental

Environmental factors associated with conduct disorder include parental rejection and neglect, inconsistent parenting with harsh discipline, early institutional living, chaotic home life, large family size, absent or alcoholic father, and antisocial and drug-dependent family members. Social factors include peer rejection, violent neighborhoods, and association with delinquent peers.

CONSIDERING CULTURE

The Boy from India with Oppositional Defiant Disorder Who Sweated Blood

A middle-class fourth-grader in India was referred to a hospital by a dermatologist. The 10-year-old boy had been having repeated episodes of blood oozing from his navel, eyes, ear lobes, and nose. Issues such as upcoming exams, fights with parents, and parents not satisfying his demands preceded the episodes of bleeding. As the only male child in the entire family, all the other family members pampered him.

Clinicians diagnosed him with oppositional defiant disorder and hematohidrosis. The two problems are connected because hematohidrosis is associated with intense emotion. They started him on a dose of lorazepam (Ativan), which is an antianxiety agent, along with propranolol (Inderal), a beta-blocker that would slow and regulate his heart rate.

The child was taught how to use relaxation techniques. Adamant, stubborn, and defiant behaviors were targeted by behavioral interventions such as decreasing contact between parents and child, cutting down secondary gain, and empowering the parents to deal with episodes. The parents were also taught the use of positive reinforcement, time out, and using a token economy that rewarded positive behavior and ignored undesirable behavior.

After 20 days in the hospital, he was discharged. The strange and dramatic bleeding stopped and his behavior had improved markedly.

Deshpande, M., Indla, V., Kumar, V., & Reddy, I. R. (2014). Child who presented with hematohidrosis (sweating blood) with oppositional defiant disorder. *Indian Journal of Psychiatry, 56*(3), 289–291.

TREATMENT APPROACHES

Psychosocial Interventions

Conduct disorder is treated similarly to oppositional defiant disorder. Treatment methods are selected based on the behaviors being targeted. For example, anger management might be targeted for one individual, while helping to improve a dysfunctional parent-child relationship might be the goal for another. Parent management skills, problem-solving skills, and multisystemic therapy—discussed later in the chapter—are useful in conduct disorder. The most successful treatments require parental participation. However, if the parents have antisocial traits as well, they are less likely to be involved in treatment (Taylor et al., 2014).

Pharmacological Treatment

Children and adolescents with conduct disorders may have behaviors (i.e., anger, aggression, etc.) that are so disruptive that families are unable to implement change. Psychopharmacological intervention may help decrease the intensity of outbursts. This, in turn, may help those with conduct disorders better respond to psychotherapeutic interventions (Wu et al., 2015, p. 135).

As with oppositional defiant disorder and intermittent explosive disorder, comorbid conditions can exacerbate the symptoms. Treating the comorbid conditions often improves conduct disorder symptoms. Medications for conduct disorder are directed at problematic behaviors such as aggression, impulsivity, hyperactivity, and mood symptoms. Five classes of medications are used for children and adolescents with conduct disorder: antidepressants, mood stabilizers, stimulants, antipsychotics, anticonvulsants, and adrenergic medications all show some efficacy (Taylor et al., 2014). Aripiprazole (Abilify) and risperidone (Risperdal) are two second-generation antipsychotics that have some proven efficacy in diminishing aggression associated with conduct disorder.

Pyromania and Kleptomania

Two problems related to impulse control disorders should be mentioned in this chapter. They are pyromania and kleptomania. **Pyromania** is described as repeated deliberate fire setting. The person experiences tension or becomes excited before setting a fire and shows a fascination with or unusual interest in fire and its contexts such as matches. The person also experiences pleasure or relief when setting a fire, witnessing a fire, or participating in the aftermath of a fire. The fire setting is done solely to satisfy this relief pleasure and not for other reasons such as to conceal a crime.

Pyromania occurs more often in males, particularly those who have poor social skills and learning difficulties (APA, 2013). Individuals with pyromania often have a history of alcohol dependence or abuse. Juvenile fire setting is usually associated with conduct disorder or attention-deficit/hyperactivity disorder.

Kleptomania is a repeated failure to resist urges to steal objects not needed for personal use or monetary value. For example, a person may take books even though they cannot read or baby outfits they consider cute even though they have no children and have plenty of money to buy them. As in pyromania, the person experiences a buildup of tension before taking the object, and relief or pleasure after the theft follows. Some research has explored whether this disorder is more closely linked to others of addictive behavior, such as substance abuse disorder, as the person is acting to satisfy a compulsion (Talih, 2011).

Kleptomania is associated with other impulse control disorders and impulse control-related problems such as impulsive buying. It is also associated with mood disorders such as major depression, anxiety disorders, eating disorders (particularly bulimia nervosa), and personality disorders.

See Table 21.1 for a summary of the characteristics of impulse control disorders.

APPLICATION OF THE NURSING PROCESS

ASSESSMENT

General Assessment

Some individuals with disruptive, impulse control, and conduct disorders may be in the healthcare system based on severe symptoms and a need to stabilize them. Patients with these disorders may also be in the healthcare system based on comorbid disorders such as attention-deficit/hyperactivity disorder, anxiety, depression, or substance abuse. Careful assessment is important to separate and understand the problems. With children, interviewing the parents along with the child and then separately will enrich the value of the assessment.

Suicide Risk

To determine the cause of the distress and the risk of violence, the nurse must listen carefully to any person expressing the wish to hurt self or others. The number one predictor of suicidal risk is a past suicide attempt. Impulsivity and aggression in this population make the possibility of suicide attempts more likely. Areas to explore when assessing suicidal risk include the following:

- Past suicidal thoughts, threats, or attempts
- Existence of a plan, lethality of the plan, and accessibility of the methods for carrying out the plan
- Feelings of hopelessness, changes in level of energy
- Circumstances, state of mind, and motivation
- Viewpoints about suicide and death (e.g., Has a family member or friend attempted or completed suicide?)
- Depression and other moods or feelings (e.g., anger, guilt, rejection)
- History of impulsivity, poor judgment, or decreased decision making

TABLE 21.1 Characteristics of Impulse Control Disorders

Disorder	Age of Onset	Lifetime Prevalence	Gender	Clinical Features	Notes
Oppositional defiant disorder	Childhood/adolescence; usually diagnosed around age 8	12.6%	More males	Angry/irritable mood Argumentative defiant behavior Vindictiveness Despite behavior, recognizes that others have rights and that there are rules	May become conduct disorder in later years.
Intermittent explosive disorder	May be diagnosed at age 6; mean age of onset ranges 13-21 years.	7.3%	More males	Impulsive and unwarranted emotional outbursts, violence, destruction of property	Early treatment may prevent worsening pathology
Conduct disorder	Childhood onset (<10 years): worse prognosis. Adolescent onset (no symptoms before age 10)	6.8%	Childhood onset: More males Adolescent onset: Equal	Unimpulsive violation of the rights of others, aggression to people and animals, destruction of property, deceitfulness, rules violation	More criminal involvement May be a precursor to antisocial personality disorder

Merikangas, K. R., He, J., Burstein, M., Swanson, S. A., Avenevoli, S., Cui, L. ... Swendsen, J. (2010). Lifetime prevalence of mental disorders in U.S. adolescents: Results from the National Comorbidity Survey Replication—Adolescent supplement. *Journal of the American Academy of Adolescent Psychiatry, 49*(10), 980–989.

- Drug or alcohol use
- Prescribed medications and any recent adherence issues
- Assessment of strengths, protective factors, and effective coping skills

For the younger person with oppositional defiant disorder or conduct disorder, a distorted concept of death and immature ego functions complicate an assessment of the lethality of a suicide plan. For instance, a child who is highly suicidal may believe a few aspirin will cause death. The incorrect judgment about the lethality does not diminish the seriousness of the intent. Some teens may make a pact to kill themselves or become upset after a friend has committed suicide or died accidentally. Early intervention is essential, and parents need to understand that suicidal thoughts or self-threatening behavior (e.g., cutting, reckless driving, binge drinking) must be taken seriously and evaluated by mental health professionals as an emergency.

Assessment Tools

There are a variety of tools that you can examine to increase your understanding of the important facets of the disorders. Also, they can help you to share information with colleagues and families of patients.

Oppositional defiant and conduct disorder in young people can be examined more carefully with the questions in Fig. 21.1. They are subsets of an attention-deficit/hyperactivity disorder

Oppositional Defiant Disorder	Never	Occasionally	Often	Very Often
1. Argues with adults	0	1	2	3
2. Loses temper	0	1	2	3
3. Actively disobeys or refuses to follow an adult's request or rules	0	1	2	3
4. Bothers people on purpose	0	1	2	3
5. Blames others for his or her mistakes or misbehaviors	0	1	2	3
6. Is touchy or easily annoyed by others	0	1	2	3
7. Is angry or bitter	0	1	2	3
8. Is hateful and wants to get even	0	1	2	3

Conduct Disorder	Never	Occasionally	Often	Very Often
1. Bullies, threatens, or scares others	0	1	2	3
2. Starts physical fights	0	1	2	3
3. Lies to get out of trouble or to avoid jobs	0	1	2	3
4. Skips school without permission	0	1	2	3
5. Is physically unkind to people	0	1	2	3
6. Has stolen things that have value	0	1	2	3
7. Destroys others' property on purpose	0	1	2	3
8. Has used a weapon that can cause serious harm (bat, knife, brick, gun)	0	1	2	3
9. Is physically mean to animals	0	1	2	3
10. Has set fire on purpose to do damage	0	1	2	3
11. Has broken into someone else's home, business, or car	0	1	2	3
12. Has stayed out at night without permission	0	1	2	3
13. Has run away from home overnight	0	1	2	3
14. Has forced someone into sexual activity	0	1	2	3

FIG. 21.1 Screening for disruptive behaviors: Vanderbilt AD/HD Diagnostic Teacher Rating Scale. (From Wolraich, M. L., Feurer, I. D., Hannah, J. N., Baumgaertel, A., & Pinnock, T. Y. [1998]. Obtaining systematic teacher reports of disruptive behavior disorders utilizing DSM-IV. *Journal of Abnormal Child Psychology, 26*[2], 141–152.)

scale. For both scales individually, scores of 2 to 3 are considered to be indicative of a problem.

ASSESSMENT GUIDELINES

Oppositional Defiant Disorder

1. Identify issues that result in power struggles and triggers for outbursts—when they begin and how they are handled.
2. Assess the child's or adolescent's view of his/her behavior and its impact on others (e.g., at home, school, and with peers). Explore feelings of empathy and remorse.
3. Explore how the child or adolescent can exercise control and take responsibility, problem solve for situations that occur, and plan to handle things differently in the future. Assess barriers and motivation to change and potential rewards to engage patient.

Intermittent Explosive Disorder

a. Assess the history, frequency, and triggers for violent outbursts.
b. Identify times in which the patient was able to maintain control despite being in a situation in which the patient might normally lose control of emotions.
c. Explore actual and potential sources of support at home and socially.
d. Assess for substance use (past and present).

Conduct Disorder

1. Assess the seriousness, types, and initiation of disruptive behavior and how it has been managed.
2. Assess anxiety, aggression and anger levels, motivation, and the ability to control impulses.
3. Assess moral development, problem solving, belief system, and spirituality for the ability to understand the impact of hurtful behavior on others, to empathize with others, and to feel remorse.
4. Assess the ability to form a therapeutic relationship and engage in honest and committed therapeutic work leading to observable behavioral change (e.g., signing a behavioral contract, drug testing, and living according to "home rules").
5. Assess for substance use (past and present).

Self-Assessment

People with impulse control disorders have behaviors that are objectionable to most people. Concerns for personal emotional and physical safety may be real or exaggerated depending on the nature of the patient's behavior. These concerns should be addressed, and steps should be taken to provide for the safest environment for care.

Negative attitudes may be directed at the patient because the caretaker feels the disorder is controllable and that the patient is choosing not to get better. Our ethical and professional responsibility to provide equal care to all people extends to this population. An empathetic view of people with these disorders is necessary, particularly when considering their environments of origin and a history of constant negative responses from others.

DIAGNOSIS

Children, adolescents, and adults with oppositional defiant disorder, intermittent explosive disorder, and conduct disorder display disruptive behaviors that are impulsive, angry/aggressive, and often dangerous. They are in conflict with others, are treatment nonadherent, do not follow age-appropriate social norms, and have inappropriate ways of meeting their needs. Nursing diagnoses are focused on protection of others and self from impulsive and premeditated acts, improving coping skills, and addressing the family.

OUTCOMES IDENTIFICATION

Outcomes for impulse control disorders relate specifically to reversing the diagnosis that has been identified. Whenever possible, outcomes should be patient-centered and agreed upon by both the nurse and the patient or his/her designee.

Signs and symptoms, nursing diagnoses, and associated outcomes for people with impulse control disorders are paired in Table 21.2.

TABLE 21.2 Signs and Symptoms, Nursing Diagnoses, and Outcomes for Impulse Control Disorders

Signs and Symptoms	Nursing Diagnoses	Outcomes
History of suicide attempts, aggression and impulsivity, conflictual interpersonal relationships; states, "If I have to stay here, I'm going to kill myself."	*Risk for suicide*	Expresses feelings, verbalizes suicidal ideas, refrains from suicide attempts, plans for the future
Body posture rigid, clenches fists and jaw, paces, invades the personal space of others, history of cruelty to animals, fire setting, and frequent fights, history of childhood abuse and witnessed family violence; states, "That wimp of a roommate better stay out of my way."	*Risk for other-directed violence*	Identifies harmful impulsive behaviors, controls impulses, refrains from aggressive acts, identifies social support
Hostile laughter, projects responsibility for behavior onto others, grandiosity, difficulty establishing relationships	*Defensive coping related to impulse control problems*	Identifies ineffective and effective coping, identifies and uses support system, uses new coping strategies
Rejection of child or hostility toward the child; unsafe home environment, abusive and/or neglectful; disturbed relationship between parent/caregiver and the child	*Impaired parenting*	Parent/caregiver participates in the therapeutic program, learns appropriate parenting skills

From Herdman, T. H., & Kamitsuru, S. (Eds.). (2014). *NANDA International nursing diagnoses: Definitions and classification, 2015–2017.* Oxford, UK: Wiley-Blackwell; Moorhead, S., Johnson, M., Maas, M. L., & Swanson, E. (2013). Nursing outcomes classification (NOC) (5th ed.). St Louis, MO: Mosby.

IMPLEMENTATION

Psychosocial Interventions

Interventions for severe oppositional defiant, conduct, and intermittent explosive disorders focus on correcting firmly entrenched patterns such as blaming others and denial of responsibility for personal actions. Children, adolescents, and adults with these disorders also must generate more mature and adaptive coping mechanisms and prosocial goals, a process that is gradual and cannot be accomplished during short-term treatment.

General interventions include the following:

1. Promote a climate of safety for the patient and for others.
2. Establish rapport with the patient.
3. Set limits and expectations.
4. Consistently follow through with consequences of rule-breaking.
5. Provide structure and boundaries.
6. Provide activities and opportunities for achievement of goals to promote a sense of purpose.

Oppositional youth are generally treated on an outpatient basis, using individual, group, and family therapy, with much of the focus on parenting issues. In conduct disorder, inpatient hospitalization for crisis intervention, evaluation, and treatment planning, as well as transfer to therapeutic foster care, group homes, or long-term residential treatment, are often needed.

Unfortunately, studies indicate that many children and adolescents may be simply placed in group homes and in some residential programs and do not maintain improvements after discharge. However, intensive programs such as multisystemic therapy, therapeutic foster care, and use of multidisciplinary community-based treatment teams for children with serious emotional and behavioral disturbances have been found to improve outcome and reduce offenses over the long term. These types of programs are more promising in improving positive adjustment, decreasing negative behaviors, and improving family stability.

Box 21.1 provides a summary of techniques to manage disruptive behaviors.

Pharmacological Interventions

Specific pharmacological interventions are described along with the disorders earlier in this chapter. A variety of medications are used to control aggression. They include tricyclic antidepressants, antianxiety medications, mood stabilizers, and antipsychotics (Taylor et al., 2014). Refer to Chapter 27 for further discussion of managing aggression.

Health Teaching and Health Promotion

When the patient is a child or adolescent, ideally families are actively engaged and given support in using parenting skills to provide nurturance and set consistent limits. They can be taught techniques for behavior modification, monitoring medication for therapeutic effects, collaborating with teachers to foster academic success, and setting up a home environment that is consistent, structured, and nurturing to promote achievement of normal developmental milestones. If families are abusive, drug dependent, or highly disorganized, the child may require out-of-home placement. The following nursing interventions are helpful when working with parents and caregivers:

- Explore the impact of the child's behaviors on family life and of the other members' behavior on the child.
- Assist the immediate and extended family to access available and supportive individuals and systems.

BOX 21.1 Techniques for Managing Disruptive Behaviors

Behavioral contract: A patient-centered verbal or written agreement between the patient and nurse or other parties (e.g., family, treatment team, teacher) about behaviors, expectations, and needs. The contract is periodically evaluated and reviewed and typically coupled with rewards and other contingencies, positive and negative.

Counseling: Verbal interactions teach, coach, or maintain adaptive behavior and provide positive reinforcement. It is most effective for motivated patients and those with well-developed communication and self-reflective skills.

Modeling: A method of learning behaviors or skills by observation and imitation that can be used in a wide variety of situations. It is enhanced when the modeler is perceived to be similar (e.g., age, interests) and attending to the task is required.

Role playing: A counseling technique in which the nurse, the patient, or a group of patients acts out a specified script or role to enhance their understanding of that role, learn and practice new behaviors or skills, and practice specific situations. It requires well-developed expressive and receptive language skills.

Planned ignoring: When the staff determines behaviors not to be safe and only attention seeking, they may be ignored. Additional interventions may be used in conjunction (e.g., positive reinforcement for on-task actions).

Physical distance and touch control: While touching and closeness may have a positive effect on many patients, patients with oppositional defiant, intermittent explosive, and conduct disorders may need increased personal space and feel threatened by touch.

Redirection: A technique used after an undesirable or inappropriate behavior to engage or re-engage an individual in an appropriate activity. It may involve the use of verbal directives (e.g., setting firm limits), gestures, or physical prompts.

Positive feedback: Emotional support and positive feedback are good for anyone, but they are particularly helpful for individuals who rarely receive such attention.

Clarification as intervention: Sometimes misunderstandings are the source of frustration and potential loss of control. Helping the patient to understand the environment and what is happening can reduce feelings of vulnerability and the urge to strike out.

Restructuring: Changing an activity in a way that will decrease the stimulation or frustration (e.g., shorten the 1:1 session or change to a physical activity). This requires flexibility and planning to have an alternative in mind in case the activity is not going well.

Limit setting: Involves giving direction, stating an expectation, or telling the patient what is required. This should be done firmly, calmly, without judgment or anger, preferably in advance of any problem behavior occurring, and consistently when in a treatment setting among multiple staff.

Simple restitution: Refers to a procedure in which an individual is required or expected to correct the adverse environmental or relational effects of his or her misbehavior by restoring the environment to its prior state, making a plan to correct his or her actions with the nurse, and implementing the plan (e.g., apologizing to the persons harmed, fixing the chairs that are upturned). Simple restitution is not punitive in nature, and there are typically additional activities involved (e.g., counseling).

Physical restraint: Seclusion and restraint may be necessary.

- Discuss how to make the home a safe environment, especially with regard to weapons and drugs; attempt to talk separately to members if possible.
- Discuss realistic behavioral goals and how to set them; explore potential problems.
- Teach behavior modification techniques. Role-play them with the parents in different problem situations that might arise with their child.
- Give support and encouragement as parents learn to apply new techniques.
- Provide education about medications.
- Refer patients, parents, or other caregivers to local self-help groups.
- Advocate with the educational system if special education services are needed.

Advanced Practice Interventions

Advanced practice psychiatric-mental health registered nurses may use a variety of psychosocial interventions that target pathology associated with impulse control disorders. The overall goals are to (1) help patients maintain control of their thoughts and behaviors and (2) assist families to function more adaptively.

Cognitive-Behavioral Therapy (CBT)

Cognitive-behavioral therapy (CBT) is an evidence-based treatment approach that can be used for children, adolescents, and adults. It is a talk therapy that focuses on a patient's feelings, thoughts, and behaviors. It is based on the idea that if we change our thoughts to be more realistic and positive, we can change the way we experience life. Cognitive therapy teaches patients to recognize the onset of the impulse to explode or act aggressively, to identify circumstances or triggers associated with the onset, and to develop methods to prevent the maladaptive behaviors from occurring.

Psychodynamic Psychotherapy

One of the older treatment approaches, psychodynamic psychotherapy, continues to have relevance. Its focus is on underlying feelings and motivations and explores conscious and unconscious thought processes. In working with impulse control problems, the therapist may help the patient to uncover underlying feelings and reasons behind rage or anger. This may help patients to develop better ways to think about and control their behavior.

Dialectical Behavioral Therapy (DBT)

A specific kind of cognitive-behavioral treatment that has a focus on impulse control is **dialectical behavioral therapy (DBT)**. Skills taught include mindfulness, emotional regulation, distress tolerance, and personal effectiveness (Cooper & Parsons, 2010). Shelton and colleagues (2011) found a DBT-Corrections Modified version of this therapy to be effective in reducing physical aggression in incarcerated adolescents.

Parent-Child Interaction Therapy (PCIT)

Another evidence-based approach is **parent-child interaction therapy (PCIT).** Therapists such as advanced practice nurses sit behind one-way mirrors and coach parents through an ear audio device while they interact with their children. The advanced practice nurse or other advanced practice provider (e.g., psychiatrist, psychologist, counselor, or therapist) can suggest strategies that reinforce positive behavior in the child or adolescent. The goal is to improve parenting strategies and thereby reduce problematic behavior.

Parent Management Training (PMT)

Parent management training (PMT) has a 65% success rate in significantly improving behavioral problems in children diagnosed with oppositional defiant disorder and conduct disorder (Kazdin, 2005). This evidence-based treatment is for children aged 2 to 14 with mild to severe behavioral problems. Parents of children with oppositional defiant disorder and conduct disorder tend to engage in patterns of negative interactions, ineffective harsh punishments, emotionally charged commands and comments, and poor modeling of appropriate behaviors. This treatment targets the parents rather than the child and focuses attention on reinforcement of positive and prosocial behavior, and on brief, negative consequences of bad behavior.

Multisystemic Therapy (MST)

Of all the treatment approaches presented in this list, **multisystemic therapy (MST)** is the most extensive. This evidence-based approach is an intensive family and community-based program that takes into consideration all of the environments of violent juvenile offenders. Therapists work with caregivers who are on call 24 hours a day, 7 days a week to go where the child is. Hanging out with friends is replaced with healthy activities such as sports or recreational activities. MST can improve family functioning, school performance, and peer relationships and can build meaningful social supports (Henggeler et al., 2009).

Teamwork and Safety

Part of teamwork and the promotion of safety is the monitoring of dynamics between staff and patients. Safety is compromised when a power struggle exists between staff and patients. The term **expressed emotion** refers to the qualitative amount of emotion displayed, usually in the context of family interactions. In the context of the treatment environment, high expressed emotion is a major cause of aggressive responses from patients with impulse control disorders. Violence increases when staff act in an authoritarian or confrontational way or engage in power struggles. Body language such as standing too close and tone of voice can indicate aggression on the part of staff. Arbitrary or poorly explained denial of privileges can trigger violent retaliation. High expressed emotion includes criticisms, resentment, or annoyance about patient behavior.

Alternatively, staff who use low expressed emotion calmly communicate in a way that reduces confrontation and decreases the need for seclusion and restraint and decreases relapse in the patient (Heebner, 2007). The best way to communicate with a potentially hostile patient includes the following techniques:

- Using nonthreatening body posture and a flat neutral tone of voice (never an angry tone of voice) when correcting behavior
- Using matter-of-fact, easy-to-understand words

- Consistently setting limits
- Avoiding personal terms (such as "I" or "you") when setting a limit

Seclusion and Restraint

Seclusion and restraint may be necessary as a last resort when working with patients with impulse control disorders. The use of time-out or a quiet area may be helpful in reducing the stimuli of the environment. Refer to Chapter 6 for more information related to seclusion and restraint.

EVALUATION

Patients with impulse control disorders exhibit an inability to self-regulate. Care is aimed at providing external boundaries and a safe environment. Ideally, patients on inpatient units demonstrate increased levels of self-regulation and ability to interact appropriately with others. In outpatient and community settings, patients will progress incrementally from aggressive and impulsive behavior and move onto considering the rights of others and behaviors that are in control.

KEY POINTS TO REMEMBER

- Impulse control disorders include oppositional defiant disorder, intermittent explosive disorder, and conduct disorder. These are disorders of impulse that are seen in mental healthcare settings and in the criminal justice system.
- Chaotic and punitive environments are strongly correlated with the development of these disorders.
- Impulsivity and aggression in this population make the possibility of suicide attempts and other-directed violence more likely. Continual assessment of suicidal risk and other-directed violence is an essential component of care.
- Nurses are often attracted to healthcare to help people who want and need their assistance. Patients with impulse control disorders may create a level of discomfort as they resist help and seem to be self-defeating and unkind. Remembering the tragic etiology of these disorders may help increase empathy and therapeutic responses.
- Nursing diagnoses are focused on protection of others and self from impulsive and premeditated acts, improvement of coping skills, and development of an increased self-esteem.
- The three most important interventions with this population are to promote a climate of safety for the patient and for others, establish rapport with the patient, and set limits and expectations.
- Pharmacological treatments are generally aimed at co-occurring conditions such as attention deficit hyperactivity disorder. Some medications such as second-generation antipsychotics will target aggressive symptoms that accompany each of these disorders.
- A variety of advanced practice interventions should be considered for this population. Most of them are evidence-based and effective.
- An important concept when working with impulse control disorders is expressed emotion. To create a positive atmosphere of teamwork and safety, expressed emotion on the part of caregivers should be low to prevent emotional and behavioral reactivity.

CRITICAL THINKING

1. Jacob is a 14-year-old adolescent who has been diagnosed with conduct disorder.
   a. Explain to one of your classmates his probable behaviors in terms of (1) aggression toward others, (2) destruction of property, (3) deceitfulness, and (4) violation of rules.
   b. What are the outcomes for this disorder?
   c. List at least seven ways you could support Jacob's parents. What are some community referrals you could give them in your own locale?
2. Mallory is a 17-year-old female being admitted to the adolescent psychiatric unit after several weeks of impulsive behaviors such as extensive cutting and running away from home.
   a. Put the following areas of assessment in order of priority and provide the rationale for your choices:
      1. Suicide risk
      2. Current coping skills
      3. Skin integrity/risk for infection
      4. Childhood development
      5. Current family relationships
   b. Identify at least three appropriate nursing diagnoses for Mallory based on the previously provided information.
   c. Name three nursing interventions to support the nursing diagnosis of ineffective coping.

CHAPTER REVIEW

Questions

1. Which statement made by a 9-year-old child after hitting a classmate is a typical comment associated with childhood conduct disorder?
   a. "I'm sorry, I won't hit him again."
   b. "He deserved it for being a sissy."
   c. "I didn't think I hit him very hard."
   d. "He hit me first. You just didn't see it."
2. What assessment data would support a diagnosis of conduct disorder? *Select all that apply.*
   a. Evidence of social isolation
   b. Arrested twice for disorderly conduct
   c. Expresses difficulty in keeping employment
   d. Demonstrates objective signs of phobia

   e. Exhibits signs of chronic self-mutilation
3. Which event experienced in the patient's childhood increases the risk of the development of behaviors associated with intermittent explosive disorder?
   a. Orphaned at age 4
   b. Physically abused from ages 3 to 10
   c. Born with a chronic congenital disorder
   d. One parent was diagnosed with obsessive-compulsive disorder
4. What is a common behavior observed in a patient diagnosed with intermittent explosive disorder? *Select all that apply.*
   a. Short attention span
   b. Threatens suicide
   c. Often purges after eating
   d. Uses alcohol to excess
   e. States, "Everyone is out to get me."
5. When discussing oppositional defiant disorder with a group of parents, what information should the nurse include about the disorder? *Select all that apply*
   a. Classic symptoms include anger, irritation, and defiant behavior.
   b. Children generally outgrow the behaviors without formal treatment.
   c. Severity is considered mild when symptoms are present in only one setting.
   d. Disorder is diagnosed equally in both males and females.
   e. Argumentative and defiant are terms often used to describe the patient.
6. Tommy, a 12-year-old boy admitted to the pediatric psychiatric unit, has recently been diagnosed with conduct disorder. In the activity room, the games he wanted to play were already in use. He responded by threatening to throw furniture and to hurt his peers who had the game he wanted. Nancy, a registered nurse, recognizes that Tommy's therapy must include:
   a. Consistency in implementing the consequences of breaking rules
   b. Empathetic reasoning when Tommy acts out in the activity room
   c. Teaching Tommy the benefits of socializing
   d. Solitary time so that Tommy can think about his actions
7. Some cultures have lower rates of diagnosed conduct disorders than observed in Western societies. The lower rate of incidence may be contributed to:
   a. Strict parenting with corporal punishment
   b. Cultural expression of anger as normal behavior
   c. Parents' limited tolerance for externalizing behavior
   d. Widespread acceptance of conduct disorders
8. Larry, a middle-aged male in a treatment facility, is loudly displaying anger in the day room with a visiting family member. It is obvious to the nurse this pattern has played out before. Violence is often escalated when family members or authority figures:
   a. Use a soft tone of voice to gain control of the situation
   b. Move away from the agitated person in fear
   c. Use simple words to communicate
   d. Engage in a power struggle
9. The impulse control spectrum can begin in childhood and continue on into adulthood, often morphing into criminal behaviors. Working with patients diagnosed with these disorders, the best examples of expressed emotion by the nursing staff are:
   a. Low to prevent emotional reactions
   b. Matched to the patient's level of emotion
   c. Flat without evidence of any emotional output
   d. High expression to improve therapeutic patient emotions
10. Claude is a new nurse on the psychiatric unit. He asks a senior nurse on staff for the "best advice" when working with oppositional defiant disorder. Which statement reflects advice on solid therapeutic communication?
   a. "When correcting behavior, use a loud firm tone."
   b. "Use language beyond the patient's education level."
   c. "When setting limits, be specific and outline consequences."
   d. "An aggressive body language will make the patients respect your position."

Answers

1. **b**; 2. **a, b, c**; 3. **b**; 4. **a, b, d**; 5. **a, b, c, e**; 6. **a**; 7. **b**; 8. **d**; 9. **a**; 10. **c**

Visit the Evolve website for a posttest on the content in this chapter: http://evolve.elsevier.com/Varcarolis

Post-Test interactive review

REFERENCES

American Psychiatric Association. (2013). *DSM-5 table of contents.* Retrieved from http://www.psychiatry.org/dsm5.

Burke, J. D., Waldman, I., & Lahey, B. B. (2010). Predictive validity of childhood oppositional defiant disorder and conduct disorder: Implications for the DSM-V. *Journal of Abnormal Psychology, 119*(4), 739–751.

Burke, J. D., Rowe, R., & Boylan, K. (2013). Functional outcomes of child and adolescent oppositional defiant disorder symptoms in young adult men. *Journal of Child Psychology and Psychiatry, 44*(3), 264–272.

Byrd, A. L., Loeber, R., & Pardini, D. A. (2013). Antisocial behavior, psychopathic features and abnormalities in reward and punishment processing in youth. *Clinical Child and Family Psychology Review, 17*(2), 125–156.

Coccaro, E. F., Royce, L., & Coussons-Read, M. (2014). Elevated plasma inflammatory markers in individuals with intermittent explosive disorder and correlation with aggression in humans. *JAMA Psychiatry, 71*(2), 158–165.

Coccaro, E. F., Lee, R., McCloskey, M., Csernansky, J. G., & Wang, L. (2015). Morphometric analysis of amygdala and hippocampus shape in impulsively aggressive and healthy control subjects. *Journal of Psychiatric Research*, *69*, 80–86.

Cooper, B., & Parsons, J. (2010). Dialectical behaviour therapy: A social work intervention? *Aotearoa New Zealand Social Work Review*, *21/22*(4/1), 83–93.

Cremers, H., Lee, R., Keedy, S., Phan, K. L., & Coccaro, E. (2015). Effects of escitalopram administration on face processing in intermittent explosive disorder: An fMRI study. *Neuropsychopharmacology*, *41*(2), 590–597.

Cyr, M., Pasalich, D. S., McMahon, R. J., & Spieker, S. J. (2014). The longitudinal link between parenting and child aggression: The moderating effect of attachment security. *Child Psychiatry and Human Development*, *45*(5), 555–564.

Fahim, C., Fiori, M., Evans, A. C., & Perusse, D. (2012). The relationship between social defiance, vindictiveness, anger, and brain morphology in eight-year-old boys and girls. *Social Development*, *21*(3), 592–609.

Fairchild, G., Toschi, N., Hagan, C. C., Goodyer, I. M., Calder, A. J., & Passamonti, L. (2015). Cortical thickness, surface area, and folding alterations in male youths with conduct disorder and varying levels of callous–unemotional traits. *NeuroImage: Clinical*, *8*, 253–260.

Fanning, J. R., Meyerhoff, J. J., Lee, R., & Coccaro, E. F. (2014). History of childhood maltreatment in intermittent explosive disorder and suicidal behavior. *Journal of Psychiatric Research*, *56*, 10–17.

Fettich, K. C., McCloskey, M. S., Look, A. E., & Coccaro, E. F. (2015). Emotion regulation deficits in intermittent explosive disorder. *Aggressive Behavior*, *41*(1), 25–33.

Harvard Medical School. (2011). Options for managing conduct disorder: Treatment works best when it involves and empowers parents. *The Harvard Mental Health Letter*, *27*(9), 1–3.

Heebner, E. R. (2007). Expressed emotion and the inpatient psychiatric facility—Expressed emotion and the inpatient psychiatric facility with low functioning psychiatric patients. *International Journal of Psychiatric Nursing Research*, *13*(1), 1554–1560.

Henggeler, S. W., Cunningham, P. B., Schoenwald, S. K., Borduin, C. M., & Rowland, M. D. (2009). *Multisystemic therapy for antisocial behavior in children and adolescents*. New York, NY: Guilford Press.

Kazdin, A. E. (2005). *Parent management training: Treatment for oppositional, aggressive, and antisocial behavior in children and adolescents*. New York, NY: Oxford University.

Latvala, A., Kuja-Halkola, R., Almqvist, C., Larsson, H., & Lichtenstein, P. (2015). A longitudinal study of resting heart rate and violent criminality in more than 700 000 men. *JAMA Psychiatry*, *72*(10), 971–978.

Loeber, R., Burke, J., & Pardini, D. A. (2009). Perspectives on oppositional defiant disorder, conduct disorder, and psychopathic features. *Journal of Child Psychology and Psychiatry*, *50*(1-2), 133–142.

Mayes, S. D., Waxmonsky, J. D., Calhoun, S. L., & Bixler, E. O. (2016). Disruptive mood dysregulation disorder symptoms and association with oppositional defiant and other disorders in a general population child sample. *Journal of Child and Adolescent Psychopharmacology*, *26*(2), 101–106.

McCloskey, M. S., Noblett, K. L., Deffenbacher, J. L., Gollan, J. K., & Coccaro, E. F. (2008). Cognitive-behavioral therapy for intermittent explosive disorder: A pilot randomized clinical trial. *Journal of Consulting Clinical Psychology*, *76*(5).

McCloskey, M. S., Kleabir, K., Berman, M. E., Chen, E. Y., & Coccaro, E. F. (2010). Unhealthy aggression: intermittent explosive disorder and adverse physical health outcomes. *Health Psychology*, *29*(3), 324–332.

Michalska, K. J., Zeffiro, T. A., & Decety, J. (2015). Brain response to viewing others being harmed in children with conduct disorder symptoms. *Journal of Child Psychology and Psychiatry*, *57*(4), 510–519.

Nickerson, A., Aderka, I. M., Bryant, R. A., & Hofmann, S. G. (2012). The relationship between childhood exposure to trauma and intermittent explosive disorder. *Psychiatry Research*, *197*(1-2), 128–134.

Noordermeer, S. D., Luman, M., & Oosterlaan, J. (2016). A systematic review and meta-analysis of neuroimaging in oppositional defiant disorder (ODD) and conduct disorder (CD) taking attention-deficit hyperactivity disorder (attention-deficit/hyperactivity disorder) into account. *Neuropsychology Review*, *26*(1), 44–72.

Ploskin, D. (2012). *Treatment for intermittent explosive disorder.* Psych Central. Retrieved from http://psychcentral.com/lib/2007/treatment-for-intermittent-explosive-disorder/.

Polanczyk, G. V., Salum, G. A., Sugaya, L. S., Caye, A., & Rohde, L. A. (2015). Annual research review: A meta-analysis of the worldwide prevalence of mental disorders in children and adolescents. *Journal of Child Psychology and Psychiatry*, *56*(3), 345–365.

Raine, A. (2014). *The anatomy of violence: The biological roots of crime.* New York, NY: Vintage Books.

Shelton, D., Kesten, K., Zhang, W., & Trestman, R. (2011). Impact of a dialectic behavior therapy-corrections modified upon behaviorally challenged incarcerated male adolescents. *Journal of Child and Adolescent Psychiatric Nursing*, *24*(2), 105–113.

Speltz, M. L., McClellan, J., Deklyen, M., & Jones, K. (1999). Preschool boys with oppositional defiant disorder: Clinical presentation and diagnostic change. *Journal of the American Academy of Child Adolescent Psychiatry*, *38*, 383–845.

Talih, F. R. (2011). Kleptomania and potential exacerbating factors: A review and case report. *Innovations in Clinical Neuroscience*, *8*(10), 35–39.

Taylor, B. P., Weiss, M., Ferretti, C. J., Berlin, G., & Hollander, E. (2014). Disruptive, impulsive-control, and conduct disorders. In R. E. Hales, S. C. Yudofsky, & L. W. Roberts (Eds.), *The American psychiatric publishing textbook of psychiatry* (6th ed.) (pp. 703–734). Washington, DC: American Psychiatric Publishing.

Wu, T., Howells, N., Burger, J., Lopez, P., Lundeen, R., & Sikkenga, A. V. (2015). Conduct disorder. In G. M. Kapalka (Ed.), *Treating disruptive disorders: A guide to psychological, pharmacological, and combined therapies*. Devon, UK: Routledge.

22

Substance-Related and Addictive Disorders

Jill Espelin, Margaret Jordan Halter

Visit the Evolve website for a pretest on the content in this chapter: http://evolve.elsevier.com/Varcarolis Pre-Test interactive review

OBJECTIVES

1. Define substance use, intoxication, tolerance, and withdrawal.
2. Define addiction or substance use disorder as a chronic disease.
3. Describe the neurobiological process that occurs in the brain and neurotransmitters involved with substance use.
4. Identify potential co-occurring medical and psychological disorders.
5. Describe the major groups of substance-related and addictive disorders in terms of use, intoxication, withdrawal, overdose, and treatment.
6. Identify relevant nursing diagnoses for alcohol use disorder specifically and substance use disorders in general.
7. Identify patterns of substance use.
8. Apply the nursing process to caring for an individual using substances.

OUTLINE

OUTLINE—cont'd

KEY TERMS AND CONCEPTS

addiction
codependence
co-occurring disorders
intoxication
patient-centered care
Screening, Brief Intervention, Referral to Treatment (SBIRT)
substance use disorder
tolerance
withdrawal

Substance use disorders are not disorders of choice. They are complex diseases of the brain characterized by craving, seeking, and using regardless of consequences. Continuous substance use results in actual changes in the brain structure and brain function. Substance use disorders are chronic and relapsing. They result in compromised executive function circuits that mediate self-control and decision making.

Historically, substance use disorders and psychiatric disorders were treated in separate systems of care. Individuals received care for mental health problems in the psychiatric system while treatment for substance disorders took place in specialized chemical dependency units or separate facilities. If both mental health and substance use disorders were present, the treatment might occur concurrently in different settings or as back-to-back treatment in one system followed by the other. Currently the trend is to integrate treatment and facilities increasingly provide services for co-occurring disorders.

Due to the magnitude of substance use disorders, agencies at the national level have been created to address them. The lead federal agency devoted to research regarding drug use is the National Institute on Drug Abuse (NIDA). Its mission is to advance science on the causes and consequences of drug use and abuse and to apply that knowledge to improve individual and public health (National Institute on Drug Abuse, 2015a). The Substance Abuse and Mental Health Administration (SAMHSA, 2014a) serves a dual mission of reducing the impact of substance use and mental illness on communities in the United States.

It is important for all nurses, regardless of their practice specialty area, to develop an understanding of the complex disease of substance use disorders. In this chapter, you are provided with an overall picture of substance use disorders, concepts central to this problem, and risk factors for its development. We will review the clinical picture for each of the substances and discuss associated treatment. Finally, we focus specifically on alcohol use disorder and apply the nursing process to it.

SUBSTANCE USE DISORDERS

In 2013, the American Psychiatric Association (APA) replaced the categories of substance abuse and substance dependence with a single category: substance use disorder. A **substance use disorder** is a pathological use of a substance that leads to a disorder of use. Symptoms fall into four major groupings:

1. Impaired control
2. Social impairment
3. Risky use
4. Physical effects (i.e., intoxication, tolerance, and withdrawal)

Substance use disorders encompass a broad range of products that human beings take into their bodies through various means (e.g., swallowing, inhaling, injecting). They range from fairly innocuous and innocent-seeming substances such as caffeine to absolutely illegal mind-altering drugs such as LSD. No matter the substance, use disorders share many commonalities, intoxication characteristics, and withdrawal attributes.

The *Diagnostic and Statistical Manual of Mental Disorders, Fifth Edition* (*DSM-5;* [APA], 2013) provides diagnostic criteria for the following psychoactive substances:

- Alcohol
- Caffeine
- Cannabis
- Hallucinogen
- Inhalant
- Opioid
- Sedative, hypnotic, and antianxiety medication
- Stimulant
- Tobacco

In addition to substances, behaviors, too, are gradually being recognized as addictive. These behavioral addictions are called *process addictions.* In process addictions, there are no substances but rather a behavior or the feeling brought about by the relevant action. While the physical signs of drug addiction do not accompany these types of addictions, compulsive actions activate the reward or pleasure pathways in the brain similarly to substances (SAMHSA, 2014b). The first process addiction, gambling, was officially declared a disorder in 2013 (APA). Internet gaming, using social media, shopping, and sexual activity are also process addictions.

Concepts Central to Substance Use Disorders

Addiction

A term that people commonly use to describe substance use disorders is **addiction**. Addiction is defined as a "primary, chronic disease of brain reward, motivation, memory, and related circuitry" (American Society of Addiction Medicine, 2016, para. 1). It is a disease of dysregulation in the hedonic (pleasure-seeking) or reward pathway of the brain. Addicted individuals are unable to consistently abstain from the substance or activity. They are also unable to recognize the extent to which the addictions are creating serious problems in functioning, interpersonal relationships, and emotional responses. Like other chronic diseases, there are cycles of relapse and remission. Ultimately, without treatment, addiction is progressive and often results in disability or premature death.

Intoxication

When people are in the process of using a substance to excess, they are experiencing **intoxication**. Intoxication may manifest itself in a variety of ways depending on the physiological response of the body to the substance being used. Individuals who are using substances are considered to be under the influence, intoxicated, or high. Terminology may vary depending on the substance and the population who is using it: alcohol causes intoxication, but cocaine makes you high.

Tolerance

People with substance use disorders experience **tolerance** to the effects of the substances. Tolerance occurs when a person no longer responds to the drug in the way that the person initially responded. It takes a higher dose of the drug to achieve the same level of response achieved initially.

Withdrawal

Withdrawal is a set of physiological symptoms that occur when a person stops using a substance. Withdrawal is specific to the substance being used, and each substance will have its own characteristic syndrome. Substance-specific withdrawal can be mild or life threatening. The same substance, or one with a similar action, may be taken to avoid or relieve withdrawal symptoms. The more intense symptoms a person has, the more likely the person is to start using the substance again to avoid the symptoms. Behavioral addictions, such as gambling, seldom have clearly identifiable intoxication or withdrawal symptoms.

EPIDEMIOLOGY

The National Survey on Drug Use and Health Survey (SAMHSA, 2015a) is conducted annually. Participants 12 years or older are randomly asked to participate. Data from this survey are the primary source for national drug use statistics and trending. Based on this survey, more than 21 million individuals, or nearly 9% of the population of the United States, are estimated to have substance use disorders (SAMHSA, 2015a).

In 2014 nearly 140 million people (about 53%) of the nation's population acknowledged drinking alcohol. About 60 million people (23%) admit to binge drinking. Binge drinking is defined as five drinks on one occasion on one day in the last month. About 16 million people (about 6%) report heavy drinking. Heavy drinking is defined as five drinks on one occasion on at least five days in the last month.

According to the 2014 survey, 27 million Americans or about 10% of the population used illicit substances in the month before the survey. Illicit substances include the nonmedical or nonprescribed use of prescription drugs. Illicit drug use in 2014 for individuals 12 to 17 years old was about 9%. For individuals aged 18 to 25, the rate was highest at 22%. For adults 26 years and older, the rate was slightly more than in previous years at 8%.

In 2014 marijuana and the nonmedical prescription pain relievers were the illicit drugs of choice. About 22 million individuals reported using marijuana in the past 30 days. Although the use of most types of illicit drugs has not increased in recent years, an overall increase in illicit drug use seems to be attributable to marijuana. The percentage of people aged 12 or older in 2014 who were current marijuana users (about 8%) was greater than the percentages in 2002 to 2013. In addition, the estimate of marijuana use was greater in 2014 than the estimates in 2002 to 2009 for young adults aged 18 to 25 and in 2002 to 2013 for adults aged 26 or older.

In the 2014 survey, more than 4 million people reported nonmedical use of prescription pain relievers. It is the rise of prescription drug misuse that has prompted the greatest concern (SAMHSA, 2015a).

Nonmedical use of stimulants including amphetamine/dextroamphetamine (Adderall) and methylphenidate (Ritalin) has more than doubled in the past few years (NIDA, 2015). The use of synthetic drugs, e-cigarettes, and hookah are on the rise among young adults.

HEALTH POLICY

Government Response to Prescription Drug Misuse

In the United States, more than 120 people die every day as a result of a drug overdose. Surprisingly, deaths due to controlled prescription drugs have outpaced those for cocaine and heroin combined. The main source for these drugs are friends or relatives who have legitimate prescriptions. Ultimately, prescription drug use may also lead to the use of heroin, which is less expensive and easier to get.

Unused drugs that find their way into the hands of people with use disorders are a real problem. In response, the Drug Enforcement Administration (DEA) began hosting the National Prescription Drug Take-Back Day Initiative. This initiative provides a safe, convenient, and reliable way of disposing of unneeded prescription drugs. As of 2016, more than 6.4 million pounds of medication had been collected during the first 11 Take-Back Days.

US Department of Justice Drug Enforcement Administration. (2015). National Drug Threat Assessment Summary. Retrieved from https://www.dea.gov/docs/2015%20NDTA%20Report.pdf.

Scheduled Drugs

Drugs are classified into five categories, or schedules, based on the drug's acceptable medical use and the drug's misuse potential. The lower the schedule number, the higher the potential for abuse. The Drug Enforcement Agency (n.d.) classifies drugs in the following way:

- Schedule I drugs carry a high potential for abuse and have no acceptable medical use. Examples are heroin and lysergic acid diethylamide (LSD).
- Schedule II drugs have a high potential for abuse, are considered dangerous, and are available only by prescription. Examples include methadone, meperidine (Demerol), and methylphenidate (Ritalin).
- Schedule III drugs have a low to moderate potential for misuse and are available only by prescription. Examples are testosterone, acetaminophen/codeine (Tylenol with codeine), and buprenorphine (Suboxone)
- Schedule IV drugs are low-risk drugs and are available by prescription. Examples of schedule IV drugs are alprazolam (Xanax), lorazepam (Ativan), and propoxyphene/acetaminophen (Darvocet).
- Schedule V drugs contain limited quantities of certain narcotics for the treatment of diarrhea, coughing, and pain. Examples are atropine/dyphenoxylate (Lomotil), guaifenesin and codeine (Robitussin AC), and pregabalin (Lyrica), available over the counter.

See Table 22.1 for information on commonly abused drugs.

TABLE 22.1 Commonly Abused Drugs

Substance	Street Names	DEA Schedule/ Administration	Acute Effects/Health Risks
Tobacco			
Nicotine	Cigarettes, cigars, bidis, and smokeless tobacco (snuff, spit tobacco, chew)	Smoked, snorted, chewed	*Increased blood pressure and heart rate* Chronic lung disease, cardiovascular disease, stroke, cancers of the mouth, pharynx, larynx, esophagus, stomach, pancreas, cervix, kidney, bladder, and acute myeloid leukemia, adverse pregnancy outcomes, addiction
Alcohol			
Alcohol		Swallowed	*Low doses: Euphoria, mild stimulation, relaxation, lowered inhibitions* *High doses: Drowsiness, slurred speech, nausea, emotional volatility, loss of coordination, visual distortions, impaired memory, loss of consciousness, respiratory arrest, seizures, coma, death* Increased risk of injuries, violence, fetal damage, depression, neurological deficits, hypertension, liver and heart disease, addiction fatal overdose
Cannabinoids			
Marijuana	Blunt, dope, ganja, grass, herb, joint, bud, Mary Jane, pot, reefer, green, trees, smoke, sinsimella, skunk, weed	I Smoked, swallowed	*Euphoria, relaxation, slowed reaction time, distorted sensory perception, impaired balance and coordination, increased heart rate and appetite, impaired learning, memory, anxiety, panic attacks, psychosis/cough* Frequent respiratory infections, possible mental health decline, addiction
Hashish	Boom, gangster, hash, hash oil, hemp	I Smoked, swallowed	
Opioids			
Heroin (Diacetylmorphine)	Smack, horse, brown sugar, dope, H., junk, skag, skunk, white horse, China white, cheese	I Injected, smoked, snorted	*Euphoria, drowsiness, impaired coordination, dizziness, confusion, nausea, sedation, feeling of heaviness in the body, slowed or arrested breathing* Constipation, endocarditis, hepatitis, HIV, addiction, fatal overdose
Opium	Laudanum, paregoric, big O, black stuff, block, gum, hop	II, III, V Swallowed, smoked	
Stimulants			
Cocaine (Cocaine hydrochloride)	Blow, bump, C, candy, Charlie, coke, crack, flake, rock, snow, toot	II Snorted, smoked, injected	*Increased heart rate, blood pressure, body temperature, metabolism, feelings of exhilaration, increased energy, mental alertness, tremors, reduced appetite, irritability, anxiety, panic, paranoia, violent behavior, psychosis* Weight loss, insomnia, cardiac or cardiovascular complications, stroke, seizures, addiction Cocaine: Nasal damage from snorting Methamphetamine: Severe dental problems
Amphetamine (Biphetamine, Dexedrine)	Bennies, black beauties, crosses, hearts, LA turnaround, speed, truck drivers, uppers	II Swallowed, snorted, smoked, injected	
Methamphetamine (Desoxyn)	Meth, ice, crank, chalk, crystal, fire, glass, go fast, speed	II Swallowed, snorted, smoked, injected	

TABLE 22.1 Commonly Abused Drugs—cont'd

Substance	Street Names	DEA Schedule/ Administration	Acute Effects/Health Risks
Club Drugs			
Methylenedioxy-methamphetamine (MDMA)	Ecstasy, Adam, clarity, Eve, lover's speed, peace, uppers. Colorful capsules with imprinted logos	I Swallowed, snorted, injected	*Mild hallucinogenic effects, increased tactile sensitivity, empathic feelings, lowered inhibition, anxiety, chills, sweating, teeth clenching, muscle cramping* Sleep disturbances, depression, impaired memory, hyperthermia, addiction
Flunitrazepam (Rohypnol) Similar to benzodiazepine chemically	Forget-me pill, Mexican Valium, R2, roach, Roche, roofies, roofinol, rope, rophies	IV Swallowed, snorted	*Sedation, muscle relaxation, confusion, memory loss, dizziness, impaired coordination* Addiction
Gamma-hydroxybutyrate (GHB)	G, Georgia home boy, grievous bodily harm, liquid ecstasy, soap, scoop, goop, liquid X	I Swallowed	*Drowsiness, nausea, headache, disorientation, loss of coordination, memory loss* Unconsciousness, seizures, coma
Classic Hallucinogens			
Ayahuasca A brew that includes chacruna or chagropanga, dimethyltryptamine (DMT)-containing plants	Aya, yagé, hoasca,	Listed in the FDA's poisonous plant database Brewed as a tea	*Strong hallucinations, altered vision and auditory perceptions, increased blood pressure, vomiting, diarrhea*
Dimethyltryptamine (DMT) Synthetic drug	Dimitri	I White or yellow powder, smoked, swallowed	*30-60 minutes of intense hallucinations, depersonalization, high blood pressure, rapid eye movements, agitation, seizures*
Lysergic acid diethylamide (LSD)	Acid, blotter, cubes, microdot, yellow sunshine, blue heaven	I Swallowed, absorbed through mouth tissues	*Altered states of perception and feeling, hallucinations, nausea, increased body temperature, heart rate, blood pressure, loss of appetite, sweating, sleeplessness, numbness, dizziness, weakness, tremors, impulsive behavior, rapid shifts in emotion* Flashbacks, hallucinogen persisting perception disorder
Mescaline	Buttons, cactus, mesc, peyote	I Swallowed, smoked	*Altered states of perception and feeling, hallucinations, nausea, increased body temperature, heart rate, blood pressure, loss of appetite, sweating, sleeplessness, numbness, dizziness, weakness, tremors, impulsive behavior, rapid shifts in emotion*
Psilocybin	Magic mushrooms, purple passion, shrooms, little smoke	I Swallowed	*Altered states of perception and feeling, hallucinations, nausea, nervousness, paranoia, panic*
Dissociative Drugs			
Ketamine (Ketalar)	Ketalar SV, cat Valium, K, Special K, vitamin K, kit kat	III Injected, snorted, smoked	*Feelings of being separate from one's body and environment, impaired motor function, analgesia, impaired memory, delirium, respiratory depression and arrest, death* Anxiety, tremors, numbness, memory loss, nausea
Phencyclidine (PCP) and analogs	Angel dust, boat, hog, love boat, peace pill	I/II Swallowed, smoked, injected	*Feelings of being separate from one's body and environment, impaired motor function, analgesia, psychosis, aggression, violence, slurred speech, loss of coordination, hallucinations* Anxiety, tremors, numbness, memory loss, nausea
Salvia divinorum	Salvia, shepherdess's herb, Maria Pastora, magic mint, Sally-D	Chewed, swallowed, smoked	*Feelings of being separate from one's body and environment, impaired motor function* Anxiety, tremors, numbness, memory loss, nausea

Continued

TABLE 22.1 Commonly Abused Drugs—cont'd

Substance	Street Names	DEA Schedule/ Administration	Acute Effects/Health Risks
Dextromethorphan (DXM)	Found in some cough and cold medications Robotripping, Robo, Triple C	Swallowed	*Feelings of being separate from one's body and environment, impaired motor function, euphoria, slurred speech, confusion, dizziness, distorted visual perceptions* Anxiety, tremors, numbness, memory loss, nausea
Classic Hallucinogens			
Other Compounds			
Anabolic steroids	Roids, juice, gym candy, pumpers	III Injected, swallowed, applied to skin	*No intoxication effects* Hypertension, blood clotting and cholesterol changes, liver cysts, hostility and aggression, acne; in adolescents premature stoppage of growth; in males prostate cancer, reduced sperm production, shrunken testicles, breast enlargement; in females menstrual irregularities, development of beard and other masculine characteristics
Inhalants solvents, propellants, thinners, and fuels	Laughing gas, poppers, snappers, whippets	Inhaled through nose or mouth	*Varies by chemical – stimulation, loss of inhibition, headache, nausea or vomiting, slurred speech, loss of motor coordination, wheezing* *Cramps, muscle weakness, depression, memory impairment, damage to cardiovascular and nervous systems, unconsciousness, sudden death*
Prescription pain relievers	Codeine: captain cody, cody, Fentanyl: apache Oxycodone: oxy	II/III/V Capsules, liquid, injected, swallowed, smoked, snorted	Drowsiness, lethargy, euphoria, slow breathing, death
Prescription sedatives	Benzodiazepines: downers Barbituates: barbs Sleep aids: rophies	II/III/IV Pill, capsule, liquid, injected, swallowed	Drowsiness, slurred speech, poor concentration, low blood pressure, decrease respiratory rate
Prescription Stimulants			
Amphetamine (Adderall, Benzedrine)	Bennies, black beauties, crosses, hearts, LA turnaround, speed, truck drivers, uppers	II Tablet, chewable, liquid, swallowed, smoked, injected	*Increased alertness, increased blood pressure and heart rate, narrowed blood vessels, increased blood sugar* Long-term high doses: heart problems, psychosis, anger
Methylphenidate (Concerta, Ritalin)	JIF, MPH, R-ball, skippy, the smart drug, vitamin R	II Liquid, tablet, chewable tablet, capsule Swallowed, snorted, smoked, injected, chewed	

National Institute on Drug Abuse. (2016). *Commonly abused drug chart.* Retrieved from http://www.drugabuse.gov/drugs-abuse/commonly-abused-drugs/commonly-abused-drugs-chart.

COMORBIDITY

Comorbidity refers to two or more disorders occurring in the same person at the same time with potential interactions and exacerbation (worsening) of symptoms. **Co-occurring disorders** may include any combination of two or more substance use disorders and mental disorders identified in the *DSM-5*. In 2014, 20.2 million adults (8.4%) had a substance use disorder (SAMHSA, 2015a). Of these, 7.9 million people had a co-occurring disorder.

Major depressive disorders, bipolar disorder, and anxiety disorders are twice as likely as unaffected individuals to have a substance use disorder. Antisocial personality disorder and conduct disorder are commonly associated with substance abuse.

RISK FACTORS

Biological

Genetic

Alcohol use disorder runs in families and about 40% to 60% of the risk comes from inheritance. Monozygotic (identical) twins are more likely to share alcohol use problems than are dizygotic (fraternal) twins. Monozygotic male twins are more likely to share alcohol use disorder than are female twins. Up to a fourfold increase in risk occurs in children of affected individuals, even when the children are given up for adoption or raised in other homes.

There is some evidence to suggest that some genes may reduce the risk of alcohol consumption by impacting alcohol metabolism. For example, certain alleles of the alcohol dehydrogenase and aldehyde dehydrogenase genes can cause a buildup of acetaldehyde that creates the classic flushing response (Ebert et al., 2016).

There appears to be genetic underlying vulnerability to addiction that expresses itself in a variety of substances. Substance use disorders such as cannabis, cocaine, and opiates definitely run in families. Twin studies support heritability in substance use disorders. Estimates range from 30% to 40% for hallucinogens and stimulants, and as high as 70% to 80% for cocaine and opiates (Ebert et al., 2016)

Neurochemical

Researchers have found neurotransmitters for all the substance use disorders with the exception of alcohol (Sadock et al., 2015). The opioids, for example, act on opioid receptors. People with too little natural opioid activity or too much opioid antagonism might be prone to self-medicating through the use of opioid drugs. Even people who originally had normal opioid function will develop altered function with repeated use of external opioids, to the point where taking the drug makes them feel normal again.

The major neurotransmitters involved in developing substance use disorders are the opioid, catecholamine (especially dopamine), and gamma-aminobutyric acid (GABA) systems (Sadock et al., 2015). The dopaminergic neurons in the ventral tegmental area (VTA) are especially important in the sensation of reward.

Neurobiology of Addiction: An Epidemic of Heroin Use and the Role of Naloxone

When a person injects, smokes, or snorts heroin the drug travels quickly to the brain through the bloodstream. In the brain, the heroin is converted to morphine by enzymes.

Morphine binds to opiate receptors in certain areas within the reward pathway including the ventral tegmental area (VTA), nucleus accumbens, and cortex. Morphine also binds to areas involved in the pain pathway (including the thalamus, brainstem, and spinal cord).

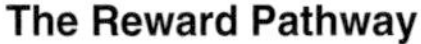

The Reward Pathway

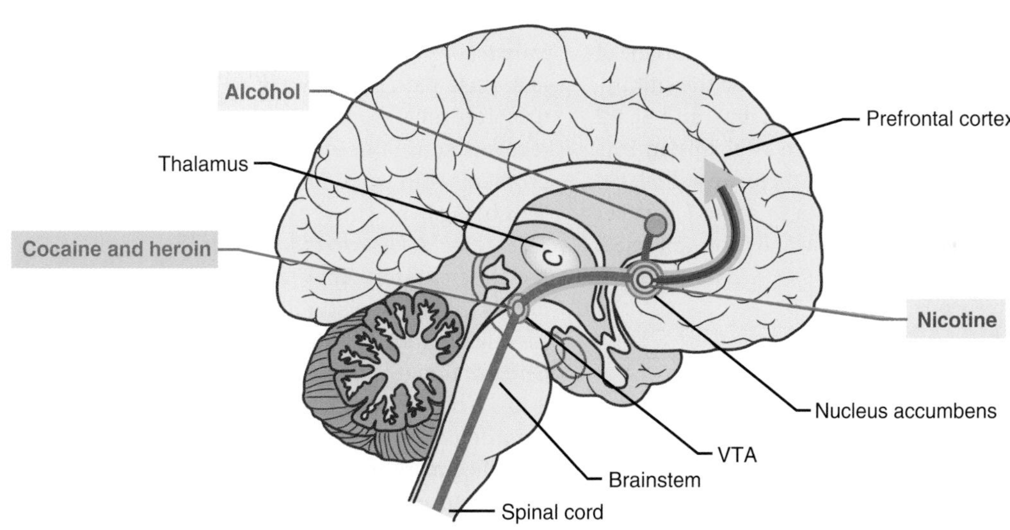

Brain Dysfunction

Tolerance to the analgesic (pain reducing) properties of heroin or morphine no longer respond to the drug in the initial way. Tolerance occurs in the pain passage pathway that includes the thalamus and the spinal cord. These areas are important in sending pain messages and are responsible for the analgesic effects of morphine. However, a person does not develop tolerance to the respiratory depressive effects of heroin/morphine.

When morphine binds to opiate receptors, it inhibits an enzyme, adenylate cyclase, that coordinates the firing of impulses. After repeated opiate receptor activation by morphine, the enzyme adapts so that the morphine can no longer cause changes in cell firing.

Addiction develops when the neurons adapt to exposure of the drug and only function normally in the presence of the drug. Many of the heroin or morphine withdrawal symptoms are generated when the opiate receptors in the thalamus and brainstem are deprived of morphine. Withdrawal can be very serious and the abuser will use the drug again to avoid the symptoms.

Naloxone's Reversal of Heroin Overdose

Overdose is particularly lethal due to respiratory depression. To reduce deaths from overdose, naloxone (trade name Narcan) is being increasingly used by both healthcare providers and the general public. This drug is a pure opioid antagonist with no pharmacological properties. After intravenous, subcutaneous, and intramuscular injection, it temporarily (1–2 hours) binds with them. Its binding ability is stronger than morphine's so it can push the morphine off and reverse the effects of morphine. A nasal spray formulation is currently available.

Environmental Factors

Many chronic stressors have their roots in socioeconomic factors. Poverty raises the risk of an unfavorable living environment, lack of parental supervision, poor educational resources, and impaired support systems. A cycle of negative environmental events often begins within disadvantaged neighborhoods, increasing stress and anxiety along with a lack of or negative social ties, which contributes to depression. Coping mechanisms may include drugs and acting out behaviors leading to destructive consequences and interaction with the legal system.

Adolescents may be strongly influenced by their peers to engage in substance use. Alcohol, which has been referred to as a "social lubricant," may increase an adolescent's feeling of belonging. Using alcohol, tobacco, and marijuana at an early age is strongly associated with coming from a home with low parental supervision.

Sociocultural

Substance use may create a sense of community and belonging in otherwise isolated individuals. The lifestyle of substance abusers may even seem alluring and dramatic to vulnerable people.

In some cultures and religions, alcohol use is not accepted, and any use would be considered deviant. In other cultures, alcohol use is a regular part of everyday life, and the amount of consumption would be alarming to people outside the culture. Muslim-majority countries such as Pakistan, Libya, and Saudi Arabia have prohibitions against alcohol. In Afghanistan it is illegal for citizens to purchase alcohol, but there are still places for foreigners to drink. In the United States some Christian denominations such as Pentecostal, Baptist, and Mormon reject the use of alcohol.

CLINICAL PICTURE

Caffeine

Caffeine is the most widely used psychoactive substance in the world. According to the APA (2013), unlike the other substances discussed in this chapter, excessive caffeine use is not an official use disorder. However, caffeine can result in intoxication and withdrawal. The half-life of caffeine in the human body is 3 to 10 hours, and the peak concentration for most people is 30 to 60 minutes (Sadock et al., 2015).

Caffeine intoxication. The prevalence of caffeine intoxication in the United States is about 7%. Caffeine intoxication is characterized by behavioral symptoms such as restlessness, nervousness, excitement, agitation, rambling speech, and inexhaustibility. Physical symptoms of intoxication are flushed face, diuresis, gastrointestinal disturbance, muscle twitching, tachycardia, or cardiac arrhythmia. These symptoms are distressing to the individual and result in impairment of normal areas of functioning. Individuals with tolerance may not experience these symptoms. Extremely high doses may result in grand mal seizures, and respiratory failure may cause death. Excessive use is associated with many psychiatric problems including bipolar disorders, eating disorders, and sleep disorders.

Caffeine withdrawal. Caffeine withdrawal is not associated with medical problems or the need for intervention. Removal of caffeine from the daily routine results in headache, drowsiness, irritability, and poor concentration. Some people experience flu-like symptoms such as nausea, vomiting, and muscle aches. Symptoms occur within 12 to 24 hours after the last dose, peak in 24 to 48 hours, and resolve within 1 week.

Cannabis Use Disorder

Cannabis, or marijuana, is the most widely used often illegal drug in the world and the fourth most commonly used psychoactive drug in the United States after caffeine, alcohol, and nicotine. It comes from the dried leaves, flowers, stems, and seeds from the hemp plant, *Cannabis sativa*. A chemical, delta-9-tetrahydrocannabinol (THC), is responsible for its mind-altering effects. The concentrated form of cannabis is known as *hashish*. Synthetic cannabinoids of THC, dronabinol (Marinol) and nabilone (Cesamet), are available by prescription for the nausea and vomiting associated with chemotherapy for cancer.

The 12-month prevalence of cannabis use disorder in adolescents is about 3.5% and about 1.5% in adults (APA, 2013). Males are more likely to have this disorder, which tends to progress slowly. Symptoms include using larger amounts over a longer period of time, craving, tolerance (needing more for intoxication), and withdrawal. Individuals with heavy marijuana use patterns may try to quit, cut down, or control its use. Too much time is spent getting cannabis, using it, and recovering from its effects. The use of this substance results in problems with work, home life, education, social, and physical well-being.

Cannabis intoxication. Cannabis intoxication heightens users' sensations. They experience brighter colors, see new details in common stimuli, and time seems to go more slowly. In higher doses, they experience depersonalization and derealization (Sadock et al., 2015). Motor skills are impacted for 8 to 12 hours, and driving and the use of machinery may be hazardous.

Delirium results in marked impairment in cognition and performance. Physical symptoms of intoxication include conjunctival injection (red eyes from vessel dilation), increased appetite, dry mouth, and tachycardia.

Cannabis withdrawal. Withdrawal from cannabis is comparatively late—within 1 week of cessation. Symptoms include irritability, anger, aggression, anxiety, restlessness, and depressed mood. Because people often use marijuana as a sleep aid, insomnia and disturbing dreams may ensue without it. A decreased appetite may lead to weight loss. Physical symptoms of marijuana withdrawal include at least one of the following: abdominal pain, shakiness, sweating, fever, chills, or headache.

Treatment. Drug screens can detect cannabis for up to 4 weeks after use (Sadock et al., 2015). Abstinence and support are the main principles of treatment for cannabis use disorder. Hospitalization or outpatient care may be required. Individual, family, and group therapies can provide support. Antianxiety medication may be useful for short-term relief of withdrawal symptoms. Patients with underlying anxiety and depression may respond to antidepressant therapy.

Hallucinogen Use Disorder

The use of hallucinogens has no medical use; by definition they are intoxicants. They cause a profound disturbance in reality. Hallucinogens are associated with flashbacks, panic attacks, psychosis, delirium, and mood and anxiety disorders (Sadock et al., 2015). They are both natural and synthetic substances. Hallucinogens are classified as schedule I controlled substances, meaning that they have no medical use and carry a high abuse potential.

Hallucinogens are found in some plants and mushrooms (or their extracts) or can be man-made. They are commonly divided into two broad categories: classic hallucinogens (e.g., LSD) and dissociative drugs (e.g., phencyclidine [PCP] and ketamine; see Table 22.1). The APA identifies two use disorders related to hallucinogens—PCP and other hallucinogens. Both problems cause a clinically significant impairment or distress within a 12-month period including craving, difficulty with role obligations, impairment, and tolerance.

Hallucinogen intoxication. Intoxication is characterized by clinically significant psychological and behavioral changes. Paranoia, impaired judgment, intensification of perceptions, depersonalization, and derealization are commonly experienced while using hallucinogens. Illusions, hallucinations, and synesthesias (e.g., hearing colors or seeing sounds) are particularly prominent with this type of intoxication. Physical symptoms include pupillary dilation, tachycardia, sweating, palpitations, blurred vision, tremors, and incoordination.

Treatment. Treatment for hallucinogen intoxication includes talking the patient down. This refers to reassurance that the symptoms are caused by the drug and that the symptoms will subside. In severe cases (Sadock et al., 2015), an antipsychotic such as haloperidol (Haldol) or a benzodiazepine such as diazepam (Valium) can be used in the short term.

Phencyclidine intoxication. PCP intoxication is a medical emergency that can result in dangerous and violent side effects. People under the influence of this drug can be belligerent, assaultive, impulsive, and unpredictable. Significant physical manifestations of this drug include nystagmus (involuntary eye movements), hypertension, tachycardia, diminished response to pain, ataxia (loss of voluntary muscle control), dysarthria (unclear speech), muscle rigidity, seizures, coma, and hyperacusis (sensitivity to sound). Hyperthermia and seizure activity may also occur. Management of individuals intoxicated by PCP is primarily supportive.

Treatment. Patients who have ingested PCP cannot be talked down and may require restraint and a calming medication such as a benzodiazepine. Mechanical cooling may be necessary for severe hyperthermia.

Hallucinogen withdrawal. There is no official withdrawal diagnosis or pattern with prolonged hallucinogen use. However, hallucinogen persisting perception disorder may be experienced during periods of sobriety, particularly from LSD. The prevalence of this problem among hallucinogen users is about 4%. The hallmark of this problem is the reexperiencing of perceptual symptoms that were experienced while intoxicated. These symptoms are distressing and impair the individual from normal functioning for weeks, months, or even years.

Inhalant Use Disorder

Volatile hydrocarbons are toxic gases inhaled through the nose or mouth to enter the bloodstream. Common household products with chemicals that share similar pharmacological properties include:

- Solvents for glues and adhesives
- Propellants found in aerosol paint sprays, hair sprays, and shaving cream
- Thinners such as paint products and correction fluids
- Fuels such as gasoline and propane

Those who use inhalants usually use them only for a short period of time. Some users continue their use despite knowing that this practice is causing serious problems. Characteristics of out-of-control inhalant use are using more and more, craving, and tolerance. Inhalants cause failure in major life roles and problems in interpersonal relationships. "Sudden sniffing death" from cardiac arrhythmias may occur with inhalants, particularly with butane and propane. This disorder occurs primarily between the ages of 12 to 17 years with a 12-month prevalence rate of about 0.4% (APA, 2013).

Inhalant intoxication. Small doses of inhalants result in disinhibition and euphoria. High doses can cause fearfulness, illusions, auditory and visual hallucinations, and a distorted body image. Apathy, diminished social and occupational functioning, impaired judgment, and impulsive and aggressive behavior accompany intoxication.

Physical responses to inhalant intoxication include nausea, anorexia, nystagmus, depressed reflexes, and diplopia. High doses and long exposure can lead to stupor, unconsciousness, and amnesia. Delirium, dementia, and psychosis are also serious possibilities from inhalant use. Although withdrawal is not a considered a disorder in the *DSM-5* (APA, 2013), some users develop a withdrawal syndrome when ceasing inhalant use.

Treatment. Inhalant intoxication usually does not require any treatment. Serious and potentially fatal responses such as coma, cardiac arrhythmias, or bronchospasm do happen. A psychotic response can be induced by inhalant intoxication. This self-limiting (a few hours to a few weeks) problem may require careful use of haloperidol (Haldol) to manage severe agitation.

CONSIDERING CULTURE

A Culture of Teenager Inhalant Use

During a 15-year period, teens in the United States abused more than 3400 different products by inhalation (also known as *huffing*). Butane, propane, and air fresheners had the highest fatality rate. The peak age for inhalant abuse was 14 years old. Inhalant use results in life-threatening symptoms, permanently disabling illnesses, and death. Adolescent use of inhalants is also associated with more sexually transmitted infections in adulthood, particularly among black men.

The most commonly abused substances are propellants, especially aerosol dusters (e.g., computer keyboard and electronics sprays), followed by gasoline and paint. Other products that are commonly inhaled are hair spray, spray deodorant, glue, correction fluid, and carburetor cleaner.

Berger, A. T., Khan, M. R., & Cleland, C. M. (2016). Racial differences in the longitudinal associations between adolescent inhalant use and young adulthood STI risk. *Journal of Substance Use, 21*(1), 14–21.

TABLE 22.2 Trends in Prevalence of Heroin Use

Time Period	Ages 12 or Older	Ages 12-17	Ages 18-25	Ages 26 or Older
Lifetime	1.80	0.10	2.00	2.00
Past year	0.30	0.10	0.80	0.30
Past month	0.20	0.10	0.20	0.20

From Substance Abuse and Mental Health Services Administration. (2015). *Behavioral health trends in the United States: Results from the 2014 National Survey on Drug Use and Health.* Retrieved from http://www.samhsa.gov/data/sites/default/files/NSDUH-FRR1-2014/NSDUH-FRR1-2014.pdf.

Opioid Use Disorder

Opioid misuse, particularly with heroin and prescription drugs, is a chronic relapsing disorder. In opioid use disorders, cravings result in larger amounts and longer periods of time being devoted to the drug and increasing tolerance to its effects. The use of this substance results in significant impairment in life roles, interpersonal conflict, and puts a person in physically hazardous situations.

The ratio of affected males to females is 1.5 to 5. In 2014 about 435,000 people aged 12 or older were current heroin users (SAMHSA, 2015a). This number corresponds to about 0.2% of the population. Opioid use problems usually begin in late teens or early 20s. Increasing age is associated with fewer affected individuals, probably due to early mortality and a cessation of use after age 40. Table 22.2 identifies the prevalence of heroin use among various age groups.

Opioid intoxication. People intoxicated on opioids exhibit psychomotor retardation, drowsiness, slurred speech, altered mood, and impaired memory and attention. They also exhibit pupillary constriction. Intense drowsiness can lead to a coma.

Opioid withdrawal. Withdrawal symptoms for opioids occur after a cessation of or reduction in heavy opioid use, or after an opioid antagonist has been administered. Symptoms of withdrawal include mood dysphoria, nausea, vomiting, diarrhea, muscle aches, fever, and insomnia. Other classic symptoms of withdrawal are lacrimation (watery eyes), rhinorrhea (runny nose), pupillary dilation, and yawning. The symptom of piloerection (bristling of hairs) or gooseflesh is the origin of the term *cold turkey* for the abstinence syndrome. Males may experience sweating and spontaneous ejaculations while awake.

Morphine, heroin, and methadone withdrawal syndrome begins 6 to 8 hours after the last dose following a period of at least a week of use. It reaches intensity during the second or third day and then subsides during the next week. Meperidine (Demerol) withdrawal begins within 8 to 12 hours from abstinence and lasts about 5 days.

See Box 22.1 for some of the signs and symptoms of intoxication and withdrawal.

Opioid overdose. Death attributable to opioids usually stems from respiratory arrest due to the respiratory depressant effect of the drug. Symptoms of overdose include unresponsiveness, slow respiration, coma, hypothermia, hypotension, and bradycardia. Three symptoms—coma, pinpoint pupils, and respiratory depression—are strongly suggestive of overdose.

BOX 22.1 Signs and Symptoms of Opioid Intoxication and Withdrawal

Opioid Intoxication	Opioid Withdrawal
Bradycardia (slow pulse)	Tachycardia (fast pulse)
Hypotension (low blood pressure)	Hypertension (high blood pressure)
Hypothermia (low body temperature)	Hyperthermia (high body temperature)
Sedation	Insomnia
Meiosis (pinpoint pupils)	Mydriasis (enlarged pupils)
Hypokinesis (slowed movement)	Hyperreflexia (abnormally heightened reflexes)
Slurred speech	Diaphoresis (sweating)
Head nodding	Piloerection (gooseflesh)
Euphoria	Increased respiratory rate
Analgesia (pain-killing effects)	Lacrimation (tearing), yawning
Calmness	Rhinorrhea (runny nose)
	Muscle spasms
	Abdominal cramps, nausea, vomiting, diarrhea
	Bone and muscle pain
	Anxiety

From Substance Abuse and Mental Health Services Administration. (2006). *TIP 45 detoxification and substance abuse treatment (DHHS Publication No. SMA 06-4224).* Washington, DC: US Government Printing Office.

Overdose treatment. Treatment for an overdose begins with promoting breathing by aspirating secretions and inserting an airway. Mechanical ventilation should be used until naloxone (Narcan), a specific opioid antagonist, can be given intramuscularly, subcutaneously, or intravenously. Increased respirations and pupillary dilation should happen quickly. Too much naloxone may produce withdrawal symptoms. Duration of action for naloxone is short compared with many opioids, so repeated administration may be required.

General treatment. Individual therapy, behavioral therapy, cognitive behavioral therapy, family therapy, and social skills training may all be helpful in the management of opioid use disorder (Sadock et al., 2015). Support groups such as Narcotics Anonymous (NA), a 12-step program, are excellent sources of help. More structure is provided in residential treatment and therapeutic communities. They work best in cases of highly motivated individuals. Confrontation in the group environment and isolation from the outside world are emphasized in these settings.

Methadone (Dolophine, Methadose) is a synthetic narcotic opioid. It is used to decrease the painful symptoms of opiate withdrawal. It also blocks the euphoric effects of opiate drugs such as heroin, morphine, and codeine, as well as semisynthetic opioids like oxycodone and hydrocodone. Methadone can only be dispensed through an opioid treatment program certified by SAMHSA. Once-a-day dosing is adequate. Methadone, too, will eventually need to be withdrawn due to dependence. In pregnant users, a low dose of methadone may be the safest course. Neonatal withdrawal is usually mild and can be managed with paregoric.

Some serious side effects may occur while taking methadone. Patients should be instructed to seek medical care if they experience difficulty breathing or shallow breathing, feel lightheaded or faint, or experience chest pain or a fast or pounding heartbeat. Hives, rash, or swelling of the face, lips, tongue, or throat could also be serious symptoms. Hallucinations or confusion should also be reported to a care provider.

Buprenorphine is used to help people reduce or quit their use of heroin or other opiates such as pain relievers like morphine. Buprenorphine is an opioid partial agonist. Like opioids, it produces effects such as euphoria or respiratory depression, but these effects are weaker than those of full drugs such as heroin and methadone. The FDA has approved the following schedule III buprenorphine products, some of which contain naloxone:

- Subutex (buprenorphine) sublingual tablets
- Bunavail (buprenorphine and naloxone) buccal film
- Suboxone (buprenorphine and naloxone) sublingual tablets
- Zubsolv (buprenorphine and naloxone) sublingual tablets
- Probuphine (buprenorphine) is supplied by four 1-inch rods surgically implanted under the skin of the upper arm for 6 months

Side effects of buprenorphine include nausea, vomiting, constipation, muscle aches and cramps, insomnia, irritability, and fever. This drug is used only after abstaining from opioids for 12 to 24 hours and in the early stages of opioid withdrawal. It can bring on acute withdrawal for patents not in the early stages of withdrawal and who have other opioids in their bloodstream. Because buprenorphine is a long-acting drug, once patients have been stabilized, they can sometimes switch to alternate-day dosing instead of dosing every day.

Naltrexone (Vivitrol) is an opioid antagonist indicated for the prevention of relapse to opioid dependence, following opioid detoxification. A long-acting injectable version of this drug, ReVia, is given once a month. If a person using naltrexone relapses and uses the misused drug, naltrexone blocks the euphoric and sedative effects. Side effects include weakness, tiredness, insomnia, increased thirst, anxiety, nervousness, restlessness, irritability, lightheadedness, fainting, muscle or joint aches, decreased sex drive, impotence, or difficulty having an orgasm.

EVIDENCE-BASED PRACTICE

Early Use of Nonmedical Prescription Opioids Linked to Subsequent Heroin Use

Problem

With a national epidemic of heroin use and its extremely dangerous consequence of overdose, researchers are trying to pinpoint which groups may be at most risk.

Purpose of the Study

(1) To explore the relationship between nonmedical use of prescription opioids in childhood and subsequent heroin use in young adulthoods and (2) to determine whether age, race/ethnicity, or income played a role in increasing risk.

Methods

Researchers examined data previously collected through the *2004–2011 National Surveys on Drug Use and Health.* The survey included 223,534 participants in the 12- to 21-year-old age group.

Key Findings

- A history of nonmedical use of prescription opioids was strongly associated with subsequent heroin initiation.
- Children using prescription opioids between the ages of 10 to 12 years had the highest risk of transitioning to heroin use.
- Race/ethnicity and income did not impact the association.

Implications for Nursing Practice

Teaching for patients who take prescription opioids should emphasize the need to safeguard these gateway drugs from friends and family who may abuse them. Knowing the serious risk for youths who experiment with opioids before adolescence should result in increased vigilance for this population.

Cerda, M., Santaella, J., Marshall, B. D. L., Kim, J. H., & Martins, S. S. (2015). Nonmedical prescription opioid use in childhood and early adolescence predicts transitions to heroin use in young adulthood: A national study. *The Journal of Pediatrics, 167*(3), 605–612.

Sedative, Hypnotic, and Antianxiety Medication Use Disorder

Drugs in this category include the benzodiazepines, benzodiazepine-like drugs (e.g., zolpidem, zaleplon), carbamates, barbiturates, (e.g., secobarbital), and barbiturate-like hypnotics (e.g., methaqualone). This class includes all prescription sleeping medications and almost all prescription antianxiety drugs. Craving is a typical feature. Use of these brain depressants negatively affects role performance and relationships. Significant tolerance and withdrawal can develop in anyone using these drugs even for their intended indication. A use disorder diagnosis is only given in the presence of additional *DSM-5* criteria such as clinically significant maladaptive behavior or psychological changes.

The 12-month prevalence of this problem is about 0.2% in adults. It occurs in males slightly more often than in females. Sedative, hypnotic, and antianxiety medication use disorders are highest among 18- to 29-year-olds (0.5%) and lowest among individuals 65 and older (0.04%).

Sedative, hypnotic, and antianxiety medication intoxication. As a group of depressants, the criteria for intoxication make sense: slurred speech, incoordination, unsteady gait, nystagmus, and impaired thinking. Coma is a dangerous possibility with this class of drugs. Inappropriate aggression and sexual behavior, mood fluctuation, and impaired judgment may also be side effects.

Overdose treatment. Overdose treatment includes gastric lavage, activated charcoal, and careful vital sign monitoring. Patients who are awake after overdosing should be kept awake to prevent a loss of consciousness. If unconscious, an intravenous fluid line should be established. An endotracheal tube may be required to provide a patent airway, and mechanical ventilation can be used if necessary.

Sedative, hypnotic, and antianxiety medication withdrawal. Repeated depressing of the central nervous system, along with the body's daily attempt to return to homeostasis, results in rebound hyperactivity with the removal of the substance. Hence, we may see symptoms such as autonomic hyperactivity, tremor, insomnia, psychomotor agitation, anxiety, and grand mal seizures. The degree and timing of the withdrawal syndrome depends on the specific substance. Half-life is an important predictor of time.

Withdrawal treatment. Gradual reduction of benzodiazepines will prevent seizures and other withdrawal symptoms. Barbiturate withdrawal can be aided by using a long-acting barbiturate such as phenobarbital.

Stimulant Use Disorder

Amphetamine-type, cocaine, or other stimulant drugs are second only to cannabis as the most widely used illicit substances in the United States. They typically produce a euphoric feeling and high energy. Long distance truckers, students studying for exams, soldiers in wartime, and athletes in competition use these drugs. As with all the use disorders, increased use, craving, and tolerance are accompanied by reduced ability to function in major roles. Stimulants represent a significant problem as a use disorder pattern can occur in as little as 1 week.

The estimated 12-month prevalence for amphetamine-type stimulants is about 0.2% in adults. Both genders are affected equally. Intravenous stimulant use is greater in males, around 4:1. Cocaine use disorder is higher, 0.3%, with more male users.

Stimulant intoxication. People feel superhuman while using stimulants. They feel elated, euphoric, and sociable. Unfortunately, they are also hypervigilant, sensitive, anxious, tense, and angry. Physical symptoms include two or more of the following: chest pain, cardiac arrhythmias, high or low blood pressure, tachycardia or bradycardia, respiratory depression, dilated pupils, perspiration, chills, nausea or vomiting, weight loss, psychomotor agitation or retardation, weakness, confusion, seizures, or coma.

Stimulant withdrawal. Withdrawal symptoms begin within a few hours to several days. Symptoms include tiredness, vivid nightmares, increased appetite, insomnia or hypersomnia, and psychomotor retardation or agitation. Functionality is impaired during this withdrawal process. Depression and suicidal thoughts are the most serious side effects of stimulant withdrawal.

See Box 22.2 for some of the signs and symptoms of intoxication and withdrawal.

Withdrawal treatment. For amphetamines, an inpatient setting is usually necessary. Individual, family, and group therapy are helpful. Depending upon the amphetamine used, specific drugs may be used short term. Antipsychotics may be prescribed for a few days. If there is no psychosis, diazepam (Valium) is useful in treating agitation and hyperactivity. Once the patient has been withdrawn from the amphetamine, depression can be treated with antidepressants such as bupropion (Wellbutrin).

The 1- to 2-week cocaine withdrawal period is distinct because there are no physiological disturbances that require inpatient care. Outpatient settings may be tried as a first approach. Some patients experience fatigue, mood changes, disturbed sleep, craving, and depression. There are no drugs that reliably reduce the intensity of these symptoms. The intense craving associated with cocaine withdrawal may require hospitalization to remove the affected individual from the usual social settings and drug sources. Unscheduled urine drug testing is usually warranted.

Tobacco Use Disorder

Craving, persistent and recurrent use, and tolerance are all symptoms of tobacco use disorder. Dependence happens quickly. Cigarettes are the most commonly used tobacco product. The 12-month prevalence of tobacco use disorder is about 13% in adults. Rates are slightly higher in males as compared with females. Most people who use tobacco begin before the age of 18.

Tobacco withdrawal. Tobacco withdrawal is distressing. At least four of the following symptoms occur: irritability, anxiety, depression, difficulty concentrating, restlessness, and insomnia. Within days after smoking cessation, heart rates decrease by 5 to 12 beats per minute. Within the first year after smoking cessation, people increase their weight by an average of 4 to 7 pounds.

Withdrawal treatment. Behavioral therapy is useful to teach the patient to recognize cravings and respond to them appropriately. Hypnosis has been used successfully to treat tobacco withdrawal. Nicotine replacement therapies in the form of gum, lozenges, nasal sprays, and patches are highly successful treatments. Non-nicotine therapy options include the antidepressant bupropion (Zyban), which reduces the cravings for nicotine. Clonidine (Catapres) decreases sympathetic activity and reduces withdrawal symptoms. Varenicline (Chantix) provides some nicotine effects to ease withdrawal symptoms and blocks the effects of nicotine from cigarettes if smoking is resumed.

Gambling Disorder

Gambling is a compulsive activity that causes economic problems and significant disturbances in personal, social, or occupational functioning. Individuals with this disorder are preoccupied with the behavior, experience an increasing desire to gamble, and lie to conceal the extent of the problem. They may try to control the behavior, cut back, or stop gambling. Otherwise honest people may commit illegal acts to finance

BOX 22.2 Signs and Symptoms of Stimulant Intoxication and Withdrawal

Stimulant Intoxication	Stimulant Withdrawal
Short Term	Depression
Increased energy	Hypersomnia (or insomnia)
Decreased appetite	Fatigue
Mental alertness	Anxiety
Increased heart rate/pressure	Irritability
Dilated pupils	Poor concentration
Long Term	Psychomotor retardation
Irregular heartbeat	Increased appetite
Chest pains	Paranoia
Increased risk of heart attack	Drug craving
Panic attacks	
Depression	
Delusions/hallucinations	
"Cocaine bugs" (skin sensation)	

From Substance Abuse and Mental Health Services Administration. (2006). *TIP 45 detoxification and substance abuse treatment (DHHS Publication No. SMA 06-4224)*. Washington, DC: US Government Printing Office.

their addiction. They may rely on others to help pay off debts and gamble to recoup losses.

The 1-year prevalence rate in females is about 0.2%, and for males it is about 0.6%. The lifetime prevalence of gambling disorder is about 0.4% to 1%. Early expression of gambling disorder is more common among males, although the progression is more rapid for females. This problem usually develops over the course of years. Gambling may be regular or episodic. Heavy gambling may be interspersed with abstinence. Stress and depression may increase this behavior.

Treatment. Legal problems, pressure from family, and other psychiatric problems may bring the person who gambles excessively into treatment. Gamblers Anonymous (GA) is a 12-step program modeled on Alcoholics Anonymous. It involves public confession, peer pressure, and peer counselors who are reformed gamblers. Hospitalization may help by removing patients from gambling environments. Individual, group, and family therapy are useful in supporting the patient.

Medications such as selective serotonin reuptake inhibitors, bupropion (Wellbutrin), mood stabilizers (lithium), and anticonvulsants such as topiramate (Topamax) may be helpful. Second-generation antipsychotics have also been used in the treatment of gambling disorder. Naltrexone, an opioid antagonist, may be given to individuals with the most severe symptoms of gambling disorder.

ALCOHOL USE DISORDER

Although alcohol is a sedative, it creates an initial feeling of euphoria. This is probably related to decreased inhibitions.

DSM-5 CRITERIA FOR ALCOHOL USE DISORDER

A. A problematic pattern of alcohol use leading to clinically significant impairment or distress, as manifested by at least two of the following, occurring within a 12-month period:
  1. Alcohol is often taken in larger amounts or over a longer period than was intended.
  2. There is a persistent desire or unsuccessful efforts to cut down or control alcohol use.
  3. A great deal of time is spent in activities necessary to obtain alcohol, use alcohol, or recover from its effects.
  4. Craving or a strong desire or urge to use alcohol.
  5. Recurrent alcohol use resulting in a failure to fulfill major role obligations at work, school, or home.
  6. Continued alcohol use despite having persistent or recurrent social or interpersonal problems caused or exacerbated by the effects of alcohol.
  7. Important social, occupational, or recreational activities are given up or reduced because of alcohol use.
  8. Recurrent alcohol use in situations in which it is physically hazardous.
  9. Alcohol use is continued despite knowledge of having a persistent or recurrent physical or psychological problem that is likely to have been caused or exacerbated by alcohol.
  10. Tolerance, as defined by either of the following:
     a. A need for markedly increased amounts of alcohol to achieve intoxication or desired effect.
     b. A markedly diminished effect with continued use of the same amount of alcohol.
  11. Withdrawal, as manifested by either of the following:
     c. The characteristic withdrawal syndrome for alcohol.
     d. Alcohol (or a closely related substance such as a benzodiazepine) is taken to relieve or avoid withdrawal problems.

Specify if:

In early remission: After full criteria for alcohol use disorder were previously met, none of the criteria for alcohol use disorder have been met for at least 3 months but for less than 12 months (with the exception that Criterion A4 may be met).

In sustained remission: After full criteria for alcohol use disorder were previously met, none of the criteria for alcohol use disorder have been met at any time during a period of 12 months or longer (with the exception that Criterion A4 may be met).

Specify if:

In a controlled environment: This additional specifier is used if the individual is in an environment where access to alcohol is restricted.

From the American Psychiatric Association. (2013). *Diagnostic and statistical manual of mental disorders* (5th ed.). Washington, DC: Author.

A cluster of behavioral and physical symptoms characterizes alcohol use disorder. The full criteria for alcohol use disorder are listed in the *DSM-5* box. Severity is based on the number of symptoms: mild (two or three symptoms), moderate (four or five symptoms), and severe (presence of six or more symptoms).

Types of Problematic Drinking

Amounts of alcohol that are considered safe vary depending upon individual factors. Table 22.3 identifies the numbers of drinks that are considered acceptable depending on the gender, age, and pregnancy.

Excessive drinking is described by two different terms. **Binge drinking** refers to drinking too much alcohol quickly. For women this amount is four or more drinks within 2 hours; for men this amount is five or more drinks within 2 hours. **Heavy drinking** is characterized by drinking too much, too often. Eight or more

TABLE 22.3 Maximum Safe Number of Drinks Based on Population

	Men	Women	Pregnant	Adolescent	Elderly
Day	4	3	0	0	3
Week	14	7	0	0	7

US Department of Health and Human Services. (2015). *2015–2020 dietary guidelines for Americans* (8th ed.). Retrieved from http://health.gov/dietaryguidelines/2015/guidelines/.

drinks in a week constitutes heavy drinking in women. Men who drink more than 14 drinks in a week are considered heavy drinkers.

Alcohol Intoxication

The legal definition of intoxication in most states requires a blood concentration of 80 or 100 mg ethanol per deciliter of blood (mg/dL). This concentration may also be expressed as 0.08 to 0.10 g/dL. Signs and symptoms of alcohol intoxication based on blood alcohol are:

- 20 mg/dL (0.02 g/dL)—Two alcoholic drinks: Slower motor performance, decreased thinking ability, altered mood, and reduced ability to multitask.
- 50 mg/dL (0.05 g/dL)—Three alcoholic drinks: Impaired judgment, exaggerated behavior, euphoria, and lower alertness.
- 80 mg/dL (0.08 g/dL)—Four alcoholic drinks: Poor muscle coordination, altered speech and hearing, difficulty detecting danger, impaired judgment, poor self-control, and decreased reasoning.
- 100 mg/dL (0.10 g/dL)—Five alcoholic drinks: Slurred speech, poor coordination, and slowed thinking.
- 150 mg/dL (0.15 g/dL)—Six alcoholic drinks: Vomiting (unless high tolerance) and major loss of balance.
- 200 mg/dL (0.20 g/dL)—Eight to 10 alcoholic drinks: Memory blackouts, nausea, and vomiting.
- 300 mg/dL (0.30 g/dL)—More than 10 alcoholic drinks: Reduction of body temperature, blood pressure, respiratory rate, sleepiness, and amnesia.
- 400 mg/dL (0.40 mg/dL)—Impaired vital signs and possible death.

Intoxication is based on a number of factors including how quickly the alcohol is consumed. Quicker ingestion results in higher levels of blood alcohol. In the United States, a standard drink is one that contains about 14 grams of pure alcohol (National Institute on Alcohol Abuse and Alcoholism, 2005). This amount is found in 12 ounces of beer with 5% alcohol content, 5 ounces of wine with 12% alcohol content, and 1.5 ounces of distilled spirits with 40% alcohol content.

Alcohol Withdrawal

Alcohol withdrawal occurs after reducing or quitting alcohol after heavy and prolonged use. The classic sign of alcohol withdrawal is tremulousness, commonly called the *shakes* or the *jitters,* that begins 6 to 8 hours after alcohol cessation (Sadock et al., 2015). Mild to moderate alcohol withdrawal includes agitation, lack of appetite, nausea, vomiting, insomnia, impaired cognition, and mild perceptual changes. Both systolic and diastolic blood pressure increases, as does pulse and body temperature. Chlordiazepoxide (Librium) is useful for tremulousness and mild to moderate agitation.

Psychotic and perceptual symptoms may begin in 8 to 10 hours. If your patient is undergoing withdrawal to the point of psychosis, it should be considered a medical emergency because of the risks of unconsciousness, seizures, and delirium. The benzodiazepines lorazepam (Ativan) or chlordiazepoxide (Librium) can be given either orally or intramuscularly and tapered over the following 5 to 7 days.

Withdrawal seizures may occur within 12 to 24 hours after alcohol cessation. These seizures are generalized and tonic-clonic. Additional seizures may occur within hours of the first seizure. Diazepam (Valium) given intravenously is a common treatment for withdrawal seizures.

Alcohol withdrawal delirium, also known as *delirium tremens (DTs)*, is a medical emergency that can result in death in 20% of untreated patients, usually as a result of medical problems such as pneumonia, renal disease, hepatic insufficiency, or heart failure (Sadock et al., 2015). Alcohol withdrawal delirium may happen anytime in the first 72 hours. Autonomic hyperactivity may result in tachycardia, diaphoresis, fever, anxiety, insomnia, and hypertension. Delusions and visual and tactile hallucinations are common in alcohol withdrawal delirium.

Delusions and hallucinations may result in unpredictable behaviors as patients try to protect themselves from what they believe are genuine dangers. Patients on any medical floor are at risk for this condition after cessation of heavy drinking for 3 days and are a danger to themselves and others. Serious physical illness such as hepatitis or pancreatitis may increase the likelihood of alcohol withdrawal delirium. It is rare to see this syndrome in individuals in good physical health.

Prevention of alcohol withdrawal delirium is the goal. Oral diazepam (Valium) may be useful in the symptomatic relief of acute agitation, tremor, impending or acute delirium tremens, and hallucinosis. Chlordiazepoxide (Librium) may keep your patient out of danger. However, once delirium appears, intravenous lorazepam (Ativan) is used to treat these severe symptoms. Seclusion may be necessary. Dehydration, often exacerbated by diaphoresis and fever, can be corrected with oral or intravenous fluids.

Alcohol-Induced Persisting Amnestic Disorder

Wernicke-Korsakoff Syndrome

People with a heavy use of alcohol for many years may suffer from short-term memory disturbances. One memory-reducing problem is Wernicke's (alcoholic) encephalopathy, an acute and reversible condition. Another problem is Korsakoff's syndrome, a chronic condition with a recovery rate of only about 20%. The pathophysiological connection between the two problems is a thiamine deficiency, which may be caused by poor nutrition associated with alcohol use or by the malabsorption of nutrients.

Wernicke's encephalopathy is characterized by altered gait, vestibular dysfunction, confusion, and several ocular motility abnormalities (horizontal nystagmus, lateral orbital palsy, and gaze palsy). These eye-focused signs are bilateral but not necessarily symmetrical. Sluggish reaction to light and anisocoria (unequal pupil size) are also symptoms. Wernicke's may clear up within a few weeks or may progress into Korsakoff's syndrome, the more severe and chronic version of this problem.

Wernicke's encephalopathy responds rapidly to large doses of intravenous thiamine two to three times daily for 1 to 2 weeks. Treatment of Korsakoff's syndrome is also thiamine for 3 to 12 months. Most patients with Korsakoff's syndrome never fully recover, although cognitive improvement may occur with thiamine and nutritional support.

Blackouts

An extremely disturbing aspect of alcohol use is blackouts. Blackouts are caused by excessive consumption of alcohol

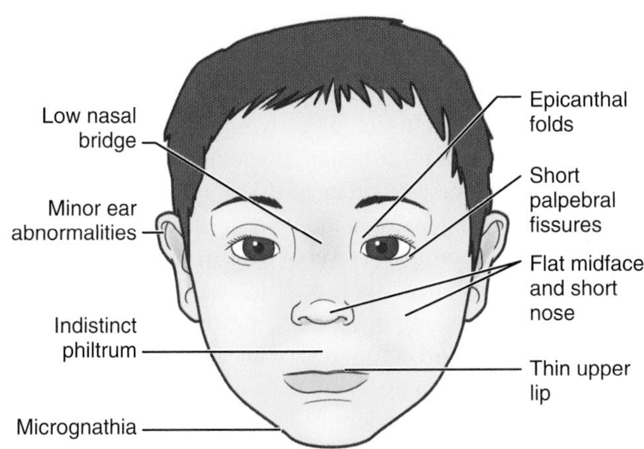

FIG. 22.1 Facial features of fetal alcohol syndrome. (From National Institute on Alcohol Abuse and Alcoholism. [2011]. *Fetal alcohol spectrum disorders.* Retrieved from http://pubs.niaaa.nih.gov/publications/AA82/AA82.htm.)

followed by episodes of amnesia. During these periods of time, a person actively engages in behaviors, can perform complicated tasks, and appears normal. This phenomenon is due to alcohol's ability to block the consolidation of new memories into ones through the hippocampus and related temporal lobe structures.

Fetal Alcohol Syndrome

Fetal alcohol syndrome is the leading cause of intellectual disability in the United States (Sadock et al., 2015). Alcohol during pregnancy inhibits intrauterine growth and postnatal development resulting in microcephaly, craniofacial malformations, and limb and heart defects. As adults, affected individuals tend to have a short stature. Women with alcohol-related disorders have a 35% risk of having a child with defects. Fig. 22.1 illustrates the facial features of fetal alcohol syndrome.

Systemic Effects

Peripheral Neuropathy

Chronic alcoholism leads to nutritional deficiencies, particularly thiamine, due to drinking rather than eating, leading to damage to the peripheral nervous system. The feeling of "pins and needles" in the lower extremities is a common symptom of peripheral neuropathy. Other symptoms include numbness, muscle weakness, sensitivity to touch, and burning. Discontinuation of alcohol will prevent further deterioration.

Alcoholic Myopathy

Binge drinking may cause a sudden acute alcoholic myopathy with muscle weakness and myonecrosis (muscle damage). Chronic alcoholic myopathy develops gradually. The characteristic symptom of this problem is a significant reduction in muscle mass and resulting muscle weakness. Recovery is possible if alcohol is avoided, but the time to recovery varies from rapid (days to weeks) with the acute form to lengthy (weeks to months) with the chronic form.

Alcoholic Cardiomyopathy

Direct toxic effects of alcohol can weaken and thin the muscles of the heart leading to enlargement and eventual heart failure. Symptoms of alcoholic cardiomyopathy are similar to other types of heart failure including fatigue, shortness of breath, and edema of the legs and feet.

Esophagitis

Inflammation of the esophagus is a direct result of the toxic effects of alcohol on the esophageal mucosa. The vomiting related to alcohol overuse is also contributory to this condition. Esophageal varices are distended veins within the esophagus or the upper part of the stomach that result from heavy drinking. These veins are at risk for bursting, which results in a medical emergency.

Gastritis

As a toxin, alcohol irritates and erodes the mucosal stomach lining. Symptoms of gastritis include nausea, vomiting, loss of appetite, belching, and bloating. Damage to the stomach lining may lead to ulcers and bleeding.

Pancreatitis

Prolonged and hazardous drinking may result in pancreatic damage. Excessive drinking, usually more than 5 years, may result in an acute attack of pancreatitis. Continued alcohol misuse eventually results in chronic pancreatitis in a minority of misusers. Abdominal pain, nausea, and vomiting are the major symptoms of acute pancreatitis. Withdrawal of alcohol in the early stages will reverse the condition. The chronic condition results in malnutrition, weight loss, and diabetes mellitus. Withdrawal of alcohol in the chronic condition may reduce inflammatory episodes and allow for better control of diabetes.

Alcoholic Hepatitis

Alcohol gets processed by the liver and produces highly toxic chemicals. Excessive alcohol over an extended period of time may result in a diseased and inflamed liver. Alcoholic hepatitis only occurs in a minority of heavy users. Genetic factors such as how the body processes alcohol, other liver disorders (e.g., hepatitis C), malnutrition, and being female increases the risk of this disorder. Symptoms of alcoholic hepatitis include appetite changes, dry mouth, weight loss, nausea and vomiting, pain or swelling in the abdomen, jaundice, fever, confusion, and fatigue.

Cirrhosis of the Liver

Cirrhosis is a slowly progressing disease in which healthy liver tissue is replaced by scar tissue. Eventually the liver can no longer function properly because the scar tissue blocks the flow of blood through the liver. This slows the processing of nutrients, hormones, drugs, and naturally produced toxins. Cirrhosis is the twelfth leading cause of death of disease (National Institutes of Health, 2014). Symptoms of cirrhosis of the liver include easy bleeding and bruising, pruritus, jaundice, ascites, leg edema, weight loss, confusion, spider-like blood vessels on the skin (petechiae), and testicular atrophy. No treatment will cure cirrhosis or repair scarring. Liver transplantation may be necessary. Low-salt diets will reduce ascites.

Leukopenia

When there is liver damage, alcoholism may cause low white blood cells due to vitamin deficiencies and low protein intake. Low white blood cells predispose individuals to infection and disease. Symptoms of leukopenia include periodontitis and gingivitis, fatigue, weakness, fever, and abdominal pain. Improved nutrition and alcohol cessation are indicated for this condition.

Thrombocytopenia

Thrombocytopenia is a complication of liver cirrhosis characterized by a low platelet count. This is caused by platelet pooling in an enlarged spleen and decreased thromboprotein production in the liver. Symptoms of thrombocytopenia include excessive bruising (purpura), petechiae (particularly on lower legs), and prolonged bleeding from cuts. Platelet count begins to rise within 2 to 5 days of abstaining from alcohol.

Cancer

Alcohol consumption is a major risk factor for head and neck cancers, especially in the oral cavity, pharynx, and larynx (National Cancer Institute, 2013). Alcohol use is also associated with liver, breast, and colorectal cancers.

APPLICATION OF THE NURSING PROCESS

SCREENING

Alcohol is a major contributing factor in:

- Increased mortality and deaths
- Morbidity and disease
- Harm to others and injury
- Increased economic loss and disabilities (SAMHSA, 2015b).

Alcohol can be fatal as a result of its severe withdrawal symptoms. Screening is essential to intervene early and provide treatment for people with substance use disorders and for those at risk of developing these disorders.

The **Screening, Brief Intervention, and Referral to Treatment (SBIRT)** is a comprehensive, integrated, public health approach to the delivery of early intervention and treatment services for persons with substance use disorders, as well as those who are at risk of developing these disorders. SBIRT identifies at-risk substance users for early intervention (SAMHSA, 2015) and consists of three major components:

- **Screening:** A nurse or other healthcare professional in any healthcare setting assesses the severity of substance use and identifies the appropriate level of treatment.
- **Brief Intervention:** A nurse or other healthcare professional focuses on increasing insight and awareness regarding substance use and motivation toward behavioral change.
- **Referral to Treatment:** A nurse or other healthcare professional provides those identified as needing more extensive treatment with access to specialty care.

A variety of other screening tools are available to assist healthcare practitioners in gaining important information on which to base plans of care. Additional screening tools are:

- AUDIT (The **A**lcohol **U**se **D**isorders **I**dentification **T**est)
- CAGE (Questions: Have you felt you needed to **c**ut down on your drinking? Are people **a**nnoyed by your drinking? Have you felt **g**uilty about your drinking? Have you ever had a drink in the morning (**e**ye-opener)? Score of 2 or more is significant, although a score of 1 requires further assessment.
- CAGE-AID (Questions are the same as CAGE but refers to **A**dapted to **I**nclude **D**rugs.)
- T-ACE (**T**olerance, **A**nnoyance, **C**ut down, **E**ye-opener)

Formalized alcohol screening is as simple as using the Alcohol Use Disorders Identification Test (AUDIT) developed for the World Health Organization. AUDIT has been effective for decades and continues to be used today (Babor et al., 2001; Table 22.4). The clinician can administer this tool or the patient can self-report.

During the screening process, instructions need to be clear and followed carefully. Nonjudgmental attitudes help with

TABLE 22.4 The Alcohol Use Disorders Identification Test (AUDIT): Self-Report Version

Patient: Because alcohol use can affect your health and interfere with certain medications and treatments, it is important that we ask some questions about your use of alcohol. Be honest, confidentiality will be upheld.
Mark the frequency that best describes your answer to each question.

Questions	0	1	2	3	4	Score
1. How often do you have a drink containing alcohol?	Never	Monthly or less	2-4 times a month	2-3 times a week	4 or more times a week	
2. How many drinks containing alcohol do you have on a typical day when you are drinking?	1 or 2	3 or 4	5 or 6	7 to 9	10 or more	
3. How often do you have six or more drinks on one occasion?	Never	Less than monthly	Monthly	Weekly	Daily or almost daily	
4. How often during the last year have you found that you were not able to stop drinking once you had started?	Never	Less than monthly	Monthly	Weekly	Daily or almost daily	
5. How often during the last year have you failed to do what was normally expected of you because of drinking?	Never	Less than monthly	Monthly	Weekly	Daily or almost daily	
6. How often during the last year have you needed a first drink in the morning to get yourself going after a heavy drinking session?	Never	Less than monthly	Monthly	Weekly	Daily or almost daily	

TABLE 22.4 **The Alcohol Use Disorders Identification Test (AUDIT): Self-Report Version—cont'd**

Questions	0	1	2	3	4	Score
7. How often during the last year have you had a feeling of guilt or remorse after drinking?	Never	Less than monthly	Monthly	Weekly	Daily or almost daily	
8. How often during the last year have you been unable to remember what happened the night before because of your drinking?	Never	Less than monthly	Monthly	Weekly	Daily or almost daily	
9. Have you or someone else been injured because of your drinking?	No		Yes, but not in the last year		Yes, during the last year	
10. Has a relative, friend, doctor, or other healthcare worker been concerned about your drinking or suggested you cut down?	No		Yes, but not in the last year		Yes, during the last year	
					Total	___

Score: 8 or more in men; 7 or more in women needs further assessment.
Babor, T. F., Higgins-Biddle, J. C., Saunders, J. B., & Monteiro, M. (2001). *The alcohol use disorders identification test* (2nd ed.). Retrieved from http://apps.who.int/iris/bitstream/10665/67205/1/WHO_MSD_MSB_01.6a.pdf.

objectivity regardless of what the individual reveals. Several trends are important such as the appearance of progression or loss of control and whether or not tolerance or withdrawal is present. Once the screening process identifies a potential problem, a more complete assessment is warranted.

ASSESSMENT

An alcohol use assessment is part of a more comprehensive assessment that evaluates the individual holistically. Ideally, this assessment involves an addictions professional with specialized knowledge and skills to make a diagnosis. The assessment will include a clinical examination of background, pattern of substance use, and any mental health symptoms. The nurse will make special note of any history of trauma, a family history of substance use or mental health problems and any disabilities, as well as the individual's strengths and level of willingness to change. As a result of this assessment, the individual may be identified as having a substance-related disorder.

Family Assessment

Understanding the process of addiction from a holistic perspective requires careful attention to the family. Living with an individual who misuses alcohol or other substances is a source of stress and requires family system adjustments. Codependence is a cluster of behaviors originally identified through research involving the families of alcoholic patients. People who are codependent often exhibit overly responsible behavior—doing for others what others could just as well do for themselves. People who are codependent often define their self-worth in terms of caring for others to the exclusion of their own needs.

Self-Assessment

Alcohol use is self-inflicted. You should carefully assess personal thoughts, opinions, and feelings as the first step to remaining objective and establishing a therapeutic relationship with a person who misuses alcohol. Most of us have been impacted in some way by someone whose life has been torn apart by substance use. Recognizing and dealing with our responses by practicing **introspection** is essential to the provision of patient-centered care protected from bias or countertransference.

You may be aware that registered nurses themselves might have personal substance use problems. For those nurses who become aware that they are engaging in risk-taking behaviors or that one of their colleagues may be experiencing difficulties, there are nonpunitive alternatives to discipline programs in the form of **peer assistance**. Many State Boards of Nursing have developed an alternative to discipline program to help impaired nurses. To determine if your state has this model, check with your state's Board of Nursing.

DIAGNOSIS

Once the comprehensive substance use assessment has been completed in a thorough, objective manner, the data are analyzed and potential or actual problems and needs are identified. Clinical decision-making skills will be used to determine which of the identified problems requires a priority intervention.

OUTCOMES IDENTIFICATION

The goals for treatment planning arise from the preferred outcome for each problem. Outcome measures may include immediate detox and stabilization for individuals experiencing withdrawal, abstinence if individuals are actively drinking, motivation for treatment and engagement in early abstinence, and pursuit of a recovery lifestyle for after discharge. Table 22.5 identifies signs and symptoms commonly experienced with substance use disorders, offer potential nursing diagnoses, and suggests outcomes.

PLANNING

The treatment plan will be developed based on the assessment and diagnoses. For treatment to be successful, a patient-centered approach includes the patient's goals. The plan should take

TABLE 22.5 Signs and Symptoms, Nursing Diagnoses, and Outcomes for Substance-Related and Addictive Disorders

Signs and Symptoms	Nursing Diagnoses	Outcomes
Impulsiveness, loss of relationships and occupation due to focus on substances or gambling, legal problems, social isolation	*Risk for suicide*	Expresses feelings, verbalizes suicidal ideas, refrains from suicide attempts, plans for the future
Impairment from substances, overdose, withdrawal from substances, hallucinations, elevated temperature, pulse, respirations, agitation	*Risk for injury*	Remains free from injury
Reports not feeling well rested, decreased ability to function, reports awakening multiple times	*Disturbed sleep pattern*	Minimal awakening, feels restored after sleep
Substitutes substances for healthy foods, lack of appetite, aversion to food	*Nutrition: less than body requirements*	Maintains a nutrient intake to meet metabolic needs
Increased appetite from cannabis use, dysfunctional eating pattern, weight 20% over ideal for height and frame, excessive intake in relation to metabolic need	*Nutrition: more than body requirements*	Maintains a nutrient intake to meet metabolic needs
Inadequate environmental hygiene, inadequate personal hygiene, nonadherence to health activity	*Self-neglect*	Obtains stable health status, adheres to medication and treatment regimen
Substance use or gambling, decreased use of social support, destructive behavior toward self and others, difficulty organizing information, inadequate problem-solving, poor concentration, reports inability to cope	*Ineffective coping*	Modifies lifestyle as needed to maintain sobriety, maintains abstinence from substances, engages in satisfying relationships
Does not perceive danger of substance use or gambling, minimizes symptoms, refuses healthcare attention, unable to admit impact of disease on life pattern	*Ineffective denial*	Accepts responsibility for behavior, maintains abstinence from substances
Substance use or gambling, lack of initiative, passivity, social isolation, reports seeing no alternatives or personal control, anger, sees no meaning in life	*Hopelessness*	Expresses feelings of self-worth, verbalizes sense of personal identity, expresses meaning in life, sets goals, believes that actions impact outcomes
Substance use leads to vulnerability to decreased liver function	*Risk for impaired liver function*	Abstains from substance use
Substance use edema, loss of appetite, fatigue, shortness of breath, decreased concentration, cough, decreased urine output, palpitations, irregular or rapid pulse	*Decreased cardiac output*	Abstains from substance use, cardiac pump supports systemic perfusion pressure
Blaming, broken promises, chaos, denial of problems, enabling maintenance of substance use pattern, immaturity, inability to accept help or express feelings, loneliness, lying, manipulation, rationalization, refuses to get help social isolation, worthlessness, deterioration of family relationships	*Dysfunctional family processes*	Family members attain cohesion and emotional bonding

From Herdman, T. H., & Kamitsuru, S. (Eds.). (2014). *Nursing diagnoses—Definitions and classification 2015-2017.* Copyright © 2014, 1994–2014 by NANDA International. Used by arrangement with John Wiley & Sons Limited; Moorhead, S., Johnson, M., Maas, M. L., & Swanson, E. (2013). *Nursing outcomes classification (NOC)* (5th ed.). St. Louis, MO: Mosby.

into account the patient's ability to recognize the problem and readiness or motivation for change.

IMPLEMENTATION

Psychosocial Interventions

Basic nursing interventions are useful in providing a supportive environment for managing substance use disorders. Promoting safety and sleep are essential first-line interventions. Also, patients with alcohol use disorder may have severely compromised nutritional status due to choosing substance over sustenance. Gradually reintroducing healthy food and hydration helps support body systems and neurological functioning. Support and encouragement for self-care (hygiene) will help improve self-esteem in individuals who may have long neglected themselves.

The development of a therapeutic relationship sets the stage for exploring harmful thoughts, anxiety, hopelessness, and spiritual distress. An understanding of current coping skills along with identification of new skills provides tools to test in a safe setting. Assistance in goal setting helps a patient to see beyond the current situation and instills hope and direction.

Psychobiological Interventions

Pharmacological

With the completion of the Human Genome Project and ongoing genetic research, it is only a matter of time before the nurse's responsibility will include not only review of laboratory data, but also a review of the patient's genetic profiles (Cheek et al., 2015). In addition to adding to the body of knowledge, this research will provide alternative options for treatment.

Nurses administer medications and provide ongoing assessment of their efficacy and side effects after administration. Nurses need to monitor vital signs frequently since an increase in pulse, blood pressure, and body temperatures are clear signs of withdrawal. The goal is to keep the patient safe and comfortable and stay ahead of withdrawal so the patient does not suffer.

Previously in the chapter we discussed medications used for other substances. Table 22.6 identifies medications used in the treatment of alcohol use disorder.

Health Teaching and Health Promotion

By 2020, substance use disorders and mental health disorders are predicted to surpass all physical diseases as the major causes

TABLE 22.6 Common Medications Used for Treatment of Alcohol Use Disorder

Generic (Brand Name)	Uses	Implications for the Therapeutic Process
Disulfiram (Antabuse)	Maintenance, relapse prevention, aversion therapy	Physical effects when alcohol is used: Intense nausea and vomiting, headache, sweating, flushed skin, respiratory difficulties, and confusion. Avoid all alcohol and substances such as cough syrup and mouthwash containing alcohol.
Naltrexone (Vivitrol—injectable, ReVia, Depade—oral)	Withdrawal, relapse prevention, decreases pleasurable feelings and cravings	Oral or long acting (once a month) injectable form. Nausea usually goes away after first month; headache, sedation Pain at injection site, patient needs to be opiate free 10 days before initiation of medication.
Acamprosate calcium (Campral)	Relapse-prevention	Begin taking on the fifth day of abstinence from alcohol. Tablets are taken three times a day. Side effects include diarrhea, gastrointestinal upset, appetite loss, dizziness, anxiety, and difficulty sleeping. Contraindicated in patients with renal impairment.
Benzodiazepines		
Lorazepam (Ativan), Chlordiazepoxide (Librium), Diazepam (Valium)	Withdrawal	Sedation, decreased anxiety, and blood pressure. Use CIWA-AR scale to assess dose according to agency policies. Assess for seizures that could lead to delirium tremens (DTs). If not treated, coma and ultimately death.
Anticonvulsants (Tegretol)	Withdrawal	Older treatments still used today. Other treatments have proven more effective and safer.
Barbiturates (Phenobarbital)		Assess for seizures that could lead to delirium tremens if not treated, coma and ultimately death.
Clonidine *(Catapres)*	Mild-moderate withdrawal	Alpha-agonist antihypertensive agent. Give every 4-6 hours as needed. Side effects dizziness, hypotension, fatigue, and headache.

CIWA-AR, Clinical Institute Withdrawal Assessment for Alcohol.
Substance Abuse and Mental Health Services Administration and National Institute on Alcohol Abuse and Alcoholism. (2015). *Medication for the treatment of alcohol use disorder: A brief guide. HHS Publication No. (SMA) 15-4907.* Rockville, MD: Author.

of disability worldwide (SAMHSA, 2015c). If genetic vulnerability accounts for 40% to 60% of an individual's risk, prevention may be the best answer to the increasing problem of substance use and addiction (NIDA, 2014). Health teaching is a part of the school curriculum, and schools may offer classes on understanding addiction as a brain disorder, its risk factors, and ways to prevent or limit exposure to psychoactive substances. Promoting classes for developing healthy coping and stress management skills and activities for increasing self-confidence and self-efficacy would also lower the risks for use of psychoactive substances.

Social activities that increase supportive relationships reduce the impact of stressful life events and provide a venue for community activities that provide health education and promotion. Pay special attention to understanding the particular impact of trauma as a risk factor. Physical, sexual, or emotional abuse at any age; physical trauma from accidents; natural disasters; or acts of violence or war can all be predisposing factors for the use of psychoactive substances or processes.

Advanced Practice Interventions

Psychotherapy. Advanced practice nurses and other substance use and addiction treatment professionals use a number of psychotherapies. Cognitive behavioral therapy and motivational interviewing are commonly used evidence-based therapies.

Destructive and negative thinking patterns play into the development of maladaptive behavioral patterns like substance use disorders. Cognitive behavioral therapy helps patients to explore thinking patterns so that the core belief system and any irrational core beliefs can be identified. Positive and negative consequences of alcohol use are explored. Patients learn to self-monitor their cravings and challenge these cravings realistically.

Motivational interviewing is an approach based on the transtheoretical or stages of change theory. It has gained popularity in its use as a brief, long-term, and supplementary intervention, particularly in the treatment of substance use disorders. It uses a person-centered approach to strengthen motivation for change (Tan et al., 2015). The advanced practice nurse and patient usually meet for an hour at a time.

Individuals may be at stage one, *precontemplation*, and need assistance in admitting there is a problem. If they have acknowledged the problem, *contemplation*, they may still not be ready to commit to addressing it. The goal of treatment is to assist in the development of awareness and a commitment. *Preparation* or getting ready, and *action* or changing take place in early treatment phases. The *maintenance* stage is the ongoing commitment to a recovery program. Without continuing action, the individual will likely return to previous behavior, *relapse*.

EVALUATION

Evaluation occurs on several levels: assessing the effectiveness of the treatment plan, using objective data to check whether nursing actions addressed the patient's symptoms, and measuring the changes in the patient's behaviors for progress toward meeting stated goals. Problematic behaviors, patterns of expression, or perceptions may improve or only undergo change in small increments, requiring alterations in the action steps or even the goals of the treatment plan to meet the patient's needs.

During the treatment experience, conduct ongoing evaluation of the process to ensure that any transference or countertransference is managed and that the goals and outcomes of treatment remain patient-centered. Evaluation will also make it possible to ensure that the patient acquires the necessary skills and competencies for continued reflection and maintenance of the new lifestyle identification.

CASE STUDY AND NURSING CARE PLAN

Alcohol Use Disorder

Mr. Stewart, aged 49 years, and his wife arrive in the emergency department. They are fearful that Mr. Stewart has had a stroke. His right hand is limp, and he is unable to hyperextend his right wrist and cannot feel his fingertips.

Ms. Winkler, the admitting nurse, begins the assessment. Mr. Stewart looks much older than his stated age. His complexion is ruddy and flushed. History taking is difficult. Mr. Stewart answers only what is asked, volunteering no additional information. He states that he took a nap that afternoon. When he woke up, he noticed the problems with his right arm.

Mr. Stewart has been unemployed for 4 years because the company he worked for went bankrupt. He has been unable to find a job but has an interview in 10 days. His wife is now working full time. They have two grown children who no longer live at home. As he talks about his children, his lips start to tremble and his eyes fill with tears.

Meanwhile, a nurse practitioner has examined Mr. Stewart. The diagnosis is radial nerve palsy. Mr. Stewart most likely passed out while lying on his arm. Because Mr. Stewart was intoxicated, he did not feel the signals (numbness and tingling) that his nerves sent out to warn him to move. He was in this position for so long that the resultant cutoff of circulation was sufficient to cause some temporary nerve damage.

Mr. Stewart's blood alcohol level is 0.31 mg/dL. This is three times the legal limit for intoxication in many states (0.1 mg/dL). Despite the high alcohol level, Mr. Stewart is alert and oriented, not slurring his speech or giving any other outward signs of intoxication. This incongruence is likely due to tolerance, a symptom of physical addiction.

Self-Assessment

Ms. Winkler has seen many patients with the disease of alcoholism make radical changes in their lives, and she has learned to view alcoholism as a treatable disease. She is aware also that it is the patient who makes the changes, and she no longer feels responsible when a patient is not ready to make that change.

Assessment

Subjective Data

- Complains of limpness in his right hand, inability to hyperextend his right wrist, and cannot feel his fingertips.
- Noticed the problems with his arm after a nap
- Unemployed for 4 years
- Upcoming job interview

Objective Data

- Appears older than age
- Complexion ruddy and flushed
- Short responses, volunteers little information
- Tearful when talking about children
- Blood alcohol level is 0.31 mg/dL
- Alert and oriented

Priority Diagnosis

Ineffective coping related to alcohol use as evidenced by increased alcohol use and impairment in life functioning.

Outcomes Identification

Client will demonstrate mild to no change in health status and social functioning due to substance addiction.

Planning

Mr. Stewart's plan of care is personalized as follows:

Short-Term Goal	Intervention	Rationale	Evaluation
1. Client will acknowledge consequences associated with alcohol use.	1a. Identify with patient those factors (genetics, stress) that contribute to chemical addiction.	1a. Emphasis on alcoholism as a disease can lower guilt and increase self-esteem.	**GOAL MET** Client admits that he cannot find a new job when he is intoxicated.
	1b. Assist patient to identify negative effects of chemical dependency.	1b. Begins to decrease denial and increase problem solving.	
2. Client will commit to alcohol-use control strategies.	2a. Determine history of alcohol use.	2a. Identifies high-risk situations.	**GOAL MET** After 3 weeks, patient states that he attends AA every day. He is learning about his triggers and new coping skills. His wife attends Al-Anon.
	2b. Identify support groups in community for long-term substance use treatment (for wife also).	2b. Alcohol addiction requires long-term treatment; Alcoholics Anonymous (AA) is effective.	

Evaluation

See individual outcomes and evaluation in the care plan.

The Care Continuum for Substance Use Disorders

Continuity of care occurs through a continuum starting with detoxification (detox), rehabilitation, halfway houses, partial programs, intensive outpatient (IOP), and outpatient settings. Mutual support groups such as Alcoholics Anonymous (AA) are strongly encouraged throughout the treatment process.

Detoxification (Detox)

Detox is warranted when the individual quits using a psychoactive substance known to cause withdrawal or when the individual is already in withdrawal. This is a medically managed inpatient program with 24-hour medical coverage while the patient's body clears itself of drugs. This process is accompanied by uncomfortable and even fatal side effects caused by withdrawal. Detox is also available as a medically monitored program with 24-hour professional supervision based on the severity of symptomatology and the presence of comorbid conditions.

Rehabilitation

Residential rehabilitation programs are available as medically managed and medically monitored inpatient programs. The medically managed programs usually employ 24-hour medical staff and provide intensive and specialized care for those individuals with either biomedical or psychiatric comorbid conditions. Medically monitored programs are also available for individuals with less complex conditions. They offer professionally directed evaluation and treatment in short-term settings for those with acute distress and moderate impairment and long-term settings for those with chronic distress or severe impairment. Short-term rehabilitation offers rehabilitation (learning lost skills) while long-term rehabs offer habilitation (learning new skills).

Halfway Houses

Halfway houses offer residential treatment in a substance-free communal or family environment that provides opportunities for independent growth. Individuals continue the work started in other treatment programs, usually in a long- or short-term residential rehabilitation center. The focus is on extending the period of sobriety; getting case management assistance in addressing educational, economic, and social needs; and integrating new life skills into a solid modeled recovery program. Most residents live in these halfway houses, but work outside.

Other Housing

Opportunities for community reintegration are also available in supportive housing units that are not part of treatment. Three-quarter-way houses, therapeutic communities, and housing programs offer drug-free living environments, peer support, and classes to assist or remediate skills needed for daily living. Residents usually attend some type of outpatient substance use treatment to continue in their recovery program.

Partial Hospitalization Program

Partial hospitalization program is an intensive form of outpatient programming for those individuals who do not need a 24-hour residential treatment, but who benefit from a structured treatment setting. Partial programs tend to run 5 days a week for about 6 hours a day with planned programming. This combination of psychotherapy and educational groups does not require the individual to have previous treatment experience. Participants may live in some type of supportive housing program or at an independent home. Medication management is available but it is not usually medically monitored or managed in this setting.

Intensive Outpatient Programs

An alternative to a partial hospitalization program is an intensive outpatient program (IOP). This is a nonresidential program, highly structured with scheduled treatment groups and at least one individual session regularly. Medication management is usually available, but it will not be monitored. Participants attend at least 3 days a week for about 3 hours per day.

Outpatient Treatment

The least-intensive form of substance use treatment is outpatient. Treatment may be a mix of individual sessions and educational or psychotherapy groups as determined by the individual's needs and the treatment goals. It is structured, drug-free, and nonresidential. Programming consists of not more than 5 contact hours a week. Web-based interventions are also available for self-paced, anonymous collective participation in treatment efforts.

Alcoholics Anonymous

Alcoholics Anonymous (AA) was founded in 1930 and is the oldest and best known of the 12-step programs. Anyone with the desire to quit drinking or using substances is welcome to attend meetings. Individuals learn how to be sober through the support of other members and the 12 steps. In most suburban and urban areas, meetings can be found every day and around the clock. Meetings are even available online and are structured for confidentiality and anonymity. Family members and other support are often welcome.

The 12-step model has been adopted worldwide. Specific groups may focus on specific addictions and/or include specific populations such as women, men, and certain groups. The size of meetings ranges from small (around 15) to large (more than 50). There are also meetings to address the special needs of family and significant others, such as Al-Anon for friends and family members of alcohol abusers, Alateen for teenage relatives of alcohol abusers, and Nar-Anon for family and friends of drug users.

Relapse Prevention

To maintain long-term sobriety, each individual must prepare for and anticipate the possibility of relapse. This includes identifying potential triggers to substance use, learning skills to regain abstinence in the event of use, and adopting healthy coping, identity, and stress management skills to address triggers before they threaten sobriety. Advances in technology have expanded options for maintaining long-term sobriety. Applications for smartphones, for example, offer a way to monitor behavioral patterns for relapse clues.

KEY POINTS TO REMEMBER

- Substance-related and addictive disorders are complex brain diseases characterized by craving, seeking, and using regardless of consequences.
- Most substance use disorders are characterized by addiction, intoxication, tolerance, and withdrawal.
- The cause of substance use is a combination of biological and environmental factors.
- Assessment of patients with substance use problems needs to be comprehensive and aimed at identifying common medical and psychiatric comorbidities.
- Clients with a co-occurring diagnosis have more severe symptoms, experience more crises, and require longer treatment for successful outcomes.
- Substance use affects the family system of the patient and may lead to codependent behavior in family members.
- Relapse is an expected complication of substance use, and treatment includes a significant focus on teaching relapse prevention.
- Successful treatments include an integrated approach, self-help groups, psychotherapy, therapeutic communities, and psychopharmacotherapy.
- Nurses need to be aware of their own feelings about substance use so that they can provide empathy and hope to patients.
- Nurses are at higher risk for substance use disorders and should be vigilant for signs of impairment in colleagues to ensure patient safety and referral to treatment for the chemically dependent nurse.
- A variety of settings are helpful in meeting the needs of individuals who are trying to maintain recovery from alcohol.

CRITICAL THINKING

1. Write a paragraph describing your possible reactions to a drug-dependent patient to whom you are assigned.
   a. Would your response be different depending on the substance (e.g., alcohol versus heroin or marijuana versus cocaine)? Give reasons for your answers.
   b. Would your response be different if the substance-dependent person were a professional colleague? How?
2. Rosetta Seymour is a 15-year-old who has started using heroin nasally.
   a. Briefly discuss the trend in heroin use among teenagers.
   b. When Ms. Seymour asks you why she needs to take more and more to get "high," how would you explain to her the concept of tolerance?
   c. If she had just taken heroin, what would you find on assessment of physical and behavioral-psychological signs and symptoms?
   d. If she came into the emergency department with an overdose of heroin, what would be the emergency care? What might be effective long-term care?
3. Tony Garmond is a 45-year-old mechanic. He has a 20-year history of heavy drinking, and he says he wants to quit but needs help.
   a. Role-play an initial assessment with a classmate. Identify the kinds of information you would need to have to plan holistic care.
   b. Mr. Garmond tried stopping by himself but is in the emergency department in alcohol withdrawal. What are the dangers for Mr. Garmond? What are the likely medical interventions?
   c. What are some possible treatment alternatives for Mr. Garmond when he is safely detoxified? How would you explain to him the usefulness and function of AA? What are some additional treatment options that might be useful to Mr. Garmond? What community referrals for Mr. Garmond are available in your area?

CHAPTER REVIEW

Questions

1. A patient with a history of alcohol use disorder has been prescribed disulfiram (Antabuse). Which physical effects support the suspicion that the patient has relapsed? *Select all that apply.*
   a. Intense nausea
   b. Diaphoresis
   c. Acute paranoia
   d. Confusion
   e. Dyspnea
2. Which assessment data confirm the suspicion that a patient is experiencing opioid withdrawal? *Select all that apply.*
   a. Pupils are dilated
   b. Pulse rate is 62 beats/min
   c. Slow movements
   d. Extreme anxiety
   e. Sleepy
3. The nursing diagnosis *ineffective denial* is especially useful when working with substance use disorders and gambling. Which statements describe this diagnosis? *Select all that apply.*
   a. Reports inability to cope
   b. Does not perceive danger of substance use or gambling
   c. Minimizes symptoms
   d. Refuses healthcare attention
   e. Unable to admit impact of disease on life pattern
4. What action should you take when a female staff member is demonstrating behaviors associated with a substance use disorder?
   a. Accompany the staff member when she is giving patient care.
   b. Offer to attend rehabilitation counseling with her.

c. Refer her to a peer assistance program.
d. Confront her about your concerns and/or report your concerns to a supervisor immediately.

5. A patient diagnosed with opioid use disorder has expressed a desire to enter into a rehabilitation program. What initial nursing intervention during the early days after admission will help ensure the patient's success?
   a. Restrict visitors to family members only.
   b. Manage the patient's withdrawal symptoms well.
   c. Provide the patient a low stimulus environment.
   d. Advocate for at least 3 months of treatment.
6. Lester and Eileen have always enjoyed gambling. Lately, Eileen has discovered that their savings account is down by $50,000. Eileen insists that Lester undergo therapy for his gambling behavior. The nurse recognizes that Lester is making progress when he states:
   a. "I understand that I am a bad person for depleting our savings."
   b. "Gambling activates the reward pathways in my brain."
   c. "Gambling is the only thing that makes me feel alive."
   d. "We have always enjoyed gaming. I do not know why Eileen is so upset."
7. Opioid use disorder is characterized by:
   a. Lack of withdrawal symptoms
   b. Intoxication symptoms of pupillary dilation, agitation, and insomnia
   c. Tolerance
   d. Requiring smaller amounts of the drug to achieve a high over time
8. Terry is a young male in a chemical dependency program. Recently he has become increasingly distracted and disengaged. The nurse concludes that Terry is:
   a. Bored
   b. Depressed
   c. Bipolar
   d. Not ready to change
9. Maxwell is a 30-year-old male who arrives at the emergency department stating, "I feel like I am having a stroke." During the intake assessment, the nurse discovers that Maxwell has been working for 36 hours straight without eating and has consumed eight double espresso drinks and 12 caffeinated sodas. The nurse suspects:
   a. Fluid overload
   b. Dehydration and caffeine overdose
   c. Benzodiazepine overdose
   d. Sleep deprivation syndrome
10. Donald, a 49-year-old male, is admitted for inpatient alcohol detoxification. He is cachexic, has multiple scabs on his arms and legs, and has lower extremity edema. An appropriate nursing diagnosis for Donald along with an expected outcome is:
   a. Risk for injury/Remains free from injury
   b. Ineffective denial/Accepts responsibility for behavior
   c. Nutrition: Less than body requirements/Maintains nutrient intake for metabolic needs
   d. Risk for suicide/Expresses feelings, plans for the future

Answers

1. **a, b, d, e**; 2. **a, d**; 3. **b, c, d, e**; 4. **d**; 5. **b**; 6. **b**; 7. **c**; 8. **d**; 9. **b**; 10. **c**

Visit the Evolve website for a posttest on the content in this chapter: http://evolve.elsevier.com/Varcarolis

Post-Test interactive review

REFERENCES

American Psychiatric Association. (2013). *Diagnostic and Statistical Manual of Mental Disorders* (5th ed.). Washington, DC: Author.

American Society of Addiction Medicine. (2016). *Definition of addiction.* Retrieved from http://www.asam.org/quality-practice/definition-of-addiction.

Cheek, D., Bashore, L., & Braceau, D. (2015). Pharmacogenomics and implications for nursing practice. *Journal of Nursing Scholarship, 47*(6), 496–504.

Ebert, D. H., Finn, C. T., & Smoller, J. W. (2016). Genetics and psychiatry. In T. A. Stern, M. Fava, T. E. Wilens, & J. F. Rosenbaum (Eds.), *Massachusetts General Hospital comprehensive clinical psychiatry* (2nd ed.) (pp. 677–701). St. Louis, MO: Elsevier.

National Cancer Institute. (2013). *Alcohol and cancer risk.* Retrieved from http://www.cancer.gov/about-cancer/causes-prevention/risk/alcohol/alcohol-fact-sheet.

National Institute on Alcohol Abuse and Alcoholism. (2005). *A pocket guide for alcohol screening and brief intervention* Retrieved from https://pubs.niaaa.nih.gov/publications/practitioner/pocketguide/pocket_guide.htm.

National Institute on Drug Abuse. (2014). *Drugs, brains, and behavior: The science of addiction.* Retrieved from http://www.drugabuse.gov/publications/drugs-brains-behavior-science-addiction/introduction.

National Institute on Drug Abuse. (2015a). *Strategic plan 2016–2020.* Retrieved from http://www.drugabuse.gov/about-nida/strategic-plan.

National Institute on Drug Abuse. (2015b). *NIDA highlights drug use trends among college-age and young adults in a new on-line resource.* Retrieved from http://www.drugabuse.gov/news-events/news-releases/2015/05/nida-highlights-drug-use-trends-among-college-age-young-adults-in-new-online-resource.

National Institutes of Health. (2014). *Cirrhosis.* Retrieved from https://www.niddk.nih.gov/health-information/health-topics/liver-disease/cirrhosis/Pages/facts.aspx.

Sadock, B. J., Sadock, V. A., & Ruiz, P. (2015). *Kaplan & Sadock's synopsis of psychiatry* (11th ed.). Philadelphia, PA: Wolters Kluwer.

Substance Abuse and Mental Health Services Administration. (2014a). About us. Retrieved from https://www.samhsa.gov/about-us

Substance Abuse and Mental Health Services Administration. (2014b). *Gambling problems: An introduction for behavioral health services providers.* Retrieved from http://www.ncpgambling.org/wp-content/uploads/2014/04/Gambling-Addiction-An-Introduction-for-Behavioral-Health-Providers-SAMHSA-2014.pdf.

Substance Abuse and Mental Health Services Administration. (2015a). *Behavioral health trends in the United States: Results from the 2014 National Survey on Drug Use and Health. (HHS Publication No. SMA 15-4927, NSDUH Series H-50).* Retrieved from http://www.samhsa.gov/data/sites/default/files/NSDUH-FRR1-2014/NSDUH-FRR1-2014.pdf.

Substance Abuse and Mental Health Services Administration. (2015b). *Mental and substance abuse disorders.* Retrieved from http://www.samhsa.gov/disorders.

Substance Abuse and Mental Health Services Administration. (2015c). *Prevention of substance abuse and mental illness: Continuum of care.* Retrieved from http://www.samhsa.gov/prevention.

Tan, S., Lee, M., Lim, G., Leong, J., & Lee, C. (2015). Motivational interviewing approach used by a community mental health team. *Journal of Psychosocial Nursing and Mental Health Services, 53*(12), 28–37.

23

Neurocognitive Disorders

Jane Stein-Parbury

Visit the Evolve website for a pretest on the content in this chapter: http://evolve.elsevier.com/Varcarolis Pre-Test interactive review

OBJECTIVES

1. Compare and contrast the clinical picture of delirium with that of dementia.
2. Discuss three critical needs of a person with delirium, stated in terms of nursing diagnoses.
3. Identify three outcomes for patients with delirium.
4. Summarize the essential nursing interventions for a patient with delirium.
5. Recognize the clinical picture of mild and major neurocognitive disorders.
6. Give an example of the following symptoms assessed during the progression of major neurocognitive disorders: (a) amnesia, (b) apraxia, (c) agnosia, and (d) aphasia.
7. Formulate three nursing diagnoses suitable for a patient with a major neurocognitive disorder and define two outcomes for each.
8. Formulate a teaching plan for a caregiver of a patient with major neurocognitive disorder including interventions for (a) communication, (b) health maintenance, and (c) safe environment.
9. Compose a list of appropriate referrals in the community—including a support group, hotline for information, and respite services—for individuals with dementia and their caregivers.

OUTLINE

KEY TERMS AND CONCEPTS

agnosia
agraphia
Alzheimer's disease
aphasia
apraxia
confabulation
delirium
dementia
executive function
hallucinations
hypermetamorphosis
hyperorality
hypervigilance
illusions
major neurocognitive disorder
mild neurocognitive disorder
perseveration
social cognition
sundowning

The clarity and purpose of an individual's personal journey through life depends on the ability to reflect on its meaning. Unfortunately, for far too many people, profound disturbances in cognitive processing cloud or destroy the meaning of the journey. Cognition represents a fundamental human feature that distinguishes living from existing. This mental capacity has a distinctive personalized impact on the individual's physical, psychological, social, and spiritual conduct of life. For example, the ability to remember the connections between related actions and how to initiate them depends on cognitive processing. This cognitive processing has a direct relationship to activities of daily living.

Cognitive functioning involves a variety of domains. Attention and orientation are basic lower-level cognitive domains. Higher-level cognitive domains are more complex and include an ability to do the following:

- Plan and problem solve (executive function)
- Learn and retain information in long-term memory
- Use language
- Visually perceive the environment
- Read social situations (social cognition)

The three main neurocognitive classifications are delirium, mild neurocognitive disorders, and major neurocognitive disorders. The first syndrome, delirium, tends to be short-term and reversible. Mild neurocognitive disorders may or may not progress to being major. Major neurocognitive disorders are commonly referred to as dementia, which is progressive and irreversible. In both mild and major neurocognitive disorders, there is a decline in cognitive functioning from a previous level, although they differ in how much they interfere with independence in everyday activities (American Psychiatric Association [APA], 2013).

DELIRIUM

EPIDEMIOLOGY

Delirium is a common complication of hospitalization, especially in older patients. The reported incidence of delirium in all hospitalized patients is up to 22% in general medical patients, between 11% and 35% in surgical patients, and up to 80% in patients in intensive care units (van Munster & Rooij, 2014). In patients over 65 years of age, delirium occurs in up to 50% (Inouye et al., 2014). The high degree of variability in the reported incidence of delirium is most likely due to its underrecognition.

RISK FACTORS

Delirium is always due to underlying physiological causes that are usually multifactorial and involve a dynamic interplay of factors. There are underlying causes that place a patient at risk for developing delirium, and there are immediate factors that precipitate the syndrome. It is the interaction of the two that results in delirium. Some of the risk factors listed in Box 23.1 are modifiable.

The key to helping patients avoid the consequences of delirium is recognizing and investigating potential causes as soon as possible. Early recognition and diagnosis are challenging for clinicians due to lack of knowledge about cognitive impairment and its clinical assessment and failure to interpret the signs and symptoms. The best evidence for the prevention and management of delirium in hospitalized patients is having clinical protocols for minimizing modifiable risk factors. Early detection of delirium may be improved by consultation with geriatric specialists (Reston & Schoelles, 2013).

CLINICAL PICTURE

Delirium is an acute cognitive disturbance and often-reversible condition that is common in hospitalized patients, especially older patients. It is characterized as a syndrome, that is, a constellation of symptoms rather than a disorder. The cardinal

BOX 23.1 Risk Factors for Delirium

- Cognitive impairment
- Older age
- Severity of disease
- Infection
- Multiple comorbidities
- Polypharmacy
- Intensive care units
- Unaddressed orientation, visual, or hearing issues
- Fractures
- Surgery
- Stroke
- Aphasia
- Vision impairment
- Restraint use
- Change in hospital rooms

symptoms of delirium are an inability to direct, focus, sustain, and shift attention; an abrupt onset with clinical features that fluctuate with periods of lucidity; and disorganized thinking and poor executive functioning. Other characteristics include disorientation (often to time and place, but rarely to person), anxiety, agitation, poor memory, and delusional thinking. When hallucinations are present they are usually visual. The *DSM-5* box identifies criteria for delirium.

DSM-5 CRITERIA FOR DELIRIUM

A. A disturbance in attention (i.e., reduced ability to direct, focus, sustain and shift attention) and awareness (reduced orientation to the environment).
B. The disturbance develops over a short period of time (usually hours to a few days), represents a change from baseline attention and awareness, and tends to fluctuate in severity during the course of a day.
C. An additional disturbance in cognition (e.g., memory deficit, disorientation, language, visuospatial ability, or perception).
D. The disturbances in Criteria A and C are not better explained by another preexisting, established, or evolving neurocognitive disorder and do not occur in the context of a severely reduced level of arousal such as coma.
E. There is evidence from the history, physical examination, or laboratory findings that the disturbance is a direct physiological consequence of another medical condition, substance intoxication or withdrawal (i.e., due to a drug of abuse or to a medication), or exposure to a toxin, or is due to multiple etiologies.

Specify whether:

Substance intoxication delirium: This diagnosis should be made instead of substance intoxication when the symptoms in Criteria A and C predominate in the clinical picture and when they are sufficiently severe to warrant clinical attention.

From the American Psychiatric Association. (2013). *Diagnostic and statistical manual of mental disorders* (5th ed.). Washington, DC: Author.

Delirium is a medical emergency that requires immediate attention to prevent irreversible and serious damage (Caplan et al., 2016). Delirium is associated with increased morbidity and mortality and can have lasting long-term consequences such as permanent cognitive decline (Inouye et al., 2014). In hospitalized patients, delirium is associated with longer hospital stays and increased complications (Anand & MacLullich, 2013).

EVIDENCE-BASED PRACTICE

Detecting Delirium in Older Adults

Problem

Delirium is the most frequent complication of hospitalization in older adults. Not only is this problem costly, but delirium is also associated with morbidity and mortality. Timely recognition is essential to offset these negative outcomes.

Purpose of Study

The purpose of the study was to identify factors associated with the recognition of delirium among registered nurses.

Methods

Researchers conducted a literature search for quantitative studies regarding nurses recognizing delirium.

Key Findings

Seven major factors related to poor recognition of delirium by nurses were identified. The factors included:

- Fluctuating nature of delirium
- Lack of delirium education
- Communication barriers
- Insufficient use of assessment tools
- Poor understanding of delirium
- Perception of delirium as burdensome
- Poor differentiation between dementia and delirium

Implications for Nursing Practice

As a future nurse, you will be in a prime position to notice delirium. Any time a patient experiences an acute onset of confusion, you should consider delirium. Nurses need to be aware of the nature of delirium, especially how it differs from dementia. Standardized assessment scales can improve your ability to detect delirium.

El Hussein, M., Hirst, S., & Salyers, V. (2014). Factors that contribute to under-recognition of delirium by registered nurses in acute care settings: A scoping review of the literature to explain this phenomenon. *Journal of Clinical Nursing, 24,* 906–915.

APPLICATION OF THE NURSING PROCESS

ASSESSMENT

Nurses who suspect delirium should perform mental and neurological status examinations, as well as a physical examination. If possible, additional information should be obtained from a person who knows the patient such as a family member or friend. The patient's medication regimen should be reviewed carefully for drug interactions or toxicity profiles. Results of laboratory data such as blood work and urinalysis should be reviewed. If no recent laboratory information exists, nurses can be instrumental in recommending an order for them.

Overall Assessment

You should consider delirium when a patient abruptly demonstrates a reduced clarity of awareness of the environment. The patient's ability to direct, focus, sustain, or shift attention becomes impaired. You may have to repeat questions because the individual's attention wanders, and the person might easily get off track and need to be refocused. Conversation is more difficult because irrelevant stimuli may easily distract the person. You may notice that the patient is no longer interacting meaningfully, staring straight through you and not recalling who he or she is.

The person may have difficulty with orientation—first to time, then to place, and last to person. For example, a man with delirium may think that the year is 1972, that the hospital is home, and that the nurse is his wife. Orientation to person is usually intact. Disorientation and confusion are usually markedly worse at night and during the early morning. In fact, some patients may be confused or delirious only at night and may be lucid during the day.

Because nurses have the most frequent contact with hospitalized patients, they are in a prime position to be the first to detect the possibility of delirium. Nursing assessment includes observation of cognitive and perceptual disturbances, physical needs, and moods and behaviors.

Cognitive and Perceptual Disturbances

It may be difficult to engage patients experiencing delirium in conversation because they are distracted, unable to focus, and exhibit memory impairment. In mild delirium, memory deficits are noticeable only on careful questioning. In more severe delirium, memory problems usually take the form of obvious difficulty in processing and remembering recent events. For example, the person might ask when a son is coming to visit even though the son left only an hour earlier.

Perceptual disturbances are also common. Perception is the processing of information about one's internal and external environment. Various misinterpretations of reality may take the form of illusions or hallucinations.

Illusions are errors in perception of sensory stimuli. A person may mistake folds in the blanket for white rats or the cord of a window blind for a snake. The stimulus is a real object in the environment. However, the individual misinterprets it, and it often becomes the object of the patient's projected fear. Unlike delusions or hallucinations, you can explain and clarify illusions for the individual.

Hallucinations are false sensory stimuli (refer to Chapter 12). Visual hallucinations are common in delirium, although tactile hallucinations may also be present. For example, individuals experiencing delirium may become terrified when they see giant spiders crawling over the bedclothes or feel bugs crawling on or under their bodies. Auditory hallucinations occur more often in other psychiatric disorders such as schizophrenia.

The individual with delirium generally is aware that something is very wrong. Statements like "My thoughts are all jumbled" may signal cognitive problems. When perceptual disturbances are present, the emotional response is often one of fear and anxiety. When this happens, the individual may show signs of psychomotor agitation.

Physical Needs

A person with delirium becomes disoriented and may try to go home. Alternatively, a person may think that the care facility *is* home. Wandering, pulling out intravenous lines and indwelling catheters, and falling out of bed are common dangers that require nursing interventions.

An individual experiencing delirium has difficulty processing stimuli in the environment, and confusion magnifies the inability to recognize reality. Make the physical environment as simple and clear as possible. Objects such as clocks and calendars can maximize orientation to time. Eyeglasses, hearing aids, and adequate lighting without glare can maximize the person's ability to interpret more accurately what is going on in the environment. The nurse should interact with the patient whenever the patient is awake. Short periods of social interaction help reduce anxiety and misperceptions.

Self-care deficits, injury, or hyperactivity or hypoactivity may lead to skin breakdown and possible infection. Often this is compounded by poor nutrition, forced bed rest, and possible incontinence. These areas require nursing assessment and intervention.

Autonomic signs, such as tachycardia, sweating, flushed face, dilated pupils, and elevated blood pressure, are often present in delirium. Monitor and document these changes carefully as they may require immediate medical attention.

You may also notice changes in the sleep-wake cycle. In some cases, a complete reversal of the day and night sleep-wake cycle can occur. The patient's level of consciousness may range from lethargy to stupor or from semi-coma to hypervigilance. In **hypervigilance**, patients are extraordinarily alert, and their eyes constantly scan the room. They may have difficulty falling asleep or may be actively disoriented and agitated throughout the night.

You should always suspect medications as a potential cause of delirium. This is especially true when there is polypharmacy and/or use of psychoactive agents. To recognize drug reactions or anticipate potential interactions before delirium actually occurs, it is important to assess all medications, prescription *and* over-the-counter, the patient is taking.

Moods and Behaviors

The individual's moods and physical behaviors may change dramatically within a short period. A person with delirium may display motor restlessness (agitation), or he or she may be "quietly delirious" and appear calm and settled. When there is agitation, delirium is considered hyperactive; when there is no agitation, delirium is considered hypoactive. Moods may swing back and forth between fear, anger, anxiety, euphoria, depression, and apathy. A person may strike out from fear or anger or may cry, call for help, curse, moan, and tear off clothing one minute and become apathetic or laugh uncontrollably the next. In short, behavior and emotions are erratic and fluctuating. The following vignette illustrates the fear and confusion a patient may experience during and after an episode of delirium.

VIGNETTE: Peter Wright, age 43, survived numerous life-threatening complications after open-heart surgery to replace his mitral valve. He spent 3 weeks in an ICU and then was moved to a general medical unit.

Peter became suspicious about his bed being moved. "Why are you taking me to another country?" He expressed concern that his organs would be removed and donated for transplantation. He began to yell for his wife. Peter knew that the very people who had saved his life were now out to get him.

When he was sure nobody was looking, he climbed out of bed and attempted to leave the unit. The nurses responded by calling security personnel to escort him back to bed. Once he was safely in bed, the nurses applied mechanical restraints and sedated him.

Peter's confusion disappeared the next day. While he realized how distorted his thinking had been during the episode, the anxiety and fear he experienced remained with him for months after discharge from the hospital.

Self-Assessment

Because the behaviors exhibited by the patient with delirium can be directly attributed to temporary medical conditions, intense personal reactions in staff are less likely to arise. In fact, intense conflicting emotions are less likely to occur in nurses working with a patient with delirium than in nurses working with a patient with dementia. Nonetheless, it can be anxiety provoking to interact with these patients, especially given the unpredictability of their condition.

ASSESSMENT GUIDELINES

Delirium

1. Do not assume that acute confusion in an older person is due to dementia.
2. Assess for acute onset and fluctuating levels of awareness.
3. Assess the person's ability to attend to the immediate environment including responses to nursing care.
4. Establish the person's usual level of cognition by interviewing family or other caregivers.
5. Assess for past cognitive impairment—especially an existing dementia diagnosis—and other risk factors.
6. Identify disturbances in physiological status, especially infection, hypoxia, and pain.
7. Identify any physiological abnormalities documented in the patient's record.
8. Assess vital signs, level of consciousness, and neurological signs.
9. Assess potential for injury, especially in relation to potential for falls and wandering.
10. Maintain comfort measures, especially in relation to pain, cold, or positioning.
11. Monitor situational factors that worsen or improve symptoms.
12. Assess for availability of immediate medical interventions to help prevent irreversible brain damage.

NURSING DIAGNOSIS

Safety needs are a priority in nursing care. Patients with delirium often perceive the environment in a distorted way, and objects are often misperceived. For example, if feeling threatened or thinking that common medical equipment is harmful, the patient may pull off an oxygen mask, pull out an intravenous or nasogastric tube, or try to flee. In such a case, the person demonstrates a *Risk for injury* as evidenced by sensory deficits or perceptual deficits.

Hallucinations, distractibility, illusions, disorientation, agitation, restlessness, and/or misperception are major aspects of the clinical picture. When some of these symptoms are present, *Acute confusion* related to delirium is an appropriate nursing diagnosis.

If fever and dehydration are present, you will need to manage fluid and electrolyte balance. If the underlying cause of the patient's delirium results in fever, decreased skin turgor, decreased urinary output or fluid intake, and dry skin or mucous membranes, then the nursing diagnosis of *Risk for deficient fluid volume* is appropriate. Fluid volume deficit may be related to fever, electrolyte imbalance, reduced intake, or infection.

Because disruption in the sleep-wake cycle may be present, the patient may be less responsive during the day and may become disruptively wakeful during the night. *Disturbed sleep pattern* or *Sleep deprivation* related to impaired cerebral oxygenation or disruption in consciousness is a likely nursing diagnosis.

Engaging in communication with a delirious patient is difficult. An example of a nursing diagnosis addressing this problem is *Impaired verbal communication* related to cerebral hypoxia or decreased cerebral blood flow as evidenced by confusion or clouding of consciousness may be diagnosed.

Fear is one of the most common of all nursing diagnoses and may be related to illusions, delusions, or hallucinations as evidenced by verbal and nonverbal expressions of fearfulness. Other nursing concerns include *Self-care deficits* and *Impaired social interaction*.

OUTCOMES CRITERIA

The overall outcome is that the person experiencing delirium will return to the premorbid level of functioning. Appropriate outcomes include the following:

- Patient will remain safe and free from injury while in the hospital.
- During periods of clarity, patient will be oriented to time, place, and person with the aid of nursing interventions such as the provision of clocks, calendars, maps, and other types of orienting information.
- Patient will remain free from falls and injury while confused with the aid of nursing safety measures.

PLANNING

Planning nursing care for a patient who is experiencing delirium involves special attention to the safety and security of the environment. You should address the following questions:

- Does the person have the necessary visual and auditory aids?
- Are there family members available to stay with the patient?
- Does the environment provide visual cues as to time of day and season of the year?
- Has the person experienced continuity of care providers?

INTERVENTION

The priorities of treatment are to keep the patient safe while attempting to identify the cause. If the underlying disorder is corrected, complete recovery is possible. If, however, the underlying disorder is not corrected and persists, irreversible neuronal damage can occur. Nursing concerns therefore center on the following:

- Preventing physical harm due to confusion, aggression, or electrolyte and fluid imbalance
- Minimizing use of restraints because they increase confusion
- Assisting with proper health management to eradicate the underlying cause
- Using supportive measures to relieve distress

The *Nursing Interventions Classification (NIC*; Bulechek et al., 2013) can be used as a guide to develop interventions for a patient with delirium (Box 23.2). Medical management of delirium involves treating the underlying organic causes. If the underlying cause of delirium is not treated, permanent brain damage may ensue. Judicious use of antipsychotic or antianxiety agents may also be useful in controlling behavioral symptoms.

BOX 23.2 *NIC* Interventions for Delirium Management

Definition: Provision of a safe and therapeutic environment for the patient experiencing an acute confusional state.

- Initiate therapies to reduce or eliminate factors causing delirium.
- Monitor neurological status on an ongoing basis. However, avoid frustrating the patient by quizzing with orientation questions that cannot be answered.
- Administer prn (as needed) medications for anxiety or agitation with caution.
- Assist with needs related to nutrition, elimination, hydration, and personal hygiene.
- Physical restraints may increase symptoms and should be avoided if at all possible. Family members can assist in maintaining safety to avoid restraint use.
- Acknowledge patient's fears and feelings.
- Provide optimistic but realistic reassurance.
- Provide patient with information about what is happening and what can be expected.
- Limit need for decision making, if frustrating or confusing to patient.
- Accept patient's perceptions or interpretation of reality and respond to the theme or feeling tone.
- Inform patient of person, place, and time, as needed.
- Approach patient slowly and from the front and address patient by name.
- Always introduce self to patient when approaching.
- Communicate with simple, direct, descriptive statements.
- Encourage significant others to remain with patient.
- Maintain a well-lit, hazard-free environment.
- Place identification bracelet on patient.
- Provide a consistent physical environment, daily routine, and caregivers.
- Use environmental cues (e.g., signs, pictures, clocks, calendars, and color coding of environment) to stimulate memory, reorient, and promote appropriate behavior.
- Provide a low-stimulation environment for patient in whom disorientation is increased by overstimulation.
- Encourage use of aids that increase sensory input (e.g., eyeglasses, hearing aids, and dentures).

From Bulechek, G. M., Butcher, H. K., Dochterman, J. M., & Wagner, C. (2013). *Nursing interventions classification (NIC,* 6th ed.). St. Louis, MO: Elsevier.

Never leave a patient in acute delirium alone. Because most hospitals and health facilities are unable to provide one-to-one supervision of the patient, you may need to encourage family members to stay with the patient.

EVALUATION

Long-term outcome criteria for a person experiencing delirium include the following:

- Patient will remain safe.
- Patient will be oriented to time, place, and person by discharge.
- Underlying cause will be treated and ameliorated.

MILD AND MAJOR NEUROCOGNITVE DISORDERS

Dementia is a broad term used to describe progressive deterioration of cognitive functioning and global impairment of intellect. It is a term that does not refer to specific disease, but rather a collection of symptoms. The *DSM-5* (APA, 2013) incorporates dementia into the diagnostic categories of mild and major neurocognitive disorders. These disorders are characterized by cognitive impairments that signal a decline from previous functioning.

When mild, the impairments do not interfere with essential activities of daily living although the person may need to make extra efforts. While such impairments may be progressive, a mild cognitive impairment does not necessarily mean that it will progress to a major neurocognitive disorder (Alzheimer's Association, 2014).

When progressive, these disorders become major neurocognitive disorders because they interfere with daily functioning and independence. While often characterized by memory deficits, neurocognitive disorders affect other areas of cognitive functioning, for example, problem solving (executive functioning) and complex attention. The *DSM-5* box describes the criteria for major neurocognitive disorders.

DSM-5 CRITERIA FOR MAJOR NEUROCOGNITIVE DISORDER

A. Evidence of significant cognitive decline from previous level of performance in one or more cognitive domains (complex attention, executive function, learning and memory, language, perceptual-motor, or social cognition) based on:
   1. Concern of the individual, a knowledgeable informant, or clinician that there has been significant decline in cognitive function; and
   2. A substantial impairment in cognitive performance, preferably documented by standardized neuropsychological testing or, in its absence, another quantified clinical assessment.

B. The cognitive deficits interfere with independence in everyday activities (i.e., at a minimum, requiring assistance with complex instrumental activities of daily living such as paying bills or managing medications).

C. The cognitive deficits do not occur exclusively in the context of delirium.

D. The cognitive deficits are not better explained by another mental disorder (e.g., major depressive disorder, schizophrenia).

From the American Psychiatric Association. (2013). *Diagnostic and statistical manual of mental disorders* (5th ed.). Washington, DC: Author.

Mild and major neurocognitive disorder criteria are general. Specific disorders such as Alzheimer's disease are listed in Table 23.1.

While the underlying etiology varies in neurocognitive disorders, nursing care is based on their behavioral manifestations. Therefore approaches to care are not necessarily different for various etiologies. It is for this reason that the remainder of this chapter focuses on the most frequently occurring major neurocognitive disorder, Alzheimer's disease.

ALZHEIMER'S DISEASE

EPIDEMIOLOGY

Alzheimer's disease attacks indiscriminately. It strikes men and women, people of various ethnicities, rich and poor, and individuals with varying degrees of intelligence. Although the disease can occur at a younger age (early onset), most of those with the disease are 65 years of age or older (late

TABLE 23.1 Types of Neurocognitive Disorders

Type of Dementia	Symptoms
Alzheimer's disease	Early: Difficulty with recent memory, impaired learning, apathy, and depression. Moderate to severe: Visual/spatial and language deficits, psychotic features, agitation, and wandering. Late: Gait disturbance, poor judgment, disorientation, confusion, incontinence, and difficulty speaking, swallowing, and walking.
Frontotemporal dementia	Impaired social cognition, disinhibition, apathy, compulsive behavior, poor comprehension, and language difficulties.
Dementia with Lewy bodies	Fluctuating cognition, early changes in attention and executive function, sleep disturbance, visual hallucinations, muscle rigidity, and other parkinsonian features.
Vascular	One or more documented cerebrovascular events. Impaired judgment, poor decision making, planning and organizing (executive functions), personality, and mood changes.
Traumatic brain injury	Trauma to the head with loss of consciousness, posttraumatic amnesia, disorientation and confusion, and/or neurological signs.
Substance/medication-induced	Symptoms of neurocognitive impairment persist beyond the usual duration of intoxication and acute withdrawal. Substances include alcohol, inhalants, sedative, hypnotic, or antianxiety agents.
HIV infection	A documented infection with HIV. Impaired executive function, slowing of processing, problems with attention, difficulty learning new information, aphasia. Symptoms dependent on area of brain affected by HIV pathogenic processes.
Prion	Insidious onset, and rapid progression of impairment. Motor features such as myoclonus or ataxia. Memory, coordination behavior changes, rapidly fatal.
Parkinson's disease	Progression of Parkinson's disease results in dementia with symptoms similar to dementia with Lewy bodies or Alzheimer's disease, and apathetic, depressed or anxious mood, sleep disorder.
Huntington's disease	Abnormal involuntary movements, severe decline in thinking and reasoning, mood changes such as irritability and depression, due to genetic defect.

onset). It is estimated that 5.3 million Americans have Alzheimer's disease (Alzheimer's Association, 2014). Two-thirds of people with dementia are women since women tend to live longer.

It is estimated that one in eight people under 65 years has Alzheimer's disease. Of the people with Alzheimer's disease:

- 4% are younger than 65 years old
- 15% are between 65 and 74 years old
- 44% are between 75 and 84 years old
- 38% are 85 years old or older (Alzheimer's Association, 2014)

RISK FACTORS

Biological Factors

Genetics

There is an increased risk for those people with an immediate family member who has or had dementia. There are three known genetic mutations that guarantee that a person will develop Alzheimer's disease, although these account for less than 1% of all cases. These mutations lead to the devastating early-onset form of Alzheimer's disease, which occurs before the age of 65 and as young as 30 years (Alzheimer's Association, 2014).

A susceptibility gene has been identified for late-onset Alzheimer's disease as well. It is a gene that makes the protein apolipoprotein E (APOE), which supports lipid transport and injury repair in the brain. Individuals carrying the ε4 allele are at increased risk of Alzheimer's disease compared with those carrying the most common ε3 allele, whereas the ε2 allele decreases risk (Liu et al., 2013).

Neurobiological

In the brains of people with Alzheimer's disease, there are signs of neuronal degeneration that begin in the hippocampus, the part of the brain responsible for recent memory. It then spreads into the cerebral cortex, the part of the brain responsible for problem-solving and higher-order cognitive functioning.

There are two processes that contribute to cell death. The first is the accumulation of the protein β-amyloid outside the neurons, which interferes with synapses. The second is an accumulation of the protein tau inside the neurons, which forms tangles that block the flow of nutrients. Interestingly, some people who have these brain changes do not go on to develop Alzheimer's disease (Alzheimer's Association, 2014).

Cardiovascular Disease

The health of the brain is closely linked to overall heart health, and there is evidence that people with cardiovascular disease are at greater risk of Alzheimer's disease. Likewise, lifestyle factors associated with cardiovascular disease, such as inactivity, high cholesterol, diabetes, and obesity, are risk factors for Alzheimer's disease (Alzheimer's Association, 2014).

Head Injury and Traumatic Brain Injury

Brain injury and trauma are associated with a greater risk of developing Alzheimer's disease and other dementias. People who suffer repeated head trauma, such as boxers and football players, may be at greater risk (Alzheimer's Association, 2014).

Environmental Factors

Social Engagement and Diet

There is some evidence that brain health is affected by modifiable factors, such as remaining mentally and socially active and consuming a healthy diet. The research regarding environmental factors is limited by few studies and low number of participants (Alzheimer's Association, 2014).

TABLE 23.2 Memory Deficit: Normal Aging Versus Dementia

Typical Age-Related Changes	Signs of Alzheimer's
Sometimes forgetting names or appointments, but remembering them later	Memory loss that disrupts daily life
Making occasional errors when balancing a checkbook	Challenges in planning or solving problems
Occasionally needing help to use the settings on a microwave or to record a television show	Difficulty completing familiar tasks
Forgetting the day of the week but figuring it out later	Confusion with time or place
Vision difficulties related to cataracts or worsening night vision	Trouble understanding visual images or spatial relationships
Sometimes having difficulty finding the correct word	New problems with words in speaking or writing
Misplacing things from time to time and retracing steps to find them	Misplacing things and losing the ability to retrace steps
Making a bad decision once in a while	Decreased or poor judgment
Sometimes feeling weary of work, family, and social obligations	Withdrawal from social and work activities
Developing specific ways of doing things and becoming irritable when routine is disrupted	Changes in mood and personality

From Alzheimer's Association. (2016). *10 early signs and symptoms of Alzheimer's disease.* Retrieved from http://www.alz.org/national/documents/checklist_10signs.pdf.

CLINICAL PICTURE

Alzheimer's disease accounts for 60% to 80% of all dementias (Alzheimer's Association, 2014). It is a devastating disease that not only affects the person who has it but also places an enormous burden on the families and caregivers of those affected. Nurses practicing in most any setting will care for patients with Alzheimer's disease and must be prepared to respond.

It is important to distinguish between normal forgetfulness and the memory deficit of Alzheimer's disease and other dementias. Severe memory loss is *not* a normal part of growing older. Slight forgetfulness is a common phenomenon of the aging process (age-associated memory loss) but not memory loss that interferes with one's activities of daily living. Table 23.2 outlines memory changes in normal aging and memory changes seen in dementia.

Many people who live to a very old age never experience significant memory loss or any other symptom of dementia. Most of us know of people in their 80s and 90s who lead active lives with their intellect intact. The slow, mild cognitive changes associated with aging should not impede social or occupational functioning.

Although dementia often begins with a worsening of ability to remember new information, it is marked by progressive deterioration in other cognitive functions such as problem-solving and learning new skills and a decline in the ability to perform activities of daily living. A person's declining intellect often leads to emotional changes such as anxiety, mood lability, and depression as well as neurological changes that produce hallucinations and delusions.

Progression of Alzheimer's Disease

Alzheimer's disease is classified according to the stage of the degenerative process. Table 23.3 outlines the three stages. These stages can be used as a guide to understand the progressive deterioration seen in those diagnosed with Alzheimer's disease. The three stages are mild, moderate, and severe. The first stage roughly corresponds to the *DSM-5* criteria for mild neurocognitive disorders. Stages two and three relate to the *DSM-5* criteria for major neurocognitive disorder .

The loss of intellectual ability is insidious. The person with mild Alzheimer's disease loses energy, drive, and initiative and has difficulty learning new things. Because personality and social behavior remain intact, others tend to minimize and underestimate the loss of the individual's abilities. The individual may continue to work, but the extent of the dementia becomes evident in new or demanding situations. Depression may occur early in the disease but usually resolves over time.

More severe symptoms appear as Alzheimer's disease progresses. The person experiences agnosia, which is the inability to identify familiar objects or people, even a spouse. Apraxia is a common symptom where a person needs repeated instructions and directions to perform the simplest tasks: "Here is the wash cloth. Pick up the soap. Now, put water on the face cloth, and rub the face cloth with soap."

Often the individual cannot remember the location of the toilet or is unaware of the process of urinating and defecating resulting in incontinence. It is usually at this point that total care is necessary. For the family, this burden can be emotionally, financially, and physically devastating. For the individual with Alzheimer's disease, the world is very frightening and nothing makes sense. In response, agitation, paranoia, and delusions are common.

VIGNETTE: Mrs. White, 78 years old, a retired teacher, has always enjoyed an active life and good health other than an underactive thyroid, which has been successfully controlled. Remarkably, her only hospitalizations were for the births of her two children, now grown and married. She is a vibrant person who takes pride in her appearance and in her beautiful home. She is beginning to forget things that she previously has taken for granted, but jokes about her failing memory as "senior moments."

Recently, her daughter found Mrs. White quite distressed as she attempted to make her famous specialty, lasagna. The ingredients were strewn all over the kitchen, and Mrs. White was frantically searching for a recipe. Her daughter was surprised because neither of them had ever used a written recipe. Her daughter managed to help Mrs. White with step-by-step instructions in the construction of the lasagna. Her daughter was worried about her mother's failing memory, fearing that it was more than usual aging. She tried to broach the subject with her dad, a loving and loyal companion to Mrs. White. His reply was simply, "I don't know what you're talking about."

The situation reached a crisis point when her daughter discovered that Mrs. White was no longer taking her thyroid medication. Since Mrs. White had taken medication for her thyroid for 30 years and could not remember now, this signaled a progression in her condition.

It was painful, but her husband, too, began to realize that Mrs. White was not functioning properly. Her once-clean house was in a state of disarray. She could no longer coordinate her clothing and usually wore the same outfit for a number of days. Often, her clothes were dirty, and her makeup was applied in a disorganized manner.

VIGNETTE: Mrs. White would stare at both the paper and television, attempting to understand but unable to retain any information. She was often restless during the day, going from one random activity to another, often rearranging her favorite knickknacks in her curio cupboard. She would attempt to wash clothes but forget to put laundry detergent in the machine. She would empty half-filled drinking glasses onto the gas range top. If these mistakes were pointed out, she would become angry, stating, "I have always done it this way."

Eating became difficult as she did not seem to recognize food on her plate, and she was unable to use a knife and fork to cut her food. Sometimes, she would pick up a spoon and ask what it was. Her weight began to decrease.

While Mrs. White always slept well throughout her adult life, she began to wander at night, often waking her husband to ask questions. She would go to the kitchen and empty the cupboards. She would enter her wardrobe and rearrange her clothing, often leaving articles of clothing lying on the floor.

When she set kitchen paper towels on fire on the gas range, her husband and family realized that she could no longer function safely at home. Her husband was unable to leave her alone, even for short periods of time, as she would be become extremely distressed, almost to the point of panic. She and her husband moved into an assisted-living facility.

APPLICATION OF THE NURSING PROCESS

ASSESSMENT

Overall Assessment

Alzheimer's disease is commonly characterized by progressive deterioration of cognitive functioning. Initial deterioration may be so subtle and insidious that others may not notice. In the early stages of the disease, the affected person may be able to compensate for loss of memory. Family members may also unconsciously deny that anything is wrong as a defense against the painful awareness that a loved one is deteriorating. As time goes on, symptoms become more obvious, and other defense mechanisms become evident.

Confabulation is the creation of stories or answers in place of actual memories to maintain self-esteem. For example, the nurse addresses a patient who has remained in a hospital bed all weekend:

Nurse: Good morning, Ms. Jones. How was your weekend?

Patient: Wonderful. I discussed politics with the president, and he took me out to dinner.

or

Patient: I spent the weekend with my daughter and her family.

Confabulation is not the same as lying. When people are lying, they are aware of making up an answer. Confabulation is unconscious.

TABLE 23.3 Stages of Alzheimer's Disease

Stage	Hallmarks
Mild Alzheimer's disease (early-stage)	The person and their loved ones notice memory lapses. The person may still be able to function independently but will experience: • Difficulties retrieving correct words or names, previously known • Trouble remembering names when introduced to new people • Greater difficulty performing tasks in social or work settings • Forgetting material that one has just read • Losing or misplacing a valuable object • Trouble with planning or organizing
Moderate Alzheimer's disease (middle-stage)	The person confuses words, gets frustrated or angry, or acts in unexpected ways such as refusing to bathe. Symptoms become noticeable to others and the person may: • Forget events or own personal history • Become moody or withdrawn, especially in socially or mentally challenging situations • Be unable to recall their own address or telephone number or the high school or college from which they graduated • Become confused about where they are or what day it is • Need for help choosing proper clothing for the season or the occasion • Have trouble controlling bladder and bowels • Change sleep patterns, such as sleeping during the day and becoming restless at night • Be at risk of wandering and becoming lost • Become suspiciousness and delusional or compulsive, for example, repetitive behavior like hand-wringing or tissue shredding
Severe Alzheimer's disease (late-stage)	The person loses the ability to respond to their environment, to carry on a conversation and, eventually, to control movement. They may still say words or phrases, but communicating pain becomes difficult. Personality changes may take place and individuals need extensive help with daily activities. The person may: • Require full-time, around-the-clock assistance with daily personal care • Lose awareness of recent experiences and of their surroundings • Require high levels of assistance with daily activities and personal care • Experience changes in physical abilities, including the ability to walk, sit and, eventually, swallow • Have increasing difficulty communicating • Become vulnerable to infections, especially pneumonia

Adapted from Alzheimer's Association. (2016). *Stages of Alzheimer's*. Retrieved from http://www.alz.org/alzheimers_disease_stages_of_alzheimers.asp?type=alzFooter.

Perseveration is the persistent repetition of a word, phrase, or gesture. This repetition continues after the original stimulus is stopped. For example, you may ask the patient where she was born and her response is Akron. Subsequently you ask her to spell the word world backward and her response is, again, Akron.

Agraphia occurs early in Alzheimer's disease. It is the diminished ability and eventual inability to read or write.

Aphasia is the loss of language ability. Initially, the person has difficulty finding the correct word, then is reduced to a few words, and finally is reduced to babbling or mutism.

Apraxia is the loss of purposeful movement in the absence of motor or sensory impairment. This results in the inability to perform once-familiar and purposeful tasks. For example, in apraxia of dressing, the person is unable to put clothes on properly (may put arms in trousers or put a jacket on upside down).

Agnosia is the loss of sensory ability to recognize objects. For example, a person may lose the ability to recognize familiar sounds (auditory agnosia) such as the ring of the telephone. Loss of this ability extends to the inability to recognize familiar objects (visual or tactile agnosia) such as a glass, magazine, pencil, or toothbrush.

Hyperorality refers to the tendency to taste, chew, and put everything in the mouth. **Hypermetamorphosis** refers to the urge to touch everything.

Sundowning is the tendency for mood to deteriorate and agitation increase in the later part of the day or at night.

Other symptoms observed in Alzheimer's disease include the following:

- Memory impairment: Initially, the person has difficulty remembering recent events. Gradually, deterioration progresses to include both recent and remote memory.
- Disturbances in executive functioning (planning, organizing, abstract thinking): The degeneration of neurons in the brain results in the wasting away of the brain's working components. These cells contain memories, receive sights and sounds, cause hormones to secrete, produce emotions, and command muscles into motion.
- Emotions, like all other cognitively based abilities, begin to diminish. At the most extreme end of the disorder, there seems to be a complete absence of emotion. This absence is manifested in a flat facial affect and unresponsiveness.

Diagnostic Tests

A wide range of problems may be mistaken for Alzheimer's disease. Depression in the older adult is the disorder frequently confused with disease. In fact, many individuals diagnosed with Alzheimer's disease also meet the diagnostic criteria for a depressive disorder. In addition, dementia and depression or dementia and delirium *can* coexist. It is important that nurses and other healthcare professionals be able to assess some of the important differences between depression, dementia, and delirium. Table 23.4 outlines important differences among these three phenomena.

CONSIDERING CULTURE

Cultural Beliefs Regarding Dementia

A timely diagnosis provides an opportunity to discuss care options before the person with dementia becomes too cognitively impaired to make decisions. Such an investigation may also result in identifying underlying treatable conditions.

Cultural barriers may result in delays in diagnosis, treatment, and care for dementia. Individuals from racial and ethnic minorities have longer treatment delays and higher levels of cognitive impairment, behavioral issues, and psychological problems when compared with their non-Hispanic white counterparts. There are a variety of reasons for these delays:

- Low levels of acculturation (i.e., adopting of values and customs of a culture)
- Cultural beliefs about memory loss and dementia (i.e., memory loss is normal with age)
- Lack of accurate knowledge about dementia
- Language barriers
- Religious and spiritual beliefs such as possession by evil spirits
- Cultural shame and stigma (e.g., the person's behavior reflects on the entire family)
- Social isolation and poor education
- Financial limitations (i.e., health insurance)

It is difficult for anyone to care for a family member with dementia. Adding the problems listed here makes a bad situation even worse. Healthcare workers, especially nurses, can provide education in the context of cultural awareness to reduce treatment delays.

Sayegh, P., & Knight, B. G. (2013). Cross-cultural differences in dementia: The Sociocultural Health Belief Model. *International Psychogeriatrics, 25*(4), 517–530.

Brain imaging with a computed tomography scan (CT), positron emission tomography (PET), and other developing scanning technologies have diagnostic capabilities because they reveal brain atrophy and rule out other conditions such as neoplasms. The use of mental status questionnaires, such as the Mini-Mental State Examination and various other tests to identify deterioration in mental status and brain damage, is an important part of the assessment.

In addition to performing a complete physical and neurological examination, it is important to obtain a complete medical and psychiatric history, description of recent symptoms, review of medications used, and nutritional evaluation. The observations and history provided by family members are invaluable to the assessment process.

Self-Assessment

Working with cognitively impaired people in any setting should make us aware of the enormous responsibility placed on caregivers. The behavioral problems these patients may display can cause tremendous stress for professionals and family caregivers alike. Caring for people unable to communicate and who have lost the ability to relate and respond to others is extremely difficult. Because stress is common when working with individuals with cognitive impairments, be proactive in minimizing its effects by:

- Having an understanding of the disease so that expectations for the person are realistic.

TABLE 23.4 **Comparison of Delirium, Dementia, and Depression**

	Delirium	Dementia	Depression
Onset	Sudden (over hours to days) and fluctuating during the course of the day.	Slowly, over months and years	May have been gradual with exacerbation during crisis or stress
Cause or contributing factors	Underlying medical condition such as a urinary tract infection, substance intoxication, or effects of medications	Alzheimer's disease, vascular disease, human immunodeficiency virus infection, neurological disease, chronic alcoholism, head trauma	Lifelong history, losses, loneliness, crises, declining health, medical conditions
Cognition	Impaired attention span, memory deficit, disorientation, disturbances in perception, not related to other cognitive disorders or reduced level of arousal	Impaired memory, judgment, calculations, attention span, abstract thinking and agnosia	Difficulty concentrating, forgetfulness, inattention
Activity level	Can be increased or reduced; restlessness, behaviors may worsen in evening (sundowning); sleep-wake cycle may be reversed	Not altered; behaviors may worsen in evening (sundowning)	Usually decreased; lethargy, fatigue, lack of motivation; may sleep poorly and awaken in early morning
Emotional state	Rapid swings; can be fearful, anxious, suspicious, aggressive, have hallucinations and/or delusions	Flat; agitation	Extreme sadness, apathy, irritability, anxiety, paranoid ideation
Speech and language	Rapid, inappropriate, incoherent, rambling	Incoherent, slow (sometimes due to effort to find the right word), inappropriate, rambling, repetitious	Slow, flat, low
Prognosis	Reversible with proper and timely treatment	Not reversible; progressive	Reversible with proper and timely treatment

ASSESSMENT GUIDELINES

Alzheimer's Disease

1. Evaluate the person's current level of cognitive and daily functioning.
2. Identify any threats to the person's safety and security and arrange their reduction.
3. Evaluate the safety of the person's home environment if possible (e.g., with regard to wandering, eating inedible objects, falling, engaging in provocative behaviors toward others).
4. Review medications (including herbs, complementary agents) the patient is taking.
5. Interview the family to gain a complete picture of the person's background and personality.
6. Explore how well the family is prepared for and informed about the progress of the person's dementia, depending on cause (if known).
7. Discuss with the family members how they are coping with the patient.
8. Review the resources available to the family. Determine if caregivers are aware of community support groups and resources.
9. Identify the needs of the family for teaching and guidance such as understanding sundowning.

- Establishing attainable outcomes for the person and recognizing when they are achieved. These outcomes may be as minor as *patient feeds self with spoon.*

NURSING DIAGNOSIS

One of the most important areas of concern is the patient's safety. Many people with Alzheimer's disease wander and can put themselves in danger. Injuries from falls and accidents can occur during any stage as confusion and disorientation progress. The potential for burns exists if the person is a smoker or is unattended when using the stove. The individual can take prescription drugs incorrectly or mistakenly drink from bottles of caustic fluids. *Risk for injury* is always a priority diagnosis in this population.

As the person's ability to recognize or name objects decreases, *Impaired verbal communication* becomes a problem. As memory diminishes and disorientation increases, *Impaired environmental interpretation syndrome, Impaired memory,* and *Confusion* occur.

Perhaps some of the most crucial aspects of the patient's care are support, education, and referrals for the family. Family members lose the love, the function, the support, the companionship, and the warmth that this person once provided. *Caregiver role strain* is always present and planning with the family and offering community support is an integral part of appropriate care. *Anticipatory grieving* is also an important phenomenon to assess and may be an important target for intervention. Helping the family grieve can make the task ahead somewhat clearer and at times less painful. Review Table 23.5 for examples of the types of everyday problems faced by people with dementia as these provide potential nursing diagnoses for confused patients.

OUTCOMES CRITERIA

Families who have a member with dementia face an exhaustive list of issues that need to be addressed. Self-care needs, impaired environmental interpretation, chronic confusion, ineffective individual coping, and caregiver role strain are just a few of the areas nurses and other healthcare members will need to target. Table 23.6 identifies signs and symptoms, nursing diagnoses, and associated outcomes for delirium and dementia.

PLANNING

Planning care for a person with dementia focuses on the person's immediate needs. Identifying the level of functioning and assessing caregivers' needs help focus planning.

TABLE 23.5 Problems that May Affect People with Dementia and Their Families

Problem	Examples
Memory impairment	Forgets appointments, visits, etc.
	Forgets to change clothes, wash, go to the toilet
	Forgets to eat, take medications
	Loses things
Disorientation	Time: Mixes night and day, mixes days of appointments, wears summer clothes in winter, forgets age
	Place: Loses way around house
	Person: Has difficulty recognizing visitors, family, spouse
Need for physical help	Dressing
	Washing, bathing
	Toileting
	Eating
	Performing housework
	Maintaining mobility
Risks in the home	Falls
	Fire from cigarettes, cooking, heating
	Flooding
	Admission of strangers to home
	Wandering out
Risks outside the home	Competence, judgment, and risks at work
	Driving, road sense
	Getting lost
Apathy	Little conversation
	Lack of interest
	Poor self-care
Poor communication	Dysphasia
Repetitiveness	Repetition of questions or stories
	Repetition of actions
Uncontrolled emotion	Distress
	Agitation
	Anger or aggression
	Demands for attention
Uncontrolled behavior	Restlessness day or night
	Vulgar table or toilet habits
	Undressing
	Sexual disinhibition
Incontinence	Urine
	Feces
	Urination or defecation in the wrong place
Emotional reactions	Depression
	Anxiety
	Frustration and anger
	Embarrassment and withdrawal
Other reactions	Suspiciousness
	Hoarding and hiding
Mistaken beliefs	Still in paid work
	Parents or spouse still alive
	Hallucinations
Decision making	Indecisive
	Easily influenced
	Refuses help
	Makes unwise decisions
Burden on family	Disruption of social life
	Distress, guilt, rejection
	Family discord

INTERVENTION

The attitude of unconditional positive regard is the nurse's single most effective tool in caring for people with dementia. It induces patients to cooperate with care, reduces catastrophic outbreaks, and increases family members' satisfaction with care. Box 23.3 lists *NIC* interventions related to the management of dementia.

Person-Centered Care Approach

The conventional construction of dementia, based on a biological model and focusing on deficits, has been that the person is eventually lost to the disease. When viewed in this way, people with dementia can be isolated into a social death by being treated as if they are already dead.

These views are challenged by a model of care that focuses on the preservation of the personhood of people with dementia. **Patient-centered care** is based on an ethical position that personhood in dementia remains and should be honored. The patient-centered approach is focused on forming meaning relationships with the person who has dementia and also their caregivers. Developing meaningful relationships maintains the unique identity of the person and promotes well-being (Smebye & Kirkevold, 2013). To achieve a person-centered approach to care, relationships must take priority over tasks. This can be challenging in many healthcare systems that are task-focused.

There is evidence that a person-centered approach to care can significantly decrease agitation in people with dementia living in residential care settings (Chenoweth et al., 2014; Stein-Parbury et al., 2012). By approaching people with dementia in a manner that attempts to enter their world and provide care based on their unique life story, they became more calm and relaxed. The conclusion is that distressing behavior such as agitation is not simply a result of dementia but rather how they are being treated in their social-psychological world.

Health Teaching and Health Promotion

Educating families who have a cognitively impaired member is one of the most important health-teaching duties nurses encounter. Families who are caring for a member in the home need to know about strategies for communicating and for structuring self-care activities (Table 23.7).

Referral to Community Supports

The Alzheimer's Association is a national agency that provides various forms of assistance to individuals with the disease and their families. The Alzheimer's Association has a Community Resource Finder that is useful in locating local resources. Additional resources that might be available in some communities are in Table 23.8.

Some families manage the care of their loved one until death. Other families eventually find that they can no longer deal with the labile and aggressive behavior, incontinence, wandering, unsafe habits, or disruptive nighttime activity. Family members

TABLE 23.6 Symptoms, Diagnoses, and Outcomes for Delirium and Dementia

Symptoms	Nursing Diagnoses	Outcomes
Wanders, has unsteady gait, acts out fear from hallucinations or illusions, forgets things (leaves stove on, doors open), falls	*Risk for injury*	Remains safe in hospital or at home
Awake and disoriented during the night *(sundowning)*, frightened at night	*Disturbed sleep pattern*	Sleep pattern is regular, balances rest and activity
Unable to take care of basic needs, incontinence, imbalanced nutrition, insufficient fluid intake	*Self-care deficit (bathing/hygiene, dressing, feeding, toileting)*	Self-care needs are met with optimal participation by the patient
Sees frightening things that are not there *(hallucinations)*, mistakes everyday objects for something frightening *(illusions)*, may become paranoid and think that others are doing bad things *(delusions)*	*Anxiety (severe/panic)*	Anxiety is reduced to a mild-moderate level, acknowledges the reality of an object or sound after it is pointed out
Does not recognize familiar people or places, has difficulty with short- and/or long-term memory, forgetful, confused	*Acute/chronic confusion*	Reports feeling safe, responds well to orientation interventions
Difficulty with communication, cannot find words, has difficulty in recognizing objects and/or people, incoherent	*Impaired verbal communication* *Impaired social interaction*	Communicates needs, connects with other patients, visitors, and staff at an optimal level with a variety of verbal and nonverbal methods
Devastated over losing place in life (during lucid moments), fearful and overwhelmed by what is happening	*Hopelessness* *Grieving*	Expresses feelings, demonstrates a decreased preoccupation with loss
Family and loved ones overburdened and overwhelmed, unable to care for patient's needs	*Disabled family coping* *Interrupted family processes* *Caregiver role strain*	Family members: express feelings in a supportive environment, have access to counseling and support groups, participate in care, utilize respite care

Herdman, T. H., & Kamitsuru, S. (Eds.). *Nursing diagnoses—Definitions and classification 2015–2017*. Copyright © 2014, 1994-2014 by NANDA International. Used by arrangement with John Wiley & Sons Limited; Moorhead, S., Johnson, M., Maas, M. L., & Swanson, E. (2013). *Nursing outcomes classification (NOC*, 5th ed.). St. Louis, MO: Mosby.

BOX 23.3 *NIC* Interventions for Dementia Management

Definition: Provision of a modified environment for the patient experiencing a chronic confusional state.

- Include family members in planning, providing, and evaluating care, to the extent desired.
- Determine and monitor cognitive deficit(s), using standardized assessment tool.
- Identify usual patterns of behavior for such activities as sleep, medication use, elimination, food intake, and self-care.
- Ascertain what is important to the patient, their values and beliefs, as well as their life history.
- Provide rest periods to prevent fatigue and reduce stress.
- Monitor nutrition and weight.
- Place identification bracelet on patient.
- Introduce self and address patient by name when initiating interaction and speak slowly.
- Give one simple direction at a time in a respectful tone of voice.
- Avoid frustrating patient by quizzing with orientation questions that cannot be answered.
- Use distraction, rather than confrontation, to manage behavior.
- Provide consistent caregivers, physical environment, and daily routine.
- Provide a low-stimulation environment with adequate lighting.
- Identify and remove potential dangers in environment for patient.
- Provide cues—such as current events, seasons, location, and names—to assist orientation.
- Seat patient at small table in groups of three to five for meals as appropriate.
- Provide finger foods to maintain nutrition for patient who will not sit and eat.
- Select television or radio programs based on cognitive processing abilities and interests.
- Select one-to-one and group activities geared to patient's cognitive abilities and interests.
- Limit number of choices patient has to make so as not to cause anxiety.
- Place patient's name in large block letters in room and on clothing, as needed.
- Use symbols, rather than written signs, to assist patient in locating room, bathroom, or other area.

From Bulechek, G. M., Butcher, H. K., Dochterman, J. M., & Wagner, C. (2013). *Nursing interventions classification (NIC*, 6th ed.). St. Louis, MO: Mosby.

need to know where and how to place their loved one for care if this becomes necessary. Families need information, support, and legal and financial guidance at this time. When the nurse is unable to provide the relevant information, proper referrals by the social worker are needed. Include information regarding advance directives, durable power of attorney, guardianship, and conservatorship in the communication with the family. Useful guidelines for families in structuring a safe environment and planning appropriate activities at home are listed in Table 23.9.

Pharmacological Interventions

The US Food and Drug Administration (FDA) has approved several medications for the treatment of Alzheimer's disease. Although these medications are used widely and have shown to have statistically significant effects when compared with placebos, they produce only a clinically marginal improvement on cognition and functioning. The benefits of these medications wane after 1 to 2 years so patients should weigh the potential side effects against the potential benefits.

TABLE 23.7 Patient and Family Teaching: Guidelines for Self-Care in Dementia

Intervention	Rationale
Dressing and Bathing	
Have the person perform all tasks within his or her present capacity.	Maintains the person's self-esteem and uses muscle groups; impedes staff burnout; minimizes further regression.
Have the person wear own clothes, even if in the hospital.	Helps maintain the person's identity and dignity.
Use clothing with elastic and substitute fastening tape (Velcro) for buttons and zippers.	Minimizes the person's confusion and eases independence of functioning.
Label clothing items with the person's name and name of item.	Helps identify the person if he or she wanders and gives the person additional clues when aphasia or agnosia occurs.
Give step-by-step instructions whenever necessary (e.g., "Take this blouse. Put in one arm…now the other arm. Pull it together in front. Now….")	The person can focus on small pieces of information more easily; allows the person to perform at optimal level.
Make sure that water in faucets is not too hot.	Judgment is lacking in the person; the person is unaware of many safety hazards.
If the person is reluctant to performing self-care, come back later and ask again.	Moods may be labile, and the person may forget but often complies after short interval.
Nutrition	
Monitor food and fluid intake.	The person may have anorexia or be too confused to eat.
Offer finger food that the person can take away from the dinner table.	Increases input throughout the day; the person may eat only small amounts at meals.
Weigh the person regularly (once a week).	Monitors fluid and nutritional status.
During periods of hyperorality, watch that the person does not eat nonfood items (e.g., ceramic fruit or food-shaped soaps).	The person puts everything into mouth; may be unable to differentiate inedible objects made in the shape and color of food.
Bowel and Bladder Function	
Begin bowel and bladder program early; start with bladder control.	Establishing same time of day for bowel movements and toileting—in early morning, after meals and snacks, and before bedtime—can help prevent incontinence.
Evaluate use of disposable diapers.	Prevents embarrassment.
Label bathroom door, as well as doors to other rooms.	Additional environmental clues can maximize independent toileting.
Sleep	
Because the person may awaken, be frightened, or cry out at night, keep area well lighted.	Reinforces orientation, minimizes possible illusions.
Maintain a calm atmosphere during the day.	Encourages a calming night's sleep.
Order nonbarbiturates (e.g., chloral hydrate) if necessary.	Barbiturates can have a paradoxical reaction, causing agitation.
If medications are indicated, consider neuroleptics with sedative properties, which may be the most helpful (e.g., haloperidol [Haldol]).	Helps clear thinking and sedates.
Avoid the use of restraints.	Can cause the person to become more terrified and fight against restraints until exhausted to a dangerous degree.

TABLE 23.8 Types of Services that May Be Available to People with Dementia

Type of Service	Services Provided	Type of Service	Services Provided
Family/caregiver Some people may live by themselves in the community; active case management is vital	Caregivers have a right to: Easy access to services Respite care Full involvement in decision making Assessment of the needs of both the caregiver and the person with dementia Information and referral Case management: Coordination of community resources and follow-up	Home care	Meals on Wheels Home health aide services Homemaker services Hospice services Occupational therapy Paid companion or sitter services Physical therapy Skilled nursing Personal care services: assistance in basic self-care activities Social work services Telephone reassurance: regular telephone calls to individuals who are isolated and homebound* Personal emergency response systems: telephone-based systems to alert others that a person who is alone is in need of emergency assistance*
Community services	Adult day care: Provides activities, socialization, supervision Physician services Protective services: Prevent, eliminate, and/or remedy effects of abuse or neglect Recreational services Transportation Mental health services Legal services		

*Vital for those living alone.

Cholinesterase Inhibitors

Because a deficiency of acetylcholine has been linked to Alzheimer's disease, medications aimed at preventing its breakdown have been developed. Drugs in this classification work by preventing an enzyme called acetylcholinesterase or, more simply, cholinesterase from breaking down acetylcholine in the brain. As a result, an increased concentration of acetylcholine leads to temporary improvement of some symptoms of Alzheimer's disease.

There is little evidence that giving cholinesterase inhibitors to individuals who have the mild version of neurocognitive disorders slows the progression to dementia (Buckley & Salpeter, 2015). The cholinesterase inhibitors produce small, but short-lived, improvements in cognitive functioning. There is minimal benefit after 1 year, and the risk of side effects doubles in people over 85 years of age.

The FDA approved the first cholinesterase inhibitor, Tacrine (Cognex), in 1993 for the treatment of mild to moderate symptoms of Alzheimer's disease. Unfortunately, tacrine was associated with a high frequency of side effects including gastrointestinal effects, elevated liver transaminase levels, and liver toxicity. As a result, it was withdrawn from the US market in 2012.

The most commonly prescribed cholinesterase inhibitor, donepezil (Aricept), was approved by the FDA in 1996. Indications for donepezil include mild, moderate, and severe Alzheimer's disease. It also appears to improve cognitive functions without the potentially serious liver toxicity attributed to tacrine. Some individuals may experience diarrhea and nausea while taking the drug. These side effects are dose-related so a decreased dose helps minimize them.

Rivastigmine (Exelon) was approved for use in 2000. The most common side effects are nausea, vomiting, loss of appetite, and weight loss. In most cases, these side effects are temporary. Patients should always take rivastigmine with food to reduce gastrointestinal side effects. The Exelon transdermal patch is applied once a day and has no food requirement. It is useful for people who have trouble swallowing pills. Patients and families should be cautioned to always remove the old patch before applying the new one to prevent serious side effects.

Galantamine (Razadyne [formerly known as *Reminyl*]) gained FDA approval in 2001. It is prescribed in the early stages of dementia.

TABLE 23.9 Patient and Family Teaching: Guidelines for Care at Home

Intervention	Rationale
Safe Environment	
Gradually restrict use of motor vehicles.	As judgment becomes impaired, the person may be dangerous to self and others.
Remove throw rugs and other objects in person's path.	Minimizes tripping and falling.
Minimize sensory stimulation.	Decreases sensory overload, which can increase anxiety and confusion.
If the person becomes verbally upset, listen and be supportive, allowing the person to be upset. Gradually try to redirect and change the topic.	Goal is to prevent escalation of anger. When attention span is short, the person can be distracted to more productive topics and activities.
Label all rooms and drawers. Label often-used objects (e.g., hairbrushes and toothbrushes).	May keep the person from wandering into other people's rooms. Increases environmental clues to familiar objects.
Install safety bars in bathroom.	Prevents falls.
Supervise the person when he or she smokes.	Danger of burns is always present.
Wandering	
If the person wanders during the night, put mattress on the floor.	Prevents falls when the person is confused.
Have the person wear medical alert bracelet that cannot be removed (with name, address, and telephone number). Provide police department with recent pictures.	The person can easily be identified by police, neighbors, or hospital personnel.
Alert local police and neighbors about wandering.	May reduce time necessary to return the person to home or hospital.
If the person is in hospital, have him or her wear brightly colored vest with name, unit, and phone number printed on back.	Makes the person easily identifiable.
Put complex locks on door.	Reduces opportunity to wander.
Place locks at top of door.	In moderate and late Alzheimer's-type dementia, ability to look up and reach upward is lost.
Encourage physical activity during the day.	Physical activity may decrease wandering at night.
Explore the feasibility of installing sensor devices.	Provides warning if the person wanders.
Useful Activities	
Provide picture magazines and children's books when the person's reading ability diminishes.	Allows continuation of usual activities that the person can still enjoy; provides focus.
Provide simple activities that allow exercise of large muscles.	Exercise groups, dance groups, and walking provide socialization, as well as increased circulation and maintenance of muscle tone.
Encourage group activities that are familiar and simple to perform.	Activities such as group singing, dancing, reminiscing, and working with clay and paint all help increase socialization and minimize feelings of alienation.

Despite slight variations in the mode of action of the cholinesterase inhibitors, there is no evidence of any differences between them with regard to effectiveness. All of the cholinesterase inhibitors have the potential to cause nausea, diarrhea, and vomiting, depending on the dosage level. Bradycardia and syncope have been associated with this class of drugs. They should be used with caution when patients are taking nonsteroidal anti-inflammatory drugs (NSAIDs).

N-methyl-D-aspartate (NMDA) Receptor Antagonist

Memantine (Namenda) was approved for use in Alzheimer's disease patients in 2003. This medication is typically added after trying the cholinesterase inhibitors. It regulates the activity of glutamate, a neurotransmitter that plays a role in information processing, storage, and retrieval. Memantine blocks NMDA receptors to protect against excessive neuronal stimulation by glutamate. It is approved for use in moderate to severe dementia, and not mild dementia.

Refer to Chapter 3 for a more-detailed discussion of psychotropic medications. Drugs approved by the FDA for treatment of Alzheimer's disease are described in Table 23.10.

Medications for Behavioral Symptoms of Alzheimer's Disease

Other medications are often useful in managing the behavioral symptoms of individuals with dementia, but these need to be used with extreme caution. The rule of thumb for older adults is "start low and go slow." Another is to use the smallest dose for the shortest duration possible and discontinue if they are not effective. In addition, because people with dementia are at high risk of developing delirium, always add medications with caution.

Most people with dementia will experience behavioral symptoms that reduce their quality of life, are distressing to them and their caregivers, and may lead to placement in a residential care facility. Some of the troubling behaviors are psychotic symptoms (hallucinations, paranoia), severe mood swings (depression is common), wandering, anxiety, agitation, and verbal or physical aggression (combativeness). Not only are these behaviors distressing, but they may also lead to injuries from falls, infections, and incontinence.

Psychotropic medications may be prescribed. Drug classifications that are used off-label include antidepressants, antipsychotics, antianxiety agents, and anticonvulsants. Of these, antipsychotics have been used most often. These medications are associated with risk of mortality, mostly from cardiovascular and infectious causes. As a result, the FDA (2008) warns that the use of all antipsychotics, both first- and second-generation, is no longer approved for dementia-related psychosis.

TABLE 23.10 FDA Approved Drugs for Alzheimer's Disease

Generic (Trade)	Action	Indications	Side Effects
Cholinesterase Inhibitors			
Donepezil (Aricept) Rivastigmine (Exelon, Exelon Patch) Galantamine (Razadyne, Razadyne ER)	Inhibit acetylcholinesterase, thereby increasing available acetylcholine.	Modestly improves cognition in mild to moderate dementia of Alzheimer's disease. Donepezil is also approved for severe Alzheimer's disease Exelon Patch approved for mild to moderate dementia of Parkinson's disease No evidence to support use in mild neurocognitive disorders, as no significant difference in progression to dementia.	Side effects are dose-related. Nausea, vomiting, diarrhea, insomnia, fatigue, muscle cramps, incontinence, bradycardia, and syncope.
***N*-methyl-D-aspartate (NMDA) Receptor Antagonist**			
Memantine (Namenda, Namenda XR-slow release)	Regulates glutamate activity by blocking NMDA receptors, thereby decreasing excitatory neurotoxicity caused by over stimulation of NMDA receptors by glutamate.	Moderate to severe Alzheimer's disease; no evidence that it modifies underlying disease.	Dizziness, agitation, headache, constipation, and confusion.
NMDA Receptor Antagonist/Cholinesterase Inhibitor			
Memantine/donepezil (Namzaric)	See memantine and donepezil.	Moderate to severe Alzheimer's disease currently stabilized on a combination of memantine and donepezil.	See side effects listed under memantine and donepezil.

US Food and Drug Administration. (2016). *Drugs.* Retrieved from http://www.fda.gov/Drugs/.

Neurobiology of Alzheimer's and the Effects of Medication on the Brain

Two essential neurotransmitters implicated in Alzheimer's disease are acetylcholine and glutamate.
Acetylcholine: is involved with learning, memory, and mood. As Alzheimer's disease progresses the brain produces less and less acetylcholine. What little acetylcholine is left is rapidly destroyed by the enzyme acetylcholinesterase.
Cholinesterase: inhibitors keep the acetylcholinesterase enzyme from breaking down acetylcholine, thereby increasing both the level and duration of action of the neurotransmitter acetylcholine.
Glutamate: is involved with cell signaling, learning, and memory. Glutamate binds to cells at the *N*-methyl-D-aspartate (NMDA) receptor and allows calcium to enter the cell. In Alzheimer's disease, excess glutamate from damaged cells leads to chronic overexposure to calcium.
NMDA: antagonists helps reduce excess calcium by blocking some NMDA receptors.

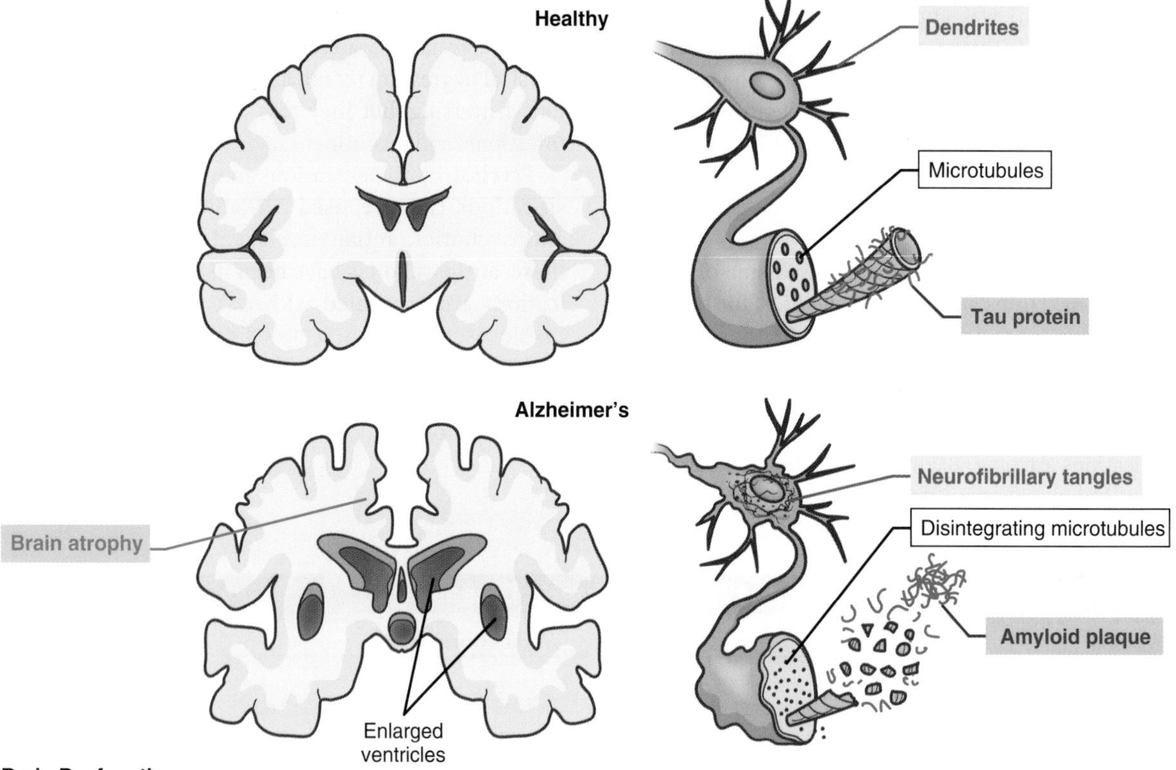

Brain Dysfunction

Amyloid plaques are sticky clumps found between nerve cells that may either cause or be the result of the disease. The clumps block communication at synapses that is normally protected by tau proteins and healthy microtubules. They may also activate immune system cells that trigger inflammation and devour disabled cells.

Neurofibrillary tangles are abnormal collections of protein threads inside nerve cells. They are comprised mainly of a protein called tau. Tangles disrupt the transport of food molecules, cell parts, and other key elements. This disruption results in cell death.

Brain atrophy is the cerebral cortex shriveling up, damaging areas involved in thinking, planning, and remembering. The hippocampus, an area of the cortex that is essential for memory, experiences severe shrinkage. Ventricles, the fluid-filled spaces within the brain, grow larger.

FDA-Approved Drugs for the Treatment of Alzheimer's Disease

Drug Name	Brand Name	Classification	Approved For
galantamine	Razadyne	Cholinesterase inhibitor	Mild to moderate
donepezil	Aricept	Cholinesterase inhibitor	All stages
rivastigmine	Exelon	Cholinesterase inhibitor	All stages
memantine	Namenda	Namenda, an NMDA antagonist, helps reduce excess calcium by blocking some NMDA receptors	Moderate to severe
donepezil and memantine	Namzaric	Cholinesterase inhibitor and NMDA receptor antagonist combination	Moderate to severe

Integrative Therapy

Aromatherapy, the use of essential oils from fragrant plants such as lavender, peppermint, and sweet marjoram, has been used with people with dementia to promote relaxation and sleep, provide pain relief, and improve mood. At present, there is limited evidence as to the effectiveness of aromatherapy in people with dementia. A recent systematic review (Forrester et al., 2014) of seven controlled trials demonstrated that there are inconsistent effects of aromatherapy on quality of life, agitation, and behavioral challenges in people with dementia.

EVALUATION

Outcome criteria for people with cognitive impairments need to be measurable, within the capabilities of the individual person, and evaluated frequently. As the person's condition continues to deteriorate, outcomes should reflect the person's diminished functioning. Frequent evaluation and reformulation of outcome criteria and short-term indicators also help reduce staff and family frustration and minimize the patient's anxiety by ensuring that tasks are not more complicated than the person can accomplish.

The overall outcomes for treatment are to promote the person's optimal level of functioning and to delay further regression whenever possible. Working closely with family members and providing them with the names of available resources and support sources may help increase the quality of life for both the family and the patient with Alzheimer's disease (see the Case Study and Nursing Care Plan).

CASE STUDY AND NURSING CARE PLAN

Cognitive Impairment

During the past 4 years, Mr. Sloane has demonstrated progressive memory impairment, disorientation, and deterioration in functioning related to Alzheimer's disease. He is 67 years old and retired at age 62 to spend some of his remaining "youth" with his wife and to do the things they always wanted to do. At age 63, he was diagnosed with Alzheimer's disease.

Mr. Sloane is incontinent when he cannot find the bathroom. He wanders away from home, despite close supervision. The police and neighbors bring him home an average of four times a week. He has fallen while getting out of bed at night, thinking he is in a sleeping bag, camping out in the mountains. The family makes the painful decision to place him in a care facility for people with Alzheimer's disease.

Brian Jackson, a registered nurse, notices that Mr. Sloane becomes frustrated when he has difficulty finding the right words for things (aphasia). At one point Mr. Sloane asked, "Who is this woman?" and pointed to his wife (agnosia).

Mrs. Sloane tells Brian that her husband can sometimes participate in dressing himself; at other times, he needs total assistance. At this point, Mrs. Sloane begins to sob, saying, "I can't bear to part with him...but I can't do it anymore. I feel as if I've betrayed him."

Brian states, "This is a difficult decision for you." Brian suggests a support group. "It might help you to feel that you are not alone" One of the groups he suggests is the Alzheimer's Association, a well-known self-help group.

Self-Assessment

Brian has worked on this unit for 4 years. He applied for this position shortly after his own father died of complications secondary to Alzheimer's disease. Brian refers to the process of living and dying with this disease as horrifying. His goal is to help others go through this with caring, dignity, and the highest level of functioning possible.

Caring for Mr. Sloane and his family is especially personal. Mr. Sloane is about the same age his father had been, looks similar to him, and has many of his mannerisms. He shared these feelings with his wife, and the two of them spent some time talking about his father and all they had been through together, good and bad. In the end, Brian sat back, breathed a deep sigh of relief, and thanked his wife for being there for him.

When Brian returned to work, he nearly walked right into Mr. Sloane. He was standing at the doorway wearing two shirts, a pair of pajama bottoms, and a baseball cap. "Are you the man who's taking me to pick up my car?" he asks. Brian smiles and says, "It looks like you have quite a day planned. Let's start with a cup of coffee," and redirects him to the day hall.

Assessment

Subjective Data

- Wanders away from home about four times a week
- "I can't bear to part with him."
- "I feel as if I've betrayed him."

Objective Data

1. Incontinent
2. Aphasia
3. Agnosia
4. Difficulty dressing himself
5. Falls out of bed
6. Impaired memory
7. Frequently disoriented

Priority Diagnosis

- Risk for injury

Supporting Data

- Wandered away from home about four times a week
- Wanders despite supervision
- Falls out of bed at night

Outcome Criteria

Although Mr. Sloane has many unmet needs that require nursing interventions, Brian decides to focus on physical safety. Criteria for successful outcome are:

- Highest level of functioning will be supported
- Optimal health will be maintained (nutrition, sleep, elimination).
- Patient will be free from fractures, bruises, contusions, burns, and falls

Short-Term Goal	Intervention	Rationale	Evaluation
Patient will remain free from injury with the aid of environmental manipulation and family or nursing precautions and interventions.	1. Minimize sensory stimulation.	1. Minimizing sensory stimulation decreases sensory overload which increases anxiety and confusion.	**GOAL MET** During his first week in the facility, Mr. Sloane remained free from injury.

Continued

CASE STUDY AND NURSING CARE PLAN—cont'd

Cognitive Impairment

Short-Term Goal	Intervention	Rationale	Evaluation
	2. If patient is upset, listen, give support, and then change the topic.	2. When attention span is short, patients can be briefly distracted to more productive topics and activities.	
	3. Label all rooms and drawers with pictures. Label often-used objects (e.g., hairbrushes and toothbrushes).	3. Labeling can keep the patient from wandering into other patient's rooms and increases environmental clues to familiar objects.	
	4. Encourage physical activity during the day.	4. Physical activity during the day might decrease wandering at night.	
	5. Provide a low bed.	5. Low beds will prevent injuries in case of falling out of the bed.	
	6. Provide adequate lighting in the bathroom at night.	6. While darkness is important for sleep, light in the bathroom will decrease wandering and promote continence.	

Evaluation

Although Mr. Sloane continues to display wandering behaviors, his wandering is contained to safe areas of the unit except for one instance when he wandered to the lobby. He was stopped by security and safely returned to the unit within 45 minutes. He has not fallen out of bed. Nursing interventions, such as placing his mattress on the floor and ensuring adequate lighting, increase his safety while at the same time acknowledging that he continues to exhibit wandering behaviors.

KEY POINTS TO REMEMBER

- *Neurocognitive disorder* is a term that refers to disorders resulting from changes in the brain and marked by disturbances in orientation, memory, intellect, judgment, and affect.
- Delirium and dementia are discussed in this chapter because they are the neurocognitive disorders most frequently seen by healthcare workers.
- Delirium has an acute onset, noticeable disturbances in consciousness, and symptoms of disorientation and confusion that change by the minute, hour, or time of day.
- Delirium is always secondary to an underlying condition. Therefore it is usually temporary, transient, and may last from hours to days once the underlying cause is treated. If the cause is not treated, permanent damage to the brain can result.
- Dementia usually has a more insidious onset than delirium. Global deterioration of cognitive functioning (e.g., memory, judgment, ability to think abstractly, and orientation) is often progressive and irreversible, depending on the underlying cause.
- All types of dementia are diagnosed as either mild or major neurocognitive disorders, differentiated by the person's functional ability.
- Signs and symptoms change according to the three stages of Alzheimer's disease: stage 1 (mild), stage 2 (moderate), and stage 3 (severe).
- Behavioral manifestations of Alzheimer's disease include confabulation, perseveration, agraphia, aphasia, apraxia, agnosia, hyperorality, hypermetamorphosis, and sundowning.
- No known cause or cure exists for Alzheimer's disease, although a number of drugs that increase the brain's supply of acetylcholine (a nerve-communication chemical) or regulate glutamate are helpful in slowing the progression of the disease.
- People with Alzheimer's disease have many unmet needs and present numerous management challenges to both their families and healthcare workers.
- Specific nursing interventions for cognitively impaired individuals can increase communication, safety, and self-care. The need for family teaching and support is crucial.

CRITICAL THINKING

1. Mrs. Kendel is an 82-year-old woman who has Alzheimer's disease. She lives with her husband, who has been trying to care for her in their home. Mrs. Kendel is having trouble dressing. She has put her blouse on backward and sometimes puts her bra on over her blouse. She often forgets where things are. She makes an effort to cook but has recently attempted to "put out" the electric burners of the stove with pitchers of water. Once in a while, she cannot find the bathroom in time, often mistaking it for a closet. At times, she cries because she is aware that she is losing her sense of her place in the world. She and her husband have always been close loving companions, and he wants to keep her at home as long as possible.
   a. Assist Mr. Kendel by writing out a list of suggestions that he can try at home that might help facilitate (a) communication, (b) activities of daily living, and (c) maintenance of a safe home environment.

b. Identify at least three interventions appropriate to this situation for each of the areas previously cited.
c. Identify resources available for maintaining Mrs. Kendel in her home for as long as possible. Provide the name of a self-help group that you would urge Mr. Kendel to join.

2. Share with your class or clinical group the name and function of at least three community agencies in your area that could be an appropriate referral for a family with a member with dementia. (For one, you can contact the Alzheimer's Association to find a local chapter; www.alz.org.)

CHAPTER REVIEW

Questions

1. Which statement made by the primary caregiver of a patient diagnosed with dementia demonstrates accurate understanding of providing the patient with a safe environment?
   a. "The local police know that he has wandered off before."
   b. "I keep the noise level low in the house."
   c. "We've installed locks on all the outside doors."
   d. "Our telephone number is always attached to the inside of his shirt pocket."
2. Which statement made by a family member tends to support a diagnosis of delirium rather than dementia?
   a. "She was fine last night but this morning she was confused."
   b. "Dad doesn't seem to recognize us anymore."
   c. "She's convinced that snakes come into her room at night."
   d. "He can't remember when to take his pills or whether he's bathed."
3. When considering the pathophysiology responsible for both delirium and dementia, which intervention is appropriate for delirium specifically?
   a. Assist with needs related to nutrition, elimination, hydration, and personal hygiene.
   b. Monitor neurological status on an ongoing basis.
   c. Place identification bracelet on patient.
   d. Give one simple direction at a time in a respectful tone of voice.
4. What side effects should the nurse monitor for when caring for a patient prescribed donepezil (Aricept)? *Select all that apply.*
   a. Insomnia
   b. Constipation
   c. Bradycardia
   d. Signs of dizziness
   e. Reports of headache
5. What is the rationale for providing a patient diagnosed with dementia easily accessible finger foods thorough the day?
   a. Increases input throughout the day
   b. The person may be anorexic
   c. Assists with monitoring food intake
   d. Helps prevent constipation
6. Ophelia, a 69-year-old retired nurse, attends a reunion of her former coworkers. Ophelia is concerned because she usually knows everyone, and she cannot recognize faces today. A registered nurse colleague recognizes Ophelia's distress and "introduces" Ophelia to those attending. The nurse practitioner recognizes that Ophelia seems to have a deficit in:
   a. Lower-level cognitive domain
   b. Delirium threshold
   c. Executive function
   d. Social cognition
7. Nancy is a nurse. After talking with her mother, she became concerned enough to drive over and check on her. Her mother's appearance is disheveled, words are nonsensical, smells strongly of urine, and there is a stain on her dressing gown. Nancy recognizes that her mother's condition is likely temporary due to:
   a. Early onset dementia
   b. A mild cognitive disorder
   c. A urinary tract infection
   d. Skipping breakfast
8. Darnell is an 84-year-old widower who has lived alone since his wife died 6 years ago. A neighbor called Darnell's son to tell him that Darnell was trying to start his car from the passenger's side. He became angry and aggressive when the car would not start. After a medical assessment, Darnell was diagnosed with a major neurocognitive disorder. The nurse realized additional family teaching is necessary when Darnell's son states:
   a. "My father's diagnosis is interfering with his daily functioning."
   b. "This neurocognitive disorder will probably progress."
   c. "Advancing age is a risk factor in my father's diagnosis."
   d. "With person-centered care, my father will be able to remain in his home."
9. In the 2 months after his wife's death, Aaron, aged 90 and in good health, has begun to pay less attention to his hygiene and seems less alert to his surroundings. He complains of difficulty concentrating and sleeping and reports that he lacks energy. His family sometimes has to remind and encourage him to shower, take his medications, and eat, all of which he then does. Which response is most appropriate?
   a. Reorient Mr. Smith by pointing out the day and date each time you have occasion to interact with him.
   b. Meet with family and support them to accept, anticipate, and prepare for the progression of his stage 2 dementia.
   c. Avoid touch and proximity; these are likely to be uncomfortable for Mr. Smith and may provoke aggression when he is disoriented.
   d. Arrange for an appointment with a therapist for evaluation and treatment of suspected depression.
10. Nurses caring for patients who have neurocognitive disorders are exposed to stress on many levels. Specialized skills training and continuing education are helpful to diffuse nursing stress, as well as: *Select all that apply.*
   a. Expressing emotions by journaling
   b. Describing stressful events on Facebook
   c. Engage in exercise and relaxation activities
   d. Having realistic patient expectations
   e. Happy hour after work to blow off steam

Answers

1. **c**; 2. **a**; 3. **b**; 4. **a, c, d, e**; 5. **a**; 6. **d**; 7. **c**; 8. **d**; 9. **d**; 10. **a, c, d**

ⓔ Visit the Evolve website for a posttest on the content in this chapter: http://evolve.elsevier.com/Varcarolis

Post-Test interactive review

REFERENCES

Alzheimer's Association. (2014). Alzheimer's Association Report: 2014 Alzheimer's disease facts and figures. *Alzheimer's and Dementia, 10*, e47–e92.

Alzheimer's Association. (2015). *FDA-approved treatments for Alzheimer's*. Retrieved from http://www.alz.org/dementia/downloads/topicsheet_treatments.pdf.

American Psychiatric Association. (2013). *Diagnostic and statistical manual of mental disorders (DSM 5)* (5th ed.). Washington, DC: Author.

Anand, A., & MacLullich, A. M. J. (2013). Delirium in hospitalized older adults. *Medicine, 41*(1), 39–42.

Buckley, J. S., & Salpeter, S. R. (2015). A risk-benefit assessment of dementia medications: Systematic review of the evidence. *Drugs and Aging, 32*, 453–467.

Bulechek, G. M., Butcher, H. K., Dochterman, J. M., & Wagner, C. (2013). *Nursing interventions classification (NIC)* (6th ed.). St. Louis, MO: Mosby.

Caplan, J. P., Cassem, N. H., Murray, G. B., Park, J. M., & Stern, T. A. (2016). Delirium. In T. A. Stern, M. Fava, T. E. Wilkens, & J. F. Rosenbaum (Eds.), *Massachusetts General Hospital comprehensive clinical psychiatry* (pp. 173–183). St. Louis, MO: Elsevier.

Chenoweth, L., Forbes, I., Fleming, R., King, M. T., Stein-Parbury, J., Luscombe, G., et al. (2014). PerCEN: A cluster randomized controlled trial of person-centered residential care and environment for people with dementia. *International Psychogeriatrics, 26*(7), 1147–1160.

Forrester, L. T., Maayan, N., Orrell, M., Spector, A. E., Buchan, L. D., & Soares-Weiser, K. (2014). Aromatherapy for dementia. *Cochrane Database of Systematic Reviews, 2014*(Issue 2). Art. No.: CD003150.

Inouye, S. K., Westendorp, R. G. J., & Saczynski, J. S. (2014). Delirium in elderly people. *Lancet, 383*, 911–922.

Liu, C., Kanekiyo, T., Xu, H., & Bu, G. (2013). Apolipoprotein E and Alzheimer disease: Risk, mechanisms, and therapy. *Nature Reviews Neurology, 9*(2), 106–118.

Reston, J. T., & Schoelles, K. M. (2013). In-facility delirium prevention programs as a patient safety strategy: A systematic review. *Annals of Internal Medicine, 158*, 375–380.

Smebye, K. L., & Kirkevold, M. (2013). The influence of relationships on personhood in dementia care: A qualitative, hermeneutic study. *BMC Nursing, 12*, 29. Retrieved from http://www.biomedcentral.com/1472-6955/12/29.

Stein-Parbury, J., Chenoweth, L., Jeon, Y.-H., Brodaty, H., Haas, M., & Norman, R. (2012). Implementing person-centered care in residential dementia care. *Clinical Gerontologist, 35*(5), 404–424.

US Food and Drug Administration. (2008). FDA requests boxed warnings on older class of antipsychotic drugs. Retrieved from https://www.fda.gov/NewsEvents/Newsroom/PressAnnouncements/2008/ucm116912.htm.

van Munster, B. C., & de Rooij, S. E. (2014). Delirium: A synthesis of current knowledge. *Clinical Medicine, 14*(2), 192–195.

24

Personality Disorders

Christine A. Tackett, Margaret Jordan Halter, and Claudia A. Cihlar

Visit the Evolve website for a pretest on the content in this chapter: http://evolve.elsevier.com/Varcarolis Pre-Test interactive review

OBJECTIVES

1. Identify characteristics of each of the 10 personality disorders.
2. Analyze the interaction of biological determinants and psychosocial risk factors in the development of personality disorders.
3. Describe the emotional and clinical needs of nurses and other staff when working with patients who have personality disorders.
4. Formulate a nursing diagnosis for each of the personality disorders.
5. Discuss two nursing outcomes for patients with antisocial and borderline personality disorder.
6. Plan basic interventions for a patient with impulsive, aggressive, or manipulative behaviors.
7. Identify the role of the advanced practice nurse when working with patients with personality disorders.

OUTLINE

OUTLINE—cont'd

KEY TERMS AND CONCEPTS

callousness
dialectical behavior therapy (DBT)
diathesis-stress model
emotional dysregulation
emotional lability
impulsivity
personality
personality disorder
separation-individuation
splitting

We may often meet someone and think, "She's quite a dramatic person" or "What an detail-oriented character he is." When we make evaluations such as these about other individuals, we are reacting to their personalities. Personality comes from the Latin word *persona,* which means "mask," and it may refer to what other people see.

Personality is an individual's characteristic pattern of relatively permanent thoughts, feelings, and behaviors that define his or her quality of experiences and relationships. A personality is considered unhealthy when interpersonal and social relationships and functioning are consistently maladaptive, complicated, or dysphoric. We know that personality can be protective for a person in times of difficulty but may also be a liability if one's personality results in ongoing relationship problems or leads to emotional distress on a regular basis.

Until quite recently, we believed that personalities were fairly fixed entities. This belief was based on William James' (1892, p. 124) view, "By the age of 30, the character has set like plaster and will never soften again." More contemporary views challenge this notion. Rather than being set like plaster, the rate of personality's change slows over time but does not cease (Newton-Howes et al., 2015). If personality traits evolve continually across the lifespan, we have an opportunity to develop and support more adaptive functioning and social relationships.

CLINICAL PICTURE

Personality disorders are among the most challenging and complex group of disorders to treat. Individuals who meet criteria for these disorders display significant challenges in self-identity or self-direction, and they have problems with empathy or intimacy within their relationships.

People with these disorders have difficulty recognizing or owning that their difficulties are problems of their personality. They may truly believe the problems originate outside of themselves. Still others may be unaware that their behavior is unusual, and they may not experience any distress.

Judgments about an individual's personality functioning must take into account the person's ethnic, cultural, and social background. Patients who differ from the majority culture or the culture of the clinician may be at risk for overdiagnosis of a personality disorder. Therefore it is important to obtain additional information from others knowledgeable of the particular cultural or ethnic norms before determining the presence of a personality disorder.

According to the American Psychiatric Association (APA, 2013), there are 10 personality disorders. These 10 disorders are grouped into clusters of similar behavior patterns and personality traits. These clusters are:

Cluster A: Behaviors described as odd or eccentric.
- Paranoid personality disorder
- Schizoid personality disorder
- Schizotypal personality disorder

Cluster B: Behaviors described as dramatic, emotional, or erratic.
- Borderline personality disorder
- Narcissistic personality disorder
- Histrionic personality disorder
- Antisocial personality disorder

Cluster C: Behaviors described as anxious or fearful.
- Avoidant
- Dependent
- Obsessive-Compulsive

In this chapter, we begin with an overview of personality disorders including epidemiology, comorbidity, and risk factors. Afterward, eight of the personality disorders are presented along with the prevalence, characteristic pathological responses, nursing care guidelines, and medical treatments. A vignette is provided to illustrate each of these disorders. After reviewing these eight disorders, two of the most common and challenging personality disorders—antisocial and borderline—will be described in more depth along with an application of the nursing process.

EPIDEMIOLOGY AND COMORBIDITY

While studies vary in their estimates of prevalence depending upon methodologies, personality disorders affect about 6% of the global population (Huang et al., 2009). In the US population, the overall prevalence rate of personality disorders among community samples is higher—around 10% (Sansone & Sansone, 2011).

Culture has a definite influence on the rate of diagnosing personality disorders. For example, Australian and North American studies reflect higher prevalence rates (Samuels, 2011). Differences may reflect personality and behavior as being viewed as deviant rather than normative in a particular culture and study methods. It is generally agreed that there are insufficient studies to address the role that ethnicity and race have on the prevalence of personality disorders (McGilloway et al., 2010).

Most referrals to mental health providers tend to be for mental state problems such as major depressive disorder or generalized anxiety disorder. Yet personality disorders are present in up to half of patients with mental state disorders, making it one of the most common psychiatric disorders (Zimmerman et al., 2008). The presence of personality disorders results in poorer outcomes in the treatment of other psychiatric disorders and may underlie treatment-resistant cases.

Personality disorders frequently co-occur with disorders of mood and eating, anxiety, and substance misuse. Personality disorders often amplify **emotional dysregulation**, a term that describes poorly modulated mood characterized by mood swings. Individuals with emotion regulation problems have ongoing difficulty managing painful emotions in ways that are healthy and effective.

The aging process has some affect on the prevalence of personality disorders. The dramatic, emotional, or erratic Cluster B disorders may mute with age as individuals become less impulsive. This dampening may be due to a general tuning down of neurotransmitters (Rosowsky et al., 2013). Other disorders such as obsessive-compulsive personality disorder or paranoid personality disorder may worsen with age, perhaps due to anxiety regarding declining sensory and cognitive capacity.

RISK FACTORS

Personality disorders are the result of complex biological and psychosocial phenomena that are influenced by multifaceted variables involving genetics, neurobiology, chemistry, and environmental factors. An overview of the possible causes of personality disorders is provided.

Biological Factors

Genetic

Genetics are thought to influence the development of personality disorders (Skodol et al., 2014). It is the personality traits and not the personality disorders themselves that are inherited. Personality disorders may represent extreme variations of normal personality traits in four areas: anxious-dependency traits, psychopathy-antisocial, social withdrawal, and compulsivity (Svrakic et al., 2008).

Neurobiological

The neurotransmitter theory proposes that certain neurotransmitters, including neurohormones, may regulate and influence temperament. Research in brain imaging has also revealed some differences in the size and function of specific structures of the brain in people with some personality disorders (Coccaro & Siever, 2005).

Psychological Factors

In the 19th century, Sigmund Freud hypothesized that personality emerged from childhood experiences rather than one's chemistry. Psychoanalytic theory focuses on the use of primitive defense mechanisms by individuals with personality disorders. Defense mechanisms such as repression, suppression, regression, undoing, and splitting have been identified as dominant. The role of Freud's psychoanalytic theory, while historically relevant and interesting, is not supported by evidence-based research.

Learning theory emphasizes that children learn maladaptive responses based on modeling or reinforcement by significant others. Cognitive theories emphasize the role of beliefs and assumptions in creating emotional and behavioral responses that influence one's experiences within the family environment.

Environmental Factors

Behavioral genetics research has shown that about half of the variance accounting for personality traits emerges from the environment (Paris, 2005). These findings suggest that, while the family environment is influential on development, there are other environmental factors besides family upbringing that shape an individual's personality. One need only think about the individual differences among siblings raised together to illustrate this point.

Childhood neglect or trauma has been established as a risk factor for personality disorders (Samuels, 2011). This association has been linked to possible biological mechanisms involving corticotropin-releasing hormones in response to early life stress and emotional reactivity (Lee et al., 2011).

Diathesis-Stress Model

The **diathesis-stress model** is a general theory that explains psychopathology using a systems approach. This theory helps us understand how personality disorders emerge from the multifaceted factors of biology and environment (Paris, 2005). **Diathesis** refers to genetic and biological vulnerabilities and includes personality traits and temperament. **Temperament** is our tendency to respond to challenges in predictable ways. Descriptors of temperament may be "laid back," referring to a calm temperament, or "uptight," as an example of an anxious temperament. These characteristics remain stable throughout a person's life.

In this model, **stress** refers to immediate influences on personality such as the physical, social, psychological, and emotional environment. Stress also includes what happened in the past such as growing up in one's family with exposure to unique experiences and patterns of interaction. Under conditions of stress, the diathesis-stress model proposes that personality development becomes maladaptive for some people, resulting in the emergence of a personality disorder (Paris, 2005).

There is a two-way directionality among stressors and diatheses. Genetic and biological traits are believed to influence the way an individual responds to the environment, while at the same time, the environment is thought to influence the expression of inherited traits. Many studies have suggested a strong correlation between trauma, neglect, and other dysfunctional family or social patterns of interaction on the development of personality disorders among individuals with certain personality traits and temperament.

CLUSTER A PERSONALITY DISORDERS

Paranoid Personality Disorder

Paranoid personality disorder is characterized by a longstanding distrust and suspiciousness of others based on the belief, which is unsupported by evidence, that others want to exploit, harm, or deceive the person. These individuals are hypervigilant, anticipate hostility, and may provoke hostile responses by initiating a counterattack.

The prevalence of paranoid personality disorder has been estimated at about 2% to 4% (APA, 2013). Slightly more men than women are diagnosed with this disorder. Relatives of patients with schizophrenia are more frequently affected with this disorder. A diagnosis of paranoid personality disorder often precedes a schizophrenia diagnosis.

Symptoms may be apparent in childhood or adolescence. Parents may notice that their child doesn't have friends and experiences social anxiety. Young people with this disorder are frequently teased due to their odd behavior.

As adults, relationships are difficult due to jealousy, controlling behaviors, and unwillingness to forgive. Projection is the dominant defense mechanism whereby people attribute their own unacknowledged feelings to others. For example, they may accuse their partner of being hypercritical when they themselves are attentively fault finding.

Guidelines for Nursing Care

- Considering the degree of mistrust, promises, appointments, and schedules should be strictly adhered to.
- Being too nice or friendly may be met with suspicion. Instead, give clear and straightforward explanations of tests and procedures beforehand.
- Use simple language and project a neutral but kind affect.
- Limit setting is essential when threatening behaviors are present.

Treatment

Individuals with paranoid personality disorder tend to reject treatment. If they somehow end up in a psychiatric treatment setting, they may appear puzzled and obviously suspicious about why this is happening. Paranoid people are difficult to interview because they are reluctant to share information about themselves for fear that the information will be used against them.

Psychotherapy is the first line of treatment for paranoid personality disorder (Sadock et al., 2015). Individual therapy focuses on the development of a professional and trusting relationship. Due to their fears, patients may behave in a threatening manner. Therapists should respond by setting limits and dealing with delusional accusations in a realistic manner without humiliating the patients.

Group therapy is threatening to people with paranoid personality disorder. However, the group setting may be useful in improving social skills. Role playing and group feedback can help reduce suspiciousness. For example, if the patient says, "I think the therapist is singling me out," other groups members may provide a reality check or describe similar feelings in the past.

An antianxiety agent such as diazepam (Valium) may be used to reduce anxiety and agitation (Sadock et al., 2015). More severe agitation and delusions may be treated with antipsychotic medication such as haloperidol (Haldol) in small doses for brief periods of time to manage the mildly delusional thinking or severe agitation. The first-generation antipsychotic medication pimozide (Orap) may be useful in reducing paranoid ideation.

VIGNETTE: Ms. Alonzo is a 54-year-old unemployed female who comes to a mental health clinic complaining of depression and pain. She believes that her health maintenance organization has circulated her medical record to all healthcare providers to prevent her from being treated. She refuses to give any social history and is reluctant to share her telephone number. When the nurse indicates that the psychiatrist does not prescribe pain medications, she smiles bitterly and says, "So they already got to you."

Schizoid Personality Disorder

People with **schizoid personality disorder** exhibit a lifelong pattern of social withdrawal. They are somewhat expressionless and operate with a restricted range of emotional expression. Others tend to view them as odd or eccentric due to their discomfort with social interaction.

The prevalence rate may be nearly 5% of the population (APA, 2013). Males are more often affected. Symptoms of schizoid personality disorder appear in childhood and adolescence. These young people tend to be loners, do poorly in school, and are the objects of ridicule by their peers for their odd behavior. There is increased prevalence of the disorder in families with a history of schizophrenia or schizotypal personality disorder. Abnormalities in the dopaminergic systems may underlie this problem.

Relationships are particularly affected due to the prominent feature of emotional detachment. People with this disorder do not seek out or enjoy close relationships. Neither approval nor rejection from others seems to have much effect. Friendships, dating, and sexual experiences are rare. If trust is established, the person may divulge numerous imaginary friends and fantasies.

Employment may be jeopardized if interpersonal interaction is necessary. Individuals with this disorder may be able to function well in a solitary occupation such as being a security guard on the night shift. They often endorse feelings of being an observer rather than a participant in life. The patient may describe feelings of depersonalization or detachment from oneself and the world.

Guidelines for Nursing Care

- Nurses should avoid being too "nice" or "friendly."
- Do not try to increase socialization.
- Patients may be open to discussing topics such as coping and anxiety.
- Conduct a thorough assessment to identify symptoms the patient is reluctant to discuss.
- Protect against ridicule from group members due to patient's distinctive interests or ideas.

Treatment

Patients with schizoid personality disorder tend to be introspective (Sadock et al., 2015). This trait may make them good, if distant, candidates for psychotherapy. As trust develops, these patients may describe a full fantasy life and fears, particularly of dependence. Psychotherapy can help improve sensitivity to others' social cues. Group therapy may also be helpful even though the patient may frequently be silent. Group therapy provides experience in practicing interactions and feedback from others. Group members may become quite important to the person with schizoid personality disorder and may be the only form of socialization he has.

Antidepressants such as bupropion (Wellbutrin) may help increase pleasure in life. Second-generation antipsychotics, such as risperidone (Risperdal) or olanzapine (Zyprexa), are used to improve emotional expressiveness.

VIGNETTE: Mr. Gray, a 30-year-old single male, is a graduate student in mathematics at a large state university. He lives alone and has never been married. He works as an assistant in a math classroom in which the professor teaches the course remotely via television. Mr. Gray wears thick glasses, and his clothing is inconspicuous. He rarely smiles and seldom looks directly at the students even when answering questions. He does get somewhat animated when he writes lengthy solutions to math problems on the blackboard. He is content with his low-paying job and has never been in psychiatric treatment.

Schizotypal Personality Disorder

People with **schizotypal personality disorder** do not blend in with the crowd. Their symptoms are strikingly strange and unusual. Magical thinking, odd beliefs, strange speech patterns, and inappropriate affect are hallmarks of this disorder.

Estimates on the prevalence of schizotypal personality disorder vary from 0.6% to 4.6% (APA, 2013). It is more common in men than women. Like the other Cluster A personality disorders, symptoms are evident in young people. People who have first-degree relatives with schizophrenia are at more of a risk for this disorder. Abnormalities in brain structure, physiology, chemistry, and functioning are similar to schizophrenia. For example, both disorders share reduced cortical volume.

The *Diagnostic and Statistical Manual of Mental Illness,* fifth edition (*DSM-5;* APA, 2013) identifies this problem as both a personality disorder and also the first of the schizophrenia spectrum disorders. The *International Classification of Diseases and Related Health Problems, 10th Revision – clinical modification* (World Health Organization, 2016), used throughout the world, classifies schizotypal along with schizophrenia and no longer lists schizotypal as a personality disorder. Chapter 12 discusses the schizophrenia spectrum disorders in greater detail.

Like schizoid personality disorder, individuals with schizotypal personality disorder have severe social and interpersonal deficits. They experience extreme anxiety in social situations. Contributions to conversations tend to ramble with lengthy, unclear, overly detailed, and abstract content. An additional feature of this disorder is paranoia. Individuals with schizotypal personality disorder are overly suspicious and anxious. They tend to misinterpret the motivations of others as being out to get them and blame others for their social isolation. Odd beliefs (e.g., being overly superstitious) or magical thinking (e.g., "He caught a cold because I wished he would") are also common.

Psychotic symptoms seen in people with schizophrenia, such as hallucinations and delusions, might also exist with schizotypal personality disorder, but to a lesser degree and only briefly. A major difference between this disorder and schizophrenia is that people with schizotypal personality disorder can be made aware of their suspiciousness, magical thinking, and odd beliefs. Schizophrenia is characterized by far stronger delusions.

Guidelines for Nursing Care

- Respect patient's need for social isolation.
- Nurses should be aware of patient's suspiciousness and employ appropriate interventions.
- Perform careful assessment as needed to uncover any other medical or psychological symptoms that may need intervention (e.g., suicidal thoughts).
- Be aware that strange beliefs and activities, like strange religious practices or peculiar thoughts, may be part of the patient's life.

Treatment

The principles of psychotherapy are similar to that of schizoid personality disorder (Sadock et al., 2015). However, clinicians should be aware that these patients may also be actively involved in groups such as cults, unusual religious groups, and engage in occult activities.

While there is no specific medication for schizotypal personality disorder, associated conditions may be treated. People with schizotypal personality disorder seem to benefit from low-dose antipsychotic agents for psychotic-like symptoms and day-to-day functioning (Ripoll et al., 2011). These agents help with such symptoms as ideas of reference or illusions. Depression and anxiety may be treated with antidepressants and antianxiety agents.

VIGNETTE: Raymond is a 55-year-old single male who lives with his mother. He is the youngest of seven children raised in a farming community. Three of his siblings are deaf, and Raymond also has some hearing loss. Raymond started therapy with Jenny, an advanced practice psychiatric-mental health registered nurse, after he suffered a career-ending injury from which he is completely disabled. Jenny and Raymond have been working together for several years.

Raymond is distressed by his belief that everyone in his hometown greets him with sexual gestures. "They obviously think I'm gay." He thinks that truck drivers talk about his sexuality on their CB radios. These beliefs create great distress and anxiety for him. He occasionally yells at or gestures at the truck drivers. Jenny has been helping Raymond to understand how his perceptions may be faulty and how his hearing loss may contribute to his perceptual difficulties and anxiety.

CLUSTER B PERSONALITY DISORDERS

Histrionic Personality Disorder

People with **histrionic personality disorder** are excitable and dramatic yet are often high functioning. They may be referred to in terms of "drama queen" or "drama major." Classic characteristics of this population include extroversion, flamboyancy, and colorful personalities. Despite this bold exterior, they tend to have limited ability to develop meaningful relationships.

Histrionic personality disorder occurs at a rate of nearly 2% in community samples (APA, 2013). In clinical settings, it tends to be diagnosed more frequently in women than men. Symptoms begin by early adulthood. Inborn character traits such as emotional expressiveness and egocentricity have also been identified as predisposing an individual to this disorder.

This disorder is characterized by emotional attention-seeking behaviors including self-centeredness, low frustration tolerance, and excessive emotionality. The person with histrionic personality disorder is often impulsive and may act flirtatiously or provocatively. Relationships do not last because the partner often feels smothered or reacts to the insensitivity of the histrionic person. The individual with histrionic personality disorder does not have insight into a personal role in breaking up relationships.

In general, individuals with this disorder do not think they need psychiatric help. They may go into treatment for associated problems such as depression that may be precipitated by losses such as the end of a relationship.

Guidelines for Nursing Care

- Nursing care should reflect an understanding that seductive behavior is a response to distress.
- Keep communication and interactions professional.
- Patients may exaggerate symptoms and have difficulty in functioning.
- Encourage and model the use of concrete and descriptive rather than vague and impressionistic language.
- Assist the patient to clarify feelings because they often have difficulty identifying them.
- Teach and role model assertiveness.
- Assess for suicidal ideation. What was intended as a suicide gesture may inadvertently result in death.

Treatment

Individuals with histrionic personality disorder may be out of touch with their feelings (Sadock et al., 2015). Psychotherapy may promote clarification of inner feelings and appropriate expression. Group therapy may be useful in this population, although distracting symptoms may be disruptive to group functioning.

There are no specific pharmacological treatments available for people with histrionic personality disorder. Medications such as antidepressants can be used for depressive or somatic symptoms. Antianxiety agents may be helpful in treating anxiety. Antipsychotics may be used if the patient exhibits derealization or illusions.

VIGNETTE: Ms. Lombard is a 35-year-old twice-divorced female admitted to an inpatient unit after an overdose of asthma medications and antibiotics. She took all of her pills after her primary care provider refused to order a sleeping pill for her. On the first night, she is withdrawn and tearful in her room. By the next morning, she is neatly groomed, even wearing makeup, and is socializing with everyone. She denies thoughts of self-harm. Over the next 2 days, Ms. Lombard monopolizes the community meetings by talking about how unappreciated she is by her family. She seeks special attention from a male evening-shift registered nurse, asking if he can stay late after his shift to sit with her. When he refuses, she demands to be placed back on one-to-one precautions because she feels suicidal again.

Narcissistic Personality Disorder

Narcissistic personality disorder is characterized by feelings of entitlement, an exaggerated belief in one's own importance, and a lack of empathy. In reality, people with this disorder suffer from a weak self-esteem and hypersensitivity to criticism. Narcissistic personality disorder is associated with less impairment in individual functioning and quality of life than the other personality-based disorders.

The prevalence of narcissistic personality disorder ranges from 0% to about 6% in community samples (APA, 2013). It tends to be more common in males than females. Age of onset is difficult to determine due to the narcissistic traits that are typically found in adolescents. There may be a familial tendency for this disorder as parents with narcissism may attribute an unrealistic sense of talent, importance, and beauty to their children. These attributions put the children at higher risk.

People with narcissistic personality disorder come across as arrogant and as having an inflated view of their self-importance. The individual with this disorder has a need for constant admiration along with a lack of empathy for others, a factor that strains most relationships over time. They are very sensitive to rejection and criticism and can be disparaging to others. A sense of personal entitlement paired with a lack of social empathy may result in the exploitation of other people.

Underneath the surface of arrogance, people with narcissistic personality disorder feel intense shame and have a fear of abandonment. In keeping with these descriptions, the main pathological personality trait of narcissism is antagonism, represented by the grandiosity and attention-seeking behaviors. They tend to tolerate rejection poorly. As a result, narcissistic individuals may seek help for depression or may seek to be validated by therapists and/or loved ones for their emotional pain of not being appreciated by others for their efforts or special qualities.

Guidelines for Nursing Care

- Nurses should remain neutral and recognize the source of narcissistic behavior—shame and fear of abandonment.
- Use the therapeutic nurse-patient relationship as an opportunity to practice how to engage in meaningful interaction.
- Avoid engaging in power struggles or becoming defensive in response to the patient's disparaging remarks.
- Role model empathy.

Treatment

Because patients need to confront their problem to make progress, treating people specifically for this disorder is difficult (Sadock et al., 2015). Because individuals are not likely to seek help for their own problems, they are more likely to be involved in couples or family therapy than individual treatment. In these family-oriented approaches, narcissistic individuals are likely to deflect suggestions that they contribute to family problems, and will instead blame others.

If a person with narcissistic personality disorder somehow seeks treatment, individual cognitive-behavioral therapy is helpful for deconstructing faulty thinking. Group therapy can also assist the person in sharing with others, seeing their own qualities in others, and learning empathy.

Lithium (Eskalith, Lithobid) has been used in patients with narcissism who demonstrate mood swings. Antidepressants can also be used if the person has symptoms of depression.

> **VIGNETTE:** Dr. Andrew McLaughlin is a 40-year-old attending psychiatrist at a university outpatient center. He is twice divorced and has no children. His grooming is impeccable, and he likes to describe his expensive shopping habits. He is usually late to staff meetings, and when he is not speaking, yawns and shifts noisily in his seat. He has a reputation for exhibiting angry outbursts at therapists in the hallway for minor mistakes such as a scheduling error. Dr. McLaughlin becomes impatient when waiting in lines and often moves to the front of the line, which has led to angry confrontation.

CLUSTER C PERSONALITY DISORDERS

Avoidant Personality Disorder

People with **avoidant personality disorder** are extremely sensitive to rejection, feel inadequate, and are socially inhibited. They avoid interpersonal contact due to fears of rejection or criticism.

Avoidant personality disorder occurs in 2.4% of the US population (APA, 2013). It is found equally among men and women. Early symptoms of the disorder are often evident in infants and children. These symptoms include shyness and avoidance that, unlike common shyness, increase during adolescence and early adulthood.

The main pathological personality traits are low self-esteem associated with functioning in social situations, feelings of inferiority compared with peers, and a reluctance to engage in unfamiliar activities involving new people. Some can function in a protective environment. However, if their support system fails, they can suffer from depression, anxiety, and anger. They are especially sensitive to and preoccupied with rejection, humiliation, and failure. They often avoid new interpersonal relationships or activities due to their fears of criticism or disapproval (APA, 2013).

Guidelines for Nursing Care

- Nurses should use a friendly, accepting, and reassuring approach.
- Remember that being pushed into social situations can cause severe anxiety for these patients.
- Convey an attitude of acceptance toward patient fears.
- Provide the patient exercises to enhance new social skills but use with caution because any failure can increase feelings of poor self-worth.
- Assertiveness training can assist the person to learn to express needs.

Treatment

Individual and group therapy is useful in processing anxiety-provoking symptoms and in planning methods to approach and handle anxiety-provoking situations (Sadock et al., 2015). Psychotherapy focuses on trust and assertiveness training.

Antianxiety agents can be helpful. Beta-adrenergic receptor antagonists (e.g., atenolol) help reduce autonomic nervous system hyperactivity. Antidepressant medications such as selective serotonin reuptake inhibitors (SSRIs) like citalopram (Celexa) and serotonin norepinephrine reuptake inhibitors (SNRIs) such as venlafaxine (Effexor) may reduce social anxiety (Ripoll et al., 2011). Serotonergic agents may help individuals with avoidant personalities feel less sensitive to rejection.

> **VIGNETTE:** Ms. Lowell is a 35-year-old single female who works for a computer repair company. As a child, she had few friends and never participated in extracurricular activities. She lives alone in her own apartment and has never had an adult intimate relationship. On the job, she rarely talks to co-workers and prefers to work alone. If she has any questions, she asks the supervisor and carefully follows directions. Although she has 7 years of experience and a good work record, she refuses the offer of a promotion because it would require her to interact with customers.

Dependent Personality Disorder

Dependent personality disorder is characterized by a pattern of submissive and clinging behavior related to an overwhelming need to be cared for. This need results in intense fears of separation.

The prevalence rate of dependent personality disorder is fairly rare with an estimate of about 0.5% (APA, 2013). Dependent personality disorder may be the result of chronic physical illness or punishment for independent behavior in childhood. The inherited trait of submissiveness may also be a factor.

People with dependent personality disorder have a high need to be taken care of. This need can lead to patterns of submissiveness with fears of separation and abandonment by others. Because they lack confidence in their own ability or judgment, they may manipulate others to assume responsibility for such activities as finances or child rearing. This may create problems by leaving them more vulnerable to exploitation by others because of their passive and submissive nature. Feelings of insecurity about their self-agency and lack of self-confidence may interfere with attempts at becoming more independent. They may experience intense anxiety when left alone for even brief periods of time (APA, 2013).

Guidelines for Nursing Care

- Nurses can help the patient identify and address current stressors.
- Be aware that strong countertransference may develop because of patient's demands for extra time and crisis states.
- The therapeutic nurse-patient relationship can provide a testing ground for increased assertiveness through role modeling and teaching of assertive skills.

Treatment

Psychotherapy is the treatment of choice for dependent personality disorder (Sadock et al., 2015). Cognitive-behavioral therapy can help patients develop more healthy and accurate thinking by examining and challenging automatic thoughts that result in fearful behavior. This process can help in developing new perspectives and attitudes about the need for other people.

There are no specific medications indicated for this disorder, but symptoms of depression and anxiety may be treated with the appropriate antidepressant and antianxiety agents. Panic attacks can be helped with the tricyclic antidepressant imipramine (Tofranil).

VIGNETTE: Ashley is a 32-year-old, married, former engineer, and she is the mother to two young children, aged 3 years and 11 months. Ashley's depression and anxiety have been more severe since she stopped working. She feels inadequate and overwhelmed by her responsibilities, so her mother moved in with the young family at her daughter's request. Her therapist, an advanced practice psychiatric-mental health registered nurse, recommended that she receive brief treatment for depression and anxiety at the partial hospitalization program. Ashley quickly bonded with the advanced practice nurse, who is an older woman. She frequently asks her for reassurance that she is doing the right thing by coming to treatment and seeks her out frequently for extra individual sessions. Gradually, as the result of individual and group therapy, Ashley begins to realize that excessive dependence on her mother contributes to longstanding feelings of ineffectiveness, helplessness, and invalidation of her own parenting skills.

Obsessive-Compulsive Personality Disorder

Obsessive-compulsive personality disorder is characterized by limited emotional expression, stubbornness, perseverance, and indecisiveness. Preoccupation with orderliness, perfectionism, and control are the hallmarks of this disorder.

Obsessive-compulsive personality disorder is one of the most prevalent personality disorders. Prevalence rates range from about 2% to 8% (APA, 2013). It is more common in men than women. Oldest siblings tend to be affected more often than subsequent siblings. Risk factors for this disorder include a background of harsh discipline and having a first-degree relative with this disorder. Obsessive-compulsive personality disorder has been associated with increased relapse rates of depression and an increase in suicidal risks in people with co-occurring depression.

The main pathological personality traits are rigidity and inflexible standards of self and others. They rehearse over and over how they will respond in social situations. They persist in goal-seeking long after it is necessary even if it is self-defeating or relationship-defeating. The preoccupation often results in losing the major point of the activity. Projects are often incomplete due to overly strict standards.

A distinction should be made between obsessive-compulsive disorder and obsessive-compulsive personality disorder. Obsessive-compulsive disorder is characterized by obsessive thoughts and repetition or adherence to rituals. They are aware that these thoughts and actions are unreasonable. Obsessive-compulsive personality disorder is characterized more by an unhealthy focus on perfectionism. They think their actions are right and feel comfortable with such self-imposed systems of rules.

People with obsessive-compulsive personality disorder often do feel genuine affection for friends and family. Yet, leisure activities and friendship are dropped in favor of excessive devotion to work and productivity.

Guidelines for Nursing Care

- Nurses should guard against power struggles with these patients as their need for control is very high.
- Patients with this disorder have difficulty dealing with unexpected changes.
- Provide structure, yet allow patients extra time to complete habitual behavior.
- Assist patients to identify ineffective coping and to develop effective coping techniques.

Treatment

Typically, patients seek help for obsessive-compulsive personality disorder, as they are aware of their own suffering. They may also seek treatment for anxiety or depression. The treatment course is often long and complicated. Both group therapy and behavioral therapy can be helpful so that patients can learn new coping skills for their anxiety and see direct benefits for change from feedback within the group.

Clomipramine (Anafranil) may help reduce the obsessions, anxiety, and depression associated with this disorder. Other serotonergic agents such as fluoxetine (Prozac) may also be effective.

VIGNETTE: Mr. Wright is a 45-year-old single male postal worker in a small town. He lives alone and has never married. He is well groomed and wears a clean, neatly ironed uniform every day. He carefully follows all policies and procedures and is quite resistant whenever there is any update or change. He frequently challenges the supervisor about policy details and has been referred to the regional personnel office countless times for resolution of these conflicts. In staff meetings, he gives excessive circumstantial details and writes extra material on the back of any required report form. When dealing with the public, he sometimes gets into arguments with customers about postal rules or the schedule. The other staff members do not consider him to be a team player because he seldom volunteers to help others. Even if he is asked to help someone, he is quick to criticize his peer's performance. Although he has worked in the same office for 10 years, he has never advanced beyond the front-line position.

CONSIDERING CULTURE

Did Northern Climates Favor People with Obsessive-Compulsive Personality Disorder?

People with obsessive-compulsive personality disorder are on a constant quest for perfectionism. They tend to forgo pleasurable activities with friends and family in favor of work and productivity. Could such behaviors be adaptive? Hertler (2015) contends that this may be the case for people who migrated to northern climates with the associated cold and seasonal scarcity.

He contends that obsessive-compulsive personality features of (1) future-oriented thought, (2) parsimoniousness, and (3) compulsive conscientiousness are essential in struggling with harsh elements. According to Hertler, these three traits are more commonly distributed in individuals within northerly latitudes.

Source: Hertler, S. C. (2015). *Evolutionary psychological science, 1*(52).

ANTISOCIAL PERSONALITY DISORDER

CLINICAL PICTURE

In this section we turn our attention to a Cluster B personality disorder that has a significant social impact. **Antisocial personality disorder** is a pattern of disregard for, and violation of, the rights of others. People with this disorder may be more commonly referred to as sociopaths. This diagnosis is reserved for adults, but symptoms are evident by the mid-teens. Symptoms tend to peak during the late teenage years and into the mid-20s. By around 40 years of age, the symptoms may abate and improve even without treatment.

The main pathological traits that characterize antisocial personality disorder are antagonistic behaviors such as being deceitful and manipulative for personal gain or hostile if needs are blocked. The disorder is also characterized by disinhibited behaviors such as high risk taking, disregard for responsibility, and impulsivity. Criminal misconduct and substance misuse are common in this population.

People with this disorder are mostly concerned with gaining personal power or pleasure, and in relationships they focus on their own gratification to an extreme. They have little to no capacity for intimacy and will exploit others if it benefits them in relationships. One of the most disturbing qualities associated with antisocial personality disorder is a profound lack of empathy, also known as **callousness**. This callousness results in a lack of concern about the feelings of others, the absence of remorse or guilt except when facing punishment, and a disregard for meeting school, family, and other obligations.

These individuals tend to exhibit a shallow, unexpressive, and superficial affect. They may also be adept at portraying themselves as concerned and caring if these attributes help them to manipulate and exploit others. A person with antisocial personality disorder may be able to act witty and charming and be good at flattery and manipulating the emotions of others. The *DSM-5* box contains criteria for antisocial personality disorder.

DSM-5 CRITERIA FOR ANTISOCIAL PERSONALITY DISORDER

A. A pervasive pattern of disregard for and violation of the rights of others, occurring since age 15 years, as indicated by three (or more) of the following:
  1. Failure to conform to social norms with respect to lawful behaviors as indicated by repeatedly performing acts that are grounds for arrest.
  2. Deceitfulness as indicated by repeated lying, use of aliases, or conning others for personal profit or pleasure.
  3. Impulsivity or failure to plan ahead.
  4. Irritability and aggressiveness as indicated by repeated physical fights or assaults.
  5. Reckless disregard for safety of self or others.
  6. Consistent irresponsibility as indicated by repeated failure to sustain consistent work behavior or honor financial obligations.
  7. Lack of remorse as indicated by being indifferent to or rationalizing having hurt, mistreated, or stolen from another.

B. The individual is at least age 18 years.

C. There is evidence of conduct disorder with onset before age 15 years.

D. The occurrence of antisocial behavior is not exclusively during the course of schizophrenia or bipolar disorder.

From the American Psychiatric Association. (2013). *Diagnostic and statistical manual of mental disorders* (5th ed.). Washington, DC: Author.

EPIDEMIOLOGY

Antisocial personality disorder is the most researched personality disorder probably due to its marked impact on society in the form of criminal activity. The prevalence of antisocial personality disorder is about 1.1% in community studies (Skodol et al., 2014). While the disorder is much more common in men (3% versus 1%), women may be underdiagnosed due to the traditional close association of this disorder with males.

ETIOLOGY

Biological Factors

Genetic

Antisocial personality disorder is genetically linked, and twin studies indicate a predisposition to this disorder. Kendler and colleagues (2012) note that there are two main dimensions of genetic risk. One is the trait of aggressive-disregard, which refers to violent tendencies without concern for others, and the trait of disinhibition, which is a lack of concern for consequences.

Neurobiological

An alteration in serotonin transmission has been implicated with the aggression and impulsivity that frequently accompany this disorder. Levels of a metabolite of serotonin, 5-hydroxyindoleacetic acid, can be measured in urine and cerebrospinal fluid. It has been found to be lower in individuals with antisocial personality disorder. Lower levels of serotonin along with dopamine hyperfunction may contribute to aggression, disinhibition, and comorbid substance use (Seo et al., 2008).

Environmental Factors

It is likely that a genetic predisposition for characteristics of antisocial personality disorder such as a lack of empathy may be set into motion by childhood maltreatment. Inconsistent parenting and discipline, significant abuse, and extreme neglect are associated with this disorder. Children reflect parental attitudes and behaviors in the absence of more prosocial influences. Virtually all individuals who eventually develop this disorder have a history of impulse control and conduct problems as children and adolescents. Chapter 21 describes impulse control and conduct disorders in greater detail.

Cultural Factors

Assigning a diagnosis of personality disorder cannot be entirely separated from the cultural context of both the individual and the person diagnosing. Cultural bias, including race, ethnicity, ageism, religion, and gender expectations, may unintentionally enter into the categorization. Some studies have found a higher prevalence rate of antisocial personality disorder in African Americans and in individuals with co-occurring substance dependence (McGilloway et al., 2010).

VIGNETTE: Richard is a 25-year-old divorced cab driver who is referred for psychiatric treatment by the court for competency evaluation after an assault charge. He told the arresting officer that he has bipolar disorder. He has a history of substance misuse and multiple arrests for disorderly conduct or assault. During his intake interview, he is polite and even flirtatious with the female psychiatric-mental health registered nurse. He insists that he is not responsible for his behavior because he is manic. The only symptom he describes is irritability. Richard points out that he cannot tolerate any psychotropic medications because of the side effects. He also notes that he has dropped out of three clinics after a few visits because "the staff don't understand me."

APPLICATION OF THE NURSING PROCESS

ASSESSMENT

People with antisocial personality disorder do not enter the healthcare system for treatment of this disorder unless they have been court-ordered to do so. Psychiatric admissions may be initiated for anxiety and depression. Entering treatment may also be a way to avoid or address legal, financial, occupational, or other circumstances. Healthcare workers also encounter this population due to the physical consequences of high-risk behaviors, such as acute injury and substance use. Keep in mind that questions asked during the assessment phase may not always result in accurate responses because the patient may become defensive or simply not tell the truth.

Self-Assessment

You may respond to a person with antisocial personality disorder in a variety of ways. Because these individuals have the capacity to be charming, you may want to defend the person as someone who is being unfairly treated and misunderstood. These feelings should be explored with your faculty or other experienced personnel. Conversely, if you are aware that your patient has a history of criminal acts, you may feel disdain or personally threatened. Again, share your concerns with individuals who are experienced in caring for this population. Awareness and monitoring of your own stress responses to patient behaviors facilitate more effective and therapeutic intervention.

ASSESSMENT GUIDELINES

Antisocial Personality Disorder

1. Assess current life stressors.
2. Assess for criminal history.
3. Assess for suicidal, violent, and/or homicidal thoughts.
4. Assess anxiety, aggression, and anger levels.
5. Assess motivation for maintaining control.
6. Assess for substance misuse (past and present).

DIAGNOSIS

This disorder presents a challenge for healthcare providers who should consider the potential for disruption in psychiatric and medical-surgical settings. Diagnoses and nursing care plans should be geared toward maintaining safety and providing structure. Nursing diagnoses are focused on the protection of the patient and others from impulsive and premeditated acts and on improving coping skills.

NANDA-I nursing diagnoses (Herdman & Kamitsuru, 2014) with the most relevance to this disorder include *Risk for other-directed violence, Defensive coping, Impaired social interaction,* and *Ineffective health maintenance.*

OUTCOMES IDENTIFICATION

Pertinent categories of nursing outcomes based on the *Nursing Outcomes Classification (NOC)* include abusive behavior self-restraint, aggression self-restraint, coping, social interaction, social isolation, health promotion knowledge, and health promoting behavior (Moorhead et al., 2013). Successfully achieving these outcomes when working with this population is extremely difficult, but maintaining safety is the priority. Small, incremental changes and progress will likely be the best outcomes. Table 24.1 lists common signs and symptoms, nursing diagnoses, and outcomes for antisocial personality disorder.

PLANNING

Distrust, hostility, and a profound inability to connect with others will impair the usual process of developing a therapeutic relationship. In the context of antisocial personality disorder, the role of the nurse will be to provide consistency, support, boundaries, and limits. Providing realistic choices (e.g., selection of a particular group activity) may enhance adherence to treatment.

IMPLEMENTATION

People with antisocial personality disorder may be involuntarily admitted to psychiatric units for evaluation. With their freedom limited they tend to be angry, manipulative, aggressive, and impulsive. Try to prevent or reduce untoward effects of manipulation (flattery, seductiveness, instilling of guilt). Set clear and realistic boundaries and consequences and ensure that all staff follow limits. Carefully document behaviors and signs of manipulation. Be aware that antisocial patients can manipulate with feelings of guilt when they are not getting what they want.

Refer to Boxes 24.1, 24.2, and 24.3 for interventions to address these behaviors based on the *Nursing Interventions Classification (NIC)* (Bulechek et al., 2013).

Teamwork and Safety

The safety of patients and staff is a prime consideration in working with individuals in this population. To promote safety, the entire treatment team should follow a solid treatment plan that emphasizes realistic limits on specific behavior, consistency in responses, and consequences for actions. Careful documentation of behaviors will aid in providing effective interventions and in promoting teamwork

Therapeutic communication techniques are valuable tools for working with individuals with antisocial personality disorder. Simply being heard can defuse an emotionally charged situation. For example, the nurse can listen to a patient's emotional complaints about the staff and the hospital without correcting errors, simply noting that the patient truly feels hurt. Showing empathy may also decrease aggressive outbursts if the patient feels that staff members are trying to understand feelings of frustration. Table 24.2 depicts a therapeutic nurse-patient interaction after an antisocial patient initiates a fight with a peer in an inpatient unit.

Pharmacological Interventions

In the United States, there are no FDA-approved medications specifically for treating antisocial personality disorder. This means that prescribers are using medications off-label until evidence-based pharmacotherapies are proven to be safe and effective. People with antisocial personality disorder respond to mood-stabilizing medications such as lithium or valproic acid (Depakote) to help with aggression, depression, and impulsivity. SSRIs such as fluoxetine (Prozac) and sertraline (Zoloft) may be used to decrease irritability and help with anxiety and depression. Benzodiazepines may help with anxiety but should be used with caution because they are addictive agents.

TABLE 24.1 Signs and Symptoms, Nursing Diagnoses, and Outcomes for Antisocial Personality Disorder

Signs and Symptoms	Nursing Diagnoses	Outcomes
Rigid posture, hyperactivity, pacing, history of child abuse, history of violence, violates rights of others, anger and aggression, impulsivity, substance misuse, negative role models	*Risk for other-directed violence*	Patient will not harm others, uses conflict resolution methods, controls impulses, expresses needs in a nondestructive manner, refrains from verbal outbursts, avoids violating others' personal space
Denial of obvious problems and weaknesses, difficulty establishing and maintaining, grandiose, hostile laughter, lack of follow-through to care, projection of blame and responsibility, rationalization of failures, ridicule of others, superior attitude toward others	*Defensive coping*	Uses effective coping strategies, uses strategies to promote safety, takes responsibility for own actions, uses strategies to avoid violent situations, obtains needed support, self-initiates goal-directed behavior, expresses belief in ability to perform actions
Unstable relationships, lacks empathy, projects hostility, shows behaviors unaccepted by dominant cultural group, grandiose, dysfunctional interactions, unaccepted social behavior	*Impaired social interaction*	Exhibits receptiveness, exhibits sensitivity to others, cooperates with others, interacts with others, exhibits consideration
History of lack of health-seeking behavior, inability to take responsibility for meeting basic health practices, impairment of personal support systems, lack of expressed interest in improving health behaviors	*Ineffective health maintenance*	Performs healthy behaviors, follows healthy diet, balances activity and rest, avoids substance use, obtains assistance from health professionals

From Herdman, T. H., & Kamitsuru, S. (Eds.) (2014). *NANDA international nursing diagnoses: Definitions and classification, 2015–2017.* Oxford, UK: Wiley-Blackwell; Used by arrangement with John Wiley & Sons Limited; Moorhead, S., Johnson, M., Maas, M. L., & Swanson, E. (2013). *Nursing outcomes classification (NOC)* (5th ed.). St. Louis, MO: Mosby.

BOX 24.1 *NIC* Interventions for Manipulative Behavior: Limit Setting

Definition: Establishing the parameters of desirable and acceptable patient behavior

Activities (partial list):

- Discuss concerns about behavior with patient.
- Identify (with patient input when appropriate) undesirable patient behavior.
- Discuss with patient, when appropriate, what is desirable behavior in a given situation or setting.
- Establish consequences (with patient input when appropriate) for occurrence or nonoccurrence of desired behaviors.
- Communicate established behavioral expectations and consequences to patient in language that is easily understood and nonpunitive.
- Refrain from arguing or bargaining with patient about established behavioral expectations and consequences.
- Monitor patient for occurrence or nonoccurrence of desired behaviors.
- Modify behavioral expectations and consequences, as needed, to accommodate reasonable changes in patient's situation.

Data from Bulechek, G. M., Butcher, H. K., Dochterman, J. M., & Wagner, C. (2013). *Nursing interventions classification (NIC)* (6th ed.). St. Louis, MO: Mosby.

BOX 24.2 *NIC* Interventions for Aggressive Behavior: Anger Control Assistance

Definition: Facilitation of the expression of anger in an adaptive nonviolent manner

Activities (partial list):

- Determine appropriate behavioral expectations for expression of anger, given patient's level of cognitive and physical functioning.
- Limit access to frustrating situations until patient is able to express anger in an adaptive manner.
- Encourage patient to seek assistance from nursing staff during periods of increasing tension.
- Monitor potential for inappropriate aggression, and intervene before its expression.
- Prevent physical harm if anger is directed at self or others (e.g., restraint and removal of potential weapons).
- Provide physical outlets for expression of anger or tension (e.g., sports, modeling clay, journal writing).
- Provide reassurance to patient that nursing staff will intervene to prevent patient from losing control.
- Assist patient in identifying source of anger.
- Identify function that anger, frustration, and rage serve for patient.
- Identify consequences of inappropriate expression of anger.

Data from Bulechek, G. M., Butcher, H. K., Dochterman, J. M., & Wagner, C. (2013). *Nursing interventions classification (NIC)* (6th ed.). St. Louis, MO: Mosby.

Methylphenidate (Ritalin) may help if there is a comorbidity of attention-deficit/hyperactivity disorder.

See Chapter 27 for a more detailed discussion on medications that target aggression.

Advanced Practice Interventions

The advanced practice psychiatric-mental health registered nurse treats patients with personality disorders in a variety of inpatient and community settings. Research shows that individuals with these disorders benefit from therapies to address other mental health conditions. Advanced practice nurses with training in psychotherapy, pharmacology, and the management of complex health challenges are in an excellent position to deliver and coordinate care. These individuals often require intense and long-term treatment.

BOX 24.3 *NIC* Interventions for Impulsive Behavior: Impulse Control Training

Definition: Assisting the patient to mediate impulsive behavior through application of problem-solving strategies to social and interpersonal situations

Activities (partial list):

- Assist patient to identify the problem or situation that requires thoughtful action.
- Assist patient to identify courses of possible action and their costs and benefits.
- Teach patient to cue himself or herself to "stop and think" before acting impulsively.
- Assist patient to evaluate the outcome of the chosen course of action.
- Provide positive reinforcement (e.g., praise and rewards) for successful outcomes.
- Encourage patient to self-reward for successful outcomes.
- Provide opportunities for patient to practice problem solving (role playing) within the therapeutic environment.
- Encourage patient to practice problem solving in social and interpersonal situations outside the therapeutic environment followed by evaluation of outcome.

Data from Bulechek, G. M., Butcher, H. K., Dochterman, J. M., & Wagner, C. (2013). *Nursing interventions classification (NIC)* (6th ed.). St. Louis, MO: Mosby.

EVALUATION

Evaluating treatment effectiveness in this patient population is difficult. Nurses may never know the real results of their interventions, particularly in acute-care settings. Even in long-term outpatient treatment, many patients with antisocial personality disorder find the relationship too intimate an experience to remain long enough for successful treatment. However, some motivated patients may be able to learn to change their behavior, especially if positive experiences are repeated.

Each therapeutic experience offers an opportunity for the patient to interact with caregivers who consistently try to teach positive coping skills. Specific short-term outcomes may be accomplished, and overall, the patient can be given the message of hope that quality of life can be improved.

BORDERLINE PERSONALITY DISORDER

CLINICAL PICTURE

Another Cluster B diagnosis, **borderline personality disorder**, is the most well known and dramatic of the personality disorders. Borderline personality disorder is characterized by severe impairments in functioning. The major features of this disorder are patterns of marked instability in emotional control or regulation, impulsivity, identity or self-image distortions, unstable mood, and unstable interpersonal relationships

TABLE 24.2 **Dialogue with a Patient with Manipulative, Aggressive, and Impulsive Traits**

Dialogue	Therapeutic Tool/Comment
Nurse: Donald, I would like to talk with you about what happened this morning.	Be clear as to purpose of interview.
Donald: OK, shoot.	
Nurse: Tell me what started the incident.	Use open-ended statements. Maintain a nonjudgmental attitude.
Donald: Well, as I told you before, I always had to fight to get what I wanted in life. My father and mother abandoned me emotionally when I was a child.	
Nurse: Yes, but tell me about this morning.	Redirect patient to present problem or situation.
Donald: OK. I disliked Richard from the first. He has it in for me, I just know it. He doesn't get along with anyone here. Just 2 days ago, he almost had a fight.	
Nurse: Donald, what do you mean, Richard has it in for you?	Explore situation.
Donald: When I'm talking to one of the nurses, he stares and makes comments under his breath.	
Nurse: What does he say?	Encourage description.
Donald: How I'm "in" with the nurses. I'm just trying to do what's expected of me here.	
Nurse: You mean that Richard is envious of your relationship with the nurses?	Validate patient's meaning.
Donald: Right. He really doesn't want to be here. He doesn't care about all that therapeutic junk.	
Nurse: You seem to know a lot about how Richard thinks. I wonder how that is.	Assist patient to make association to present situation.
Donald: He reminds me of someone I knew when I was young. His name was Joe. We called him "Bones."	
Nurse: Tell me more about Bones.	Explore situation further.
Donald: We called him Bones because he was skinny. He was into drugs and never ate. He was also called Bones because he was selfish. He never shared anything. He never even had a girl that I knew about.	
Nurse: So Richard reminds you of someone who is selfish and lonely?	Make interpretation of information. Note increasing anxiety.
Donald: That's right. I've had three marriages and girlfriends on the side. No one can take them away from me. (Angrily.) Just let them try!	
Nurse: Tell me about the anger you're experiencing now.	Identify feelings and explore threat or anxiety.
Donald: Richard! I know he wants to be like me, but he can't. I'll hurt him if he makes any more comments about me.	
Nurse: Donald, you will not hurt anyone here on the unit.	Set limits on, and expectations of, patient's behavior.
Donald: I'm sorry, I didn't mean that.	
Nurse: It's important that we examine your part in the incident this morning and ways to cope without threats or violence.	Focus on patient's responsibility and suggest alternative methods of coping with situation.
Donald: Listen, I know I've gotten into trouble because I can't control my temper, but that's because I won't get any respect until I can show them I don't fear them.	Patient exhibits rationalization.
Nurse: Who are "they"?	Clarify pronoun.
Donald: People like Richard.	
Nurse: You've told me that fighting was a way of survival as a child, but as an adult, there are other ways of handling situations that make you angry.	Show understanding and suggest other means of coping.
Donald: You're right. I've thought about this. Do you think it would help if you give me some meds to control my anger?	Patient exhibits superficial and concrete thinking—possible manipulation.
Nurse: I wasn't thinking of medications but of a plan for being aware of your anger and talking it out instead of fighting it out.	Clarify meaning toward behavior change. Start to explore alternatives Donald can use when angry instead of fighting.
Donald: I told you before, I *have* to fight.	
Nurse: What about the consequences of your fighting?	Identify results of impulsive behavior.
Donald: I feel bad afterward. Sometimes I wish it hadn't happened.	Patient continues to explore.

One of the primary features of borderline personality disorder is **emotional lability**, that is, rapidly moving from one emotional extreme to another. Typically, these emotional shifts include responding to situations with emotions that are out of proportion to the circumstances, pathological fear of separation, and intense sensitivity to perceived personal rejection.

Another disruptive trait common in people with borderline personality disorder is **impulsivity**. Impulsivity is manifested in acting quickly in response to emotions without considering the consequences. This impulsivity results in damaged relationships and even in suicide attempts.

Self-destructive behaviors are prominent in this disorder. Ineffective and often harmful self-soothing habits such as cutting, promiscuous sexual behavior, and numbing with substances are common and may result in unintentional death. Chronic suicidal ideation is also a common feature of this disorder and influences the likelihood of accidental deaths.

Co-occurring mood, anxiety, or substance disorders complicate the treatment and prognosis of the condition.

Borderline personality disorder is also characterized by feelings of antagonism, manifested in hostility, anger, and irritability in relationships. Physical violence toward intimate partners and nonintimate partners alike may occur. Rarely, a homicide of family members or others occurs. Violence is also manifested in destructive behaviors such as property damage.

An unusual feature of this disorder is the use of **splitting** as a primary defense or coping style. Splitting refers to the inability to view both positive and negative aspects of others as part of a whole. This inability results in viewing someone as either a wonderful person or a horrible person. This kind of dichotomous thinking and coping behavior is believed to be partly a result of the person's failed experiences with adult personality integration. It is likely influenced by exposure to earlier psychological, sexual, or physical trauma. For example, the individual may tend to idealize another person (friend, lover, healthcare professional) at the start of a new relationship, hoping that this person will meet all of his or her needs. But at the first disappointment or frustration, the individual's status quickly shifts to one of devaluation, and the other person is despised.

People with borderline personality disorder seek out treatment for depression, anxiety, suicidal and self-harming behaviors, and other impulsive behaviors including substance use. The person with borderline personality disorder frequently seeks repeat hospitalizations. While hospitalization may decrease self-destructive risk for patients with borderline personality disorder, it is not regarded as an effective long-term solution. The *DSM-5* box contains criteria for borderline personality disorder.

DSM-5 CRITERIA FOR BORDERLINE PERSONALITY DISORDER

A pervasive pattern of instability of interpersonal relationships, self-image, affects, and marked impulsivity, beginning by early adulthood and present in a variety of contexts, as indicated by five (or more) of the following:

1. Frantic efforts to avoid real or imagined abandonment. (Note: Do not include suicidal or self-mutilating behavior covered in Criterion 5.)
2. A pattern of unstable and intense interpersonal relationships characterized by alternating between extremes of idealization and devaluation.
3. Identity disturbances: Markedly and persistently unstable self-image or sense of self.
4. Impulsivity in at least two areas that are potentially self-damaging (e.g., spending, sex, substance abuse, reckless driving, binge eating). (Note: Do not include suicidal or self-mutilating behavior covered in Criterion 5.)
5. Recurrent suicidal behavior, gestures, or threats, or self-mutilating behavior.
6. Affective instability due to a marked reactivity of mood (e.g., intense episodic dysphoria, irritability, or anxiety usually lasting a few hours and only rarely more than a few days).
7. Chronic feelings of emptiness.
8. Inappropriate, intense anger or difficulty controlling anger (e.g., frequent displays of temper, constant anger, recurrent physical fights).
9. Transient, stress-related paranoid ideations or severe dissociative symptoms.

From American Psychiatric Association. (2013). *Diagnostic and statistical manual of disorders* (5th ed.). Washington, DC: Author.

EPIDEMIOLOGY AND COMORBIDITY

Borderline personality disorder occurs at a rate of about 1.6% in community studies (Skodol et al., 2014). It carries a high mortality rate—nearly 10%— primarily from suicide. This disorder results in extensive utilization of services from the healthcare system. This personality disorder seems to decrease with age. Over the course of a decade, people with borderline personality disorder experienced high rates of remission and low rates of relapse (Gunderson, 2011).

About 85% of individuals with borderline personality disorder also meet the diagnostic criteria for another psychiatric disorder (Lenzenweger et al., 2007). Substance use in individuals with borderline personality disorder is extremely common with some studies suggesting the rate of co-occurrence above 50% (Pennay et al., 2011). Women with this disorder are more likely to have major depressive disorder and anxiety disorders (Tadic et al., 2009). Men are more likely to have substance use disorders or antisocial personality disorder.

Nonpsychiatric diagnoses are also associated with borderline personality disorder. They include diabetes, high blood pressure, chronic back pain, fibromyalgia, and arthritis.

ETIOLOGY

Biological Factors

Genetic

Borderline personality disorder is around five times more common in first-degree biological relatives with the same disorder compared with the general population (APA, 2013). This disorder is highly associated with genetic factors such as hypersensitivity, impulsivity, and emotional dysregulation (Gunderson, 2011). A meta-analysis by Amad and colleagues (2014) identified that familial and twin studies support the potential role of genetic vulnerability at approximately 40%.

Neurobiological

There is evidence of serotonergic dysfunction that accompanies the borderline trait of impulsivity. It may also contribute to depression and aggression that commonly accompanies this disorder. The serotonin transporter gene 5-HTT may have shorter alleles, which have been associated with lower levels of serotonin and increased impulsive aggression.

Structural and functional magnetic resonance imaging have revealed abnormalities in the prefrontal cortex and limbic regions. The frontal region is implicated in regulatory control processes and the limbic region is essential for emotional processing (Krause-Utz et al., 2014). Limbic hyperreactivity and diminished control by the frontal brain may explain poor emotion processing, impulsivity, and interpersonal disturbances.

See the neurobiology of borderline personality disorder feature for more information about the neurobiology of borderline personality disorder.

Neurobiology of Borderline Personality Disorder

Borderline personality disorder (BPD) is a serious and disabling brain disorder marked by impulsivity and emotionaldysregultion.

Serotonin: Altered functioning of serotonin in the brain has been linked to depression, aggression and difficulty in controlling destructive urges. The serotonin transporter gene 5-HTT is thought to have shorter alleles in BPD which have been associated with lower levels of serotonin and increased impulsive aggression.

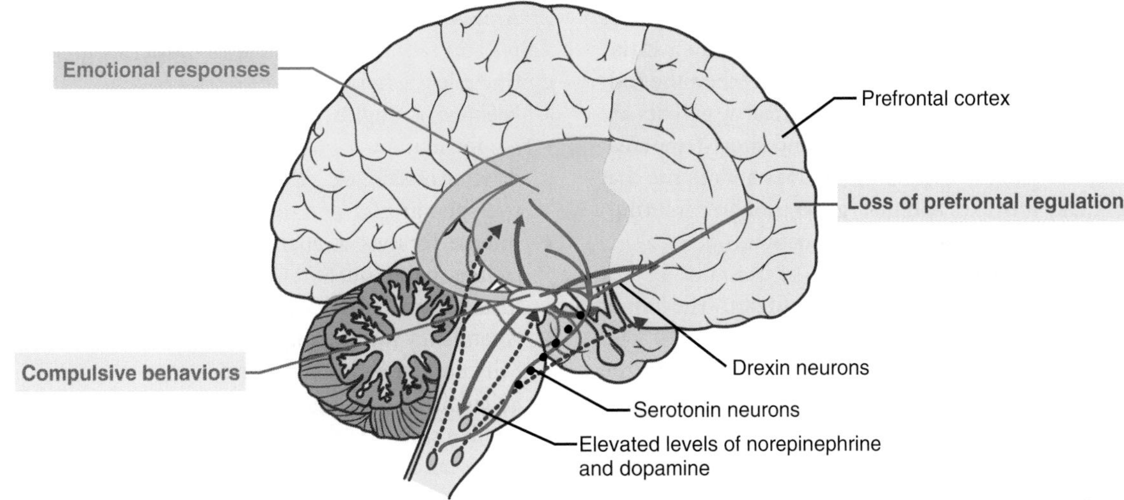

Emotional dysregulation: Emotional responses that are poorly modulated (e.g., angry outbursts, rage, marked fluctuation of mood, self-harm) that can shift within seconds, minutes, or hours

Brain Imaging (fMRI) Findings

Prefrontal cortex: In times of stress, this part of the brain helps us regulate emotions and refrain from inappropriate actions. The prefrontal cortex helps with reality testing and guides attention and thought. In people with BPD this part of the brain doesn't respond. Instead there is an extreme perception and intensity of negative emotions.

Limbic system/ amygdala: In BPD, parts of the emotional center of the brain are overstimulated and take longer to return to normal. Also, **certain neurotransmitters** that act as constraints in normal circumstances may underfunction in BPD, leaving a person in a prolonged fight-or-flight response.

Medications/Therapy to Help Individuals Regulate Their Emotions

Method	What's Involved	What It Does
Medications	Mindfulness, deep breathing, relaxation techniques	Helps brain switch from sympathetic nervous system (arousal) to the parasympathetic (relaxation mode)
Dialectic behavioral therapy (DBT)	SSRIs, anticonvulsants, second-generation antipsy-chotics, lithium	Helps dampen angry, impulsive, labile behavior

Dialectical Living. (n.d.). Emotion dysregulation. Retrieved from http://www.dialecticalliving.ca/emotion-regulation-disorder-bpd/; Ruocco, A. C., Amirthavasagam, S., Choi-Kain, L. W., & McMain, S. F. (2013). Neural correlates of negative emotionality in borderline personality disorder: An activation-likelihood-estimation meta-analysis. *Biological Psychiatry*, 73(2), 153–160; Nauert, R. (2015). Brain scans clarify borderline personality disorder. *Psych Central*. Retrieved from http://psychcentral.com/news/2009/09/04/brain-scans-clarify-borderline-personality-disorder/8184.html.

Psychological Factors

Margaret Mahler (1895–1985), a Hungarian-born child psychologist who worked with emotionally disturbed children, developed a framework that is useful in considering borderline personality disorder. Mahler and colleagues (1975) believed that psychological problems are a result of the disruption of the normal **separation-individuation** of the child from the mother.

According to Mahler, an infant progresses from complete self-absorption with an inability to separate itself from its mother to a physically and psychologically differentiated toddler. Mahler emphasized the role of the significant other (traditionally the mother) in providing a secure emotional base of support that promotes enough confidence for the child to separate. This support is achieved through a balance of holding (emotionally and physically) a child enough for the child to feel safe, while at the same time fostering and encouraging independence and natural exploration.

Problems may arise in this separation-individuation. If a toddler leaves his or her mother on the park bench and wanders off to the sandbox, ideally two things should happen. First, the child should be encouraged to go off into the world with smiles and reassurance: "Go on, honey, it's safe to go away a little." Second, the mother needs to be reliably present when the toddler returns, thereby rewarding her efforts. Clearly, parents are not perfect and are sometimes distracted and short-tempered. Mahler notes that raising healthy children does not require that parents never make mistakes and that "good enough parenting" will promote successful separation-individuation.

Stages of this process are as follows:

- **Stage 1 (birth to 1 month): Normal autism.** The infant spends most of its time sleeping.
- **Stage 2 (1 to 5 months): Symbiosis.** The infant perceives the mother-infant as a single fused entity. Infants gradually distinguish the inner from the outer world.
- **Stage 3 (5 to 10 months): Differentiation.** The infant recognizes distinctness from mother. Progressive neurological development and increased alertness draw the infant's attention away from self to the outer world.
- **Stage 4 (11 to 18 months): Practicing.** The ability to walk and explore greatly expands the toddler's sense of separateness.
- **Stage 5 (18 to 24 months): Rapprochement.** Toddlers move away from their mothers and come back for emotional refueling. Periods of helplessness and dependence alternate with the need for independence.
- **Stage 6 (2 to 5 years): Object constancy.** When children comprehend that objects (in this case, the object is the mother) are permanent even when they are not in their presence, the individuation process is complete.

Children who later develop borderline personality may have had this process disrupted. The rapprochement stage is particularly crucial and coincides with the "terrible twos" that are characterized by darting away and clinging and whining. Some experts suggest that this phase is not a desirable time for extended separation between parent and child.

Consider the previous ideal example of the child who wants to play in the sandbox. If the child wanders off to the sandbox and returns to a caregiver who is emotionally unavailable, perhaps hurt by the attempt at independence, the child feels unsafe to explore. Alternately, if the caregiver has personal issues related to dependency and abandonment, he may be threatened by the child's attempts at independence and respond with clinging and halting exploration. The child cannot safely move on to the next stage of development. A fear of abandonment from others, along with a sense of anger, carries over into adulthood.

APPLICATION OF THE NURSING PROCESS

ASSESSMENT

Assessment Tools

The preferred method for determining a diagnosis of borderline personality disorder is the semi-structured interview obtained by clinicians. Self-report inventories, such as the well-known Minnesota Multiphasic Personality Inventory (MMPI), are useful because they have built-in validity and reliability scales for the clinician to refer to when interpreting test results.

Areas of assessment that are typically included on questionnaires and rating scales related to borderline personality disorder include the following:

- Feelings of emptiness
- An inclination to engage in risky behaviors such as reckless driving, unsafe sex, substance use, binge eating, gambling, or overspending
- Intense feelings of abandonment that result in paranoia or feeling spaced out
- Idealization of others and becoming close quickly
- A tendency toward anger, sarcasm, and bitterness
- Self-mutilation and self-harm
- Suicidal behaviors, gestures, or threats
- Sudden shifts in self-evaluation that result in changing goals, values, and career focus
- Extreme mood shifts that occur in a matter of hours or days
- Intense, unstable romantic relationships

Patient History

Borderline personality disorder usually begins before adulthood. Important issues in assessment for borderline personality disorder include a history of suicidal or aggressive ideation or actions, treatment history, and medication (prescribed and illicit) use.

Significant areas about which further details must be obtained include current or past physical, sexual, or emotional abuse and level of current risk of harm from self or others. Information regarding prior use of any medication, including psychopharmacological agents, is important.

Self-Assessment

Because interpersonal difficulties are central to the problems faced by people diagnosed with borderline personality disorder, it is understandable that these problems surface in the treatment milieu and within the relationships between these patients and their caregivers. The therapeutic relationship often follows an initial hesitancy on the part of patient, then an upward curve of idealization by the patient toward the caregiver. This idealization is invariably followed by a devaluation of the staff member when the patient is disappointed by unmet—frequently impossible—expectations.

For example, a female patient may briefly idealize her male nurse on the inpatient unit, telling staff and patients alike that she is "the luckiest patient because [she has] the best nurse in the hospital." The rest of the team understands that this comment is an exaggeration. After days of constant dramatic praise for the nurse, with subtle insults to the rest of the staff, some members of the team may start to become annoyed. A similar scenario can occur if the patient constantly complains about one staff member. Staff may be torn between defending and criticizing the targeted staff member.

EVIDENCE-BASED PRACTICE

How Do Psychiatric Nurses Respond to Patients with Borderline Personality Disorder?

Problem

People diagnosed with borderline personality disorder have problems relating to people in their everyday lives. There is anecdotal evidence that they are also unpopular among mental health nurses.

Purpose of Study

To determine whether mental health nurses respond to people with borderline personality disorder in problematic ways.

Methods

A systematic integrated literature review of quantitative and qualitative studies was conducted. Forty articles through April 2015 were included. Papers were gathered describing primary research focused on psychiatric nurses' attitudes, behavior, experience, and knowledge regarding adults with borderline personality disorder.

Key Findings

- Psychiatric nurses find patients with this diagnosis very challenging to work with.
- Psychiatric nurses report poorer attitudes than other healthcare professionals toward this population.
- Psychiatric nurses hold poorer attitudes toward patients with borderline personality disorder than other diagnostic groups.
- Nurses who utilize a coherent therapeutic framework to guide their practice experience improvement in caregiving.

Implications for Nursing Practice

Mental health nurses have all heard a dismissive, "Oh, she's just a borderline" in response to certain patients. We need a fresh approach to this problem. The authors conclude that developing nurses to lead in the design, implementation, and teaching of coherent therapeutic frameworks will improve the therapeutic relationship.

Dickens, G. L., & Lamont, E. (2016). Mental health nurses' attitudes, behaviour, experience and knowledge regarding adults with a diagnosis of borderline personality disorder: Systematic, integrative literature review. *Journal of Clinical Nursing, 25*(13-14).

ASSESSMENT GUIDELINES

Borderline Personality Disorder

1. Assess for suicidal or violent thoughts toward others. If these are present, the patient will need immediate attention.
2. Determine whether the patient has a medical disorder or another psychiatric disorder (especially a substance use disorder) that may be responsible for the symptoms.
3. View the assessment about personality functioning from within the person's ethnic, cultural, and social background.
4. Has the patient experienced a recent important loss? Borderline personality disorder is often exacerbated after the loss of significant supporting people or in a disruptive social situation.
5. Evaluate for a change in personality in middle adulthood or later, which signals the need for a thorough medical workup or assessment for unrecognized substance use disorder.

Clinical supervision and additional education are helpful and supportive to staff on the front lines of care. Awareness and monitoring of one's own stress responses to patient behaviors facilitate more effective and therapeutic intervention, regardless of the specific approach to their care.

DIAGNOSIS

People with borderline personality disorder are usually admitted to psychiatric treatment programs because of symptoms with comorbid disorders or dangerous behavior. Emotions such as anxiety, rage, and depression, and behaviors such as withdrawal, paranoia, and manipulation are among the most frequent that healthcare workers must address.

The nursing diagnosis *Self-mutilation* is most often associated with this disorder. It is defined as "deliberate self-injurious behavior causing tissue damage with the intent of causing nonfatal injury to attain relief of tension" (Herdman & Kamitsuru, 2014, p. 412). Characteristics include:

- Disturbed interpersonal relationships
- Feels threatened with loss of significant relationship
- History of self-directed violence
- Impulsivity
- Irresistible urge to cut self
- Labile behavior
- Mounting tension that is intolerable
- Use of manipulation to obtain nurturing relationship with others

Other nursing diagnoses directly relevant to borderline personality disorder are *Risk for suicide, Risk for self-directed violence, Risk for other-directed violence, Social isolation, Impaired social interaction, Disturbed personal identity,* and *Ineffective coping.*

OUTCOMES IDENTIFICATION

Realistic outcomes are established for individuals with borderline personality disorder based on the perspective that personality change occurs with one behavioral solution and one learned skill at a time. This can be expected to take a lot of time and repetition. In the acute-care setting, the focus is on the presenting problem, which may be depression or severe anxiety. Healthcare providers do not expect resolution of chronic behavior problems during the hospital stay but rather to be met with appropriate therapeutic feedback and incremental steps toward recovery in an outpatient setting.

The *Nursing Outcomes Classification (NOC)* provides useful scales for measuring improvement in mutilation self-restraint, suicide self-restraint, aggression self-control, impulse self-control, social interaction skills, abusive behavior self-restraint, social interaction, social isolation, identity, self-awareness, coping, and stress level (Moorhead et al., 2013). Table 24.3 lists common signs and symptoms associated with borderline personality disorder, suggests nursing diagnoses, and identifies potential outcomes.

TABLE 24.3 Signs and Symptoms, Nursing Diagnoses, and Outcomes for Borderline Personality Disorder

Signs and Symptoms	Nursing Diagnoses	Outcomes
Impulsivity, abrading, biting, cuts on body, hitting, ingestion of harmful substances, inhalation of harmful substances, insertion of object into body orifice, picking at wounds, scratches on body, self-inflicted burns	*Self-mutilation*	Patient refrains from intentional self-inflicted injury, maintains self-control without supervision, obtains assistance as needed, uses support groups, follows treatment regimen
History of self-mutilation and suicide attempts, family history of self-destructive behavior, disturbed interpersonal relationships, isolation, impulsivity, manipulation to obtain nurturing relationships	*Risk for suicide* *Risk for self-directed violence*	Patient remains free from harm, maintains healthy connections, maintains control without supervision, uses social support group, plans for the future
Impulsivity, history of other-directed violence, threats	*Risk for other-directed violence*	Expresses needs in a constructive manner, monitors anger, maintains self-control without supervision
Behavior unaccepted by dominant cultural group, hypersensitivity to negative evaluation, unstable relationships, reports feeling rejected, experiences feelings of differences from others, inability to achieve a sense of social engagement, intense and unstable relationships	*Social isolation* *Impaired social interaction*	Exhibits receptiveness and sensitivity to others, cooperates with others, uses assertive behaviors as appropriate, interacts with others
Dependency, excessive emotional responses, attention-seeking, reports feeling emptiness, uncertainty about goals, uncertain boundaries with others	*Disturbed personal identity*	Verbalizes clear sense of personal identity, performs social roles, challenges negative images of self, establishes personal boundaries, maintains awareness of thoughts and feelings
Difficulty in relationships, manipulation, destructive behavior toward others and self, inability to meet role expectations, inadequate problem solving, uses self-mutilation to calm and summon nurturing	*Ineffective coping*	Uses effective coping strategies, expresses emotion, seeks emotional support, uses strategies to promote safety, takes responsibility for own actions, identifies available community resources, obtains needed support, self-initiates goal-directed behavior, expresses belief in ability to perform action

From Herdman, T. H., & Kamitsuru, S. (Eds.). (2014). *NANDA International nursing diagnoses: Definitions and classification, 2015–2017.* Oxford, UK: Wiley-Blackwell; Used by arrangement with John Wiley & Sons Limited; Moorhead, S., Johnson, M., Maas, M. L., & Swanson, E. (2013). *Nursing outcomes classification (NOC)* (5th ed.). St. Louis, MO: Mosby.

PLANNING

A therapeutic relationship is essential with patients who have borderline personality disorder because most of them have experienced failed relationships, including therapeutic alliances. Their distrust and hostility can be a setup for failure. When patients blame and attack others, the nurse needs to understand the context of their complaints. These attacks originate from the feeling of being threatened. The more intense the complaints are, the greater their fear of potential harm or loss is. Be aware of manipulative behaviors such as flattery, seductiveness, and instilling guilt. The Case Study and Nursing Care Plan presents a patient with borderline personality disorder.

CASE STUDY AND NURSING CARE PLAN

Borderline Personality Disorder

Brianna Drake is a 24-year-old single administrative assistant who lives alone. She has been seen in the emergency department several times for superficial suicide attempts. She is admitted because she has cut her wrists, ankles, and labia with glass and has lost a lot of blood. This event is precipitated by her graduation from a community college. States, "I feel empty inside."

Upon admission she is sweet, serene, and grateful to all the nurses, calling them "angels of mercy." Within a week, she is angry at half of the nurses and demands a new primary nurse, saying that the one she has (to whom she had grown attached) hates her.

Brianna has a history of heavy drinking and has managed to sneak alcohol onto the unit. She has been found in bed with a young male patient. She continually breaks unit rules and then pleads to have the behavior forgiven and forgotten. When angry, she threatens to cut herself again. She appears restless and tense and frequently asks for antianxiety medication several times a shift. When asked what she is anxious about, she says, "Uh…don't know…I feel so empty inside." Brianna frequently paces up and down the halls, with an angry expression.

Self-Assessment

Salma is a recent graduate and is Brianna's primary nurse. After the first week of working with Brianna, Salma is discouraged and dreads coming in to work. She confides to Nancy, a co-worker with 20 years of experience, that Brianna "just knows how to get under my skin." The two nurses discuss the biological basis of borderline personality disorder and treatment principles. Nancy also suggests that a team meeting be held to evaluate the plan of care and to focus on consistent limit-setting among the staff.

Assessment

Subjective Data

- History of superficial suicide attempts
- History of heavy drinking
- Recent graduate from a community college
- States, "I feel empty inside"
- Calls nurses "angels of mercy"
- Requests a new primary nurse because current nurse hates her
- When angry threatens to cut herself
- Asks for antianxiety medication several times a shift

CASE STUDY AND NURSING CARE PLAN—cont'd

Borderline Personality Disorder

Objective Data

- Cuts on wrists, ankles, and labia
- Calm on admission
- Snuck alcohol onto the unit
- In bed with a male patient
- Breaks unit rules
- Restless and tense
- Paces with an angry expression

Priority Diagnosis

Ineffective coping related to inadequate psychological resources, as evidenced by self-destructive behaviors

Outcomes Identification

Patient will consistently demonstrate the use of effective coping strategies.

Planning

The initial plan is to maintain patient safety and to encourage verbalization of feelings and impulses instead of action.

Implementation

Brianna's plan of care is personalized as follows:

Outcome criteria: Patient will consistently demonstrate the use of effective coping strategies.

Short-Term Goal	Intervention	Rationale	Evaluation
Brianna will consistently demonstrate a decrease in stress as evidenced by talking about feelings with staff every day and an absence of acting-out behaviors.	1. Encourage verbalization of feelings, perceptions, and fears. 2. Support the use of appropriate defense mechanisms.	1. Discussing and understanding the dynamics of frustration help reduce the frustration by helping patient take positive action. 2. Discussing and understanding the meaning of defenses help reduce the potential for acting out.	**GOAL MET** Brianna was able to experience problems and deal with them appropriately. Acting out was minimal or absent. *Example:* Patient had an appointment for a job interview. She wanted to stay in bed and avoid the interview, but instead she talked with the nurse about her fear of "growing up" and was able to get up and go to the interview.

Evaluation

See individual outcomes and evaluation in the care plan.

IMPLEMENTATION

Psychosocial Interventions

People with borderline personality disorder are impulsive and may be suicidal, self-mutilating, aggressive, manipulative, and even psychotic during periods of stress. Provide clear and consistent boundaries and limits. Use straightforward communication. When behavioral problems emerge, calmly review the therapeutic goals.

Refer to Boxes 24.1, 24.2, and 24.3 for more interventions to address these behaviors based on the *Nursing Interventions Classification (NIC)* (Bulechek et al., 2013).

A useful approach for patients with borderline personality disorder relates to the response to superficial self-destructive behaviors. Acting in accordance with unit policies, the nurse remains neutral and dresses the wound in a matter-of-fact manner. Then the patient is instructed to write down the sequence of events leading up to the injury, as well as the consequences, before staff will discuss the event. This cognitive exercise encourages the patient to think independently about his or her own behavior instead of merely ventilating feelings. It facilitates the discussion with staff about alternative actions.

Pharmacological Interventions

In the United States, there are no medications specifically approved by the FDA for treating borderline personality disorder. This means that prescribers are using the medications off-label until evidenced-based pharmacotherapies are proven to be safe and effective.

Psychotropic medications geared toward maintaining patients' cognitive function, symptom relief, and improved quality of life are available. People with borderline personality disorder often respond to antidepressants such as SSRIs, anticonvulsants, and lithium for mood and emotional dysregulation symptoms. Naltrexone (Revia, Vivitrol), an opioid receptor antagonist, has been found to reduce self-injurious behaviors. Second-generation antipsychotics may control anger and brief psychosis.

Teamwork and Safety

When individuals with borderline personality disorder are admitted to the hospital, partially hospitalized, or in day treatment settings, team management is a significant part of treatment. The primary goal is management of the patient's affect in a group context. Community meetings, coping skills groups, and socializing groups are all helpful for these patients. They have the opportunity to interact with peers and staff to discuss goals and learn problem-solving skills. Dealing with emotional issues that arise in the milieu requires a calm, united approach by the staff to maintain safety and to enhance self-control.

Common problems resulting from staff splitting can be minimized if the unit leaders hold weekly staff meetings in which staff members are allowed to ventilate their feelings about conflicts with patients and each other. Consistency and a team approach help ensure productive use of therapeutic time and structure for the patient. Patient-centered approaches allow the patient to be part of the treatment planning.

Advanced Practice Interventions

Advanced practice nurses are likely to interact with staff members regarding the treatment of individuals with borderline personality disorders as part of their practice and clinical supervision responsibilities. The advanced practice registered nurse can assist staff members in engaging these patients in a therapeutic alliance.

Psychotherapy

Advanced practice psychiatric-mental health registered nurses are often the clinical leaders in providing individual and group psychotherapy. There are three essential therapies for borderline personality disorder:

1. **Cognitive-behavioral therapy (CBT):** CBT can help individuals to identify and change inaccurate core perceptions of themselves and others and relationship problems. CBT may result in a reduction of mood and anxiety symptoms and reduce the number of self-harming or suicidal behaviors.
2. **Dialectical behavior therapy (DBT)**: DBT is an evidence-based therapy developed by Linehan (1993) to treat chronically suicidal individuals with borderline personality disorder. DBT combines cognitive and behavioral techniques with *mindfulness*, which emphasizes being aware of thoughts and actively shaping them.

   The goals of DBT are to increase the patient's ability to manage distress and improve interpersonal effectiveness skills. Treatment focuses on behavioral targets, beginning with identification of and interventions for suicidal behaviors and then progressing to a focus on interrupting destructive behaviors (Fig. 24.1). Finally, DBT addresses quality-of-life behaviors across a hierarchy of care (Fig. 24.2).
3. **Schema-focused therapy:** Schema-focused therapy combines parts of CBT with other forms of therapy that focus on the ways that individuals view themselves. This reframing of "schemas" is based on the notion that borderline personality disorder is the result of a dysfunctional self-image, probably brought about by a dysfunctional childhood. This dysfunctional self-image affects how individuals respond to stress, react to their environment, and interact with others.

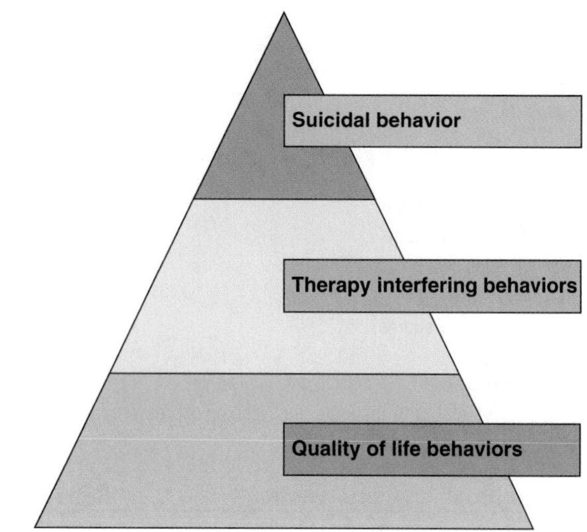

FIG. 24.1 Dialectical behavior therapy treatment targets.

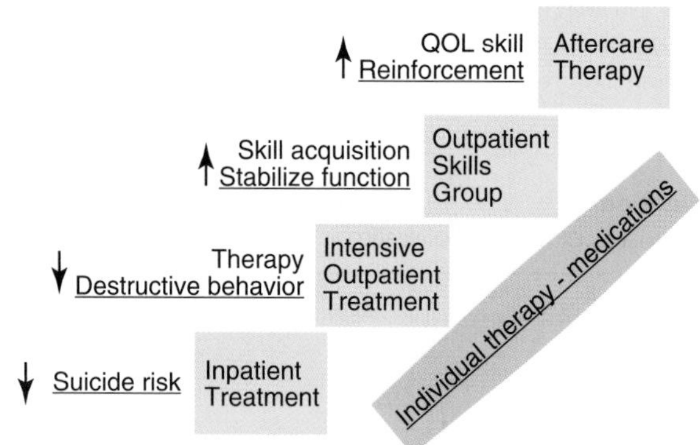

FIG. 24.2 Dialectical behavior therapy treatment hierarchy. *QOL*, Quality of life. Data from Torgersen, S. (2009). Prevalence, sociodemographics, and functional impairment. In J. M. Oldham, A. E. Skodol, & D. S. Bender (Eds.), *Essentials of personality disorders* (pp. 83–102). Washington, DC: American Psychiatric Publishing.

EVALUATION

Evaluating treatment effectiveness in this patient population is difficult. Freedom from harm to self and others is a tangible and satisfying positive evaluation. Nurses may never know the real results of their intervention, particularly in acute-care settings. Even in long-term outpatient treatment, patients with borderline personality disorder experience too many disruptions to relationships to remain long enough for successful treatment. As noted earlier, however, some motivated patients may be able to learn to change their behavior, especially if positive experiences are repeated.

Each therapeutic experience offers an opportunity for self-observation interacting with caregivers who consistently and reliably try to teach positive coping skills. Specific short-term outcomes may be accomplished, and overall, the patient can be given the message of hope that quality of life can always be improved.

KEY POINTS TO REMEMBER

- All personality disorders share characteristics of inflexibility and difficulties in interpersonal relationships that impair social or occupational functioning.
- Personality disorders are most likely caused by a combination of biological and psychosocial factors.
- Patients with personality disorders often enter psychiatric treatment because of distress from a comorbid mental illness.
- Nurses may experience intense emotional reactions to patients with personality disorders and need to make use of clinical supervision to maintain objectivity.
- Despite the relatively fixed patterns of maladaptive behavior, some patients with personality disorders are able to change their behavior over time as a result of treatment.

CRITICAL THINKING

1. Mr. Beech is undergoing surgery for a broken leg. He is suspicious of the staff and believes that the IV he is receiving for hydration and preanesthesia will be used for harmful purposes. He keeps his eyes closed and refuses to answer or look at his family who describe him as odd. He has schizotypal personality disorder.
   a. Explain how being friendly and outgoing may be threatening to Mr. Beech.
   b. Explain how being matter-of-fact and neutral and sticking to the facts would be effective to Mr. Beech.
   c. What could be done to give Mr. Beech some control over his situation as a hospitalized patient?
   d. How could you best handle his beliefs and lack of interpersonal comfort with caregivers so that both you and he would feel most comfortable?
2. Cherie is brought to the emergency department after slashing her wrist with a razor. She has previously been in the emergency department for drug overdose and has a history of addictions. Cherie can be sarcastic, belittling, and aggressive to those who try to care for her. When the psychiatric triage nurse comes in to see her, Cherie is initially adoring and compliant, telling him, "You are the best nurse I've ever had, and I truly want to change." But when he refuses to support her request for diazepam (Valium) and meperidine (Demerol) for "pain," she yells at him, "You are a stupid excuse for a nurse. I want to see the doctor immediately." Cherie has borderline personality disorder.
   a. What defense mechanism is Cherie using?
   b. How could the nurse handle this situation while setting limits and demonstrating concern?

CHAPTER REVIEW

Questions

1. Which statement made by the psychiatric nurse demonstrates an accurate understanding of the factors that affect an individual's personality?
   a. "Therapy will help her identify that her problems are personality related."
   b. "I'll need to learn more about this patient's cultural beliefs."
   c. "It's encouraging to know that personality disorders respond well to treatment."
   d. "A person's personality is fluid and adjusts to current social situations."
2. When assessing a patient diagnosed with a borderline personality disorder, which statement by the patient warrants immediate attention?
   a. "My mother died ten years ago."
   b. "I haven't needed medication in weeks."
   c. "My dad never loved me."
   d. "I'd really like to hurt her for hurting me."
3. What is the current accepted professional view of the effect of culture on the development of a personality disorder?
   a. There aren't sufficient studies to confirm the role that ethnicity and race have on the prevalence of personality disorders.
   b. The North American and Australian cultures produce higher incidences of personality disorders among their populations.
   c. Neither culture nor ethnic background is generally considered in the development of personality disorders.
   d. Personality disorders have been found to be primarily the products of genetic factors, not cultural factors.
4. Which personality disorders are generally associated with behaviors described as "odd or eccentric"? *Select all that apply.*
   a. Paranoid
   b. Schizoid
   c. Histrionic
   d. Obsessive-compulsive
   e. Avoidant
5. Which behaviors are examples of a primitive defense mechanism often relied upon by those diagnosed with a personality disorder? *Select all that apply.*
   a. Regularly attempts to split the staff
   b. Attempts to undo feelings of anger by offering to do favors
   c. Regresses to rocking and humming to sooth themselves when fearful
   d. Lashes out verbally when confronted with criticism
   e. Destroys another person's belongings when angry
6. Personality disorders often co-occur with mood and eating disorders. A young woman is undergoing treatment at an eating disorders clinic and her nurse suspects the patient may also have a Cluster B personality disorder due to the young woman's:
   a. Desire to avoid eating
   b. Dramatic response to frustration
   c. Excessive exercise routine
   d. Morose personality traits
7. Larry is from a small town and began displaying aggressive and manipulative traits while still a teenager. Now at 40 years old, Larry is serving a life sentence for the murders of his wife and her brother. John, the prison psychiatric nurse practitioner, recognizes that Larry's treatment will most likely:
   a. Transform Larry to a model prisoner
   b. Not improve Larry's coping skills
   c. Reaffirm Larry's high-risk behaviors
   d. Manifest as small incremental changes
8. Connor is a 28-year-old student, referred by his university for a psychiatric evaluation. He reports that he has no friends at the university and people call him a loner. Recently, Connor has been giving lectures to pigeons at the

university fountains. Connor is diagnosed as schizotypal, which differs from schizophrenia in that persons diagnosed as schizotypal:
   a. Can be made aware of their delusions
   b. Are far more delusional than schizophrenics
   c. Have a greater need for socialization
   d. Do not usually respond to antipsychotic medications

9. Garret's wife of 8 years is divorcing him because the marriage never developed a warm or loving atmosphere. Garrett states in therapy, "I have always been a loner," and was never concerned about what others think. The nurse practitioner suggests that Garrett try a trial of bupropion (Wellbutrin) to:
   a. Improve his flat emotions
   b. Assist in getting a good night's sleep
   c. Increase the pleasure of living
   d. Prepare Garrett for group therapy

10. Josie, a 27-year-old patient, complains that most of the staff do not like her. She says she can tell that you are a caring person. Josie is unsure of what she wants to do with her life and her "mixed-up feelings" about relationships. When you tell her that you will be on vacation next week, she becomes very angry. Two hours later, she is found using a curling iron to burn her underarms and explains that it "makes the numbness stop." Given this presentation, which personality disorder would you suspect?
   a. Obsessive-compulsive
   b. Borderline
   c. Antisocial
   d. Schizotypal

Answers

1. **b;** 2. **d;** 3. **a;** 4. **a, b;** 5. **a, b, c;** 6. **b;** 7. **d;** 8. **a;** 9. **c;** 10. **b**

Visit the Evolve website for a posttest on the content in this chapter: http://evolve.elsevier.com/Varcarolis

Post-Test interactive review

REFERENCES

Amad, A., Ramoz, N., Thomas, P., Jardri, R., & Gorwood, P. (2014). Genetics of borderline personality disorder: Systematic review and proposal of an integrative model. *Neuroscience and Behavioral Reviews, 40*, 6–19.

American Psychiatric Association. (2013). *Diagnostic and statistical manual of mental disorders* (5th ed.). Washington, DC: Author.

Bulechek, G. M., Butcher, H. K., Dochterman, J. M., & Wagner, C. (2013). *Nursing interventions classification (NIC)* (6th ed.). St. Louis, MO: Mosby.

Coccaro, E. F., & Siever, L. J. (2005). Neurobiology. In J. M. Oldham, A. E. Skodol, & D. S. Bender (Eds.), *Textbook of personality disorders* (pp. 155–169). Washington, DC: American Psychiatric Publishing.

Gunderson, J. G. (2011). Borderline personality disorder. *New England Journal of Medicine, 364*, 2037–2042.

Herdman, T. H., & Kamitsuru, S. (Eds.). (2014). *NANDA International nursing diagnoses: Definitions and classification* (pp. 2015–2017). Oxford, UK: Wiley-Blackwell.

Huang, Y., Kotov, R., de Girolamo, G., Preti, A., Angermeyer, M., Benjet, C., et al. (2009). DSM-IV personality disorders in the WHO World Mental Health Surveys. *British Journal of Psychiatry, 195*(1), 46–53.

James, W. (1892). *Psychology: The briefer course*. New York, NY: Henry Holt.

Kendler, K. S., Aggen, S. H., & Patrick, C. J. (2012). A multivariate twin study of the DSM-IV criteria for antisocial personality disorder. *Biological Psychiatry, 71*(3), 247–253.

Krause-Utz, A., Winter, D., Niedtfeld, I., & Schmah, C. (2014). The latest neuroimaging findings in borderline personality disorder. *Current Psychiatry Reports, 16*(438).

Lee, R. J., Hempel, J., TenHarmsel, A., Tianmin, L., Mathe, A. A., & Klock, A. (2011). The neuroendocrinology of childhood trauma in personality disorder. *Psychoneuroendocrinology, 37*(1), 1–9.

Lenzenweger, M. F., Lane, M. C., Loranger, A. W., & Kessler, R. C. (2007). DSM-IV personality disorders in the National Comorbidity Survey Replication. *Biological Psychiatry, 62*(6), 553–564.

Linehan, M. M. (1993). *Cognitive behavioral treatment of borderline personality disorder*. New York, NY: Guilford.

Mahler, M. S., Pine, F., & Bergman, A. (1975). *The psychological birth of the human infant*. New York, NY: Basic Books.

McGilloway, A., Hall, R. E., Lee, T., & Bhui, K. S. (2010). A systematic review of personality disorder, race, and ethnicity: Prevalence, aetiology and treatment. *BMC Psychiatry, 10*(33), 1–14.

Moorhead, S., Johnson, M., Maas, M. L., & Swanson, E. (2013). *Nursing outcomes classification (NOC)* (5th ed.). St. Louis, MO: Mosby.

Newton-Howes, G., Clark, L. A., & Chanen, A. (2015). Personality disorder across the life course. *Lancet, 385*, 727–734.

Paris, J. (2005). A current integrative perspective on personality disorders. In J. M. Oldham, A. E. Skodol, & D. S. Bender (Eds.), *Textbook of personality disorders* (pp. 119–128). Washington, DC: American Psychiatric Publishing.

Pennay, A., Cameron, J., Reichert, T., Strickland, H., Lee, N. K., Hall, K., et al. (2011). A systematic review of interventions for co-occurring substance use disorder and borderline personality disorder. *Journal of Substance Abuse Treatment, 41*, 363–373.

Ripoll, L. H., Triebwasser, J., & Siever, L. (2011). Evidence-based pharmacotherapy for personality disorders. *International Journal of Neuropsychopharmacology, 14*, 1257–1288.

Rosowsky, I., Abrams, R. C., & Zwieg, R. A. (2013). *Personality disorders in older adults*. New York, NY: Routledge.

Sadock, B. J., Sadock, V. A., & Ruiz, P. (2015). *Kaplan & Sadock's synopsis of psychiatry* (11th ed.). Philadelphia, PA: Wolters Kluwer.

Samuels, J. (2011). Personality disorders: epidemiology and public health issues. *International Review of Psychiatry, 23*(3), 223–233.

Sansone, R. A., & Sansone, L. A. (2011). Personality disorders: A nation-based perspective on prevalence. *Innovations in Clinical Neuroscience, 8*(4), 13–18.

Seo, D., Patrick, C. J., & Kennealy, P. J. (2008). Role of serotonin and dopamine system interactions in the neurobiology of impulsive aggression and its comorbidity with other clinical disorders. *Aggression and Violent Behavior, 13*(5), 383–395.

Skodol, A. E., Bender, D. S., Gunderson, J. G., & Oldham, J. M. (2014). Personality disorders. In R. E. Hales, S. C. Yudofsky, & G. O. Gabbard (Eds.), *Textbook of psychiatry* (6th ed.) (pp. 851–894). Washington, DC: American Psychiatric Publishing.

Svrakic, D. M., Leck-Tosevski, D., & Divac-Jovanovic, M. (2008). DSM axis II: Personality disorders or adaptation disorders? *Current Opinions in Psychiatry, 22*, 11–117.

Tadic, A., Wagner, S., Hoch, J., Baskaya, O., von Cube, R., Skaletz, C., et al. (2009). Gender differences in axis I and axis II comorbidity in patients with borderline personality disorder. *Psychopathology, 42*(4), 257–263.

World Health Organization. (2016). *International classification of diseases and related health problems,* 10th revision—clinical modification. Retrieved from https://www.cdc.gov/nchs/icd/icd10cm.htm.

Zimmerman, M., Chelminski, I., & Young, D. (2008). The frequency of personality disorders in psychiatric patients. *Psychiatric Clinics of North America, 31*, 405–420.

25

Suicide and Nonsuicidal Self-Injury

Faye J. Grund

Visit the Evolve website for a pretest on the content in this chapter: http://evolve.elsevier.com/Varcarolis Pre-Test interactive review

OBJECTIVES

1. Define essential terms associated with suicide including suicidal ideation, suicide attempt, and completed suicide.
2. Describe the growing problem of suicide in the United States.
3. Identify comorbid psychiatric disorders that accompany suicidality.
4. Discuss risk factors for the development of suicidal ideation and for suicide.
5. Identify evidence-based practice suicide risk assessment tools.
6. Discuss basic-level interventions to address suicidality in the hospital or in community settings.
7. Explain key elements of suicide precautions and environmental safety factors in the hospital.
8. Describe three expected reactions a nurse may experience when working with patients who have suicidal ideation.
9. Examine nursing interventions for nonsuicidal self-injury.

OUTLINE

KEY TERMS AND CONCEPTS

completed suicide
copycat suicide
lethality
nonsuicidal self-injury
postvention
primary intervention
psychological autopsies
suicidal ideation
suicide
suicide attempt

A tribute to Adam Hall on the first anniversary of his death from his loving mother…July 1, 2014:

Dearest Adam,

It's hard to believe that a year has gone by. The void created by your departure fills me with such emptiness... while echoes of your laughter linger... urging me and those whose lives you touched to press forward living life to the fullest, seizing and celebrating each moment.

I am so grateful to have been blessed with a son such as you. 26, almost 27 years were so fleeting a time. Over in what seems to have been a heartbeat. I purposed my life toward building your future, creating possibility in your life... 'living vicariously through you' as you often expressed.

So many questions remain. Golden moments flash across my mind, your warmth, your charm, the love you shared, the depth of your character, the contagious ardor with which you embraced your passions... impossible to capture in mere words. You were loved, adored, and admired. You were so ardent and able. I was so proud of you and cherished you with all my being.

Love,

Mom

(Personal communication courtesy of Carolyn Bucklen.)

Suicide is devastating for those of us who lose a family member or friend. What brings a person to such a drastic and permanent solution to life's problems? As unimaginable this act is to many of us, a human life ends every 13 minutes as the result of suicide, leading to the loss of approximately 113 American lives daily (Centers for Disease Control and Prevention [CDC], 2015).

Suicidal ideation is thinking about personal death, including the wish to be dead, considering methods of accomplishing death, and formulating plans to carry the act out. **Suicide** is the intentional act of killing oneself by any means. A **suicide attempt** is actually carrying out an act or acts with the intention of death, which may or may not prove fatal. A **completed suicide** is one in which self-injurious acts committed by an individual results in death.

As healthcare workers and clinicians, our interest is in preventing these suicides. Suicide is largely preventable and should be considered a "never event." Yet too often, we direct efforts only toward individuals who are at immediate risk (Hogan & Grumet, 2016). In the year before their deaths, 83% of individuals received either inpatient or outpatient healthcare services and approximately half of those who died by suicide did not have a mental health diagnosis (Ahmedani et al., 2014). It is critical for healthcare providers to be advocates for this problem and to mobilize the community to reduce factors that may contribute to suicide.

In the American Psychiatric Association's (APA's) *Diagnostic and Statistical Manual,* fifth edition (*DSM-5;* APA, 2013), the focus on suicidal ideation and behaviors has been increased. Characteristics that make people more vulnerable to risk for suicide are identified throughout the manual. In addition, Section III highlights disorders that require further study. Suicidal behavior disorder is among the disorders in this section. In this chapter, we will include the criteria for this proposed disorder. We will also review facts about suicide, discuss assessment and care of patients who may be suicidal, and address the needs of patient's families. Another disorder included in the *DSM-5* for further study, nonsuicidal self-injury, will also be discussed in this chapter.

EPIDEMIOLOGY

According to the CDC (2016) nearly 43,000 people died by suicide in 2014 making it the 10th-leading cause of death in the United States. In 2014 suicide was the second-leading cause of death for 10- to 34-year-olds, the fourth-leading cause of death in 35- to 54-year-olds, and the eighth-leading cause of death among 55- to 64-year-olds (CDC, 2016).

In 2014 attempted suicide or suicidal ideation led to approximately 470,000 annual visits to the emergency room, and outcomes may be catastrophic for the individual (CDC, 2016). Consider the case of a young man with schizophrenia with deep depression and confusion. He takes a medication overdose and kneels down in front of his couch to pray for forgiveness as he dies. His father finds him near death and calls the paramedics. The young man lives, but due to being in a kneeling position for so long, the circulation to his legs was severely compromised. This compromise resulted in amputation of both legs and a lifelong physical disability.

It is important to consider that the number of suicides may actually be double or triple those reported due to underreporting in general. Purposefully steering a car into a bridge abutment and crashing may look like an accident. However, many reported accidents, homicides, and deaths ruled as undetermined are actually suicides.

The military is increasingly concerned about suicide rates among enlisted service members and veterans. Until recently, service in the military was a protective factor for suicide. However, since 2008, suicide rates among active duty service members has increased and surpassed rates of civilians. Suicide rates among veterans are also increasing at higher rates than among the US general population, especially for women (Nock et al.,

BOX 25.1 Suicide Facts

General

- Suicide is the 10th-leading cause of death for all ages.
- The National Violent Death Reporting System examined toxicology tests of those who committed suicide in 16 states; 33% tested positive for alcohol, 24% for antidepressants, and 20% for opiates or prescription painkillers.

Gender Statistics

- Males take their own lives at nearly four times the rate of females and represent almost 78% of all US suicides.
- During their lifetime, women attempt suicide two to three times more often than men.
- Suicide is the seventh-leading cause of death for males and the 14th-leading cause for females.
- In 2014 men had a suicide rate of 20.7, and women had a rate of 5.8 (per 100,000).
- Firearms were the most common method of death by suicide accounting for a little less than half (49.9%) of all suicide deaths. The next most common methods were suffocation (including hangings) at 26.7% and poisoning at 15.9%.

Racial and Ethnic Statistics

- Among American Indians/Alaska Natives aged 10 to 34 years, suicide is the second-leading cause of death.
- Suicide rates among American Indian/Alaskan Native adolescents and young adults aged 15 to 34 (19.5 per 100,000) are 1.5 times higher than the national average for that age group (12.9 per 100,000).
- Of Hispanic students in grades 9 to 12, significantly more Hispanics (11.3%) attempt suicide than black and white students.

Age Statistics

- In 2013, 17% of US high school students reported that they had seriously considered attempting suicide during the 12 months preceding the survey. About 8% of students reported that they had actually attempted suicide one or more times during the same period.
- Suicide is the third-leading cause of death among 10- to 14-year-olds.
- Suicide is the second-leading cause of death among 15- to 34-year-olds.
- The rate of suicide for adults ages 75 years and older was 16 per 100,000.

Attempted Suicide

- In 2013 nearly 836,000 people were treated in emergency departments for self-inflicted injuries.
- There is one suicide for every 25 attempted suicides.

Centers for Disease Control and Prevention. (2015). *Suicide facts at a glance: 2015.* Retrieved from http://www.cdc.gov/violenceprevention/pdf/suicide-datasheet-a.pdf.

2014). Box 25.1 provides some facts about suicide including data for specific age groups.

Comorbidity

Suicidal ideation is the result of inner pain, hopelessness, and helplessness suffered by individuals. Psychiatric disorders are risk factors for suicide because these disorders are present at the time of 90% of completed suicides (American Foundation for Suicide Prevention, 2015). Depression is the diagnosis most commonly associated with suicide, and approximately 50% of those who complete suicide are experiencing depression at the time of death (American Association of Suicidology, 2014). Patients diagnosed with anorexia nervosa and posttraumatic stress disorders are also at greater risk for suicide. Loss of relationships, financial difficulty, and impulsivity are also common in this population.

TABLE 25.1 Percentage of Suicides Attributable to Psychiatric Disorders

Disorders	Percentage
Affective illnesses (major depression and bipolar disorder)	32%-47%
Drug or alcohol abuse	3%-17%
Schizophrenia	15%-20%
Personality disorders	8%-11%

From Harding, M. (2014). Suicide risk assessment and threats of suicide. *Patient.* Retrieved from patient.info/doctor/suicide-risk-assessment-and-threats-of -suicide.

Individuals with a diagnosis of schizophrenia have an eightfold increased risk than those in the general population, especially during the first few years of the illness (Goldberg, 2016). It is the leading cause of early death in this population. Twenty percent of patients diagnosed with schizophrenia will attempt suicide at least once. Up to 13% of these people die from suicide, usually related to depressive symptoms rather than to command hallucinations or delusions.

Patients with substance use disorders, who use both legal and illicit substances, have a higher suicide risk. Years of substance use and comorbidity with depression are factors associated with increased risk. Many individuals who die by suicide have alcohol in their blood at the time of death and have used an illicit substance in the days before their death. Alcohol, a depressant, tends to dull one's senses, and individuals who are otherwise ambivalent about whether to end their lives may act on suicidal thoughts. Drugs and alcohol increase the risk of suicide by decreasing inhibitions, increasing aggressiveness, and impairing the individual's judgment. Using both cocaine and alcohol simultaneously is a particularly deadly combination (Arias et al., 2016). Table 25.1 identifies the percentage of suicides attributable to psychiatric disorders.

RISK FACTORS

Biological Factors

Suicidal behavior may run in families. Margaux Hemingway's death in 1996 was the fifth suicide among four generations of writer Ernest Hemingway's (1899–1961) family. Twin and adoption studies suggest genetic factors in suicide. Concordance rates are higher among monozygotic (identical) twins than among dizygotic (fraternal) twins.

Recent studies indicate a combined effect of genetic and epigenetic (external gene altering) factors. Guintivano and colleagues (2014) found that the *SKA2* gene expression was lower in individuals with suicidal ideation. This lowered gene expression along with anxiety and stress could account for about 80% of suicidal behaviors and the progression from suicidal ideation to suicide attempt. These findings are consistent with the diathesis-stress model or the dual-risk hypothesis.

Low serotonin levels are related to depressed mood. Studies have found low levels of serotonin or its metabolites in the cerebrospinal fluid of patients who are suicidal. Postmortem examinations of individuals who complete suicide also reveal low levels of serotonin in the brainstem and/or the frontal cortex.

Psychological Factors

Sigmund Freud originally theorized that suicide resulted from unacceptable aggression toward another person that is turned inward. Karl Menninger added to Freud's work by describing three aspects of suicidal hostility: the wish to kill (revenge), the wish to be killed (guilt), and the wish to die (hopelessness). Aaron Beck identified a central emotional factor underlying suicide intent: hopelessness. Cognitive styles that contribute to higher risk are rigid all-or-nothing thinking, inability to see different options, and perfectionism.

Environmental Factors

Recent theories of suicide focus on the diathesis-stress model, the lethal combination of suicidal fantasies accompanied by loss (love, self-esteem, job, and freedom due to imminent incarceration), rage or guilt, and identification with an individual who completed suicide (copycat suicide). A **copycat suicide** follows a highly publicized suicide of a public figure, an idol, or a peer in the community. Adolescents are at especially high risk due to their immature prefrontal cortex, the portion of the brain that controls the executive functions involving judgment, frustration tolerance, and impulse control.

Cultural Factors

Cultural factors, including religious beliefs, family values, sexual orientation, gender identity, bullying behavior, and attitude toward death, have an impact on suicide rates. In 2013 ethnicity was a significant factor in the number of deaths by suicide in the United States. The suicide rate is highest among whites. In 100,000 people, 11.7 American Indians/Alaska Natives, 6 Asians/Pacific Islanders, 5.3 Hispanics, and 5.4 African Americans die by suicide (Brown & Johns, 2015).

CONSIDERING CULTURE

Suicide and Bullying in LBGT Youth

Youth bullying is on the rise in the United States, especially among the lesbian, gay, bisexual, or transgender (LGBT) community. These youth report extremely high rates of harassment including online bullying, name calling, verbal harassment, and physical harassment. They also report higher rates of suicidal thoughts, plans, and attempts than their heterosexual peers.

Mueller, James, Abrutyn, and Levin (2015) studied data collected by the CDC with an adolescent youth sample size of 75,344 from nine states: 5,541 self-reported as LGBT. They found:

- Black and Hispanic heterosexual youths were less likely to be bullied than were white heterosexual youths.
- White LGBT and Hispanic bisexual females were more likely to be bullied than white heterosexual adolescents.
- Black LGBT's vulnerability to bullying was about the same as white heterosexual youths.
- Sexual minority youths were more likely to report suicide ideation regardless of their race/ethnicity, gender, or having been bullied.

While bullying is a problem, it does not seem to explain increased suicidal ideation among LGBT youth. More research is necessary to identify risk factors. The researchers did make some recommendations. They suggest that school policymakers create safe environments for LGBT youth, promote respect for others, and include issues related to LGBT education within the school environment.

Mueller, A., James, W., Abrutyn, S., & Levin, M. (2015). Suicide ideation and bullying among US adolescents: Examining the intersections of sexual orientation, gender, and race/ethnicity. *American Journal of Public Health, 105*(5), 980–985.

Among African Americans, men complete suicide more often than women, and the peak rate occurs in young adulthood and middle age. Protective factors for this group as a whole include religion and the role of the extended family, both of which provide a strong social support system. Similarly, among Hispanic Americans, Roman Catholic religion (in which suicide is considered a sin) and the importance given to the extended family decrease the risk for suicide. There is also the philosophy of *fatalismo*, a belief that divine providence regulates the world. This philosophy removes the blame from the individual who is unable to control adverse events. Risk factors for recent Hispanic immigrants are not understanding the US healthcare system, fear of being deported, and language barriers.

Among Asian Americans, suicide rates increase with age. Beliefs that reduce suicide attempts include the adherence to religions that emphasize interdependence between the individual and society (i.e., self-destruction is seen as disrespectful to the group or selfish). The high value given to the reputation of the family, however, may lead to the conclusion that suicide is preferable if it prevents shame to the family. A belief in reincarnation may make death a potentially honorable solution to life problems for the elderly in this population.

Societal Factors

Human beings are social beings that have evolved by banding together, yet our society is becoming increasingly isolated. Texting has replaced talking on the phone. People drive to work alone. Suburban neighbors frequently do not know one another's names. Urban dwellers know that making eye contact or talking to strangers is a taboo. Isolation sets the stage for loneliness and despair.

In a more formal way, society regulates a specific suicide, namely assisted suicide. In the United States, individual states have the authority to regulate, allow, or prohibit assisted suicide. Increasingly, states are considering cases to determine the legality of assisted suicide. Other countries, including the Netherlands, Belgium, Switzerland, and Canada, have laws in place allowing physician-assisted suicide. The ethical and moral dilemmas in this evolving trend are clear.

Another societal concern is suicide bombing, which has grown exponentially since September 11, 2001. Suicide bombers believe, or are convinced by others, that it is a honor to die in defense of their faith, that real happiness exists beyond this life, and that for martyrs, dying is not real death but an honorable entrance to the afterlife.

Other Risk Factors

Risk factors for suicide include the following (American Association of Suicidology, 2014):

- **Race:** Caucasian suicides account for the highest percentage of completed suicides, approximately 85% to 90%. Caucasians (14.75 per 100,000) have higher suicide completions than Asian/Pacific Islanders (6.36 per 100,000) or Hispanics (5.36 per 100,000).
- **Religion:** Religiosity is associated with decreased rates of suicide. Protestants and Jews have higher rates of suicide than Roman Catholics.
- **Marriage:** Being married, especially with children in the home, significantly reduces the risk of suicide. Divorced men are more likely than divorced women to kill themselves.
- **Profession:** Professionals are generally considered at higher risk for suicide, particularly if there is a loss in status. Among professionals, physicians, dentists, veterinarians, and chiropractors are at highest risk. Law enforcement personnel, sales personnel, mechanics, insurance agents, and lawyers are also at higher risk. Over the past several years, there has been an increased risk in construction workers and heavy equipment operators.
- **Physical health:** Those individuals who have chronic illnesses are at increased risk of suicide. Loss of mobility, disfigurement, and chronic pain are especially associated with suicide.

Extensive data are available about risk factors for suicide, based on epidemiological studies and **psychological autopsies** (i.e., retrospective reviews of the deceased person's life within several months of death to establish likely diagnoses at the time of death). There is also evidence concerning protective factors (those that tend to reduce risk). Box 25.2 provides a description of significant psychosocial risk and protective factors for suicide.

CLINICAL PICTURE

A history of suicide attempts puts a person at a high probability of actually completing suicide in the future, particularly in the 12 months following the attempt. Han and colleagues (2014) note that, among those who attempted suicide in the past 12 months, only 56.4% received mental health treatment, and those who did not receive mental health treatment reported high rates of unmet treatment needs. Because suicide behaviors are often associated with other psychiatric disorders, especially major depression, the pathological features are similar, and similar treatment plans are appropriate no matter what other disorder is present. You should direct your attention to individuals who exhibit these behaviors because of the serious outcomes that may result.

Suicidal behavior disorder was proposed as a new disorder for the *DSM-5* (APA, 2013). Supporters for its inclusion believed that such a diagnosis would be a way to better identify and track individuals who are at greatest risk for suicide. Opponents of adding this disorder argued that such a label was unnecessary since diagnosing associated conditions such as major depressive disorder already provided a way to identify and track risk. In the end, suicidal behavior disorder was voted down, but was added to the manual in a section called "Conditions for Further Study."

BOX 25.2 Suicide Warning Factors, Risk Factors, and Protective Factors

Warning Factors (immediate risk of suicide)

- Often talking or writing about death, dying, or suicide
- Making comments about being hopeless, helpless, or worthless
- Expressions of having no reason for living; no sense of purpose in life; saying things like "It would be better if I wasn't here" or "I want out"
- Increased alcohol and/or drug misuse
- Withdrawal from friends, family, and community
- Reckless behavior or more risky activities, seemingly without thinking
- Dramatic mood changes
- Talking about feeling trapped or being a burden to others

Risk Factors (characteristics that make it more likely that an individual will consider, attempt, or die by suicide)

- Previous suicide attempt(s)
- A history of suicide in the family
- Substance use
- Mood disorders (depression, bipolar disorder)
- Access to lethal means (e.g., keeping firearms in the home)
- Losses and other events (e.g., the breakup of a relationship or a death, academic failures, legal difficulties, financial difficulties, bullying)
- History of trauma or abuse
- Chronic physical illness including chronic pain
- Exposure to the suicidal behavior of others

Protective Factors (characteristics that make it **less** likely that individuals will consider, attempt, or die by suicide)

- Effective mental healthcare; easy access to a variety of clinical interventions
- Strong connections to individuals, family, community, and social institutions
- Problem-solving and conflict resolution skills
- Contact with providers (e.g., follow-up phone call from healthcare professional)

American Psychiatric Association. (2015). *Suicide prevention.* Retrieved from http://www.psychiatry.org/patients-families/suicide-prevention.

APPLICATION OF THE NURSING PROCESS

Suicide risk assessment is based on identifying specific risk and protective factors, taking a psychosocial and health history, and establishing a therapeutic relationship with the patient during the interview. The nurse usually completes this assessment in conjunction with other clinicians because comparison of data and impressions from two or more interviewers can result in a more comprehensive evaluation.

ASSESSMENT

Assessment tools are helpful in providing a baseline evaluation that can be compared over time. One assessment tool that encompasses both risk and protective factors, provides the clinician with a tool to benchmark risk, and suggests interventions is the Suicide Assessment Five-step Evaluation and Triage (SAFE-T). This tool was established based on sponsored research outcomes from the Substance Abuse and Mental Health Services Administration. A free pocket guide can be downloaded from http://store.samhsa.gov/product/SMA09-4432. The tool allows the clinician to benchmark relative risk (high, moderate, low) and to develop a treatment plan, in consultation with the patient, to reduce current risk.

Verbal and Nonverbal Clues

Individuals considering suicide usually provide some clues to their intent, especially to people who are supportive of them such as nurses. These clues come in the form of open messages also known as overt statements, or in a concealed manner known as covert statements. Additionally, the nurse should teach family members and other support people in the community regarding these statements that may indicate risk. Examples include the following:

Overt Statements

- "I can't take it anymore."
- "Life isn't worth living anymore."
- "I wish I were dead."
- "Everyone would be better off if I died."

Covert Statements and Nonverbal Clues

- "It's okay now. Soon everything will be fine."
- "Things will never work out."
- "I won't be a problem much longer."
- "Nothing feels good to me anymore and probably never will."
- "How can I give my body to medical science?"

Most often, it is a relief for people contemplating suicide to finally talk to someone about their despair and loneliness. Asking about suicidal thoughts does not give a person the idea to commit suicide. Asking is, in fact, a professional responsibility similar to asking about chest pain in cardiac conditions. Talking openly leads to a decrease in isolation and can increase problem-solving alternatives for living. People who contemplate suicide, attempt suicide, and even those who regret the failure of their attempt are often extremely receptive to talking about their suicide crisis. Specific questions to ask about suicidal ideation include the following:

- Have you ever felt that life was not worth living?
- Have you been thinking about death recently?
- Do you ever think about suicide?
- Have you ever attempted suicide?
- Do you have a plan for completing suicide?
- If so, what is your plan for suicide?

The following dialogue illustrates how the nurse can make covert messages more open:

Nurse: You haven't eaten or slept well for the past few days, Theresa.

Theresa: No, I feel pretty low lately.

Nurse: How low are you feeling?

Theresa: Oh, I don't know. Nothing seems to matter to me anymore. It's all so meaningless…

Nurse: Tell me about it, Theresa. I want to understand how you're feeling. What is meaningless?

Theresa: Life…the whole thing…nothingness. Life is a bad joke.

Nurse: Are you saying you don't think life is worth living?

Theresa: Well…yes. It's all so hopeless anyway.

Nurse: Are you thinking of killing yourself?

Theresa: Oh, I don't know. Well, sometimes I think about it. I probably would never go through with it.

Nurse: Theresa, let's talk more about what you're thinking and feeling. This is important. I'll need to share your thoughts with other members of the staff.

The nurse should be alert for nonverbal behavioral clues including showing a sudden brightening of mood with more energy (especially after recently being prescribed an antidepressant medication), giving away possessions, writing letters, or organizing financial affairs. Individuals may be at greater risk as their mood lifts because they have enough energy to act on their feelings of ambivalence regarding suicide. The risk of suicide is highest in the first year after a suicide attempt (Han et al., 2014).

Establishing a therapeutic relationship with the patient and asking directly about suicidal feelings are essential elements of the nurse-patient relationship. Asking about suicidal ideation is the single most important assessment (and intervention). Possible reasons for hesitancy in screening include lack of personal comfort, lack of professional confidence, and time constraints. Crisis intervention techniques involve listening for the emotional feeling message underlying the verbal message, especially when the patient presents as angry, hostile, and overwhelmed. The therapeutic alliance established with a patient is a dynamic changeable interaction. Thus you should be constantly assessing and documenting it.

Lethality of Suicide Plan

The evaluation of a suicide plan is extremely important in determining the degree of suicidal risk. There are three main elements to consider when evaluating lethality: (1) Is there a specific plan with details? (2) How lethal is the proposed method? (3) Is there access to the planned method? People who have definite plans for the time, place, and means are at highest risk.

Based on the **lethality** of a method, which indicates how quickly a person would die by that mode, you can classify the method as higher or lower risk. Higher-risk methods, also referred to as *hard methods*, include:

- Using a gun
- Jumping off a high place
- Hanging
- Poisoning with carbon monoxide
- Staging a car crash

Examples of lower-risk methods, also referred to as *soft methods*, include:

- Cutting one's wrists
- Inhaling natural gas
- Ingesting pills

When the patient confirms access to the proposed method, the situation is more serious. A man who has access to a high building and states that he will jump from it or a woman who has a gun and says that she will shoot herself is at serious risk for suicide. When people are experiencing psychotic episodes, they are also at high risk—regardless of the specificity of details—because impulse control and judgment are grossly impaired. A person suffering psychosis is particularly vulnerable when depressed or having command hallucinations.

Self-Assessment

Healthcare professionals working with individuals who are suicidal need collaboration with other clinicians. Fear, grief, anger, puzzlement, and condemnation of suicidal feelings and intent are common emotions experienced. If these intense emotional responses are not acknowledged, countertransference may limit effective intervention. Understanding the patient with suicidal behavior disorder, as well as acknowledging, understanding, and accepting the emotions that arise from working with and caring for these patients, is essential.

DIAGNOSIS

The nursing diagnosis with the highest priority is *Risk for suicide.* Feelings of hopelessness, anger, frustration, abandonment, and rejection are common among people who are suicidal. Nursing diagnoses that address problems related to depressed mood, anxiety, mania, or disturbed thought include *Self-care deficit, Sleep pattern disturbance, Altered nutrition,* and *Anxiety*. See the clinical chapters focusing on depressive disorders, bipolar disorders, and schizophrenia spectrum disorders for more information.

OUTCOMES CRITERIA

Relevant *Nursing Outcomes Classification (NOC)* outcomes include *Suicide Self-Restraint, Coping, Hope, Social support, Spiritual health,* and *Self-esteem* (Moorhead et al., 2013). Table 25.2 describes signs and symptoms, potential nursing diagnoses, and outcomes for suicidal behavior.

ASSESSMENT GUIDELINES

Suicide

1. Assess risk factors including history of suicide (in family, friends), degree of hopelessness and helplessness, and lethality of plan.
2. Assess protective factors that may be built upon.
3. If there is a history of suicide attempt, assess intent, lethality, and injury, determine whether the patient's age, medical condition, psychiatric diagnosis, or current medications put the patient at higher risk.
4. A change from sad or depressed to happy and peaceful may be a red flag. Often a decision to complete suicide gives a feeling of relief and calm.
5. Always assess social supports and helpfulness of significant others, particularly if you need to manage the patient on an outpatient basis.

PLANNING

The plan of care for the patient who is suicidal is based on risk and protective factors. When there is a comorbid psychiatric disorder, the treatment plan includes appropriate nursing approaches (e.g., care for patients with depression or schizophrenia). The patient's significant others need to be involved because the patient's perception of isolation is a significant cause of hopelessness.

INTERVENTION

Nursing interventions for patients with suicidal ideation and suicide attempts focus on prevention, treatment, and postvention. Improving *overall* community mental health services may reduce the incidence of suicide more effectively than extensive efforts directed at identifying individuals who are imminently suicidal. Therefore more attention focused on prevention that involves community-wide participation will lead to improved outcomes.

Prevention is a **primary intervention** and includes activities that provide support, information, and education to prevent suicide (Box 25.3). Primary intervention is practiced in a wide variety of community settings such as schools, homes, churches, clinics, hospitals, and work settings. Elementary school children are screened using evidence-based tools that focus on both risk factors and warning signs. High schools are adopting suicide prevention curricula that involve elements of education, peer support, discussions about risk and prevention factors, and warning signs.

Nurses can learn about suicide prevention through the Question, Persuade, Refer (QPR) model (Quinnett, 2007). This model, originally developed in 1995, is a simple educational "train the trainer" program that provides ordinary citizens with education about how to recognize a mental health emergency, get individuals at risk the help they need, and provide hope through the process. The Case Study and Nursing Care Plan represents the case of a young woman with suicidal ideation treated in an outpatient setting.

TABLE 25.2 Signs and Symptoms, Nursing Diagnoses, and Outcomes for a Patient with Suicidal Ideation

Signs and Symptoms	Potential Nursing Diagnoses	Outcomes
Gives overt or covert clues (e.g., "I can't stand the pain"), has a plan (gun), is in high-risk category on assessment (elderly or teenager, isolated, depressed, had a recent loss), has a psychiatric diagnosis (substance use, depression, borderline personality disorder, anorexia nervosa, or psychosis)	*Risk for suicide*	Remains free from injury, expresses will to live, discloses plan for suicide if present, refrains from attempting suicide
Overwhelmed with situational crises, relies heavily on drugs or alcohol, has few supportive systems, shows poor problem-solving skills	*Ineffective coping*	Identifies coping mechanisms to assist with situational crisis, identifies social support within community
Lacks hope for the future, believes nothing can change intolerable situation, intense feelings of isolation, no control over the future	*Hopelessness*	Expresses willingness to call on others for help, identifies one support system within community.
Believes that he or she is no good, worthless, ineffective, a burden to others, cannot do anything right	*Chronic low self-esteem*	Describes feelings of self-worth

Herdman, T. H., & Kamitsuru, S. (Ed.). (2014). *Nursing diagnoses—Definitions and classification 2015-2017.* Copyright © 2014, 1994–2012 by NANDA International. Used by arrangement with John Wiley & Sons Limited; Moorhead, S., Johnson, M., Maas, M. L., & Swanson, E. (2013). *Nursing outcomes classification (NOC)* (5th ed.). St. Louis, MO: Mosby.

CASE STUDY AND NURSING CARE PLAN

A Patient with Suicidal Ideation in the Outpatient Setting

Olivia is a 23-year-old single waitress who comes to the emergency department by ambulance after a first suicide attempt. Her live-in boyfriend had narrowly prevented her from fatally shooting herself with their gun. She sustained a minor scalp wound and is under observation. She stares at the ground, talks softly, and looks profoundly sad. The psychiatric nurse and psychiatrist on call then interview her.

She states that she has been under increasing stress for the past 2 months since entering a management-training program at work. Olivia ultimately failed at the program and lost her job. She states, "I have tons of bills and Christmas is coming." She admits to keeping her feelings to herself. "I don't want my family to find out what a mess I've made of things…again." She denies having a social network. Olivia reports she self-medicates with drugs and alcohol. She states that she feels "like a total loser."

Because Olivia continues to state that she wants to kill herself, she is hospitalized. After careful assessment, the care team places Olivia on an antidepressant. Problems relating to her depressive state are assessed and monitored (poor appetite, insomnia, self-care deficit, and anxiety). After 3 days on suicide precautions, she is no longer acutely suicidal and agrees to continue treatment in the outpatient division of the hospital.

Self-Assessment

Mrs. Ruiz is a registered nurse with 5 years' experience. Mrs. Ruiz feels empathy for Olivia's attempt to end her life. Yet, she also feels conflicted because she believes, as a Catholic, that attempting to take your life is a sin. Mrs. Ruiz recognizes her own feelings and knows that Olivia has problems with which she can help.

Assessment

Subjective Data

- Reported first suicide attempt in a 23-year-old female
- Self-medicating with alcohol and substances
- Without a social support systems
- Recent failure at work and subsequent loss of job
- No history of bipolar disorder or related behaviors
- "I have tons of bills and Christmas is coming."
- "I don't want my family to find out what a mess I've made of things…again."

Objective Data

- Minor scalp wound
- Stares at the ground
- Talks softly
- Looks sad

Priority Diagnosis

Risk for suicide as evidenced by suicide attempt, substance use, job loss, debt, and lack of social support.

Outcomes Identification

Patient will consistently use suicide prevention resources and social support groups within the community.

Planning

The initial plan is to establish a working relationship with Olivia, involving her in planning her own treatment and identifying alternative actions for suicidal ideation in the future.

Implementation

Ms. Ruiz develops the following nursing care plan.

Short-Term Goal	Intervention	Rationale	Evaluation
1. Olivia will seek help when feeling self-destructive.	1a. Assess suicidal ideation status. 1b. Even if Olivia denies suicidal ideas, develop a future plan. 1c. Monitor effectiveness of antidepressant therapy and assess for side effects.	1a. Suicide attempts increase the rate of subsequent attempts. Ongoing periodic checks provide support and external boundaries. 1b. Demonstrates concern and offers alternatives if suicidal thoughts return. 1c. Important to assess for agitation and increase in suicidal feelings and to monitor for lifting of depressive state.	**GOAL MET** Olivia agrees to talk to the nurse about suicidal feelings, which she denied during checks. Once discharged if clinic is closed, she will call the crisis hotline. Olivia agreed to a session that included her boyfriend, and he removed the gun from her apartment. No adverse side effects. Increase in socialization, improved hygiene, reported improvement in sleep and appetite. States her mood is improving, and she feels more hopeful.
2. Olivia will talk about painful feelings by the end of the first week.	2a. Listen attentively and provide feedback. 2b. Refocus attention back to Olivia and the emotions underlying her anger. 2c. Give frequent opportunities for discussion of feelings through verbal invitation and stated concern.	2a. Support and feedback make patients feel stronger and better able to handle stress. 2b. Arguments and power struggles keep attention away from important issues. 2c. Aggressive, hostile communications cover painful feelings. When patient can express feelings in words, there is less need to act them out.	**GOAL MET** During the initial sessions, angry communication is constant. By the end of the first week, Olivia states, "You really want to understand." Olivia talks of feeling like a failure as a daughter, girlfriend, and employee.
3. Olivia will explore other employment opportunities by the end of the second week.	3. Alternative solutions can be explored once feelings and problems are identified.	3. Acceptable alternatives increase a future orientation and decrease hopelessness. Patient can experience feelings of control over situation.	**GOAL MET** By the end of the second week, Olivia talks about attending a job fair. She accepted a referral to social services for registering for unemployment benefits and debt management.

Evaluation

See individual outcomes and evaluation within the care plan.

BOX 25.3 Goals of the National Strategy for Suicide Prevention

- Integrate and coordinate suicide prevention activities across multiple sectors and settings.
- Implement research-informed communication efforts designed to prevent suicide by changing knowledge, attitudes, and behaviors.
- Increase knowledge of the factors that offer protection from suicidal behaviors and that promote wellness and recovery.
- Promote responsible media reporting of suicide, accurate portrayals of suicide and mental illnesses in the entertainment industry, and the safety of online content related to suicide.
- Develop, implement, and monitor effective programs that promote wellness and prevent suicide and related behaviors.
- Promote efforts to reduce access to lethal means of suicide among individuals with identified suicide risk.
- Provide training to community and clinical service providers on the prevention of suicide and related behaviors.
- Promote suicide prevention as a core component of healthcare services.
- Promote and implement effective clinical and professional practices for assessing and treating those identified as being at risk for suicidal behaviors.
- Provide care and support to individuals affected by suicide deaths and attempts to promote healing and implement community strategies to help prevent further suicides.
- Increase the timeliness and usefulness of national surveillance systems relevant to suicide prevention and improve the ability to collect, analyze, and use this information for action.
- Promote and support research on suicide prevention.
- Evaluate the impact and effectiveness of suicide prevention interventions and systems and synthesize and disseminate findings.

US Department of Health and Human Services (HHS) Office of the Surgeon General and National Action Alliance for Suicide Prevention. (2012). *National Strategy for Suicide Prevention: Goals and Objectives for Action*. Washington, DC: Author.

PSYCHOSOCIAL INTERVENTIONS

The key element is establishing a therapeutic alliance to encourage the patient to engage in more realistic problem solving. Helpful staff characteristics include warmth, sensitivity, interest, and consistency. After hospitalization, nurse may work with these patients in the clinic, in a partial hospitalization program, or in home care.

One particular aspect of counseling is the use of a patient **safety plan**. This is a written six-step plan that includes identification of warning signs, internal coping strategies, social settings, and people who provide distraction. It also provides instructions on people who patients can ask for help, professionals or agencies where they can find help during a crisis, and how to make the environment safe (Fig. 25.1). Additionally, this written safety plan asks the patient to identify something most important to them worth living for.

PSYCHOBIOLOGICAL INTERVENTIONS

Pharmacological Interventions

Pharmacological interventions are used to alleviate symptoms of comorbid disorders. Antidepressants are used for patients who have a depressive disorder or an anxiety disorder. Close monitoring must occur especially when patients begin medication and when the dosage changes. Strong nursing care involves careful patient (and family, if appropriate) teaching about the benefits and risks of antidepressant therapy.

There is clear evidence that long-term lithium treatment for bipolar disorder and major depression significantly reduces suicide and suicide attempts. Because lithium frequently causes serious side effects and necessitates periodic blood work to test for therapeutic levels, patient and family education is important to support adherence.

For patients experiencing psychotic or bipolar manic episodes, antipsychotic medication is usually ordered. Second-generation antipsychotics are preferable to first-generation antipsychotics because they have fewer adverse effects. Some studies have shown a reduced suicide rate among patients with schizophrenia receiving clozapine (Clozaril). Monitor the use of clozapine closely, however, because of the risk of severe side effects (e.g., agranulocytosis, myocarditis, and altered glucose metabolism).

Finally, antianxiety medication may help treat risk factors such as severe anxiety, panic, and agitation. Aggressive treatment of anxiety beyond antidepressants is advisable based on current research (Fawcett, 2013).

A significant nursing intervention to assist the patient with suicidal ideation regain self-control is the careful administration of medication. Medications prescribed to high-risk patients are monitored carefully. Lethal overdose is nearly impossible with the newer antidepressants such as selective serotonin reuptake inhibitors (SSRIs). Overdose remains a concern with tricyclic antidepressants and monoamine oxidase inhibitors. Mouth checks may be used to be sure that patients are not saving (hoarding) medications in the hospital. In the community, provision of a limited-day supply or family supervision is required.

Somatic Intervention

An alternative somatic treatment for acute suicidal risk is electroconvulsive therapy (ECT). Evidence suggests that ECT decreases acute suicidal ideation. This treatment is useful for patients with depression or psychosis whose behavior is considered life threatening and for whom waiting for medication to take effect is not feasible. It is also safe and effective for pregnant patients, patients with certain medical conditions who cannot tolerate medication, and patients who do not respond to multiple trials of medication. Refer to Chapter 14 for further discussion of ECT.

Health Teaching and Health Promotion

The nurse teaches the patient about psychiatric diagnoses, medications and complementary therapies, and age-related developmental crises. Teaching is also important regarding community resources, coping skills, stress management, and communication skills. Additionally, teaching regarding the development of a safety plan is important in the prevention of suicide. When possible, include the family or significant others to strengthen the patient's support system.

Patient Safety Plan Template

Step 1: Warning signs (thoughts, images, mood, situation, behavior) that a crisis may be developing:

1. ______
2. ______
3. ______

Step 2: Internal coping strategies—Things I can do to take my mind off my problems without contacting another person (relaxation technique, physical activity):

1. ______
2. ______
3. ______

Step 3: People and social settings that provide distractions:

1. Name ______ Phone ______
2. Name ______ Phone ______
3. Place ______ 4. Place ______

Step 4: People whom I can ask for help:

1. Name ______ Phone ______
2. Name ______ Phone ______
3. Name ______ Phone ______

Step 5: Professionals or agencies I can contact during a crisis:

1. Clinician Name ______ Phone ______
   Clinician Pager or Emergency Contact # ______
2. Clinician Name ______ Phone ______
   Clinician Pager or Emergency Contact # ______
3. Local Urgent Care Services ______
   Urgent Care Services Address ______
   Urgent Care Services Phone ______
4. Suicide Prevention Lifeline Phone: 1-800-273-TALK (8255)

Step 6: Making the environment safe:

1. ______
2. ______

The one thing that is most important to me and worth living for is:

______

FIG. 25.1 Patient Safety Plan Template. Stanley, B., & Brown, (2008). *How can a safety plan help?* National Suicide Prevention Lifeline. Retrieved from http://suicidepreventionlifeline.org/wp-content/uploads/2016/08/Brown_StanleySafetyPlanTemplate.pdf.

Case Management

Case management is an important aspect of nursing care for the patient with suicidal ideation. The patient's perception of being alone without supports often blinds them to the real support figures who are present. Reconnecting the patient with family and friends is a major focus, whether in the hospital or the community. Aftercare referrals may include information on the following resources: treatment providers, substance treatment centers, crisis hotlines, support groups for patients or families, and recreational activities to enhance socialization and self-esteem. Encouraging the patient to get reacquainted with a previous spiritual support system may also be beneficial.

Milieu Therapy

Nurses play an important role in the treatment of patients who are at risk, those who have suicidal ideation, and those who have made a suicide attempt. In the hospital or community setting, the registered nurse utilizes psychosocial and psychobiological interventions, safety and teamwork, health teaching, and case management to provide care to patients who have suicidal ideation or have attempted suicide.

An interprofessional approach that emphasizes communication involving clinicians, nurses, social workers, therapists, counselors, and support persons is essential for reducing the number of suicides. This collaborative approach maximizes patient safety and improves outcomes through timely communication and improved coordination of care.

For patients with acute suicidal intentions, suicide precautions, in accordance with hospital policy, are part of the plan of care. Nursing staff must continuously observe patients who are suicidal. Table 25.3 provides a general description of suicide

TABLE 25.3 Suicide Precautions with Constant One-to-One Observation

Staff Assessment	Possible Patient Symptoms	Nursing Responsibilities
Patient with suicidal ideation or delusions of self-mutilation who, according to assessment by unit staff, presents clinical symptoms that suggest a clear intent to follow through with the plan or delusion	1. Patient is currently verbalizing a clear intent to harm self. 2. Patient shows no insight into existing problems. 3. Patient has poor impulse control. 4. Patient has already attempted suicide in the recent past by a particularly lethal method (e.g., hanging, gun, carbon monoxide poisoning).	1. One-to-one nursing observation and interaction 24 hours a day (never let patient out of staff's sight). 2. Chart patient's whereabouts and record mood, verbatim statements, and behavior every 15 to 30 minutes per protocol. 3. Ensure that meal trays contain no glass or metal silverware. 4. When patient is sleeping, hands should always be in view, not under the covers. 5. Observe patient swallow each dose of medication.

BOX 25.4 Environmental Guidelines for Minimizing Suicidal Behavior on the Psychiatric Unit

- Use plastic utensils and count utensils when the tray is collected.
- Do not assign patient to a private room, and ensure the door remains open at all times.
- Jump-proof and hang-proof the bathrooms by installing breakaway shower rods and recessed shower nozzles.
- Keep electrical cords to a minimal length.
- Install unbreakable glass in windows. Install tamper-proof screens or partitions too small to pass through. Keep all windows locked.
- Lock all utility rooms, kitchens, adjacent stairwells, and offices. All nonclinical staff (e.g., housekeepers, maintenance workers) should receive instructions to keep doors locked.
- Take all potentially harmful gifts (e.g., flowers in glass vases) from visitors before allowing them to see patients. Search all items brought to patients by visitors.
- Go through personal belongings with patient present, and remove all potentially harmful objects (e.g., belts, shoelaces, metal nail files, tweezers, matches, razors, perfume, and shampoo).
- Ensure that visitors do not bring in or leave potentially harmful objects in patient's room (e.g., matches, nail files).
- Search patient for harmful objects (e.g., drugs, sharp objects, cords) if allowed to leave unit on pass.

precautions. This intense attention from the nurse provides for safety and allows for constant reassessment of risk.

Monitoring flow sheets for suicide precautions is more clinically useful if they include a description of the patient's affect and behavior. For example, instead of noting "Patient watching television," the nurse will describe the patient's affect (e.g., hostile, fearful, calm) at each observation. Flow sheets should also indicate clear accountability for staff starting and ending their periods of observation. In addition to observing the patient, the nurse is responsible for monitoring the environment for safety hazards. Review Box 25.4 for guidelines on how to minimize physical risks in the environment.

Studies show that acute care of patients who are suicidal is usually effective. Suicide risk is highest in the first few days of hospital admission and during times of staff rotation. Assessment of suicidal risk must be an ongoing process. You should perform an assessment particularly before a change in level of observation or upon sudden improvement or worsening of symptoms.

Documentation of Care

As for documentation, you must ensure that the record is complete and identify any late entries. Courts require that the patient be periodically evaluated for suicidal risk, that the treatment plan provide for high-level security, and that staff members follow the individual treatment plan. Despite following institution protocols, treatment plans, and the appropriate standards of practice, suicides do occasionally still happen. This is especially the case for patients in the community. Human behavior is simply not predictable.

HEALTH POLICY

Preventing Veteran Suicide

The Veterans Administration (VA) reports that approximately 22 veterans end their lives by suicide every day. Many of them are unemployed, socially isolated, homeless, or struggling with addictions. These problems are most often connected to posttraumatic stress disorder (PTSD) following deployment to Iraq or Afghanistan.

In an extraordinary demonstration of bipartisanship, both the House and Senate unanimously passed the Clay Hunt Suicide Prevention for American Veterans Act, and President Barack Obama signed the bill into law on February 3, 2015. The bill was named in honor of Clay Hunt, a marine veteran who ended his life in 2011 after struggling with PTSD. Although he sought help for his illness, he waited more than 6 months to see a psychiatrist.

The bill provides for independent reviews of the Department of Defense's programs to prevent suicide and creates peer support and community outreach pilot programs. Due to the shortage of psychiatric clinicians, the legislation provides loan debt repayment for psychiatry students who choose to work in the VA health system. Additionally, through resources provided by the legislation, a website was created that provides information about mental health services to veterans and allows the VA to collaborate with other organizations in efforts to prevent suicide.

Leonard, K. (2015). Obama signs suicide prevention law to aid veterans. *US News and World Report.* Retrieved from http://www.usnews.com/news/articles/2015/02/12/obama-signs-veterans-suicide-prevention-bill.

Postvention

Survivors of suicide, the circle of survivors of a person who has completed suicide, are the largest group of mental health casualties related to suicide. Surviving family and friends may experience overwhelming guilt and shame compounded by the difficulty of discussing the frequently taboo subject of suicide, sadness, loneliness, abandonment, and disbelief.

Adolescents who suffer traumatic grief after a friend's death by suicide are more likely to report suicidal ideation within 6 years of the suicide (Melhem et al., 2004). Family members of individuals who complete suicide develop a 4.5-times greater risk of suicide than those in families in which no suicide occurred. Despite their suffering, only approximately 25% of survivors seek treatment. Adults bereaved by suicide have a higher probability of attempting suicide than individuals bereaved by sudden natural causes of death. Based on a statistic that there are six survivors per suicide completion, there are more than 6 million Americans who are considered survivors in the United States during the past 25 years.

EVIDENCE-BASED PRACTICE

Is a Loss Due to Suicide a Risk Factor for Suicide?

Problem

Most mental health professionals agree that losing a relative or a friend to suicide is in itself a risk factor for suicide. We do not know, however, if that risk is just like any other sudden loss by death or if the risk increases when applied to relative or peer suicide.

Purpose of Study

This study was conducted to test the hypothesis that young adults bereaved by suicide have an increased risk of suicidal ideation and suicide attempts as compared with other young adults bereaved by other sudden deaths.

Methods

There were 3432 respondents aged 18 to 40 who studied or worked at higher education institutions in the United Kingdom recruited for this online survey. To be included in the study, participants had to have experienced the natural, unnatural, or suicide loss of a close friend or relative since the age of 10. Two key questions were, "Have you ever thought about taking your life?" and "Have you ever made an attempt to take your life?"

Key Findings

- Adults who were bereaved by suicide had a higher probability of attempting suicide than those bereaved by sudden natural causes.
- The effect of suicide bereavement was similar whether participants were blood-related to the deceased or not.

Implications for Nursing Practice

Bereavement by suicide is a specific risk factor for suicide attempts. Nursing assessments should always involve a screening for a history of suicide in blood relatives, nonblood relatives, and friends.

Pitman, A. L., Osborn, D. P. J., Rantell, K., & King, M. B. (2016). Bereavement by suicide as a risk factor for suicide attempt: A cross-sectional national UK-wide study of 3,432 young bereaved adults. *British Medical Journal Open, 6*(1).

One survivor wrote a personal account several years after the suicide of her daughter:

"If only I hadn't responded with anger and frustration during our last phone call...she was angry with herself and seemed to want to pick a fight with me—which was the pattern. If I could have looked past her angry words and instead tuned into the desperation behind them, maybe I could have gotten her to open up to me. Now I can only look back and consider the many, many times I should have picked up on the severity of her illness and how she struggled. If I have any advice for others based on my experience, it is to get connected, listen, and be a real part of the lives of those you love. That's the only way you'll know when something is just not right and understand their deep despair. This also applies to friends and family of survivors. Please don't treat us like we're 'contagious.' And please do talk about our loss. The worst thing possible is to avoid mention of our lost loved one."

Healthcare providers are often involved in providing mental healthcare and support to these survivors, which is referred to as **postvention**. Survivors have given the following suggestions to healthcare professionals:

- If being a survivor is the main reason an individual seeks treatment, remember that the survivor, not the deceased, is the patient. Focus on the patient's thoughts and feelings, and do a thorough assessment as you usually would.
- If you are a friend or relative of a suicide survivor, remember that the most difficult time for these survivors is not so much in the immediate aftermath of the suicide. Rather, it is in the weeks, months, and *years* following their loss. Make frequent efforts to reach out to these individuals, especially on the most difficult anniversary dates. Do not be afraid of talking about the deceased person. In fact, speak of them often. While this may seem counterintuitive and uncomfortable for most, survivors of suicide universally want their loved one to be remembered in this way. Talking reduces the hurt, isolation, and stigma.
- If being a survivor comes out as an incidental finding during an assessment, ask open-ended questions and evaluate how much the loss has been resolved.
- Recommend community resources and survivor support groups and show empathy about the loss of someone to suicide. Know about local Survivors of Suicide (SOS) support groups in your area, and refer the survivors and their families as soon as possible following the suicide.

Staff members who have cared for a patient who completed suicide within the treatment facility are similarly traumatized by suicide. Staff may also experience symptoms of posttraumatic stress disorder with guilt, shock, anger, shame, and decreased self-esteem. Group support is essential as the inpatient treatment team conducts a thorough psychological postmortem assessment. The team will carefully review the event to identify the potential overlooked clues, faulty judgments, or changes that are needed in agency protocols.

Most facilities have a clear policy about communication with families after suicide. Although some lawyers advise having no contact except through them, others recommend designating a spokesperson that can address the feelings of the family without discussing the details of the patient's care. Give referrals to family members to assist them in dealing with their grief and to address any emotional problems that develop, especially in adolescents.

Advanced Practice Interventions

The psychiatric-mental health advanced practice registered nurse may treat patients with suicidal ideation directly with psychotherapy, psychobiological interventions, clinical supervision for direct care staff, or consultation in non-psychiatric settings (e.g., healthcare unit, nursing home, or forensic site). Following hospitalization, the advanced practice nurse may provide aftercare for the patient who has coexisting psychiatric disorders. This care includes individual and family therapy and medication management.

EVALUATION

Evaluation of a patient with suicidal ideation is ongoing. The nurse must be constantly alert to changes in mood, thinking, and behavior. The nurse also looks for indications that the patient is communicating thoughts and feelings more readily and that the patient's social network is widening. If the person is able to talk about feelings and engage in problem solving with you, this is a positive sign.

Suicidal behavior is the result of interpersonal turmoil. If an episode of major depressive disorder is the main admitting diagnosis and a serious suicidal gesture resulted from this depression, both problems are initially assessed and treated. When the patient is no longer an acute suicide risk, treating the suicidal ideation and depressive disorder becomes the main focus of care. Essentially, the nurse evaluates each short-term goal and establishes new ones as the patient progresses toward the long-term goal of resolving suicidal ideation.

Once stabilized, the patient may be admitted to a partial hospitalization program (PHP). PHPs tend to be 6 hours a day, 5 days a week. An intensive outpatient (IOP) treatment program is another slightly shorter option, usually 3 hours a day, 3 days a week. Both the PHP and IOP allow patients to go home in the evening to practice new coping skills. Community-based support groups are also available that are effective and financially affordable for the patient. Nurses should be knowledgeable about, and proactive in, referring patients to these support groups.

NONSUICIDAL SELF-INJURY

A closely related problem to suicidal behavior is **nonsuicidal self-injury**. These self-injuries are deliberate and direct attempts to inflict shallow, yet painful injuries to the surface of the body without intending to end one's life. The behavior most commonly consists of cutting, burning, scraping/scratching skin, biting, hitting, skin picking, and interfering with wound healing. Often the self-injurers report multiple methods of self-injury.

For these behaviors to be considered significant, they typically last at least a year and happen repeatedly. The majority of self-injurers do not seek professional help. Even when they are not engaged in the behaviors, self-injurers tend to be thinking about self-injury. Self-injurious actions are most often done with the intent to either alleviate psychic pain or to pierce the psychic numbness these individuals describe. Other times, these actions are used to punish themselves, to connect with others, to get attention, to escape a responsibility, or to avoid a situation.

Epidemiology

The lifetime prevalence of nonsuicidal self-injury is difficult to accurately determine due to attempts to conceal the behavior. However, some have estimated that between 13% to 23% of adolescents engage in the behaviors. It is a global problem, peaking between 20 to 29 years of age with 17% to 35% reporting engaging in the behavior. There is a decline in the behavior beyond this age. Estimates are that approximately 6% of the US population has engaged in the behavior at some time in their life. Research regarding prevalence by gender is inconclusive. Some studies report that there is less discrepancy between the sexes than there is with suicidal behavior.

Comorbidity

Nonsuicidal self-injury often occurs with other mental health disorders including depression, anxiety, eating disorders, and substance use disorders. In the past, researchers thought there was a direct relationship between borderline personality disorder and nonsuicidal self-injury. However, Bracken-Minor and McDevitt-Murphy (2014) conducted research and concluded that the emotional regulation and distress tolerance found in individuals with nonsuicidal self-injury was distinctly different from characteristics found in borderline personality disorder.

Risk Factors

Biological Factors

Studies related to the physiological mechanism of action in nonsuicidal self-injury are inconclusive; however, researchers continue to investigate the neurobiological mechanisms behind the disorder. Several neurochemical pathways in the brain play a role in the development of these behaviors. Although studies are inconclusive, the neurotransmitter group of monoamines including serotonin, dopamine, and norepinephrine may play a role in the mediation of self-injury, and research is ongoing. As practitioners continue to search for an effective treatment, clinical research will seek to find the neurobiological basis of nonsuicidal self-injury.

Environmental Factors

Recent studies have investigated the prevalence of nonsuicidal self-injury behaviors internationally to determine best practices for treatment and whether culturally different approaches to care are relevant. Similar rates of the behavior occur among adolescents in the United States and among several European countries with the behavior stabilizing among youth over the past several years and no significant increases internationally. With this stabilization in occurrence rates, researchers have the opportunity to further investigate cultural differences in the behavior and whether these differences lead to different treatment modalities.

Societal Factors

Self-injurious behaviors such as cutting may be a social phenomenon that is rampant in society. Individuals often learn about the behavior from a peer who is engaging in nonsuicidal self-injury and begin using the behaviors themselves in an attempt to alleviate personal discomfort. In fact, after an individual who engages in nonsuicidal self-injury is admitted to an inpatient unit, others on the unit begin to engage in the behavior.

CLINICAL PICTURE

Nonsuicidal self-injury is not an official disorder in the *DSM-5*. It is still under review to determine whether it will become a recognized disorder by the American Psychiatric Association. However, the behaviors associated with the disorder are often seen in both inpatient and outpatient settings.

APPLICATION OF THE NURSING PROCESS

There is limited research on the effectiveness of nursing care for patients who engage in nonsuicidal self-injury. However, holistic interdisciplinary approaches to care where patients are included in planning their care will likely lead to best outcomes.

ASSESSMENT

A history from the patient regarding the self-injurious behavior includes types of self-injury, triggers for the behavior, and frequency of the behavior (Tofthagen et al., 2014). Additionally, ask the patient what has worked effectively in stopping the behaviors in the past. Appropriate physical assessment to determine the condition of wounds, if present, allows you to plan appropriate interventions.

Self-Assessment

Nurses caring for patients who engage in self-injury report that they are emotionally affected by caring for these patients. Emotions experienced include feeling defeated by relapses, discouragement, and powerlessness (Tofthagen et al., 2014). Additionally, nurses need to be aware that transference may occur through projection of the patient's emotions onto the nurse. Establishing appropriate professional boundaries with the patient is important for self-care, as is collaboration with other clinicians.

DIAGNOSIS

The nursing diagnoses with the highest priorities are *Self-mutilation* and *Risk for self-mutilation.* Patients may be experiencing feelings of anxiety, tension, and self-reproach. Consider any nursing diagnosis that is appropriate for underlying comorbid psychiatric as appropriate (see the clinical chapters dealing with these diagnoses for further information).

OUTCOMES CRITERIA

The relevant *Nursing Outcomes Classification (NOC)* is *Mutilation self-restraint,* which is defined as "personal actions to refrain from intentional self-inflicted injury" (Moorhead et al., 2013, p. 369). Measurements for this outcome include:

- Refrains from gathering means for self-injury
- Obtains assistance as needed
- Refrains from injuring self
- Uses available support groups
- Uses medication as prescribed
- Uses effective coping strategies

PLANNING

The plan of care for individuals who engage in self-injury includes demonstration of a caring attitude toward the patient, bearing hope for recovery, observing for signs of self-harm, evaluating the need for medication, and providing appropriate interventions for patients' wounds and injuries. Engage patients in their recovery plan, which encompasses a six-step approach to recovery including: (1) limit setting for safety, (2) developing self-esteem, (3) discovery of the motive for self-injury and the role it served for the patient, (4) learning that self-injury can be self-controlled, (5) replacing the self-injury with coping skills, and (6) entering a maintenance phase (Gonzales & Bergstrom, 2013).

INTERVENTIONS

Basic nursing interventions for patients with nonsuicidal self-injury include caring for the patient's wounds and injuries, establishing a therapeutic alliance, and teaching coping skills to replace the self-injurious behaviors. A therapeutic relationship will provide support and an alternative to self-injury when anxiety increases.

Advanced practice psychiatric-mental health nurses may work with patients who use self-injury to cope. Currently, there are no evidence-based practices for treating this disorder. Psychotherapeutic interventions for this population should facilitate the patient's ability to learn coping strategies. Specific therapies that are used include cognitive behavioral therapy, dialectical behavior therapy, and group therapy. Treating underlying psychiatric disorders using psychopharmacology is an additional role of the advanced practice nurse.

EVALUATION

Similar to suicidal behavior, the evaluation of patients with nonsuicidal self-injury behaviors is ongoing. The development of a therapeutic alliance with the patient allows for the patient to trust the care provider. The nurse must continue to evaluate whether the patient is communicating his or her thoughts and feelings accurately and whether the patient's perception is that engagement in the behaviors is declining while being replaced with appropriate coping skills.

KEY POINTS TO REMEMBER

- Suicide is a significant public health problem in the United States and should be approached as a "never event."
- Specific biological, psychosocial, and cultural factors increase the risk of suicide.
- Treating the coexisting psychiatric disorder may help most patients with suicidal ideation.
- Certain health conditions and psychiatric diagnoses are associated with increased risk for suicide.
- Every suicide attempt must be taken seriously even if the person has a history of multiple attempts.
- Nursing care of the patient who is suicidal is challenging but rewarding. Patients' desperate feelings evoke intense reactions in staff, but most people with suicidal behaviors respond to treatment and do not complete suicide.
- If a patient completes suicide, family, friends, and healthcare workers are traumatized and need postvention in terms of support, possibly including referrals for psychiatric treatment.
- Nonsuicidal self-injury is a problem that is becoming increasingly important, especially among young people.
- Treatment of patients with suicidal and nonsuicidal self-injury behaviors involves an interdisciplinary team working together to implement plans of care developed with support of the patient's family and friends.

CRITICAL THINKING

1. Locate and review the suicide protocol at your hospital unit or community center. Are there any steps you anticipate having difficulty carrying out? Discuss these difficulties with your peers or clinical group.
2. How would you respond to another staff member who expresses guilt over the completed suicide of a patient on your unit?
3. Identify three common and expected emotional reactions that a nurse might have when initially working with persons who manifest suicidal behavior disorder.
   a. How do you think you might react?
   b. What actions could you take to deal with the event and obtain support?

CHAPTER REVIEW

Questions

1. Which patient statement does not demonstrate an understanding of a suicide safety plan?
   a. "I know that when I start thinking about my dad, I'm going to start thinking about killing myself."
   b. "Going for a really long, hard run helps clear my mind and stops the suicidal thoughts."
   c. "My sister is always there for me when I start getting suicidal."
   d. "I keep the suicide prevention phone number in my wallet."
2. Which interventions will help make the environment on the unit safer for suicidal patients? *Select all that apply.*
   a. All windows are kept locked.
   b. Every shower has a breakaway shower rod.
   c. Eating utensils are counted when trays are collected.
   d. Patient doors are kept open.
   e. Staying within listening distance of the patient.
3. What are the nursing responsibilities to a patient expressing suicidal thoughts? *Select all that apply.*
   a. Instituting one-to-one observation.
   b. Documenting the patient's whereabouts and mood every 15 to 30 minutes.
   c. Ensuring that the patient has no contact with glass or metal utensils.
   d. Ensuring that patient has swallowed each individual dose of medication.
   e. Discussing triggers of depression.
4. When considering community suicide prevention programs, what population should the nurse plan to service with regular suicide screenings? *Select all that apply.*
   a. 10- to 34-year-olds
   b. Males
   c. College-educated adults
   d. Rural population
   e. Native American
5. Research supports which intervention implemented on a long-term basis significantly reduces the incidence of suicide and suicide attempts in a patient diagnosed with bipolar disorder?
   a. A selective serotonin reuptake inhibitor (SSRI)
   b. Electroconvulsive therapy (ECT)
   c. One-on-one observation
   d. Lithium
6. Gladys is seeing a therapist because her husband committed suicide 6 months ago. Gladys tells her therapist, "I know he was in pain, but why didn't he leave me a note?" The therapist's best response would be:
   a. "He probably acted quickly on his impulse to kill himself."
   b. "He did not want to think about the pain he would cause you."
   c. "He was not able to think clearly due to his emotional pain."
   d. "He thought you may think it was an accident if there was no note."

7. Martin is a 23-year-old male with a new diagnosis of schizophrenia, and his family is receiving information from a home health nurse. The topic of education is suicide prevention, and the nurse recognizes effective teaching when the mother says:
   a. "Persons with schizophrenia rarely commit suicide."
   b. "Suicide risk is greatest in the first few years after diagnosis."
   c. "Suicide is not common in schizophrenia due to confusion."
   d. "Most persons diagnosed with schizophrenia die of suicide."
8. Sigmund Freud, Karl Menninger, and Aaron Beck theorized that hopelessness was an integral part of why a person commits suicide. A more recent theory suggest suicide results from:
   a. Elevated serotonin levels
   b. The diathesis-stress model
   c. Outward aggression turned inward
   d. A lack of perfectionism
9. Which person is at the highest risk for suicide?
   a. A 50-year-old married white male with depression who has a plan to overdose if circumstances at work do not improve.
   b. A 45-year-old married white female who recently lost her parents, suffers from bipolar disorder, and attempted suicide once as a teenager.
   c. A young single white male who is alcohol dependent, hopeless, impulsive, has just been rejected by his girlfriend, and has ready access to a gun he has hidden.
   d. An older Hispanic male who is Catholic, is living with a debilitating chronic illness, is recently widowed, and who states, "I wish that God would take me too."
10. Kara is a 23-year-old patient admitted with depression and suicidal ideation. Which intervention(s) would be therapeutic for Kara? *Select all that apply.*
   a. Focus primarily on developing solutions to the problems leading the patient to feel suicidal.
   b. Assess the patient thoroughly and reassess the patient at regular intervals as levels of risk fluctuate.
   c. Avoid talking about the suicidal ideation as this may increase the patient's risk for suicidal behavior.
   d. Meet regularly with the patient to provide opportunities for the patient to express and explore feelings.
   e. Administer antidepressant medications cautiously and conservatively because of their potential to increase the suicide risk in Kara's age group.
   f. Help the patient to identify positive self-attributes and to question negative self-perceptions that are unrealistic.

Answers

1. **b;** 2. **a, b, c, d;** 3. **a, b, c, d;** 4. **a, b, e;** 5. **d;** 6. **c;** 7. **b;** 8. **b;** 9. **c;** 10. **b, d, e, f**

Visit the Evolve website for a posttest on the content in this chapter: http://evolve.elsevier.com/Varcarolis

Post-Test interactive review

REFERENCES

Ahmedani, B., Simon, G., Stewart, C., Beck, A., Waitzfelder, B., Rossom, R., et al. (2014). Health care contacts in the year before suicide death. *Journal of General Internal Medicine*, 29(6), 870–877.

American Association of Suicidology. (2014). *Facts and statistics.* Retrieved from http://www.suicidology.org/resources/facts-statistics.

American Foundation for Suicide Prevention. (2015). *Suicide statistics.* Retrieved from http://afsp.org/about-suicide/suicide-statistics/.

American Psychiatric Association. (2013). *Diagnostic and statistical manual of mental disorders* (5th ed.). Washington, DC: Author.

Arias, S. A., Dumas, O., Sullivan, A. F., Boudreaux, E. D., Miller, I., & Camargo, C. A. (2016). Substance use as a mediator of the association between demographics, suicide attempt history, and future suicide attempts in emergency department patients. *Crisis, 37*(4).

Bracken-Minor, K., & McDevitt-Murphy, M. (2014). Differences in features of non-suicidal self-injury according to borderline personality disorder screening status. *Archives of Suicide Research, (18)*, 88–103.

Brown, J., & Johns, D. (2015). Suicide and race. *SAMHSA*. Retrieved from http://blog.samhsa.gov/2015/07/28/suicide-and-race/#.VqvhQlInj2A.

Centers for Disease Control and Prevention. (2015). *Suicide facts at a glance: 2015.* Retrieved from http://www.cdc.gov/violenceprevention/pdf/suicide-datasheet-a.pdf.

Centers for Disease Control and Prevention. (2016). *Injury prevention and control: Data and statistics.* Retrieved from http://webappa.cdc.gov/cgi-bin/broker.exe.

Fawcett, J. (2013). Suicide and anxiety in DSM-5. *Depression and Anxiety, 30*, 898–901.

Goldberg, J. (2016). *Schizophrenia and suicide. Web MD.* Retrieved from http://www.webmd.com/schizophrenia/guide/schizophrenia-and-suicide?page=2.

Gonzales, A., & Bergstrom, L. (2013). Adolescent non-suicidal self-injury (NSSI) interventions. *Journal of Child and Adolescent Psychiatric Nursing, 26*, 124–130.

Guintivano, J., Brown, T., Newcomer, A., Jones, M., Cox, O., Maher, B., et al. (2014). Identification and replication of a combined epigenetic and genetic biomarker predicting suicide and suicidal behaviors. *American Journal of Psychiatry, 171*(12), 1287–1296.

Han, B., Compton, W., Gfroerer, J., & McKeon, R. (2014). Mental health treatment patterns among adults with recent suicide attempts in the United States. *American Journal of Public Health, 104*(12), 2359–2368.

Hogan, M., & Grumet, J. G. (2016). Suicide prevention: An emerging priority for health care. *Health Affairs, 35*(6), 1084–1090.

Melhem, N.M., Day, N., Shear, M.K., Day, R., Reynolds, CF., & Brent, D. (2004). Traumatic grief among adolescents exposed to a peer's suicide. *American Journal of Psychiatry*, 161, 1411–1416.

Moorhead, S., Johnson, M., Maas, M. L., & Swanson, E. (2013). *Nursing outcomes classification (NOC)* (5th ed.). St. Louis, MO: Mosby.

Nock, M., Stein, M., Heeringa, S., Ursano, R., Colpe, L., Fullerton, C., et al. (2014). Prevalence and correlates of suicidal behavior among soldiers: Results from the Army Study to Assess Risk and Resilience in Service members (Army STARRS). *Journal of the American Medical Association Psychiatry, 71*, 514–522.

Quinnett, P. (2007). *QPR gatekeeper training for suicide prevention: the model, rationale, and theory. Unpublished manuscript.* Retrieved from http://www.uwlax.edu/conted/pdf/2012QPRtheoryPaper.pdf.

Tofthagen, R., Talseth, A., & Lisbeth, F. (2014). Mental health nurses' experiences of caring for patients suffering from self-harm. *Nursing Research and Practice (2014), Article ID 905741.*

26

Crisis and Disaster

Margaret Jordan Halter

Visit the Evolve website for a pretest on the content in this chapter: http://evolve.elsevier.com/Varcarolis **Pre-Test** interactive review

OBJECTIVES

1. Identify the three types of crises and provide an example of each.
2. Identify six aspects of crisis that have relevance for nurses involved in crisis intervention.
3. Compare and contrast the differences among primary, secondary, and tertiary intervention including appropriate intervention strategies.
4. Explain to a classmate four potential crisis situations that patients may experience in hospital settings.
5. Provide concrete examples of interventions to minimize crisis situations.
6. List at least five resources in the community that could be used as referrals for a patient in crisis.
7. Recognize disaster occurrences and management as global concerns.
8. Differentiate among disaster types.

OUTLINE

KEY TERMS AND CONCEPTS

adventitious crisis
crisis intervention
disaster
equilibrium
homeostasis
maturational crisis
mitigation
primary care
recovery
response
secondary care
situational crisis
tertiary care

A hurricane rips into a coastline, levees fail, 80% of a major city floods, and nearly 2000 die. A 29-year-old man enters a crowded nightclub and begins shooting indiscriminately in the name of religion resulting in the deaths of 50 people. A nursing student discovers she is pregnant and the father of the baby has abandoned her. All of these situations signal the beginning of a crisis.

In this chapter, we will discuss characteristics of crisis, theoretical models regarding crisis, types of crises, and phases of crisis. Nursing care for people experiencing severe events will also be described here. This nursing care is based on the principle of **crisis intervention**, a directive, time-limited, and goal-directed strategy designed to assist individuals who are experiencing a crisis. It has been shown to be effective in helping people adaptively cope with stressful events. Knowledge of crisis intervention techniques is an important skill of all nurses no matter the practice specialty or clinical setting.

CRISIS CHARACTERISTICS

The human organism's internal environment maintains a relatively stable state while interacting with external forces. This stable state is referred to as **homeostasis** or **equilibrium**. A **crisis,** which is a major disturbance caused by a stressful event or threat, disrupts this homeostasis. In a crisis normal coping mechanisms fail resulting in an inability to function as usual. Equilibrium is replaced by disequilibrium.

A successful outcome for a crisis depends on (1) the realistic perception of the event, (2) adequate situational supports, and (3) adequate coping mechanisms.

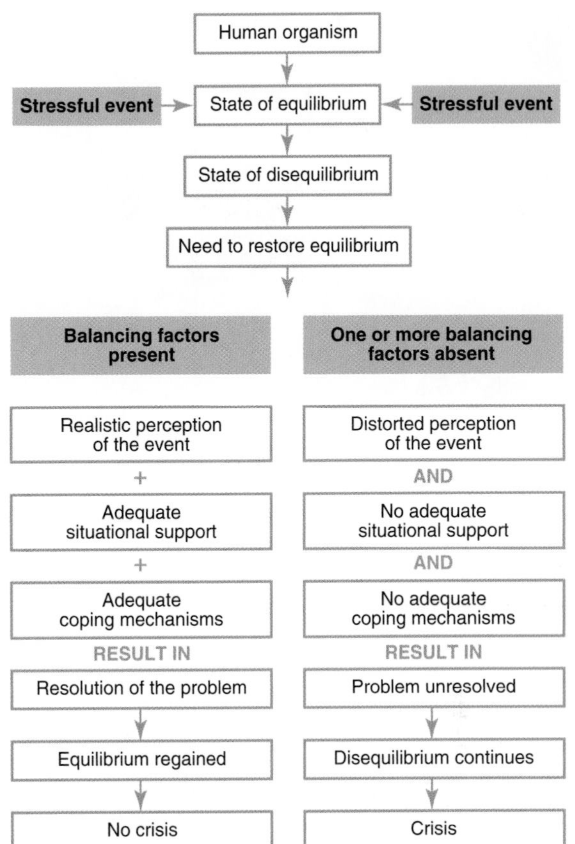

FIG. 26.1 Paradigm: The effect of balancing factors in a stressful event. (From Aguilera, D. C. [1998]. *Crisis intervention: Theory and methodology* [8th ed.]. St. Louis, MO: Mosby.)

Perception of the Event

An important concept associated with crisis is that of individual perception, which may range from realistic to distorted. The perception of threat is based on a person's unique perspective and coping abilities.

People vary in the way they absorb, process, and use information from the environment. Some people may respond to a minor event as if it were life threatening. Conversely, others may assess a life-threatening event and carefully consider options. For example, 10-year-old twins Amy and Annie's parents are divorcing. Amy's grades plummet, she becomes despondent and has trouble sleeping. Annie, on the other hand, announces to her friends, "We get to move, I'll have a new bedroom that I can paint, and we will be able to walk to school."

Situational Support

Situational support includes all the people who are available that can be depended upon to help during the time of a crisis. Nurses and other health professionals who use crisis intervention are providing situational support.

Coping Mechanisms

Coping mechanisms and skills are acquired through a variety of sources, such as cultural responses, modeling behaviors of others, and life opportunities that broaden experience and promote the adaptive development of new coping responses. Many factors compromise a person's ability to cope with a crisis event. These may include the number of other stressful life events with which the person is currently coping, other unresolved losses, concurrent psychiatric disorders or medical problems, excessive fatigue or pain, and the quality and quantity of a person's usual coping skills.

A depiction of two potential responses to a stressful event is illustrated in Fig. 26.1

A crisis may pose a threat to personality organization, but it also presents an opportunity for personal growth, development, and change. Successful crisis resolution results from the development of adaptive coping mechanisms, reflects ego development, and suggests the employment of physiological, psychological, and social resources.

CRISIS THEORY

On November 28, 1942, one of the deadliest single-building fires in history occurred. A nightclub, the Cocoanut Grove in Boston, was filled beyond capacity with more than 1000 people. When a fire broke out, people ran to the main entrance, which was a single revolving door. The door quickly became jammed with people and unusable. Other inward swinging exit doors trapped crowds as they desperately tried to escape. Laws requiring outward swinging exit doors were enacted as a result of this fire.

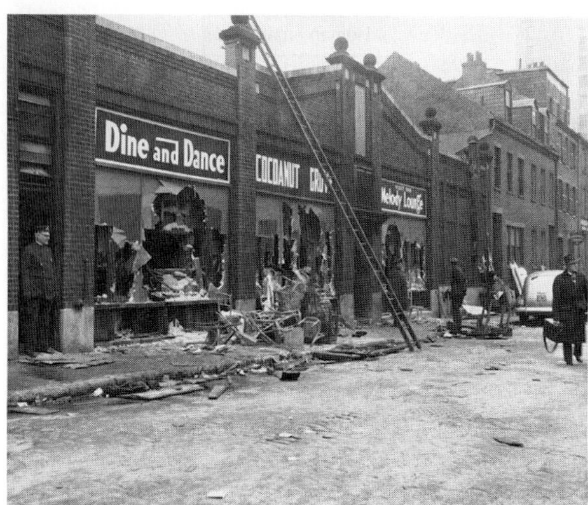

Cocoanut Grove Nightdub after the fire. (Photo by United States Army Signal Corps on November 30, 1942. Courtesy of the Trustees of the Boston Public Library/Print Department at http://www.bpl.org [CC-BY-NC-ND 2.0].)

Erick Lindemann, a Boston psychiatrist, conducted a classic study of the close relatives and friends of the 492 victims of the fire. This study formed the foundation of crisis theory and clinical intervention. He concluded that immediate behavioral responses to crisis were not abnormal or pathological. Rather, they were predictable and normal grief behaviors that consisted of:

- Preoccupation with the lost one
- Identification with the lost one
- Expressions of guilt and hostility
- Disorganization in daily routine
- Somatic complaints

Lindemann (1944) proposed that interventions could eliminate or decrease potential serious personality disorganization in the immediate aftermath of the crisis. He believed that the same interventions that were helpful in bereavement—brief therapy and grief work—would prove just as helpful in dealing with other types of stressful events.

Gerald Caplan (1964) expanded crisis theory to all traumatic events and outlined crisis intervention strategies. His theory is grounded in the concept of homeostasis and returning the individual to a state of equilibrium. He noticed that psychiatric patients dealt with crises in a maladaptive manner and ended up less healthy than before the crisis. Caplan believed that personal and social resources were the key to preventing deterioration after a time of crisis.

Numerous contemporary clinicians and theorists continue to redefine and enhance our understanding of crisis and effective intervention continues (Behrman & Reid, 2002; Roberts, 2005). The 1961 report of the Joint Commission on Mental Illness and Health addressed the need for community mental health centers throughout the country. This report stimulated the establishment of crisis services, which are now an important part of mental health programs in hospitals and communities.

Roberts's seven-stage model of crisis interventions (Fig. 26.2; Roberts & Ottens, 2005) is a useful model in helping individuals who have suffered from an acute crisis. It is also used with people who are diagnosed with acute stress disorder.

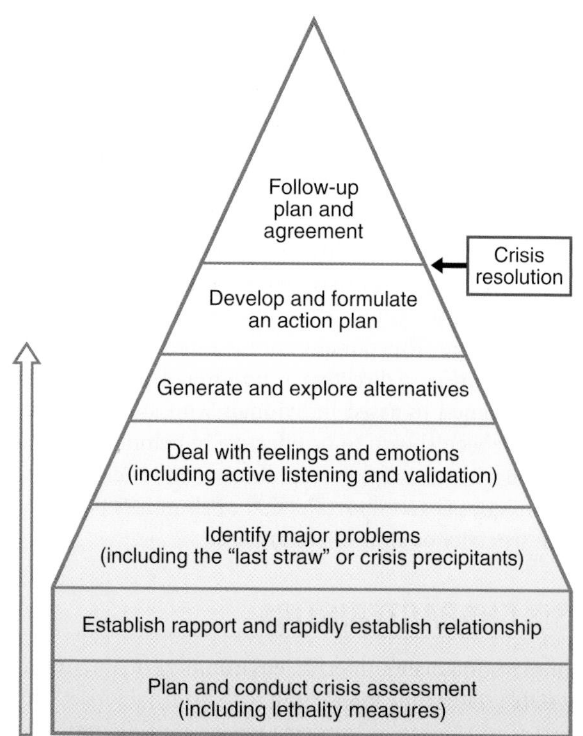

FIG. 26.2 Roberts's seven-stage model of crisis intervention. (From Roberts, A. R., & Ottens, A. J. [2005]. The seven-stage crisis intervention model: A road map to goal attainment, problem solving, and crisis resolution. *Brief Treatment and Crisis Intervention, 5,* 329–339.)

TYPES OF CRISIS

An understanding of the types and phases of crises lays the groundwork for the application of the nursing process. There are three basic types of crisis situations: (1) maturational (or developmental) crises, (2) situational crises, and (3) adventitious crises. Identifying which type of crisis the individual is experiencing or has experienced helps in the development of a patient-centered plan of care.

Maturational Crisis

A process of maturation occurs across the lifespan. Erik Erikson (1902–1994) conceptualized this process as eight stages of ego growth and development (refer to Table 2.6 in Chapter 2). Each stage represents a time when physical, cognitive, instinctual, and sexual changes prompt an internal conflict or crisis, which results in either psychosocial growth or regression. Therefore each developmental stage represents a developmental, or **maturational crisis.**

When a person reaches a new stage, coping styles are no longer effective, and new coping mechanisms have yet to be developed. Thus for a time the person is without effective defenses. This often leads to increased tension and anxiety, which may manifest as variations in the person's normal behavior. Examples of events that can precipitate a maturational crisis include leaving home for the first time, marriage, the birth of a child, retirement, and the death of a parent.

Erikson believed that the way these crises are resolved at one stage affects the person's ability to pass through subsequent stages. Each crisis provides the starting point for movement toward the next stage. If a person lacks support systems and adequate role models, successful resolution may be difficult or may not occur. Unresolved problems in the past and inadequate coping mechanisms adversely affect what is learned in each developmental stage. When a person experiences severe difficulty during a maturational crisis, professional intervention may be indicated.

Factors may disrupt individuals' progression through the maturational stages. For example, alcohol and drug addiction disrupts progression through the maturational stages. Unfortunately, this interruption occurs too often among individuals during their adolescent years. When the addictive behavior is controlled (e.g., by the late teens or mid-20s), the young person's growth and development resume at the point of interruption. For example, a young person whose addiction is arrested at 22 years of age may have the psychosocial and problem-solving skills of a 14-year-old. Often these teenagers do not receive treatment and have impaired or absent adult coping skills.

Situational Crisis

A **situational crisis** arises from events that are extraordinary, external rather than internal, and often unanticipated. Examples of events that can precipitate a situational crisis include the loss or change of a job, the death of a loved one, an abortion, a change in financial status, divorce, and severe physical or mental illness.

Whether or not these events precipitate a crisis, again, depends on factors such as the degree of support available from caring friends, family members, and others. General emotional and physical status also impacts our ability to tolerate stressful events.

Adventitious Crisis

An **adventitious crisis** is not a part of everyday life. It is caused by events that are unplanned and may be accidental, caused by nature, or human-made. This type of crisis results from (1) a natural **disaster** (e.g., flood, fire, earthquake), (2) a national disaster (e.g., acts of terrorism, war, riots, airplane crashes), or (3) a crime of violence (e.g., rape, assault or murder in the workplace or school, bombing in crowded areas, spousal or child abuse).

Serious post-trauma responses include acute stress disorder, posttraumatic stress disorder, and major depressive disorder. Psychological first aid through crisis intervention and debriefing can reduce the incidence of these disorders.

It is also possible to experience more than one type of crisis situation simultaneously, and as expected, the presence of more than one crisis further taxes individual coping skills. Consider a 51-year-old woman who may be going through a midlife crisis (maturational) when her husband dies suddenly of cancer (situational). Think about the survivors of Hurricane Katrina in 2005, many of whom were members of vulnerable groups—racial, social, and financial—and may have been experiencing maturational or situational crises prior to the hurricane. They were then confronted with the devastation of the hurricane and the simultaneous onset of multiple losses. Many of them lost family members and friends, homes and belongings, employment, the loss of jobs, community supports, and even personal identification.

PHASES OF CRISIS

Through extensive study of individuals experiencing crisis, Caplan (1964) identified behaviors that followed a fairly distinct path. These behaviors were categorized in four phases of crisis.

Phase 1

A person confronted by a conflict or problem that threatens his or her self-concept responds with increased feelings of anxiety. The increase in anxiety stimulates the use of problem-solving techniques and defense mechanisms in an effort to address the problem and lower anxiety.

Phase 2

If the usual defensive response fails and the threat persists, anxiety continues to rise and produce rising levels of discomfort. Individual functioning becomes disorganized. Trial-and-error attempts at solving the problem and restoring balance begin.

Phase 3

If the trial-and-error attempts fail, anxiety can escalate to severe and panic levels. The person mobilizes automatic relief behaviors, such as withdrawal and flight. The individual may make some form of resolution such as compromising needs or redefining the situation to reach an acceptable solution in this stage.

Phase 4

If the problem is not solved and new coping skills are ineffective, anxiety can overwhelm the person and lead to serious personality disorganization, depression, confusion, violence against others, or suicidal behavior.

APPLICATION OF THE NURSING PROCESS

Nurses, perhaps more than any other group of health professionals, deal with people who are experiencing disruption in their lives. Because people typically experience increased stress and anxiety in medical, surgical, and psychiatric situations, nurses are often positioned to initiate and participate in crisis intervention. Crisis theory defines aspects of crisis that are basic to crisis intervention and relevant for nurses (Box 26.1).

ASSESSMENT

General Assessment

Components of crisis assessment come from established crisis theory and constitute a sound knowledge base for the application of the nursing process. Data gained from the assessment guide both the nurse and the patient in setting realistic and meaningful goals and in planning possible solutions to the problem situation.

BOX 26.1 Foundation for Crisis Intervention

- A crisis is self-limiting and usually resolves within 4 to 6 weeks.
- At the resolution of a crisis, the patient will emerge at one of three different functional levels:
  - A higher level of functioning.
  - The same level of functioning.
  - A lower level of functioning.
- The goal of crisis intervention is to return the patient to at least the precrisis level of functioning.
- The form of crisis resolution depends on the patient's actions and others' interventions.
- During a crisis, people are often more receptive than usual to outside intervention. With intervention, the patient can learn different adaptive means of problem solving to correct inadequate solutions.
- The patient in a crisis situation is assumed to be mentally healthy, to have functioned well in the past, and to be presently in a state of disequilibrium.
- Crisis intervention deals only with the patient's present problem and resolution of the immediate crisis (e.g., the "here and now").
- The nurse must be willing to take an active, even directive, role in intervention, which is in direct contrast to conventional therapeutic intervention that stresses a more passive and nondirective role.
- Early intervention probably increases the chances for a good prognosis.
- Encourage the patient to set realistic goals and plan a focused intervention with the nurse.

A crisis may result in such serious disorganization and discomfort that ending the pain may feel like a reasonable solution. The nurse's initial task is to assess the patient's potential for suicide. Sample questions to ask include:

- Have you thought about hurting yourself?
- Have you thought of how you would do this?
- Do you feel you can keep yourself safe?

After assessing safety and intervening appropriately, the nurse assesses the three main areas previously discussed: (1) the patient's perception of the precipitating event, (2) the patient's situational supports, and (3) the patient's personal coping skills.

VIGNETTE: Madison, a 25-year-old woman, is brought to the emergency department by police after being beaten by her husband. Madison is seen by the medical personnel and then interviewed by the psychiatric-mental health registered nurse working in the emergency department. The nurse calmly introduces herself and tells Madison she would like to talk with her. The nurse says, "It looks as if things are overwhelming. Is that how you're feeling?" Madison is slumped in the chair, her hands in her lap, head hanging down, and has tears in her eyes. She nods.

Assessing Perception of Precipitating Event

The nurse's task is now to assess the individual's perception of the problem. The more clearly the person can define the problem, the more likely the person will identify effective solutions. Sample questions and comments that facilitate the assessment include the following:

- What leads you to seek help now?
- Has anything upsetting happened to you within the past few days or weeks?
- Describe how you are feeling right now.
- How does this situation affect your life?
- How do you see this event affecting your future?
- What do you hope to get out of this treatment?

VIGNETTE: Nurse: "Madison, tell me what happened."

Madison: "I can't go home..., I am so afraid..., No one believes me..., I can't go through it again."

Nurse: "Tell me what you can't go through again."

(Madison starts to cry, shaking with sobs. The nurse sits quietly for a moment and then speaks.)

Nurse: "Tell me what is so terrible. Let's look at it together."

After a while, Madison tells the nurse that her husband beats her regularly, and he becomes particularly brutal when he drinks. The beatings have become much worse over time. Madison states, "I'm afraid that he'll eventually kill me."

Assessing Situational Supports

Next, the nurse determines resources by assessing the patient's support systems. When available, family and friends can be involved by offering emotional or material support. If these resources are unavailable, the nurse acts as a temporary support person while assisting the patient to establish relationships with individuals or groups in the community. Sample questions include the following:

- Is there anyone—family or friends—you would like to have involved in your care?
- Have you ever used a community agency for support?
- Do you have a religious affiliation?
- Are you active in a religious group?

VIGNETTE: Nurse: "Madison, what are your options? Do you have any family who can support you?"

Madison: "No. My family is in another state."

Nurse: "How about friends?"

Madison: "I really don't have any friends. My husband's jealousy has made it impossible for me to have friends. He finds fault with everyone."

Nurse: "What about your co-workers?"

Madison: "My co-workers are nice, but I can't tell them things like this."

The nurse learns that Madison does well at her job. Madison explains that her job helps her forget her problems for a little while. Getting good job reviews also has another reward: It is the only time her husband says anything nice about her.

Assessing Coping Skills

Finally, the nurse assesses the patient's coping skills. Common positive coping mechanisms may be seeking out someone to talk to, writing feelings in a journal, or engaging in other physical activity. Ineffective coping includes overeating, drinking, smoking, withdrawing, yelling, and fighting. Sample questions to ask include the following:

- What have you been doing to relieve the anxiety you have been feeling?
- What has helped in the past to relieve stress?
- Did you try it this time? If so, what was different?
- What helped you through difficult times in the past?

VIGNETTE: Nurse: "You've been through an emotionally painful time. Your anxiety is understandable. What has helped you in the past to make you feel more calm?"

Madison: "I don't know. Probably talking."

Nurse: "Okay. While you're here, we will talk for at least 30 minutes each day. In group therapy, you will have the chance to share what you've been going through and also hear about how others cope."

Madison: "Thanks. I don't want to be in an abusive marriage. I just don't know where to turn."

Nurse: "I understand. We will work together to come up with a plan."

Self-Assessment

Nurses need to monitor and acknowledge personal feelings and thoughts when dealing with patients in crisis. Even experienced nurses working in disaster situations can become overwhelmed when witnessing catastrophic loss of human life (e.g., acts of terrorism, plane crashes, school shootings) and/or mass destruction of homes and belongings (e.g., floods, fires, tornadoes). In fact, researchers find that mental healthcare providers may experience psychological distress from working with traumatized populations and may even develop posttraumatic stress disorder.

Debriefing is an important step for staff in coming to terms with overwhelmingly violent or otherwise disastrous situations. Such an intervention helps staff put the crisis in perspective and begin their own recovery. Debriefing is discussed in detail later in the chapter.

ASSESSMENT GUIDELINES

Crisis

1. Determine whether the patient is able to identify the *precipitating event.*
2. Assess the patient's understanding of *situational supports.*
3. Identify the patient's usual *coping styles,* and determine what coping mechanisms may help the present situation.
4. Determine whether there are certain religious or cultural beliefs that need to be considered in assessing and intervening in this patient's crisis.
5. Assess whether this situation is one in which the patient needs primary intervention (education, environmental manipulation, or new coping skills), secondary intervention (crisis intervention), or tertiary intervention (rehabilitation).

DIAGNOSIS

The North American Nursing Diagnosis Association International (NANDA-I; Herdman & Kamitsuru, 2014) provides nursing diagnoses to consider for a person who is in crisis. The nursing diagnosis of *Ineffective coping* is often useful. Ineffective coping may be evidenced by inability to meet basic needs, inability to meet role expectations, alteration in social participation, use of inappropriate defense mechanisms, or impairment of usual patterns of communication. The related-to component will vary with the individual patient.

Anxiety related to a maturational, situational, or adventitious crisis is always present in moderate, severe, and panic levels. Severe and panic level anxiety will need to be addressed and reduced before learning more effective coping skills.

CONSIDERING CULTURE

Examining the Gun Culture in the United States

In 2012 Adam Lanza, 24, shot and killed his mother. He proceeded to an elementary school where he murdered 20 children and six staff members with semiautomatic weapons at Sandy Hook Elementary School in Connecticut. As police arrived, he shot himself in the head. The news videos portrayed terrified and sobbing children being led from the school holding hands. Pictures of the first-grade victims and their teachers were published in newspapers and shown on television. These innocent faces were so heartbreaking that many people could not bring themselves to look at them.

As the crisis unfolded, a debate ensued regarding gun control and the issue of a gun culture in the United States. One post on Facebook read, "Before you go blaming assault rifles for this tragedy, folks, he [Lanza] used handguns." Another said, "More people get killed by hammers and clubs than by rifles." A response to this post was, "If Lanza had walked into that school with a hammer, those six staff members could have taken him down."

The United States has a strong gun culture. The Second Amendment in the Constitution provides the legal right for the personal possession of arms. The Wild West is romanticized for its gun slinging. Wars are part of the fabric of our history. Guns are associated with strength and virility. A general argument is that if only bad people have guns, then good people cannot defend themselves.

Rights of gun owners are being challenged in unprecedented ways. In response to the shooting and ensuing crisis, President Barack Obama called for tighter regulations on assault rifles and magazines (clips) with multiple rounds and stringent background checks for people buying guns. People are paying increasing attention toward preventing people like Lanza, who was believed to have a psychiatric disorder, from having access to guns. Violent video games are associated with aggression and decreased prosocial behaviors (Greitemeyer & Mugge, 2014). These games have been on the radar for outright bans.

How this clash between the two cultures, the gun culture and gun-control culture, will play out is yet to be seen. The murders that took place in Sandy Hook Elementary dramatically energized a nation and will likely be a force for a change in laws that will impact the gun culture in the United States.

Greitemeyer, T., & Mugge, D. O. (2014). Video games do affect social outcomes. *Personality and Social Psychology Bulletin, 40*(5), 578–589.

OUTCOMES IDENTIFICATION

The planning of realistic outcomes is patient-centered and includes the patient and family, which result in outcomes congruent with the patient's cultural and personal values. Without the patient's involvement, the outcome criteria may be irrelevant or unacceptable solutions to that person's crisis. Table 26.1 identifies signs and symptoms commonly experienced in crises, offers potential nursing diagnoses, and suggests outcomes.

TABLE 26.1 Signs and Symptoms, Diagnoses, and Outcomes for Crisis Intervention

Signs and Symptoms	Nursing Diagnoses	Outcomes
Inability to meet basic needs, decreased use of social support, inadequate problem solving, inability to attend to information, isolation	*Ineffective coping*	Modifies lifestyle as needed, uses effective coping strategies, reports decrease in physical symptoms of stress, reports decrease in negative feelings
Denial, exaggerated startle response, flashbacks, horror, hypervigilance, intrusive thoughts and dreams, panic attacks, feeling numb, substance misuse, confusion, incoherence	*Posttrauma syndrome* *Rape-trauma syndrome*	Exhibits non-labile mood, impulse control; reports adequate sleep, exhibits concentration, tends to ADLs, shows interest in surroundings
Minimizes symptoms, delays seeking care, displays inappropriate affect, makes dismissive comments when speaking of distressing events	*Ineffective denial*	Recognizes reality of health situation, maintains relationships, copes with health situation, makes decisions about health, reports sense of life being worth living
Overwhelmed, depressed, states has nothing in life worthwhile, self-hatred, feelings of being ineffectual, sees limited alternatives, feels strange, perceives a lack of control	*Risk for suicide*	Remains free from harm, expresses feelings of self-worth, verbalizes sense of personal identity, expresses meaning in life, sets goals, believes that actions impact outcomes
Difficulty with interpersonal relationships, isolated, has few or no social supports	*Social isolation*	Expresses a sense of belonging, effects meaningful relationships
Changes in family relationships and functioning, difficulty performing family caregiver role	*Compromised family coping* *Caregiver role strain*	Manages family problems, expresses feelings openly among family members, respite for caregiver, sense of control for caregiver

From Herdman, T. H., & Kamitsuru, S. (Ed.). *Nursing diagnoses—Definitions and classification 2015–2017*. Copyright © 2014, 1994–2012 by NANDA International. Used by arrangement with John Wiley & Sons Limited; Moorhead, S., Johnson, M., Maas, M. L., & Swanson, E. (2013). *Nursing outcomes classification (NOC)* (5th ed.). St. Louis, MO: Elsevier.

PLANNING

Nurses are called upon to plan and intervene through a variety of crisis-intervention modalities. These modalities include disaster nursing, mobile crisis units, group work, health education and crisis prevention, victim outreach programs, and telephone hotlines. You may be involved in planning and intervention for an individual (e.g., cases of physical abuse), for a group (e.g., students after a classmate's suicide or shooting), or for a community (e.g., disaster nursing after tornadoes, shootings, and airplane crashes).

VIGNETTE: In a group meeting with the nurse and a social worker, Madison announces that she has made a decision to leave her husband and not return home. Madison, the nurse, and the social worker establish goals:
- Madison will return to her precrisis state within 2 weeks.
- Madison will find a safe environment.
- Madison will identify at least two outside supports within 24 hours.

IMPLEMENTATION

Psychosocial Interventions

Crisis intervention is a function of the psychiatric-mental health registered nurse. The focus is on the present problem only and has two initial goals:

1. **Patient safety.** You can apply external controls for protection of the patient in crisis if the patient is suicidal or homicidal.
2. **Anxiety reduction.** Use anxiety-reduction techniques so that the patient can mobilize inner resources.

During the initial interview, the patient in crisis first needs to gain a feeling of safety. Feelings of support and hope will temporarily diminish anxiety. The nurse needs to play an active role by indicating that help is available by using crisis-intervention skills competently and showing genuine interest and support.

The nurse may act as educator, advisor, and role model, always keeping in mind that it is the patient who solves the problem, not the nurse. The following are important assumptions when working with a patient in crisis:

- The patient is in charge of his or her own life.
- The patient is able to make decisions.
- The crisis counseling relationship is one between partners.

The nurse helps the patient to gain new perspectives on the situation. The nurse supports the patient during the process of finding constructive ways to solve or cope with the problem. It is important for the nurse to be mindful of how difficult it is for the patient to change behavior. Table 26.2 offers guidelines for nursing interventions and corresponding rationales.

Levels of Care

Psychotherapeutic crisis interventions are directed toward three levels of care: (1) primary, (2) secondary, and (3) tertiary.

Primary Care

Primary care promotes mental health and reduces mental illness to decrease the incidence of crisis. On this level the nurse can:

- Work with a patient to recognize potential problems by evaluating the patient's experience of stressful life events.
- Teach the patient specific coping skills, such as decision making, problem solving, assertiveness skills, meditation, and relaxation skills.
- Assist the patient in evaluating the timing or reduction of life changes to decrease the negative effects of stress as much as possible. This may involve working with a patient to plan environmental changes, make important interpersonal decisions, and rethink changes in occupational roles.

TABLE 26.2 Guidelines for Crisis Intervention

Intervention	Rationale
Assess for suicidal or homicidal thoughts or plans.	Safety is always the first consideration.
Take initial steps to make patient feel safe and less anxious.	A person who feels safe and less anxious is able to more effectively problem solve solutions with the nurse.
Listen carefully (e.g., make eye contact, give frequent feedback to verify and convey understanding, summarize what patient says).	A person who believes someone is really listening is more likely to believe that someone cares about his or her situation and that help may be available. This offers hope.
Crisis intervention calls for directive and creative approaches. Initially the nurse may make phone calls to arrange babysitters, schedule a visiting nurse, find shelter, or contact a social worker.	A person who is confused, frightened, or overwhelmed may be temporarily unable to perform usual tasks.
Identify needed social supports (with patient's input) and mobilize the priority.	Determine a person's need for shelter, help with care for children or elders, medical workup, emergency medical attention, hospitalization, food, safe housing, and self-help groups.
Identify needed coping skills (e.g., problem solving, relaxation, assertiveness, job training, newborn care, self-esteem building).	Increasing coping skills and learning new ones can help with current crisis and help minimize future crises.
Involve patient in identifying realistic, acceptable interventions.	The person's involvement in planning increases his or her sense of control, self-esteem, and adherence to plan.
Plan regular follow-up (e.g., phone calls, clinic visits, home visits) to assess patient's progress.	Evaluate the plan to see what works and what does not.

Secondary Care

Secondary care establishes intervention during an acute crisis to *prevent* prolonged anxiety from diminishing personal effectiveness and personality organization. The nurse's primary focus is to ensure the safety of the patient. After safety issues have been dealt with, the nurse works with the patient to assess the patient's problem, support systems, and coping styles. Desired goals are explored and interventions planned. Secondary care lessens the time a patient is mentally disabled during a crisis. Secondary care occurs in hospital units, emergency departments, clinics, or mental health centers, usually during daytime hours.

Tertiary Care

Tertiary care provides support for those who have experienced a severe crisis and are now recovering from a disabling mental state. Social and community facilities that offer tertiary intervention include rehabilitation centers, sheltered workshops, day hospitals, and outpatient clinics. Goals are to facilitate optimal levels of functioning and prevent further emotional disruptions. People with severe and persistent mental problems are often extremely susceptible to crisis, and community facilities provide the structured environment that can help prevent problem situations.

Box 26.2 lists the *Nursing Interventions Classification (NIC)* interventions for responding to a crisis (Bulechek et al., 2013).

Critical incident stress debriefing. **Critical incident stress debriefing (CISD)** is an example of a tertiary intervention directed toward a group that has experienced a crisis. CISD consists of a seven-phase group meeting that offers individuals the opportunity to share their thoughts and feelings in a safe and controlled environment. It is used to debrief staff on an inpatient unit following a patient suicide or an incident of violence, to debrief crisis hotline volunteers, to debrief schoolchildren and school personnel after multiple school shootings, and to debrief rescue and health care workers who have responded to a natural disaster or a terrorist attack such as that on the World Trade Center.

The phases of CISD are:

- *Introductory phase*—Meeting purpose is explained; an overview of the debriefing process is provided; confidentiality is ensured; guidelines are explained; team members are identified; and questions are answered.
- *Fact phase*—Participants discuss the facts of the incident; participants introduce themselves, tell their involvement in the incident, and describe the event from their perspective.
- *Thought phase*—Participants discuss their first thoughts of the incident.
- *Reaction phase*—Participants talk about the worst thing about the incident—what they would like to forget, what was most painful.
- *Symptom phase*—Participants describe their cognitive, physical, emotional, or behavioral experiences at the incident scene and describe any symptoms they felt following the initial experience.
- *Teaching phase*—The normality of the expressed symptoms is acknowledged and affirmed; anticipatory guidance is offered regarding future symptoms; the group is involved in stress-management techniques.
- *Reentry phase*—Participants review material discussed, introduce new topics, ask questions, and discuss how they would like to bring closure to the debriefing. Debriefing team members answer questions, inform, and reassure; provide written material; provide information on referral sources; and summarize the debriefing with encouragement, support, and appreciation.

VIGNETTE: After talking with the nurse and the social worker, Madison seems open to going to a safe house for battered women. She also agrees to talk to a counselor at a mental health facility. The nurse sets up an appointment at which she, Madison, and the counselor will meet.

BOX 26.2 Crisis Intervention

Definition: Use of short-term counseling to help the patient cope with a crisis and resume a state of functioning comparable to or better than the precrisis state.

Activities:

- Provide an atmosphere of support.
- Avoid giving false reassurances.
- Provide a safe haven.
- Determine whether the patient presents a safety risk to self or others.
- Initiate necessary precautions to safeguard the patient or others at risk for physical harm.
- Encourage expression of feelings in a nondestructive manner.
- Assist in identification of the precipitants and dynamics of the crisis.
- Encourage patient to focus on one implication at a time.
- Assist in identification of personal strengths and abilities that the patient can use in resolving the crisis.
- Assist in identification of past or present coping skills and their effectiveness.
- Assist in development of new coping and problem-solving skills as needed.
- Assist in identification of available support systems.
- Link the patient and family with community resources, as needed.
- Provide guidance about how to develop and maintain support systems.
- Introduce the patient to persons (or groups) who have successfully undergone the same experience.
- Assist in identification of alternative courses of action to resolve the crisis.
- Assist in evaluation of the possible consequences of the various courses of action.
- Assist the patient to decide on a particular course of action.
- Assist in formulating a time frame for implementation of the chosen course of action.
- Evaluate with the patient whether the crisis has been resolved by the chosen course of action.
- Plan with the patient how adaptive coping skills can be used to deal with crises in the future.

Adapted from Bulechek, G. M., Butcher, H. K., Dochterman, J. M., & Wagner, C. (2013). *Nursing interventions classification (NIC)* (6th ed.). St. Louis, MO: Mosby.

EVALUATION

NOC (Moorhead et al., 2013) includes a measurement for each outcome and for the indicators that support the outcome. Each indicator is measured on a 5-point Likert scale. When compared with a baseline measurement for the indicator, later measures help the nurse to evaluate the effectiveness of the crisis intervention. If the intervention has been successful, the patient's level of anxiety and ability to function should be at pre-crisis levels. Often, a patient chooses to follow up on additional areas of concern and is referred to other agencies for more long-term work. Crisis intervention frequently serves to prepare a patient for further treatment.

Modalities of Crisis Intervention

Crisis intervention can happen in almost any setting. Traditionally, people seeking emergency help go to hospitals. Unfortunately, not only are emergency rooms expensive, but they may also lack the time and staff with specialized training necessary to address patients' needs.

New models of providing emergency care are referred to, not surprisingly, as crisis care (Substance Abuse and Mental Health Service Administration, 2014). Examples of newer models include 23-hour observation, short-term crisis residential services, 24/7 crisis hotlines, warm lines, mobile crisis services, peer crisis services, and psychiatric advance directive plans. The evidence base for these services is growing, and research has shown that these services can have an impact on health care costs as well as quality of life.

- **23-hour crisis stabilization:** The goal of 23-hour crisis stabilization and observation is to quickly deescalate crisis situations and avoid unnecessary and costly hospitalizations. Patients are provided with specific referrals for outpatient care such as residential substance treatment or partial hospitalization programs.
- **Short-term crisis residential services:** Continuous 24-hour observation and supervision for people who do not require inpatient services are provided in short-term crisis residential services. The goal is to eliminate or reduce acute symptoms of psychiatric disorders. Participants are provided with a range of community-based resources and a safe environment for care and recovery.
- **24/7 crisis hotlines:** Telephone hotlines are an essential first-line intervention for people in acute crises. They can provide immediate responses from a variety of people—from professionals and trained volunteers. These confidential services do not require insurance and can link people with other community services.
- **Warm lines:** Similar to crisis hotlines, warm lines provide confidential telephone support. Unlike crisis hotlines, warm lines are not designed for crisis situations, but to prevent escalation of distress. This support service is provided by trained consumers, people who have experience using mental health services.
- **Mobile crisis service:** Mobile crisis teams provide acute crisis stabilization and psychiatric assessment services to people within their own homes and in other sites outside of traditional clinical settings. Staff includes a variety of mental health professionals such as counselors, social workers, and registered nurses. Typically, a psychiatrist or advanced practice psychiatric-mental health registered nurse is on-call. The goal of these mobile services is to provide a rapid response, resolve crisis situations, and prevent hospitalizations.
- **Peer crisis services:** Peer crisis services are provided by people who have had experience with living with a psychiatric disorder. Peers provide a calming environment, support, and links to psychiatric support. Services are intended to last less than 24 hours, but may be continued for several days.
- **Psychiatric advance directive plan:** A psychiatric advance directive plan is a proactive method of addressing a crisis situation before it occurs. Usually advance directives are used in end-of-life situations. In psychiatry these plans take the form of a document that is developed by the consumer to be used in crisis situations where the consumer is unable

to make decisions. It stipulates wishes such as treatment choices, treatment facilities, providers, and designates a support person who can be involved in decision making.

Sometimes crises involve people with mental illnesses interfacing with law enforcement as police officers serve on the front lines in responding to mental health crises. Many states have set up specialized **crisis intervention team** (CIT) training programs to prepare police officers to react appropriately to situations involving mental illness. In the United Kingdom, the Ride-Along Model allows a police officer and a mental health clinician to jointly respond to distressed consumers in the community (Boscarato et al., 2014).

Disaster Response

There is a growing awareness of interdependencies that exist among all members of the global community. Each successive large-scale earthquake, tsunami, hurricane, flood, or wildfire has ripple effects regardless of where in the world it occurs. Directly or remotely, we experience some element of the far-reaching depletion of human, economic, and natural resources. Consider the declining values of international stocks, illness-ravaged citizens in Haiti, or the devastation of flood victims on the US Gulf Coast.

A decade of 21st-century disaster literature supports disaster preparedness by developing resilient communities and assessing disaster risks on a local level. Considering the unique forms of devastation connected with any disaster, reducing risk within local communities should be expedient, eventually extending into networking communities then to larger societal and national programs (Federal Emergency Management Agency [FEMA], 2012).

Professional nurses regularly provide strong and dynamic core contributions to the multiple facets of disaster and recovery relief efforts around the world. Professional nurses are experienced care providers and managers of care, adaptable with critical thinking and problem-solving expertise. Also, professional nurses are visibly emerging around the world both as disaster researchers and authors and as pivotal spokespeople in disaster management planning arenas.

Each catastrophic event will set in operation a five-phase disaster management continuum including the following:

1. **Preparedness:** The protective plan designed before the event to structure the response, assess risk, and evaluate damage.
2. **Mitigation:** Attempt to limit a disaster's impact on human health and community function.
3. **Response:** Actual implementation of the disaster plan.
4. **Recovery:** Actions focus on stabilizing the community and returning it to its previous status.
5. **Evaluation:** Evaluating the response effort to prepare for the future (FEMA, 2012).

Any unexpected occurrences that create needs beyond the capabilities of victims to address without assistance will result in crisis experiences. Everyone experiences a crisis at some time.

Disaster Management Context

On November 25, 2002, the events of 9/11 prompted the creation of a government cabinet, the Department of Homeland Security (DHS). Its charge was to coordinate responses to US disasters, particularly in situations where local and state resources were inadequate to the presenting challenges. As a result, the DHS has ultimate governmental responsibility for the safety of US citizens and territories while ensuring adequate preparedness, response, and recovery protocols are immediately available.

To achieve its objectives, the DHS uses civilian first responders, local emergency response professionals who prepare for and respond to natural disasters or terrorist threats or any other large-scale event. In 2004 DHS furthered its agenda and created the National Incident Management System (NIMS) to help first responders from different disciplines and areas to effectively work together when a community exhausts its available resources in addressing a large-scale occurrence.

To understand NIMS operations, incident command system training (ICS) is required. ICS provides a common organizational structure facilitating an immediate response to occurrences by establishing a clear chain of command that supports the coordination of personnel and equipment at the event site. The DHS has developed minimal core competencies for individuals expected to participate in an event and has included these in established training programs (FEMA, 2012).

EVIDENCE-BASED PRACTICE

Who Are the People Who Call Crisis Helplines and Why Do They Call?

Problem

Crisis helplines tend to have limited funding and personnel. Frequent callers present a challenge in providing optimal outcomes for all callers by utilizing scarce resources.

Purpose of the Study

Researchers in this study hoped to describe frequent callers and compare them with non-frequent callers. They wanted this information to develop approaches that might work best in meeting the needs of frequent callers.

Methods

Australia's largest crisis helpline, Lifeline, provided an anonymous dataset for the researchers to analyze. Encrypted phone numbers made it possible to determine who were frequent callers. These were people who averaged more than half a call per day in any period from 1 week to the full 549 days for which they had data (e.g., 4.7 calls in 7 days or 40 calls in 60 days).

Key Findings

- 411,725 calls were made by 98,174 individuals
- 2594 (2.6%) met the definition of frequent caller
- Characteristics of frequent callers included being male or transgender, never married, and increasing age up until 64 years
- Calls were associated with suicidality, self-harm, mental health issues, crime, child protection, and domestic violence

Implications for Nursing Practice

The characteristics of frequent callers describe an at-risk group that is uncharacteristically reaching out. Nurses in any practice setting should be aware of subtle signs and symptoms of distress in anyone but especially unmarried or transgendered males.

Spittal, M. J., Fedyszyn, I., Middleton, A., Bassilios, B., Gunn, J., Woodward, A., & Pirkis, J. (2015). Frequent callers to crisis helplines: Who are they and why do they call? *Australian and New Zealand Journal of Psychiatry, 49*(1), 54–64.

CASE STUDY AND NURSING CARE PLAN

Crisis

Ms. Greg, the advanced practice psychiatric-mental health registered nurse, is called to the neurological unit to see Mr. Begay, a 43-year-old man with Guillain-Barré syndrome. He has severe muscle weakness and is not yet able to breathe on his own.

The nurse manager reports that Mr. Begay makes sexually suggestive remarks, uses abusive language, and has angry outbursts. The nurses state that they have tried to be patient and understanding. However, nothing seems to get through to him.

Mr. Begay, a Native American, was employed as a taxicab driver. His fiancée visits him every day. He needs assistance with every aspect of his activities of daily living. Because of his severe muscle weakness, he has to be turned and positioned every 2 hours and fed through a gastrostomy tube.

Assessment

Ms. Greg gathers data from Mr. Begay, the nursing staff, and Mr. Begay's fiancée.

Perception of the Precipitating Event

Mr. Begay expresses anger about needing a nurse to "scratch my head and help me blow my nose." He still cannot figure out how his illness developed. He says the doctors told him that it was too early to know for sure if he would recover completely but that the prognosis was hopeful.

Support System

Ms. Greg speaks with Mr. Begay's fiancée. Mr. Begay's relationships with his fiancée and with his Native American cultural group are strong. With minimal ties outside their reservation, neither Mr. Begay nor his fiancée has much knowledge of supportive agencies.

Personal Coping Skills

Mr. Begay comes from a male-dominated subculture where the man is expected to be a strong leader. His ability to be an independent person with the power to affect the direction of his life is central to his perception of being acceptable as a man.

Mr. Begay feels powerless, out of control, and enraged. He is handling his anxiety by displacing these feelings onto the environment, namely, the staff and his fiancée. This redirection of anger temporarily lowers his anxiety and distracts him from painful feelings. His behavior leads others to minimize interactions with him, which increases his sense of isolation and helplessness.

Self-Assessment

Ms. Greg meets with the staff twice. The staff discuss feelings of helplessness and lack of control stemming from their feelings of rejection by Mr. Begay. They talk of their anger about Mr. Begay's behavior and frustration about the situation. Ms. Greg points out to the staff that Mr. Begay's feelings of helplessness, lack of control, and anger at his situation are the same feelings the staff are experiencing.

The nurses make a plan to focus more on the patient, less on personal reactions, and decide on two approaches they can try as a group. First, they will not take Mr. Begay's behavior personally. Second, Mr. Begay's displaced feelings will be refocused back to him.

Priority Diagnosis

Ineffective coping related to inadequate coping methods as evidenced by inappropriate use of defense mechanisms (displacement), anger, isolation, and continued escalation of anxiety.

Outcomes Identification

Mr. Begay will state that he feels more comfortable discussing difficult feelings by discharge.

Implementation

Mr. Begay's care plan is personalized as follows:

Short-Term Goal	Intervention	Rationale	Evaluation
1. By the end of the week, Mr. Begay will be able to name and discuss at least two feelings about his illness and lack of mobility.	1a. Nurse will meet with patient daily for 15 minutes at 7:30 a.m. 1b. When patient lashes out, nurse will remain calm. 1c. Nurse will consistently redirect and refocus anger from environment back to patient (e.g., "It must be difficult to be in this situation"). 1d. Nurse will come on time each day and stay for allotted time.	1a. Night is usually the most frightening for patient; in early morning, feelings are closer to surface. 1b. Patient perceives that nurse is in control of her feelings. This can reassure patient and increase patient's sense of security. 1c. Refocusing feelings offers patient opportunity to cope effectively with his anxiety and decreases need to act out. 1d. Consistency sets stage for trust and reinforces that patient's anger will not drive nurse away.	**GOAL MET** Within 7 days, Mr. Begay speaks to nurse more openly about feelings.

CASE STUDY AND NURSING CARE PLAN—cont'd

Crisis

Dialogue	Therapeutic Tool/Comment
Nurse: "Mr. Begay, I'm here as we discussed. I'll be spending 15 minutes with you every morning. We could use this time to talk about some of your concerns."	Nurse offers herself as a resource, gives information, and clarifies her role and patient expectations. Night is Mr. Begay's most difficult time. In the early morning, he will be the most vulnerable and open for therapeutic intervention and support.
Mr. Begay: "Listen, sweetheart, my only concern is how to get a little sexual relief, get it?"	
Nurse: "Being hospitalized and partially paralyzed can be overwhelming for anyone. Perhaps you wish you could find some relief from your situation."	Nurse focuses on the process "need for relief," not the sexual content, and encourages discussion of feelings.
Mr. Begay: "What do you know, Ms. Know-it-all? I can't even scratch my nose without getting one of those fools to do it for me…"	
Nurse: "It must be difficult to have to ask people to do everything for you."	Nurse restates what the patient says in terms of his feelings and continues to refocus away from the environment back to the patient.
Mr. Begay: "Yeah… The other night a fly kept landing on my face. I had to shout for 5 minutes before one of those stupid aides came in."	
Nurse: "Having to rely on others for everything can be a terrifying experience for anyone. It sounds extremely frustrating for you."	Nurse acknowledges that frustration and anger would be a natural response for anyone in this situation. This encourages the patient to talk about these feelings instead of acting them out.
Mr. Begay: "Yeah… It's a bitch…like a living hell."	

Evaluation

After 6 weeks, Mr. Begay is able to get around with assistance, and his ability to perform his activities of daily living is increasing. Although Mr. Begay still feels angry and overwhelmed, he is able to identify his feelings and acts them out less often. He is able to talk to his fiancée about his feelings, and he lashes out at her less. He is looking forward to going home, and his boss is holding his old job. He contacted the Guillain-Barré Society to attend a support group.

Staff feel more comfortable and competent in their relationships with Mr. Begay. The goals have been met. Mr. Begay and Ms. Greg agree that the crisis is over and terminate their visits. Mr. Begay is given the number of the crisis unit and encouraged to call if he has questions or feels the need to talk.

KEY POINTS TO REMEMBER

- Crises can lead to personality disorganization but also offer opportunities for emotional growth.
- There are three types of crises: maturational, situational, and adventitious.
- Crises are usually resolved within 4 to 6 weeks.
- Crisis intervention therapy is short term, from 1 to 6 weeks, and focuses on the present problem only.
- Resolution of a crisis takes three forms: a patient emerges at a higher level, at the precrisis level, or at a lower level of functioning.
- Social support and intervention can promote successful resolution.
- Nurses take an active and directive approach with the patient in crisis.
- Whenever possible, the patient is an active participant in setting goals and planning possible solutions.
- Crisis intervention is usually aimed at the mentally healthy patient who generally is functioning well but is temporarily overwhelmed and unable to function.
- The crisis model can be adapted to meet the needs of patients in crisis who have long-term and persistent mental problems.
- Specific qualities in the nurse that can facilitate effective intervention are a caring attitude, flexibility in planning care, an ability to listen, and an active approach.
- The basic goals of crisis intervention are to reduce the individual's anxiety level and to support the effort to return to the patient's precrisis level of functioning.
- Disaster occurrences and management are global concerns that involve nurses.
- Disaster-preparedness training can optimize nursing contributions to disaster planning and management.

CRITICAL THINKING

1. List the three important areas of the crisis assessment once safety concerns have been identified. Give examples of two questions in each area that need to be answered before planning can take place.
2. Barbara, 21 years old and a junior in nursing school, tells her nursing instructor that her father (aged 45 years) has just lost his job. Her father has been drinking heavily for years, and Barbara is having difficulty coping. Because of her father's

alcoholism and the increased stress in her family, Barbara wants to leave school. Her mother has multiple sclerosis and thinks Barbara should quit school to take care of her.

a. How many different types of crises are going on in this family? Discuss the crises from the viewpoint of each family member.
b. If this family came for crisis counseling, what areas would you assess, and what kinds of questions would you ask to evaluate each member's individual needs and the needs of the family as a unit (perception of events, social supports, coping styles)?
c. Formulate some tentative goals you might set in conjunction with the family.
d. Identify—by name—appropriate referral agencies in your area that would be helpful if members of this family were willing to expand their use of outside resources and stabilize the situation.
e. How would you set up follow-up visits for this family? Would you see the family members together, alone, or in a combination during the crisis period (4 to 6 weeks)? How would you decide whether follow-up counseling was indicated?

CHAPTER REVIEW

Questions

1. Which patient statement indicates the helpfulness of the nurse-patient relationship?
   a. "I appreciate the time you spent with me. I have a better understanding of what I can do to manage my problem."
   b. "I really need to talk with you. You always give me good advice about how to address my anger issues."
   c. "If it wasn't for you and the hours we've spent talking, I don't think I would be on my way to getting my anxiety under control."
   d. "You always showed me sympathy when I was at my lowest point after the sexual assault. Knowing you had been there too was such a help."
2. A female nurse had been sexually assaulted as a teenager. She finds it difficult to work with patients who have undergone the same trauma. What is the most helpful response?
   a. Discussing these feelings with the nurse supervisor.
   b. Requesting that these patients not be a part of her patient assignment.
   c. Discussing these feelings with a mental health professional.
   d. Accepting her role in providing unbiased, respectful, and professional care to all patients.
3. A patient whose history includes experiences with abusive partners is being treated for major depressive disorder. The patient's care plan includes *rape-trauma syndrome* among its nursing diagnoses. What goal is directly associated with this diagnosis?
   a. Remains free from self-harm
   b. Wears appropriate clothing
   c. Reports feeling stronger and having a sense of hopefulness
   d. Demonstrates appropriate affect for both positive and negative emotions
4. The nurse is engaged in crisis intervention with a patient reporting, "I have no reason to keep on living." What is the nurse's initial intervention?
   a. Advise the patient about the services available to help them.
   b. Ask the patient, "Have you ever been this depressed before?"
   c. Ask the patient, "Do you have any plan to hurt yourself or anyone else?"
   d. Assure the patient that he or she is in a safe place and will be well cared for.
5. Which statement concerning a crisis experience is true and should be used as a guideline for crisis management care? *Select all that apply.*
   a. A crisis is self-limiting and usually resolves within 4 to 6 weeks.
   b. The earlier interventions are implemented, the better the expected prognosis.
   c. The nurse should maintain a nondirective role.
   d. The patient in crisis is assumed to be mentally unhealthy and in an extreme state of disequilibrium.
   e. The goal of crisis management is to return the patient to at least the precrisis level of functioning.
6. Which statement about crisis theory will provide a basis for nursing intervention?
   a. A crisis is an acute time-limited phenomenon experienced as an overwhelming emotional reaction to a problem perceived as unsolvable.
   b. A person in crisis has always had adjustment problems and has coped inadequately in the usual life situations.
   c. Crisis is precipitated by an event that enhances a person's self-concept and self-esteem.
   d. Nursing intervention in crisis situations rarely has the effect of stopping the crisis.
7. Lilly, a single mother of four, comes to the crisis center 24 hours after a fire in which all the houses within a one-block area were wiped out. All of Lilly's household goods and clothing were lost. Lilly has no other family in the area. Her efforts to mobilize assistance have been disorganized, and she is still without shelter. She is distraught and confused. You assess the situation as:
   a. A maturational crisis.
   b. An adventitious crisis.
   c. A crisis of confidence.
   d. An existential crisis.
8. When responding to the patient in question 7, the intervention that takes priority is to:
   a. Reduce anxiety.
   b. Arrange shelter.
   c. Contact out-of-area family.
   d. Hospitalize and place the patient on suicide precautions.

9. Which belief would be least helpful for a nurse working in crisis intervention?
   a. A person in crisis is incapable of responding to instruction.
   b. The crisis counseling relationship is one between partners.
   c. Crisis counseling helps the patient refocus to gain new perspectives on the situation.
   d. Anxiety-reduction techniques are used so the patient's inner resources can be accessed.

10. The highest-priority goal of crisis intervention is:
   a. Anxiety reduction.
   b. Identification of situational supports.
   c. Teaching specific coping skills that are lacking.
   d. Patient safety.

Answers

1. **a;** 2. **c;** 3. **c;** 4. **c;** 5. **a, b, e;** 6. **a;** 7. **b;** 8. **a;** 9. **a;** 10. **d**

ⓔ Visit the Evolve website for a posttest on the content in this chapter: http://evolve.elsevier.com/Varcarolis

Post-Test interactive review

REFERENCES

Behrman, G., & Reid, W. (2002). Post-trauma intervention: Basic tasks. *Brief Treatment and Crisis Intervention, 2*(1), 39–47.

Boscarato, K., Lee, S., Kroschel, J., Hollander, Y., Brennan, A., & Warren, N. (2014). Consumer experience of formal crisis-response services and preferred methods of crisis intervention. *International Journal of Mental Health Nursing, 23*(4), 287–295.

Bulechek, G. M., Butcher, H. K., Dochterman, J. M., & Wagner, C. (2013). *Nursing interventions classification (NIC)* (6th ed.). St. Louis, MO: Mosby.

Caplan, G. (1964). *Principles of preventive psychiatry*. New York, NY: Basic Books.

Federal Emergency Management Agency. (2012). *FEMA: Plan and prepare*. Retrieved from http://www.fema.gov/plan-prepare-mitigate/ and www.fema.gov/preparedness-1.

Herdman, T. H., & Kamitsuru, S. (Eds.). (2014). *NANDA International nursing diagnoses: Definitions and classification* (pp. 2015–2017). Oxford, UK: Wiley-Blackwell.

Joint Commission on Mental Illness and Health. (1961). *Action for mental health: Final report, 1961*. New York, NY: Basic Books.

Lindemann, E. (1944). Symptomatology and acute grief. *American Journal of Psychiatry, 101*, 141–148.

Moorhead, S., Johnson, M., Maas, M. L., & Swanson, E. (2013). *Nursing outcomes classification (NOC)* (5th ed.). St. Louis, MO: Elsevier.

Roberts, A. R., & Ottens, A. J. (2005). The seven-stage crisis intervention model: A road map to goal attainment, problem solving, and crisis resolution. *Brief Treatment and Crisis Intervention, 5*, 329–339.

Substance Abuse and Mental Health Service Administration. (2014). Crisis services: Effectiveness, cost-effectiveness, and funding strategies. Retrieved from http://store.samhsa.gov/shin/content//SMA14-4848/SMA14-4848.pdf.

27

Anger, Aggression, and Violence

Lorann Murphy

Visit the Evolve website for a pretest on the content in this chapter: http://evolve.elsevier.com/Varcarolis Pre-Test interactive review

OBJECTIVES

1. Compare and contrast three theories that explain the origins of anger, aggression, and violence.
2. Compare and contrast interventions for a patient with healthy coping skills with those for a patient with marginal coping behaviors.
3. Apply at least four principles of deescalation with a moderately angry patient.
4. Describe two criteria that make the use of seclusion or restraint more appropriate than verbal intervention.
5. Discuss three types assessment questions and their value in the nursing process.
6. Role-play with classmates using understandable but unhelpful responses to anger and aggression in patients.
7. Role-play with classmates using helpful responses to anger and aggression in patients.

OUTLINE

KEY TERMS AND CONCEPTS

aggression
anger
deescalation techniques
restraint
seclusion
trauma-informed care
validation therapy
violence

Anger, aggression, and violence are the subjects of daily news headlines. Due to the scope and prevalence of the problem you may notice an expanding list of terminology used to describe specific types of aggression. *Road rage* is a dangerous habit rampant in high-stress industrialized societies and is accompanied by cursing, offensive gestures, and cutting others off while driving. *Air rage* is objectionable behavior, aggressive utterances, threats, and violence within the confines of an aircraft. *Desk rage* includes lashing out while at work. Hospitals, as 24-hour-a-day high-stress environments, have even earned a term for their own brand of confrontation: *ward rage.*

CLINICAL PICTURE

Anger is an emotional response to frustration of desires, a threat to one's needs (emotional or physical), or a challenge. It is a normal emotion that can even be positive when it is expressed in a healthy way. Once anger is acknowledged, channeling anger into productive pursuits such as exercise, art, or cleaning out a closet is healthy. Anger can also be a motivator to try harder or an aid in survival when fighting is the last and only resort.

Aggression is an action or behavior that results in a verbal or physical attack. Aggression tends to be used synonymously with violence. However, aggression is not always inappropriate and is sometimes necessary for self-protection. On the other hand, **violence** is always an objectionable act that involves intentional use of force that results in, or has the potential to result in, injury to another person.

Coping with a patient's anger is a challenge. Effective nursing intervention becomes more difficult when the anger becomes personal and is directed at the nurse or nursing student. Nursing interventions should, ideally, begin before anger and aggression become a problem. Anxiety is often the precipitant for negative feelings and behaviors. Assessing and responding to this anxiety can have extremely positive returns. Refer to Chapter 15 for interventions to reduce anxiety before it becomes a crisis.

EPIDEMIOLOGY

The Centers for Disease Control and Prevention (2015) reported almost 60,000 violence-related injuries in 2014. It is likely that you will need to manage violent behavior at some point in your career. Nurses are frequent targets of violence because they have the most direct patient contact. Violence can occur anywhere in the hospital, but it is most frequent in the emergency rooms (Speroni et al., 2014). Psychiatric units, geriatric units, and intensive care units are also overrepresented in patient and patients' significant other attacks.

Examples of attacks on nurses include:

- A Texas outpatient surgery center where the son of a patient accused staff of trying to kill his mother. He fatally stabbed a nurse who was trying to protect other patients (DeMarche, 2013).
- A Maine psychiatric hospital where a patient with a chair injured a nurse's face and head. Another angry patient on the same unit stabbed a nurse with a pen (Adams, 2014).
- A Texas emergency room where a woman became enraged over being denied pain medication. When the nurse handed the patient a clipboard with discharge instructions, the patient struck the nurse in the face with the clipboard (KWTX News, 2016).

COMORBIDITY

A great deal of research has been done on aggression and violence in persons with posttraumatic stress disorders (PTSD) and substance use disorders. Johnson et al. (2016) found that persons with bipolar disorder have difficulty with anger and aggression even during remission.

Anger and hostility have effects on physical well-being. They are risk factors for hypertension and cardiovascular disease including myocardial infarctions and ischemic strokes (Mostofsky et al., 2014). Expression of anger in older adults predicted a higher prevalence of metabolic syndrome (Boylan & Ryff, 2015).

ETIOLOGY

Biological Factors

Genetics

Some individuals are biologically more predisposed than others to respond to life events with irritability, easy frustration, and anger. This predisposition may be a function of genetics or of neurological development that occurs in the context of certain infant and childhood environments. Individuals who have a history of aggression have been shown to be more acutely aware of subtle facial cues of anger (Wilkowski et al., 2012).

Neurobiological

Neurological conditions are associated with anger and aggression. Brain tumors, Alzheimer's disease, temporal lobe epilepsy, and traumatic injury to certain parts of the brain result in changes to personality that could include increased violence. Many patients with brain injury have severe behavior disorders, including aggressiveness, that disrupt their lives.

One area of the brain associated with aggression is the limbic system. It is located just beneath the cerebrum on both sides of the thalamus. It is responsible for combining higher mental functions and primitive emotions into one system, learning, and the formation of memories. Important structures within this system include the amygdala and hippocampus.

The *amygdala* is the emotional center of the brain. It helps evaluate the emotional content of our experiences. It helps the brain to recognize potential threats and whether to activate the fight-or-flight response. In animal studies, stimulation of the amygdala produces rage responses, whereas lesions in the same structure result in meekness. In humans, men with lower amygdala volume exhibit higher levels of aggression from childhood to adulthood (Pardini et al., 2014).

The *hippocampus* lies in close proximity to the amygdala and connects to it. This seahorse-shaped structure is essential to the formation of new memories. Research demonstrates that aggressive behavior may result in the formation of new cells within the hippocampus (Smagin et al., 2015). Male mice that repeatedly won fights with other mice became more aggressive and anxious. This study demonstrates that getting angry may make a person angrier, and the cycle continues.

The especially large prefrontal cortex in humans also plays an important role in aggressive behavior. This area of the brain is responsible for executive function. Executive function allows us to distinguish between good and bad, consequences of actions, goal-directed behavior, and suppressing socially unacceptable activities. According to Siever (2008), aggressive acts triggered by anger-provoking stimuli are the result of a failure of the control systems in the prefrontal cortex. Individuals with antisocial personality disorder have been shown to have less gray matter in their prefrontal cortexes (Narayan et al., 2007).

Neurotransmitters

Neurotransmitters, especially serotonin, dopamine, and gamma-amino butyric acid (GABA), play a vital role in anger and aggression (Narvaes & de Almeida, 2014). Serotonin can both inhibit and stimulate aggressive behavior, depending on the part of the brain being measured. Dopamine's impact on reward-seeking behavior may increase aggression. Like serotonin, dopamine can sometimes enhance aggression and sometimes reduce impulsivity that leads to aggression. GABA, the main inhibitory neurotransmitter, may reduce aggressiveness; its absence may increase impulsivity and aggressive responses.

Psychological Factors

Sigmund Freud (1930) wrote in *Civilization and Its Discontents* that the conflict between sexual needs and societal norms was the source of mankind's dissatisfaction, aggression, hostility, and ultimately violence. Menninger (2007) asserted that the struggle for control over our lives is a fundamental drive in every person. If that control is threatened, we experience trauma, and it is from that trauma that anger, aggression, and violence may originate.

Early behaviorists believed that emotions, including anger, were learned responses to environmental stimuli (Skinner, 1953). The stimulus is often a perceived threat, and this perception leads to the emotional and physiological arousal necessary to take action. Although the threat is usually understood as an alert to physical danger, Beck (1976) noted that other threats to areas such as values, beliefs, and moral code could also lead to anger. For example, clinic patients kept waiting for long periods of time without explanation may perceive this wait as a lack of respect. When the initial appraisal is followed by thoughts such as, "They have no right to treat me this way. I am a person too," anger may escalate and violence is possible. Patients less predisposed to anger might interpret the wait as a sign that the clinic is busy. These patients might be frustrated by the situation. However, in the absence of anger they might be proactive and ask how much longer the wait is likely to be, find distractions in the environment, or reschedule the appointment.

Social learning researchers demonstrated that children learn aggression by observing and imitating behaviors of others, especially if that behavior is rewarded (Bandura, 1973). Thus children who watch television violence or experience violence in the home learn aggressive ways of resolving problems. Not only is television violence portrayed as an option for resolving conflict, but most of those violent acts do not result in negative consequences. Bullying is another less extreme form of violence that is far more prevalent and has significant consequences. *Bullying* is any negative activity, including teasing, kicking, hitting, and spitting, intended to bother or harm someone else.

CONSIDERING CULTURE

The Anger Syndrome

Cho Hyun-Ja, a 42-year-old Korean female, comes to the clinic with complaints of anger, feelings of emptiness, insomnia, and general feelings of unfairness about her life. She also complains of dry mouth, headaches, and palpitations. Cho indicates that she will either run away from home or divorce her husband. She is tearful and sighs frequently during the interview. You suspect she may be suffering from *hwa-byung*, an anger syndrome found in nearly 5% of Koreans, mostly in middle-aged or older women. *Hwa-byung* patients are more aware of physical symptoms (which are socially acceptable) rather than psychological symptoms (which are not). Because Koreans are socialized to internalize emotion, you realize that the best approach to treating *hwa-byung* is holistic. Education can include basic coping strategies and promoting healthy lifestyle choices. Pastoral counseling, support groups, and family or marital therapy is useful. Cognitive behavioral techniques can be used as an adjunct to addressing the anger and anxiety.

Lee, J., Wachholtz, A., & Choi, K. (2015). *A review of the Korean cultural syndrome Hwa-Byung: Suggestions for theory and intervention.* Retrieved from http://www.ncbi.nlm.nih.gov/pmc/articles/PMC4232959/.

APPLICATION OF THE NURSING PROCESS

ASSESSMENT

General Assessment

When patients are experiencing anger, you often see it manifested behaviorally. Increased demands, irritability, frowning, redness of the face, pacing, twisting of the hands, or clenching and unclenching of the fists are all signs of irritation. Speech may either be increased in rate and volume or may be slowed, pointed, and quiet. You should address any change in behavior from what is typical for that patient. Box 27.1 identifies signs and symptoms that indicate the risk of escalating anger leading to aggressive behavior.

BOX 27.1 Predictors of Violence

Signs and symptoms that usually *(but not always)* precede violence:

- Hyperactivity: most important predictor of imminent violence (e.g., pacing, restlessness)
- Increasing anxiety and tension: clenched jaw or fist, rigid posture, fixed or tense facial expression, mumbling to self (patient may have shortness of breath, sweating, and rapid pulse)
- Verbal abuse: profanity, argumentativeness
- Loud voice, change of pitch; or very soft voice, forcing others to strain to hear
- Stone silence
- Intense eye contact or avoidance of eye contact
- Recent acts of violence, including property violence
- Alcohol or drug intoxication
- Possession of a weapon or object that may be used as a weapon (e.g., fork, knife, rock)
- Isolation that is uncharacteristic

Milieu characteristics conducive to violence:

- Overcrowding
- Staff inexperience
- Provocative or controlling staff
- Poor limit setting
- Arbitrary revocation of privileges

It is also important to assess the patient's history of aggression or violence. Most of our reactions to stimuli come from our previous experiences; therefore, identifying patients' triggers is essential. Initial and ongoing assessment of the patient can reveal problems before they escalate to anger and aggression. Such assessment also leads directly to the appropriate nursing diagnosis and intervention.

HEALTH POLICY

Workplace Violence

Workplace violence has been occurring in the healthcare setting for decades. The American Nurses Association's *Code of Ethics for Nurses with Interpretive Statements* states that nurses are required to:

"Create an ethical environment and culture of civility and kindness, treating colleagues, coworkers, employees, students, and others with dignity and respect" (ANA, 2015a, p. 4).

In 2015 the American Nurses Association wrote a position statement on incivility, bullying, and workplace violence. They encouraged collaboration of registered nurses and employers to create a culture of respect. Use of evidence-based strategies that prevent incivility, bullying, and workplace violence was also suggested. Other recommendations for nurses include establishing an agreed-upon code word if they are feeling threatened, developing a plan to address incivility and bullying, and becoming advocates for identification and prevention of incivility and bullying.

American Nurses Association. (2015a). *Incivility, bullying and workplace violence.* Retrieved from http://www.nursingworld.org/Bullying-Workplace-Violence; American Nurses Association. (2015b). *Code of ethics for nurses with interpretive statements.* Silver Spring, MD: NurseBooks.org.

Trauma-informed care is an older concept of providing care that has recently been reintroduced. It is based on the notion that disruptive patients often have histories that include violence and victimization (Sansone et al., 2012). These traumatic histories can impede patients' ability to self-soothe, result in negative coping responses, and create a vulnerability to coercive interventions (such as restraint) by staff. Trauma-informed care focuses on the patient's past experiences of violence or trauma and on the role these experiences currently play in their lives.

Careful assessment can reduce the potential for violence. In a study conducted at New York State Psychiatric Institute, patients filled out a questionnaire that identified things that made them upset, how they responded to being upset, and how they wanted to be treated when they became upset. Examples of how they wanted to be treated included talking with them and allowing them time out alone. Making use of the patients' suggestions resulted in a decreased amount of time in restraints and seclusion and a reduction in the number of fights and assaults on the unit (Hellerstein et al., 2007).

EVIDENCE-BASED PRACTICE

The School Nurse: Comfort for Bullied School Children

Problem

Children who have been bullied have an increased risk for anxiety, depression, and psychiatric problems as adults. Children who have been identified as aggressors also are at increased risk for psychiatric problems. Children who are either aggressors or victims of bullying display more somatic complaints and physical illnesses than other children. In the past, most emphasis has been in identifying victims of bullying. We also must be aware of the aggressors and intervene appropriately with them as well.

Purpose of Study

The purpose of the study was to examine how bullying victims and aggressors are linked to somatic complaints, physical illnesses, and injuries in elementary-aged children.

Methods

This study looked at third- to sixth-grade students from six elementary schools who had visited the school nurse during the past year. The researcher collected school nurse logs with types of complaints. The children also filled out a self-report of victimization.

Key Finding

Regardless of whether the student was a victim or a bully, both roles were associated with an increase in school nurse visits for somatic complaints, physical illnesses, and physical injury.

Implications for Nursing Practice

The school nurse is integral in the identification and intervention of peer victimization in schools. The nurse should be aware that frequent visits might be an indicator of a child's involvement in aggressive episodes either as a victim or as a perpetrator. The nurse's plan of care will focus on early intervention for the victim and for the aggressor to assist in promoting mental and physical well-being for each child.

From Vernberg, E. M., Nelson, T. D., Fonagy, P., & Twemlow, S. W. (2011). Victimization, aggression and visits to the school nurse for somatic complaints, illnesses, and physical injuries. *Pediatrics, 127*(5), 842–848.

Self-Assessment

Like patients, nurses have their own histories. The nurse's ability to intervene effectively depends on self-awareness of strengths, needs, concerns, and vulnerabilities. Without this awareness, nursing interventions can end up being impulsive or emotion-based responses. Self-awareness includes recognizing choice of words and tone of voice, as well as nonverbal communication through body posture and facial expressions.

ASSESSMENT GUIDELINES

Anger and Aggression

General risk identification includes assessing for the following:

1. A history of violence is the single best predictor of future violence.
2. Patients who are delusional, hyperactive, impulsive, or predisposed to irritability are at higher risk for violence.
3. Major factors associated with violence can be assessed with these questions:
   - Does the patient have a wish or intent to harm?
   - Does the patient have a plan?
   - Does the patient have the means available to carry out the plan?
   - Does the patient have demographic risk factors: male gender, aged 14 to 24 years, low socioeconomic status, inadequate support system, and prison time?
4. Aggression by patients occurs most often in the context of limit-setting by the nurse.
5. History of limited coping skills, including lack of assertiveness or use of intimidation, indicates a higher risk of using violence.

DIAGNOSIS

Patients may have coping skills that are adequate for day-to-day events but may be overwhelmed by the stresses of illness or hospitalization. Other patients may have a pattern of maladaptive coping that is marginally effective and coping strategies that may increase the possibility of anger and aggression. When the nursing assessment identifies potential for anger or aggression, *Risk for other-directed violence, Risk for self-directed violence, Ineffective coping* (overwhelmed or maladaptive), *Stress overload,* and *Impaired impulse control* are important nursing diagnoses to consider (Kamitsuru & Herdman, 2014).

OUTCOMES IDENTIFICATION

Clearly defined outcome criteria are important for identifying the behaviors that staff can encourage if their interventions have been successful. The *Nursing Outcomes Classification (NOC)* outlines specific outcome criteria for use with angry and aggressive patients (Moorhead et al., 2013). Table 27.1 identifies signs and symptoms commonly experienced with anger and aggression, offers potential nursing diagnoses, and suggests outcomes.

PLANNING

Planning interventions requires a sound assessment, including patient history (previous acts of violence, comorbid disorders, past triggers) and present coping skills. Patients need to be willing and able to learn alternative and nonviolent ways of handling angry feelings.

IMPLEMENTATION

Ideally, intervention begins before any sign of escalation. It is important to develop a relationship of trust with the patient by having numerous brief, nonthreatening, nondirective interactions (e.g., talking about the weather, sports, or something of interest to the patient).

In settings in which staff can reasonably expect episodes of patient anger and aggression, regular teaching and practice of verbal and nonverbal interventions are essential. This fosters nurses' increased confidence in their own abilities and those of co-workers.

Psychosocial Interventions

If you can attempt to determine what the patient is feeling, you have already begun to intervene. Frequently, you can accomplish this by telling the patient that you are concerned and want to listen. It is essential to acknowledge the patient's needs, regardless of whether the expressed needs are rational or possible to meet. It is equally as important to clearly state your expectations for the patient's behavior: "I expect that you will stay in control."

However, patient behavior may escalate quickly, or the patient may mask early signs of distress. Nurses may be distracted and miss those early signs. Some agitated patients may be so acutely upset that they do not respond to early nursing interventions. In these situations, the problem with anger may not be resolved before the risk for violence arises. Pharmacological intervention, seclusion, or restraint may be necessary to ensure the safety of patients and staff.

Approach the patient in a controlled, nonthreatening, and caring manner. If you are experiencing fear, you may find that this is quite challenging. Maintaining a calm exterior while your interior is in an upheaval requires considerable self-discipline and will come with experience.

Patients who are at risk for violence need much more personal space than those who are not. Allow the patient enough space so that you are perceived as less of a threat. Always stay about 1 foot farther than the patient can reach with arms or legs. Be sure you have left yourself an escape route if necessary, that is, make sure that the patient is not between you and the door.

While you are giving the patient space, the patient may be invading your space with verbal abuse and profanity. As uncomfortable as this may be, you cannot take the patient's words personally or respond in kind. It is also important not to end the conversation because of the patient's verbal abusiveness or to forbid the patient from communicating in this way.

When anger is escalating, a patient's ability to process decreases. It is important to speak to the patient slowly and in short sentences, using a low and calm voice. Never yell but continue to model controlled behavior.

Use open-ended statements and questions such as "You think people are treating you unfairly?" rather than challenging statements such as "What is going on right now?" Avoid ending statements with "Okay?" because it may give the impression that choices exist. Find out what is behind the angry feelings and behaviors. Identify the patient's options and encourage the

TABLE 27.1 Signs and Symptoms, Nursing Diagnoses, and Outcomes for Aggression

Signs and Symptoms	Nursing Diagnoses	Outcomes
Body language (rigid posture, clenching of fists and jaw, hyperactivity, pacing), history of violence, history of family violence, history of substance use	*Risk for other-directed violence*	Identifies when angry, identifies alternatives to aggression, refrains from verbal outbursts, avoids violating others' personal space, maintains self-control
Impulsivity, suicidal ideation (has plan, ability to carry it out), overt or covert statements regarding killing self, feelings of worthlessness, hopelessness, helplessness	*Risk for self-directed violence*	Expresses feelings, verbalizes suicidal ideas, refrains from suicide attempts, plans for the future
Difficulty with simple tasks, inability to function at previous level, poor problem solving, poor cognitive functioning, verbalizations of inability to cope	*Ineffective coping*	Identifies ineffective and effective coping, uses support system, uses new coping strategies, engages in personal actions to manage stressors effectively
Demonstrates feelings of anger, impatience; reports feelings of pressure, tension, difficulty in functioning, anger, impatience; experiences negative impact from stress; reports problems with decision making	*Stress overload*	Expresses feelings constructively, reports feelings of calmness and acceptance; physical symptoms of stress are reduced or absent; decision making is optimal

From Kamitsuru, S., & Herdman, T. H. (Eds.). (2014). *NANDA International nursing diagnoses: Definitions and classification, 2015–2017*. Oxford, UK: Wiley-Blackwell; Moorhead, S., Johnson, M., Maas, M. L., & Swanson, E. (2013). *Nursing outcomes classification (NOC)* (5th ed.). St. Louis, MO: Elsevier.

individual to assume responsibility for choices made. You may want to give two options such as, "Do you want to go to your room or to the quiet room for a while?" This approach decreases the sense of powerlessness that often precipitates violence.

Pay close attention to the environment. Choose a quiet place to talk to the patient but one that is visible to staff. This is most beneficial in helping a patient regain control. Staff should know you are working with the patient, keep an eye on the interaction, and be prepared to intervene if the situation escalates. At this point, move other patients away and, as much as possible, remove any objects in the area that could be used as a weapon.

Considerations for Staff Safety

There are six basic considerations for ensuring safety:

1. Avoid wearing dangling earrings, necklaces, and scarves in acute care environments. The patient may become focused on these and grab at them, causing serious injury.
2. Ensure that there is enough staff for backup. Only one person should talk to the patient, but staff need to maintain an unobtrusive presence in case the situation escalates.
3. Always know the layout of the area. Correct placement of furniture and elimination of obstacles or hazards are important to prevent injury if the patient requires physical interventions.
4. Do not stand directly in front of the patient or in front of the doorway. The patient may consider this position as confrontational. It is better to stand off to the side and encourage the patient to have a seat.
5. If a patient's behavior begins to escalate, provide feedback: "You seem to be very upset." Such an observation allows exploration of the patient's feelings and may lead to deescalation of the situation.
6. Avoid confrontation with the patient, either through verbal means or through a "show of support" with security guards. Verbal confrontation and discussion of the incident must occur when the patient is calm. A show of force by security guards may serve to escalate the patient's behavior. Security personnel are better kept in the background until they are needed to assist.

Box 27.2 lists some principles underlying **deescalation techniques.**

BOX 27.2 Deescalation Techniques: Practice Principles

- Maintain the patient's self-esteem and dignity
- Maintain calmness (your own and the patient's)
- Assess the patient and the situation
- Identify stressors and stress indicators
- Respond as early as possible
- Use a calm clear tone of voice
- Invest time
- Remain honest
- Determine what the patient considers to be needed
- Identify goals
- Avoid invading personal space; in times of high anxiety, personal space increases
- Avoid arguing
- Give several clear options
- Use genuineness and empathy
- Be assertive (not aggressive)
- Do not take chances; maintain personal safety

From Mason, T., & Chandley, M. (1999). *Management of violence and aggression* (p. 73). Philadelphia, PA: Churchill Livingstone.

Pharmacological Interventions

When a patient is showing increased signs or symptoms of anxiety or agitation, it is perfectly appropriate to offer the patient an as-needed medication to alleviate symptoms. When used in conjunction with psychosocial interventions and deescalation techniques, this can prevent an aggressive or violent incident.

Antianxiety agents and antipsychotics are used in the treatment of acute symptoms of anger and aggression. These agents,

TABLE 27.2 Drugs Used for Acute Management of Violent Behavior

Generic (Trade)	Forms	Considerations
Antianxiety Agents (Benzodiazepines)		
Lorazepam (Ativan)	PO, SL, IM, IV	Drug of choice in this class Use with caution with hepatic dysfunction
Alprazolam (Xanax)	PO	Paradoxical (opposite response) with personality disorders and elderly
Diazepam (Valium)	PO, IM, IV	Rapid onset of calming and sedating Long half-life; use with caution in elderly
First-Generation Antipsychotics		
Haloperidol (Haldol)	PO, IM, IV	Favorable side-effect profile. Due to risk of neuroleptic malignant syndrome, keep hydrated, check vital signs, and test for muscle rigidity
Perphenazine	PO	Risk of neuroleptic malignant syndrome increases, keep hydrated. Frequent vital sign checks and testing for muscular rigidity are recommended.
Chlorpromazine (Thorazine)	PO, PR, IM	Very sedating Injections can cause pain; watch for hypotension
Loxapine (Adasuve)	Inhalation	Rapid systemic delivery. Available only through a restricted program. Risk for fatal bronchospasm – contraindicated for individuals with breathing disorders.
Second-Generation Antipsychotics		
Risperidone (Risperdal)	PO, orally disintegrating tablet	Calms while treating underlying condition Watch for hypotension with reflex tachycardia Increased risk of stroke in elderly
Olanzapine (Zyprexa, Zydis)	PO, IM, disintegrating tablet	Useful in patients unresponsive to haloperidol Calms while treating underlying condition Avoid IM combination with lorazepam Increased risk of stroke in elderly
Ziprasidone (Geodon)	PO, IM	Use cautiously with QT prolongation Less sedating
Combinations		
Haloperidol (Haldol), lorazepam (Ativan), and diphenhydramine (Benadryl) or benztropine (Cogentin)	IM	Commonly used in the acute setting Men who are young and athletic are at increased risk of dystonia Consider akathisia if agitation increases
Perphenazine, lorazepam (Ativan), and diphenhydramine (Benadryl), or benztropine (Cogentin)	IM	Consider this combination if patient has difficulty taking haloperidol

From Gerken, A. T., Gross, A. F., & Sanders, K. M. (2016). Aggression and violence. In T. A. Stern, M. Fava, T. E. Wilens, & J. F. Rosenbaum (Eds.), *Massachusetts General Hospital comprehensive clinical psychiatry* (2nd ed.) (p. 716.). St. Louis, MO: Elsevier.

their form of delivery, and considerations are in Table 27.2. During aggressive or violent incidents, haloperidol (Haldol) has historically been the most widely used first-generation antipsychotic. Second-generation antipsychotics such as olanzapine (Zyprexa) and ziprasidone (Geodon) have become more common due to reduced side effects compared with first-generation drugs. A dissolving tablet version of olanzapine (Zydis) was introduced recently as an alternative to injectable medication with effects being seen within 10 minutes of administration. An inhaled first-generation antipsychotic loxapine (Adasuve) has been approved for use in limited settings due to the potential for a fatal bronchospasm.

Antianxiety benzodiazepines such as lorazepam (Ativan) may reduce the amount of antipsychotic that is needed to control agitation. You may also have orders to administer a combination of an antipsychotic (haloperidol or perphenazine) and a benzodiazepine (lorazepam) intramuscularly. Diphenhydramine or benztropine (Cogentin) added to the injection reduces extrapyramidal side effects.

It is the nurse's role to assess for appropriateness of as-needed medications. The nurse also educates the patient about the medication, the reason it is being given, and the potential side effects of the medication, even if the patient is out of control.

The long-term treatment of anger, aggression, and violence is based on treating the underlying psychiatric disorder. Selective serotonin reuptake inhibitors (SSRIs), lithium, anticonvulsants, benzodiazepines, second-generation antipsychotics, and beta-blockers are all used successfully for specific patient populations. Anger and aggression related to attention-deficit disorder and attention-deficit/hyperactivity disorder may be reduced through the use of psychostimulants. Table 27.3 gives an overview of the drugs used to treat chronic aggression.

Health Teaching and Health Promotion

One of the most important roles a nurse plays in a patient's recovery is that of role model and educator. You can model appropriate responses and ways to cope with anger, teach patients a variety of methods to appropriately express anger,

TABLE 27.3 Drugs Used for Long-Term Management of Chronic Aggression

Class	Population	Considerations
Selective serotonin reuptake inhibitors (SSRIs)	Depression, anxiety, personality disorder, dementia, and intellectual disability	Reduces irritability, impulsivity, and aggression Stabilizes mood Use cautiously with bipolar disorder
Lithium	Intellectual disability, conduct disorder, antisocial personality, bipolar disorder, and prison inmates	TSH levels measured before treatment Due to anti-aggressive properties, blood levels can be lower than those necessary to treat bipolar mania
Anticonvulsants	Schizophrenia, prison inmates, antisocial/borderline personality, conduct disorders, and bipolar disorders	Significantly reduces impulsive aggression Similar doses with bipolar disorder Multiple drug interactions Periodic blood levels Monitor CBC and LFTs
Gabapentin	Patients with co-existing anxiety disorder and personality disorders	No interactions with other anticonvulsants
Benzodiazepines	Should have underlying component of anxiety	Potential for abuse, dependence, and withdrawal May cause paradoxical aggression
Second-generation antipsychotics	Schizophrenia, psychosis, and mania	Clozapine superior to other second-generation drugs but must monitor ANC monthly Fewer side effects and greater adherence than first-generation antipsychotics
Beta-blockers	Organic brain disease, brain injury, dementia, intellectual disability	Propranolol contraindicated with asthma, COPD, and IDDM Sedation side effects may explain anti-aggressive effects
Psychostimulants	ADD/ADHD in children and adults	Potential for addiction and abuse

From Gerken, A. T., Gross, A. F., & Sanders, K. M. (2016). Aggression and violence. In T. A. Stern, M. Fava, T. E. Wilens, & J. F. Rosenbaum (Eds.), *Massachusetts General Hospital comprehensive clinical psychiatry* (2nd ed.) (p. 716.). St. Louis, MO: Elsevier.

and educate patients regarding coping mechanisms, deescalation techniques, and self-soothing skills to manage behavior. It is also helpful to assist the patient in identifying triggers for angry or aggressive behavior. One method that can be used if the patient is not out of control is a "do over." The patient who responds inappropriately can try again to respond in a more appropriate way while being coached by the nurse.

Interest in using alternative interventions such as forgiveness and compassion in healthy patients has been gaining interest (Griffin et al., 2015). Nurses may introduce these concepts and educate the patient on how to incorporate them into their lives.

Teamwork and Safety

A multidisciplinary approach is important for all patients but especially for a patient with behavioral issues. All team members must implement a plan of care and execute that plan. During team meetings, staff should discuss intervention strategies. The plan for discharge with appropriate follow-up, possibly with an anger-management course, must be put into place. The consistency of intervention among all team members is key to the patient's success.

A thorough consideration of the environment is important when considering anger and aggression on the unit. It is important to be proactive and not reactive. It is hard to imagine how the stimulation of a psychiatric unit might be experienced by someone whose anxiety is extremely high or who is delusional or confused. If the patient has enough control, sometimes simply taking a timeout in his or her own room is sufficient. A multisensory room is another form of timeout. It is also known as a *Snoezelen*, named partly from the Dutch word for "dozing." This quiet room is partially lit, has relaxing music available, and comfortable furniture and soft pillows. It promotes feelings of security and safety.

Realize that behavior rarely occurs in a vacuum. The nurse must examine the milieu as a whole and identify the stressors patients have to deal with, especially patients who have an antisocial personality disorder. These individuals have a tendency to create havoc and make it appear that another patient is at fault, either for their own pleasure or for their own purposes (e.g., escaping the unit or getting into the medication room). So even while dealing with an incident, staff must be aware of what could be happening in the surrounding environment.

Use of Seclusion or Restraints

Occasionally, despite numerous interventions, a patient will become violent and require seclusion or restraint. When this happens, it is essential to have an organized approach to the seclusion or restraint. Legally, most courts hold that seclusion and restraint be implemented only when a patient creates a risk of harm to self or others and no less restrictive alternative is available. These measures should never be used for punishment or for the convenience of staff. Seclusion or physical restraint is used only after alternative interventions have been tried. These interventions include verbal interventions, offering an as needed medication, decreasing sensory stimulation, presence of a significant other, frequent observation, or one-on-one observation of the patient.

According to the US Department of Health & Human Services [HHS], Centers for Medicare and Medicaid Services (2008), **seclusion** refers to "the involuntary confinement of a patient alone in a room, or area from which the patient is physically prevented from leaving" (p. 96). The goal of seclusion is never punitive. Rather, the goal of seclusion is safety of the patient and others. Seclusion is less restrictive than restraint and may be helpful in reducing sensory overstimulation.

Restraint is defined as "any manual method, physical or mechanical device, material, or equipment that immobilizes or reduces the ability of a patient to move his or her arms, legs, body, or head freely" (HHS, 2008, p. 90).

There are several contraindications for the use of seclusion and restraint (Sadock et al., 2015). Patients who have extremely unstable medical and psychiatric conditions are not considered safe candidates for these treatments. Chronic obstructive pulmonary disease, spinal injury, seizure disorder, and pregnancy are examples of contraindicated problems. Delirium or dementia may make seclusion and restraint intolerable due to the absence of stimulation. These restrictive measures should be avoided in patients who are overtly suicidal and those who require monitoring for severe drug reactions or overdoses.

A patient may not be held in seclusion or restraint without an order from a licensed practitioner, although in emergency situations, the order may be received after the fact. Once in restraint, a patient must be directly observed and formally assessed at frequent regular intervals for level of awareness, level of activity, safety within the restraints, hydration, toileting needs, nutrition, and comfort. Licensing and accreditation agencies mandate how frequently you need to observe patients in seclusion and restraint.

Each team member is trained in the correct use of seclusion and restraint. The team should be organized before approaching the patient so that there is a clear leader and each team member knows his or her individual responsibility. The team leader is the only person talking to the patient to decrease stimuli. The patient must be given every opportunity to regain control so that the least restrictive method can be used. If restraints are to be used, the patient is informed at this point of the team's intent and the reason for the actions. The team remains calm and acts as quickly as possible.

Once the patient is placed in seclusion or restrained, the nurse must get an order from the appropriate healthcare provider. The nurse may also get an order for medication and administer it to the patient. The team leader continues to communicate with the patient in a calm steady voice indicating decisiveness, consistency, and control. Guidelines for the use of mechanical restraints are in Box 27.3.

While the patient is in seclusion or restraint, close monitoring to determine the patient's ability to reintegrate into unit activities is mandatory. Reintegration should be gradual and geared toward the patient's ability to handle increasing amounts of stimulation. If the reintegration proves to be too much for the patient and results in increased agitation, the individual is returned to the room or another quiet area. Patients must be able to follow commands and control behaviors before reintegration can occur.

BOX 27.3 Guidelines for Use of Mechanical Restraint

Indications for Use

- To protect the patient from self-harm
- To prevent the patient from assaulting others

Legal Requirements

- Multidisciplinary involvement
- Appropriate healthcare provider's signature according to state law
- Patient advocate or relative notification
- Seclusion/restraint discontinued as soon as possible

Documentation

- Patient's behavior leading to restraint/seclusion
- Least-restrictive measures used before restraint
- Interventions used and patient's response interventions
- Plan of care for restraint/seclusion use implemented
- Ongoing evaluations by nursing staff and appropriate healthcare providers

Clinical Assessments

- Patient's mental state at time of restraint
- Physical examination for medical problems possibly causing behavioral changes
- Need for restraints

Observation

- Staff in constant attendance
- Complete written record every 15 minutes
- Monitor vital signs
- Assess range of movement
- Observe blood flow in hands/feet
- Observe that restraint is not rubbing
- Provide for nutrition, hydration, and elimination

Release Procedure

- Patient must be able to follow instructions and stay in control
- Termination of restraints
- Debrief with patient

Restraint Tips

- Physical holding of a patient against will is a restraint
- Four side rails up is a restraint except in seizure precautions
- Keeping a patient in his or her room by physical intervention is seclusion
- Tucking sheets in so tightly patient cannot move is a restraint
- Orders for seclusion/restraint cannot be prn ("as needed")

Generally, a structured reintegration is the best approach. Once the patient no longer requires the locked seclusion room or restraints and is able to exercise self-control, he or she can be returned to the unit. Afterward, the patient should be observed carefully to maintain safety. In some cases, the patient may require further seclusion or restraint for which you would have to obtain another order.

Immediately after the seclusion or restraint episode, the staff must engage in debriefing with one another. Staff analysis of the episode of violence, referred to as *critical incident debriefing*, is crucial for a number of reasons. First, a review is necessary to ensure that quality care was provided to the patient. Staff members need to critically examine their response to the patient. Questions to be answered include the following:

- Could we have done anything that would have prevented the episode? If yes, then what could have been done, and why was it not done in this situation?
- Did the team respond as a team? Were team members acting according to the policies and procedures of the unit? If not, why not?
- How do staff members feel about this patient? About this situation? Feelings of fear and anger are discussed and handled. Employee morale, productivity, use of sick leave time, transfer requests, and absenteeism are all affected by patient violence, especially if a staff member has been injured. Staff members must feel supported by their peers and by the organizational policies and procedures established to maintain a safe environment.
- Is there a need for additional staff education regarding how to respond to violent patients?
- How did the actual restraining process go? What could have been done differently? Do not focus only on whether staff members were acting like a team.
- If injury occurred, has it been reported and cared for? It has been shown that there is vast underreporting of violence against healthcare staff.

When the patient is reintegrated into the unit, discussion with the patient is an important part of the therapeutic process. Going over what occurred allows the patient to learn from the situation, to identify the stressors that precipitated the out-of-control behavior, and to plan alternative ways of responding to these stressors in the future.

The nurse must provide documentation in situations in which violence was either averted or actually occurred including the following:

- Behaviors that occurred as the patient was escalating
- Nursing interventions and the patient's responses
- Evaluation of the interventions used
- Detailed description of the patient's behaviors during the assaultive stage
- All nursing interventions used to defuse the crisis
- Patient's response to those interventions
- Observations of the patient and interventions performed while the patient was in restraints and/or seclusion
- The way the patient was reintegrated into the unit milieu

Box 27.4 lists selected *Nursing Interventions Classifications (NIC)* for *Anger Control Assistance* (Bulechek et al., 2013).

Let's take a closer look at intervening in different settings with patients who are exhibiting anger and have the potential for aggression and violence.

BOX 27.4 NIC Interventions for Anger-Control Assistance

Definition: Facilitation of the expression of anger in an adaptive, nonviolent manner

Activities (partial list):

- Establish basic trust and rapport with patient.
- Use calm, reassuring approach.
- Determine appropriate behavioral expectations for expression of anger, given patient's level of cognitive and physical functioning.
- Limit access to frustrating situations until patient is able to express anger in an adaptive manner.
- Encourage patient to seek assistance from nursing staff or responsible others during periods of increasing tension.
- Monitor potential for inappropriate aggression and intervene before its expression.
- Prevent physical harm if anger is directed at self or others (e.g., restrain and remove potential weapons).
- Provide reassurance to patient that nursing staff will intervene to prevent patient from losing control.
- Use external controls (e.g., physical or manual restraint, timeouts, and seclusion) as needed to calm patient who is expressing anger in a maladaptive manner.

Adapted from Bulechek, G. M., Butcher, H. K., Dochterman, J. M., & Wagner, C. (2013). *Nursing interventions classification (NIC)* (6th ed.). St. Louis, MO: Mosby.

Caring for Patients in General Hospital Settings

Patients with Healthy Coping Who Are Overwhelmed

A patient loses autonomy and control when hospitalized, which can cause a great deal of related distress. When this stress is combined with the uncertainty of illness, a patient may respond in ways that are not usual for him or her. A careful nursing assessment, with history and information from family members, helps evaluate whether a patient's anger is a usual or an unusual way of managing stress.

Interventions for patients whose usual coping strategies are healthy involve finding ways to reestablish or substitute similar means of dealing with the hospitalization. This problem solving occurs in collaboration with the patient in interactions that demonstrate the nurse acknowledges the patient's distress, validates it as understandable under the circumstances, and indicates a willingness to search for solutions. Validation includes making an apology to the patient when appropriate, such as when a promised intervention (e.g., changing a dressing by a certain time) has not been delivered, or sympathizing with the patient about the "horrible food" by assisting with menu selections.

Patients who have become angry may be unable to moderate this emotion enough to problem solve with their nurses. Others may be unable to communicate the source of their anger. Often, the nurse—knowing the patient and the context of the anger—can make an accurate guess at what feeling is behind the anger. Naming this feeling can lead to a dissipation of the anger, help the patient to feel understood, and lead to a calmer discussion of the distress. Some of the feelings that can precipitate anger are listed in Box 27.5. The following vignette provides an example of nursing interventions that are helpful in dissipating anger in a hospital situation.

VIGNETTE: Rachel, a 41-year-old woman with a history of peripheral vascular disease, surgeries for vascular grafts, and repair of graft occlusions is admitted to the hospital with severe pain in her left foot. Tests reveal that vessels to the foot are occluded. Additional surgery is ruled out, and medication is prescribed. Unfortunately, the medication is ineffective, and the foot begins to necrotize. Physicians discuss amputation with the patient. Rachel refuses the surgery, demands a series of unproven alternative therapies, and is extremely angry with all members of the hospital staff. The treatment team becomes increasingly impatient to schedule surgery before the tissue death worsens

Continued

and because the patient is beginning to exhibit signs of systemic infection. This impatience aggravates the patient's feelings of being out of control and erodes her belief that she is a competent partner in her treatment.

The nurse is aware that before Rachel became disabled by progressive vascular disease, she had been employed for many years as a buyer at a local department store. The nurse knows too that the patient's family lives some distance from the hospital and is unable to visit regularly. Nursing intervention is twofold. First, Rachel's anger and unwillingness to discuss her condition ends when the nurse empathizes with her feelings of fear and being out of control. Once the anger is reduced, the nurse is able to help Rachel negotiate more time for the final decision; this allows her to process anticipatory grieving (including stages of denial, anger, and bargaining). In this interval, the patient's wish to explore alternative therapies is addressed via second and third medical opinions. Rachel is also able to spend more time discussing her concerns with her family.

BOX 27.5 Feelings that May Precipitate Anger

- Discounted
- Embarrassed
- Frightened
- Found out
- Guilty
- Humiliated
- Hurt
- Ignored
- Inadequate
- Insecure
- Unheard
- Out of control of the situation
- Rejected
- Threatened
- Tired
- Vulnerable

Patients with Marginal Coping Skills

Patients whose coping skills were marginal before hospitalization need a different set of interventions than those with basically healthy ways of coping. Patients with maladaptive coping are poorly equipped to use alternatives when their initial attempts to cope are unsuccessful or are inappropriate. Such patients frequently manifest anger that moves quickly from anxiety to aggression. For some people, anger and intimidation are primary strategies used to obtain their short-term goals of feelings of control or mastery. For others, the anger occurs when limited or primitive attempts at coping are unsuccessful and alternatives are unknown. For these patients, anger and violence are particular risks in inpatient settings.

This is especially true for hospitalized patients with chemical dependence who may be anxious about being cut off from their substance of choice. They may have well-founded concerns that any physical pain will be inadequately addressed. Many patients with marginal coping also have personality styles that externalize blame. That is, they see the source of their discomfort and anxiety as being outside themselves; relief must therefore also come from an outside source (e.g., the nurse, medication).

Interventions begin with attempts to understand and meet the patient's needs. For instance, you can moderate baseline anxiety by the provision of comfort items before they are requested (e.g., decaffeinated coffee, deck of cards). This can build rapport and acts symbolically to reassure. Reducing ambiguity or uncertainty can also help minimize anxiety. This strategy includes clear and concrete communication. Nurses should be clear about what is within the nurse's power to provide, such as "I can't order Vicodin for you, but I will talk with your nurse practitioner about what we can do." Most hospitals have some sort of withdrawal protocol assuring the patient that he or she will not go through withdrawal without medication. This can be very anxiety relieving if the patient has a chemical dependency problem.

Interventions for anxiety might also include the use of distractions such as magazines, action comics, and video games. Generally, distractions that are colorful and do not require sustained attention work best, although this varies according to the patient's interests and abilities. Finally, patients with a high level of baseline anxiety and limited coping skills are helped when their interactions with the treatment team are predictable. This may include speaking with the physician at a specific time each day and consistency in nursing assignments. Individuals from outside the unit such as a chaplain or a volunteer may help by giving the patient more attention.

Because these patients have limited coping skills, once anxiety is moderated, nursing interventions include teaching alternative behaviors and strategies. For patients who externalize blame, it is best to precede such teaching by a gentle challenge. The challenge serves to engage the patient's interest in teaching that might otherwise be seen as irrelevant. This intervention is also important in that the nurse has (1) avoided a punitive or demeaning response that might have fueled escalation of the patient's anger, (2) taught a number of strategies, and (3) provided the patient with choices and thus with more control.

Often, others communicate anger through long-term verbal abuse. If attempts to teach alternatives have not been successful, you can use three interventions:

1. The first is to leave the room as soon as verbal abuse begins. The patient can be informed that the nurse will return in a specific amount of time (e.g., 20 minutes) when the situation is calmer. A matter-of-fact, neutral manner is important because fear, indignation, and arguing are gratifying to many verbally abusive patients. Alternatively, if the nurse is in the middle of a procedure and cannot leave immediately, the nurse can break off conversation and eye contact, completing the procedure quickly and matter-of-factly before leaving the room. The nurse avoids chastising, threatening, or responding punitively to the patient.
2. Withdrawal of attention of verbal abuse is successful only if a second intervention is also used. This step requires attending positively to, and thus reinforcing, nonabusive

communication by the patient. Interventions can include discussing non–illness-related topics, responding to requests, and providing emotional support.

3. Patients who are verbally abusive may respond best to the predictability of routine such as scheduled contacts with the nurse (e.g., every 30 or 60 minutes). Use of such contacts provides nursing attention that is not contingent on the patient's behavior and therefore does not reinforce the abuse. Of course, the patient's illness or injury may sometimes require nursing visits for assessment or intervention outside the scheduled contact times. These visits can be carried out in a calm, brief, matter-of-fact manner.

Implementing appropriate interventions can be difficult when the nurse is feeling threatened. Remaining matter-of-fact with patients who habitually use anger and intimidation can be difficult; these patients are often skillful at making personal and pointed statements. It is important to remember that patients do not know their nurses personally and thus have no basis on which they can make judgments. Nurses can also vent their own responses elsewhere with other staff or family members (while maintaining confidentiality) or by critical incident debriefing.

VIGNETTE: A 21-year-old man who was in an automobile accident is bedridden with a pelvic fracture. During his first day of admission, he yells at each nurse who walks by his room, using expletives in his demands that the nurse enter the room.

The nurse who is assigned to the patient for the evening stops in his doorway after he yells at her and asks in mild disbelief, "Is this working for you? Do nurses really come in here when you yell at them that way?" The patient responds sullenly, justifying his behavior by complaining about his care. However, the nurse's challenge has caught his attention, and she goes on to suggest alternative strategies for contacting her and other nurses. The strategies are immediately put into use by the patient.

Caring for Patients in Inpatient Psychiatric Settings

It is important to know that not all psychiatric patients are violence-prone, and aggression appears to be correlated less with certain illnesses than with certain patient characteristics. The two most significant predictors of violence are a history of violence and a history of impulsivity.

Situational factors contribute to patient anger and aggression. For instance, feelings of vulnerability and powerlessness resulting from trying to come to grips with depersonalized hospital routines, intrusive procedures, and restrictions on freedom can lead to anger and possibly aggression. Additional causes of patients' anger include (1) unrealistic expectations that their nurses will be angels of mercy, (2) the feeling that care providers are ignoring their physical and psychological needs, and (3) the feeling that healthcare providers fail to recognize the uniqueness and wholeness of the patient.

If staff can identify patients who have a potential for violence, early intervention becomes possible. Nurses can work with these patients to recognize early signs of anger and can teach them strategies to manage the anger and prevent aggression.

VIGNETTE: A 19-year-old man has a 2-year history of quadriplegia. He also has a history of drug misuse that began in grade school, an inability to set or work toward long-term goals, and a primary coping style of anger and intimidation. The patient is admitted to an inpatient psychiatric unit because of increasing suicidal ideation. He clearly communicates to staff that his preferred means of coping with anger is to "cuss people out" and run into them with his wheelchair. In the hospital, however, the consequence of wheelchair assaults is that the patient is secluded in his room, which he finds intolerable. The patient asks the staff to help him manage his anger.

The nurse assigned to this young man sets aside time to interview him regarding the triggers for his anger. He identifies several issues that "make him angry." These typically relate to feeling unheard and controlled by the staff. Together, the nurse and patient examine alternative ways for him to deal with these situations. Two coping strategies are telling the staff he doesn't feel they are listening to him and letting them know he needs to be involved in planning his care.

The patient and nurse also role-play a situation in which the staff member tells the patient that he must attend a group session. Such a situation would usually result in the patient's becoming angry and aggressive. In the role-play he is willing to "try out" alternative responses to communicate his feelings and thus to handle his anger. In addition, the patient is willing to enter into a behavioral contract with the nurse, stating that he will not curse at staff or assault anyone with his wheelchair. Instead, he will let the staff know when he is feeling angry and what the triggering issue is so that he can find a nonaggressive resolution.

Because the patient is motivated to gain personal control, he responds positively to these suggestions. In addition, once it becomes clear that his issues of feeling unheard and out of control underlie most episodes of anger, the patient is able to target these issues for problem solving. He develops effective and appropriate ways to make himself heard and understood. The patient's suicidal impulses, which occur when he is frustrated, also diminish.

Caring for Patients with Cognitive Deficits

Patients with cognitive deficits are particularly at risk for acting aggressively. Such deficits may result from delirium, dementias (e.g., Alzheimer's disease, multi-infarct dementia), or brain injury (refer to Chapter 23). Traditional approaches to disorientation and to the agitation it can cause have relied heavily on reality orientation and medication. Reality orientation consists of providing the correct information to the patient about place, date, and current life circumstances. For many patients, this is comforting because it reminds them of pertinent information and helps them feel grounded. For others, reality orientation does not work. Because of their cognitive disorder, they can no longer "enter into our reality." They become frightened and more agitated and may become aggressive. Orientation aids, such as a calendar and a clock, can provide easy reference and increased autonomy. Such aids must be prominent and easily read by patients with diminished eyesight. Sedating medication may calm agitation, but the risks often outweigh the benefits. Sedation only further clouds a patient's sensorium, which makes disorientation worse and increases the risk of falls and injuries. It is better to examine alternative interventions.

Typically, patients experiencing delirium will be in and out of reality. At times they will appear perfectly fine, and at others they will have a clouded sensorium. They will sometimes fall asleep as you are talking to them. Often, patients with delirium have visual hallucinations, commonly of children, animals, or bugs. Occasionally, they will show periods of paranoia. The best intervention for delirium is to find and treat the medical cause. The next choice is to medicate the symptoms with a low-dose antipsychotic and discontinue it as the delirium clears.

Patients with any clouding of the sensorium have difficulty interpreting environmental stimuli. Another set of interventions involves making the environment as simple, predictable, and comfortable as possible. Simplicity includes decreasing sensory stimuli. In the hospital, this might include placing the patient's bed away from doorways that enter onto the hall and choosing not to turn on the television. Establishing a routine of activities for each day and displaying the day's schedule prominently in the patient's room can provide predictability. You can enhance the comfort of the patient by providing familiar photographs and objects from home. The availability of a rocking chair can provide a rhythmic source of self-soothing.

Sometimes the patient with a cognitive disorder experiences such severe agitation and aggression that it is referred to as a *catastrophic reaction*. The patient may scream, strike out, or cry because of overwhelming fear. Adopting a calm and unhurried manner is the best approach to take with such a patient. To respond effectively to episodes of agitation, it is crucial to identify the antecedents (i.e., what preceded the episode) and the consequences of such episodes. Once antecedents are understood, interventions are often obvious.

VIGNETTE: An 81-year-old woman with Alzheimer's disease always becomes agitated during her morning care. Her caregivers begin to dread this responsibility. Careful observation of antecedents to the episodes of agitation reveals a natural course to the morning problems. The patient is initially calm when care begins. However, one staff person gives morning care to the patient and her roommate at the same time, moving between the two. Observation of the process reveals that the patient becomes distracted by cues being given to her roommate and often startles when the caregiver returns to her. As this process continues over several minutes, the patient becomes increasingly distressed and then agitated. The patient's morning agitation ends when a change is made so that one person who remains with her throughout the process provides the patient's care.

Patients who misperceive their setting or life situation can use **validation therapy** to calm themselves. Some disoriented older patients believe that they are young and feel the need to return to important tasks that were a significant part of those earlier years. For example, a woman may insist that she must go home to take care of her babies. Telling the patient that her babies have grown up and there is no home to return to is not only cruel but nontherapeutic and will result in increased agitation. It is often more helpful to reflect back to the patient the feelings behind her demand and to show understanding and concern for her worry.

Rather than attempting to reorient the patient, the nurse should ask the patient to further describe the setting or situation reported to be a problem (e.g., the need to return home). During the conversation, the nurse can comment on what appears to be underlying the patient's distress thus validating it. In the earlier example, the woman who believes that she needs to return home to care for her children is asked to tell the nurse more about her children. The nurse may note that the patient misses her children and that the current setting gets lonely at times:

Nurse: "Mrs. Green, you miss your children, and this can be a lonely place."

As the nurse shows interest in aspects of the patient's life, the nurse establishes himself or herself as a safe understanding person. In turn, the patient often becomes calmer and more open to redirection. As patients reminisce in this fashion, they often bring themselves into the present:

Patient: "Of course, they're all grown and doing well on their own now."

Refer to Chapter 23 for a more detailed discussion of interventions for people with cognitive impairments. Refer to Chapter 31 for a more detailed discussion of the use of validation and reminiscent therapeutic modalities for older adults.

EVALUATION

Evaluation of the care plan is essential for patients who are potentially angry and aggressive. A well-considered plan has specific outcome criteria (see Table 27.1). Evaluation provides information about the extent to which the interventions have achieved the outcomes. Revision focuses on all aspects of the nursing process:

- Was the assessment accurate and thorough?
- Were the nursing diagnoses applicable to the assessment data?
- Did the nursing diagnoses accurately drive nursing interventions?
- Was the plan comprehensive and individualized?

The initial plan may have included assessment of the environmental stimuli that precede a patient's agitation. Once these are identified, the plan provides interventions specific to those stimuli. However, the plan can work only if staff members evaluate the effectiveness of the approach by noting the extent to which agitation is decreased. Evaluation may reveal that the patient's agitation has decreased except in specific situations. You then revise the plan to include these situations.

KEY POINTS TO REMEMBER

- Violence in the United States is widespread. Nurses are particularly likely to come across anger, aggression, and violence if they work in the emergency room, psychiatric units, geriatric units, and intensive care units.
- Understanding patient cues to escalating aggression, appropriate goals for intervention for individuals in a variety of situations, and helpful nursing interventions is important for nurses in any setting.
- The expression of anger can lead to increased anger and to negative physiological changes.
- Biological factors and psychological factors provide explanations for anger, aggression, and violence.

- It is helpful for providers of care to know what cues to look for and what to assess verbally and nonverbally when a patient's anger is escalating.
- A patient's past aggressive behavior is the most important indicator of future aggressive episodes.
- Working with angry and aggressive patients is a challenge for all nurses, and a careful understanding and recognition of one's personal responses to angry or threatening patients can be crucial.
- Many approaches are effective in helping patients deescalate and maintain control.
- Different interventions are used, depending on the patient's coping abilities, cognitive status, and potential for violence.
- Specific medications such as antipsychotics, mood stabilizers, and antianxiety medications may be useful in treating acute episodes of agitation in the long term.
- Seclusion and restraints may be necessary to ensure the safety of the patient, other patients, and the staff. They should be used only when other less restrictive measures such as verbal intervention, offering as needed medication, and reducing stimuli have failed.
- Each unit should have a protocol for the safe use of restraints and for the humane management of care during the time the patient is restrained and clear guidelines for understanding and protecting the patient's legal rights.
- Patients who are overwhelmed, possess marginal coping skills, or have cognitive deficits require special attention to reduce and prevent episodes of anger, aggression, and violence.

CRITICAL THINKING

1. Jennifer admits a 24-year-old man with mania to an inpatient unit. She notes that the patient is irritable, has trouble sitting during the interview, and has a history of assault.
   a. Identify appropriate responses the nurse can make to the patient.
   b. What interventions should be built into the care plan?
   c. Identify at least three long-term outcomes to consider when planning care.
2. What are the two indicators for the use of seclusion and restraint rather than verbal interventions? Give rationales for your answers.
3. Discuss the use of restraint and seclusion with your clinical group or in class. Choose a side and defend it (even if you do not necessarily believe it) regarding the following:
   a. There are always better alternatives to seclusion and restraint.
   b. Seclusion and restraint are underutilized; people who have tried to limit their use have gone too far.
   c. Using chemical restraint with medication is/is not preferable to seclusion and restraint.

CHAPTER REVIEW

Questions

1. Which individuals are most at risk for displaying aggressive behavior? *Select all that apply.*
   a. An adolescent embarrassed in front of friends.
   b. A young male who feels rejected by the social group.
   c. A young adult depressed after the death of a friend.
   d. A middle-aged adult who feels that concerns are going unheard.
   e. A patient who was discovered telling a lie.
2. A newly admitted male patient has a long history of aggressive behavior toward staff. Which statement by the nurse demonstrates the need for more information about the use of restraint?
   a. "If his behavior warrants restraints, someone will stay with him the entire time he's restrained."
   b. "I'll call the primary provider and get an as needed (prn) seclusion/restraint order."
   c. "If he is restrained, be sure he is offered food and fluids regularly."
   d. "Remember that physical restraints are our last resort."
3. Which intervention(s) should the nurse implement when helping a patient expresses anger in an inappropriate manner? *Select all that apply.*
   a. Approach the patient in a calm, reassuring manner.
   b. Provide suggestions regarding acceptable ways of communicating anger.
   c. Warn the patient that being angry is not a healthy emotional state.
   d. Set limits on the angry behavior that will be tolerated.
   e. Allow any expression of anger as long as no one is hurt.
4. Which guidelines should direct nursing care when deescalating an angry patient? *Select all that apply.*
   a. Intervene as quickly as possible
   b. Identify the trigger for the anger
   c. Behave calmly and respectfully
   d. Recognize the patient's need for increased personal space
   e. Demands are agreed to as long as they won't result in harm to anyone
5. Which comorbid condition would result in cautious use of a selective serotonin reuptake inhibitors for a patient with chronic aggression?
   a. Asthma
   b. Anxiety disorder
   c. Glaucoma
   d. Bipolar disorder

6. John Patrick is a widower with four daughters. He has enjoyed a healthy relationship with all of them until they reached puberty. As each girl began to mature physically, he acted in an aggressive manner, beating her without provocation. John Patrick is most likely acting on:
   a. Self-protective measures
   b. Stress of raising four daughters
   c. Frustration of unhealthy desire
   d. Motivating his daughters to be chaste
7. A nurse named Darryl has been hired to work in a psychiatric intensive care unit. He has undergone training on recognizing escalating anger. Which statement indicates that he understands danger signs in regard to aggression?
   a. "I need to be aware of patients who are withdrawn and sitting alone."
   b. "An obvious change in behavior is a risk factor for aggression."
   c. "Patients who seek constant attention are more likely to be violent."
   d. "Patients who talk to themselves are the most dangerous."
8. An effective method of preventing escalation in an environment with violent offenders is to develop a level of trust through:
   a. A casual authoritative demeanor
   b. Keeping patients busy
   c. Brief, frequent, nonthreatening encounters
   d. Threats of seclusion or punishment
9. Twenty-four-hour observation is a good choice for restraint in which of the following patients?
   a. An inmate with suicidal ideation on hospice care
   b. A sex offender in the psychiatric intensive care unit
   c. An aggressive female with antisocial personality disorder
   d. An inmate diagnosed with paranoid schizophrenia
10. Chronic obstructive pulmonary disease, spinal injury, seizure disorder, and pregnancy are conditions that:
    a. Frequently result in out of control behavior.
    b. Respond well to therapeutic holding.
    c. Necessitate the use of only two-point restraint.
    d. Contraindicate restraint and seclusion.

Answers

1. **a, b, d, e**; 2. **b**; 3. **a, b, d**; 4. **a, b, c, d**; 5. **d**; 6. **c**; 7. **b**; 8. **c**; 9. **a**; 10. **d**

Visit the Evolve website for a posttest on the content in this chapter: http://evolve.elsevier.com/Varcarolis

Post-Test interactive review

REFERENCES

Adams, B. (2014). *Riverview nurse hospitalized after attack by angry patient*. Retrieved from http://www.pressherald.com/2014/08/18/riverview-nurse-hospitalized-after-attack-by-angry-patient/.

Bandura, A. (1973). *Aggression: A social learning analysis*. New York, NY: Prentice Hall.

Beck, A. (1976). *Cognitive therapy and the emotional disorders*. New York, NY: International Universities Press.

Boylan, J. M., & Ryff, C. D. (2015). High anger expression exacerbates the relationship between age and metabolic syndrome. *Journals of Gerontology*, *70*(1), 77–82.

Bulechek, G. M., Butcher, H. K., Dochterman, J. M., & Wagner, C. (2013). *Nursing interventions classification (NIC)* (6th ed.). St. Louis, MO: Mosby.

Centers for Disease Control and Prevention. (2015). Surveillance for violent deaths—national violent death reporting system, 16 states. *Morbidity and Mortality Weekly Report*, *59*(SS04), 1–50. Retrieved from http://www.cdc.gov/mmwr/pdf/ss/ss5904.pdf.

DeMarche, E. (2013). *Houston nurse fatally stabbed in hospital attack hailed as hero for saving patient*. Retrieved from http://www.foxnews.com/us/2013/11/27/houston-nurse-fatally-stabbed-in-hospital-attack-hailed-hero-for-saving.html.

Freud, S. (1930). *Civilization and its discontents*. Austria: Internationaler Psychoanalytischer Verlag Wien.

Griffin, B. J., Worthington, E. L., Lavelock, C. R., Wade, N. G., & Hoyt, W. T. (2015). Forgiveness and mental health. In L. Toussaint, E. Worthington, & D. R. Williams (Eds.), *Forgiveness and health* (pp. 77–90). Netherlands: Springer.

Hellerstein, D. J., Staub, A. M., & Lequesne, E. (2007). Decreasing the use of restraint and seclusion among psychiatric inpatients. *Journal of Psychiatric Practice*, *13*(5), 1–16.

Herdman, T.H., & Kamitsuru, S. (Eds.). (2014). *NANDA International nursing diagnoses: Definitions and classification*, 2015–2017. Oxford, UK: Wiley Blackwell.

Johnson, S. L., & Carver, C. S. (2016). Emotion-relevant impulsivity predicts sustained anger and aggression after remission in bipolar I disorder. *Journal of Affective Disorders*, *189*, 169–175.

KWTX News. (2016). *Local woman jailed after ER nurse attacked over pain medication*. Retrieved from http://www.kwtx.com/content/news/Local-woman-jailed-after-ER-nurse-attacked-over-pain-meds-383298321.html.

Menninger, W. W. (2007). Uncontained rage: A psychoanalytic perspective on violence. *Bulletin of the Menninger Clinic*, *71*(2), 115–131.

Moorhead, S., Johnson, M., Maas, M. L., & Swanson, E. (2013). *Nursing outcomes classification (NOC)* (5th ed.). St. Louis, MO: Elsevier.

Mostofsky, E., Penner, E. A., & Mittleman, M. A. (2014). Outbursts of anger as a trigger of acute cardiovascular events: A systematic review and meta analysis. *European Heart Journal*, *35*(21), 1404–1410.

Narayan, K. L., Narr, V., Kumari, R. P., Woods, P. M., Thompson, A. W., Toga, T., et al. (2007). Regional cortical thinning in subjects with violent antisocial personality disorder or schizophrenia. *American Journal of Psychiatry*, *164*, 1418–1427.

Narvaes, R., & de Almeida, R. M. M. (2014). Aggressive behavior and three neurotransmitters: Dopamine, GABA, and serotonin–A review of the last 10 years. *Psychology and Neuroscience*, *7*(4), 601–607.

Pardini, D. A., Raine, A., Erickson, K., & Loeber, R. (2014). Lower amygdala volume in men is associated with childhood aggression, early psychopathic traits, and future violence. *Biological Psychiatry*, *75*(1), 73–80.

Sadock, B.J., Sadock, V.A., & Ruiz, P. (2015). *Kaplan and Sadock's synopsis of psychiatry* (11th ed.). Philadelphia, PA: Wolters Kluwer.

Sansone, R. A., Farukhi, S., & Wiederman, M. W. (2012). History of childhood trauma and disruptive behaviors in the medical setting. *International Journal of Psychiatry in Clinical Practice, 16*(1), 68–71.

Siever, L. J. (2008). Neurobiology of aggression and violence. *The American Journal of Psychiatry, 165*(4), 429–442.

Skinner, B. (1953). *Science and human behavior*. New York, NY: Macmillan.

Smagin, D. A., Park, J., Michurina, T. V., Peunova, N., Glass, Z., Sayed, K., et al. (2015). Altered hippocampal neurogenesis and amygdalar neuronal activity in adult mice with repeated experience of aggression. *Frontiers in Neuroscience,* 9. Retrieved from http://journal.frontiersin.org/article/10.3389/fnins.2015.00443/full.

Speroni, K. G., Fitch, T., Dawson, E., Dugan, L., & Atherton, M. (2014). Incidence and cost of nurse workplace violence perpetrated by hospital patients or patient visitors. *Journal of Emergency Nursing, 40*(3), 218–228.

US Department of Health and Human Services, Centers for Medicare and Medicaid Services. (2008). *Revised interpretive guidelines for seclusion and restraint*. Retrieved from http://www.cms.hhs.gov/EOG/downloads/EO%.

Wilkowski, B. M., & Robinson, M. D. (2012). When aggressive individuals see the world more accurately: The case of perceptual sensitivity to subtle facial expressions of anger. *Personality and Social Psychology Bulletin, 38*(1), 540–543.

28

Child, Older Adult, and Intimate Partner Violence

Margaret Jordan Halter, Judi Sateren

Visit the Evolve website for a pretest on the content in this chapter: http://evolve.elsevier.com/Varcarolis Pre-Test interactive review

OBJECTIVES

1. Identify the nature and scope of family violence and factors contributing to its occurrence.
2. Identify three indicators of (a) physical abuse, (b) sexual abuse, (c) neglect, and (d) emotional abuse.
3. Describe risk factors for both victimization and perpetration of family violence.
4. Describe four areas to assess when interviewing a person who has experienced abuse.
5. Identify two common emotional responses the nurse might experience when faced with a person subjected to abuse.
6. Formulate four nursing diagnoses for the survivor of abuse and list supporting data from the assessment.
7. Write out a safety plan for a victim of intimate partner abuse.
8. Discuss the legal and ethical responsibilities of nurses when working with families experiencing violence.
9. Compare and contrast primary, secondary, and tertiary levels of intervention, giving two examples of intervention for each level.
10. Describe at least three possible referrals for an abusive family including the telephone numbers of appropriate agencies in the community.
11. Discuss three therapeutic modalities useful in working with abusive families.

OUTLINE

OUTLINE—cont'd

KEY TERMS AND CONCEPTS

act of commission
act of omission
crisis situation
economic abuse
emotional abuse
family violence
neglect
perpetrator
physical abuse
primary prevention
safety plan
secondary prevention
sexual abuse
shelters or safe houses
survivor
tertiary prevention
vulnerable person

There's no place like home. This is a statement familiar to most of us, and home is a source of refuge and peace for many. Yet for some children, adults, and elders, the home is a dangerous place where family members or intimate partners demonstrate disregard for the rights of others. Family violence, also called domestic violence, is among the most important public health issues in the United States. Nurses are in a unique position to respond to family violence and are educated to identify, evaluate, and treat both victims and perpetrators of violence.

Types of Abuse

Legal definitions of family or domestic violence vary from state to state. Forty-six states have specific definitions in their civil statutes. Generally speaking, the major types of abuse include the following:

- Physical abuse is the infliction of physical pain or bodily harm such as slapping, punching, hitting, choking, pushing, restraining, biting, throwing, and burning.
- Sexual abuse is any form of sexual contact or exposure without consent or in circumstances in which the victim is incapable of giving consent. Sexual abuse is also referred to as *sexual assault* or *rape* and is discussed in Chapter 29.
- Emotional abuse is the undermining of a person's self-worth. This may include constant criticism, humiliating, diminishing one's abilities, name-calling, intimidating, isolating, and damaging relationships with others.
- Neglect is the failure to provide for physical, emotional, educational, and medical needs.
- Economic abuse is controlling a person's access to economic resources making an individual financially dependent. Forbidding school attendance or employment keeps a person dependent.

Crisis Situation

Anyone may be at risk for abuse in a crisis situation, or a situation that puts stress on a family with a violent member. A person with effective impulse control, problem-solving skills, and a healthy support system is less likely to resort to violence. However, stressful life events tax coping skills, leaving the perpetrator incapable of dealing with the situation. Social isolation caused by frequent moves or an inability to make friends contributes to ineffective coping during crisis situations.

Perpetrator and the Vulnerable Person

The term perpetrator applies to any member of a household who is violent toward another member such as parents, partners, siblings, and extended family members. Perpetrators often consider their own needs to be more important than anyone else's and look toward others to meet their needs. Both male and female perpetrators perceive themselves as having poor social skills. They describe their relationships with their partners as being the closest they have ever known, and they typically lack supportive relationships outside the relationship.

The vulnerable person is the family member upon whom abuse is perpetrated. This individual is variously referred to as the *victim, survivor*, or *victim/survivor*. Using the term survivor recognizes the recovery and healing process that follows victimization and does not have the connotation of passivity that victim has.

CHILD ABUSE

In 2014 there were 3.6 million referrals for child abuse and neglect (US Department of Health and Human Service [HHS], 2016). The most common form of abuse was neglect (78%), followed by physical abuse (18%) and sexual abuse (9%). Other types of abuse including emotional and threatened abuse, parent's drug/alcohol abuse, or lack of supervision made up the remaining 11% of cases.

Child abuse can take the form of something improper that is done to a child, which is an act of commission (Centers for Disease Control and Prevention [CDC], 2016). Acts of commission are deliberate and intentional. They include physical, sexual, and emotional abuse. An act of omission, or neglect, occurs when a child's basic physical, emotional, or educational needs are not met or when a child is not protected from harm. Acts of omission include physical neglect, emotional neglect, medical and dental neglect, educational neglect, inadequate supervision, and exposure to violence.

Epidemiology

Girls are slightly more likely to be abused and make up 51% of the victims. In general, the younger children are, the more vulnerable they are to abuse. Tragically, children under the age of 1 account for about 24% of all abuse cases (HHS, 2016). Approximately 80% of children who die are younger than 4 years of age, and boys die at a slightly higher rate than girls. In 2014 nearly 1600 children died of abuse and neglect.

The prevalence of sexual abuse in children is difficult to determine due to the fact that children are often unable to describe their experience. About 40% do not exhibit clear symptoms of sexual abuse (American Psychological Association, 2014). Relatively uncommon in infants, sexual abuse increases with age. By age 17, sexual abuse and sexual assault occur in nearly 27% of all girls and about 5% of all boys (Finkelhor et al., 2014). Adults are responsible for these cases of abuse and assault about 11% of the time for girls and about 2% for boys. Females are at most risk in late adolescence.

About 92% of child abuse perpetrators are the victim's parents (HHS, 2016). Females are somewhat more likely to abuse children. Women make up 51% of the perpetrators.

The prevalence of child abuse varies within ethnic communities. Table 28.1 gives statistics related to abuse rates and fatalities within various ethnicities.

Risk Factors

Children are most likely to be abused if they are younger than 4 years of age (CDC, 2015a). Other risk factors for child abuse include being perceived as being different due to temperamental traits, congenital abnormalities, or chronic disease. Perhaps the child reminds the parents of someone they do not like such as an ex-spouse. Children who do not live up to the parents' fantasy of what the child should be like are at risk. Children who are the result of unwanted pregnancies are at higher risk.

TABLE 28.1 Victims of Abuse and Fatalities Among Different Ethnicities: 2014

Race or Ethnicity	Total Abuse Cases	Total Child Fatalities
African American	21.4%	30.3%
American Indian or Alaska Native	1.6%	0.6%
Children of multiple races	7.5%	3.8%
Hispanic	22.7%	15.1%
White	44%	43%
Asian	0.9%	1.1%

Data from the US Department of Health & Human Services. (2016). *Child maltreatment 2014*. Washington, DC: US Government Printing Office.

Interference with emotional bonding between parents and child, which can occur because of a premature birth or prolonged illness requiring hospitalization, has also been found to increase the risk for future abuse. Adolescents are abused at least as frequently as younger children. However, such abuse is often overlooked, perhaps because society views adolescents as capable of defending themselves.

Box 28.1 identifies characteristics of parents who abuse their children.

Comorbidity

The occurrence of one type of abuse is a fairly strong predictor of the occurrence of another type. The secondary effects of abuse, such as anxiety, depression, and suicidal ideation, are healthcare issues that can last a lifetime. Major depressive disorder and posttraumatic stress disorder (PTSD) are two of the most prevalent disorders resulting from childhood trauma.

Family violence is common in the childhood histories of juvenile offenders, runaways, violent criminals, prostitutes, and those who in turn are violent toward others. Exposure to abuse can adversely affect a child's development because the energy needed to successfully accomplish developmental is instead devoted to coping with abuse.

Abused adolescents exhibit more psychopathological changes, poorer coping and social skills, a higher incidence of dissociative identity disorder, and poorer impulse control than do other adolescents. Women who are victims of prolonged childhood sexual abuse are more likely to develop major psychiatric distress.

INTIMATE PARTNER VIOLENCE

Intimate partner violence includes physical violence, rape, and/or stalking and psychological aggression by a current or former intimate partner (CDC, 2015b). The intimate partner may be a spouse, boyfriend/girlfriend, dating partner, or ongoing sexual partner.

BOX 28.1 Characteristics of Abusive Parents

- A history of abuse, neglect, or emotional deprivation as a child
- Family authoritarianism
- Low self-esteem, feelings of worthlessness, depression
- Poor coping skills
- Social isolation (may be suspicious of others)
- Involvement in a crisis situation
- Unrealistic expectations of child's behavior
- Frequent use of harsh punishment
- History of severe mental illness, such as schizophrenia
- Violent temper outbursts
- Expects the child to satisfy needs for love, support, and reassurance
- Projection of blame onto the child for parents' "troubles"
- Inability to seek help from others
- Perception of the child as bad or evil
- History of drug or alcohol abuse
- Feeling of little or no control over life
- Low tolerance for frustration
- Poor impulse control

Four of five victims of intimate partner violence are women (Bureau of Justice Statistics, 2012). Females between the ages of 18 and 34 experience the highest rate of intimate partner violence.

Nearly half of married couples have instances of abuse. Evidence suggests that intimate partner violence affects same-sex relationships at about the same rates as heterosexual relationships (Stephenson et al., 2011). One out of 10 homicides is due to spousal murder, and about a third of females who are killed are or were in an intimate relationship with their killer.

Cycle of Violence

Walker (1979) describes a pattern of behavior that perpetrators of violence may use to control their partners. This cycle consists of three stages: the tension-building stage, the acute battering stage, and the honeymoon stage.

- The **tension-building stage** begins with minor incidents such as pushing, shoving, and verbal abuse. During this time, the victim often ignores or accepts the behavior due to fear of escalation. Abusers then rationalize that their behavior is acceptable. As the tension builds, both participants may try to reduce it. The abuser may try to reduce the tension with the use of alcohol or drugs, and the victim may try to reduce the tension by minimizing the importance of the incidents ("I should have had the house neater…dinner ready").
- The **acute battering stage** occurs when the tension peaks. It is usually triggered by an external event or by the abuser's emotional state. Some experts believe that the victim may actually provoke the incident to remove the tension and fear and to move on to the honeymoon phase.
- After the abuse occurs, the abuser and victim enter a period of calm known as the **honeymoon stage.** During this stage, the abuser usually demonstrates kindness and loving behaviors. The abuser, at least initially, feels remorseful and apologetic and may bring presents, make promises, and tell the victim how much she is loved and needed. The victim usually feels needed and loved and hopes for change. Legal proceedings or plans to leave initiated during the acute battering stage may be abandoned.

Unfortunately, without intervention, the cycle will repeat itself. Over time, the periods of calmness and safety become briefer, and the periods of anger and fear are more intense. Each repeat of the pattern erodes the victim's self-esteem. The victim either believes the violence was deserved or accepts the blame for it. This can lead to feelings of depression, hopelessness, immobilization, and self-deprecation. Fig. 28.1 illustrates the cycle of violence.

Risk Factors

Men who abuse may believe in male dominance and need to be in charge. Physically acting out makes them feel more in control, more masculine, and more powerful. Parent-child interactions, peer group experiences, observations of the partner dyad, and the influence of the media (television, comics, video games, movies) support the same message: Males can expect to be in a position of power in relationships and may use physical aggression to maintain that position.

Pathological jealousy is a characteristic of an intimate partner abuser. Many perpetrators refuse to allow their partners

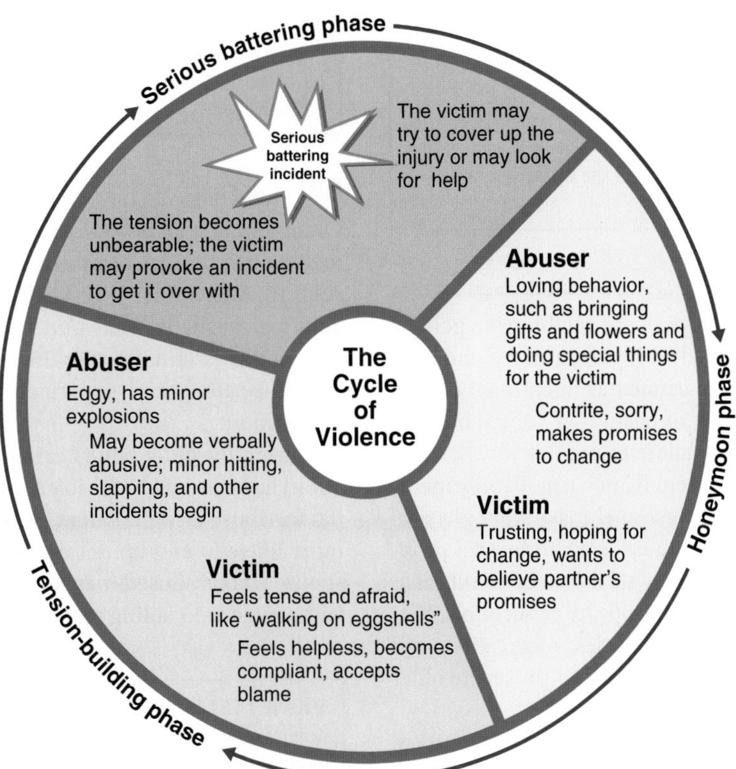

FIG. 28.1 The cycle of violence. (Redrawn from YWCA of Annapolis and Anne Arundel County, 1517 Ritchie Highway, Arnold, MD 21012.)

to work outside the home. Some demand that their partners work in the same place as they do so that they can monitor activities and friendships. It is common for abusers to accompany their partners to and from activities. They may forbid the victim from having personal friends or to participate in activities outside the home. Perpetrators may restrict mobility by monitoring an odometer and keeping stopwatches. Even after imposing such restrictions, abusers often accuse their partners of infidelity or other acts of betrayal. Controlling finances and expenditures is an additional means of limiting the freedom of the abused.

Individuals are more likely to engage in family violence when they use substances. Alcohol and other drugs (illicit or prescribed) tend to weaken inhibitions and lead to a disregard of social rules prohibiting violence. The victim may rationalize that alcohol and drugs cause the abuse, saying, "He was drunk and didn't know what he was doing." However, even when drug and alcohol use is reduced or eliminated, family violence usually still occurs.

Pregnancy may trigger or increase violence. The partner may resent the added responsibility a baby entails, or he may resent the relationship the baby will have with his mate. Violence also escalates when the woman makes a move toward independence such as visiting friends without permission, getting a job, or going back to school. Victims are at greatest risk for violence when they threaten to or actually leave the relationship.

VIGNETTE: The nurse in a walk-in clinic assesses Janet for bilateral corneal abrasions. The nurse becomes suspicious as she notes the patient's vague responses to history questions and her unrelenting checking of the clock, followed by the urgent statement, "I've got to get home." On further questioning, Janet reveals that she is often quite fatigued due to caring for her five children, all under the age of 7. Her husband, who works until 2 a.m., expects her to be awake when he comes home from work and have a warm meal ready. "He hits me if I'm asleep." She had taped her eyes open so that even if she were lying down when he came home she would look awake. "I didn't even think about taking my contacts out."

OLDER ADULT ABUSE

For many older adults, the golden years are anything but golden. It can be a sad, stressful time filled with pain, anxiety, and poverty. Older adult mistreatment is defined as intentional actions that cause harm or creates a risk of harm to a vulnerable person. This mistreatment includes failure to provide for the older adults' basic needs or to protect them from harm. Family member, custodians, and care facility personnel may inflict physical abuse and sexual abuse. Financial abuse is an additional problem in this population. Caretakers may steal cash or credit cards or coerce the older person to transfer property or accounts. Victims also lose personal belongings, vehicles, medication, and food stamps. All 50 states have enacted laws to prosecute older adult abuse.

Abuse of older adults is too commonly found in the news. Recent examples include:

- An 87-year-old woman in Missouri died 2 days after being found naked and lying in a bed soaked with urine and fecal matter (Farley, 2017). Her daughter was charged in the incident. She said she'd have taken better care of her, but she was too tired.
- New Jersey healthcare workers wearing floral scrubs were caught on camera as they lashed out, striking helpless patients (Sullivan, 2016). Workers were seen roughly force-feeding a 91-year-old Alzheimer's patient and ignoring a woman who fell to the floor.
- A 26-year-old man who worked at a senior living center in Illinois faced charges of aggravated criminal sexual assault after he tried to pay other men to sexually assault patients (Eades, 2016). He allegedly wanted to capture the abuse on videos or pictures.

Epidemiology

The Centers for Disease Control and Prevention (CDC, 2015c) estimate that about 1 out of every 10 adults older than age 60 are victims of abuse. This number may be far higher in that for every case reported, five go unreported. This lack of reporting may be due to isolation, dependency, and fear of retaliation. Further complicating the picture is that the older adult may be caring for him- or herself, which creates the potential for self-neglect. Elder abuse occurs in both institutional and family settings. Family members are often the perpetrators in most of the incidents.

VIGNETTE: Walter, a 73-year-old man, came to the ambulatory care clinic looking very fatigued and complaining of pain in his left shoulder "since last night." Holding his left arm close to his side, Walter averted his eyes from those of the receptionist, nurse, and doctor. When asked if anything had occurred that might have caused the pain, he answered, "I fell." When asked why he did not seek care the previous night, Walter stated, "I…I…thought it would go away overnight." X-rays revealed a fractured clavicle. After additional direct, supportive questioning, the patient admitted his son had shoved him to the floor.

Risk Factors

Older adults may become vulnerable because they are in poor mental or physical health or are disruptive due to disorders such as Alzheimer's disease. The dependency needs of older adults are usually what put them at risk for abuse. The typical victim is female, over 75 years of age, Caucasian, living with a relative, and experiencing a physical and/or mental impairment.

Caring for older adults can be stressful in the best of cases, but in families in which violence is a coping strategy, the potential for abuse is high. Parents who abuse their own children are more likely to end up as targets for abuse by their offspring. A spouse who is abused may retaliate in later years by responding with violence to failing physical or cognitive health.

VIGNETTE: Ms. Randall, 83-years-old, is admitted from an adult foster home for evaluation of deterioration in her mental status. She is confused and disoriented as to time and place and is unable to give a coherent history. Blood and urine are collected for diagnostic evaluation. The laboratory report notes semen in the urine. Adult Protective Services is called to begin an investigation into the adult family home.

APPLICATION OF THE NURSING PROCESS

ASSESSMENT

General Assessment

You will encounter victims of violence in every healthcare setting. Therefore you should screen all patients for possible abuse. Symptoms may be vague and can include chronic pain, insomnia, hyperventilation, or gynecological problems. Attention to the interview process and setting are important to facilitate accurate assessment of physical and behavioral indicators of family violence. All assessments should include questions to elicit a history of sexual abuse, family violence, and drug use or abuse. Any assessment should be completed with the victim alone, and it is helpful to have an institutional policy that facilitates screening in private.

Interview Process and Setting

You can gather important and relevant information about the family situation by conducting a routine assessment with tact, understanding, and a relaxed attitude. When interviewing, sit near the patient and spend some time establishing trust and rapport before focusing on the details of the violent experience. Establishing trust is crucial if the patient is to feel comfortable enough to self-disclose. The interview should be nonthreatening and supportive.

It is better to ask about ways of solving disagreements or methods of disciplining children rather than to use the words *abuse* or *violence*. It is also important not to assume a person's sexual orientation. Use the term *partner* when asking about the relationship. Key interviewing guidelines are listed in Box 28.2.

The person who experienced the violence should be allowed to tell the story without interruption. Reassure the patient that he or she did nothing wrong. Verbal approaches may include the following:

- Tell me about what happened to you.
- Who takes care of you? (for children and dependent older adults)
- What happens when you do something wrong? (for children) *or* How do you and your partner/caregiver resolve disagreements? (for women and dependent older adults)
- What do you do for fun?
- Who helps you with your child(ren)/parent?
- What time do you have for yourself?

Questions that are open-ended and require a descriptive response can be less threatening and elicit more relevant information than questions that are direct or can be answered with *yes* or *no*:

- What arrangements do you make when you have to leave your child alone?
- How do you discipline your child?
- When your infant cries for a long time, how do you get him/her to stop?
- What about your child's behavior bothers you the most?

When trust has been established, openness and directness about the situation can strengthen the relationship with those experiencing or perpetrating violence. A five-question assessment tool developed by Soeken and colleagues (1998) has been used extensively to assist in the routine identification of intimate partner abuse (Fig. 28.2).

BOX 28.2 Interview Guidelines

Do

- Conduct the interview in private.
- Be direct, honest, and professional.
- Use language the patient understands.
- Ask the patient to clarify words not understood.
- Be understanding.
- Be attentive.
- Inform the patient if you must make a referral to Children's or Adult Protective Services, and explain the process.
- Assess safety and help reduce danger (at discharge).

Do Not

- Try to "prove" abuse by accusations or demands.
- Display horror, anger, shock, or disapproval of the perpetrator or situation.
- Place blame or make judgments.
- Allow the patient to feel "at fault" or "in trouble."
- Probe or press for answers the patient is not willing to give.
- Conduct the interview with a group of interviewers.

VIGNETTE: Charlene Peters is a 42-year-old married woman in a relationship she describes as "bad for a long time." She is brought to the emergency department by ambulance with swollen eyes, lips, and nose and lacerations to her face. She tells the nurse that her husband had been asleep for an hour before she joined him. When she got into bed, Charlene tried to redistribute the blankets. Suddenly he leaped from the bed and began pummeling her face with his fists. He screamed, "Don't you ever wake me up again" and threw her against the wall. She cried out to her 11-year-old son to call 911. The police arrived, called an ambulance, and took Mr. Peters to jail.

The nurse takes Charlene to a private examination room for a full assessment. Mrs. Peters states that her relationship with her husband has always been stormy. The beatings began 5 years earlier when she was pregnant with their second child. The beatings had increased in intensity, and this emergency department visit is the fifth in a year. Tonight was the first time she ever called the police.

Charlene is shaken. Periods of crying alternate with periods of silence. She appears apathetic and in a moderate level of anxiety. The nurse explores alternatives designed to help her reduce the danger when she is discharged. "I'm concerned that you will be hurt again if you go home. What options do you have?" Charlene agrees that she is in danger. Along with the nurse, Charlene makes arrangements with a women's shelter for her and her two children. She also plans to file for a restraining order.

The nurse charts the abuse referrals. Keeping careful and complete records helps ensure that Charlene will receive proper follow-up care and will assist her when and if she pursues legal action.

Assessing Various Types of Abuse

Physical Abuse

A series of minor complaints, such as headaches, back trouble, dizziness, and accidents (especially falls), may be a covert indicator of violence. Overt signs of battering include bruises, scars, burns, and other wounds in various stages of healing, particularly around the head, face, chest, arms, abdomen, back, buttocks, and genitalia. Injuries that should arouse the nurse's suspicion are listed in Box 28.3.

If the explanation does not match the injury seen or if the patient minimizes the seriousness of the injury, you should

ABUSE ASSESSMENT SCREEN

1. Within the last year, have you been hit, slapped, kicked, or otherwise physically hurt by someone?

   ☐ Yes ☐ No

   If yes, by whom? ____________________

   Total number of times: ____________________

2. Since you've been pregnant, have you been hit, slapped, kicked, or otherwise physically hurt by someone?

   ☐ Yes ☐ No

   If yes, by whom? ____________________

   Total number of times: ____________________

   Mark the area of injury on the body map below.

3. Within the last year, has anyone forced you to have sexual activities?

   ☐ Yes ☐ No

   If yes, who? ____________________

   Total number of times: ____________________

4. Have you ever been emotionally or physically abused by your partner or someone important to you?

   ☐ Yes ☐ No

   If yes, by whom? ____________________

   Total number of times: ____________________

5. Are you afraid of your partner or anyone listed above?

   ☐ Yes ☐ No

Score each incident according to the following scale:

1 = Threats of abuse including use of a weapon

2 = Slapping, pushing; no injuries and/or continuing pain

3 = Punching, kicking, bruises, cuts, and/or continuing pain

4 = Beating up, severe contusions, burns, broken bones

5 = Head injury, internal injury, permanent injury

6 = Use of weapon, wound from weapon

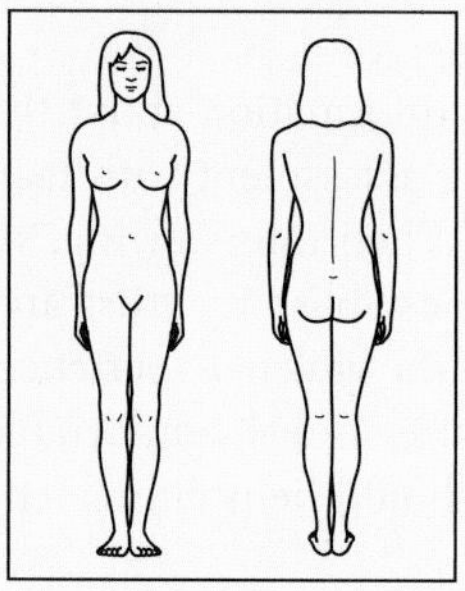

SCORE

____

____

____

____

____

____

FIG. 28.2 Abuse assessment screen. (From Soeken, K., McFarlane, J., Parker, B., & Lominack, M. [1998]. The abuse assessment screen: A clinical instrument to measure frequency, severity and perpetrator of abuse against women. In J. Campbell [Ed.], *Empowering survivors of abuse: Health care for battered women and their children* [pp. 575–579]. New Brunswick, NJ: Transaction.)

BOX 28.3 Common Presenting Problems of Victims of Abuse

Emergency Department

- Bleeding injuries, especially to head and face
- Internal injuries, concussions, perforated eardrum, abdominal injuries, severe bruising, eye injuries, strangulation marks on neck
- Back injuries
- Broken or fractured jaw, arms, pelvis, ribs, clavicle, legs
- Burns from cigarettes, appliances, scalding liquids, acids
- Psychological trauma, anxiety, attacks of hyperventilation, heart palpitations, severe crying spells, suicidal tendencies
- Miscarriage

Ambulatory Care Settings

- Perforated eardrum, twisted or stiff neck and shoulder muscles, headache
- Depression, stress-related conditions (e.g., insomnia, violent nightmares, anxiety, extreme fatigue, eczema, loss of hair)
- Talk of having "problems" with husband or son, describing person as very jealous, impulsive, or an alcohol or substance user
- Repeated visits with new complaints
- Bruises of various ages and specific shapes (fingers, belt)

Any Setting

- Signs of stress due to family violence: emotional, behavioral, school, or sleep problems and increase in aggressive behavior
- Injuries in a pregnant woman
- Recurrent visits for injuries attributed to being "accident-prone"

suspect abuse. Ask patients directly in a nonthreatening manner if someone close to them has caused the injury. Observe the nonverbal response such as hesitation or lack of eye contact. Then ask specific questions such as: "When was the last time it happened? How often does it happen? In what ways are you hurt?" Inconsistent explanations serve as a warning that further investigation is necessary. Vague explanations should also alert the nurse to possible abuse. "She fell from a chair [from a lap, down the stairs]." "He was running away." "The hot water was turned on by mistake."

Nonspecific bruising in older children is common. Any bruises on an infant younger than 6 months of age should be considered suspicious. **Shaken baby syndrome**, the leading cause of death as a result of physical abuse, usually occurs in children younger than 2 years old. Injuries are a result of the brain moving in the opposite direction as the baby's head. A baby who has been shaken may have respiratory problems, bulging fontanels, retinal hemorrhages, and central nervous system damage resulting in seizures, vomiting, and coma.

Sexual Abuse

Sexualized behavior is one of the most common symptoms of sexual abuse in children. Younger children may have precocious sexual knowledge, may draw sexually explicit images, or demonstrate sexual aggression. One telling clue is when a child acts out sexual interactions in play, for example, with dolls.

Masturbation may be excessive in sexually abused children. In older children, sexual promiscuity is one of the most common symptoms of sexual abuse, and there is a strong connection between sexual abuse and later promiscuity.

PTSD symptoms, such as nightmares, somatic complaints, and feelings of guilt, are also common in children who are sexually abused. There are a variety of emotional, behavioral, and physical consequences of sexual abuse with depression being the most commonly reported symptom by adults who were sexually abused as children. Other consequences include anxiety, suicide, aggression, chronic low self-esteem, chronic pain, obesity, substance misuse, self-mutilation, and PTSD.

Emotional abuse

Emotional abuse may exist on its own or in conjunction with physical or sexual abuse. Although it is less obvious and more difficult to assess than physical violence, you can identify it through indicators such as low self-esteem, reported feelings of inadequacy, anxiety and withdrawal, learning difficulties, and poor impulse control.

Neglect

Neglected children and older adults often appear undernourished, dirty, and poorly clothed. Neglect is also manifested by inadequate medical care such as lack of immunizations and untreated medical or dental conditions.

Economic Abuse

Economic abuse may take the form of failure to provide for the needs of the victim when adequate funds are available. Bills may be left unpaid by the person in charge of finances, which may result in disconnection of the heat or electricity. In the case of spousal abuse, the perpetrator may prevent the victim from pursuing education or finding a job, thereby ensuring dependency.

Level of Anxiety and Coping Responses

Nonverbal responses to the assessment interview may indicate of the victim's anxiety level. Agitation and anxiety bordering on panic are often present in victims experiencing violence. Because they live in terror, abused individuals remain vigilant and unable to relax or sleep. Signs and somatic symptoms of living with chronic stress and severe levels of anxiety include hypertension, irritability, and gastrointestinal disturbances. Hesitation, lack of eye contact, and use of vague statements such as "It's been rough lately" indicate that the situation is difficult to talk about.

Coping mechanisms used by many victims to endure living in violent and terrifying situations often prevent the termination of the relationship. These coping mechanisms may take the form of flawed beliefs or myths (Table 28.2). Because of feelings of confusion, shame, despair, and powerlessness, victims may withdraw from interaction with others, increasing their isolation.

Family Coping Patterns

To effectively assess abuse, the nurse must show a willingness to listen and avoid any judgmental tone. It is important to assess family strengths as well as stressors. Questioning about memories of early family relationships can provide additional information about attitudes in the home and the way they might influence coping. Asking parents about how they were disciplined as children may provide insight into their child-rearing attitudes and practices.

Living with and caring for children and older adults can cause frustration, stress, and anger. Unless there are appropriate outlets for stress, abuse can occur. Box 28.4 is a useful guide for assessing the risk of child and/or older adult abuse in the home.

TABLE 28.2 Myth Versus Fact Abuse

Myth	Fact
The victim's behavior causes violence.	The victim's behavior is *not* the cause of the violence. Violence is the abuser's pattern of behavior.
Men have the right to keep their wives and/or children in line.	No person has the right to beat or hurt another person.
Intimate partner abuse is a minor problem.	There is a *real* danger that abusive partners may kill victims.
Battered women are masochistic and like to be beaten. They could leave if they really wanted to.	Women do not like, ask, or deserve to be abused. Factors influencing a decision to leave include fear of injury or death, financial dependence, and welfare of children.
Family abuse occurs in poorly educated people from poor, working-class backgrounds.	Abuse can happen in a tenement or a mansion in families of all socioeconomic, religious, cultural, and educational backgrounds.
Family matters are private, and families should be allowed to take care of their own problems.	Intervention in family abuse is justified; abuse always escalates in frequency and intensity, can end in death, and is passed on to future generations.
Myths victims commonly believe: "I can't live without him/her." "If I hadn't done ____, it wouldn't have happened." "She/he will change." "I stay for the sake of the children." "He's jealous because he loves me."	These myths are coping mechanisms used to allay panic in a situation of random and brutal violence. They give the illusion of control and rationality.
Alcohol and stress are the causes of physical and verbal abuse.	There are no excuses and abuse is not acceptable behavior. People are abusive because they have acquired the belief that violence and aggression are acceptable and effective responses to real or imagined threats.
Violence occurs only between heterosexual partners.	Gay and lesbian partners experience violence for reasons similar to those in heterosexual relationships.
Pregnancy protects a woman from battering.	Battering frequently begins or escalates during pregnancy.

Support Systems

The person experiencing abuse is usually in a dependent position, relying on the perpetrator for basic needs. This dependence, along with the isolation the perpetrator imposes on the person, limits the victim's access to support systems. Children's options are especially limited, as are those of the physically and mentally disabled. Assessing for support should focus on intrapersonal, interpersonal, and community resources.

Suicide Potential

A person experiencing violence may feel desperate to leave, yet be trapped in an abusive relationship. Suicide may seem like the only option. In fact, victims of intimate partner violence are twice as likely to attempt suicide (Clay, 2014). Horrifying cases of murder-suicide are most likely to occur in the context of this type of abuse. Elder abuse and neglect are strongly associated in cases of suicide in the older adult population.

Children who were subjected to abuse are at increased risk for suicide as adults. Sexual abuse and, to a lesser degree, physical abuse create this risk. The identity of the abuser and the frequency of the abuse influence the degree of suicide risk. When the abuser is an immediate family member and when the abuse is repeated, the risk is increased.

BOX 28.4 Factors to Assess During a Home Visit

For a Child

- Responsiveness to infant's signals
- Caregiver's facial expressions in response to infant
- Playfulness of caregiver with infant
- Nature of physical contact during feeding and other caretaking activities
- Temperament of infant
- Caregiver's history of harsh discipline or abuse as a child
- Parental attitudes:
  - Feelings of inadequacy as a parent
  - Unrealistic expectations of child
  - Fear of "doing something wrong"
  - Attribution of negative qualities to newborn
  - Misdirected anger
  - Continued evidence of isolation, apathy, anger, frustration, projection
  - Adult conflict
- Environmental conditions:
  - Sleeping arrangements
  - Child management
  - Home management
  - Use of supports (formal and informal)
- Need for immediate services for situational (economics, child care), emotional, or educational information:
  - Information about hotlines, baby-sitters, homemakers, parent groups
  - Information about child development
  - Information about child care and home management services

For an Older Adult

- Absence of or lack of access to basic necessities (food, water, medications)
- Unsafe housing
- Lack of or inadequate utilities, ventilation, space
- Poor physical hygiene
- Lack of assistive devices, such as hearing aids, eyeglasses, wheelchair
- Medication mismanagement (outdated prescriptions, unmarked bottles)

A suicide attempt may be the presenting problem in the emergency department. With sensitive questions conducted in a caring manner, the nurse can elicit the history of violence. Often the means of attempted suicide is overdose with a combination of alcohol and other central nervous system depressants or sleeping medications.

When the crisis of the immediate suicide attempt has been resolved, careful questioning to determine lethality is in order. For example, if the patient still feels that life is not worth living, has a suicide plan, and has the means to carry it out, you must consider admission to an inpatient psychiatric unit. On the other hand, if the patient is talking about future plans and about staying "for the sake of the children," outpatient referrals are appropriate.

Homicide Potential

When working with an abused spouse, ask whether the patient feels safe going home and if so, whether a safety plan is in place for when the violence recurs. Always assess the potential for lethality. Certain factors place a vulnerable person at greater risk for homicide including the following:

- The presence of a gun in the home
- Alcohol and drug misuse
- History of violence on the part of the perpetrator in other situations
- Extreme jealousy and obsessiveness on the part of the perpetrator

The perpetrator of violence may eventually become the victim. Therefore, always ask individuals victimized by violence if they have ever felt like killing the perpetrator. If yes, ask whether they have the means to do so. If the answer is yes, intervention is required.

Drug and Alcohol Use

A person experiencing violence may self-medicate with alcohol or other drugs as a way of escaping an intolerable situation. The drugs are usually central nervous system depressants, such as benzodiazepines, prescribed by physicians for stress-related symptoms (e.g., insomnia, gastrointestinal upsets, anxiety, and difficulty concentrating). Assess for a chronic alcohol or drug problem (refer to Chapter 22) and provide appropriate treatment referrals. The patient should not be discharged to the abuser. Treatment choices can include both inpatient and outpatient options.

Maintaining Accurate Records

Because of the possibility of future legal action, it is essential that the healthcare record contain an accurate and detailed description of the victim's medical history, the psychosocial history of the family, and observations of the family interactions during the interviews. Especially important in documentation of findings from the initial assessment are:

1. Verbatim statements of who caused the injury and when it occurred.
2. A body map to indicate size, color, shape, areas, and types of injuries with explanations (see Fig. 28.2).
3. Physical evidence of sexual abuse, when possible.

Follow procedures for evidence collection carefully as this can impact legal action. If the abuse has just occurred, ask the patient to return in a day or two for more photographs as bruises may be more evident at that time. You must assure the patient of the confidentiality of the record and of its power should legal action be initiated. Even if intervention does not occur at this time, begin the record. The next provider will be aware of the problem and will be in a better position to offer support.

ASSESSMENT GUIDELINES

Family Violence

Assess:

1. Signs and symptoms of victims of abuse
2. Potential for abuse in vulnerable families. For example, some indicators of vulnerable parents who might benefit from education and instruction in effective coping techniques
3. Physical, sexual, and/or emotional abuse and neglect and economic maltreatment of older adults
4. Family coping patterns
5. Patient's support system
6. Drug or alcohol use
7. Suicidal or homicidal ideas
8. Posttrauma syndrome

Self-Assessment

Working with those who experience violence may arouse intense and overwhelming feelings. Strong negative feelings toward abuse may cloud your judgment and interfere with objective assessment and intervention, no matter how you try to cover or deny personal bias. Common responses of healthcare professionals to violence are listed in Table 28.3.

A personal history of abuse may cause you to identify too closely with the victim, and personal issues connected with the abuse may surface, further clouding judgment. Sharing perceptions and feelings with other professionals can help reduce feelings of isolation and discomfort.

DIAGNOSIS

Focus your nursing diagnoses on the underlying causes and symptoms of family violence. While many of the diagnoses are directed toward protecting vulnerable family members, you can also include the perpetrator in plans of care. Safety is the number one concern and is addressed in *Risk for violence* (other-directed or self-directed), *Risk for suicide, Pain,* and *Risk for infection. Rape-trauma syndrome* is addressed in Chapter 29.

Living in a situation where vulnerable individuals feel unsafe and helpless warrants the nursing diagnoses of *Anxiety, Fear, Hopelessness,* and *Powerlessness.* Constant negative messages and being treated in a disrespectful manner suggest the diagnoses of *Situational* and *Chronic low self-esteem.* Deficits in managing day-to-day responsibilities are addressed in *Ineffective individual coping.* The family as patient gets focus with diagnoses of *Dysfunctional family process, Impaired parenting, Disabled family coping, Caregiver role strain,* and *Ineffective role performance.*

OUTCOMES IDENTIFICATION

The *Nursing Outcomes Classification* (*NOC*; Moorhead et al., 2013) provides an overall outcome where the individual is free from being hurt or exploited, which is called abuse cessation. The following indicators address specific types of abuse:

- Physical abuse has ceased.
- Emotional abuse has ceased.
- Sexual abuse has ceased.
- Financial exploitation has ceased.

Ratings that you may find quite useful in determining the degree to which an outcome has been met are available in *NOC* (pp. 71–76). These scales include abuse cessation, abuse protection, abuse recovery, abuse recovery (emotional, financial, physical, or sexual). An additional outcome addresses the perpetrator with abusive behavior self-restraint (p. 77). Other outcomes focus on addressing the nursing diagnoses described in the previous section.

You should make the identification of desired outcomes patient-centered and therefore developed in conjunction with the survivor and primary support person. Continually reassess these outcomes and revise them as new information about the survivor's needs emerges.

Table 28.4 identifies signs and symptoms, potential nursing diagnoses, and outcomes for victims of child, intimate partner, and elder abuse, as well as for abusers.

TABLE 28.3 Common Responses of Healthcare Professionals to Violence

Response	Source
Anger	Anger may be felt toward the person responsible for the abuse, toward those who allowed it to happen, and toward society for condoning its occurrence through attitudes, traditions, and laws.
Embarrassment	The victim is a symbol of something close to home: the stress and strain of family life unleashed as uncontrollable anger.
Confusion	The view of the family as a haven of safety and privacy is challenged.
Fear	A small percentage of perpetrators are dangerous to others.
Anguish	The nurse may have experienced abuse.
Helplessness	The nurse may want to do more, eliminate the problem, or cure the victim and/or perpetrator.
Discouragement	Discouragement may result if no long-term solution is achieved.
"Blame the victim" mentality	Healthcare workers can get caught up in blaming the victim for behaviors they see as provoking the abuse.

TABLE 28.4 Signs and Symptoms, Nursing Diagnoses, and Outcomes for Family Violence

Signs and Symptoms	Potential Nursing Diagnoses	Outcomes
History of abuse, history of violence, substance use	*Risk for violence*	Family members remain free of harm
Bruises, cuts, broken bones, lacerations, scars, burns, wounds in various phases of healing, vaginal-anal bruises, sores, discharge, peritoneal pain	*Pain* *Risk for infection*	Timely treatment of injuries, healing of physical injuries, absence of pain, protection from further injuries
Restlessness, scanning, vigilance, uncertainty, isolation, fear, depression, feelings of helplessness, decreased control over environment, abuse	*Fear* *Powerlessness*	Behavioral manifestations of anxiety absent, reports a decrease in anxiety, reports feeling safe, expresses expectations of a positive future, sets goals
Poor eye contact and body posture, lack of respect from significant others, traumatic situation, neglect, feelings of shame and low self-esteem, feelings of worthlessness	*Chronic low self-esteem*	Maintains eye contact and erect posture, describes positive level of confidence, expects positive responses from others, describes feelings of success and self-worth
Poor coping skills, hostility, impulsivity, inadequate problem solving, substance abuse	*Ineffective individual coping*	Discusses the abusive behavior, obtains needed treatment, controls impulses, refrains from substance abuse

From Herdman, T. H. (Ed.). *Nursing diagnoses—Definitions and classification, 2012–2014*. Copyright © 2012, 1994–2012 by NANDA International. Used by arrangement with John Wiley & Sons Limited; Moorhead, S., Johnson, M., Maas, M. L., & Swanson, E. (2013). *Nursing outcomes classification (NOC)* (5th ed.). St. Louis, MO: Mosby.

PLANNING

Nurses and other healthcare workers encounter abuse frequently, not only in healthcare settings but also in their communities and families. The nurse is often the first point of contact for people experiencing abuse and thus is in an ideal position to contribute to prevention, detection, and effective intervention. The Joint Commission requires staff education in family violence and abuse, as well as the development of standards of care to guide clinical practice.

Most hospitals and community centers provide protocols for dealing with child, intimate partner, or elder abuse. Unless it is a case of child abuse in which the child has been removed from the home, most interventions performed after necessary emergency care will take place within the community. Plans should center on the patient's safety first. Whenever it is possible or in the best interests of the patient, plans should be discussed with the patient. Planning should also take into consideration the needs of the abuser(s) (e.g., parents, caretakers, spouse, or partner) if they are motivated to learning alternatives to abuse and violence.

IMPLEMENTATION

Reporting Abuse

Nurses are legally mandated to report suspected or actual cases of child and vulnerable adult abuse. The appropriate agency may be the state or county child welfare agency, law enforcement agency, juvenile court, or county health department. Each state has specific guidelines for reporting, including whether the report can be oral, written, or both, and within what time period the suspected abuse or neglect must be reported (immediately, within 24 hours, or within 48 hours). Every abused person is a crime victim, and assault with a weapon is reportable in most states. All 50 states have marital rape statutes. The following vignette gives an example of a child-abuse case that requires reporting.

VIGNETTE: Two nurses who work in a family practice clinic are suspicious of child abuse. Hannah, 12 years old, has recurrent urinary tract infections. Her father, who accompanies her into the bathroom when she is providing urine samples, always brings her to clinic visits. He answers all questions for Hannah even when providers direct the questions to her.

After pressure by the nurses, the physician agrees to ask Hannah some questions in private. The nurses think the physician has minimized the problem, asked superficial questions, and dismissed their concerns. They decide to report their concerns to Children's Protective Services. They inform the father who becomes outraged at their accusations and threatens to change doctors.

Subsequent investigation confirms the likelihood of sexual abuse, and Hannah is placed in temporary foster care with follow-up counseling. The father refuses treatment and threatens to sue the nurses. Four months later, the father leaves the family.

The case in the preceding vignette illustrates that a reasonable basis for suspecting abuse, not proof, is all that is required to report. Nurses must attempt to maintain both an appropriate level of suspicion and a neutral, objective attitude. One can be too concerned and jump to conclusions, which is what the physician in this case thought the nurses were doing. On the other hand, too little concern can result in an incomplete examination to avoid confrontation, which is what the nurses thought the physician was doing. Given these opposing stances, the case was reported as required by law and ethical standards, and Children's Protective Services was given the opportunity to investigate.

Culture

Culture is important because it is central to how people organize their experience. Even the most acculturated people have a tendency to revert to their cultural past in organizing coping strategies after a stressful event. If there is a language barrier, the nurse should speak slowly and clearly in English, without using jargon, and allow time for the response. If the patient speaks no English, provide a trained medical interpreter. A family member should *not* be used as an interpreter to ensure confidentiality and protect the person from future retaliation.

BOX 28.5 Personalized Safety Guide

Suggestions for Increasing Safety While in the Relationship

- I will have important phone numbers available to my children and myself.
- I can tell ______ and ______ about the violence and ask them to call the police if they hear suspicious noises coming from my home.
- If I leave my home, I can go to (list four places) _______, _______, ______, or _______.
- I can leave extra money, car keys, clothes, and copies of documents with _______.
- If I leave, I will bring ________ (see checklist).
- To ensure safety and independence, I will open my own savings account, rehearse my escape route with a support person, and review safety plan on ________ (date).

Suggestions for Increasing Safety When the Relationship Is Over

- I can change the locks; install steel or metal doors, a security system, smoke detectors, and an outside lighting system.
- I will inform _______ and ________ that my partner no longer lives with me and ask them to call the police if he or she is observed near my home or my children.
- I will tell people who take care of my children the names of those who have permission to pick them up. The people who have permission are ______, _______, and _______.
- I can tell _______ at work about my situation and ask _______ to screen my calls.
- I can avoid stores, banks, and ________ that I used when living with my battering partner.
- I can obtain a protective order from ________. I can keep it on or near me at all times, as well as have a copy with ________.
- If I feel down and ready to return to a potentially abusive situation, I can call _______ for support or attend workshops and support groups to gain support and strengthen my relationships with other people.

Important Phone Numbers

- Police _____________
- Hotline _____________
- Friends _____________
- Shelter _____________

Checklist of Items to Take

- Identification
- Birth certificates for me and my children
- Social Security card
- School and medical records
- Money, bank books, credit cards
- Keys to house, car, office
- Driver's license and registration
- Medications
- Change of clothes
- Welfare identification
- Passport(s), green card, work permit
- Divorce papers
- Lease or rental agreement, house deed
- Mortgage payment book, current unpaid bills
- Insurance papers
- Address book
- Pictures, jewelry, items of sentimental value
- Children's favorite toys and/or blankets

Counseling

Counseling includes crisis intervention measures. It is important to emphasize that people have a right to live without fear of violence, physical harm, or assault. Telling an abused person that "no one deserves to be hit" can be a powerful statement in and of itself. The role of the nurse is to support the victim, counsel about safety, and facilitate access to other resources as appropriate.

You should counsel individuals experiencing intimate partner violence about developing a **safety plan**, a plan for a rapid escape when abuse recurs. Ask patients to identify the signs of escalation of violence and to pick a particular sign that will tell them that "now is the time to leave." If children are present, they can all agree on a code word that, when spoken by the parent, means "It is time to go." If the individual plans ahead, it may be possible to leave before the violence occurs. It is important that the plan include a destination and transportation. The nurse should suggest packing the items listed in Box 28.5 ahead of time. The person should keep the packed bag in a place where the perpetrator will not find it.

If a survivor of intimate partner violence chooses to leave, **shelters or safe houses** (for both sexes) are available in most communities. They are open 24 hours a day and can be reached through hotline information numbers, hospital emergency departments, YWCAs, or the local office of the National Organization for Women. The address of the house is usually kept secret to protect abused individuals from attack by the perpetrator. Besides offering protection, many of these shelters and safe houses serve important educational and consciousness-raising functions. Patients should be given the number of the nearest available shelter even if they decide for the present to stay with their partners.

Case Management

Community mental health centers are becoming increasingly involved in the delivery of services to victims and perpetrators of abuse. Nurses working in these settings have the opportunity to coordinate community, medical, criminal justice, and social services to provide comprehensive assistance to families in crisis.

A nurse functioning in a case manager role can assist the patient in choosing the best options and coordinating the interventions of several agencies. Box 28.6 lists selected *NIC* interventions for *Abuse protection support* for children, intimate partners, and older adults (Bulechek et al., 2013).

Promotion of Community Support

An important intervention is to support help seeking. You may provide referral numbers and even stand by as the patient makes a phone call for an appointment. Make specific referrals regarding emergency financial assistance and legal counseling available to each patient. Vocational counseling is another referral that may be appropriate. Give patients referrals to parenting resources that enable them to explore alternative approaches to discipline (e.g., no hitting, slapping, or other expressions of violence).

BOX 28.6 Interventions for Abuse Protection Support for Children, Intimate Partners, and Older Adults

Abuse Protection Support: Children

Definition: Identification of high-risk, dependent child relationships and actions to prevent possible or further infliction of physical, sexual, or emotional harm or neglect of basic necessities of life

Activities:*

- Identify mothers who have a history of late (4 months or later) or no prenatal care.
- Identify parents who have had another child removed from the home or have placed previous children with relatives for extended periods.
- Identify parents with a history of domestic violence or a mother who has a history of numerous "accidental" injuries.
- Determine whether a child demonstrates signs of physical abuse, including numerous injuries in various stages of healing; unexplained bruises and welts; unexplained pattern, immersion, and friction burns; facial, spiral, shaft, or multiple fractures; unexplained facial lacerations and abrasions; human bite marks; intracranial, subdural, intraventricular, and intraocular hemorrhaging; whiplash shaken infant syndrome; and diseases that are resistant to treatment and/or have changing signs and symptoms.
- Encourage admission of child for further observation and investigation as appropriate.
- Monitor parent-child interactions and record observations.
- Report suspected abuse or neglect to proper authorities.

Abuse Protection Support: Intimate Partners

Definition: Identification of high-risk, dependent domestic relationships and action to prevent possible or further infliction of physical, sexual, or emotional harm or exploitation of a domestic partner

Activities:*

- Screen for risk factors associated with domestic abuse (e.g., history of domestic violence, abuse, rejection, excessive criticism, or feelings of being worthless and unloved; difficulty trusting others or feeling disliked by others; feeling that asking for help is an indication of personal incompetence; high physical care needs; intense family care responsibilities; substance abuse; depression; major psychiatric illness; social isolation; poor relationships between domestic partners; multiple marriages; pregnancy; poverty; unemployment; financial dependence; homelessness; infidelity; divorce; or death of a loved one).
- Document evidence of physical or sexual abuse using standardized assessment tools and photographs.
- Listen attentively to individual who begins to talk about own problems.
- Encourage admission to a hospital for further observation and investigation, as appropriate.
- Provide positive affirmation of worth.
- Report any situations in which abuse is suspected in compliance with mandatory reporting laws.

Abuse Protection Support: Older Adults

Definition: Identification of high-risk, dependent elder relationships and actions to prevent possible or further infliction of physical, sexual, or emotional harm; neglect of basic necessities of life; or exploitation

Activities:*

- Identify older patients who perceive themselves to be dependent on caretakers due to impaired health status, functional impairment, limited economic resources, depression, substance abuse, or lack of knowledge of available resources and alternatives for care.
- Identify family caretakers who have a history of being abused or neglected in childhood.
- Monitor patient-caretaker interactions and record observations.
- Report suspected abuse or neglect to proper authorities.

*Partial list.

Adapted from Bulechek, G. M., Butcher, H. K., Dochterman, J. M., & Wagner, C. (2013). *Nursing interventions classification (NIC)* (6th ed.). St. Louis, MO: Mosby.

Health Teaching and Health Promotion

In families at risk for abuse, health teaching and health promotion include meeting with both the individual and the family to help them learn to recognize behaviors and situations that might trigger violence.

Explain normal developmental and physiological changes to enable family members to gain a more positive view of the victim and the crisis situation. Gaining a more complete understanding can help family members broaden their insight and thus increase their compassion. They may then begin to anticipate new stress situations and be able to prepare for them before a crisis occurs.

Nurses who work on a maternity unit are often in a position to identify risk factors for abuse between new parents and initiate appropriate interventions including education about effective parenting and coping techniques. Share information about these interventions with the patient's healthcare team for appropriate monitoring and follow-up. Parents who are candidates for special attention include the following:

- New parents whose behavior toward the infant is rejecting, hostile, or indifferent.
- Teenage parents who require special help in handling the baby and discussing their expectations of the baby and their support systems.
- Parents with cognitive deficits for whom careful, explicit, and repeated instructions on caring for the child and recognizing the infant's needs are indicated.
- Parents who grew up watching their mothers be abused. This is a significant risk factor for perpetuation of family violence.

Nurses can also recognize when children are at risk and make referrals to community resources including emergency child care facilities, emergency telephone numbers, numbers of 24-hour crisis centers or hotlines, and respite programs in which volunteers take the child for an occasional weekend so that parents can get some relief. Community health nurses can make home visits to identify risk factors for abuse in the crucial first few months of life during which the style of parent-child interactions is established. See Box 28.4 for important factors for the community health nurse to assess during a home care visit. Such observations made by nurses in clinic and public health settings are fundamental in case findings and evaluation.

Prevention of Abuse

Primary Prevention

Primary prevention consists of measures taken to prevent the occurrence of abuse. Identifying individuals and families at high risk, providing health teaching, and coordinating supportive services to prevent crises are examples of primary prevention. Specific strategies include:

1. Reducing stress
2. Reducing the influence of risk factors
3. Increasing social support
4. Increasing coping skills
5. Increasing self-esteem

Community health nurses are in a unique position to assess family functioning in the home during visits for other medical problems. In addition, the community health nurse and clinic nurse maintain contact with the family over time, which allows for assessment of changes. They are also in an excellent position to connect parents to appropriate resources in the community that can meet their needs. All nurses can work to reduce society's acceptance of violence by working toward social policy change.

Secondary Prevention

Secondary prevention involves early intervention in abusive situations to minimize their disabling or long-term effects. Nurses can establish screening programs for individuals at risk, participate in the medical treatment of injuries resulting from violent episodes, and coordinate community services to provide continuity of care. Healthcare professionals can help reduce stress and depression by providing supportive therapy, support groups, pharmacotherapy, and contact information for community resources. Social dysfunction or lack of information can be addressed by counseling and education. You can reduce caregiver burden by arranging assistance in caring for the family member, housekeeping, or, in cases in which caregiving needs exceed even optimal caregiver capacity, by placing the patient in a more appropriate setting. The following vignette illustrates a successful secondary prevention effort.

VIGNETTE: Six-year-old Gavin is brought to the school nurse by his teacher who said he had complained of an upset stomach. When the nurse examines Gavin, she notices bruises on his arms and abdomen. Gavin appears frightened and hesitant to speak.

Nurse: "How did you hurt yourself, Gavin?" *(Gavin looks down and starts to cry.)* "It's OK if you don't want to talk about it."

Gavin: *(Does not look at the nurse and speaks softly.)* "My mom hit me."

Nurse: "Tell me what happened before that."

Gavin: "Mom was mad because I didn't put my toys away."

Nurse: "What does your mom usually do when she gets mad?"

Gavin: "She yells mostly. Sometimes she hits me."

Nurse: "Tell me about the hitting."

Gavin: "Mom hits me a lot since my dad left." *(Gavin starts to cry to himself.)*

Gavin appears well nourished and properly dressed. He is at his approximate developmental age except for some language delay; however, because of the physical evidence and history, the nurse notifies Children's Protective Services, and the family situation is evaluated for possible placement of Gavin in protective custody. The initial evaluation concludes that there is no indication of serious potential harm to the child and that Gavin should return home. The mother, who is initially defensive, starts to cry and states, "I can't cope with being alone, and I don't know where to turn."

Nursing interventions center on caring for Gavin's immediate health needs, finding supports for the mother to help her cope with crises, providing a counseling referral for the mother to learn alternative ways of expressing anger and frustration, and informing the mother of parents' groups.

Tertiary Prevention

Tertiary prevention, which often occurs in mental health settings, involves nurses facilitating the healing and rehabilitative process by counseling individuals and families, providing support for groups of survivors, and assisting survivors of violence to achieve their optimal level of safety, health, and well-being. Legal advocacy programs for survivors of intimate partner violence are an example of tertiary prevention. Complementary therapies, such as mindfulness-based stress reduction, can also assist survivors in the healing process.

Advanced Practice Interventions

A nurse who is educated at the master's or doctoral level and is certified in advanced practice psychiatric nursing is qualified to conduct psychotherapy. This type of therapy is most effective after crisis intervention when the situation is less chaotic and tumultuous. A variety of therapeutic modalities are available for treatment of abusive families.

Individual Psychotherapy

The goals of individual therapy for a survivor are empowerment, the ability to recognize and choose productive life options, and the development of a solid sense of self. People who have experienced abuse as a child or have left a violent relationship may choose individual therapy to address symptoms of depression, anxiety, somatization, or PTSD.

Many of the psychological symptoms shown by women who have been abused can be understood as complex survival strategies and responses to violence. Nurses must address the guilt, shame, and stigmatization experienced by survivors of abuse. It is helpful for nurses to understand that the individual's feelings and behaviors may be reflective of the grieving process because he or she has experienced numerous losses as a result of the abusive relationship. Helping the survivor work through the stages of grieving can promote healing.

Individual psychotherapy is often indicated for the perpetrator particularly when an individual psychopathological process is identified. Therapy for the perpetrator is most effective when it is court-mandated because the perpetrator is more likely to complete the course of treatment. Nurses engaged in therapy with perpetrators have a duty to warn potential victims if they conclude that the perpetrator is a danger. Refer to Chapter 6 for a more detailed discussion of the duty to warn and duty to protect.

Family Psychotherapy

Because abuse is a symptom of a family in crisis, each part of the family system needs attention. Also, because change in one member of the family system affects the whole system, all members need support and understanding. Interventions may maximize positive interactions among all family members. Couples therapy can put the abused partner at increased risk of harm or even death. Conjoint therapy should take place *only* if the perpetrator has had individual therapy and has demonstrated change as a result and if both parties agree to participate.

Expected outcomes are that the perpetrator will recognize destructive patterns of behavior, learn alternative responses, control impulses, and refrain from abusive behavior. Intermediate goals are that members of the family will openly communicate and learn to listen to one another. Refer to Chapter 35 for a more detailed discussion of family therapy.

Group Psychotherapy

Participation in therapy groups provides assurances that one is not alone and that change is possible. Because many survivors of abuse have been isolated, they have been deprived of validation and positive feedback from others. Working in a group can help diminish feelings of isolation, strengthen feelings of self-esteem and self-worth, and increase the potential for realistic problem solving in a supportive atmosphere.

Groups often use cognitive-behavioral techniques to help the abuser see abusive actions as behavioral patterns that they can change. In therapy groups, perpetrators learn to recognize the thoughts preceding an abusive incident, the responses to the thoughts, and how to interrupt negative feelings about their partners. Perpetrators who have never discussed problems with anyone before are encouraged to discuss their thoughts and feelings. Group therapy can help create a community of healing and restoration. Refer to Chapter 34 for a more detailed discussion of group therapy.

EVALUATION

Failures of interventions with abusive families often are due to problems within the social, economic, and political systems in which we live. Nurses can direct their interventions to the social environment. Questions that nurses should consider are:

- Is corporal punishment an acceptable technique for guiding behavior in children?
- How do we address the unequal burden of caregiving responsibilities placed on women?
- Why is a low priority given to education and preparation for parenthood?
- How can we change the belief that older adults have little social value?

CASE STUDY AND NURSING CARE PLAN

Family Violence

Mrs. Robb, a recently widowed 84-year-old woman, moved to her son's apartment 3 months ago. She had been living in her third-floor walk-up in the city. Because of her declining health and crime in the neighborhood, she went to live with her son, John. He and his wife, Judy, who have been married for 20 years, have five children 6 to 18 years of age, all living in a rather cramped three-bedroom apartment.

Ms. Green, a visiting nurse, monitors Mrs. Robb's blood pressure. Over a series of visits, the nurse notices that Mrs. Robb is looking unkempt, pale, and withdrawn. While taking her blood pressure, Ms. Green observes bruises on Mrs. Robb's arms. When questioned about the bruises, Mrs. Robb appears anxious. She says that she slipped in the bathroom. Mrs. Robb stiffens in her chair when her daughter-in-law, Judy, enters the room. The nurse notices that Judy avoids eye contact with Mrs. Robb.

When the nurse asks about the injuries, Judy responds with anger, blaming Mrs. Robb for causing so many problems. She will not explain the reason for the change in Mrs. Robb's behavior or the origin of the bruises to the nurse. She merely comments, "I have had to give up my job since my mother-in-law came here. It's been difficult and crowded. The kids are complaining. We are having trouble making ends meet since I gave up my job, and my husband is no help at all."

Self-Assessment

Ms. Green has worked with violent families, but this is the first time she has encountered older adult mistreatment. She discusses her reactions with the other team members. She is especially angry with Judy although she is able to understand the daughter-in-law's frustration. The team concurs with Ms. Green that this family could use some support. If abuse does not stop, they will need to take more drastic measures and contact legal services.

Assessment

Subjective Data

- Stressful crowded living conditions
- Economic hardships leading to stress
- No support for the daughter-in-law from the rest of the family for the care of Mrs. Robb
- Mrs. Robb states she slipped in the bathroom, but physical findings do not support this explanation.
- Judy states, "It's been difficult and crowded."

Objective Data

- Physical symptoms of violence (bruises, unkempt appearance).
- Withdrawn and apprehensive behavior.
- No eye contact between Mrs. Robb and her daughter-in-law

Diagnosis

On the basis of the data, the nurse formulates the following nursing diagnosis:

- *Risk for injury* related to increase in family stress as evidenced by signs of violence

Outcomes Identification

Overall outcome: Abuse cessation: Evidence that the victim is no longer hurt or exploited

Short-term indicators:

- Evidence that physical abuse has ceased
- Evidence that emotional abuse has ceased

CASE STUDY AND NURSING CARE PLAN—cont'd

Family Violence

Planning

Ms. Green discusses several possible outcomes with members of her team, giving attention to the priority of outcomes and to whether they are realistic in this situation. She also plans to report the elder abuse to Adult Protective Services and to work with Mrs. Robb, Judy, and the rest of the family to improve this situation for everyone.

Implementation

Mrs. Robb's plan of care is personalized as follows:

Short-Term Goal	Intervention	Rationale	Evaluation
1. On each visit made by the nurse, the patient will state that abuse has decreased, using a scale from 1 to 5 (1 being the least abuse).	1a. Assess severity of signs and symptoms of abuse. 1b. Do a careful home assessment to identify other areas of abuse and neglect. 1c. Discuss with patient factors leading to abuse and concern for safety.	1a. Accurate charting (body map, pictures with permission, verbatim statements) helps follow progress and provides legal data. 1b. Check for inadequacy of food, presence of vermin, blocked stairways, medication safety issues, etc. All indicate abuse and neglect. Determine the kinds of problems in the home, and plan intervention. Identify community resources that could help the elder and caregivers. 1c. Allows family stressors and potential areas for intervention to be identified. Validates that situation is serious and increases patient's knowledge base.	**GOAL MET** Patient states that after family talked to the nurse and planned strategies, physical abuse no longer occurs.
2. Within 2 weeks, patient will be able to identify at least two supportive services to deal with emergency situations.	2. Discuss with patient supportive services such as hotlines and crisis units to call in case of emergency situations and develop a written list	2. Maximizes patient's safety through use of support services.	**GOAL MET** Patient has a list with important phone numbers. She has called the hotline once to get information on transportation to the senior center in town.
3. Within 3 weeks, family members will identify difficult issues that increase their stress levels.	3. Discuss with family members their feelings, and identify at least four areas that are most difficult for the various family members.	3. Listening to each family member and identifying unmet needs helps both family and nurse identify areas that require changing and appropriate interventions.	**GOAL MET** Family members identify areas such as overwork, lack of free time, lack of privacy, and financial difficulties, all of which increase their stress levels.
4. Within 3 weeks, family will seek out community resources to help with anger management, need for homemaker support, and other needs.	4. Identify potential community supports, skills training, respite places, homemakers, financial aids, etc., that might help meet family's unmet needs.	4. When stressed, individuals solve problems poorly and do not know about or cannot manage to organize outside help. Finances are often a problem.	**GOAL MET** Judy is responding well to anger management groups. Both Judy and her husband are attending a support group for caregivers.

Evaluation

Eight weeks after Ms. Green's initial visit, Mrs. Robb appears well groomed, friendly, and more spontaneous in her conversation. She comments, "Things are better with my daughter-in-law." No bruises or other signs of physical violence are noticeable. She is considerably more outgoing and has even taken the initiative to contact an old friend. Mrs. Robb has talked openly to her son and daughter-in-law about stress in the family. Mrs. Robb says that she went for a walk when her daughter-in-law Judy appeared tense and returned to find that the tension had lessened. Neither Mrs. Robb nor her family has initiated plans for alternative housing.

KEY POINTS TO REMEMBER

- Abuse can occur in any family and can be predicted with some accuracy by examining the characteristics of perpetrators and vulnerable people in which violence is likely.
- Abuse can be physical, sexual, emotional, economic, or can be caused by neglect.
- The most common form of child abuse is neglect.
- Risk factors for child abuse include being younger than 4, being a child who is somehow different, and an impairment in the emotional bond between parent and child.
- Intimate partner violence tends to become progressively worse and can end in death.

- A cycle of violence with tension-building, acute battering, and honeymoon stages is commonly present in cases of intimate partner violence.
- Older adult abuse is far too common and is often difficult to uncover due to dependency.
- Family members and custodial healthcare workers are most often implicated in abuse of older adults.
- Assessment includes identifying indicators of abuse, levels of anxiety, coping mechanisms, support systems, suicide and homicide potential, and alcohol and drug misuse.
- Registered nurses are legally mandated to report suspected or actual abuse in the case of children and vulnerable adults.
- Community referral and support are essential in helping individuals and families with abusive situations.

CRITICAL THINKING

1. A colleague who has witnessed a child being abused states, "I don't think it's any of our business what people do in the privacy of their own homes."
   a. What would you be legally required to do?
   b. What are your ethical responsibilities?
2. You successfully convinced your colleagues to assess routinely for abuse, and now they want to know how to do it. How would you go about teaching them to assess for child abuse? Intimate partner abuse? Elder abuse?
3. Your health maintenance organization's routine health screening form for adolescents, adults, and older adults has just been changed to include questions about family abuse. How would you respond to patients who indicate on this form that abuse occurs in their home?
4. Write out a safety plan that could be adopted by individuals who are being abused.
   a. Identify at least four referrals in your community for a victim of family violence.
   b. Identify two referrals in your community for a perpetrator of family violence.

CHAPTER REVIEW

Questions

1. Which statement made by a new mother should be explored further by the nurse?
   a. "I have three children, that's enough."
   b. "I think the baby cries just to make me angry."
   c. "I wish my husband could help more with the baby."
   d. "Babies are a blessing, but they are a lot of work."
2. Which problem is observed in children who regularly witness acts of violence in their family? *Select all that apply.*
   a. Phobias
   b. Low self-esteem
   c. Major depressive disorder
   d. Narcissistic personality disorder
   e. Posttraumatic stress disorder
3. What situation associated with a caregiver presents the greatest risk that an older adult will experience abuse by that caregiver?
   a. The caregiver is a single male relative.
   b. The caregiver was neglected as a child.
   c. The caregiver is under the age of 30.
   d. The caregiver has little experience with the elderly.
4. What safety-related responsibility does the nurse have in any situation of suspected of abuse?
   a. Protect the patient from future abuse by the abuser.
   b. Inform the suspected abuser that the authorities have been notified.
   c. Arrange for counseling for all involved parties but especially the patient.
   d. Report suspected abuse to the proper authorities.
5. The nurse is assisting a patient to identify safety issues that may occur now that she has left an abusive partner. What telephone numbers should be available to the patient? *Select all that apply.*
   a. The police department
   b. An abuse hotline
   c. A responsible friend or family member
   d. A domestic violence shelter
   e. The hospital emergency department
6. Secondary effects of abuse often manifest as arrested development in children due to the fact that:
   a. Coping is easier than emotional growth
   b. Energy for development is diverted to coping
   c. Children cannot differentiate love from abuse
   d. Abuse fosters a sense of belonging, even if dysfunctional
7. The use of a patient-centered interview technique works well for gathering information about abusive situations. It is a good use of clinical time to sit near the patient and:
   a. Establish trust and rapport
   b. Ask lots of questions
   c. Interrupt the patients' story to allow for decompression
   d. Utilize closed-ended questions
8. The abused person is often in a dependent position, relying on the abuser for basic needs. At particular risk are children and the elderly due to:
   a. The love they have for parents or children.
   b. Their limited options.
   c. The need to feel safe at home.
   d. Other relatives do not want them.
9. An appropriate expected outcome in individual therapy regarding the perpetrator of abuse would be:
   a. A decrease in family interaction so that there are fewer opportunities for abuse to occur.
   b. The perpetrator will recognize destructive patterns of behavior and learn alternate responses.
   c. The perpetrator will no longer live with the family but have supervised contact while undergoing intensive inpatient therapy.

d. A triad of treatment modalities, including medication, counseling, and role-playing opportunities.

10. Perpetrators of domestic violence tend to: *Select all that apply.*

a. Have relatively poor social skills and to have grown up with poor role models.

b. Believe they, if male, should be dominant and in charge in relationships.

c. Force their mates to work and expect them to handle the financial decisions.

d. Be controlling and willing to use force to maintain their power in relationships.

e. Prevent their mates from having relationships and activities outside the family.

Answers

1. **b;** 2. **a, b, c, e;** 3. **b;** 4. **d;** 5. **a, b, c, d;** 6. **b;** 7. **a;** 8. **b;** 9. **b;** 10. **a, b, d, e**

ⓔ Visit the Evolve website for a posttest on the content in this chapter: http://evolve.elsevier.com/Varcarolis

Post-Test interactive review

REFERENCES

American Psychological Association. (2014). Child sexual abuse: What parents should know. Retrieved from http://www.apa.org/pi/families/resources/child-sexual-abuse.aspx.

Bulechek, G. M., Butcher, H. K., Dochterman, J. M., & Wagner, C. (2013). *Nursing interventions classification (NIC)* (6th ed.). St. Louis, MO: Mosby.

Bureau of Justice Statistics. (2012). *Intimate partner violence 1993-2010.* Retrieved from http://www.bjs.gov/index.cfm?ty=pbdetail&iid=4536.

Centers for Disease Control and Prevention. (2015a). *Child maltreatment: Risk and protective factors.* Retrieved from http://www.cdc.gov/violenceprevention/childmaltreatment/riskprotectivefactors.html.

Centers for Disease Control and Prevention. (2015b). *Intimate partner violence surveillance uniform definitions and recommended data elements.* Retrieved from https://www.cdc.gov/violenceprevention/pdf/intimatepartnerviolence.pdf.

Centers for Disease Control and Prevention. (2015c). *Elder abuse prevention.* Retrieved from http://www.cdc.gov/features/elderabuse/.

Centers for Disease Control and Prevention. (2016). *Child abuse and neglect: Definitions.* Retrieved from https://www.cdc.gov/violenceprevention/childmaltreatment/definitions.html.

Clay, R. A. (2014). *Suicide and intimate partner violence.* Retrieved from http://www.apa.org/monitor/2014/11/suicide-violence.aspx.

Eades, A. (2016, January 19). *Nursing home employee accused of sexual abuse of seniors.* Retrieved from http://www.illinoishomepage.net/news/local-news/nursing-home-employee-accused-of-sexual-abuse-of-seniors/332590041.

Farley, D. (2017, January 3). *Victim of suspected elderly abuse dies.* Retrieved from http://www.semissourian.com/story/2373464.html.

Finkelhor, D., Shattuck, A., Turner, H. A., & Hamby, S. L. (2014). The lifetime prevalence of child sexual abuse and sexual assault assessed in late adolescence. *Journal of Adolescent Health, 55*(3), 329–333.

Moorhead, S., Johnson, M., Maas, M. L., & Swanson, E. (2013). *Nursing outcomes classification (NOC)* (5th ed.). St. Louis, MO: Mosby.

Soeken, K., McFarlane, J., Parker, B., & Lominack, M. (1998). The abuse assessment screen: A clinical instrument to measure frequency, severity and perpetrator of abuse against women. In J. Campbell (Ed.), *Empowering survivors of abuse: Health care for battered women and their children* (pp. 575–579). New Brunswick, NJ: Transaction.

Stephenson, R., Rentsch, C., Salazar, L., & Sullivan, P. (2011). Dyadic characteristics and intimate partner violence among men who have had sex with men. *Western Journal of Emergency Medicine, 12*(3), 324–332.

Sullivan, S. P. (2016, December 22). *Elder abuse caught on video.* Retrieved from http://www.nj.com/news/index.ssf/2016/12/elder_abuse_caught_on_video_ag_announces_free_home.html.

US Department of Health & Human Services. (2016). *Child maltreatment 2014.* Retrieved from https://www.acf.hhs.gov/cb/resource/child-maltreatment-2014.

Walker, L. E. (1979). *The battered woman* (2nd ed.). New York, NY: Springer.

29

Sexual Assault

Jodie Flynn

Visit the Evolve website for a pretest on the content in this chapter: http://evolve.elsevier.com/Varcarolis Pre-Test interactive review

OBJECTIVES

1. Define sexual assault, sexual violence, completed rape, and attempted rape.
2. Discuss the implications for the underreporting of sexual assault.
3. Describe the profile of the victim and the perpetrator of sexual assault.
4. Distinguish between the acute and long-term phases of the rape-trauma syndrome, and identify some common reactions during each phase.
5. Identify five areas to assess when working with a person who has been sexually assaulted.
6. Analyze personal thoughts and feelings regarding rape and its impact on survivors.
7. Formulate two long-term outcomes and two short-term goals for the nursing diagnosis posttrauma syndrome.
8. Identify six overall guidelines for nursing interventions related to sexual assault.
9. Describe the role of the sexual assault nurse examiner to a colleague.
10. Discuss the long-term psychological effects of sexual assault that might lead a person to seek psychiatric care.
11. Identify three outcome criteria that would signify successful interventions for a person who has suffered a sexual assault.

OUTLINE

KEY TERMS AND CONCEPTS

acquaintance (or date) rape
attempted rape
completed rape
rape-trauma syndrome
revictimization
sexual assault
sexual violence
spousal (or marital) rape

In 2008 a 42-year-old Austrian woman, Elisabeth Fritzl, reported to police that she had been imprisoned in the soundproofed, windowless cellar of her family home since the age of 18. Her own father, Josef Fritzl, lured her there, locked her in, and raped her repeatedly for the next 24 years. This abuse resulted in seven children, one of whom died shortly after birth. Three of the surviving children were taken upstairs to be raised by Fritzl and his wife. He explained to his wife that their daughter, Elisabeth, had run away to join a cult and had left the children on the doorstep. The other three children remained in the cellar with their mother, never seeing the light of day. They were forced to witness the continual rape of their mother by their father/grandfather.

When the moldy, dark conditions caused the eldest daughter, Kersten, 19, to become mortally ill, Elisabeth begged Fritzl to get her treatment. Fritzl relented and took her to a hospital where Elisabeth would later be taken to visit. It was there that Elisabeth revealed the nature of her daughter's illness and her own abuse on the condition that she would never have to see her father again. Elisabeth was reunited with all of her children. Fritzl was sentenced to life in prison for the criminally insane.

SEXUAL ASSAULT AND SEXUAL VIOLENCE

This story is horrific and demonstrates some of the most contemptible violations that can be perpetrated by one human being on another. In this chapter, we will further explore these types of violations. **Sexual assault** and **sexual violence** are broad terms that encompass unwanted sexual advances and sexual harassment to stranger rape, marital rape, date rape, and drug-facilitated sexual assault. Incest, human sex trafficking, and female genital mutilation are other examples of sexual assault.

Although sexual assault generally involves adult males assaulting adult females, it includes any combination of females, males, adults, and children. Vulnerable individuals such as the disabled and the elderly are often targets. Sexual violence also includes denying emergency contraception or measures to prevent sexually transmitted infections, organized rape during conflict or war, and sexual homicide.

Rape

The Federal Bureau of Investigation (FBI, 2012) considers rape to be the second-most violent crime in a group of crimes that includes murder, robbery, and aggravated assault. Victims are traumatized, both physically and emotionally, and are often seen in healthcare settings. Nurses are instrumental in providing holistic care for those who have been sexually assaulted and also in helping to preserve evidence. Preservation of evidence can lead to the prosecution of a crime or the exoneration of an innocent person of interest. Therefore it is essential that nurses be informed adequately about their roles and responsibilities with regard to providing both medical and legal care.

Rape is classified into two categories: completed rape and attempted rape.

Completed Rape

Completed rape is defined as "penetration, no matter how slight, of the vagina or anus with any body part or object, or oral penetration by a sex organ of another person, without the consent of the victim" (FBI, 2016). This revised definition will lead to a more uniform statistical reporting of rape. It replaces a decades-old definition that did not account for crimes against men, threats of violence, as well as all rapes in which the victim is a child and unable to consent. The term "forcible" rape was removed because the term rape clearly implies force. Examples of completed rape include (FBI, 2014):

- A female high school student was drinking with a male classmate at her house. The male gave her a pill that he said would make her feel "really good." After taking the pill, the woman did not recall what happened. A rape kit indicated semen from sexual penetration.
- A man working in a residential facility led a woman with a severe mental disability to the woods behind the facility. There he fondled her and sexually penetrated her. Because of the woman's disability, she was unable to understand and consent to the sexual act.
- One night, a woman's husband was very drunk, and he accused her of sleeping around. He became enraged, pushed her onto the bed, and penetrated her with an object. She was too afraid to fight back.

Attempted Rape

Threats of rape or intention to rape that is unsuccessful are referred to an **attempted rape**. Examples of rape attempts include (FBI, 2014):

- A man attacked a woman on the street, knocked her down, and attempted to rape her. A pedestrian frightened the man away before he could complete the attack.
- At a local bar, a man slipped gamma-hydroxybutyrate acid (GHB), a drug sometimes used to facilitate sexual assault, into the drink of his date. He could not convince the woman to leave her friends and go home with him. After an investigation, detectives concluded that the man intended to rape the woman.

Laws and Sexual Assault

Because state laws vary in regard to sexual assault, it is important for you to identify how sexual acts are medically and legally defined within your community. Based on your jurisdiction and legal mandates, healthcare providers may be required to report a sexual assault to law enforcement. Patient identification may be withheld if the individual wishes to remain anonymous. Evidence can be stored until the individual decides whether or not to report the assault.

Regardless of whether individuals report the sexual assault to police, states and tribal governments are required to pay for or reimburse for sexual assault examinations. Most states (32) pay through the victim compensation program; six states require the county where the offense occurred to pay for the examination; six states require that the law enforcement agency that requests the examination pay for it; and six states designate a sexual assault reimbursement program to pay for forensic examinations

TABLE 29.1 Lifetime Prevalence of Rape, Stalking, and Sexual Assault by Sex and Race/Ethnicity of Victim

	Rape		Stalking		Sexual Assault*	
	Women	Men	Women	Men	Women	Men
All races, non-Hispanic, Hispanic	19.3	1.7	15.2	5.7	—	—
White, non-Hispanic	20.5	1.6	15.9	4.7	46.9	22.2
Black, non-Hispanic	21.2	—	13.9	9.1	38.2	24.4
Hispanic	13.6	—	14.2	8.2	35.6	26.6
American Indian/Alaskan Native	27.5	—	24.5	—	55.0	24.5
Asian or Pacific Islander	—	—	—	—	31.9	15.8
Multiracial	32.3	—	22.4	9.3	64.1	39.5

*Includes being made to penetrate a perpetrator, sexual coercion, unwanted sexual contact, and noncontact unwanted sexual experiences.
Data from Breiding, M. J., Smith, S. G., Basile, K. C., Walters, M. L., Chen, J., & Merrick, M. T. (2014). *Prevalence and characteristics of sexual violence, stalking, and intimate partner violence victimization. National Intimate Partner and Sexual Violence Survey, United States, 2011. Morbidity and Mortality Weekly Report.* Retrieved from https://www.cdc.gov/mmwr/preview/mmwrhtml/ss6308a1.htm.

(AEquitas, 2012). Failure to comply with this reimbursement mandate results in loss of funding from the Violence Against Women grant initiatives. This mandate is patient-centered and gives control back to individuals who should be the primary decision makers in personal health and legal matters.

For the remainder of this chapter, victims of sexual assault will be referred to using the female pronoun in recognition of the fact that women are more frequently sexually assaulted. However, the principles discussed apply to anyone. In healthcare settings, victims of sexual assault are referred to as *patients,* advocacy groups use the term *survivor,* and legal systems use the term *victim.* Within this chapter, individuals will often be referred to as *patients* because those individuals are cared for in healthcare settings.

EPIDEMIOLOGY

Rape

In the United States, an estimated 19.3% of women and 1.7% of men have been raped at some time in their lives (Breiding et al., 2014). The 12-month prevalence is estimated at 1.6% in women. Among female victims of completed rape, the first rape experience happened before age 25 years in nearly 79% of victims. The first rape experience happened before age 18 in 40% of females. Both males and females are more likely to be raped by a male. The lifetime prevalence and 12-month prevalence of intimate partner rape is estimated at nearly 9% and around 1%, respectively.

Almost half of female victims have been raped by an acquaintance. Intimate partners accounted for about 45% of female victims (Breiding et al., 2014). Nearly 60% of women who experience alcohol/drug facilitated penetration were victims of acquaintances. About 45% of male victims were raped by an acquaintance, and intimate partners raped 29% of male victims.

A male who is raped is more likely to experience physical trauma and to have been victimized by several assailants. Reports of male-to-male rape occur primarily in locked institutions such as prisons and maximum-security hospitals. Males experience the same devastation, physical injury, and emotional consequences as females. Although they may cover their responses, they too benefit from care and treatment.

Race and ethnicity are associated with rape. Women who identify themselves as multiracial are the most likely to be raped, followed by American Indian/Alaskan Native and Black non-Hispanic.

Stalking

About 15% of women and nearly 6% of men have been victims of stalking at some point in their lifetimes (Breiding et al., 2014). The 12-month prevalence of stalking is about 4% of women and 2% of men. Most female victims (about 54%) and nearly half of male victims (nearly 50%) were first stalked before 25 years of age.

Sexual Violence

Precise estimates of sexual violence are impossible because this crime is greatly underreported. According to the FBI (2016) Uniform Crime Reporting Program, for the first 6 months of 2015 there was an overall increase of 1.7% in the number of violent crimes reported when compared with statistics reported for the same time in 2014. The violent crime category includes murder, rape, robbery, and aggravated assault.

Table 29.1 summarizes the lifetime prevalence of rape, stalking, and sexual violence.

Sexual Offenders and Relationships with Victims

While we often think of a stranger lurking in the shadows of parking lots as the typical sexual offender, this is not true. The terms **spousal (or marital) rape** and **acquaintance (or date) rape** describe the nature of the relationship between victim and rapist. In recent years, courts have recognized spousal rape in which the perpetrator (nearly always the male) is married to the person raped. In acquaintance rape, the perpetrator is known to, and presumably trusted by, the person raped. The psychological and emotional outcomes of rape seem to vary depending on the level of intimacy between the victim and the perpetrator. Sexual distress is more common among women who have been

TABLE 29.2 Lifetime Reports of Sexual Violence by Type of Perpetrator

	Intimate Partner	Family Member	Person of Authority	Acquaintance	Stranger
Women					
Rape	45.4	12.1	2.6	46.7	12.9
Forced penetration	48.1	14.9	—	38.8	11.0
Alcohol or drug facilitated penetration	40.4	—	—	58.4	12.4
Made to penetrate	53.2	—	—	—	—
Sexual coercion	74.1	8.1	6.1	25.5	—
Unwanted sexual contact	23.4	22.1	8.9	47.2	21.1
Noncontact unwanted sexual experiences	26.6	15.1	3.7	33.5	49.3
Men					
Rape	29.0	—	—	44.9	—
Forced penetration	—	—	—	32.2	—
Alcohol or drug facilitated penetration	—	—	—	51.0	—
Made to penetrate	54.5	—	—	43.0	8.6
Sexual coercion	69.5	—	—	26.7	—
Unwanted sexual contact	22.6	6.1	6.7	51.8	23.7
Noncontact unwanted sexual experiences	30.9	7.2	7.0	39.2	30.9

Data from Breiding, M. J., Smith, S. G., Basile, K. C., Walters, M. L., Chen, J., & Merrick, M. T. (2014). *Prevalence and characteristics of sexual violence, stalking, and intimate partner violence victimization. National Intimate Partner and Sexual Violence Survey, United States, 2011. Morbidity and Mortality Weekly Report.* Retrieved from https://www.cdc.gov/mmwr/preview/mmwrhtml/ss6308a1.htm.

sexually assaulted by intimates, and fear and anxiety are more common in those assaulted by strangers. Depression occurs in both groups. Table 29.2 summarizes perpetrator, sex of victims, and type of assault.

Acquaintance (or date) rape has increased in the United States with drugs, often combined with alcohol, being used to commit sexual assault. Date-rape drugs may render a woman incapable of resisting an attack and facilitate acquaintance rape. Once the drugs are ingested, victims lose their ability to fight off attackers, develop amnesia, and become unreliable witnesses. Because the symptoms mimic those of alcohol, victims are not always screened for these drugs.

The increase in prevalence and incidence of drug-assisted rape led to the passage of the Drug-Induced Rape Prevention and Punishment Act in 1996. This law allows up to 20 years' imprisonment and fines for anyone who intends to commit a violent crime by administering a controlled substance to an unknowing individual (US Department of Justice, 1997). Table 29.3 provides information about date-rape drugs.

CLINICAL PICTURE

Just as there is no typical patient presentation after a sexual assault, emotional responses will vary from person to person. However, many survivors experience criteria for the diagnoses of acute stress disorder and posttraumatic stress disorder following this type of crime. Chapter 16 provides a complete description of these disorders.

Acute stress disorder is a psychiatric reaction to a serious trauma such as witnessing a death, suffering a serious injury, or a sexual violation. Symptoms usually begin immediately after the sexual assault, persist at least 3 days, and can extend for up to 1 month. Symptoms are grouped into five categories (American Psychiatric Association, 2013):

1. Intrusive symptoms. Recurrent and intrusive memories, dreams, flashbacks, and psychological or physiological distress in response to cues that remind the individual of the assault.
2. Negative thoughts and mood or feelings. For example, feelings may vary from a persistent and distorted sense of blame of self or others, to estrangement from others or markedly diminished interest in activities, to an inability to remember key aspects of the event.
3. Dissociative symptoms. Altered sense of reality and an inability to remember parts of the traumatic event.
4. Avoidance. Changing routines to escape situations similar to the trauma. Victims might avoid places, events, or objects that remind them of the experience. Emotions related to avoidance are numbness, guilt, and depression. Some have a decreased ability to feel certain emotions such as happiness. They also might be unable to remember major parts of the trauma. They feel that their future offers fewer possibilities than other people have.
5. Arousal symptoms. Difficulty concentrating or falling asleep, being easily startled, feeling tense, and angry outbursts. These can combine to make it difficult for victims to complete normal daily tasks.

If symptoms extend beyond 1 month, the diagnosis of acute stress disorder will no longer apply. A person's diagnosis may change to posttraumatic stress disorder (PTSD). The symptoms are similar with the two diagnoses. PTSD may be diagnosed in children less than 6 years of age, school-age children, adolescents, and adults.

TABLE 29.3 **Drugs Associated with Date Rape**

Drug, Alternate Names, and Status in the United States	Form, Mechanism of Action, and Onset	Effect on Victim	Overdose Symptoms and Treatment
GHB (gamma-hydroxybutyric acid) Also known as *G, Georgia home boy, liquid ecstasy, salty water, scoop,* and many others Legal in the United States for narcolepsy Schedule III central nervous system depressant Often made in home labs	Liquid, white powder, or pill with a salty taste; newer pills are oval and green-gray in color. A dye in these commercial pills makes clear liquids turn bright blue and dark drinks turn cloudy. A metabolite of gamma-aminobutyric acid Onset within 5-20 minutes; duration is dose related and from 1-12 hours	Produces relaxation, euphoria, and disinhibition Incoordination, confusion, deep sedation, and amnesia Tolerance and dependence exhibited by agitation, tachycardia, insomnia, anxiety, tremors, and sweating	Respiratory depression, seizures, nausea, vomiting, bradycardia, hypothermia, agitation, delirium, unconsciousness, and coma Intubation for severe respiratory distress; atropine for bradycardia, and benzodiazepines for seizure activity. Vomiting should be induced when possible.
Rohypnol (flunitrazepam)* Also known as *forget-me pill, roofies, club drug, roachies, R2, and rophies* Schedule IV potent benzodiazepine Not legal in the United States	Pill that dissolves in liquids 10 times stronger than diazepam Impact is within 10-30 minutes and lasts 2-12 hours	More potent when combined with alcohol; causes sedation, psychomotor slowing, muscle relaxation, and amnesia Dependence and tolerance may develop	Overdose unlikely Airway protection and gastrointestinal decontamination
Ketamine Also known as *black hole, bump, K, kit kat, purple, and Special K* Legal in the United States for anesthesia, mainly in animals	Comes as a liquid or a white powder An anesthetic frequently used in veterinary practice; also a hallucinogenic substance related to PCP (phencyclidine) Onset within 30 seconds intravenously and 20 minutes orally; duration only 30-60 minutes; amnesia effects may last longer	Causes dissociative reaction, with a dreamlike state leading to deep amnesia and analgesia and complete compliance of the victim May become confused, paranoid, delirious, combative, with drooling and hallucinations	Airway maintenance and use of anticholinergics such as atropine and benzodiazepines

*Two other benzodiazepines, clonazepam (Klonopin) and alprazolam (Xanax), are also used.
Data from Office of Women's Health. (2012). *Date rape drugs fact sheet.* Retrieved from http://womenshealth.gov/publications/our-publications/fact-sheet/date-rape-drugs.html.

Some individuals who are diagnosed with PTSD may be given an additional specifier of "with dissociative symptoms." These dissociative symptoms are:

1. **Depersonalization:** Feeling detached from one's mental processes or body. For example, affected individuals may feel like they are in a dream, that their bodies are not real, or that time is moving slowly.
2. **Derealization:** Feeling like surroundings are unreal. This symptom is characterized by a feeling that the world around the individual is unreal, dreamlike, distant, or distorted.

Psychological Effects of Sexual Assault

Most people who are raped suffer severe and long-lasting emotional trauma. Long-term effects of sexual assault may include depression, suicide, anxiety, and fear. Other consequences of this horrific offense include difficulties with daily functioning, low self-esteem, sexual dysfunction, and somatic (physical) complaints.

Victims of incest may experience a negative self-image, depression, eating disorders, personality disorders, self-destructive behavior, and substance misuse. A history of sexual abuse in psychiatric patients is associated with a characteristic pattern of symptoms that may include depression, anxiety disorders, chemical dependency, suicide attempts, self-mutilation, compulsive sexual behavior, and psychosis-like symptoms.

Specialized Sexual Assault Services

Facilities may have trained sexual assault nurse examiners (SANEs) or other specially trained clinicians to provide care to patients who have been sexually assaulted. A SANE is a registered nurse who has specialized training in caring for sexual assault patients, has demonstrated competency in conducting medical and legal evaluations, and has the ability to be an expert witness in court.

The SANE uses the nursing process with a patient-centered approach during the examination process. A SANE is a member of the Sexual Assault Response Team (SART), a multidisciplinary team approach to caring for victims of sexual assault. Members include nurses, physicians, attorneys, social service workers, advocates, mental health professionals, forensic laboratory personnel, and other collaborative agencies that provide services for sexual assault patients. If a SANE or specially trained clinician is not available in your facility, nurses should be prepared to provide both the medical and legal aspects of care.

Guidelines for Medical Forensic Examinations

In 2013 the US Department of Justice published the second edition of *A National Protocol for Sexual Assault Medical Forensic Examinations for Adults/Adolescents.* This document assists healthcare facilities in establishing protocols in caring for adolescent and adult sexual assault survivors. This protocol offers guidance and best practice recommendations specific to patient-centered procedures related to the examination process. The protocol highlights:

- Providing patient-centered care, include prioritizing these patients.
- Ensuring patient privacy.
- Providing culturally responsive care.

- Accommodating support people as needed.
- Using age-appropriate language.
- Assessing and respecting patient priorities.
- Integrating medical and evidence collection procedures.

The Emergency Nurses Association (2010) position statement on care of sexual assault and rape victims recommends:

1. An individualized, multidisciplinary, and multiagency approach.
2. A physical and social environment conducive to private, empathetic, and unbiased care by healthcare providers, family members, law enforcement officers, and members of the justice system.
3. A private and safe environment with personnel limited to healthcare providers during sexual assault care. Interpreters must be available if needed. With the consent of the patient, a specially trained advocate also may be present.
4. Comprehensive, competent, and sensitive emergency healthcare.
5. Employment of SANE nurses in the emergency department is highly recommended.
6. Emergency nurses should collaborate to promote and establish ongoing community education focused on preparing the public and emergency nurses to better identify, prevent, care for, and report incidents of sexual assault and rape.
7. Emergency nurses should be involved in research concerning the identification, assessment, and treatment of victims of sexual assault and rape.

Historically, patients who were sexually assaulted and went to healthcare facilities for medical care and evidence collection had to wait for long periods of time to be evaluated. Often they were not considered in need of acute care because they lacked visible physical injuries. Now, a patient who is sexually assaulted is considered a priority due to the intense psychological impact and potential hidden physical injury. Collecting legal evidence is also a priority, and delays may result in its destruction or contamination.

The care of sexual assault victims varies from facility to facility. Patel and colleagues (2013) surveyed 582 emergency departments for comprehensive medical care management of female sexual assault patients. They found that less than one-fifth of US hospitals provide comprehensive services to sexual assault patients. All emergency departments provided acute medical care. Most provided care for sexually transmitted infection (77%), human immunodeficiency virus (**HIV**) management (65%), and emergency contraception (60%). Rape crisis counseling was provided in only 234 of the 582 emergency departments.

APPLICATION OF THE NURSING PROCESS

ASSESSMENT

General Assessment

The nurse should talk with the patient, the family, or friends who accompany the patient to gather as much objective data as possible for assessing the crisis. The nurse then assesses the patient's (1) level of anxiety, (2) coping mechanisms, (3) available support systems, (4) signs and symptoms of emotional trauma, and (5) signs and symptoms of physical trauma. Information obtained from the assessment is then analyzed, and nursing diagnoses are formulated.

Level of Anxiety

Patients experiencing severe-to-panic levels of anxiety will not be able to problem solve or process information. Support, reassurance, and appropriate therapeutic techniques can lower the patient's anxiety and facilitate mutual goal setting and the assimilation of information. Refer to Chapters 10 and 15 for more detailed discussions of the levels of anxiety and therapeutic interventions.

Coping Mechanisms

The same coping skills that have helped the survivor through other difficult problems in her lifetime will be used in adjusting to the rape. In addition, new ways of getting through the difficult times may be developed for both the short- and long-term adjustment. Behavioral responses include crying, withdrawing, smoking, using alcohol and drugs, talking about the event, becoming extremely agitated, confused, disoriented, incoherent, and even laughing or joking.

Cognitive coping mechanisms are the thoughts people have that help them deal with high anxiety levels. A positive cognitive response might be "At least I am alive and will get to see my children again." Not-so-positive responses may become generalized as a way to sum up the situation: "It's my fault this happened; my mother warned me about working in such a trashy place" may develop into an ego-damaging refrain. If such thoughts are verbalized, the nurse will know what the patient is thinking. If not, the nurse can ask questions such as "What are you thinking and feeling?"; "What can I do to help you in this difficult situation?"; or "What has helped in the past?"

Available Support Systems

The availability, size, and usefulness of a patient's social support system should be assessed. Often partners or family members do not understand the survivor's feelings about the sexual assault, and they may not be the best supports available. Pay careful attention to verbal and nonverbal cues of the patient that may communicate the strength of the social network.

Involve the patient, family, or friends, who accompany the patient, or other healthcare providers in collaborative holistic data collection. Obtaining information from others is particularly important if the patient is unable to provide details surrounding the sexual assault (i.e., the patient is unconscious, nonverbal, or has a disability). If interpreting services are needed a certified medical interpreter should be contacted.

VIGNETTE: Celia, a home care provider, brings Ms. Smith, a 64-year-old woman with a history of schizophrenia, to the emergency department. Celia tells the triage nurse that Ms. Smith, who is also a paraplegic, has been reclusive for the past few days and behaving strangely. According to Celia, Ms. Smith does not eat, sleeps all day, and repeatedly says that she is pregnant.

The triage nurse asks Ms. Smith, "Can you tell me why you are here?" She begins to sob, stares at the floor, rocks back and forth in her wheelchair, and mutters, "Someone is hurting me, and I am pregnant." A physical assessment reveals bruises on her upper thighs and breasts. The triage nurse has been trained as a sexual assault nurse examiner (SANE) and immediately recognizes that Ms. Smith needs a sexual assault evaluation. She states, "I believe you, and I will help you. You are safe here." Ms. Smith responds quietly, "Thank you."

Signs and Symptoms of Emotional Trauma

The first challenge for any healthcare provider is to identify if the patient is a forensic patient. A forensic patient is anyone who seeks treatment and also needs to interact with the legal system or has the potential to interact with the legal system. Patients may disclose a history of sexual assault or report a history that is inconsistent with physical findings. Others may demonstrate a behavioral change that causes a concern for family, friends, caregivers, or other healthcare providers. Patients may seek help at a healthcare facility after a sexual assault occurs, visit their primary care provider, or contact law enforcement.

A nursing history should be obtained and carefully recorded. When taking a history, the nurse determines only the details of the assault that will be helpful in addressing the immediate physical and psychological needs of the patient. The nurse allows the patient to talk at a comfortable pace and poses questions in nonjudgmental descriptive terms. Always avoid asking "why" questions because they are inherently evaluative. For example, "Why did you walk home alone?" or "Why didn't you run?"

Suicidal ideation may be present and should be assessed. Ask direct questions such as "Are you thinking of harming yourself?" or "Have you ever tried to kill yourself before or after this attack occurred?" If the answer is yes, the nurse conducts a thorough suicide assessment (i.e., plan, means to carry it out), as described in Chapter 25.

Signs and Symptoms of Physical Trauma

It is essential that nurses provide psychological support while collecting and preserving legal evidence. The nurse should be conscientious of the patient's reactions during the physical examination and advise her to report any signs of pain or discomfort immediately.

During the examination, the nurse will inspect and palpate for any signs of injury. Recent injuries may not show visible bruising. Palpating the skin and finding tender spots can improve evidence collection and further documentation of an injured site. Physical signs of injury post-sexual assault can include injuries to the face, head, neck, extremities, and anogenital areas. Physical injuries should be carefully documented (i.e., size, color, description, and location of injury), both in narrative and pictorial form using preprinted body maps, hand-drawn copies, or photographs. If an injury is present, ask the patient if she knows how that injury occurred. It is important to recognize that many reported cases of sexual assault have no physical signs of injury.

The nurse will collect and preserve legal evidence such as blood; hair samples; oral swabs; nail swabs or scrapings; and anal, genital, or penile swabs. Facilities may have standardized sexual assault evidence collection kits that provide direction on how to collect and preserve evidence. This can be helpful to nurses and other clinicians who do not have specialized training in evidence collection and preservation.

The nurse takes a gynecological history, including the date of the last menstrual period and the likelihood of current pregnancy, and assesses for a history of sexually transmitted infections. A detailed genital examination, with a speculum, is needed to observe for signs of injury for the female patient. If the patient has never undergone a genital examination, the steps of the examination will need to be explained. The nurse plays a crucial role in reducing **revictimization**, which refers to the trauma of the examination itself because the patient may experience it as another violation of her body. Recognizing this, the nurse can explain the examination procedure in a way that will be reassuring and supportive.

Best Practice Guidelines

The examination involves five steps:

1. Head-to-toe physical assessment, observing for signs of injury
2. Detailed genital examination, observing for signs of injury
3. Evidence collection and preservation
4. Documentation of physical findings (both written and photo documentation)
5. Treatment, discharge planning, and follow-up care

The patient has the right to decline parts of the legal or medical examination. Informed consent must be provided and consent forms signed before photographs are taken, a physical examination occurs, and any other procedures that might be needed to collect evidence and provide treatment. A shower and change of clothing should be made available to the patient as soon as possible after the examination and collection of evidence.

According to guidelines by the Centers for Disease Control and Prevention (2015), providing prophylactic treatment for sexually transmitted diseases is common practice. Sexually transmitted diseases, including HIV and hepatitis exposure, are often a concern of patients who are sexually assaulted. This worry should always be addressed and the patient given information needed to evaluate the likelihood of risk and follow-up care. With this information, the person and her sexual partner(s) can make educated choices about testing and safer sex practices until further testing can be done and results communicated.

About 5% of women who are raped become pregnant as a result (Rape, Abuse, and Incest National Network, 2008). Pregnancy prevention is offered in the emergency department once pregnancy tests establish that the patient was not already pregnant before the assault. Emergency contraception or morning-after pills are contraceptives that do not cause abortion. They act on follicular development and inhibit ovulation. If there is no egg available to the sperm, then pregnancy cannot occur.

Assessment data are carefully documented including verbatim statements by the patient, detailed observations of emotional and physical status, and results of the physical examination. Laboratory tests are noted and findings recorded as soon as they are available.

Self-Assessment

Nurses' attitudes influence the physical and psychological care received by rape survivors. Knowing the myths and facts surrounding sexual assault can increase your awareness of your personal beliefs and feelings regarding rape. If you examine your

TABLE 29.4 Myth Versus Fact: Rape

Myth	Fact
Many women really want to be raped.	Women do not ask to be raped—no matter how they are dressed, what their behavior is, or where they are at any given time. Studies show that violence toward women in the media leads to attitudes that foster tolerance of rape.
Most rapes occur for the purpose of sex.	Sex is used as an instrument of violence in rape. Rape is an act of aggression, anger, or power.
In most cases it is strangers who rape women.	The majority (69%) of rape victims are raped by someone they know.
An unarmed man cannot rape a healthy adult female who resists.	Most men can overpower most women because of differences in body build. Also, the victim may panic, which makes her actions less effective than usual.
Most charges of rape are unfounded.	There is no evidence to show that there are more false reports for rape than for other crimes. Most rape victims do not even report the rape.
Rapes usually occur in dark alleys.	Over 50% of all rapes occur in the home.
Rape is usually an impulsive act.	Most rapes are planned; over 50% involve a weapon.
Nice girls don't get raped.	Any woman is a potential rape victim. Victims range in age from 6 months to 90 years.
There was not enough time for a rape to occur.	There is no minimal time limit that characterizes rape. It can happen very quickly.
Do not fight or try to get away, because you will just get hurt.	There are no verifiable data to substantiate the theory that a victim will be injured if he or she tries to get away.
Only females are raped.	There are a growing number of male rape victims.

personal feelings and reactions *before* encountering a patient who has been sexually assaulted, you will be better prepared to give empathetic and effective care. Examining your feelings about abortion is also important because a patient might choose an abortion if a pregnancy results from rape. Table 29.4 compares rape myths and facts.

DIAGNOSIS

Several domains of functioning are impacted by sexual assault and rape. Specific to rape, the coping/stress tolerance domain is the most relevant. Within this domain, the nursing diagnosis of *Rape-trauma syndrome* applies to the physical and psychological effects of rape. **Rape-trauma syndrome** is defined as "sustained and maladaptive response to a forced, violent sexual penetration against the victim's will and consent" (Herdman & Kamitsuru, 2014, p. 318). Defining characteristics of rape-trauma syndrome are listed in Box 29.1.

ASSESSMENT GUIDELINES

Sexual Assault

1. Assess psychological trauma and document the patient's verbatim statements.
2. Assess level of anxiety. If in a severe-to-panic level of anxiety, the patient will not be able to problem solve or process information.
3. Assess physical trauma. Use a preprinted body map and ask permission to take photographs.
4. Assess available support system. Often partners or family members do not understand the trauma of rape, and they may not be the best supports to draw on at this time.
5. Identify community supports (e.g., attorneys, support groups, therapists) that work in the area of sexual assault.
6. Encourage, but not pressure, the patient to talk about the experience.

BOX 29.1 Defining Characteristics of Rape-Trauma Syndrome

Shame	Mood swings	Anxiety	Dissociation
Guilt	Aggression	Fear	Disorganization
Helplessness	Anger	Disturbed sleep	Shock
Powerlessness	Agitation	Nightmares	Confusion
Dependence	Revenge	Sexual dysfunction	Phobias
Low self-esteem	Substance abuse	Muscle tension	Paranoia
Depression	Suicide attempts	Hyperalertness	

A variety of diagnoses would also apply to the victim of sexual assault. They include, but are not limited to, the following:

- *Disturbed personal identity*
- *Situational low self-esteem*
- *Interrupted family processes*
- *Sexual identity*
- *Sexual dysfunction*
- *Anxiety*
- *Fear*
- *Social isolation*

OUTCOMES IDENTIFICATION

The long-term outcome includes the absence of any residual symptoms after the trauma. *Sexual abuse recovery* is specifically linked to sexual assault. It is defined as the "extent of healing of physical and psychological injuries due to sexual abuse or exploitation" (Moorhead et al., 2013, p. 76). Indicators for improvement include the following:

- Expressions of the right to have been protected from abuse
- Healing of physical injuries
- Relief of anger in nondestructive ways

- Feelings of empowerment and expressions of hope
- Evidence of comfort in relationships

PLANNING

Unless the patient has sustained serious physical or psychological injury, treatment is offered, and the patient is released. Because the ramifications of rape are experienced for an extended time after the acute phase, the plan of care includes information for follow-up care. The patient needs information about available community supports and how to access them. Nurses may also encounter rape survivors in other settings when they are no longer in acute distress but still dealing with the aftermath of rape. Such settings include inpatient facilities, the community, and the home. A comprehensive plan of care addresses the continuing needs of the rape survivor in any setting.

IMPLEMENTATION

Timely intervention can reduce the aftermath of rape. The occurrence of rape can be the most devastating experience in a person's life and constitutes an acute situational (unexpected) crisis. Typical crisis reactions reflect cognitive, affective, and behavioral disruptions. For survivors to return to their previous level of functioning, it is necessary for them to fully mourn their losses, experience anger, and work through their fears. Box 29.2 identifies interventions for rape-trauma syndrome.

Counseling

The sexual assault patient may be too traumatized, ashamed, or afraid to go to the hospital. Cultural definitions of what constitutes rape may also affect the decision to seek treatment. For these reasons, 24-hour telephone and chat lines—such as the Rape, Abuse, and Incest National Network (RAINN)—provide direct communication with volunteers trained in rape crisis support. These types of support services focus on helping the person through the period of acute distress by assessing what has happened and determining what kind of assistance is needed. Counselors provide empathetic listening, the survivor is encouraged to go to the emergency department, and the main focus is on the immediate steps the person may take.

The most effective approach for counseling in the emergency department or crisis center is to provide nonjudgmental care and optimal emotional support. Conveying the confidential nature of the visit is crucial. Simply listening and letting the patient talk is a powerful intervention. A patient who feels listened to and understood is no longer alone and feels more in control of the situation.

It is especially important to help the survivor and significant others to separate issues of vulnerability from blame. Although the person may have made choices that made her more vulnerable, she is not to blame for the rape. She may, however, decide to avoid some of those choices in the future (e.g., walking alone late at night or excessive use of alcohol). Focusing on one's behavior (which is controllable) allows the survivor to believe that similar experiences can be avoided in the future.

VIGNETTE: Ms. Smith comes to see that it was not her fault that she was raped and feels comfortable that she is believed. Ms. Smith is now verbal and able to recall the events of the sexual assault to the healthcare providers and SANE before discharge.

With the patient's consent, the nurse involves her support system, which includes her family, friends, and group home providers. The nurse discusses with them the nature and trauma of sexual assault and possible delayed reactions that may occur. Ms. Smith expressed the aftermath of her assault, "It takes a few days to hit you. It was bad. It was really rough for my mom. I needed to be reassured. I needed to be told that there was nothing I could have done to prevent it. Understanding helps."

BOX 29.2 Interventions for Rape-Trauma Syndrome

Definition: Provision of emotional and physical support immediately after a reported rape

Activities:

- Provide support person to stay with patient.
- Explain legal proceedings available to patient.
- Explain rape protocol and obtain consent to proceed through protocol.
- Document whether patient has showered, douched, or bathed since incident.
- Document mental state, physical state (clothing, dirt, and debris), history of incident, evidence of violence, and prior gynecological history.
- Determine presence of cuts, bruises, bleeding, lacerations, or other signs of physical injury.
- Implement rape protocol (e.g., label and save soiled clothing, vaginal secretions, and vaginal hair combings).
- Secure samples for legal evidence.
- Implement crisis intervention counseling.
- Offer medication to prevent pregnancy, as appropriate.
- Offer prophylactic antibiotic medication against sexually transmitted disease.
- Inform patient of availability of human immunodeficiency virus testing, as appropriate.
- Give clear, written instructions about medication use, crisis support services, and legal support.
- Refer patient to rape advocacy program.
- Document according to agency policy.

From Bulechek, G. M., Butcher, H. K., Dochterman, J. M., & Wagner, C. (2013). *Nursing interventions classification (NIC)* (6th ed.). St. Louis, MO: Mosby.

Social support is tremendously beneficial. The survivor who is able to confide comfortably in one or two friends or family members, especially immediately after the assault, is likely to experience fewer somatic manifestations of stress. In many cases, family and friends need support and reassurance as much as the survivor does. This is especially true for those from traditional cultures, particularly those cultures that believe that sexual assault brings shame to the entire family. The longstanding cultural myth that women are the property of men still prevents some people from empathizing with the woman's severe emotional wound and from being supportive. Instead, in these cases, the woman is devalued.

CASE STUDY AND NURSING CARE PLAN

Rape

Kayla is a 36-year-old single mother of two. One evening she and her friends go bowling. Later in the evening, *Kayla* is tired and wants to go home before her friends. A man at the bowling alley offers to take her home. Not in the habit of going home alone with men she does not know, she hesitates. A friend whom she trusts encourages her to go with John and says "he's a good guy."

John drives *Kayla* home. He asks if he can use the bathroom before driving home. She hesitantly agrees. After using the bathroom, John approaches *Kayla* and forcibly kisses her. As she protests, John becomes more aggressive. She manages to get away from him briefly, but he caught her and began to pummel her with his fists and bite her. He tells her angrily, "If you don't do what I say, I'll break your neck" and proceeds to rape her. A neighbor hears the commotion and calls the police. When the police arrive, John is gone and they take *Kayla* to the emergency department. The neighbor meets them there.

In the emergency department, *Kayla* is visibly shaken. She keeps saying over and over, "I shouldn't have let him take me home. I should have fought harder. I shouldn't have let him do this."

The nurse takes *Kayla* to a quiet room. The nurse then notifies the advanced practice registered nurse practitioner and the rape-victim advocate. When the nurse comes back, she tells *Kayla* that she would like to talk to her before the doctor comes. *Kayla* glances at her neighbor and then stares at the floor. The nurse asks the neighbor to wait outside.

Kayla: "It was horrible. I feel so dirty."

Nurse: "You have had a traumatic experience."

Kayla: "I feel so ashamed. I never should have let that man take me home."

Nurse: "You think that if you hadn't gone home with a stranger, this wouldn't have happened?"

Kayla: "Yes…I shouldn't have let him do it; I shouldn't have let him rape me."

Nurse: "You mentioned that he said he would break your neck if you didn't do as he said."

Kayla: "Yes, he said that…he was going to kill me. It was awful."

Nurse: "It seems you did the right thing to stay alive."

As the nurse continues to talk with *Kayla*, her anxiety level seems to decrease. The nurse talks to *Kayla* about the kinds of symptoms rape victims often have after a rape and explains that the reactions she might have 2 or 3 weeks from now are normal.

The nurse says that the nurse practitioner will want to examine her and explains the procedure. *Kayla* signs a consent form. While preparing *Kayla* for examination, the nurse notices bite marks and bruising on both breasts. She also notes *Kayla's* lower lip, which is cut and bleeding. The nurse keeps detailed notes of her observations and draws a body map depicting the injuries. After the examination, *Kayla* is given clean clothes and a place to shower.

Self-Assessment

The nurse has worked with rape survivors before and has helped develop the hospital's protocol for sexual assault victims. It took a while for her to be able to remain both neutral and responsive because of her own anger at this type of violence. She recalls a time when a woman came in stating that she was raped but was so calm, smiling, and polite that the nurse initially did not believe her story. She had not at that point examined her own feelings or dealt with the popular societal myths regarding rape. It was only later when she had talked to more experienced healthcare personnel that she learned that crisis reactions could seem bizarre, confusing, and contradictory.

Assessment

Subjective Data

- "It was horrible. I feel so dirty."
- "I shouldn't have let him rape me."
- "He said that he was going to kill me."
- Guilt
- Self-blame

Objective Data

- Crying and sobbing
- Stares at the floor
- Bruising and bite marks on breasts
- Lip cut and bleeding
- Rape reported to the police

Priority Diagnosis

Rape-trauma syndrome related to sexual assault

Outcomes Identification

Patient will begin the healing of physical and psychological injuries caused by the sexual assault.

Planning

The nurse plans to provide emotional and physical support to Kayla while she receives care in the emergency setting and to make sure that Kayla is aware of the importance of follow-up care.

Implementation

Kayla's plan of care is personalized as follows:

Short-Term Goal	Intervention	Rationale	Evaluation
1. Patient will begin to express reactions and feelings about the assault before leaving the emergency department.	1a. Remain neutral and nonjudgmental and assure patient of confidentiality.	1a. Lessens feelings of shame and guilt and encourages sharing of painful feelings.	**GOAL MET** Patient was able to share feelings and express guilt. She realizes that she is not to blame. Anxiety was reduced to mild-moderate.
	1b. Do not leave patient alone.	1b. Deters feelings of isolation and escalation of anxiety.	
	1c. Allow the patient negative expressions and behavioral self-blame while using reflective techniques.	1c. Fosters feelings of control.	
	1d. Assure patient she did the right thing to save her life.	1d. Decreases burden of guilt and shame.	
	1e. When anxiety level decreases to moderate, encourage problem solving.	1e. Increases survivor's feeling of control in her own life. (When in severe anxiety, a person cannot problem solve.)	
	1f. Teach common reactions experienced by people in long-term reorganization phase (e.g., phobias, flashbacks, insomnia, increased motor activity).	1f. Helps survivor anticipate reactions and understand them as part of recovery process.	

Continued

CASE STUDY AND NURSING CARE PLAN—cont'd

Rape

Short-Term Goal	Intervention	Rationale	Evaluation
2. Patient will receive appropriate interventions to protect her physical status and support future legal proceedings.	2a. Explain rape protocol procedures and why they are being done.	2a. To decrease anticipatory anxiety and reduce revictimization.	**GOAL MET** Patient underwent a thorough physical examination, received prophylactic treatment to prevent sexually transmitted diseases and pregnancy, and will have the evidence she needs for legal proceedings.
	2b. Provide as much privacy as possible during the examination. Have as few people as necessary to provide care.	2b. Posttrauma patients are extremely vulnerable. Additional people in the environment will increase anxiety.	
	2c. Document physical injuries, collect evidence, and record verbatim statements by the patient.	2c. Careful documentation and data collection will support the patient in pursuing legal action.	
	2d. Provide prophylactic treatment for sexually transmitted diseases, assess for pregnancy, and offer pregnancy prevention.	2d. Sexually transmitted diseases and pregnancy are unnecessary possibilities after a rape.	

Evaluation

Kayla is able to express her feelings in the emergency department and talk about the possible reactions she might experience as she moves through the reorganization phase. Her anxiety level is reduced to mild-moderate.

Promotion of Self-Care Activities

When preparing the patient for discharge, the nurse provides all referral information and printed follow-up instructions. Printed instructions include potential physical concerns and emotional reactions, legal matters, victim compensation (state financial assistance paid through perpetrators' fines and fees), and online resources (e.g., support groups) can help. This is important because the amount of verbal information the patient can retain likely will be limited due to high levels of anxiety. Written material can be referred to repeatedly over time. Healthcare referrals are provided for continuity of care, and victim assistance program information can also be given.

Case Management

The emotional state and other psychological needs of the patient should be reassessed by telephone or personal contact within 24 to 48 hours of discharge from the hospital. Make sure you discuss this with the patient before discharge. Also, the most up-to-date contact information should be on file in the medical record. Referrals should be made for resources or support services. Effective crisis intervention and continuity of care require outreach activities and services beyond the emergency medical setting.

Survivors may avoid seeking treatment from psychiatric-mental healthcare providers due to stigma. Therefore the outpatient nurse should make a more focused assessment of stress-related symptoms and/or depression and ascertain the need for mental health referral. Reporting symptoms and seeking medical treatment are adaptive coping behaviors and can be reinforced.

Follow-up visits should occur at least 2, 4, and 6 weeks after the initial evaluation. At each visit, the patient should be assessed for psychological progress, the presence of sexually transmitted diseases, and pregnancy. Follow-up examinations provide an opportunity to (1) detect new infections acquired during or after the assault; (2) complete hepatitis B vaccination, if indicated; (3) complete counseling and treatment for other STDs; and (4) monitor side effects and adherence to postexposure prophylactic medication, if prescribed.

Advanced Practice Interventions

Psychotherapy

The psychiatric-mental health advanced practice registered nurse may offer individual or group psychotherapy for either the rape survivor or the perpetrator.

Survivors. Most of those who have been raped are eventually able to resume their previous lifestyle and level of functioning after supportive services and crisis counseling. However, many continue to experience emotional trauma including flashbacks, nightmares, fear, phobias, and other symptoms associated with PTSD (refer to Chapter 16). Depression and suicidal ideation often follow a sexual assault. Some people who survive rape may be susceptible to a psychotic episode or an emotional disturbance so severe that hospitalization is required. Others whose emotional lives may be overburdened with multiple internal and external pressures may require individual psychotherapy.

Rape victims benefit from group therapy or support groups. Group therapy can make the difference between a person's coming out of the crisis at a lower level of functioning or gradually adapting to the experience with an increase in coping skills. Support groups are available locally or online. There are support groups specific to rape, acquaintance rape, and incest.

Perpetrators. Psychotherapy is essential for perpetrators of sexual assault if behavioral change is to occur. Unfortunately, most perpetrators do not acknowledge the need for behavioral change, and no single method or program of treatment has been found to be totally effective. The nurse's awareness of personal feelings and reactions will be crucial to avoid interference with the therapeutic process.

EVALUATION

We consider **sexual assault** survivors to be in recovery if they are relatively free of any signs or symptoms of acute stress disorder and PTSD. Signs of recovery include the following:

- Sleeping well with few instances of episodic nightmares or broken sleep
- Eating as they did before the rape
- Being calm and relaxed or only mildly suspicious, fearful, or restless
- Getting support from family and friends
- Generally positive self-regard about themselves
- The absence or only mild instances of somatic reactions
- Returning to pre-rape sexual functioning and interest

In general, the closer the survivor's lifestyle is to the pattern that was present before the rape, the more complete the recovery has been.

CONCLUSION

Nurses need to review hospital-based policy and procedures manuals to determine if protocols have been established in how to care for a sexual assault patient. If your facility does not have a policy, consider establishing one for your area. The International Association of Forensic Nurses (IAFN, 2015) provides SANE Education Guidelines for the evaluation of adult/adolescent and pediatric patients. Certification is provided by the IAFN for nurse providers (i.e., SANE-A, SANE-P).

KEY POINTS TO REMEMBER

- Sexual assault is a common and often underreported crime of violence.
- Females are far more likely to be victims of sexual assault and tend to know their perpetrators. Sexual assault of males tends to be underreported due to the humiliation and stigma attached to such victimization.
- Psychoactive substances play a major role in sexual assault, and alcohol is the most commonly used date-rape drug. Other disinhibiting and amnestic substances play a role in forcible sex acts.
- A rape survivor experiences a wide range of feelings, which may or may not be exhibited to others.
- Sexual assault is often followed by feelings of fear, degradation, anger, and rage. Helplessness, anxiety, sleep disturbances, disturbed relationships, flashbacks, depression, and somatic complaints are also common.
- The initial medical evaluation may be frightening and stressful. A police interview, repeated questioning by health professionals, and the physical examination itself all have the potential to add to the trauma and revictimization of the sexual assault.
- Nurses can minimize repetition of questions and support the patient as she goes through the medical and legal evaluation.
- Survivors require long-term healthcare that can include counseling to minimize long-term effects of the rape and assisting in an early return to a normal living pattern.
- Telephone and online resources are available to assist sexual assault and rape survivors.

CRITICAL THINKING

1. Jonah, 18 years of age, is brutally beaten and sexually assaulted by an unidentified male as he makes his way home from a party in an unfamiliar part of town. He is found semiconscious by a passerby and taken to the emergency department. Isaac has bite marks on his neck; extensive bruises around his head, chest, and buttocks; and has sustained a cracked rib and anal tears. Ms. Santinez, a nurse and rape counselor in the emergency department, works with Jonah using the hospital's sexual assault protocol and evidence collection kit. Jonah appears stunned and confused and has difficulty focusing on what the nurse says. He states repeatedly, "This is crazy, this can't be happening…I can't believe this has happened to me…Oh, my God, I can't believe this."
   a. What areas of Jonah's assessment should be given highest priority by Ms. Santinez and her staff while he is in the emergency department?
   b. Chart the signs and symptoms of Jonah's physical and emotional trauma and verbatim statements in as much detail as you can.
   c. Identify the short-term outcome criteria for Jonah that ideally would be met before he leaves the emergency department.
   d. What information does Jonah need to have regarding potential signs and symptoms that may occur in the near future? Why is this important for him to understand at present?
   e. Identify specific indicators that will be met if Jonah recovers with minimal trauma from the event. How would you evaluate these criteria?
   f. If Jonah wishes not to report the sexual assault to police, would you still complete the examination?

CHAPTER REVIEW

Questions

1. Which statement made by a sexually assaulted patient strongly suggests the drug gamma-hydroxybutyrate acid (GHB) was involved in the attack?
   - **a.** "I remember everything that happened, but felt too tired to fight back."
   - **b.** "The drink I was given had a salty taste to it."
   - **c.** "They tell me I was unconscious for 24 hours."
   - **d.** "I heard that I was fighting the nursing staff and saying that they were trying to kill me."
2. Considering the guilt that women feel after being sexually assaulted, which nursing assessment question has priority?
   - **a.** "Do you want the police to be called?"
   - **b.** "Did you recognize the person who assaulted you?"
   - **c.** "Do you have someone you trust that can stay with you?"
   - **d.** "Do you have any thoughts about harming yourself?"
3. Which statement is an accurate depiction of sexual assault?
   - **a.** Rape is a sexual act.
   - **b.** Most rapes occur in the home.
   - **c.** Rape is usually an impulsive act.
   - **d.** Women are usually raped by strangers.
4. Which signs and symptoms are associated with acute stress disorder and often observed in patients who have been sexually assaulted? *Select all that apply.*
   - **a.** Outbursts of anger
   - **b.** Depression
   - **c.** Auditory hallucinations
   - **d.** Flashbacks
   - **e.** Amnesia for the event
5. Which racial identification places a woman at the greatest risk of being sexually assaulted in her lifetime?
   - **a.** Multiracial
   - **b.** American Indian
   - **c.** Black non-Hispanic
   - **d.** Caucasian
6. The stress of being raped often results in suffering similar to people who have witnessed a murder or had a physiological reaction to trauma, resulting in:
   - **a.** Posttraumatic stress disorder
   - **b.** Anxiety
   - **c.** Depression
   - **d.** All of the above
7. A young woman named Carly was raped behind the restaurant where she works after closing shift. Six months have passed and Carly has not been able to return to work, refuses to go out to eat, and feels that she has less value as a woman now that she has been raped. Carly's clinical presentation suggests:
   - **a.** Re-experiencing
   - **b.** Hyperarousal
   - **c.** Avoidance
   - **d.** Physical effects
8. Ron is a victim of assault and has revealed to his family and friends the fact that he was raped. The family reacts with horror and disgust, and the nurse caring for Ron recognizes:
   - **a.** Ron's family is being judgmental.
   - **b.** Ron's family should leave the hospital.
   - **c.** Ron's family will also need support.
   - **d.** Dysfunctional family dynamics.
9. Perpetrators of sexual assault are often incarcerated but frequently do not undergo therapy. Samuel, convicted of rape and sentenced to 15 years in prison, has requested to see a therapist. The psychiatric nurse practitioner is surprised to learn of the request as many perpetrators:
   - **a.** Boast of their assault history
   - **b.** Feel regret and remorse
   - **c.** Do not acknowledge the need for change
   - **d.** Are unable to recognize rape as a crime
10. You are working at a telephone hotline center when Abby, a rape victim, calls. Abby states she is afraid to go to the hospital. What is your best response?
    - **a.** "I'm here to listen, and we can talk about your feelings."
    - **b.** "You don't need to go to the hospital if you don't want to."
    - **c.** "If you don't go to the hospital, we can't collect evidence to help convict your rapist."
    - **d.** "Why are you afraid to seek medical attention?"

Answers

1. **b**; 2. **d**; 3. **b**; 4. **a, b, d, e**; 5. **a**; 6. **d**; 7. **c**; 8. **c**; 9. **c**; 10. **a**

Visit the Evolve website for a posttest on the content in this chapter: http://evolve.elsevier.com/Varcarolis

Post-Test interactive review

REFERENCES

AEquitas. (2012). *Summary of laws and guidelines: Payment of sexual assault forensic examinations.* Retrieved from http://www.aequitasresource.org/Summary_of_Laws_and_Guidelines-Payment_of_Sexual_Assault_Forensic_Examinations_2.6.12.pdf.

American Psychiatric Association. (2013). *Diagnostic and statistical manual of mental disorders* (3rd ed.). Arlington, VA: Author.

Breiding, M. J., Smith, S. G., Basile, K. C., et al. (2014). *Prevalence and characteristics of sexual violence, stalking, and intimate partner violence victimization. National Intimate Partner and Sexual Violence Survey, United States, 2011. Morbidity and Mortality Weekly Report.* Retrieved from https://www.cdc.gov/mmwr/preview/mmwrhtml/ss6308a1.htm.

Centers for Disease Control and Prevention. (2015). *Sexually transmitted diseases treatment guidelines.* Retrieved from http://www.cdc.gov/std/tg2015/sexual-assault.htm.

Drug-Induced Rape Prevention and Punishment. Drug-Induced Rape Prevention and Punishment Act, 21 U.S.C. 1996 § 841(b)(7).

Emergency Nurses Association. (2010). *Emergency Nurses Association position statements: Care of sexual assault victims.* Retrieved from http://www.ena.org/SiteCollectionDocuments/Position%20Statements/SexualAssault RapeVictims.pdf.

Federal Bureau of Investigation. (2012). *Crime in the United States.* Retrieved from https://www.fbi.gov/about-us/cjis/ucr/crime-in-the-u.s/2012/crime-in-the-u.s.-2012/violent-crime/violent-crime.

Federal Bureau of Investigation. (2014). *Reporting rape in 2013.* Retrieved from https://www.fbi.gov/about-us/cjis/ucr/recent-program-updates/reporting-rape-in-2013-revised.

Federal Bureau of Investigation. (2016). *Preliminary crime stats for the first half of 2015.* Retrieved from https://www.fbi.gov/about-us/cjis/ucr/crime-in-the-u.s/2015/preliminary-semiannual-uniform-crime-report-januaryjune-2015/home.

Herdman, T. H., & Kamitsuru, S. (Eds.). (2014). *NANDA International nursing diagnoses: Definitions and classification 2015–2017.* Oxford, UK: Wiley-Blackwell.

International Association of Forensic Nurses. (2015). *Sexual assault nurse examiner (SANE) education guidelines.* Retrieved from http://c.ymcdn.com/sites/www.forensicnurses.org/resource/resmgr/2015_SANE_ED_GUIDELINES.pdf.

Moorhead, S., Johnson, M., Maas, M. L., & Swanson, E. (2013). *Nursing outcomes classification (NOC)* (5th ed.). St. Louis, MO: Mosby.

Patel, A., Roston, A., Tilmon, S., et al. (2013). Assessing the extent of provision of comprehensive medical care management for female sexual assault patients in U.S. hospital emergency departments. *International Journal of Gynecology and Obstetrics, 123*(1), 24–28.

Rape, Abuse and Incest National Network. (2008). *Who are the victims?* Retrieved from http://www.rainn.org/get-information/statistics/sexual-assault-victims.

US Department of Justice; Office of the Attorney General. (1997). *September 23 memorandum for all United States attorneys.* Retrieved from http://www.usdoj.gov/ag/readingroom/drugcrime.htm.

US Department of Justice. (2013). *A national protocol for sexual assault medical forensic examinations: Adults/adolescents (No. NCJ 206554.).* Washington, DC: Office on Violence Against Women. Retrieved from https://www.ncjrs.gov/pdffiles1/ovw/241903.pdf.

30

Dying, Death, and Grieving

Sandra Snelson Yaklin, Natalie Boysen

Visit the Evolve website for a pretest on the content in this chapter: http://evolve.elsevier.com/Varcarolis Pre-Test interactive review

OBJECTIVES

1. Describe the evolution of life-saving measures and their impact on end-of-life issues.
2. Discuss the role of palliative care and hospice in supporting patients and families facing chronic diseases and terminal illnesses.
3. Identify stages of the dying process as described by Kübler-Ross.
4. Explain the controversy around facilitating death.
5. Describe the components of advance care planning for death.
6. Distinguish nursing care at the end of life including communication, presence, and symptom management.
7. Discuss the process of death and associated care for the patient and the family.
8. Explain the distinction between the terms grief, bereavement, and mourning.
9. Differentiate anticipatory grief, complicated grieving, disenfranchised grief, and dysfunctional grieving.
10. Describe nursing care for individuals who are grieving and are experiencing complicated grieving.

OUTLINE

KEY TERMS AND CONCEPTS

advance directive
anticipatory grief
artificial nutrition and hydration
bereavement
complicated grieving
disenfranchised grief
euthanasia
grieving
hospice
mourning
palliative care
persistent complex bereavement disorder
physician-assisted suicide

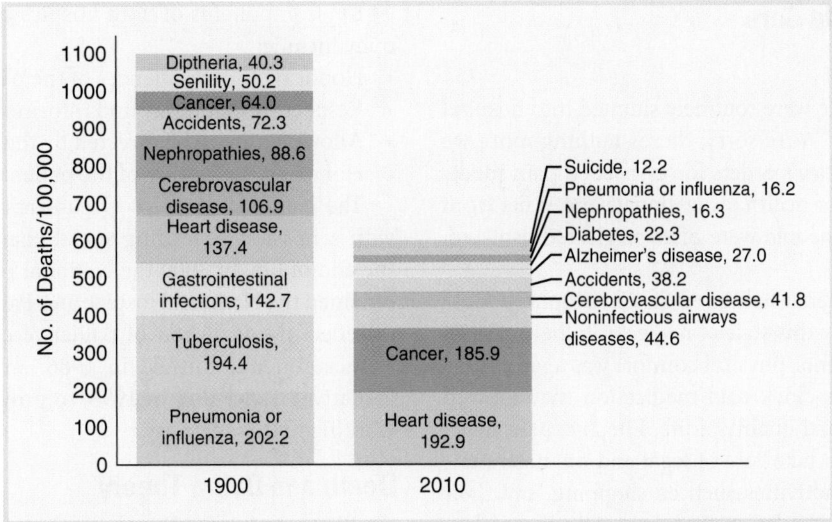

FIG. 30.1 Primary causes of death in America. From Jones, D.S., Podolsky, S.H., & Greene, J.A. (2012). The burden of disease and the changing task of medicine. *New England Journal of Medicine, 366,* 2,333–2,338.

There will be no one like us when we are gone, but there is no one like anyone else, ever. When people die, they cannot be replaced. They leave holes that cannot be filled, for it is the fate—the genetic and neural fate—of every human being to be a unique individual, to find his own path, to live his own life, to die his own death.

Oliver Sacks (2015)

Caring for patients with terminal illnesses or who are near death due to other conditions challenges and rewards nurses in deep and personal ways. In caring for individuals who are dying and grieving nurses may grow personally by both accepting their patients' deaths and by developing a richer understanding of their own mortality. Nurses also have the opportunity to bring dignity to dying and death and to help shape an enduring, positive memory for family members and caregivers. Nurses also work with individuals who have been impacted by the loss of another person or people and are grieving this loss.

In this chapter we will explore some of the most intimate of subjects that any of us will face. We will begin by discussing the process of dying and death and then turn our attention to the grieving process.

DEATH AND DYING

One hundred and fifty years ago, the primary cause of death was infectious diseases. Most of those diseases have been eradicated. Chronic health problems are now the primary causes of death in the United States (Fig. 30.1). We have become accustomed to having tools such as surgery, medications, and diagnostic technologies to combat life-threatening conditions. Advances in technology have blurred the line between life and death. We can artificially feed those who cannot eat. We can breathe for those who cannot breathe. We can filter blood when kidneys fail. We can restart hearts, kill cancers, and transplant organs. In spite of all our skills and technology, we all still die.

In some ways, dying has become more complex precisely because there is so much we can do to sustain and prolong life. In fact, the medical model is based on the prolongation of life. When should we stop having one more surgery, trying one more round of chemotherapy, seeing one more doctor? These are profound questions for individuals facing the prospect of death. Their families wrestle deeply with the uncertain quest to do what is right when they have no idea what is right.

An Aging Population

The United States experienced an unprecedented birth rate in the 18 years after the end of World War II (1946–1964). This generation of children is known as the baby boomer generation. The 79 million baby boomers account for a staggering 26% of the total US population. In 2014 the US Census Bureau released a report projecting that the number of Americans over the age of 65 is expected to almost double from 43.1 million in 2012 to 83.7 million by 2050 (Hogan & Hogan, 2014). Every day for the next 19 years, 10,000 baby boomers will turn 65.

This burgeoning sector of the population will place unprecedented strains on a healthcare system where health spending is growing faster than the overall economy (Martin et al., 2011). At this rate of growth, by the year 2040 one of every three dollars will be spent on healthcare. By the year 2080, spending on healthcare will rise to one of every two dollars.

Medicare is the federal government's national program that provides health insurance for older adults. Medicare is a fee-for-service system, which means that more medical services result in more reimbursement for healthcare providers. One astounding Medicare statistic is that only 5% of people who die each year account for approximately 25% of all Medicare dollars spent (Riley & Lubitz, 2010). Aggressive medical care at the end of life is undoubtedly driving up the cost of end-of-life care. Another huge Medicare expenditure is in providing care for elderly patients living with multiple chronic conditions and functional limitations (Aldridge & Kelley, 2015).

*Special thanks to Natalie Boysen for her contributions to this chapter.

Models for End-of-Life Care

Hospice

In the 1960s, dying people were routinely shunted into hospital rooms with phrases like "We're sorry, there's nothing more we can do for you," with doctor's orders for as-needed pain medication. Despite the care of health professionals and visits from helpless relatives, dying people were often neglected, isolated, and left to die in pain.

In 1967, Cicely Saunders established St. Christopher's Hospice in London to remedy this state of neglect (Stolberg, 1999). At St. Christopher's, patients' physical comfort was aggressively pursued with around-the-clock pain medication that allowed them to experience optimal quality of life. Effective pain management enabled them to take care of legal and financial matters, engage in normal activities such as shopping, say their goodbyes, restore damaged relationships, and align themselves spiritually.

Hospice is a model of care that supports and cares for patients facing death. It is available to everyone, regardless of age, diagnosis, or the ability to pay. A physician must certify hospice patients with a life expectancy of 6 months or less. In addition, the patient must choose hospice care rather than curative treatments.

Hospice is a multidisciplinary team approach that focuses on patient care not cures. This approach meshes well with values in nursing. Physicians, nurses, chaplains, and social workers collaborate to navigate the questions, concerns, and decisions faced by those who are dying. The hospice care extends beyond caring for the patient to include caring for the family. Hospice care is often delivered in the patient's home. In addition, there are some freestanding inpatient facilities. Hospice services can also be delivered in nursing homes and even in hospitals. Hospice care both saves money and improves quality of life (Kelley et al., 2013).

Nonprofit and for-profit hospice organizations have proliferated, and there are currently over 6,000 hospice organizations in the United States. These hospices served approximately 1.6 to 1.7 million people in 2014. The majority of hospice-enrolled patients (58.9%) died at home (National Hospice and Palliative Care Organization, 2015). Unfortunately, 75% of non-hospice patients die in an institutional settings such as a hospital or a nursing home (Wilson et al., 2013).

Palliative Care

Patients may not be eligible for hospice care because it is not always possible to determine when a patient's life expectancy is less than 6 months. More commonly, older individuals have a constellation of chronic diseases that result in a gradual decline over several years. Caring for those with incurable chronic diseases such as diabetes, heart disease, and dementia requires long-term palliative support. **Palliative care** is patient- and family-centered care that optimizes quality of life anticipating, preventing, and treating suffering. Palliative care addresses physical, intellectual, emotional, social, and spiritual needs. Palliative caregivers promote patient autonomy, access to information, and choice.

Key components of both hospice and palliative care philosophy include:

- Honoring the experiences of the patient and family
- Respecting autonomy and informed choice
- Allowing care to be directed by the patient (and family)
- Honoring the dignity of the patient and family.

The National Hospice Organization was founded in 1978 with a mission of leading social change for improved care at the end of life. In 2000 the National Hospice Organization was renamed the National Hospice and Palliative Care Organization to reflect the inclusion of palliative care. The Hospice Nurses Association was formed in 1986, and renamed Hospice and Palliative Association in 1998, to provide a network for nurses working in this specialty.

Death and Dying Theory

Dr. Elisabeth Kübler-Ross began actively listening to the terminally ill, and out of her groundbreaking work came a construct of the human response to death and loss that has entered the mainstream. Kübler-Ross (1969) identified distinctive phases, or cycles, in people's responses to terminal illness:

- **Denial and Isolation:** Denial is typically a brief reaction, in which the patient is in disbelief or shock about their situation. This phase functions as a buffer after receiving shocking news and allows the patient to regroup. This phase can also result in "doctor shopping," in which the patient will seek advice from other specialists in hopes that their diagnosis will indeed be a mistake. Examples of expressions in this phase include, "There has been a mix-up with my test results" or "No, it can't be true. That's impossible."
- **Anger:** This phase typically surfaces when the patient is ready to acknowledge their illness, when they come to terms with the fact that they are in fact seriously ill. The patient becomes pessimistic and very unhappy. An example of a question in this phase is, "Why me? Why not someone else?" This phase is particularly difficult for the family and medical personnel to deal with because the anger is often projected unpredictably on to whomever happens to be around. The most important things the angry patient needs are respect, understanding, attention, and time.
- **Bargaining:** As the patient attempts to deal with overwhelming feelings of vulnerability and helplessness, they may secretly try to make deals with a higher power to prolong their life. Examples of this include, "I'll stop smoking if I can just stay alive long enough to attend my daughter's wedding" or "If only I had gone to the doctor sooner."
- **Depression:** This phase arises when the patient can no longer avoid a sense of great loss. They can feel guilty because of the strain they feel they're putting on their family and a deep sadness for experiences they may miss out on. Kübler-Ross defines two phases of depression: preparatory and reactive. Preparatory refers to the patient preparing themselves for their final separation from this world, while reactive encompasses the unrealistic guilt or shame the patient feels about their illness. In this phase, it is imperative that the patient is allowed to express their justified sadness.

- **Acceptance:** Although this phase should not be confused with happiness, it does warrant a quiet peacefulness in the end of life. It is a final time for resting, free of pain and struggle. The patient may wish for solitude and may not be as talkative. Times of silence during visits may be the most meaningful mode of communication for these patients. This phase can be notably difficult for loved ones of the patient, as they may not have accepted the impending loss and view the patient's ambivalence with their death as "giving up."

Kübler-Ross also realized that personal growth did not necessarily cease in the last stages of life. On the contrary, it often accelerated.

FACILITATING DEATH

As previously discussed, there is so much we can do to sustain and prolong life. How far is going too far? Are we ever obligated to end the suffering of people who are tormented by tremendous pain or who are unable to end their own lives due to conditions such as Lou Gehrig's disease (amyotrophic lateral sclerosis)?

Conditions that result in hotly contested legal battles frequently reside in the brain. A persistent vegetative state is a chronic condition that preserves the brain's ability to maintain blood pressure, respiration, and cardiac function, but not cognitive function. Hypothalamic and medullary brainstem functions remain intact to support cardiorespiratory and autonomic functions and are sufficient for survival if care is adequate. The cortex is severely damaged (eliminating cognitive function), but the reticular activating system (RAS) remains functional (making wakefulness possible). Patients have no awareness of self and interact with the environment only through reflexes. Seizure activity may be present but not be clinically evident (Maiese, 2016).

One famous case that happened in 1976 was when Karen Anne Quinlan suffered a severe anoxic brain injury and fell into a persistent vegetative state. She was not able to breathe on her own. She was intubated and placed on a ventilator. Karen's family petitioned the State of New Jersey for the right to remove the ventilator. Karen had made her wishes known to her family that she would not want to be kept alive artificially. However, by the time the court allowed the family to remove Karen's ventilator she had stabilized and continued to breathe on her own for 10 more years.

Brain death is the loss of function of the entire cerebrum and brainstem, resulting in coma, no spontaneous respiration, and loss of all brainstem reflexes. Spinal reflexes, including deep tendon, plantar flexion, and withdrawal reflexes, may remain. Recovery does not occur (Maiese, 2016). Cases of brain death have resulted in court cases where, despite the family's wish to keep a loved one alive, the ruling is to remove life support since the person is considered dead.

Artificial Nutrition and Hydration

The provision of food and water are emotionally charged activities. Disagreements about the best course of action can result in deep fractures within families. On the one hand, is disinterest in eating and drinking a sign of impending death? On the other hand, would sustenance and hydration increase the quality of life and chance of living?

BOX 30.1 HPNA Position Statement on Artificial Nutrition and Hydration

Artificial nutrition and hydration interventions were originally developed to provide short-term support for patients who were acutely ill and are often used to provide a bridge to recovery, or to meet therapeutic goals of prolonging life. There are few well-designed studies that have examined the effectiveness of artificial nutrition and hydration in meeting these goals. One of the most important aims of hospice and palliative care is to minimize suffering and discomfort. When artificial nutrition and hydration is used in patients with advanced illness in the terminal phase, the evidence suggests that these measures are seldom effective in preventing suffering. Artificial nutrition and hydration is a medical intervention that should be evaluated for each individual, utilizing evidenced-based practices reflecting the benefits and burdens, the clinical circumstances, and the overall goals of care.

From Hospice and Palliative Nurses Association. (2011). *HPNA position statement: Artificial nutrition and hydration in advanced illness.* Retrieved from http://hpna.advancingexpertcare.org/wp-content/uploads/2015/08/Artificial-Nutrition-and-Hydration-in-Advanced-Illness.pdf.

Artificial nutrition and hydration through feeding tubes or intravenous fluids is legally considered a medical intervention and not a comfort measure. Supplementation of food and water is therefore not a component of basic care for the actively dying. It does not generally benefit people who are dying. In fact, providing artificial hydration by such means as intravenous fluids can increase edema, pulmonary congestion, ascites, nausea, and vomiting. Generally, the unwillingness or inability to eat and drink is caused by the impending death of the patient.

According the US Patient Self Determination Act (PSDA) (H.R. 4449, 1990), an individual patient or designated surrogate can decide whether or not to refuse life-sustaining or life-prolonging treatments. The PSDA also affirms the right to withhold artificial nutrition or hydration, as well as the right to withdraw these support measures.

Several high-profile legal battles in the United States have arisen in the past 35 years regarding food and hydration. Laws were created to help both families and medical institutions determine the circumstances under which nutrition and artificial hydration may be removed from patients.

The Hospice and Palliative Nurses Association suggests that the decision to use artificial nutrition and hydration be made on a case-by-case basis. Their position statement is in Box 30.1.

Euthanasia

Often called mercy killing, **euthanasia** is the act of putting someone to death. Euthanasia means that someone other than the patient commits an action with the intent to end the patient's life. Three types of euthanasia exist:

- Voluntary euthanasia is typically performed when a person is suffering from a terminal illness and is in great pain. When the patient performs this procedure with the help of a doctor, the term physician-assisted suicide is often used and is discussed below.

- When individuals are unable to consent, passive euthanasia may be used. Examples of passive euthanasia include discontinuing a medication that is keeping a patient alive or not performing a life-saving procedure on a person.
- An involuntary euthanasia is actively ending a person's life, typically by the injection of a lethal drug. This active form of euthanasia is used in cases of the death penalty.

Physician-Assisted Suicide

In **physician-assisted suicide**, the means, such as medication or a weapon, to end a patent's life is provided to the patient. Unlike euthanasia, in assisted suicide, someone else makes the means of death available, but does not act as the direct agent of death.

The federal government allows each state to legislate its own laws about the legality of physician-assisted suicide. In Montana, physicians will not be prosecuted for assisting patients in death, but there is no law permitting the practice. New Mexico asserts that mentally competent terminally ill patients have a constitutional right to seek a physician's assistance in ending their own lives, however this law is being contested. The following states allow physician-assisted suicide:

- Oregon—1997
- Washington—2009
- Montana—2010
- Vermont—2013
- California—2015
- Colorado—2016

Dr. Jack Kevorkian was a Michigan pathologist who claimed to have assisted at least 130 terminally ill patients to die. Juries acquitted Dr. Kevorkian three times on charges of assisted suicide. Dr. Kevorkian was convicted of second-degree murder after filming and broadcasting his administration of a lethal dose of medication to a terminally ill patient. He served 8 years in prison.

The American Medical Association, disability-rights advocates, and most major religious groups oppose physician-assisted suicide. The American Nurses Association (ANA) and the National Hospice and Palliative Care Organization have also published position statements in opposition to physician-assisted suicide (Box 30.2).

BOX 30.2 Nurses Position Statements on Physician-Assisted Suicide

The American Nurses Association prohibits nurses' participation in assisted suicide and euthanasia because these acts are in direct violation of *Code of Ethics for Nurses with Interpretive Statements*, the ethical traditions and goals of the profession, and its covenant with society. Nurses have an obligation to provide humane, comprehensive, and compassionate care that respects the rights of patients but upholds the standards of the profession in the presence of chronic debilitating illness and at the end of life.

The National Hospice and Palliative Care Organization does not support the legalization of physician-assisted suicide. The National Hospice and Palliative Care Organization looks forward to participating in and guiding the ongoing dialogue and debate to continuously improve upon and promote comfort and dignity in life closure, and affords the highest regard for patient choice and self-determination.

From American Nurses Association. (2013). *Ethics position statements/euthanasia assisted suicide and aid in dying.* Retrieved from http://www.nursingworld.org/MainMenuCategories/EthicsStandards/Ethics-Position-Statements/Euthanasia-Assisted-Suicide-and-Aid-in-Dying.pdf; National Hospice and Palliative Care Organization. (2005). Commentary and resolution on physician assisted suicide. Retrieved from http://www.nhpco.org/sites/default/files/public/PAS_Resolution_Commentary.pdf.

Arguments Surrounding Physician-Assisted Suicide

Advocates of physician-assisted suicide believe that misuse of this practice can be prevented through state regulations that ensure informed, competent, and freely made decisions. Opponents believe that opening the door to assisted suicide will result in a slippery slope where people other than competent terminally ill patients are assisted to die. For example, during the discussion of the Affordable Care Act, a rumor circulated that death panels would be set up to determine when older adults would be allowed or assisted to die.

Why aren't all states taking similar positions? There are legal and ethical arguments both for and against euthanasia and assisted suicide (Prince-Paul & Daily, 2015).

Individual liberty. One argument concerns individual liberty compared with the state's responsibility to protect its citizens. Under the law, individuals have the right to refuse or withdraw treatment. However, this is counterbalanced by the notion that the government has a constitutional power to override certain rights to protect citizens from irrevocable acts.

Autonomy. A primary value of citizens of the United States is individualism. The ethical concept of autonomy supports self-determination. Every competent person has the right to make momentous decisions based on personal convictions. An opposing argument notes that human beings are the stewards but not the absolute masters of the gift of life.

Quality of care. Removal of legal bans on assisted suicide would likely enhance the opportunity for excellent end-of-life care for all patients. Legislation could be enacted to require that patients receive the best in palliative care. Opponents of this position cite that the aim of medicine should be to facilitate a death that is pain-free, but one that is also a human experience. A good natural death contributes to a strong society.

Nonmaleficence. Another ethical concept relevant to euthanasia is that of nonmaleficence or doing no harm. Is helping to end life harmful? From the patient's perspective, there may be no difference between ending life by providing a lethal injection and by stopping treatment that prolongs life. On the other hand, as nurses, we have been taught that the role of the nurse is to promote, preserve, and protect human life. Assisted death violates the oath to do no harm and may be considered the ultimate betrayer of trust between the patient and the nurse.

Beneficence. Beneficence is the other side of the coin of nonmaleficence and means to do good. Patients could benefit from relief that is now legally available to people who have physicians who are willing to risk assisting them to die. On the other hand, a misdiagnosis of the illness, inadequate assessment of competence, or pressure from the family or the physician might place the patient in jeopardy. Doing good means to preserve and support life.

ADVANCE CARE PLANNING

Advance care planning helps patients and their families achieve end-of-life goals, avoid hospitalization, and increase hospice and palliative care use (Brinkman-Stoppelenburg et al., 2014). Because three in ten US adults are family caregivers, conversations about end-of-life care should include the patients, life-partners, and other family members. A staggering 70.3% of patients who faced treatment decisions in the final days of their lives were incapable of participating in their own decisions (Silveira et al., 2010).

Caregivers who face the prospect of making end-of-life decisions for a loved one without the benefit of these conversations are more likely to suffer from depression, anxiety, and stress in the months after the death. Encouraging patients to talk about end-of-life issues and complete paperwork to support their wishes is an important intervention for basic level registered nurses. Nurse practitioners and physicians are now able to bill Medicare for advance care planning services including time spent in end-of-life conversations (Centers for Medicare and Medicaid Services, 2016).

The advance directive and durable power of attorney for healthcare discussed below are legal documents. Websites with fairly simple instructions and minimal costs can make the process of completing these documents doable for most people.

Advance Directive

One in five Americans over the age of 75 (22%) say they have neither written down nor talked with anyone about their wishes for medical treatment at the end of their lives (Pew Research Center, 2013). Fifty-seven percent of Americans, however, reported that they would wish to refuse treatment if they were in intractable pain or had an incurable disease.

A written document stating how you want medical decisions to be made if you lose the ability to make them for yourself is called an **advance directive**. It may also be called a living will. This document spells out what sort of life-prolonging measures should be taken if there's no hope for recovery.

Durable Power of Attorney for Healthcare

A durable power of attorney for healthcare covers all healthcare decisions, and lasts only as long as the individual is incapable of making decisions. A trusted person, called an agent, is named in this legal document to carry out the wishes of the incapacitated individual.

NURSING CARE AT THE END OF LIFE

For patients and family members to make informed choices and goals, conversations between healthcare providers, patients, and families need to occur. The focus should be on supporting patients' informed choices and goals of care. According to the American Nurses Association's Code of Ethics (2016), nurses have a moral duty to help patients determine these preferences and goals at the end of life.

Communication

Despite being trained to discuss difficult and sensitive issues with patients and families, nurses are often afraid to talk about death. Talking about death is difficult because of the emotions involved including our own fear, uncertainty, lack of control, lack of information, and conflict. To minimize the role of these emotions, it is important for the nurse to establish a therapeutic relationship before asking patients or families to make difficult decisions at the end of life.

Art of Presence

Caring for patients who are terminally ill requires some shifts in professional expectations. Whole-person care involves seeing the patient first and foremost as a human being and being attentive to all aspects of suffering. As front-line caregivers, nurses usually help patients get better, stronger, and more independent. Patients who are terminally ill are going to grow weaker, sicker, and ultimately die. There are often ways nurses can take action to make a patient feel better such as pain medication, bathing, and turning. Sometimes, however, the best action is simply being present with the dying and their families.

To use the art of presence, two essential skills are listening and observing. Reflect back to the speaker by restating or summarizing the message. Ask the patient and family open-ended questions such as:

- Would you tell me what this is like for you?
- How do you see your condition right now?
- Where do you see things going?
- Are you worried about anything?
- What are you hoping for?

Sometimes saying little or nothing is also a good approach. You can practice staying silent and giving the patient or family member time to respond. The presence of a caring nurse can invite and permit the patient to discover new dimensions of his or her own experiences, bringing greater wholeness.

Symptom Management

Excellent symptom management is a hallmark of palliative nursing. The patient and/or the patient's advance directives and medical proxy determine the goals of care. Palliative care offers a wide spectrum of interventions to alleviate symptoms guided by patients' own reports and careful assessment. Some of the most commonly reported end-of-life symptoms are constipation, dyspnea, fatigue, depression, and delirium. Each symptom must be assessed individually.

It is easy to confuse treatable, reversible, and temporary conditions by attributing them to the terminal diagnosis. For example, if a patient reports feeling depressed, it is important not assume that symptoms are due to the dying process. Depression, pain, or other treatable problems must be addressed and treated. If a patient becomes confused or lethargic, it is essential to rule out such things as medication effects, dehydration, delirium, urinary tract infections, or constipation.

Pain involves the whole person with physical, spiritual, and emotional components. Pain is also considered the fifth vital sign alongside heart rate, respiratory rate, blood pressure,

BOX 30.3 HPNA Position on Pain Management

Most ethical concerns about causing harm (i.e., hastening death) through administration of opioids can be resolved through thoughtful application of established facts regarding the physiology of pain, the mechanism of drug action, and by careful ongoing assessment and reassessment of the patient's condition. Administering the specific drug or combination of drugs—no more and no less—required to relieve symptoms, using well-validated treatment guidelines, is a fundamental responsibility of the nurse caring for any patient experiencing distressing symptoms.

From Hospice and Palliative Nurses Association. (2013). HPNA *position statement: Ethics of opioid use at the end-of-life.* Retrieved from http://hpna.advancingexpertcare.org/wp-content/uploads/2015/08/The-Ethics-of-Opioid-Use-at-End-of-Life.pdf.

and temperature (Morone & Weiner, 2013). Unlike the other vital signs, clinicians have no way of verifying or validating a patient's subjective pain. Therefore pain is accepted to be what the patient says it is. Assessing pain includes site, character, onset, duration/frequency, intensity, exacerbating/palliating factors, physical examination, and rating of pain using a pain scale.

VIGNETTE: You are caring for a 42-year-old man dying of lung cancer. He patient is agitated, grimacing, and clutching the bed sheets. When you ask him if he needs pain medication, he averts his gaze and looks out the window. His wife says, "I think he's worried that the medication will make him so sleepy that he will miss the visit of my daughter and me." You respond, "Perhaps we can use the lower dose of morphine that's been ordered for now, and give him more after your visit." The wife gratefully replies, "Yes, let's try that."

Clinical difficulties arise as patients begin the process of dying. Patients and families look to the nurse to help answer these questions. Families are often concerned that pain medication might shorten their loved one's life. The Hospice and Palliative Nurses Association (HPNA, 2013) provides a position statement on this topic in Box 30.3.

Anticipatory Grief

Once a life-threatening diagnosis has been received or curative efforts are stopped, people begin a period of grieving called **anticipatory grief** or anticipatory mourning. This type of grief is anticipatory in the sense that a future loss is being mourned in advance. It happens as people acknowledge the importance of the dying person, adjust their lives to accommodate the intervening time, and foresee how their futures will be altered by the loss.

The experience of anticipatory grief varies by individual, family, and culture. Aspects of finalizing the connection include spending time together, talking, making memories, life review, saying goodbye (often indirectly or metaphorically), touch, communication, taking care of business, and detaching from one another. A common emotional experience is anger—at the disease, the medical community, others, life—in addition to sadness, hurt, fear, anxiety, and hidden grief.

Sustenance

Encourage families to offer water orally as often as their actively dying loved one desires and is able to swallow. Take great care, however, to listen to patients and their family members and to include the interdisciplinary team in this decision. One important distinction to keep in mind is that the patient is not dying of dehydration or lack of food, but rather from their illness.

Palliative Care for Patients with Dementia

According to the World Health Organization (2015), dementia is a leading cause of disability. Therefore all caregivers should receive education on the unique elements of palliative dementia care to increase comfort and enhance quality of life. Individuals with advanced dementia experience significant impairments in insight, language, and judgment, which limit their ability to communicate unmet needs and desires. Imagine not being able to convey that you were uncomfortable, had to urinate, or wanted to be someplace quiet rather than a crowded day hall. Difficult behaviors, such as irritability or refusal to cooperate with care, are often forms of communication indicating discomfort in body, mind, or spirit. When caregivers use an *anticipatory* approach to care, they can frequently prevent or reduce behaviors that result when a person with dementia is unable to communicate important unmet needs.

It helps if caregivers can focus on the person rather than the disease. We can recognize the numerous opportunities to affirm the meaning of the individual's life, uphold dignity, and provide pleasurable sensory and spiritual experiences. The goal is to create meaningful connections for these patients.

It is also important to address healthcare decisions for advanced dementia such as resuscitation, hospitalizations, antibiotics, and nutrition/hydration. Healthcare providers should: (1) identify the patient's goals for care and consider educating the family to minimize aggressive medical interventions, (2) eliminate medications that may detract from safety or quality of life, and (3) proactively manage issues such as pain and depression.

Families and friends spend a significant amount of time, finances, and emotions caring for a loved one with dementia. It is important to recognize and support the role of family caregivers as they navigate the day-to-day challenges and cope with losses. The Marwit-Meuser Caregiver Grief Inventory (Marwit & Meuser, 2002) is a tool developed to identify the unique forms of grief experienced by caregivers of those with dementia. High scores may indicate a need for intervention and formal support. Low scores indicate either denial of distress or positive adaptation. This tool is easily searchable and available online.

Developmental Tasks in Dying

Ira Byock (1996), an American palliative care physician, believes that the final stage of life has its own developmental tasks. Human beings are social beings with individual and shared dreams, pasts, and future hopes. The process of dying remains filled with opportunities for growth, reconciliation, and meaning. Task work at the end of life is not just a *to do* list, it is the person's choice to do—or not to do. See Table 30.1 for a list of some of the tasks a patient may move through at the end of life.

TABLE 30.1 Developmental Landmarks and Tasks for the End of Life

Sense of completion with worldly affairs	Transfer of fiscal, legal, and formal social responsibilities
Sense of completion in relationships with community	Closure of multiple social relationships (employment, commerce, organizational, congregational). Components include: expressions of regret, expressions of forgiveness, acceptance of gratitude and appreciation Leave taking; the saying of goodbye
Sense of meaning about one's individual life	Life review The telling of "one's stories" Transmission of knowledge and wisdom
Experienced love of self	Self-acknowledgement Self-forgiveness
Experienced love of others	Acceptance of worthiness
Sense of completion in relationships with family and friends	Reconciliation, fullness of communication and closure in each of one's important relationships. Component tasks include: expressions of regret, expressions of forgiveness and acceptance, expressions of gratitude and appreciation, acceptance of gratitude and appreciation, expressions of affection Leave taking; the saying of goodbye
Acceptance of the finality of life and of one's existence as an individual	Acknowledgement of the totality of personal loss represented by one's dying and experience of personal pain of existential loss Expression of the depth of personal tragedy that dying represents Decathexis (emotional withdrawal) from worldly affairs and cathexis (emotional connection) with an enduring construct or acceptance of dependency
Sense of a new self (personhood) beyond personal loss	
Sense of meaning about life in general	Achieving a sense of awe Recognition of a transcendent realm Developing/achieving a sense of comfort with chaos
Surrender to the transcendent, to the unknown; "letting go"	

From Byock, I. R. (1996). The nature of suffering and the nature of opportunity at the end-of-life. *Clinics in Geriatric Medicine, 12*(2), 237.

THE DYING PROCESS

The process of dying varies based upon the underlying cause. Some general signs of approaching death include:

- Growing weakness (asthenia)
- Loss of appetite
- Increasing drowsiness
- Change in mentation (shortening attention span, difficulty processing information)
- Circulatory changes (increased heart rate, decreased blood pressure)
- Mottling of skin (grayish-blue splotches on knees, ankles, feet)
- Decrease in urine production
- Breathing changes (Cheynes-Stokes respirations)

Agitation and delirium are not uncommon at the end of life. One of the more disturbing changes that sometimes accompany the dying process is the presence of a death rattle, which is caused by pooling of saliva in the upper airway.

Provide families with information about what to do when their loved one dies. If the patient dies at home, instruct the family to telephone their hospice provider. After the phone call is received by hospice, a registered nurse will be sent to the home. Upon arrival, the nurse should enter the home respectfully and provide introductions to each family member present and state, "I am the registered nurse on call. I am so sorry for your loss."

Invite family members to remain at the bedside if they desire. Confirm the identity of the patient. Use a stethoscope to listen for a heartbeat for 2 minutes while feeling for a pulse and watching for respirations. After 2 minutes without a heartbeat or breath, the nurse will pronounce the time of death, stating, "I am pronouncing the time of death at (time/date)." Sometimes family members are confused by the fact that the official time of death is the pronouncement time rather than the time that the patient stopped breathing. It might be important to clarify for family members that this is the time that is used for the death certificate.

Each facility or hospice program will have a policy regarding the kind of postmortem care that is provided. Families will remember the actions of the nurse, so take care to communicate deep respect for both the dead and for the bereaved. The nurse should also offer to contact a social worker or chaplain, if desired. Family members should be invited to participate in this care, if they desire. Care may vary according to culture but may include bathing, combing hair, or dressing in a special outfit.

The nurse may call the medical examiner to see if an autopsy is necessary. The laws regarding notification vary from state to state. Typically, autopsies are only required if the death is unexpected, unusual, or there is suspected abuse (e.g., broken bones or falls). Once the medical examiner releases the patient, the nurse will then contact the funeral home to come and pick the body up.

GRIEVING

Loss is part of the human experience, and grieving is the response that enables people to accept and reconcile with the loss and adapt to change. **Grieving** is a normal and complex process in response to loss. We grieve the commonplace losses in our lives—loss of a relationship (e.g., divorce, separation, death, abortion), health (e.g., a body function or part, mental or physical capacity), a friendship, status or prestige, security (e.g., occupational, financial, social, cultural), or a dream. Other normal losses include changes in circumstances such as retirement, promotion, marriage, and aging. These losses can promote growth through adaptation or may result in apathy, anger, and resentment.

Losing a significant person through death is a major life crisis. Long-term relationships bond us to each other deeply, shaping our world and our identity in it. The loss of a love one can diminish aspects of our own self-concept. Grief is experienced holistically, affecting us emotionally, cognitively, spiritually, and physically. Those who grieve sometimes describe the death of a loved one feeling like an amputation.

While grief is a reaction to a loss, **bereavement**, derived from the Old English word *berafian* meaning, "to rob," is the period of grieving after a death. **Mourning** refers to things people do to cope with grief including shared social expressions of grief such as viewing hours, funerals, and bereavement groups. Everyone grieves but not everyone engages in the work of mourning. The length of time, degree, and ritual for mourning are often typically determined by cultural, religious, and familial factors.

The goals of mourning have evolved from doing the grief work, getting over it, and moving on with life. Mourning is a complex, individual, culturally embedded process of accepting the death. It involves confronting the painful experience of grief, constructing an identity and a life in a transformed environment, and finding an enduring relationship with the deceased based not on physical presence but on accurate memory.

Depending on many factors, this process can take months to a number of years. Losses transform lives, and we are never quite the same person again. Over time, people move from pain defining who they are and constant preoccupation with their loss to living with the residual pain and forever carrying the memory of the loved one.

Grieving Theories

A variety of theories exist to explain the process of grieving. Freud (1961) introduced the concept of "grief work," which referred to the process of looking at the past, reliving memoires, and detaching from the deceased. Freud believed that grief need to be confronted; this concept continued to be useful for later theory and therapy.

Most early theories are based on stages such as described by Kübler-Ross (1969) and Bowlby (1980) by which individuals progress toward the resolution of the loss. Later theorists such as Worden (2009) took a more dynamic approach by viewing the grieving process as tasks. All stage theories follow a similar pattern and are similarly useful.

As previously discussed, Kübler-Ross's groundbreaking work provides a framework for understanding reactions to dying (Kübler-Ross, 1969). Her stage theory was eventually applied to the grieving process as well. Denial, anger, bargaining, depression, and acceptance are used to explain responses to loss.

John Bowlby (1980), a British psychologist, relied on childhood attachment experiences to explain bereavement reactions in adulthood. He believed that grief is an instinctive universal response to separation. According to Bowlby, grief evolves through a sequence of four overlapping and flexible phases: shock and numbness, yearning and protest, despair and disorganization, and reorganization and recovery.

J. William Worden (2009) identifies tasks that have to be worked through if grief is to be resolved. His model emphasizes moves from passive phases of grief to four active tasks of mourning.

- **Task 1**: Accepting the reality of loss.
- **Task 2:** Working through and experiencing the pain of grief.
- **Task 3:** Adjusting to an environment without the deceased person. The bereaved person must embrace new roles and adjust to the changing dynamics of the environment. Often the full extent of what this involves, and what has been lost, is not realized until some time after the loss.
- **Task 4:** Withdrawing emotionally from or relocating the deceased and moving on. Relocation requires that the bereaved person forms an ongoing relationship with his or her memories of the deceased in such a way that he or she is able to continue with his or her life.

Worden notes that every loss must be assessed in the context of mediating factors. These factors include the nature of the person who died, the nature of the attachment, the circumstances of the death, personality factors, family history, social circumstances, and life changes resulting from the death. His model can help to empower the mourner and serve as a specific guide for the nurse providing counseling.

While viewing the grieving process as linear—from denial to eventual acceptance—is attractive, grieving is just not that neat. In reality, these stages overlap and may be non-sequential. Strobe (1998) suggests a dual process model of coping and bereavement. It incorporates the stage/phase models of loss-oriented processes with the restoration of a new lifestyle. The restoration process involves coping with everyday life, building a new identity, and developing new relationships. Table 30.2 summarizes the dual process model.

Grief and Technology

As minute details of our lives emerge in social media, so does grief. During or after the loss of a loved one, social media can serve as an outlet for a grieving person to express thoughts and feelings and get positive supportive feedback. In one study, Facebook profiles of deceased individuals were reviewed for the posts made by loved ones. Results indicate a potential for loved ones to continue a bond with the deceased by sharing memories, expressing sorrow, and gaining social support (Getty et al., 2011). Social networking technologies can help people make sense of death and maintain a relationship with the deceased.

Grief Versus Major Depressive Disorder

An individual who is grieving is clinically different from a person who has major depressive disorder. The previous edition of the *Diagnostic and Statistical Manual of Psychiatry Fourth Edition Text Revision* (*DSM-IV-TR*) encouraged clinicians to avoid diagnosing an individual with major

TABLE 30.2 Dual Process Model of Coping

Loss-Oriented Processes	Restoration-Oriented Process
Grief work	Attending to life changes
Intrusion of grief	Distraction from grief
Denial/avoidance of restoration changes	Doing new things
Breaking bonds/ties	Establishing new roles/identitifies/relationships

depressive disorder within 2 months of the loss of a loved one. This clinical guideline was referred to as the bereavement exclusion. The fifth edition of the manual, the *DSM-5*, however, removed this exclusion. Table 30.3 clarifies the difference between symptoms in grief and major depressive disorder.

Types of Grieving and Associated Nursing Care

Grieving

Grieving, also known as acute grieving, is the painful experience after a loss. Herdman and Kamitsuru (2014) define *grieving* as "A normal complex process that includes emotional, physical, spiritual, social and intellectual responses and behaviors by which individuals, families, and communities incorporate an actual, anticipated, or perceived loss into their daily lives" (p. 338).

There is no clear ending for grieving. Gradually the sadness diminishes, the pain subsides, and the individual moves on. According to the American Psychiatric Association (APA, 2013), grief is considered persistent if it extends beyond 12 months in adults and 6 months in children. Signs that grief is subsiding include:

- Accepting that the loved one has died.
- Distressing memories of the deceased are under control.
- Anger over the loss is no longer present.
- Experiencing adaptive appraisals of oneself in relation to the deceased.
- Avoidance of reminders of the loss is no longer present.
- Belief that life is worth living without the deceased.
- Increased sense of identity apart from the lost relationship.
- Engaging in activities, pursuing relationships, or planning for the future.

Nursing care for individuals who are experiencing grieving supports positive expectations for the future and re-engaging in activities and interests. As discussed previously in the dying and death section, the art of presence will reduce isolation in the grieving individual. Eye contact, the suitable use of touch, and a posture of attentiveness express warmth and provide comfort.

Listening is the absolute best nursing interventions that a nurse can employ. People need to tell their stories, usually over and over, and move through the storyline in their own time. Sincere expression of sympathy such as "I am so sorry for your loss. You must be devastated," shows engagement, interest, and empathy. Avoid clichés, and minimizing expressions, which may actually be damaging. Saying "Have you considered having another child?," or "She is no longer suffering" suggest that the patient move on or wanted the loved one to suffer. Table 30.4 describes some examples of communication to avoid and communication to use with grieving individuals.

Spiritual care is important to people with spiritual convictions and religious beliefs. Assess the role of faith in your patient's life and the perspective of death that accompanies religious beliefs. Offer support and referrals to pastoral counseling (when available) or community resources.

Grief support groups are available for every type of loss (e.g., spouse, child, pet), age group, and special conditions (e.g., disease, suicide, casualty of war). Hearing from others in various levels of grief, sharing the story of loss with others and receiving feedback, and being part of a group who really understands are powerful tools for healing. People may choose to attend local groups or online support groups depending on what works best and feels most comfortable.

Complicated Grieving

The APA (2013) proposes a condition for further study that is not yet an actual diagnosis, but is useful in our discussion on grieving. This medical diagnosis is persistent complex bereavement disorder. **Persistent complex bereavement disorder** would apply to individuals whose bereavement persists beyond 12 months in adults and 6 months in children.

TABLE 30.3 Symptoms of Grief Versus Major Depressive Disorder

Symptom	Grief	Major Depressive Disorder
Feelings	Emptiness and loss	Depressed mood and anhedonia (inability to experience pleasure)
Physical	Insomnia, poor appetite, weight loss, decreased energy that gradually improves	Insomnia, poor appetite, weight loss, decreased energy
Intensity	Intense sadness and anger that occurs in waves and gradually subsides	Depressed mood is constant, most of the day, nearly every day
Thoughts	Focused on the deceased and reminders of the deceased	Self-critical, pessimistic ruminations, accompanied by thoughts of death
Mood	Depressed mood intermittent; increasingly positive emotions such as humor	Pervasive unhappiness and misery
Guilt	May experience guilt over failing the deceased (e.g., not visiting enough, not expressing love enough)	Continual, excessive, and inappropriate guilt
Self-esteem	Intact; reorganization tasks may impact sense of self (e.g., "Who am I without him?")	Worthlessness and self-loathing
Thoughts of death	May focus on someday reuniting with the deceased	Focused on ending the pain of depression; may develop a plan for death

Data from American Psychiatric Association: *Diagnostic and Statistical Manual of Mental Disorders*, ed. 5, Washington, DC, 2013, Author.

TABLE 30.4 Communication and Grief

What Not To Say	What To Say	Rationale
"I know how you feel."	"Your loss must be devastating. I can't imagine how you must be feeling right now."	Unfortunately, you cannot really know how that person feels.
"When my mother died, I cried for months and could hardly eat… [*and proceed with long story*]."	"When I lost my mother, I was in a fog for days. This must be difficult for you right now."	While it is helpful to know that others have experienced loss, during the acute grief period the focus should be on the griever. Sharing lengthy stories is not helpful.
After a sudden and unexpected death: "At least he didn't suffer."	"It must have been so shocking to lose your husband so suddenly. Did he have any symptoms?"	No one wants suffering for a loved one, yet sudden deaths are also highly traumatizing. Chances to prepare and say goodbye are lost.
"Have you thought about getting another ____ [wife, pet, job]?"	"Your loved one was irreplaceably special."	The griever is not interested in a replacement; they want their loved one back.
"She is with God now."	"I can only imagine how much you are missing her now."	Implying that the loss is God's doing may make the griever feel betrayed or punished by God. This statement also assumes that the griever believes in God.
"You can be grateful for the time you had together."	"You were married for 36 years."	This implies that the griever is ungracious. The griever is probably gracious but still wants his or her loved one back.
"Let me know if there is anything I can do for you."	"I would like to take the flowers from the funeral home to your house."	The grieving person is overwhelmed. Suggesting that they find something for you to do is an additional burden. Make a concrete offer of assistance.

In addition to the timing, interference with normal functioning is the hallmark symptom that distinguishes typical grieving from a psychiatric disorder. Suicidal ideation and disinterest in living make this bereavement disorder particularly dangerous.

The prevalence of this problem is about 2% to 5%. It is more common in females than in males, perhaps because females tend to outlive their spouses. High degrees of dependency on the deceased person and the death of a child are risk factors.

Care for the individual who is experiencing complicated grieving begins with a nursing diagnosis of *risk for complicated grieving* if risk factors exist, or *complicated grieving* if the problem has already occurred. Herdman and Kamitsuru (2014) define *risk for complicated grieving* as being "vulnerable to a disorder that occurs after death of a significant other in which the experience of distress accompanying bereavement fails to follow normative expectations and manifests in functional impairment, which may compromise health" (p. 340).

Herdman and Kamitsuru (2014) define **complicated grieving** as "A disorder that occurs after the death of a significant other, in which the experience of distress accompanying bereavement fails to follow normative expectations and manifests in functional impairment" (p. 339). The outcome for both the risk and actual diagnosis is grief resolution (Moorhead et al., 2012).

Symptoms of complicated grieving include preoccupation with thoughts of the deceased person, feelings of emptiness, anger, depression, disbelief, detachment, and rumination. Self-blame may be a prominent symptom. For example, a widow may obsessively blame herself for her spouse not seeking help for chest pain.

Nursing care for complicated grieving includes the care previously discussed for grieving. Protection from self-harm is an additional nursing intervention for this population. See Chapter 25 for care associated with suicidal ideation. Encouraging the patient to talk and helping him or her integrate the good and bad aspects of the deceased into a unified whole is an important aspect of care. Assisting with aspects of everyday life, such as encouraging adequate nutrition and hydration, monitoring sleep, and encouraging physical activity may be required.

Disenfranchised Grief

Sometimes, an individual experiences an intense loss that is not congruent with a socially recognized relationship. Examples are a lover, a divorced spouse, a caregiver, an abortion, or a pet. We call this **disenfranchised grief**. This could also include the grief felt by healthcare workers over the loss of a patient. Typically, these mourners do not have the opportunity to publicly grieve the loss. Expressing grief would be viewed as unacceptable. To acknowledge and recognize such losses can help the griever begin the work of mourning.

When taking care of a patient who has experienced an unconventional loss, it is important to provide support and guidance. Seeking individual psychotherapy may be instrumental in working through conflicting feelings and issues. Local support groups may be of benefit, but there is always concern about anonymity and disclosure outside the group. Another good source of support is an anonymous virtual support group. There are actually many online support groups for disenfranchised grief.

Grief Caused by Public Tragedy

Public tragedies can cause another kind of loss. Public tragedies involve a loss whose impact is felt broadly across a community or the general public. Entire communities and nations are shocked by genocide, war, assassinations, natural disasters, and school shootings. The 24-hour cycle of media coverage gives us all constant access to tragedies across the world. It is important to explore the impact of public tragedies. As with other losses, acknowledging and validating the personal impact of the loss is therapeutic.

SELF-CARE

Nurses are on the forefront of caring for the sick and dying. Nurses should model good self-care because daily exposure to grief and dying can lead to increased vulnerability to emoctional attachments and compassion fatigue. Nurses often grow attached to some patients and may experience both anticipatory grieving and bereavement. To maintain emotional balance and health, it is essential to rely on the support of others and practice good self-care. This is a journey that promotes greater self-understanding, wisdom, and compassion.

Nurses should practice conscious self-care in both their professional and private lives. The ANA Code of Ethics Provision 5.2 states that nurses should model the same care for their own health that they teach to their patients (Box 30.4).

BOX 30.4 Guidelines for Self-Care When Caring for the Dying

1. Remind yourself that what is happening to your patients and their families is not happening to you. This is their life drama right now but not your own.
2. When you notice that you are having a particularly strong emotional reaction, either positive or negative (countertransference), take it as a signal to explore your deeper issues or needs by talking with a trusted friend, counselor, or colleague.
3. Protect your private life by practicing time management, avoiding working outside of normal hours, protecting your pager or home telephone number, and taking regular days off and vacations.
4. Clearly state what you can and cannot do for your patients so your human and professional limitations are known upfront.
5. Practice humility. There is much you can do, but there is also much that is unknown and unknowable.
6. Do your own mourning when your heart is touched and you need to acknowledge the importance of others in your life. Even after a person has died, you can honor the relationship you had in your memory. Attend funerals or create grieving rituals when this happens.
7. Create a healthy, balanced private life by exercising regularly, eating a balanced diet, sleeping adequately, and leaving time for vacations and nurturing friendships.

KEY POINTS TO REMEMBER

- The hospice movement offers compassionate care for those who are dying, generally during the last 6 months of life. Hospice and palliative care both focus on patients' physical and emotional comfort and offer holistic support for dying people and their families.
- More hospitals are offering palliative end-of-life care, but conflict continues to exist between the wishes of dying people and their families and the medical model of treatment that focuses on the prolongation of life.
- When providing end-of-life care to people with dementia, challenging behaviors may communicate discomfort in mind, body, or spirit. Care should focus on providing meaningful connections with patients and between family members and their loved one.
- People who work with the dying need to maintain their own emotional health. Multidisciplinary teams usually deliver end-of-life care. Nurses need to draw on team support, protect their private lives by setting clear personal boundaries, and recognize their human and professional limitations.
- Providing timely and ongoing information about the disease and its effects and about physical and psychological signs of death can help the family deal with anticipatory mourning.
- Grief and mourning are distinct holistic processes and normal reactions to a loss, real or perceived, including the loss of a person, loss of security, loss of self-confidence, and loss of a dream.
- Common phenomena are evident during the experience of grief, and mourning is greatly influenced by cultural norms. However, everyone's experience of grieving is shaped by mediating factors such as the relationship to the person who died and the capacities of the mourner.
- Indicators of the potential for complicated or unresolved grief include social isolation, extensive dependency on the deceased person, unresolved interpersonal conflicts, loss of a child, violent and senseless death, and/or a catastrophic loss.
- Grief work is successful when the relationship to the deceased person has been restructured, energy is available for new relationships and life pursuits, and the mourner can remember realistically both the pleasures and the disappointments of the lost relationship.

CRITICAL THINKING

1. George is dying of pancreatic cancer. His wife and adult children are asking about using hospice. Help George's family make an informed decision by describing hospice care.
2. What are some concrete ways in which you can help another to cope with loss? Identify specific components in the following areas:
   a. How can you let the person tell his or her story and what is the potential therapeutic value of doing so?
   b. What are some things you might say that could offer comfort?

CHAPTER REVIEW

Questions

1. Which statement made to the grieving patient demonstrates effective therapeutic communication? *Select all that apply.*
   a. "Your loved one was irreplaceably special."
   b. "It must be comforting to know they are with God now."
   c. "You can be very grateful for the time you had together."
   d. "I would like to take the flowers from the funeral home to your house."
   e. "Your loss must be devastating. I can't imagine how you must be feeling right now."
2. Considering the subject of medically assisted death, which statements identify the pros and cons of the argument associated with the issue of nonmaleficence? *Select all that apply.*
   a. From the patient's perspective, there is no difference between ending life by providing a lethal prescription and by stopping treatment that prolongs life.
   b. Assisted death violates the oath to "do no harm" and destroys trust between patient and nurse.
   c. There is equal protection under the law that allows the right to refuse or withdraw treatment and to commit suicide.
   d. Every competent person has the right to make decisions based on personal convictions.
   e. Human beings are the stewards but not the absolute masters of the gift of life.
3. Which statement made by a patient demonstrates acceptance of criteria required of hospice care?
   a. "I want my family to be with me."
   b. "There is no cure for my illness. I've accepted that."
   c. "It's important to me that I die in my own home."
   d. "I don't want my family to bear the burden of caring for me."
4. Which statement made by a widow demonstrates that her grief work has been effective? *Select all that apply.*
   a. "I can remember how much my deceased husband loved chocolate chip ice cream."
   b. "Painting is my new passion, and I really enjoy learning the various strokes."
   c. "Jim could be very stubborn when he thought he was right."
   d. "I don't know why he had to die."
   e. "I just can't believe he's gone."
5. Which factor has the greatest influence on the hospice nurse's ability to provide respectful professional care?
   a. Acceptance that death is a natural part of life.
   b. Possession of excellent care giving nursing skills.
   c. The existence of a healthy, well-balanced personal life.
   d. The desire to work with both the patient and the family.
6. There is conflict surrounding the dying experience in modern medicine. The medical model of treatment in the United States has traditionally been focused on the prolongation of life. What intrinsic factor plays into this medical model?
   a. Healthcare works do not want their patients to die.
   b. Medicare is a fee-for-service model.
   c. Palliative care is expensive to administer.
   d. Keeping people alive as long as possible is the ethical thing to do.
7. Holly is a 53-year-old female with terminal breast cancer. Holly's nurse in the hospital brings up the subject of hospice care. Holly becomes upset and states, "I am not ready to give up and die." You respond that hospice is:
   a. A model of healthcare that emphasizes quality of life for you and your family.
   b. The end of curative treatments and pain management.
   c. A multidisciplinary team providing curative and therapeutic treatment.
   d. An aggressive medical plan to end suffering and hasten death.
8. Guadalupe is the matriarch of a large family. She is terminally ill and none of her family members know her end-of-life wishes. The best action for the nurse is to:
   a. Discuss durable power of attorney.
   b. Organize a family meeting with Guadalupe's permission to discuss her goals and wishes.
   c. Have a family meeting without Guadalupe so as not to upset her.
   d. Ask the doctor to tell Guadalupe that she is dying.
9. A bereavement group run by a local hospice includes a woman who is distraught over her supervisor's death. The woman appears severely distressed. She has trouble functioning with activities of daily living and making the simplest of decisions. The group facilitator recognizes that this woman is suffering from disenfranchised grief after learning:
   a. The woman was in love with her married supervisor.
   b. She has not taken enough time off work to grieve properly.
   c. The supervisor died over a year ago.
   d. Her family is not involved enough to support her.
10. The dying patient with a neurocognitive disorder such as Alzheimer's disease is especially challenging to provide care for. They may have symptoms or pain that they are unable to adequately describe or define. Reversible conditions that respond to treatment that may affect level of consciousness, anxiety, or agitation include:
    a. Inability to communicate
    b. Distended bladder, constipation, or nausea
    c. Reduced urinary output
    d. Weakness due to the dying process

Answers

1. **a, d, e**; 2. **a, b**; 3. **b**; 4. **a, b, c**; 5. **c**; 6. **d**; 7. **a**; 8. **b**; 9. **a**; 10. **b**

ⓔ Visit the Evolve website for a posttest on the content in this chapter: http://evolve.elsevier.com/Varcarolis

Post-Test interactive review

REFERENCES

Aldridge, M. D., & Kelley, A. S. (2015). The myth regarding the high cost of end-of-life care. *American Journal of Public Health, 105*(12), 2411–2415.

American Nurses Association. (2016). *Code of ethics for nurses with interpretive statements.* Retrieved from http://nursingworld.org/DocumentVault/Ethics-1/Code-of-Ethics-for-Nurses.html.

American Psychiatric Association. (2013). *Diagnostic and statistical manual of mental disorders* (5th ed.). Washington, DC: Author.

Bowlby, J. (1980). *Attachment and loss.* New York, NY: Basic Books.

Brinkman-Stoppelenburg, A., Rietjens, J. A., & Van der Heide, A. (2014). The effects of advance care planning on end-of-life care: A systematic review. *Palliative Medicine, 28*(8), 1000–1025.

Byock, I. R. (1996). The nature of suffering and the nature of opportunity at the end-of-life. *Clinics in Geriatric Medicine, 12*(2), 237.

Centers for Medicare and Medicaid Services. (2016). *Frequently asked questions about billing the physician fee schedule for advance care planning services.* Retrieved from https://www.cms.gov/Medicare/Medicare-Fee-for-Service-Payment/PhysicianFeeSched/Downloads/FAQ-Advance-Care-Planning.pdf.

Freud, S. (1961). Mourning and melancholia. In J. Strachy (Ed.), *The complete psychological works (pp. 243–258).* London, ENG: Hogarth.

Getty, E., Cobb, J., Gabeler, M., et al. (2011). I said your name in an empty room: Grieving and continuing bonds on Facebook. *Proceedings of the SIGCHI Conference on Human Factors in Computer Systems,* 997–1000.

Herdman, T. H., & Kamitsuru, S. (Eds.). (2014). *NANDA International nursing diagnoses: Definitions and classification* (pp. 2015–2017). Oxford, UK: Wiley-Blackwell.

Hogan, J. M., & Hogan, H. (2014). *An aging nation: The older population in the United States.* Retrieved from https://www.census.gov/prod/2014pubs/p25-1140.pdf.

H.R. 4449. (1990). Patient self-determination act of 1990. Retrieved from https://www.congress.gov/bill/101st-congress/house-bill/4449.

Kelley, A. S., Deb, P., Du, Q., Carlson, M. D. A., & Morrison, R. S. (2013). Hospice enrollment saves money for Medicare and improves care quality across a number of different lengths-of-stay. *Health Affairs, 30*(3), 552–561.

Kübler-Ross, E. (1969). *On death and dying.* New York, NY: Macmillan.

Maiese, K. (2016). *Vegetative state and minimally conscious state - neurologic disorders.* Retrieved from http://www.merckmanuals.com/professional/neurologic-disorders/coma-and-impaired-consciousness/vegetative-state-and-minimally-conscious-state.

Martin, A., Lassman, D., Whittle, L., & Catlin, A. (2011). Recession contributes to slowest annual rate of increase in health spending in five decades. *Health Affairs, 30*(1), 11–22.

Marwit, S. J., & Meuser, T. M. (2002). Development and initial validation of an inventory to assess grief in caregivers of people with Alzheimer's disease. *The Gerontologist, 42,* 751–765.

Moorhead, S., Johnson, M., Maas, M. L., & Swanson, E. (2013). *Nursing outcomes classification (NOC)* (5th ed.). St. Louis, MO: Mosby.

Morone, N. E., & Weiner, D. K. (2013). Pain as the fifth vital sign: Exposing the vital need for pain education. *Clinical Therapeutics, 35*(11), 1728–1730.

National Hospice and Palliative Care Organization. (2015). *The Medicare hospice benefit.* Retrieved from http://www.nhpco.org/sites/default/files/public/communications/Outreach/The_Medicare_Hospice_Benefit.pdf.

Pew Research Center. (2013). *Views on end-of-life medical treatment.* Retrieved from http://www.pewforum.org/2013/11/21/views-on-end-of-life-medical-treatments/.

Prince-Paul, M., & Daly, B. (2015). Ethical considerations. In B. Ferrell & N. Coyle (Eds.), *Textbook of palliative nursing* (4th ed.) (p. 1043). Oxford, London: Oxford University Press.

Riley, G., & Lubitz, J. (2010). Long-term trends in Medicare payments in the last year of life. *Health Services Research, 45*(2), 565–576.

Sacks, O. (2015). *Gratitude.* New York, NY: Alfred A. Knopf.

Silveira, M. J., Kim, S. Y., & Langa, K. M. (2010). Advance directives and outcomes of surrogate decision making before death. *New England Journal of Medicine, 362*(13), 1211–1218.

Stolberg, S. G. (1999, May 11). A conversation with Dame Cicely Saunders: Reflecting on a life of treating the dying. *New York Times,* Health and Fitness Section.

Stroebe, M. S. (1998). New directions in bereavement research: Exploration of gender differences. *Palliative Medicine, 12*(2), 5–12.

Wilson, D. M., Cohen, J., Deliens, L., et al. (2013). The preferred place of last days: Results of a representative population-based public survey. *Journal of Palliative Medicine, 16*(5), 502–508.

Worden, J. W. (2009). *Grief counseling and grief therapy* (4th ed.). New York, NY: Springer.

World Health Organization. (2015). *Dementia factsheet 362.* Retrieved from http://www.who.int/mediacentre/factsheets/fs362/en/.

31

Older Adults

Leslie A. Briscoe

Visit the Evolve website for a pretest on the content in this chapter:
http://evolve.elsevier.com/Varcarolis Pre-Test interactive review

OBJECTIVES

1. Describe mental health disorders that may occur in older adults.
2. Discuss the importance of pain assessment and tools used to assess pain in older adults.
3. Explain the importance of a comprehensive geriatric assessment.
4. Recognize the significance of healthcare costs for older adults.
5. Compare the facts and myths about aging.
6. Analyze how ageism may affect attitudes and willingness to care for older adults.
7. Explore issues related to the use of physical and chemical restraints in long-term care.
8. Identify legislation, advanced directives, and their impact on nursing care.
9. Describe the role of the nurse in various geriatric care settings.

OUTLINE

KEY TERMS AND CONCEPTS

adult day care
advance directives
ageism
agnosia
aphasia
apraxia
late-life mental illness
medication reconciliation
Patient Self-Determination Act (PSDA)
polypharmacy
prescribing cascade

An aging population is a global phenomenon that is occurring at a record-breaking rate, especially in developing countries. In the United States, this increase in the proportion of older adults affects the economy, health, and social services. According to the Administration on Aging (2013), the number of individuals over 65 years old has grown by 24.7% between 2003 and 2013. Those individuals over 85 years old are projected to more than double from 6 million in 2013 to 14.6 million in 2040. Among this cohort, the fastest-growing subgroups are racial and ethnic minorities. Individuals in minority groups represent about 21% of those who are 65 years or older. This number is expected to increase to nearly 29% by 2030. The number of centenarians, those individuals 100 years and older, has more than doubled since 1980, to over 67,000 in 2013. Fig. 31.1 shows the projected rate of growth in people 65 and older until 2060.

As people live longer, they are more likely to deal with chronic illness and disability. At least 92% of older adults have at least one chronic disease, and 77% have at least two (National Council on Aging, n.d.). The most common chronic illnesses are heart disease, cancer, stroke, and diabetes, which are responsible for almost two-thirds of all deaths each year. The risk of developing a chronic illness dramatically increases with age. Individuals 75 and older are the most prone to chronic illnesses and functional disabilities. After age 85, there is a one in three chance of developing dementia, immobility, incontinence, or another age-related disability. Fig. 31.2 illustrates selected medical conditions in residential care residents based on facility size.

Women generally outlive men. This has significant ramifications for society at large and for the healthcare system in particular. Not only do women make up the largest proportion of older adults, they also use healthcare services more frequently than men and seek services earlier, even for minor conditions.

Chronological age is an arbitrary indicator of function, because there are significant variables that contribute to the health and functioning of older adults. For example, individuals who live beyond 100 years old experience a progressive delay in the age of onset of impaired physical and cognitive functioning, age-associated diseases, and overall morbidity (Anderson et al., 2012). Common classifications for people 65 years and older is:

- **Young-old:** 65 to 74 years
- **Middle-old:** 75 to 84 years
- **Old-old:** 85 to 100 years
- **Centenarians:** 100 to 104 years
- **Semisupercentenarians:** 105 to 109 years
- **Supercentenarians:** 110 to 119 years

Aging is accompanied by limited regenerative abilities and increased susceptibility to disease, syndromes, and sickness. The last years of life are often punctuated by losses, some obvious and some subtler. While retirement may be welcome, it still represents the loss of a career and possibly self-identity. Losses may be people—a spouse, children, and friends. As the ability to care for themselves becomes more difficult, familiar surroundings and independence may be lost in favor of assisted living or residential care. Older adults experience diminished senses—taste, smell, hearing, and sight. Cognitive decline and physical health problems weigh on an individual's day-to-day function.

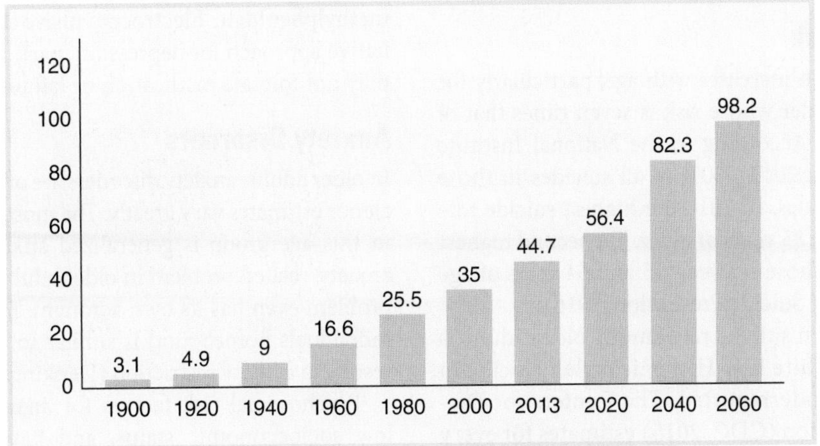

FIG. 31.1 Number of persons 65 and older: 1900–2060. Note: Increments in years are uneven. Source: US Census Bureau. (2015). *Population estimates and projections*. Retrieved from http://www.census.gov/content/dam/Census/library/publications/2015/demo/p25-1143.pdf.

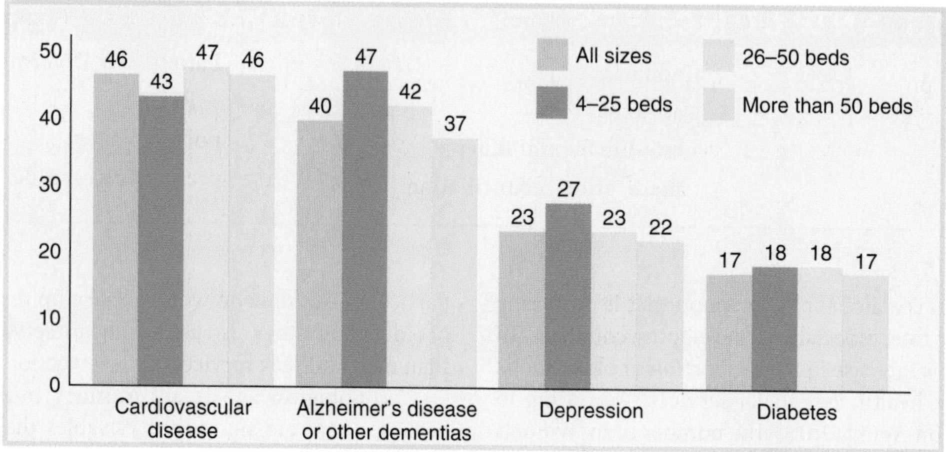

FIG. 31.2 Medical conditions among residential care residents by community size. Centers for Disease Control and Prevention. (2015). *Variation in residential care community resident characteristics.* Retrieved from http://www.cdc.gov/nchs/products/databriefs/db223.htm.

MENTAL HEALTH ISSUES RELATED TO AGING

Late-Life Mental Illness

Older adults who develop late-life mental illness are less likely than young adults to be accurately diagnosed and receive mental health treatment. Psychiatric issues such as depression, cognitive deficits, and prolonged grieving are not a normal part of aging. Diagnosing and treating psychiatric disorders prolongs the individual's ability to remain independent and increases the ability to take the lead in personal choices.

Depression

Mood disorders are often underidentified because of comorbid medical conditions. Depression is quite common after cardiac events and strokes, but care providers can confuse it with dementia or delirium. A careful systematic assessment is necessary to properly distinguish among the three. The cardinal differences include the following:

- Onset of mental-status change and course of illness
- Level of consciousness
- Attention span

Aging and Suicide Risk

The risk of suicide for men increases with age, particularly for white men ages 65 and older whose risk is seven times that of females of the same age. According to the National Institute of Mental Health (NIMH; 2015), 80% of all suicides in those 65 and older are white males. In 2014 the highest suicide rate (19.3%) was among people 85 years or older. The second highest rate (19.2%) occurred in those between 45 and 64 years of age (American Foundation for Suicide Prevention, 2016).

Even though the known suicide rate among older adults is high, especially among white non-Hispanic males, suicide in this group is probably underreported. The Centers for Disease Control and Prevention (CDC, 2015) estimates for every one completed suicide, there are four suicide attempts in the older adult population. The numbers also do not reflect those who passively or indirectly commit suicide by abusing alcohol, starving themselves, overdosing or mixing medications, stopping life-sustaining drugs, getting into auto accidents, or simply losing the will to live. Treating depression is cost effective, saves lives, and decreases healthcare expenditures. Chapter 25 provides an in-depth discussion of suicide.

Early identification of risk factors and treatment for depression are key measures for suicide prevention. Risks for suicide include:

- Diagnosable psychiatric illness (psychosis, anxiety, substance use, previous suicide attempts)
- Psychological alterations (personality, emotional reactivity, impulsiveness)
- Stressful life events

Other risk factors include access to weapons, access to large doses of medications, and chronic or terminal illness. Some protective factors include spiritual beliefs, being married, personal resilience, perception of social/family support, and having children.

Selective serotonin reuptake inhibitors (SSRIs) are the first-line of treatment for depression. This category is often helpful if anxiety, worry, or rumination is problematic. If pain or diabetic neuropathy is a comorbid condition, serotonin norepinephrine reuptake inhibitors (SNRIs) are often prescribed. Treatment-resistant depression can be treated with psychostimulants such as methylphenidate. Electroconvulsive therapy is also a good alternative approach for depression, particularly in older adults who may not tolerate medication or fail to improve.

Anxiety Disorders

In older adults, anxiety disorders are often undiagnosed and prevalence estimates vary greatly. The most common anxiety disorder in this age group is generalized anxiety disorder. One unique anxiety-related problem in older adults is the fear of falling. This problem even has its own acronym: FOF. Its impact on keeping individuals homebound is similar to agoraphobia because FOF results in activity restriction (Denkinger et al., 2015).

Psychosocial risk factors for anxiety include childlessness, low socioeconomic status, and having experienced trauma. Other risk factors include being female, single, and having multiple medical conditions. Protective factors include social support, spiritual beliefs, physical activity, cognitive stimulation, and having coping strategies.

First-line treatment for anxiety disorders in all age groups, including older adults, is SSRIs along with cognitive behavioral therapy. Benzodiazepines such as lorazepam (Ativan), alprazolam (Xanax), or diazepam (Valium) are also used to treat anxiety, but are often prescribed inappropriately in older adults. Using this class of drugs may result in increased falls, fractures, mental decline, and delirium. When used in low doses, these problems are less likely, but it is better to avoid the drugs in this class if at all possible. Benzodiazepines have recently been implicated in an increased risk of Alzheimer's disease for individuals with chronic use (De Gage et al., 2014). Chapter 15 discusses anxiety disorders in greater detail.

Delirium

Delirium is a time-limited medical condition caused by physiological changes usually due to an identifiable underlying pathology. Fluctuations in consciousness and changes in cognition develop over a short period of time (hours to days). Unfortunately, disorientation in older adults may be labeled as dementia and disregarded. It is crucial to obtain data from family or caregivers about a baseline level of functioning. A patient who is newly confused, falling, disrobing, and fighting with staff should be assessed for delirium. Asking family members questions such as "Has your mother been shopping and cooking for herself?"; "Does she pay her own bills?"; or "Does she ever get lost when driving?" may give subtle clues about whether changes are acute or have been coming on slowly.

Treatment of delirium begins with identifying the cause. You may ask, "Is your father taking any new medication?" or "Has your father fallen or hit his head recently?" The delirium may be due to drug reactions or toxicity, infections, electrolyte or metabolic imbalances, anemia, thyroid dysfunction, vitamin deficiencies, stroke, and a multitude of other problems. A multidisciplinary approach is often helpful to identify causation. Pharmacists are helpful in identifying possible drug-related effects. Geriatricians provide a comprehensive approach to physical assessment. Psychiatric consultation can provide mental status evaluation and recommendations for treatment of behaviors.

Neurocognitive Disorders

The most common neurocognitive disorders are Alzheimer's disease and vascular disease. Both are characterized by a functional decline, **aphasia** (difficulty finding words), **apraxia** (difficulty carrying out motor functions), **agnosia** (failure to recognize objects), and disturbances in executive functioning (organizing, planning, abstracting, insight, judgment). Changes in executive functioning may result in forgetting how to make old family recipes or the inability to pay bills. Tragically, limited insight and judgment often lead to increased vulnerability to exploitation. Chapter 23 presents a more complete picture of delirium and dementia and associated care.

Alcohol Use Disorder

Although heavy drinking tends to decline with age, it continues to be a serious problem that may result in serious problems for older adults. The antecedents to late-onset alcohol use problems are often related to environmental conditions and may include retirement, widowhood, and loneliness. Previous work, family responsibilities, and marriage may have been protective in keeping a person with vulnerability from drinking too much. Once these demands are gone and the structure of daily life is removed, there may be little impetus to stay sober.

Risk factors for heavy drinking in older adults are being male and single, having less than a high school education, low income, and cigarette smoking (Karlamangla et al., 2006). Additionally, depression often plays a role in increased alcohol consumption in the older adult (National Institute on Aging, 2015). Identifying alcohol and substance use problems is often difficult because the personality and behavioral changes frequently go unrecognized. Whenever there is a suspicion or indication that an older adult is misusing alcohol, the healthcare provider should conduct a screening test. The Michigan Alcoholism Screening Test–Geriatric version (MAST-G; Box 31.1) is an instrument commonly used to assess older adults' alcohol use.

The older person who misuses alcohol exhibits confusion, malnutrition, self-neglect, weight loss, depression, and falls. Diarrhea, urinary incontinence, decreased functional status, failure to thrive, and dementia may also be present. Long-term excessive alcohol use can lead to alcohol-induced dementia. Symptoms include impaired executive functioning and significant lack of insight. This is in contrast to the memory or language problems of Alzheimer's disease.

Moos and colleagues (2010) conducted a study where 719 participants were followed over a 20-year span. Excessive drinking late in life was found in about 33% of participants. Indicators of excessive use were past drinking history, reliance on substances for stress reduction, and support of peers in drinking behavior. There is evidence that older adults respond to treatment as well as, if not better than, younger adults. Intentional brief interventions by a healthcare provider or participation in a group setting can support older adults in decreasing alcohol consumption. Group therapy along with self-help groups like Alcoholics Anonymous can be effective. It is important that healthcare providers recognize and recommend these options.

EVIDENCE-BASED PRACTICE

Why Do Older Adults Attempt Suicide?

Problem

Suicide rates increase with age, particularly in white males. There is limited understanding regarding the reasons older people attempt suicide.

Purpose of the Study

The purpose of this study was to gain an understanding about the reasons for late-life suicide.

Methods

Researchers interviewed 103 participants age 70 years and older. Subjects were older adults who were seen in emergency rooms after a suicide attempt in Sweden over a 3-year period. Multiple tools were used to measure cognition, illness rating, psychiatric symptoms, and depression. In addition, there was a clinical interview and medical record review. Participants were followed for 1 year through continued review of their records.

Key Findings

- The most common method for suicide attempt was overdose (N = 73).
- About a third of participants had previous suicide attempts.
- About 70% lived alone.

Continued

EVIDENCE-BASED PRACTICE—cont'd

- Reasons for the attempt included: To escape (29%), reduced functioning and autonomy (24%), psychological problems (24%), somatic problems and physical pain (16%), feeling like a burden (13%), social problems and family conflict (13%), and a lack of meaning in life (8%).
- Lethal means of suicide attempt and reattempts were associated with a sense of not belonging.

Implications for Nursing Practice

It is important to understand and recognize potential risk factors for suicide in the older adult. Nurses have the ability to screen for and identify those who may be at greatest risk. Targeting those at greater risk may guide interventions such as increasing socialization, interpersonal therapy, or an environmental change.

From Van Orden, K., Wiktorsson, S., Duberstein, P., Berg, A., & Waern, M. (2015). Reasons for attempted suicide in later life. *American Journal of Geriatric Psychiatry, 23*(5), 536–544.

Pain

Pain is common among older adults and affects their sense of well-being and quality of life. Up to 85% of the older population is believed to have conditions that predispose them to pain (Mailis-Gagnon et al., 2008). These conditions include arthritis, peripheral vascular disease, and diabetic neuropathy. Depression may cause or increase the perception of pain. Pain can affect the older adult's functioning and ability to perform activities of daily living (ADLs) such as walking, toileting, and bathing, especially if the pain is from musculoskeletal disease. Pain can lead to increased stress, delayed healing, decreased mobility, disturbances in sleep, decreased appetite, and agitation with accompanying aggressive behaviors. Chronic pain is linked to depression, low self-esteem, social isolation, and feelings of hopelessness. There is mounting evidence that treatment of pain improves mood and treatment of mood improves pain (Goesling et al., 2013).

Barriers to Accurate Pain Assessment

The appropriate assessment and treatment of pain in older adults may have complications. They may believe that pain is a punishment for past behaviors, an inevitable part of aging, indicative of impending death, relates to serious illness, expensive to test and diagnose, or a sign of weakness. External obstacles to pain management include inadequate assessment by health professionals, complicated clinical presentation, assumptions by healthcare professionals that pain is part of aging, and communication deficits due to cognitive impairment.

The use of open-ended questions such as "Tell me about your pain, aches, soreness, or discomfort" yields significantly more information than use of a pain scale alone. Assess changes in behavior that indicate pain, especially in patients who have language impairment (e.g., dementia, stroke). Unlike younger adults, older adults may understate pain using milder words such as *discomfort, hurting,* or *aching.* Multiple painful problems may occur together, making differentiation of new pain from preexisting pain difficult. Sensory impairments, memory loss, dementia, and depression can add to the difficulty of obtaining an accurate pain assessment. Interviews with family members, caregivers, or friends may be helpful.

BOX 31.1 Michigan Alcoholism Screening Test—Geriatric Version (Mast-G)

Please answer "Yes" or "No" to each question by marking the line next to the question. When you finish answering the questions, please add up how many "Yes" responses you checked and put that number in the space provided at the end.

1. After drinking, have you ever noticed an increase in your heart rate or beating in your chest? _____ Yes _____ No
2. When talking to others, do you ever underestimate how much you actually drank? _____ Yes _____ No
3. Does alcohol make you sleepy so that you often fall asleep in your chair? _____ Yes _____ No
4. After a few drinks, have you sometimes not eaten or been able to skip a meal because you didn't feel hungry? _____ Yes _____ No
5. Does having a few drinks help you decrease your shakiness or tremors? _____ Yes _____ No
6. Does alcohol sometimes make it hard for you to remember parts of the day or night? _____ Yes _____ No
7. Do you have rules for yourself that you won't drink before a certain time of the day? _____ Yes _____ No
8. Have you lost interest in hobbies or activities you used to enjoy? _____ Yes _____ No
9. When you wake up in the morning, do you ever have trouble remembering part of the night before? _____ Yes _____ No
10. Does having a drink help you sleep? _____ Yes _____ No
11. Do you hide your alcohol bottles from family members? _____ Yes _____ No
12. After a social gathering, have you ever felt embarrassed because you drank too much? _____ Yes _____ No
13. Have you ever been concerned that drinking might be harmful to your health? _____ Yes _____ No
14. Do you like to end an evening with a nightcap? _____ Yes _____ No
15. Did you find your drinking increased after someone close to you died? _____ Yes _____ No
16. In general, would you prefer to have a few drinks at home rather than go out to social events? _____ Yes _____ No
17. Are you drinking more now than in the past? _____ Yes _____ No
18. Do you usually take a drink to relax or calm your nerves? _____ Yes _____ No
19. Do you drink to take your mind off your problems? _____ Yes _____ No
20. Have you ever increased your drinking after experiencing a loss in your life? _____ Yes _____ No
21. Do you sometimes drive when you have had too much to drink? _____ Yes _____ No
22. Has a doctor or nurse ever said he or she was worried or concerned about your drinking? _____ Yes _____ No
23. Have you ever made rules to manage your drinking? _____ Yes _____ No
24. When you feel lonely, does having a drink help? _____ Yes _____ No

TOTALS: _____ Yes _____ No

Scoring: A score of 3 points or less is considered to indicate no alcoholism; a score of 4 points is suggestive of alcoholism; a score of 5 points or more indicates alcoholism.

From Blow FC, Brower KJ et al.: The Michigan Alcoholism Screening Test-Geriatric Version (MAST-G): A new elderly specific screening instrument. *Alcoholism: Clinical and Experimental Research 16*:372, 1992.

Assessment Tools

When pain is suspected, the nurse begins with a physical assessment for medical origins of the pain and assesses the level of pain. The Wong-Baker FACES Pain Rating Scale (Fig. 31.3) is an active assessment instrument. The FACES scale shows facial

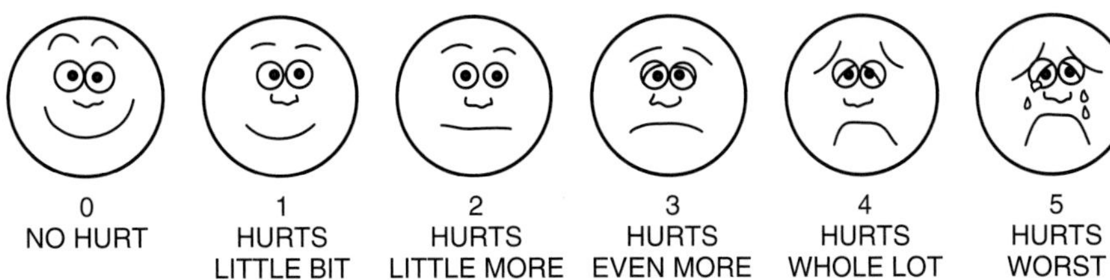
0
NO HURT
1
HURTS
LITTLE BIT
2
HURTS
LITTLE MORE
3
HURTS
EVEN MORE
4
HURTS
WHOLE LOT
5
HURTS
WORST

FIG. 31.3 Wong-Baker FACES Pain Rating Scale. (From Hockenberry, M., & Wilson, D. [2013]. *Wong's essentials of pediatric nursing* [9th ed.]. St. Louis, MO: Mosby.) Explain to the patient that the first face represents a person who feels happy because he has no pain, and that the other faces represent people who have pain, ranging from a little to a lot. Explain that face 10 represents a person who hurts as much as you can imagine, but you don't have to be crying to be in that much pain. Ask the patient to choose the face that best reflects how he or she is feeling.

	0	1	2	Score
Breathing Independent of vocalization	Normal	Occasional labored breathing; short period of hyperventilation	Noisy, labored breathing; long period of hyperventilation; Cheyne-Stokes respirations	
Negative Vocalization	None	Occasional moan or groan; low-level speech with a negative or disapproving quality	Repeated troubled calling out; loud moaning or groaning; crying	
Facial Expression	Smiling or inexpressive	Sad; frightened; frown	Facial grimacing	
Body Language	Relaxed	Tense; distressed pacing; fidgeting	Rigid; fists clenched; knees pulled up; pulling or pushing away; striking out	
Consolability	No need to console	Distracted or reassured by voice or touch	Unable to console, distract, or reassure	
			TOTAL	

FIG. 31.4 Pain Assessment in Advanced Dementia (PAINAD) scale. (From Warden, V., Hurley, A. C., & Volicer, L. [2003]. Development and psychometric evaluation of the Pain Assessment in Advanced Dementia [PAINAD] scale. *Journal of the American Medical Directors Association, 4*(1), 9–15.)

expressions on a scale from 0 (a smile) to 5 (crying grimace). Respondents choose the face that depicts the pain they feel.

People with cognitive deficits often act-out due to pain. The Pain Assessment in Advanced Dementia (PAINAD) scale evaluates the presence and severity of pain in patients with advanced neurocognitive disorders who no longer have the ability to communicate verbally (Fig. 31.4). The scale evaluates five domains: breathing, negative vocalization, facial expression, body language, and consolability (Box 31.2). The score assists the caregiver in the development of appropriate pain intervention.

Pain Management

Pharmacological pain treatments. Pain can be managed with pharmacological and alternative measures. Pharmacological pain management relies on the use of nonprescriptive and prescriptive medications, frequently based on the recommendation of the healthcare provider. Persistent pain is common among seniors. Yet, older adults may experience adverse drug reactions due to age- and disease-related changes in pharmacodynamics and pharmacokinetics. Careful monitoring of medication effects will help aid in avoiding overmedication or undermedication. Hepatic and renal functioning should be evaluated periodically.

Non-opioids. Non-opioids are useful for mild-to-moderate pain (Horgas et al., 2012). Acetaminophen is the preferred non-opioid medication. However, while it relieves pain, it does nothing to reduce inflammation. Acetaminophen can be toxic to the liver. The maximum dose should be reduced to 50% to 75% in adults with a history of alcohol use problems or reduced hepatic function.

Nonselective nonsteroidal anti-inflammatory drugs (NSAIDs) work by inhibiting one or both of two enzymes involved in the production of inflammation, pain, and

BOX 31.2 Pain Assessment in Advanced Dementia Scale (PAINAD)

Instructions: Observe the patient for 5 minutes before scoring his or her behaviors. Score the behaviors according to the following chart. The patient can be observed under different conditions (e.g., at rest, during a pleasant activity, during caregiving, after the administration of pain medication).

Behavior	0	1	2	Score
Breathing Independent of vocalization	Normal	Occasional labored breathing Short period of hyperventilation	Noisy labored breathing Long period of hyperventilation Cheyne-Stokes respirations	
Negative vocalization	None	Occasional moan or groan Low-level speech with a negative or disapproving quality	Repeated troubled calling out Loud moaning or groaning Crying	
Facial expression	Smiling or inexpressive	Sad Frightened Frown	Facial grimacing	
Body language	Relaxed	Tense Distressed pacing Fidgeting	Rigid Fists clenched Knees pulled up Pulling or pushing away Striking out	
Consolability	No need to console	Distracted or reassured by voice or touch	Unable to console, distract, or reassure	
			TOTAL SCORE	

Scoring: The total score ranges from 0-10 points. A possible interpretation of the scores is: 1-3 = mild pain; 4-6 = moderate pain; 7-10 = severe pain. These ranges are based on a standard 0-10 scale of pain, but have not been substantiated in the literature for this tool.

Source: Warden V, Hurley AC, & Volicer L. (2003). Development and psychometric evaluation of the Pain Assessment in Advanced Dementia (PAINAD) scale. *Journal of the American Medical Directors Association, 4*(1):9–15.

fever—cyclooxygenase-1 and cyclooxygenase-2 (COX-1 and COX-2). COX-1 functions to protect the lining of the stomach and intestines from the damaging effects of acid, promote blood clotting, and regulate normal kidney function. When these enzymes are inhibited, gastrointestinal bleeding and nephrotoxicity are dangerous potential side effects of nonselective NSAIDs. Nonselective NSAIDs include drugs such as ibuprofen (Motrin, Advil), naproxen (Aleve), and aspirin.

A newer group of NSAIDs that selectively inhibits only one COX enzyme is called a COX-2 inhibitor. Because this classification of drugs does not block COX-1, they do not cause ulcers or increase the bleeding as much as the older NSAIDs. Celecoxib (Celebrex) is the only COX-2 inhibitor available in the United States.

In 2015 the US Food and Drug Administration (FDA) strengthened an existing warning in prescription drug labels and over-the-counter labels. This warning indicates that NSAIDs can increase the chance of a heart attack, stroke, and potentially life-threatening gastrointestinal bleeding. These serious side effects can occur as early as the first weeks of using these drugs. The risk may increase the longer NSAIDs are used and increase with higher doses. Although aspirin is also an NSAID, this warning does not apply to aspirin.

Chronic pain may be treated with pain modulators such as gabapentin (Neurontin), pregabalin (Lyrica), SNRIs, and tricyclic antidepressants. Consultation with a pain-management specialist is often helpful with chronic pain syndromes. Some considerations in pharmacological pain management in older adults are listed in Box 31.3.

Opioids. Opioids may be indicated for treating moderate-to-severe acute pain. Opioids are metabolized in the liver and excreted by the kidneys either unchanged or as metabolites (American Society of Pain Management Nursing, 2016). As the result of normal aging, renal insufficiency often occurs, making older adults susceptible to drug effects and metabolite accumulation. Initial doses of opioids should be reduced in senior patients and longer dosing intervals should be scheduled.

The trend is to avoid opioids for non–cancer-related chronic pain due to evidence that the risks are significant including increased risk of fractures, hospitalization, and mortality. Furthermore, they may not even be beneficial for long-term pain. Prescribers also reported concern about misuse of opioids by family and friends.

Older adults' response to pain treatment is improved when the patient actively participates in treatment decisions. A trusting and mutually respectful relationship with providers reduces anxiety and associated pain. Being understood supports the goal of patient-centered care.

Nonpharmacological pain treatments. Nonpharmacological treatments for pain include physical therapy, vagal nerve stimulation, exercise, hydrotherapy, heat and cold packs, chiropractic, and transcutaneous electrical nerve stimulation (TENS). Yoga, biofeedback, hypnosis, acupuncture, massage, Reiki, guided imagery, reflexology, and therapeutic touch

BOX 31.3 Tips for Pharmacological Pain Management in Older Adults

- Remember that older adults often receive pain medication less often than younger adults, which results in inadequate pain relief. Compensate for this.
- Safe administration of analgesics is complicated because of possible interactions with drugs used to treat multiple chronic disorders, nutritional alterations, and altered pharmacokinetics in older adults.
- Analgesics reach a higher peak and have a longer duration of action in older adults than in younger individuals. Start with one-fourth to one-half the adult dose and titrate up carefully.
- Give oral analgesics around the clock when initiating pain management. Administer on an as-needed basis later on as indicated by the patient's pain status.
- If acute confusion occurs, assess for other contributing factors before changing the medication or stopping analgesic use. Confusion in postoperative patients is associated with unrelieved pain rather than with opiate use.
- *Acetaminophen* is an effective analgesic in older adults, although it is ineffective in reducing inflammation. There is an increased risk of end-stage renal disease with long-term use. It does not produce the increased stroke and myocardial infarction risk or gastrointestinal bleeding seen with nonsteroidal anti-inflammatory drugs (NSAIDs).
- Opioids have a greater analgesic effect and longer duration of action for moderate-to-severe pain than non-opioid analgesics. Opioids should be avoided for non-cancer-related chronic pain due to evidence that risks may outweigh the benefits. Risks include increased risk of fractures, hospitalization, and mortality.
- Assess bowel function daily because constipation can be a frequent side effect of opioid use.

Data from Davis, M., & Srivastava, M. (2003). Demographics, assessment and management of pain in the older adult. *Drugs and Aging, 20*(1), 23–35.

are integrative therapies for managing pain. Herbal remedies include cayenne, capsaicin, ginger extract, echinacea, kava, and willow bark. It is important to ask older adults if they are utilizing any alternative treatments for pain relief. Pain-management education is important for both the patient and caregivers. Refer to Chapter 36 for a full discussion of integrative therapies.

It is critical for nurses to evaluate the effectiveness of pain interventions at regular intervals and to be attentive to behavioral changes or verbal responses that indicate that the patient is experiencing pain. It is a common misconception to assume that the ability to perceive pain decreases with aging. No physiological changes in pain perception in older adults have been demonstrated.

HEALTHCARE CONCERNS OF OLDER ADULTS

Financial Burden

Healthcare expenses for older adults are nearly four times higher than the expenses for the rest of the population. With the predicted growth in this population, illness prevention and maintenance of functional ability must be priorities. According to the US Census Bureau (2014), 10% of those 65 and older live below the poverty level ($11,173). There are much higher poverty rates in Hispanic and African American older adults (28% and 22%, respectively) in 2013 (Cubanski et al., 2015).

Medicare Part D has reduced the financial burden of paying for medications. In 2016, Medicare Part D paid 75% of total drug costs after a deductible of up to $360 and a monthly premium are paid (Medicare.gov, 2016). Depending upon the plan chosen by the individual, co-payments (e.g., $10 per prescription) or coinsurance (e.g., 10% of the drug cost) is required. Once out-of-pocket and covered medication expenses reach $3310, the coverage gap (or so-called "donut hole") starts. People are still required to pay monthly premiums during the coverage gap period. Once expenses reach $4850 (not including monthly premiums), catastrophic coverage kicks in. During this period, people pay either a 5% coinsurance for covered drugs or a copay of $2.95 for covered generic drugs and $7.40 for covered brand-name drugs, whichever is greater.

Nurses need to be aware of these financial burdens that impact health practices. Education for seniors regarding availability and use of other resources such as patient assistance programs for expensive medications is crucial. Encourage seniors to ask their physicians and pharmacists about financial assistance for medications. Local advocacy agencies like the AARP or Area Agency on Aging often have free assistance for seniors to help them select a Medicare insurance plan that will best cover their specific medications.

Caregiver Burden

Another phenomenon with the aging population is the increase in caregiver burden. Caregiver burden is the amount of physical, emotional, financial, and psychosocial support provided to a loved one with a chronic illness. One common scenario is a two-income family in the middle of raising children and planning for retirement who are faced with assisting aging parents. This family is sometimes referred to as a sandwich family—sandwiched between two generations. Another is one older adult spouse taking care of the other. Dwindling healthcare benefits, shorter hospital stays, limited home-care options, greater life expectancy, and complicated procedures to access care have increased the need for adult children and aging spouses to provide uncompensated care to loved ones. Due to the stress of this burden, caregivers are at risk for depression and caregiver burnout.

Resources for caregivers include the following the books:

- Mace and Rabins, *The 36-Hour Day*
- Lustbader, *Taking Care of Aging Family Members*

Agencies and associations provide helpful and up-to-date information including medication information, resources, and support groups. These rich resources can be found online. They include:

- AARP
- Alzheimer's Association
- US National Library of Medicine
- Family Caregiver Alliance
- US Department of Veterans Affairs
- Caregiver Action Network
- National Institute on Aging
- Administration on Aging

Unfortunately, having family caregivers is not common for older adults who have a chronic psychiatric disorders. Schizophrenia and bipolar disorders often take a toll on family members and intimate relationships, and it is not uncommon for those with severe mental illness to have no family available for support as they age. Grown children may be estranged because of a parent's frequent hospitalization, poor parenting ability, or paranoid symptoms. The support system of those aging with chronic mental illness often becomes case managers, community nurses, and mental health providers.

Ageism

Western cultures do not generally view growing older as a privilege, and old age does not tend to confer a revered social status upon those who have attained it. **Ageism** is a bias against older people based on advanced age. Ageism differs from other forms of discrimination in that it cuts across gender, race, religion, and socioeconomic status.

Ageism and Public Policy

You can observe the results of ageism in every level of society. Financial and political support for programs geared toward older adults are difficult to obtain. However, groups such as the Gray Panthers and the AARP are powerful governmental lobbying groups that fight to change this disturbing attitude.

Ageism and Research

Traditionally, researchers have used subjects between the ages of 18 and 65. Older adults have been excluded from clinical trials for medication being tested due to polypharmacy or having a chronic illness. Information about medications obtained from a younger, healthier population may not be generalizable to older, sicker adults. In 2012 the FDA issued guidelines that recommended geriatric population be included in clinical trials of medications. The rationale for this recommendation included:

- Trial participants should represent the patient population receiving the therapy.
- People over age 65 make up the majority of patients being treated for chronic conditions.
- This population has age-related physiological changes that can affect the pharmacokinetics of the drug and the pharmacodynamics the drug, which may influence the drug response the dose.

HEALTHCARE DECISION MAKING

Advance Directives

Since the 1960s, people have increasingly sought to participate in decision making about healthcare. In 1990 Congress passed the **Patient Self-Determination Act (PSDA)** (H.R. 4449, 1990) requiring that healthcare facilities provide clearly written information for every patient including legal rights to make healthcare decisions, especially the right to accept or refuse treatment.

PSDA also establishes the right of a person to provide directions, or **advance directives**, for clinicians to follow in the event of a serious illness. Such a directive indicates preferences for the types and amount of medical care desired. The directive comes into effect should physical or mental incapacitation prevent the patient from making healthcare decisions. Patients can communicate these wishes through one or more of the following instruments: (1) a living will, (2) a directive to physician, and (3) a durable power of attorney for healthcare. These documents must be in writing, and the patient's signature must be witnessed. Depending on state and institutional provisions, signatures may need to be documented by a notary.

Every healthcare facility receiving federal funds is required to have written policies, procedures, and protocols in compliance with the PSDA. The law does not specify who talks with patients about treatment decisions, but nurses often discuss these issues with patients. If the advance directive of a patient is not being followed, the nurse is required to intervene on the patient's behalf. Although nurses may discuss options with their patients, they may not assist patients in writing advance directives because this is considered a conflict of interest (Box 31.4).

BOX 31.4 Nurses' Responsibilities and the Patient Self-Determination Act of 1990

Part of Nursing Admission Assessment

- Nurses should know the laws of the state in which [they] practice...and should be familiar with the strengths and limitations of the various forms of the advance directive.
- The American Nurses Association recommends that the following questions be part of the nursing admission assessment:
  1. Do you have basic information about advance care directives, including living wills and durable power of attorney?
  2. Do you wish to initiate an advance care directive?
  3. If you have already prepared an advance care directive, can you provide it now?
  4. Have you discussed your end-of-life choices with your family or designated surrogate and healthcare workers?

Responsibilities of Healthcare Workers Under the Patient Self-Determination Act of 1990

- Hospitals, skilled nursing facilities, home health agencies, hospice organizations, and health maintenance organizations serving Medicare and Medicaid patients must:
  1. Maintain written policies and procedures for providing information to their patients for whom they provide care.
  2. Give written material to patients concerning their rights under state law to make decisions about medical care including the right to accept or refuse surgical or medical care and to formulate advance directives and provide written policies and procedures for the realization of these rights.
  3. Document in patients' records whether they have advance directives.
  4. Not discriminate in care or in other ways against patients who have or have not prepared advance directives.
  5. Make sure that policies are in place to ensure compliance with state laws governing advance directives.

From Schlossberg, C., & Hart, M. A. (1992). Legal perspectives. In M. Burke & M. Walsh (Eds.), *Gerontologic nursing care of the frail older adult* (p. 469). St. Louis, MO: Mosby; American Nurses Association. (1992). Position statement on nursing and the patient self-determination act. Washington, DC: Author.

Living Will

A **living will** is a personal statement of how and where one wishes to die. It is activated only when the person is terminally ill and incapacitated, and a competent patient may alter a living will at any time. The question of whether an incompetent person can change a living will is addressed on a state-by-state basis. Executing a living will does not always guarantee its application.

Directive to Physician

In a **directive to physician**, a physician is appointed to serve as a surrogate medical decision maker, particularly in cases of terminal illness when an individual has no family. There needs to be verification of terminal illness by two physicians, and the patient must be competent at the time of signing. The physician must agree in writing to be the patient's agent and must also be one of the two physicians who made the original determination that the patient is terminally ill. Unlike the living will, the patient can revoke the directive to physician orally at any time without regard to patient competency.

Durable Power of Attorney for Healthcare

The **durable power of attorney for healthcare** is the designation of a person to act as the patient's medical decision maker. The patient must be competent when making the appointment and must also be competent to revoke the power. Individuals do not have to be terminally ill or incompetent to allow the empowered individual to act on their behalf.

Guardianship

A **guardianship** is a court-ordered relationship in which one party, the guardian, acts on behalf of an individual, the ward. For a guardianship to be enacted, the ward must be lacking capacity to manage personal and/or financial affairs. After an evaluation, usually by a physician or psychologist, probate court determines if guardianship is necessary. Many people with mental illness, mental retardation, traumatic brain injuries, and organic brain disorders such as dementia have guardians. It is important that healthcare workers identify patients who have guardians and communicate with the guardians when healthcare decisions are being made.

The Nurse's Role in Decision Making

The nurse is often responsible for explaining the legal policies of the institution to both the patient and family and can help them understand advance directives. There are usually three common approaches to care:

1. **Full code:** All life-saving measures are initiated.
2. **Do not resuscitate–comfort care arrest (DNR-CCA):** All life-saving measures are initiated except in the case of a full cardiac arrest and intubation.
3. **Do not resuscitate–comfort care only (DNR-CCO):** Medical care focuses on providing pain-free quality of life and comfort free of invasive procedures and intubation.

Ethical dilemmas can occur in regard to these life or death decisions. For example, when a patient has a feeding tube and a DNR–CCO status is later initiated, do we remove the feeding tube? Hospital bioethics committees can assist by looking at the situation objectively.

NURSING CARE OF OLDER ADULTS

Nurses encounter older adults in a variety of settings. In each of these settings, the nurse is responsible for applying the nursing process in a patient-centered way. Some nursing students are not given adequate information and are not exposed to older patients, and they may hold ageist views when beginning nursing careers (Chippendale, 2015). It is vital for nurses to provide respect to older patients and appreciate their wisdom and life experience. Positive attitudes toward older adults and their care can be promoted and instilled during basic nursing education.

There are many theories about the process of aging from biological, genetic, psychological, and psychosocial perspectives (Box 31.5). Substantial literature is available regarding what shortens the life expectancy and on behaviors that predispose

BOX 31.5 Major Theories of Aging

Biological

- **Cellular functioning:** Cells accumulate damage resulting in errors of replication.
- **Error theory:** Error in protein synthesis results in impaired cellular function.
- **Oxidative stress theory:** Production of free radicals increases and the body's ability to remove them decreases, resulting in DNA damage.
- **Wear-and-tear theory:** Internal and external stressors harm cells.
- **Programmed aging theory:** Biological or genetic clock plays out on genes.
- **Neuroendocrine theory:** A programmed decline in the functioning of the nervous, endocrine, and immune systems where cells lose their ability to reproduce.
- **Immunity theory:** An accumulation of damage and decline in the immune system.

Developmental

- **Jung's theory of personality:** Individuals move from outward achievement to self-acceptance.
- **Erikson:** Integrity is built on morality and ethics.
- **Peck:** Redefining self, letting go of occupational identity, rising above body discomforts, and establishing meaning, accompanies successful aging.
- **Maslow:** Self-actualization and the evolution of developmental needs occur as the individual ages.
- **Tornstam:** Disengagement with the world can be a time of introspection leading to wisdom.

Psychosocial

- **Role theory:** The ability of an individual to adapt to changing roles predicts adjustment to aging.
- **Activity theory:** Actions, roles, and social pursuits are important for satisfactory aging.
- **Disengagement theory:** Mutual withdrawal occurs between the aging person and others.
- **Continuity theory:** Life satisfaction and activity are expressions of enduring personality traits.
- **Age-stratification theory:** Individuals are viewed as members of an age group (e.g., young, middle-age, old) with similarities to others in the group.
- **Modernization theory:** Modern society devalues the contributions of elders and elders themselves.

Data from Jett, K. (2015). Theories of aging. In E. A. Touhy & K. Jett (Eds.). *Ebersole & Hess' toward healthy aging: Human needs and nursing response* (9th ed.) (pp. 31–39). St. Louis, MO: Elsevier.

BOX 31.6 Facts and Myths About Aging

Facts

- The senses of vision, hearing, touch, taste, and smell decline with age.
- Muscular strength decreases with age. Muscle fibers atrophy and decrease in number.
- Regular sexual expressions are important to maintain sexual capacity and effective sexual performance.
- At least 50% of restorative sleep is lost as a result of the aging process.
- Older adults are major consumers of prescription drugs because of the high incidence of chronic diseases in this population.
- Older adults have a high incidence of depression.
- Many individuals experience difficulty when they retire.
- Older adults are prone to become victims of crime.
- Older widows appear to adjust better than younger ones.

Myths

- Most adults past the age of 65 have dementia.
- Sexual interest declines with age.
- Older adults are unable to learn new tasks.
- As individuals age, they become more rigid in their thinking and set in their ways.
- The aged are well off and no longer impoverished.
- Most older adults are infirm and require help with daily activities.
- Most older adults are socially isolated and lonely.

humans to disease. Current trends center on the concept of aging well and how aging well can be accomplished. Nursing is about maintenance of health, prevention of illness, and helping individuals with their response to disease. There is a growing focus on healthy eating, exercise, socialization, spirituality, effective coping skills, avoiding alcohol/tobacco, and healthy relationships as a basis for aging well. Nurses can play a vital role in this movement as educators and advocates for health.

Box 31.6 provides some facts and myths about aging that influence how society perceives the older adult.

Assessment

Nurses who work with older adults need specific knowledge about normal aging, drug interactions, and chronic disease. Those who work with older patients who have mental health problems or cognitive deficits need to have additional skills in effective communication, behavioral intervention, and recognition of how the care setting affects the older individual. The National Institutes of Health recommends a comprehensive geriatric assessment. This comprehensive assessment includes a focus on physical and mental health; functional, economic, and social status; and environmental factors that might impinge on the person's well-being. Fig. 31.5 provides an example of a comprehensive geriatric assessment.

Assessment Strategies with Older Adults

An examination and interview of an older adult conducted in unfamiliar surroundings can produce anxiety. Unlike younger patients who may be comfortable discussing personal issues—family conflicts, feelings of sadness, sexual practices, finances, and bodily functions—older adults may view these topics as private or taboo. As a result, they may be uncomfortable discussing them. It is important to respect these feelings while reviewing essential history by:

- Conducting the interview in a private area.
- Introducing oneself and asking the patient what he or she would like to be called (unless you are an older adult, the use of the first name is rarely appropriate unless you are invited to do so).
- Establishing rapport and putting the patient at ease by sitting or standing at the same level as the patient.
- Ensuring that lighting is adequate and noise level is low in recognition of the fact that hearing and vision may be impaired.
- Using touch (with permission) to convey warmth while at the same time respecting the patient's comfort level with personal touch.
- Summarizing the interaction, inviting feedback and questions, and thanking patients for giving their time and information.

Physical Assessment

A thorough assessment, including a physical assessment and diagnostic testing, must precede any treatment and/or diagnosis of a mental illness in older adults. Common tests include thyroid, kidney, and liver function; complete blood count; comprehensive metabolic panel; vitamin B_{12}, folic acid, and therapeutic drug levels; urinalysis; serology (RPR); β-type natriuretic peptide (BNP); HIV testing; and computed tomography (CT) of the head when indicated.

Medication Reconciliation

In older adults, it is important to perform a systematic review of current medication use known as **medication reconciliation**. Medication reconciliation is the process of developing the most accurate list possible of all medications a patient is taking. This list should include drug name, dose, frequency, and route. The purpose of this process is to reduce adverse incidents, side effects, and potentially lethal combinations.

Assessing the use of multiple medications (**polypharmacy**) includes prescription, over-the-counter drugs, and herbal agents. **Adverse drug reactions** or negative responses to drugs are common among the older adult. Older adults are at greater risk for these events due to multiple medical problems and memory issues that may result in taking too little or too much medication. Renal and liver impairment affect excretion and are associated with dose-related adverse reactions.

Metabolic changes and decreased drug clearance compound the risk of drug-drug interactions. The risk of adverse drug reactions doubles for people taking five to seven medications as compared with those taking fewer than five medications (Onder et al., 2010). For people taking eight or more medications, the risk of adverse drug reactions increases by four times. The American Geriatrics Society (2015) recently updated the criteria for and list of potentially inappropriate medications for older adults. Many psychiatric medications appear on the list including benzodiazepines, anticholinergics, antipsychotics, antidepressants, antiepileptics, and antiparkinson drugs. Nurses must be diligent in reviewing senior's medication lists for completeness.

COMPREHENSIVE GERIATRIC ASSESSMENT				
Name:		Date of birth:		Gender:
Physical Health				
Chronic disorder				
Vision	Adequate Inadequate	Eyeglasses: Y N		Needs evaluation
Hearing	Adequate Inadequate	Hearing aids: Y N		
Mobility	Ambulatory: Y N	Assistive device:		
	Falls: Y N			Needs evaluation
Nutrition	Albumin:	TLC:	HCT:	
	Weight:	Weight loss or gain: Y N		Needs evaluation
Incontinence	Y N	Treatment:	Y N	Needs evaluation
Medications	Total number:	Reviewed & revised:	Y N	
	Adverse effects/allergy:			
Screening	Cholesterol:	TSH:	B_{12}:	Folate:
	Colonoscopy: Date:		N/A	
	Mammogram: Date:		N/A	
	Osteoporosis: Date:		N/A	
	Pap smear: Date:		N/A	
	PSA: Date:		N/A	
Immunization	Influenza: Date:			
	Pneumonia: Date:			
	Tetanus: Date:		Booster:	
Counseling	Diet Exercise	Calcium	Vitamin D	
	Smoking Alcohol	Driving	Injury prevention	
Mental Health				
Dementia	Y N	MMSE score:	Date:	Cause (if known):
Depression	Y N	GDS score:	Date:	Treatment: Y N
Functional Status				
ADL	Bathing: I D	Dressing: I D		Toileting: I D
	Transferring: I D	Feeding: I D		Continence: Y N

FIG. 31.5 Comprehensive geriatric assessment. *ADL,* Activities of daily living; B_{12}, vitamin B_{12}; *D,* dependent; *GDS,* Geriatric Depression Scale; *HCT,* hematocrit; *I,* independent; *MMSE,* Mini-Mental State Examination; *N,* no; *PSA,* prostate-specific antigen; *TLC,* total lymphocyte count; *TSH,* thyroid-stimulating hormone; *Y,* yes.

Prescribing cascades happen when drug-induced symptoms are treated with another drug. The provider may assess the side effect of the first drug as part of the original medical problem or a new one. Prescribing cascades are particularly problematic and complicated. One of the most common examples is when a person begins antiparkinson therapy for symptoms brought about by antipsychotics. Antiparkinson drugs may bring about new and dangerous symptoms such as delirium and orthostatic hypotension. Anticholinesterase inhibitor drugs used to treat dementia (e.g., donepezil, rivastigmine, and galantamine) may cause urinary incontinence and diarrhea. These symptoms may result in a prescribing cascade with use of an anticholinergic such as oxybutynin, which can cause cognitive dulling and confusion.

Pharmacists have begun to play a critical role in reviewing and advising on matters of prescribing for the older adult. The American Geriatrics Society (2015) has updated the Beers List and Criteria, which was developed in 1991 to identify inappropriate medications for the older adult. Maher et al. (2014) identify how polypharmacy affects the older adult. They cite nine negative clinical consequences of inappropriate drug use:

1. Increased healthcare costs
2. Adverse drug reactions
3. Drug interactions
4. Nonadherence
5. Decline in functional status
6. Increased cognitive impairment
7. Increased falls
8. Increased urinary incontinence
9. Increased risk of malnutrition

Common problems associated with medication include confusion, which can be caused by anticholinergics, antihistamines, and benzodiazepines. Psychosis has been linked to the use of levodopa, steroids, and even cholesterol-lowering medications. Depressive symptoms have been linked with alpha-adrenergics and opiates.

Mental Status Exam

Assessment of the cognitive, behavioral, and emotional status of the older adult is important in managing the nursing care of the patient. The periodic repetition of screening tools serves to evaluate the effectiveness of interventions targeting mood problems. The Geriatric Depression Scale (Short Form; Box 31.7) is a subjective yes/no questionnaire and the Cornell Scale for Depression in Dementia is an objective behavioral checklist for caregivers to help identify the presence of depressive symptoms (Alexopoulos, 1988). It's also important to recognize that having thoughts or wishes of death may occur during times of acute medical illness or emotional distress. So it is essential to further assess for suicidal intent and/or plans by asking questions such as:

- Have you ever thought about ending your life or wish you didn't wake up?
- Have you ever felt that life is not worth living?
- Have you ever tried to hurt yourself in the past?
- Are you looking for ways to harm yourself?
- Do you have thoughts of harming others?
- Do you have any means to harm yourself or others? Weapons? Large amounts of medication? (This may need to be asked to family members, as well.)

At times when individuals—older adults included—are sick or are in significant pain, they may verbalize a death wish by saying "I just wish I would die" or "If I had a gun, I'd shoot myself." This should never be ignored; rather it needs to be explored. Often people just feel frustrated, desperate, ignored, unheard, or disrespected, but they aren't able to articulate these emotions. Encourage the individual to say more about what he or she is experiencing, get more information, provide active listening, and offer support. These types of statements and data need to be documented and reported to the care provider. If there are active

BOX 31.7 Geriatric Depression Scale (Short Form)

Geriatric Depression Scale: Short Form: Choose the best answer for how you have felt over the past week:

1. Are you basically satisfied with your life? YES / **NO**
2. Have you dropped many of your activities and interests? **YES** / NO
3. Do you feel that your life is empty? **YES** / NO
4. Do you often get bored? YES / **NO**
5. Are you in good spirits most of the time? YES / **NO**
6. Are you afraid that something bad is going to happen to you? **YES** / NO
7. Do you feel happy most of the time? YES / **NO**
8. Do you often feel helpless? **YES** / NO
9. Do you prefer to stay at home, rather than going out and doing new things? **YES** / NO
10. Do you feel you have more problems with memory than most? **YES** / NO
11. Do you think it is wonderful to be alive now? YES / **NO**
12. Do you feel pretty worthless the way you are now? **YES** / NO
13. Do you feel full of energy? YES / **NO**
14. Do you feel that your situation is hopeless? **YES** / NO
15. Do you think that most people are better off than you are? **YES** / NO

Answers in bold indicate depression. Score 1 point for each bolded answer. A score > 5 points is suggestive of depression. A score ≥ 10 points is almost always indicative of depression. A score > 5 points should warrant a follow-up comprehensive assessment.

From Greenberg, S. H. (2012). *Geriatric Depression Scale (GDS)*. Hartford Institute for Geriatric Nursing, NYU College of Nursing. Retrieved from https://consultgeri.org/try-this/general-assessment/issue-4.pdf.

suicidal thoughts and intent, the individual should not be left alone. Elicit help from other staff and the mental health team.

Interventions for the prevention of suicide in older adults are discussed in greater depth later in this chapter. Also refer to Chapter 25 for a more detailed discussion of suicide assessment and intervention.

Driving and the Older Adult

Older adults living in the community may still be driving, which can become a safety concern for caregivers, family, and the public. If there is evidence an older adult can no longer safely drive a vehicle (e.g., failing visual acuity, hearing loss, cognitive deficits, impaired mobility, or movement disorders such as Parkinson's disease) or if there have been occurrences of frequent small collisions or getting lost, it is appropriate to consult with medical providers about further assessment. At times, it's appropriate to notify the state bureau of motor vehicles for a driving evaluation to determine ability for safe operation of a vehicle. Other times, family can be encouraged to facilitate having seniors give up the keys to the car or disable a car so it won't run in the best interest of public safety.

CONSIDERING CULTURE

Keeping Jose at Home

Jose is a 75-year-old married man born and raised in Puerto Rico. He came to the United States in his 20s, served in the military, and worked in the steel industry until retirement. Jose was active in his church and served as the treasurer for many years. He was head of a family with five daughters in a traditional patriarchal home. Jose's wife never worked outside the home, did not drive, and spoke little English, despite having been in the United States most of her adult life.

The family began to notice significant changes in Jose's behavior and function. His primary care provider ruled out physical illness, and Jose was referred for Alzheimer's disease evaluation.

His wife and eldest daughter, Maria, accompanied him for the evaluation. Jose was pleasant and cooperative. His daughter helped to interpret when necessary.

Jose's wife and Maria were most alarmed by Jose's withdrawal from church activities after experiencing an inability to manage his treasurer duties. He also lost interest in activities, had difficulty organizing his day, and needed reminders to shave and shower. Evaluation revealed a moderate to severe cognitive impairment.

Despite being instructed not to drive, his daughters were not willing to take the keys as this would be disrespectful. Eventually, Jose was pulled over by police due to erratic driving. He was agitated at the time and was briefly hospitalized.

Recognizing the potential danger in driving, his family devised a solution. They disabled the car. This allowed Jose to maintain his authority, keep the keys, yet prevented him from driving.

Jose's wife and daughters made sure Jose took his medication, had proper nutrition, and was able to maintain his daily routine. Jose eventually stopped speaking English and reverted to his primary language. Although the dementia progressed over the next 5 years, he was never placed in long-term care. His family continued to care for him until the end.

Older Adult Abuse

Abuse or exploitation is another area to explore during a nursing assessment. Questions about being hit, pushed, kicked, and slapped are important. It is also imperative to inquire about care being withheld. Not being fed, cleaned, helped, or cared for is also abuse. Asking "How are you being treated at home?" or "Are you afraid of anyone?" may encourage further exploration. Financial exploitation is another issue that is difficult to uncover. Older adults may feel ashamed or embarrassed to admit they have been taken advantage of by family, friends, or strangers. Box 31.8 provides helpful interview techniques to use with older adults. The topic of older adult violence is discussed in depth in Chapter 28.

Intervention

The trend for patient-centered care, relationship-based care, and the patient as a participant in care may be foreign concepts to the older adult. Most have experienced medical care as "listening to the doctor" regardless of whether or not they agree. This shift in approach may need much reinforcement with the older adult who has been socialized as a passive recipient of healthcare.

Certain psychotherapeutic methods are especially useful for older adults:

- Providing empathetic understanding and active listening
- Encouraging ventilation of feelings and normalizing emotional responses
- Reestablishing emotional equilibrium when anxiety is moderate to severe
- Providing health education, discussing alternative solutions, and encouraging questions
- Assisting in the use of problem-solving approaches
- Allowing adequate time to process information
- Ensuring hearing aids are working or using an amplifier to facilitate good communication
- Providing written information in large print

BOX 31.8 Helpful Techniques for Interviewing Older Adults

- Gather preliminary data before the session and keep questionnaires relatively short.
- Ask about often-overlooked problems such as difficulty sleeping, incontinence, falling, depression, dizziness, or loss of energy.
- Pace the interview to allow the patient to formulate answers; resist the tendency to interrupt prematurely.
- Use yes-or-no or simple-choice questions if the older patient has trouble coping with open-ended questions.
- Begin with general questions such as, "How can I help you most at this visit?" or "What's been happening?"
- Be alert for information on the patient's relationships with others, thoughts about families or co-workers, typical responses to stress, and attitudes toward aging, illness, occupation, and death.
- A request such as, "Tell me about how you spend your days" often provides important information.
- Assess mental status for deficits in recent or remote memory and determine if confusion exists.
- Be aware of all medications the patient is taking, and assess for side effects, efficacy, and possible drug interactions.
- Determine how fast the condition of the patient has been changing to assess the extent of the patient's concerns.
- Include the family or significant other in the interview process for added input, clarification, support, and reinforcement.

From National Institute on Aging. (2012). *Talking with your older patient: A clinician's handbook.* Retrieved from http://www.nia.nih.gov/health/publication/talking-your-older-patient-clinicians-handbook.

Psychosocial Interventions

The nurse uses counseling skills to assist the patient with exploring the present situation, looking at alternatives, and planning for the future. Sometimes counseling is provided in a group setting. This approach helps build relationships, provides focus on the here and now, and reduces feelings of isolation.

There is growing evidence that physical and mental exercise helps maintain and improve cognitive function. Nurses can encourage this activity with cognitive stimulation activities, which may be conducted individually or in groups of five to eight people (Woods et al., 2012). This evidence-based approach may result in significant improvement in language skills. Examples of cognitively stimulating activities are word games, puzzles, music, and discussion of past events.

Reminiscence is a cognitive stimulation activity that engages seniors in socialization and rapport building. In groups or individually, the nurse can encourage discussion about past pleasant events or memories such as first car, favorite memory from school, favorite band or song, or seasonal activities growing up. Assisting to evoke pleasant feelings or memories is an effective method to improve mood particularly in those with memory impairment.

Psychobiological Interventions

Pharmacological. Evidence about the biology of mental illness and the discovery of new psychotropic medications has expanded the role of the geropsychiatric nurse. Nurses play a vital role in monitoring, reporting, and managing medication side effects such as acute dystonia, akathisia, pseudoparkinsonism, neuroleptic malignant syndrome (NMS), serotonin syndrome, and anticholinergic effects. Physical assessment of response to medication is also important; this includes monitoring vital signs, pain, laboratory work, elimination (bowel and bladder), changes in gait, prevention of falls, and neurological checks when appropriate. Teaching patients and/or family about management of medications is a vital part of nursing care (Box 31.9).

Advanced-Practice Interventions

Psychiatric-mental health advanced practice registered nurses may provide individual and/or group psychotherapy to older adults. Individual modalities such as cognitive-behavioral therapy, motivational interviewing, interpersonal therapy, and psychodynamic therapy are commonly used. Group therapy focuses on instilling hope by diminishing social isolation and loneliness. Group members can learn creative ways to improve mood and increase quality of life.

Treatment Settings for Older Adults

Care for older adults may become unmanageable at home. Medical providers are responsible for determining an appropriate level of care. This may range from acute hospitalization, to skilled nursing care facility, to adult day care, to community-based programs, or to respite care. A discussion of several care settings follows.

Geropsychiatric Units

An older adult may require acute inpatient psychiatric healthcare for conditions such as acute mental status changes with agitation, psychotic symptoms, major depression with suicidal intent, bipolar disorder, and schizophrenia. Inpatient treatment is recommended when the patient is at risk of self-harm, whether intentional or unintentional, or poses a risk of harm to other people.

BOX 31.9 Patient and Family Teaching: Drug Safety

- Learn about your medicines: Read medicine labels and package inserts and follow the directions.
- If you have questions, ask your nurse, pharmacist, or primary care provider.
- Talk to your team of healthcare professionals about your medical conditions, health concerns, and all the medicines you take (prescription and over-the-counter medicines), as well as dietary supplements, vitamins, and herbal supplements. The more they know, the more they can help.
- Keep track of side effects or possible drug interactions, and let your doctor know right away about any unexpected symptoms or changes in the way you feel.
- Be sure to keep all care provider appointments.
- Use a calendar, pillbox, or something to help you remember what medications you need to take and when.
- Write down information your healthcare provider gives you about your medicines or your health condition.
- Take a friend or relative to your doctor's appointments if you think you need help to understand or remember what the doctor tells you.
- Have a "medicine check-up" at least once a year. Go through your medicine cabinet to get rid of old or expired medicines.
- Ask your healthcare provider or pharmacist to go over all the medicines you now take. Remember to tell them about all the over-the-counter medicines, vitamins, dietary supplements, and herbal supplements you take.

Hospitalization may be an opportunity for the patient to receive much-needed assessment of the skin, feet, hair, mouth, and perineal areas. These assessments often can uncover hidden infections, unhealed wounds, and growths that may otherwise have been missed and can lead to needed medical attention.

Specialized geropsychiatric units provide a comprehensive and specialized approach to care. These units utilize a multidisciplinary approach to assessment, treatment planning, implementation, and evaluation of care. Ideally, the team consists of registered nurses, geriatric psychiatrists, geriatricians, social workers, pharmacists, psychologists, dietitians, occupational therapists, and physical therapists.

One of the major roles of the nurse is milieu management. This involves assisting in adjustment to the environment, keeping the unit safe by making sure roommates are compatible, call lights are within reach, and patients at risk for falling are close to the nurses' station.

Recognizing the tone of the unit and making modifications when needed, such as reducing noise levels and de-cluttering areas, are critical roles of the staff nurse. Another vital aspect of nursing is the prevention and reduction of agitation by maintaining a visible presence on the unit and anticipating the patient's needs. Crisis intervention techniques may be necessary if an agitated patient does not respond to redirection or verbal attempts to deescalate agitation. As a crisis situation unfolds, staff response will largely determine the outcome, and a well-trained crisis team improves these outcomes. The crisis team leader is usually a nurse for several reasons:

1. Nurses provide professional care 24 hours a day, 7 days a week, and have detailed knowledge of patients and the milieu.
2. The nurse is aware of the patient's medical condition.
3. The nurse is able to guide the team and help prevent injury to patients who may need physical restraint.

After the crisis has been deescalated, the team leader, the team, and other patients (as indicated) need to discuss the situation; this will help restore a sense of safety and calm. As the agitated patient gains control, it is important to help the individual ease back into the milieu with dignity.

Skilled Nursing Facilities

As acute hospital care of older adults with psychiatric illnesses is decreasing, the use of long-term skilled nursing facilities is increasing. The use of these facilities to treat older adults with severe mental illness is controversial. Opponents fear that skilled nursing facilities will become the psychiatric institutions of the 21st century, providing little more than custodial care.

Whereas some long-term care settings provide specialized psychiatric-mental healthcare or behavioral units, most do not. There may be little consistency in the education of nurses and nursing assistants in appropriate psychiatric assessment and intervention. Staff may believe that patients who refuse personal hygiene, medication, or wound care are exercising their rights to refuse care rather than recognizing the negative symptoms of schizophrenia or depression. Nurses who repeatedly accept these refusals without further evaluation may inadvertently contribute to a patient's deterioration.

Federal legislation has had a significant impact on the treatment of older adults in extended-care facilities. The PSDA of 1990 declared that nursing-home residents have the right to be free from unnecessary drugs and physical restraints. Clinicians have begun to focus on the use of nonpharmacological interventions for the treatment of agitation, wandering, confusion, yelling, and aggression. Drugs that are avoided include antipsychotics, antidepressants, antianxiety agents, and sedatives.

Nurses can play an important role in advocating for psychiatric evaluation and intervention to assist with (1) medication management, (2) monitoring and documenting behavioral issues, (3) notifying the physician of behavioral changes, and (4) planning care for the needs of those residents with mental illness.

Due to past inappropriate use of restraints, which led to injuries and deaths, federal legislation regarding their safe use was put into place. The requirements governing the use of restraints include the following:

1. Consultation with a physical and/or occupational therapist.
2. The least restrictive measures must be considered and documented.
3. A physician's order is required.
4. Consent of the resident or family must be obtained.
5. Documentation must be provided that the restraint enables the resident to maintain maximum functional and psychological well-being.

Assisted Living

This setting is utilized when a resident needs minimal assistance with ADLs. Meals are provided as well as 24-hour assistance as needed. Care is tailored to the needs of the resident, and care is paid for based on needs. This level of care is usually not covered by insurance and can be quite expensive. There are waiver programs in some states that provide for Medicaid reimbursement.

Respite Care

Family caregivers are at great risk for burnout. Respite care is designed to allow caregivers to have a break for a specific number of days. During this time, the patient is admitted to a nursing facility for a planned number of days. Family can then go on vacation, travel, or just have a needed break from caregiving. Respite care can also be provided in the home as well.

Residential Care

As discussed in Chapter 4, the psychiatric care system has increasingly become focused on the goal of community living rather than institutional living, but resources necessary to meet this goal have been chronically underfunded. Patients who would benefit from residential care are often moved from the most structured environment (inpatient care) to unstructured environments. These settings vary greatly and families and guardians should be educated to investigate what specific services will be provided.

Partial Hospitalization

Partial hospitalization programs are recommended for ambulatory patients who do not need 24-hour nursing care. They provide structured activities along with nursing and medical supervision, intervention, and treatment. These programs tend to be located within general hospitals, in psychiatric hospitals, or as part of the community mental health system.

Day Care Programs

Multipurpose senior centers provide a broad range of services including: (1) health promotion and wellness programs; (2) health screening; (3) social, educational, and recreational activities; (4) meals; and (5) information and referral services. For those in need of mostly custodial care services, **adult day care** is an appropriate choice. Older adults are cared for during the day and stay in a home environment at night. The programs allow older adults to continue their present living arrangements and maintain their social ties to the community; they also relieve families of the burden of 24-hour-a-day care for older adult dependents.

Home Healthcare

Home-based healthcare assists the homebound older adult to adjust to and manage illness and disability either before or after hospitalization. It is often the role of the health homecare nurse to help a person affected by a cognitive disorder, medical illness, or a severe and persistent mental illness to remain in the home. The National Association of Area Agencies on Aging assists in providing local home care services, such as housekeeping, meal preparation, and assistance with ADLs, to increase the older adult's ability to live independently. Chapter 4 discusses home psychiatric-mental healthcare in greater detail.

Community-Based Programs

Community-based programs are an alternative to promote the older adult's independent functioning and reduce the stress on the family system. These programs provide specialized case management services that assist older adults with coordination of care and other supports, such as Meals on Wheels and transportation.

KEY POINTS TO REMEMBER

- The older adult population is increasing exponentially.
- The increase in the number of older adults poses a challenge not only to nurses but also to the entire healthcare system to respond to the special needs of this population.
- Attitudes toward older adults are often negative, reflecting ageism—a bias against older adults based solely on age. Ageism occurs at all levels of society and even among healthcare providers, which affects the way we render care to our older patients.
- Maintaining a positive regard that demonstrates respect will improve interactions with older adults.
- Nurses who care for older adults in various settings may function at different levels. All should be knowledgeable about the process of aging and be aware of the differences between normal and abnormal aging changes.
- The Patient Self-Determination Act established guidelines and a philosophy of care that call for patients to be free from unnecessary use of drugs and physical restraints.

- The use of more than five medications doubles the risk of an adverse reaction.
- Accurate pain assessment is important, and the nurse must remember that older adults tend to understate their pain.
- Nurses working with older adult patients with concurrent mental health problems should be knowledgeable about psychotherapeutic approaches relevant for the older adult.
- When it comes to dying and death, older adults' wishes and those of their families are frequently ignored. The implementation of the Patient Self-Determination Act, passed in 1990, allows patients autonomy and dignity in death.
- A variety of treatment settings are available to older adults. The level of disability, cognitive abilities, and psychiatric disorders influence the choice of setting.

CRITICAL THINKING

1. Mr. Jackson, a 70-year-old African American, has received treatment for alcohol withdrawal. He is quiet, refuses to eat, does not sleep at night, and admits to wishing he would die. He also confides that he attempted suicide when his wife died 5 years earlier, and that is when he started drinking heavily.
   - **a.** Culturally, what may be helpful to know about older African Americans' response to depression?
   - **b.** Which depression assessment tool is appropriate to use in assessing the severity of Mr. Jackson's condition? Explain your answer.
2. Mrs. Duff is 75 years old and lives with her daughter's family. She has moderate-advanced Alzheimer's disease. Although Mrs. Duff's family wants to keep her at home for as long as possible, they are overwhelmed by her needs and unable to leave her alone.
   - **a.** What community supports might be best for Mrs. Duff? Explain your answer.

CHAPTER REVIEW

Questions

1. During an interview with a patient, which question asked of an older adult is associated with the Patient Self-Determination Act?
   - **a.** "Who besides yourself may have access to your medical information?"
   - **b.** "Have you discussed your end-of-life choices with your family or designated surrogate?"
   - **c.** "Do you have the information you need to make an informed decision about your treatment?"
   - **d.** "How can I help you feel comfortable about this interview and any decisions you need to make?"
2. Which statement made by a nurse requires immediate correction by the supervisor?
   - **a.** "Many older patients are depressed."
   - **b.** "Retirement is a difficult time for older patients."
   - **c.** "Cognitive decline is normal in patients who are 65 and older."
   - **d.** "Sleep-related problems are often reported by older adults."
3. Considering psychosocial role theory, which patient demonstrates healthy adjustment to aging?
   - **a.** The 70-year-old who is training for a 5-mile running race
   - **b.** The older adult who controls diabetes with diet and exercise
   - **c.** The retiree who volunteers 3 days a week at the local library
   - **d.** The 80-year-old who is upbeat and hopeful during chemotherapy for lung cancer
4. The older patient is discussing chronic pain and asks the primary care provider for a prescription. Which medication should the nurse anticipate being ordered rather than an opioid?
   - **a.** Gabapentin
   - **b.** Acetaminophen
   - **c.** Morphine
   - **d.** Fentanyl
5. Which statement by an older patient with a mild neurocognitive disorder demonstrates a safe response to beginning a new medication?
   - **a.** "I read the information the pharmacist gave me when I got the prescription filled."
   - **b.** "My daughter comes with me to appointments so that we get all the information we need."
   - **c.** "I know I can call my doctor if I think of any questions later."
   - **d.** "I always follow the instructions on the medication bottle."
6. Anxiety problems in older adults can manifest as a fear of falling, greatly influencing an older adult's personal freedom. A home health nurse checking on a patient with mild dementia and anxiety related to falling should question which new order?
   - **a.** Yoga and tai-chi
   - **b.** Xanax
   - **c.** Relaxation techniques
   - **d.** Electric wheelchair
7. Fred is an older adult with spinal stenosis and who is being treated with a short-term prescription of opioids for an acute episode of back pain. His nurse recognizes additional teaching is necessary when Fred states:
   - **a.** "Sitting up straight seems to reduce the pain."
   - **b.** "Sometimes I use a heating pad on my back."
   - **c.** "Once I get moving for the day my pain gets better."
   - **d.** "My wife and I share my Norco for our aches and pains."
8. Ling works as a registered nurse in an Alzheimer's care home. Ling has a specialized rapport-building technique she uses called reminiscence. She uses this technique by:
   - **a.** Telling the residents stories about her grandparents' lives.
   - **b.** Playing music from the residents' formative years.
   - **c.** Reviewing movies that the residents enjoy.
   - **d.** Encouraging the residents to talk about pleasurable past events.

9. Marco, age 83, has dementia and difficulty feeding himself despite the fact that there is nothing wrong with his motor functions. Which term should the nurse use to document this finding?
   a. Aphasia
   b. Apraxia
   c. Agnosia
   d. Disinhibition anergia
10. You are caring for Ellie, age 91, whose provider has written a "DNR-CCO" order. Which nursing action would be appropriate if Ellie were to go into cardiac arrest?
   a. Immediately call for the code team
   b. Notify the attending physician and family of the change in status
   c. Administer prescribed medication morphine for pain control
   d. Initiate cardiopulmonary resuscitation

Answers

1. **b**; 2. **c**; 3. **c**; 4. **a**; 5. **b**; 6. **b**; 7. **d**; 8. **d**; 9. **b**; 10. **b**

Visit the Evolve website for a posttest on the content in this chapter: http://evolve.elsevier.com/Varcarolis

Post-Test interactive review

REFERENCES

Administration on Aging. (2013). *A profile of older Americans: 2014*. Retrieved from http://www.aoa.acl.gov/aging_statistics/profile/2014/docs/2014-profile.pdf.

Alexopoulos, G. S. (1988). Cornell scale for depression in dementia. *Biological Psychiatry*, *23*(3), 271–284.

American Foundation for Suicide Prevention. (2016). *Suicide statistics*. Retrieved from http://afsp.org/about-suicide/suicide-statistics/.

American Geriatrics Society. (2015). Updated Beers criteria for potentially inappropriate medication use in older adults. *Journal of American Geriatric Society*, *63*, 2227–2246.

American Society of Pain Management Nursing. (2016). *Prescribing and administering opioid doses based solely on pain intensity*. Retrieved from http://www.aspmn.org/Documents/Position%20Statements/Dose_Numbers_PP_Final.pdf.

Anderson, S. L., Sebastiani, P., Dworkis, et al. (2012). Health span approximates life span among many supercentenarians: Compression of morbidity at the approximate limit of life span. *Journals of Gerontology*, *67A*(4), 395–405.

Centers for Disease Control and Prevention. (2015). *Suicide: Facts at a glance*. Retrieved from http://www.cdc.gov/violenceprevention/pdf/suicide-datasheet-a.PDF.

Chippendale, T. (2015). Factors associated with interest in working with older adults: implications for educational practices. *Journal of Nursing Education*, *54*(9), S89–93.

Cubanski, J., Casillas, G., & Damico, A. (2015). *Poverty among seniors: Updated analysis of national and state level poverty rates under the official and supplemental poverty measures. Kaiser Family Foundation Issue Brief*. Retrieved from http://files.kff.org/attachment/issue-brief-poverty-among-seniors-an-updated-analysis-of-national-and-state-level-poverty-rates-under-the-official-and-supplemental-poverty-measures.

De Gage, S. B., Moride, Y., Duccruet, T., et al. (2014). Benzodiazepine use and risk of Alzheimer's disease: Case-control study. *BMJ*, *349*, g5205.

Denkinger, M. D., Lukas, A., Nikolaus, T., & Hauer, K. (2015). Factors associated with fear of falling and associated activity restriction in community-dwelling older adults. *The American Journal of Geriatric Psychiatry*, *23*(1), 72–86.

Goesling, J., Clauw, D., & Hassett, A. (2013). Pain and depression: An integrated review of neurobiological and psychological factors. *Current Psychiatry Reports*, *15*, 421.

Horgas, A. L., Yoon, S. L., & Grall, M. (2012). Pain management. In M. Boltz, E. Capezuti, T. Fulmer, & D. Zwicker (Eds.), *Evidence-based geriatric nursing protocols for best practice* (4th ed.). New York, NY: Springer.

H.R. 4449. (1990). *Patient self-determination act of 1990*. Retrieved from https://www.congress.gov/bill/101st-congress/house-bill/4449.

Karlamangla, A., Zhou, K., Reuben, D., et al. (2006). Longitudinal trajectories of heavy drinking in adults in the United States of America. *Addiction (Abingdon, England)*, *101*(1), 91–99.

Maher, R., Hanlon, J., & Hajjar, E. (2014). Clinical consequences of polypharmacy in older adult. *Expert Opinion on Drug Safety*, *13*(1), 57–65.

Mailis-Gagnon, A., Nicholson, K., Yegneswaran, B., & Zurowski, M. (2008). Pain characteristics of adults 65 years of age and older referred to a tertiary care pain clinic. *Pain Research and Management*, *13*(5), 389–394.

Medicare.gov. *Costs in the coverage gap*. (2016). Retrieved from https://www.medicare.gov/part-d/costs/coverage-gap/part-d-coverage-gap.html.

Moos, R. H., Schutte, K. K., Brennan, P. L., & Moos, B. S. (2010). Late-life and life history predictors of older adults of high-risk alcohol consumption and drinking problems. *Drug Alcohol Dependency*, *108*(102), 13–20.

National Council on Aging. (n.d.). *Facts about aging*. Retrieved from https://www.ncoa.org/news/resources-for-reporters/get-the-facts/healthy-aging-facts/.

National Institute of Mental Health. (2015). *Suicide statistics, anxiety statistics*. Retrieved from https://www.nimh.nih.gov/health/topics/suicide-prevention/index.shtml.

National Institute on Aging. (2015). *Alcohol use in older adults*. Retrieved from https://www.nia.nih.gov/health/publication/alcohol-use-older-people.

Onder, G., Petrovic, M., Tangiisuran, B., et al. (2010). Development and validation of a score to assess risk of adverse drug reactions among in-hospital patients 65 years or older: The GerontoNet ADR risk score. *Archives of Internal Medicine*, *170*(13), 1142–1148.

United States Census Bureau. (2014). *Poverty*. Retrieved from www.census.gov/hhes/www/poverty.

United States Food and Drug Administration. (2012). *Guidance for industry E7 studies in support of special populations: Geriatrics*. Retrieved from http://www.fda.gov/downloads/Drugs/GuidanceComplianceRegulatoryInformation/Guidances/UCM189544.pdf.

United States Food and Drug Administration. (2015). *FDA drug safety communication: Nonsteroidal anti-inflammatory drugs can cause heart attacks and strokes*. Retrieved from http://www.fda.gov/Drugs/DrugSafety/ucm451800.htm.

Woods, B., Aquirre, E., Spector, A. E., & Orrell, M. (2012). Cognitive stimulation to improve cognitive functioning in people with dementia. *Cochrane Database System Review*. Retrieved from http://www.ncbi.nlm.nih.gov/pubmed/22336813.

32

Serious Mental Illness

Edward A. Herzog

Visit the Evolve website for a pretest on the content in this chapter: http://evolve.elsevier.com/Varcarolis Pre-Test interactive review

OBJECTIVES

1. Discuss the effects of serious mental illness on daily functioning, interpersonal relationships, and quality of life.
2. Describe three common problems associated with serious mental illness.
3. Discuss five evidence-based practices for the care of individuals with serious mental illness.
4. Explain the role of the nurse in the care of people with a serious mental illness.
5. Develop a nursing care plan for an individual with serious mental illness.
6. Discuss the causes of treatment nonadherence and plan interventions to promote treatment adherence.

OUTLINE

KEY TERMS AND CONCEPTS

anosognosia
assertive community treatment (ACT)
consumer
deinstitutionalization
guardianship
insurance parity
National Alliance on Mental Illness
outpatient commitment
peer support specialist
psychoeducation
psychiatric advance directives
recovery model
severe mental illness (SMI)
social skills training
stigma
supported employment
supportive psychotherapy
transinstitutionalization
vocational rehabilitation

The term severe mental illness (SMI) refers to a group of psychiatric disorders, most of which are primarily biological in origin, that can significantly affect functioning and one's quality of life, especially if they go untreated. Other terms used interchangeably with SMI are:

- Broad-based mental illness—any commonly accepted mental health diagnosis
- Severe and persistent mental illness (SPMI)—similar to SMI, but emphasizing chronicity
- Biologically based mental illness—illnesses that have been determined to be due to biological differences in the brain

SMIs include major depressive disorder, bipolar disorder, schizophrenia, schizoaffective disorder, panic disorder, posttraumatic stress disorder, borderline and antisocial personality disorder, and obsessive-compulsive disorder. In 2014 almost 10 million adults (about 4% of all adults) in the United States lived with SMI (National Institute of Mental Health, 2014). Fig. 32.1 illustrates the prevalence of SMI based on demographic characteristics.

SMIs are usually lifelong disorders. Some patients experience remissions interrupted by exacerbations of varying lengths. Sometimes the remissions are essentially symptom-free, but more typically there is some degree of residual symptoms. For others, the illness follows a chronic and sometimes deteriorating course during which symptoms wax and wane but never remit.

SMIs are devastating. Individuals with SMI are more likely to be victims of crime, have medical illnesses (often undertreated or untreated), and die prematurely. They are also more likely to experience homelessness, be incarcerated, be unemployed or underemployed, live in poverty, and engage in substance misuse. People with SMI often struggle with activities of daily living (ADLs), functioning at work or school, relationships, social interaction, coping, communication, and task completion. They may also experience impairment related to leisure activities,

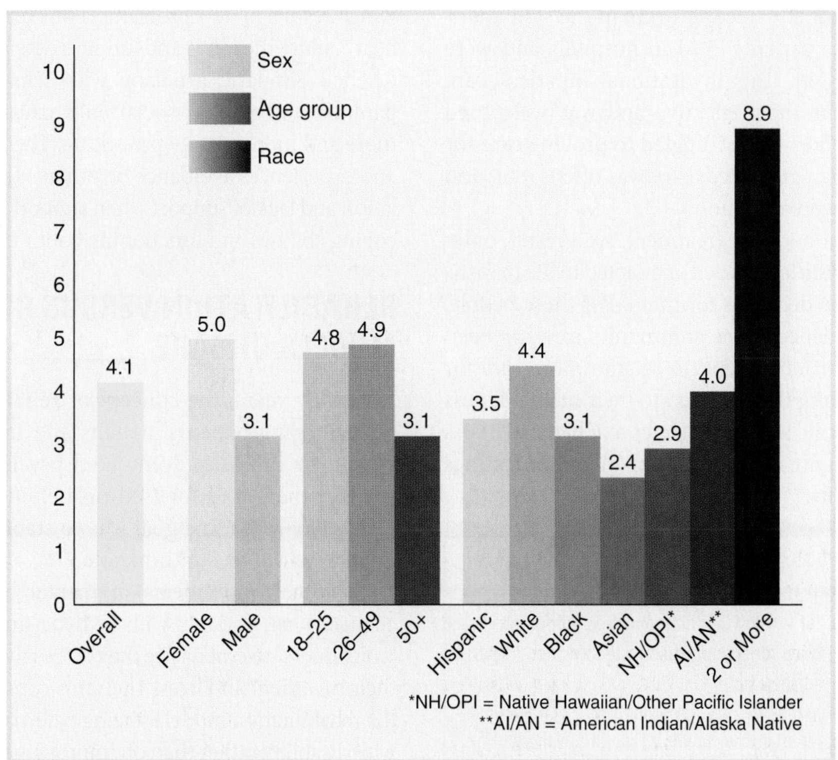

FIG. 32.1 Prevalence of serious mental illness in the United States. National Institute of Mental Health. (2014). *Serious mental illness among US adults.* Retrieved from http://www.nimh.nih.gov-/health/statistics/prevalence/serious-mental-illness-smi-among-us-adults.shtml

health maintenance, vocational and academic activities, remaining safe in the community, and managing finances. They can experience difficulty exercising sound judgment, controlling impulses, concentrating, and coping with everyday stressors.

These impairments, along with related factors such as poverty, stigma, unemployment, and living in high-crime areas reduce access to healthcare. Inadequate housing can significantly impact quality of life and can cause people with SMI to live in a parallel universe separate from "normals" or "neurotypicals," names sometimes used to describe people without mental illnesses. Stigma, others' irrational fear of mental illness, and the patient's residual symptoms or socially inappropriate behavior can cause others to avoid the patient and refuse them housing or employment.

In this chapter we refer to people with serious mental illness as consumers. The term **consumers** indicates the potential for active participation in treatment and an empowerment of the individual for this participation.

SERIOUS MENTAL ILLNESS ACROSS THE LIFESPAN

SMI can affect individuals of any gender, age, educational level, culture, or location. However, those living with SMIs can be separated into two groups based on their experiences with the mental health system: (1) those old enough to have experienced long-term institutionalization (usually before 1980) and (2) those young enough to have been hospitalized only for brief acute care and receiving most of their care in the community.

Older Adults

Older adults with SMI probably received care in the state mental hospital system where patients lived in hospitals and were treated by professional staff. This institutional inpatient care model was considered the most effective and was welcomed by communities and families who struggled to provide care for this population. Care was regimented, care was often poor, and human rights violations were common.

Patients had little say about their treatment. As a result, older adults may have become *institutionalized* or adapted to life in institutions where others made decisions for them. For these people, the transition to independence in the community care has been difficult. In addition, older adults tend to require more care for medical conditions including those related to their mental illness such as diabetes or metabolic syndrome (refer to Chapter 12). As a result, many older adults are cared for in nursing home settings instead of in the community.

VIGNETTE: During adolescence and early adulthood, Marianne lived in a state hospital. When she was discharged, she moved to a group home. She spent long periods staring out her window but did not ask to go out into the garden. She rarely initiated or asked for anything and instead waited for others to approach her or provide for her. Her caregivers worked for months to help her to become more independent. One day, Marianne spontaneously walked into the kitchen and made a sandwich, which she ate in the garden. Her progress had begun as the dependency caused by institutionalization gave way to growing independence.

Younger Adults

People without a history of institutionalization usually do not have problems of passivity and dependency. Instead, most experience a series of short-term hospitalizations. These hospital stays stabilize the illness but often fail to overcome issues such as not recognizing the need for treatment and resultant treatment nonadherence. This has contributed to a cycle of treatment, brief recovery, nonadherence, and relapse. Intermittent treatment puts young adults with SMI at particular risk for additional problems. These problems include increased frequency of relapse, arrest and incarceration, homelessness, substance use, unemployment, and poorer long-term prognosis.

VIGNETTE: Christopher served in the army for 5 years. Afterward, he accepted a job at the post office. His problems began when he accused a coworker of poisoning his lunch. He gradually became more paranoid, developed auditory hallucinations, and began threatening coworkers. These symptoms led to his first hospitalization, treatment, and improvement. After discharge, Christopher stopped his medication and dropped out of treatment. Unable to function, he lost his job and later his housing. For the next 10 years, Christopher worked only intermittently, was homeless off and on, and drank heavily whenever he had money. Treatment came during periodic involuntarily hospitalizations when his behavior became dangerous to himself or others. He resisted community care and denied having an illness. One day, Christopher simply vanished. His family eventually learned that he had been struck by a car and died in a veterans hospital in another state shortly after disappearing.

DEVELOPMENT OF SERIOUS MENTAL ILLNESS

SMI has much in common with chronic physical illness: the original problem increasingly overwhelms and erodes the ability to cope, which results in new problems. For example, in chronic congestive heart failure the lungs and kidneys deteriorate due to cardiac insufficiency. Similarly, a person with schizophrenia may experience paranoia and a loss of social skills, causing interactions to become more and more anxiety provoking. The patient begins to withdraw and experiences avoidance by others. This results in increased isolation and lack of support when support is most needed. As a result, coping abilities and functioning continue to deteriorate.

REHABILITATION VERSUS RECOVERY: TWO MODELS OF CARE

For many years, the concept of **rehabilitation**, which focused on managing patients' deficits and helping them learn to live with their illnesses, dominated psychiatric care. Staff directed the treatment and focused on helping patients to function in their daily roles. The goal was to stabilize the disability. Recovery from SMI was unthinkable.

Advocacy movements in mental health produced sweeping change. First, patients with SMI began to refer to themselves as "consumers" to emphasize the choices they have or seek to have over their treatment and lives. Then this consumer movement criticized the rehabilitation model as being paternalistic and focused on living with disability rather than on improving quality of life and achieving recovery. The **recovery model**, which has its roots in the substance abuse community, developed out of this consumer movement.

The recovery model is supported by the National Alliance on Mental Illness (NAMI), the leading mental health consumer support and advocacy organization in the United States.

The recovery model:

- Is patient/consumer-centered.
- Is hopeful and empowering.
- Emphasizes the person and the future rather than the illness and the present.
- Involves an active partnership between patient and care providers.
- Focuses on strengths and abilities rather than dysfunction and disability.
- Encourages independence and self-determination.
- Focuses on achieving goals of the patient's choosing (not staff's).
- Emphasizes staff working collaboratively with consumers, building on strengths to help consumers achieve the highest possible quality of life.
- Aims for increasingly productive and meaningful lives for those with SMI.

ISSUES CONFRONTING THOSE WITH SERIOUS MENTAL ILLNESS

Establishing a Meaningful Life

Finding meaning in life and establishing goals can be difficult for people living with SMI, particularly if they also experience poor self-esteem. Patients struggle with the possibility that they may never be the person they once expected to be. It is helpful to find ways to reset goals so that meaning can be found in new directions such as helping others, volunteering, or even successfully managing their illness. This reset is important to achieve a satisfactory quality of life and to avoid despair.

If a person cannot work or attend school, there is a significant amount of free time to fill. This free time can result in boredom and stagnation. Options for constructive use of leisure time are limited if a person doesn't have transportation or lacks money. Helping the patient discover affordable options to structure free time and bring pleasure to life is important. Helpful options include borrowing movies, magazines, or books from the library (also usually a nice environment to spend time); going for walks to nearby parks or in malls; and going to free or low-cost concerts. Joining a clubhouse or day program can counter social withdrawal, increase social skills, and help build support systems.

Comorbid Conditions

Physical Disorders

People with SMI are at greater risk from co-occurring physical illnesses, particularly hypertension, obesity, cardiovascular disease, and diabetes. The risk of premature death is over three times greater than the general population, and on average, patients with SMI die more than 25 years prematurely (Olfson et al., 2015). Contributing factors include failing to provide for their own health needs (e.g., forgetting to take medicine), inability to access or pay for care, higher rates of smoking, poor diet, criminal victimization, and stigma.

A mental illness can distract healthcare staff from the patient's real medical needs. They may feel or be told that they are unwelcome in clinic waiting rooms because of their behaviors, appearance, or hygiene. Also, expressing health concerns in an eccentric or unclear manner can influence the quality of care received.

One patient with schizophrenia experienced priapism—a medically dangerous extended period of erection—as a side effect. Due to psychotic thinking, he interpreted the pain to emergency department staff as "demons sticking needles in my [penis]." The resident did not assess for priapism partly because of the bizarre description, his assumption that the patient's distress was due to his mental illness, and possibly his own discomfort working with this population.

There is strong support for integrating mental and physical healthcare in a single setting to enhance access, improve coordination, and facilitate staff understanding and communication. One example is for mental health centers partnering with primary care providers so that their consumers can receive both forms of care in a single coordinated delivery setting.

Depression and Suicide

Suicide occurs 12 times more frequently in people with SMI. For example, half of those with schizophrenia attempt suicide, and one in 10 succeeds. Consider a successful premed student who develops SMI, then 3 years later finds herself unemployed and living in a group home. There is a significant disconnect between her former life path and her current situation. This loss of what might have been can lead to acute or chronic grief that, along with the chronicity of the illness and its demands and impact on daily life, can contribute to despair, depression, and risk of suicide. Helping the patient find support, caring, meaning, and value to life can avert suicide.

Substance Use

In 2013, 1% of all adults age 18 or over in the United States (2.3 million adults) had a co-occurring substance use disorder and SMI (Substance Abuse and Mental Health Services Administration, 2014). Substance use in this population is primarily alcohol and marijuana. It can be a maladaptive response to boredom or a form of self-medication, countering the dysphoria, anxiety, or other symptoms caused by illness or its treatment (e.g., the sedation caused by one's medications). Substance use significantly increases the risk of relapse and impairs judgment and impulse control.

While cigarette smoking has declined among the general population over the past decade, there has been little change among people with SMI (Weinberger, 2016). For example, more than 80% of people with schizophrenia are nicotine dependent. The prevailing belief that nicotine is a form of self-medication that improves cognitive ability has not been supported by research. Nicotine can, however, reduce the effectiveness of certain psychotropic medications. Cigarette smoking contributes to comorbid physical health problems and reduced quality of life.

Social Problems

Stigma

Stigma is the perception that an individual is flawed. The perception is covertly or overtly linked to some personal defect in the person being stigmatized. A lack of understanding and incorrect beliefs about mental illness result in stigma about SMI. For example, some may believe that people with SMI are violent when in fact violence is rare. Nonetheless, the result of this stigmatizing belief is fear and avoidance of people with SMI, particularly those who have psychotic disorders. Stigma can cause shame, anger, and isolation in the consumer and can lead to discrimination in healthcare, housing, and employment.

It is often hard to grasp that individuals can recover from mental illness. This is mostly due to stereotypical images of mental illness and limited corrective contact with people with SMIs. Initiatives such as NAMI's (2016b) *#Iamstigmafree* program seeks to improve understanding and acceptance through public education and reduction of stigma.

Isolation and Loneliness

Social isolation and loneliness are concerns with SMIs. Stigma, poor self-image, passivity, impaired hygiene, and similar factors reduce interaction and interfere with relationships. Romantic relationships and opportunities for sexual expression are usually desired, but isolation, which may be compounded by sexual dysfunction from medications, reduces the chances. Dating services specifically for people with SMI can be helpful. Support groups such as NAMI provide for interaction in a supportive low-stigma environment and provide opportunities to practice social skills, develop social comfort, and establish relationships.

Victimization

Stereotypes suggest that people with SMI are more likely to be violent than people without mental illness, but the reverse is actually true. People with mental illness are more likely to be *victims* of violence than *perpetrators* (De Mooij et al., 2015). Sexual assault or coerced sexual activity also occurs in this vulnerable population. Impaired judgment, impaired interpersonal skills (e.g., unknowingly acting in ways that might provoke others such as standing too close), impaired facial recognition (e.g., not recognizing irritation), poor self-esteem, dependency, and appearing more vulnerable to criminals may contribute to victimization. Drug use and poor living conditions in high-crime neighborhoods increase the risk of victimization and can worsen the psychiatric condition.

Economic Challenges

Unemployment and Poverty

Most people get at least part of their identity and sense of value from the work they do. Many people with SMI would like to work. However, symptoms such as cognitive slowing or disorganization interfere with obtaining or succeeding at work. Eighty-five percent of people with SMI are unemployed, and disability entitlements do not provide much income (NAMI, 2014). Finding an employer open to hiring a person with SMI can be difficult, and antidiscrimination laws do not guarantee a job. Fig. 32.2 illustrates the employment rates of people with SMI.

Newer medications can be extremely expensive (over $1000/month). Copays or Medicaid "spend-downs" (the monthly need to exhaust personal funds to continue Medicaid eligibility) are obstacles to treatment. Individuals with insurance may find that their share of costs is prohibitively high or that their insurance provider limits mental healthcare coverage or does not cover it at all. Providing mental healthcare coverage equal to that for physical healthcare or **insurance parity** is required under the Affordable Care Act. Yet insurers still treat mental illness differently such as requiring preauthorization for care when preauthorization is not required for comparable physical healthcare.

Housing Instability

People with SMIs often have limited funds and thus limited housing options. Affordable housing may require living far from resources such as stores, healthcare, and support people or

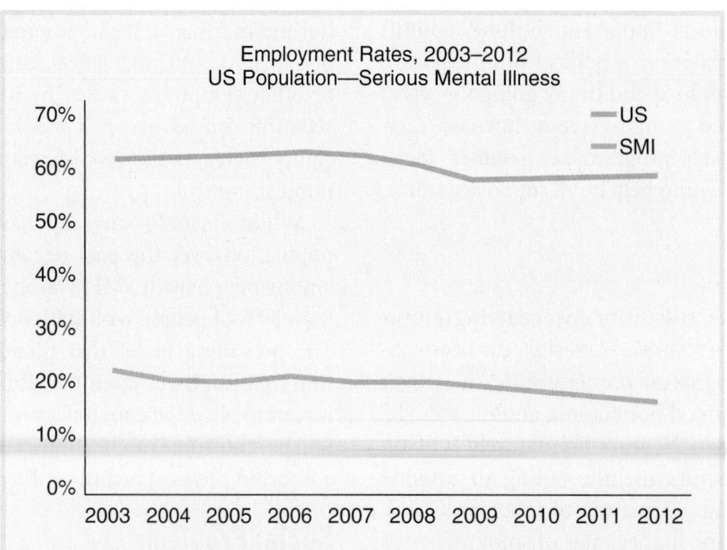

FIG. 32.2 Employment rates for people with serious mental illness. National Alliance on Mental Illness. (2014). *Road to recovery: Employment and mental illness.* Retrieved from http://www.nami.org/work

living in unsafe neighborhoods. As an adult who expects autonomy, living with parents can be extremely challenging and may result in conflict and volatility. Behaviors such as nonadherence and impaired self-care can disrupt housing with family and lead to estrangement.

An episode of inappropriate behavior could lead to eviction and a negative reputation among landlords, closing doors to future housing. Police may not recognize symptoms of mental illness, leading to arrest. Imagine a consumer who is experiencing hallucinations. She becomes disruptive and is arrested instead of the police de-escalating the situation. This arrest can potentially leave the woman ineligible for housing subsidies or public housing. Even with a subsidy, waiting lists might be several years long. Finding and keeping good housing can be challenging. Consumers can also lose housing due to extended hospitalization. Fortunately, options such as "no reject, no eject" housing is becoming common. These are group homes that hold the consumer's room even if hospitalized. Medicaid will now cover housing in some cases (NAMI, 2015b).

Caregiver Burden

Caregivers, particularly family members, are challenged to cope with the persistent needs of people with SMI and may find themselves unable to shoulder the burden. They report that navigating the mental health system is challenging and stressful. Due to stigma or isolation, caregivers carry this burden with little support, emotionally and financially.

Ensuring that caregivers are connected with resources and connecting the patient with services that will increase independence (such as vocational and housing support) are essential nursing interventions (National Alliance for Caregiving, 2016). Caregivers also age, become ill, and require care themselves, often creating a difficult adjustment when a caregiver can no longer provide care or housing. Planning for the transition from family caregivers to independence before a crisis occurs and making arrangements for financial support (such as living trusts) when finances allow can preserve stability and avert relapse.

Box 32.1 recounts a family member's difficulty in living with a brother who has an SMI.

Treatment Issues

Anosognosia

Anosognosia (uh-no-sog-NOH-zee-uh), the inability to recognize one's illness due to illness itself, affects most of those with SMI. In SMI, the illness affects the one organ needed to have insight and make good decisions: the brain. As a result it can take months or years for a person with SMI to recognize and acknowledge his or her mental illness. Some may assume that the patient is in denial. While this can happen, anosognosia is much more likely in SMI. Table 12.3 in Chapter 12 includes interventions for anosognosia.

Nonadherence

More than half of all people with mental illness are not receiving treatment or are nonadherent to treatment. This can quadruple the likelihood of relapse. Anosognosia, side effects, medication costs, lack of trust in providers, and the stigma of mental illness also cause nonadherence. Factors that promote adherence, such as establishing a trusting therapeutic alliance, can be neglected. Healthcare providers often respond primarily with medication education and pointing out the consequences of nonadherence, but patients faced with repetitive medication groups and exhortations to take medications often become *more* resistant rather than insightful. Box 32.2 describes more effective nursing interventions that promote adherence.

Medication Side Effects

Psychotropic medications can produce a range of distressing side effects, from involuntary movements to increased risk of diabetes. Some side effects (e.g., dystonias) are treatable. Others may diminish over time or the individual can compensate for these through behavioral changes. For example, one simple response is to changing position slowly to reduce dizziness from hypotension. Addressing side effects is essential to promote adherence and maximize quality of life. Refer to Chapter 3 for a detailed discussion of drugs used in the treatment of SMI and to chapters on individual disorders for nursing care–related to side effects.

Treatment Inadequacy

NAMI evaluates services provided to those with SMI and finds most states lacking. The most recent ratings gave below-average ratings to 27 states. The highest grade of a B went to only six states. NAMI cited the following problems (2010):

BOX 32.1 My Brother with a Severe Mental Illness

In ordinary circumstances, family relationships are challenging. Adding a sibling with serious mental illness can create challenges that are, at times, insurmountable. In my family's case, my younger brother began exhibiting odd behavior in late adolescence, mostly walking the street at night and making irrational statements. He claimed that he was switched at birth with my youngest brother.

John, the sixth of seven children, was intelligent, entertaining, and well liked in school. When John's symptoms began to surface, my parents did not attribute the behaviors to a psychiatric disorder. However, when John suffered a freak head injury involving a garbage dumpster lid and was subsequently treated for the injury, the focus shifted to mental illness.

Now 60 years old, my brother has had intense psychiatric care including forced hospitalizations and periods of being legally judged incompetent. Our father tried to care for him and meet his needs while my brother's delusions caused his son to deny him as his natural father. He is convinced he has a Russian mother, even though our non-Russian mother passed away nearly 30 years ago. In addition to losing all of his childhood friends long ago, his behavior has served to alienate nearly all of his siblings.

Since our father passed away, we are trying to help John, but it is difficult. The Privacy Rules associated with the Health Insurance Portability and Accountability Act of 1996 (HIPAA) restrict sharing his healthcare information. So far he has been unwilling to sign a release. The hospitalizations are occurring more frequently, and the medications seem to be losing their effectiveness. Recently he indicated that he is considering suicide. As a result, we have been forced to seek a court-appointed guardian for him.

BOX 32.2 Interventions to Improve Adherence to Treatment

- Encourage careful selections of medications that are most likely to be effective, well tolerated, and acceptable to the patient.
- Actively help the patient to manage side effects to avert/minimize distress that could cause nonadherence.
- Simplify treatment regimens to make them more acceptable and understandable to the patient (e.g., once-a-day dosing instead of twice).
- Tie treatment adherence to achieving the *patient's* goals (not staff's or society's) to increase motivation. Reinforce improvements (e.g., such as living in the community without rehospitalization), connecting them to treatment adherence.
- Assign consistent committed caregivers skilled at building trusting therapeutic relationships and who will be able to work with the patient for extended periods of time.
- To improve patient insight and motivation, educate the patient and family about SMI and the role of treatment in recovery. However, education alone will not lead to adherence, particularly for people with anosognosia.
- Minimize obstacles to treatment by providing assistance with treatment costs and access.
- Involve the patient and family in support groups with members who have greater insight and firsthand experience with illness and treatment—people whose viewpoints the patient may be more likely to appreciate and accept. Peer support specialists could be especially helpful here.
- Provide culturally sensitive care. Not attending to cultural beliefs and practices (e.g., mistrust of healthcare and authority figures or valuing self-sufficiency or privacy above healthcare) can result in rejection of treatment.
- When other interventions have not been successful, use medication monitoring and long-acting forms of medication (depot injections or sustained-release forms) to increase the likelihood that needed medication will be in the patient's system. Note: Mouth checks may not find pills hidden in the patient's mouth, engaging the patient in conversation for several minutes after he takes the pills is also of limited benefit. For people on oral medications, fast-dissolving or liquid forms are the best option for ensuring their ingestion.
- Never reject, blame, or shame the patient when nonadherence occurs. Instead, label it as simply an issue for continuing focus, and accept that achieving adherence often requires numerous tries. Remind yourself that nonadherence is common and often is due to anosognosia from the illness itself.

- Fragmented and inadequately funded services
- Inadequate housing
- Excessive institutionalization

Although standards of care now exist for most SMIs, providers do not always follow them. Instead, consumers must be informed and diligent in ensuring that they are receiving the most effective treatment, and agencies and staff must be diligent in updating their programs and practice (NAMI, 2015c).

Residual Symptoms

Residual symptoms are those that do not improve completely or consistently with treatment. This can be frustrating, and patients may feel that these symptoms mean they will not get better or that treatments are not working. This leads to helplessness and despair, and the patient may discontinue treatment in response, worsening the illness.

Relapse, Chronicity, and Loss

The majority of patients with an SMI face the possibility of relapse even when exactly adhering to treatment, which may contribute to hopelessness and helplessness. Living with an SMI paradoxically requires *more* effort and emotional resources from people *less* able to cope with such demands. Each relapse can cause loss of relationships, employment, and housing, adding that much more loss to the patient's life and making discharge planning significantly more complicated.

SERIOUS MENTAL ILLNESS RESOURCES

Comprehensive Community Treatment

Ideally, the community-based mental healthcare system provides comprehensive, coordinated, and cost-effective care for the consumer with mental illness. However, in 2003, the President's New Freedom Commission on Mental Health concluded that services—particularly for serious mental illness—were fragmented and inefficient with blurring of responsibility among agencies, programs, and levels of government. Many consumers "fall through the cracks," and those who received treatment had difficulty achieving financial independence because of limited job opportunities and the fear of losing health insurance in the workplace (becoming employed and having an income may cause ineligibility for Medicaid or Medicare; President's New Freedom Commission on Mental Health, 2003).

The goal of community psychiatric treatment is to improve the consumer's ability to function independently and achieve a satisfying quality of life. Community mental health centers, private providers (psychiatrists, psychologists, counselors, social workers, and advanced practice registered nurses [APRNs]), and other private, public, and governmental agencies provide outpatient care. Community services vary with local needs and resources.

Rural communities or those with limited finances may provide only mandated services (and limited access to them), whereas other communities may have a broad array of accessible services. Needed services may be unavailable or have long waiting lists due to funding cutbacks, and consumers may have difficulty finding the services they need amid the maze of agencies and services.

Community Services and Programs

The public healthcare system provides most care to those with SMIs. This system uses tax support to provide services even to those who are indigent and without adequate (or any) health insurance. Community mental health centers typically provide psychiatric or medical-somatic services and prescribe and monitor medications. Psychiatrists, advanced practice psychiatric-mental health registered nurses, and sometimes physician assistants provide these services along with support from basic-licensure nurses.

Case management helps patients with day-to-day needs, treatment coordination, and access to services. Paraprofessional staff (people trained to assist professionals) usually provide this care. They work in the patient's home, school, and vocational settings and coordinate overall care, facilitating access to services while providing basic education, guidance, and support. Case managers may provide **medication monitoring**, observing and facilitating the patient's use of medications to promote adherence. One evidence-based model of case management for patients with SMIs is assertive community treatment (ACT), discussed later in this chapter.

Day programs provide structure and therapeutic activities to patients who attend the program 1 or more days a week. Services often include education regarding social skills, ADLs, and prevocational skills (the fundamentals needed before one can be successfully employed [e.g., interviewing, dressing for work]). Day programs also provide social contact and peer support. Staff monitor the patient's status so that they can detect and address concerns quickly. A variety of staff, and sometimes consumers themselves, provide day program services. Peer support specialists, that is, other consumers who are in recovery, may provide some of the services.

Individual and group psychotherapy includes counseling and therapy based on a variety of models, usually provided by independently licensed mental health professionals (e.g., licensed independent social workers or APRNs). Psychotherapy approaches for SMI include (1) family therapy (helping family members function more effectively by providing skills and knowledge necessary to support loved ones with mental illnesses), (2) psychoeducation groups (educating about mental health topics [e.g., psychotropic drugs] and skills [e.g., conflict resolution]), and (3) support groups (providing support related to daily challenges of living with chronic illness). This chapter discusses three other approaches: cognitive therapy, cognitive-behavioral therapy (CBT), and supportive psychotherapy.

The following services may be provided by community mental health centers or through other public and private agencies:

Crisis intervention services focus on helping patients regain their ability to cope when facing overwhelming stress such as psychological trauma or relapse. Impaired cognition and problem solving increase the risk of crisis in people with SMI. Stressors, such as changes in routines at home or work, physical or financial problems, victimization, or anniversaries of traumatic events, may overwhelm coping and result in crises. A person with SMI and limited coping abilities may respond to a small stressor first by seeking hospitalization. Crisis intervention seeks to help that person manage the stressor in less restrictive settings and avoid more-disruptive inpatient care.

Crisis intervention emphasizes finding new support or calling on existing resources for additional support. Crisis services range from staff on call who provide direct support 24 hours a day by phone or in person, to support lines (or "warm" lines, for lower levels of distress) or hotlines (for crises and high levels of distress) providing phone-based screening, support, crisis intervention, and referral services. Crisis residential or stabilization programs in some communities typically provide a stay of several days to 2 weeks when acuity is too great to remain in a community residence but not high enough to require hospitalization.

Emergency psychiatric services provide emergency assessments, crisis intervention, and sometimes emergency medications or adjustments. Individuals with SMI may be unable to recognize that their illness is worsening or that they are becoming unsafe. Therefore most communities provide a 24-hour emergency psychiatric evaluation program that can initiate emergency inpatient admissions on an involuntary basis. An additional emergency service is a **mobile crisis team.** It is composed of mental health professionals who go to residences, jails, or even street corners. In some communities, law-enforcement officers are responsible for initiating involuntary emergency psychiatric evaluations. Local probate courts can also order such evaluations upon petition by family members or other interested parties.

Housing services help people progress toward independent living and to maintain stability and avoid homelessness. Settings include supervised or unsupervised group homes. Board-and-care homes provide room, board, and limited supervision by laypeople in their homes. Housing services includes independent community housing such as apartments and houses. Programming may target special populations such as individuals with a forensic history. This group includes criminal offenders who may have been found not guilty by reason of insanity who no longer require inpatient care, but require special or intensive monitoring and programming in the community.

Partial hospitalization programs (PHPs), often affiliated with inpatient programs, typically provide most of the services available to inpatients but on an outpatient basis. Patients usually attend PHPs Monday through Friday for most of the day. Inpatients may be stepped down to PHP programs from inpatient units for further stabilization before being released to other community services. Outpatients may use PHP services to control symptoms in order to avoid inpatient care. **Intensive outpatient programs (IOPs)** are similar, but tend to be less lengthy. Patients may attend 3 to 5 days a week, usually for half a day.

Community outreach programs often focus on homeless individuals or people who do not seek care on their own. Professional or paraprofessional teams work in the community to engage people with mental illness who are in need of services and to provide patient advocacy. **Multiservice centers** collaborate with outreach programs to supply hot meals, laundry, and shower facilities. They can also provide clothing, social activities, and transportation to and from services. For SMI people who are homeless or living in drop-in shelters, these centers provide access to phones and a mailing address, usually essential when seeking work or benefits.

Substance Use Treatment

A variety of services exist for those who have a dual diagnosis of SMI and alcohol-related or drug-related problems. Substance disorder clinics provide therapeutic and rehabilitative services and medication-assisted treatments such as detoxification or methadone. They also provide psychosocial interventions and psychotherapy. Help for families is also available. Most clinicians endorse integrated treatment that is delivered by a single provider rather than split between a mental health agency and a drug/alcohol agency. Refer to Chapter 22 for a detailed discussion of treatment settings for patients with substance use disorders.

VIGNETTE: Christopher, who has a history of SMI, is causing a disturbance in the public library. He is arrested when he refuses a police officer's order to leave. Charged with disorderly conduct, he is subsequently found to be "guilty but insane" and conditionally released to mandatory psychiatric treatment. At a local clinic he receives a long-acting intramuscular antipsychotic medication due to his history of nonadherence. He also joins a day program and is assigned to a case manager who helps him apply for Supplemental Security Income. When his aging parents state that he can no longer live with them, he moves to a group home. Because Christopher wants to work, he is referred to Goodwill Industries where he receives job training and coaching, leading to a job unloading trucks. The stable housing and the requirements of his conditional release lead to consistent treatment and prevent nonadherence. He remains stable and employed for the next 5 years.

EVIDENCE-BASED TREATMENT APPROACHES

Assertive Community Treatment

Assertive community treatment (ACT) involves consumers working with a multidisciplinary team that provides a comprehensive array of services. This team approach eliminates the need for multiple departments or agencies to provide services. Research supports this model for improving the quality of life and reducing inpatient admissions, incarceration, and homelessness among people with SMI (Benthe, 2015). At least one member of the team is available 24 hours a day for crisis care. The emphasis is on treating the patient within his or her own environment. Although ACT programs cost more to operate, proponents believe those costs are offset by reduced care costs elsewhere.

Cognitive-Behavioral Therapy

Cognitive-behavioral therapy (CBT) has been effective in helping individuals with SMI reduce and cope with symptoms such as delusions and impaired social functioning (Zagorski, 2015). The cognitive component of CBT focuses on patterns of thinking and "self-talk" (i.e., what one says to oneself internally). It identifies distorted thinking and negative self-talk and guides patients to substitute more effective ways of thinking. The behavioral component of CBT uses natural consequences and positive reinforcers (rewards) to shape the person's behavior in a more positive or adaptive manner. Refer to Chapter 2 for a more detailed discussion of CBT.

VIGNETTE: Christopher has done well in a group home and decides to move to his own apartment. Over the next 2 months, his mental status remains stable. However, his nurse, who weighs him monthly, notices that he has lost 12 pounds. Christopher denies any change in his eating habits, and he doesn't follow up with the primary care provider to whom he's been referred. During the next 6 weeks he loses another 10 pounds. Christopher's work supervisor noticed that Christopher is talking out loud to himself, is more isolated, and today, smelled of alcohol. The supervisor dismisses him for the day and requires him to get treatment before returning to work. At his appointment, the psychiatrist, nurse, and nurse-therapist discuss these changes and recommend that Christopher go into the partial hospitalization program for support and medication reevaluation. Although he denies that he has a problem, Christopher reluctantly agrees.

Cognitive Enhancement Therapy

Cognitive enhancement therapy (CET) is based on the principle of neuroplasticity, that healthier areas of the brain can assume neurological functions for the compromised areas of the brain. CET is a lengthy process of structured computer-based drills and group exercises (e.g., 60 or more) that incrementally challenge and strengthen functions such as focusing attention and processing and recalling information. It can also help with interpreting social and emotional information such as judging a person's mood from his or her expression or tone of voice. Research has shown that CET leads to sustained improvement in cognition and improves social and vocational functioning (Keefe et al., 2016).

Family Support and Partnerships

Families and significant others can face significant stresses related to the mental illness of a loved one, and both may suffer from insufficiencies in empathy and understanding. Sound **family support** is one of the strongest predictors of recovery. When treatment providers work as empathic partners with patients and significant others, this enhances treatment and reduces conflict. NAMI's Family-to-Family program focuses on understanding SMI, coping skills, and the recovery process (NAMI, 2016a). NAMI meetings and support groups specific to various SMIs, for example, the Depression and Bipolar Support Alliance, serve as excellent sources of support and practical guidance for primary consumers (patients) and secondary consumers (their significant others).

Social Skills Training

Social skills training is an evidence-based practice that focuses on teaching a wide variety of social and ADL skills. People with SMI often have social deficits that cause functional impairment. For example, a person may not realize that standing too close causes discomfort to others and can lead to negative outcomes such as rejection or a poor job evaluation. Care providers break down complex interpersonal skills, such as resolving a conflict, into more manageable subcomponents. They then teach them how to deal with the problem step by step. They also use role-playing and group interaction to practice skills.

VIGNETTE: Christopher is admitted to the partial hospitalization program (PHP). He attends groups on medication, living with SMI, substance use, and symptom management. The clinicians notice odd behavior. Christopher will only eat or drink out of unopened containers and seems guarded. He discloses that he has not taken any medication since he moved out of his group home. The psychiatrist changes his prescription to a quick-dissolving oral and a long-acting injectable medication. He begins to eat normally and gains 4 pounds in 2 weeks.

He is discharged from the PHP a month later. He again attends the day program at the community mental health center. There he is provided with structure, supportive group therapy, socialization, case management, and medication management. His case manager finds him a room in a family care home with a supportive caregiver. Over the next 3 months, Christopher gradually returns to his baseline functioning. He returns to work 2 days a week and also attends the day program 2 days a week.

Vocational Rehabilitation and Related Services

Consumers with SMI who are employed experience improved socialization, confidence, organizational abilities, socialization, income, and quality of life. Vocational services, or vocational rehabilitation, typically include training skills to enhance employment and financial support for attaining employment. Day programs may use a **clubhouse model** in which consumers run the programing. Consumer-run businesses, such as a coffee shop or housekeeping service, teach all members to perform a job in the business. Such programs have led to the supported employment model, which has been shown to be more effective in helping individuals with SMI achieve employment. Elements of this approach include:

1. Financial incentives to employers to employ people with SMI
2. Rapid placement in a competitive job preferred by the patient
3. Continuing individualized support on the job (e.g., a coach at the worker's side providing support, guidance, and training in coordination with supervisors)
4. Integration of mental health and employment services

EVIDENCE-BASED PRACTICE

Is Weight Loss Possible for People Taking Antipsychotic Medication?

Problem

Adults with SMI represent the greatest and least recognized health disparity problem and have up to a 30-year reduced life expectancy. This is mainly due to cardiovascular disease related to obesity, largely due to medication-related weight gain, and smoking.

Purpose of Study

To determine whether a lifestyle intervention for people with SMI would reduce weight and diabetes risk.

Methods

Participants (n = 200) were over 18 years old, taking antipsychotics agents for more than 30 days, and had a body mass index over 27. They were randomly assigned to usual care (n = 96) or a 6-month weekly group intervention plus six monthly maintenance sessions (n = 104). The intervention emphasized moderate calorie reduction, a Dietary Approaches to Stop Hypertension (DASH) diet, and physical activity. Data were collected at baseline, again after 6 months, and again after 12 months.

Key Findings

- Intervention participants lost 4.4 kg more than control participants from baseline to 6 months, and 2.6 kg more from baseline to 12 months.
- At 12 months, fasting glucose levels in the control group had increased from 106 to 109, and the intervention group decreased from 106 to 100.

Implications for Nursing Practice

Weight gain and metabolic problems are not inevitable. People taking antipsychotics can lose weight and improve fasting glucose levels. Nurses can share the results of this study to motivate patients taking this class of medications.

From Green, C. A., Yarborough, B. J. H., Leo, M. C., Yarborough, M. T., Stumbo, S. P., Janoff, S. L., ... Stevens, V. J. (2015). The STRIDE weight loss and lifestyle intervention for individuals taking antipsychotic medications: A randomized trial. *American Journal of Psychiatry, 172*(1), 71–81.

OTHER TREATMENT APPROACHES

Court-Involved Intervention

Psychiatric advance directives are legal documents that allow an individual whose disorder is in remission to direct how to manage treatment if judgment becomes impaired during a relapse. For example, when well, a consumer can agree to accept hospitalization or medications should he or she experience a relapse. This proactive plan helps the consumer maintain control over treatment and avoid the need for involuntary admission and court involvement.

Guardianship involves the appointment of a person (guardian) to make decisions for the consumer during times when judgment is impaired or is disabled with anosognosia. Guardians may be significant others or attorneys. They are typically appointed during a court process addressing the issue of whether or not a patient is competent to provide for his or her own needs.

Individuals who have been appointed a guardian typically may not enter into contracts, consent to sexual activity, or authorize their own treatment. All of those actions require the guardian's approval. In some cases, the guardian's authority is limited to the person's finances, as when a consumer is functional in most respects but unable to manage money, placing basic needs for food and shelter at risk. The guardian is responsible for using the consumer's funds to meet such needs. An alternative is the use of a **payee**, often a volunteer or staff member, whom the consumer agrees to allow to manage his finances, usually via a contract.

Consumer-Run Programs

As previously discussed with vocational rehabilitation, **consumer-run programs** may be informal clubhouses, which offer socialization, recreation, and sometimes other services. They may also be competitive businesses, such as snack bars or janitorial services, which provide needed services and consumer employment while encouraging independence and building vocational skills. In Cincinnati, Ohio, for example, consumers working with a food service professional run a restaurant open to the public, both learning skills and developing experience in the food service industry. Community mental health centers typically have consumer-run programming as part of day programs.

Peer Support

Peer support involves receiving support from one's peers. This can be from untrained peers in a peer support group or by specially trained and sometimes certified **peer support specialists**. NAMI and other programs offer training that enables consumers to assist peers effectively in their recovery process. Peer support specialists may work in hospitals or day programs to encourage and help their peers. They draw on firsthand experience with SMI to enhance their effectiveness. People with SMI are often more open to accepting information from people who have experienced what they are going through.

Wellness and Recovery Action Plans

Wellness and recovery action plans (Copeland & Jonikas, 2014) and similar programs are psychoeducational programs that empower and train consumers in skills that promote recovery and prepare them to deal with stressors and crises. Training focuses on daily maintenance plans with actions and resources needed to maintain wellness such as adequate rest and sleep. These programs help individuals to identify and manage triggers that could provoke a relapse, early identification of impending relapse, and crisis plans for managing crises or impending relapse. Typically, they provide a wide variety of useful tools, templates, and techniques.

Technology

Technology can reduce costs and improve treatment access and outcomes. Electronic records available in multiple locations can assist in assessments or promote continuity of care anywhere in the community. Those who cannot afford electronic access often have, or can be provided with, a cell phone, allowing for improved monitoring and faster response if, for example, a patient misses an appointment. Smartphone applications can help consumers manage stress, prevent weight gain through exercise or dietary means, and remember their treatments. Text reminders can promote treatment adherence by tracking medications or appointment. Medication dispensers that track when medications are taken are also helpful. Personnel in remote locations are now able to speak with patients by telephone or internet-based video when patients cannot otherwise access distant services or specialists.

Exercise

Exercise holds benefits for people with SMI including improved coping with symptoms, reduced anxiety and depression, and enhanced self-esteem. Exercise helps with weight control, which is essential for people with weight-related comorbidities such as diabetes and hypertension. Exercise is a cost-effective intervention that can be done almost anywhere. While SMI symptoms such as avolition are obstacles to exercise, motivational and group interventions can improve exercise participation (Göhner et al., 2015).

NURSING CARE OF PATIENTS WITH SERIOUS MENTAL ILLNESS

Nurses encounter patients with SMI in a variety of medical and psychiatric settings. All roles and techniques used by psychiatric-mental health nurses in inpatient psychiatric settings also apply in the community and other healthcare settings.

Assessment Strategies

Important aspects of assessment include:

- Intentional risk to self or others: Suicidality or homicidality
- Unintentional risk: Inadequate nutrition, clothing inadequate for the weather, neglect of medical needs, or carelessness while driving, smoking, or cooking
- Depression or hopelessness
- Anxiety
- Signs of impending relapse: Decreased sleep, increased impulsivity or paranoia, diminished reality testing, increased delusional thinking, or command hallucinations
- Physical health problems that can cause psychiatric symptoms and be mistaken for mental illness or relapse (e.g., brain tumors or drug toxicity)
- Comorbid illnesses: To ensure that the patient provides appropriate self-care and receives adequate healthcare
- Treatment nonadherence: Signs such as worsening of symptoms, unused medications, missed appointments, or reluctance to discuss these issues.

Table 32.1 lists selected signs and symptoms of problems associated with SMI, potential nursing diagnoses that apply to the patient with SMI, and examples of specific nursing outcomes.

Intervention Strategies

Box 32.3 outlines two relevant *Nursing Interventions Classification (NIC)* interventions for the management of serious mental illness. Basic nursing interventions for patients with SMI are listed in the following text. Additional interventions are in Table 13.3 in Chapter 13 and other chapters covering individual mental illnesses.

- Involve the patient in goal-setting and treatment planning. This increases treatment adherence and improves treatment outcomes.
- Emphasize quality of life rather than simply focusing on symptoms as this conveys an interest in the person rather than the illness and promotes recovery.
- Maintain sustained therapeutic relationships; trust in providers is key to overcoming anosognosia and achieving treatment adherence. People with SMI often require extended periods to form these connections.
- Focus on coping with current issues rather than past difficulties.
- Encourage reality testing to enable consumers to recognize and counter hallucinations and delusional thinking. For instance, if a person experiences frightening hallucinations while in public, he can learn to scan the room and determine if others seem frightened. If not, he can learn to attribute his experience to his illness and to ignore the hallucinations.
- Enable consumers to recognize and respond to stigma. Stigma predisposes SMI people to isolation and social discomfort. The resulting isolation contributes to loneliness and reduces access to support.
- Promote social skills and provide opportunities for socialization, especially with positive role models, such as other patients who are further along in recovery.
- Involve consumers in support groups such as NAMI that expose them to members who "have been there." Such groups provide support, socialization opportunities, and practical suggestions for issues and problems facing patients and significant others. Peer support specialists are another excellent resource for this purpose.
- Educate consumers about their illness and recovery. Understanding the illness enhances coping, treatment adherence, and quality of life.

TABLE 32.1 Signs and Symptoms, Nursing Diagnoses, and Outcomes for Serious Mental Illness

Signs and Symptoms	Nursing Diagnoses	Outcomes
Absence of eye contact, difficulty expressing thoughts, difficulty in comprehending usual communication pattern, inappropriate verbalization	*Impaired verbal communication*	Exchanges messages accurately with others, uncompromised spoken language, accurately interprets messages received
Withdrawal, inappropriate interpersonal behavior, social discomfort, lack of belonging	*Impaired social interaction*	Engages others, appears relaxed, cooperates with others, uses assertive behaviors as appropriate, exhibits sensitivity to others
Absence of supportive significant other(s), preoccupation with own thoughts, shows behaviors unaccepted by dominant cultural group, withdrawn, reports feeling alone, feels different from others, feels rejected	*Social isolation*	Interacts with others (e.g., family, friends, neighbors, mental health consumers), participates in community activities (e.g., church, volunteer work, clubs), participates in leisure activities with others
Failure to keep appointments, missing medication dosages, evidence of exacerbation of symptoms, failure to progress	*Nonadherence**	Discusses prescribed treatment regimen with health professional, performs treatment regimen as prescribed, keeps appointments with health professionals, monitors own treatment response
Self-negating verbalization, lacks success in life events, hesitant to try new situations, indecisive behavior, lack of eye contract, nonassertive behavior	*Chronic low self-esteem*	Describes feelings of self-worth, fulfills personally significant roles, maintains eye contact, accepts compliments from others
Apprehension about care receiver's care if caregiver is unable to provide care, apprehension about possible institutionalization of care receiver, lack of time to meet personal needs, anger, stress, frustration, impatience, limited social life	*Caregiver role strain*	Caregiver receives adequate respite, social support, opportunities for leisure activities, supplemental services to assist with care; caregiver reports sense of control and certainty about future

*NANDA-I diagnosis is *noncompliance*.

From Herdman, T. H., & Kamitsuru, S. (Eds.). (2014). *Nursing diagnoses—Definitions and classification 2015-2017*. Copyright © 2014, 1994–2014 by NANDA International. Used by arrangement with John Wiley & Sons Limited; Moorhead, S., Johnson, M., Maas, M., & Swanson, E. (2013). *Nursing outcomes classification (NOC)* (5th ed.). St. Louis, MO: Mosby.

- Care for the whole person. SMI patients have more physical illness; poorer hygiene and health practices; less access to effective medical treatment; increased risk for victimization, STDs, and undesired pregnancies. They also have more premature mortality than the general population. Avoiding obesity through exercise and good nutritional practices can reduce the risk of comorbidities such as metabolic syndrome. Sound physical health conserves energy and resources for use in coping with SMI.
- Involving individuals with co-occurring substance use disorders in Alcoholics Anonymous and Narcotics Anonymous (AA/NA) and other dual-diagnosis services. Substance use disorder rates are high in SMI populations. They increase relapse and interfere with recovery. Achieving sobriety is most associated with AA and integrated treatment programs.

Evaluation

Identified outcomes serve as the basis for evaluation. Each *NOC* outcome has a built-in rating scale that helps the nurse to measure improvement.

BOX 32.3 *NIC* Interventions for Serious Mental Illness

Self-Care Assistance: ADLs*

- Teach the individual the appropriate and safe storage of medications.
- Assist the individual to understand how to use public transportation (e.g., buses and bus schedules, taxis, city or county transportation for disabled people).
- Assist individual in establishing safe methods and routines for cooking, cleaning, and shopping.

Family Support*

- Help family to share concerns, feelings, and questions.
- Accept the family's values in a nonjudgmental manner.
- Provide emotional support and connect to support resources such as NAMI and respite providers.
- Promote congruence among patient, family, and staff expectations.

*Partial list.

From Bulecheck, G. M., Butcher, H. K., & Dochterman, J. M. (2013). *Nursing interventions classification (NIC)* (6th ed.). St. Louis, MO: Mosby.

CURRENT ISSUES AFFECTING THOSE WITH SMI

Outpatient Commitment

Involuntary inpatient care has long been used to treat those who are unable to recognize their illness (anosognosia) and the need for treatment. **Outpatient commitment**, which provides mandatory treatment in the community, is relatively new. Typically ordered by a court when a patient leaves a hospital or prison, it is for people who would otherwise be unlikely to continue treatment, resulting in their becoming a danger to self or society.

The practice of outpatient commitment is controversial. On the one hand, individuals who do not recognize having a mental illness are provided with healthcare and, potentially, a better quality of life. They are allowed maximum freedom and are able to live in the community and avoid institutionalization. On the other hand, this approach is paternalistic and is at odds with the recovery model of mental healthcare. Research on the effectiveness of outpatient commitment has demonstrated results that both support and reject this approach.

Criminal Offenses and Incarceration

People with SMIs may commit crimes due to desperation, impaired judgment, or impulsivity. Most often they are nonviolent crimes such as petty theft or disorderly conduct. Police may also become involved with people who seem unable to care for themselves, have become a public nuisance, or cannot be persuaded to accept treatment but do not meet criteria for involuntary treatment (usually imminent danger to self or others). For example, a patient with impaired judgment without shelter in cold weather may stay in a laundromat for warmth. The presence of an unkempt person who is talking to herself and is not using appropriate personal space will cause the other patrons to feel uncomfortable. If expelled, she is at risk of hypothermia. In such a case, the risk to self may not be "imminent," and emergency hospitalization is not a legal option. Significant others or police may then seek the person's arrest simply for the patient's own safety.

Most mental illness advocates believe that incarceration, even if "for the patient's own good," is harmful. Imprisonment can lead to victimization, despair, relapse due to stress or overstimulation, loss of housing or employment, and inadequate treatment. Criminal convictions may make consumers ineligible for most housing or employment, trapping them in a cycle of release and reincarceration. Advocates instead support diversion from jail to clinical care. Interventions to achieve this include (1) **educating police** so that they can identify mental illness, distinguish it from criminal intent, and connect people with SMI to help instead of jailing them and (2) establishing special **mental health courts** designed to intercept people whose crimes are secondary to mental illness. These courts employ specially trained officials with authority to order treatment in lieu of conviction thereby avoiding the stigma and other consequences of conviction and incarceration.

Deinstitutionalization and Transinstitutionalization

Prior to the 1960s people often lived long term in state psychiatric hospitals (refer to Chapter 4). The newer treatments available in the 1960s improved many patients' conditions enough that they no longer needed to be institutionalized and could live instead in the community. **Deinstitutionalization**, the mass shift of patients from state hospitals into the community, began in the 1960s and has continued since. However, planned systems of community care needed by individuals with SMI did not always materialize, leaving them to fend for themselves without access to the services they needed. It was also common for patients to experience difficulty in adjusting to independence after years of being institutionalized.

As a result, former patients ended up being readmitted to state hospitals or cared for in other kinds of institutions. **Transinstitutionalization** is the shifting of a person or population from one kind of institution to another such as a state hospital, jail, prison, nursing home, or shelter. For example, people who were discharged from state hospitals ended up homeless and subsequently were arrested for a variety of crimes. Now there are more people with SMI in prisons than in hospitals.

Inadequate Access to Care

SMI often makes it difficult for individuals to work or find well-paying jobs and jobs with health insurance benefits. As a result, people with SMI tend to rely on the public mental health system, which is run by state and local governments, with services delivered largely by state hospitals and community mental health centers. One consequence of deinstitutionalization was that 90% of state hospital beds were eliminated, making it difficult to provide hospital care to many who continue to need it (Torrey, 2106). Further, most public mental health services rely on state and local funding, and the economic recession that began in 2007 has resulted in funding cutbacks that have reduced already-overwhelmed mental health and related services.

Inpatient and outpatient services for children and adolescents are in especially short supply. The result is that delayed admissions and waiting lists for outpatient care are now commonplace. The Affordable Care Act and Medicaid expansion have resulted in dramatically more people with SMI having health insurance (NAMI, 2015a). However, even those with insurance, who can use private care providers, often find that there are still barriers to getting needed care such as burdensome preauthorization requirements (required for psychiatric care but not for medical care) that discourage or delay access to needed services (Funkenstein et al., 2016; Box 32.4).

BOX 32.4 Resources

Organizations

Mental Health America is a nonprofit organization of advocates, consumers, and significant others who work to strengthen mental health services and educate the nation about mental health issues. Its website provides resources pertaining to recovery, wellness, and severe mental illness.

The **National Alliance on Mental Illness** is a support and advocacy organization for those with SMI and those who care about them. It has national, state, and local chapters and provides a wealth of educational materials and services.

NAMI Family-to-Family is a class for families and friends of people with mental illness. It helps participants better understand mental illness, increase coping skills, and become advocates for their loved ones.

NAMI Peer-to-Peer is a free 10-session educational program for adults with SMI who want to better understand their illness and move toward recovery. It is taught by trained peers who themselves are recovering from SMI. Everything is confidential.

The **National Institute of Mental Health** is the main national research organization for mental illness. Its website contains information about research findings, proposals and grants, as well as a variety of educational resources on mental illness.

The **Substance Abuse and Mental Health Services Administration** (SAMHSA) seeks to reduce the impact of substance misuse and mental illness and works to move research findings into practice. Its website offers much useful information, including a mental health services locator to help consumers find local services.

BOX 32.4 Resources—cont'd

Video Resources

Frontline: The New Asylums details the societal factors that have led to the incarceration of hundreds of thousands of people with severe mental illness in American jails and prisons. The video chronicles the financial and human consequences of this unintended and disastrous policy.

Frontline: The Released is a companion video to *The New Asylums* that follows inmates with mental illness as they are released to the community. The inadequacies and strengths of the community mental health system become apparent as the inmates struggle to establish a life outside institutions.

Kings Park: Stories from an American Mental Institution This documentary follows a group of former New York state hospital patients as they visit the now-closed state hospital where they spent months or years of their lives. Interviews chronicle the lives and experiences of those deinstitutionalized from the state hospital system, sometimes only to experience still sadder fates.

Minds on the Edge: Facing Mental Illness features a fast-moving panel discussion of issues facing the individuals with severe mental illness in our communities. Using hypothetical situations and featuring mental health professionals, advocates, policy makers, and consumers, the panel looks at the problems plaguing our mental health system and offers keen insights into ways that this population could be helped much more effectively.

Out of the Shadow, a documentary about a family's efforts to find care for a loved one with schizophrenia that captures well the issues that can occur when children are raised by a parent with severe mental illness. It also documents the obstacles to treatment created by an underfunded mental health system.

The Soloist (2009, Dreamworks SKG and Universal Studios), based on a true story, is a movie that chronicles the life of a man whose schizophrenia interrupted a promising musical career. It accurately portrays severe mental illness and many of the issues experienced by consumers and those who attempt to help them.

KEY POINTS TO REMEMBER

- Patients with SMI often suffer from multiple impairments in thinking, emotions, perception, and interaction with others.
- The course of SMI involves exacerbations and remissions; these can be discouraging and lead a patient to believe he or she cannot recover.
- Social problems related to SMI include stigmatization, isolation, and victimization.
- One of the most difficult symptoms of SMI is anosognosia, the inability to recognize one's illness due to the illness itself.
- People with SMI often suffer complications due to insufficient housing, nonadherence to treatment, comorbid medical or substance use problems, and the stigma of mental illness.
- Coordinated comprehensive community services help people with SMI to function at an optimal level, but such services may not be available or accessible to those who need them.
- The recovery model stresses hope, strengths, quality of life, patient involvement as an active partner in treatment, and eventual recovery.
- The family and support systems play a major part in the care of many people with SMI, so you should include them as much as possible in planning, education, and treatment activities.

CRITICAL THINKING

1. John Yang, 42, dually diagnosed with schizophrenia and cannabis (marijuana) use disorder, is brought to the clinic by his mother, Mrs. Yang. Because they are new in town, she does not know what is available in the community. John takes haloperidol (Haldol), but Mrs. Yang says he often refuses it because of muscle rigidity and sexual side effects. They have tried several first-generation antipsychotic drugs without success.
   a. What areas of John's life might you want to explore in your assessment? Consider relationships, employment history, cognitive abilities, coping, and behavior. How would you use this information for long-term planning?
   b. As a patient advocate, how might you respond to John's medication nonadherence with first-generation antipsychotics?
   c. What obstacles to adherence exist for a dually diagnosed patient? What approach or change in treatment would offer John the best chance of success?
   d. Which resources mentioned in this chapter might be appropriate for John?
   e. Identify three areas of psychoeducation you'd provide for John and his mother.
2. In your psychiatric rotation in a state hospital, many of the patients are diagnosed with schizophrenia. Although you had been apprehensive about this rotation, you are surprised that patients respond well to you, that you are fascinated by this specialty, and that you're considering it as a career. A fellow student remarks, "You must be crazy to want to work with these people."
   a. What social and other issues might be reflected in this student's remark?
   b. Identify other social prejudices that have been significant problems in the United States. What responses were effective in countering these and reducing their impact?

CHAPTER REVIEW

Questions

1. Which statement made by a patient diagnosed with a serious mental illness reflects a common situation associated with this disorder in *today's* healthcare system? *Select all that apply.*
   - **a.** "I have been in a state institution most of my life."
   - **b.** "I've been homeless for years."
   - **c.** "Once a care provider knows my psychiatric history, my physical problems are not taken seriously."
   - **d.** "No one wants to hire a person with mental issues."
   - **e.** "My family doesn't want to be around me because I hear voices."
2. What is the primary reason the nurse should include the family of a patient with a serious mental illness in treatment planning?
   - **a.** They know the patient better than anyone.
   - **b.** The patient is likely willing to listen to them.
   - **c.** They are likely the patient's support system.
   - **d.** The patient will turn to them first when needing help.
3. A 73-year-old man was diagnosed with a serious mental illness at age 20. Subsequently, he was frequently hospitalized. Two years ago, he was transferred to a group home. When considering the effects of institutionalization, which behavior demonstrates adaptation to the new environment?
   - **a.** Willingly takes his medications
   - **b.** Keeps his room neat and clean
   - **c.** Makes himself lunch when he is hungry
   - **d.** Enjoys spending the afternoon watching television
4. Due to the need to self-medicate for anxiety, a patient diagnosed with schizophrenia smokes two packs of cigarettes a day. What unique risk does nicotine pose to this patient's health?
   - **a.** Lung cancer
   - **b.** Cardiovascular constriction
   - **c.** Impaired psychotropic medication therapy
   - **d.** Increased incidence of lung-reacted disorders
5. Which functions are often simultaneously impaired when a patient is experiencing a serious mental illness? *Select all that apply.*
   - **a.** Cognition
   - **b.** Emotions
   - **c.** Perceptions
   - **d.** Social interactions
   - **e.** Self-care
6. Charlie is coping well with a severe mental illness diagnosis. He and his 91-year-old father live together on the family farm. This stable and secluded life has allowed Charlie to live with minimal stimulation, and his relapses have been few. Charlie's caseworker makes a visit to open up a conversation on where Charlie will live when his father can no longer care for him. By bringing up the topic now, the caseworker is hoping to:
   - **a.** Arrange housing for Charlie for when his father dies.
   - **b.** Avert a relapse and preserve stability in Charlie's life.
   - **c.** Rescue Charlie when the crisis occurs.
   - **d.** Make Charlie realize he will soon live independently.
7. Jimmy has been hospitalized three times for schizophrenia. Typically, he is very disorganized, spends his money irresponsibly, and loses his housing when he does not pay the rent. In turn, Jimmy cannot be located by his case manager, which leads to treatment nonadherence and relapse. Which response would be most therapeutic? *Select all that apply.*
   - **a.** Advise Jimmy that if he does not pay his rent, he will be placed in a group home instead of independent housing.
   - **b.** Discuss with Jimmy the option of having a guardian who will ensure that the rent is paid and that his money is managed to meet his basic needs.
   - **c.** Suggest to Jimmy and his prescribing clinician that he be placed on a long-acting injectable form of antipsychotic medication to improve treatment nonadherence.
   - **d.** Encourage Jimmy's case manager to hold him responsible for the outcomes of his poor decisions by allowing periods of homelessness to serve as a natural consequence.
8. Individuals with severe mental illness (SMI) diagnoses can suffer from ineffective healthcare. Providers may be unaccustomed to working with this population or not comprehend obscure details described by the person seeking medical attention. This hurdle can be overcome by:
   - **a.** Seeking medical attention at the emergency department.
   - **b.** Having a community clinic in the area where the SMI live.
   - **c.** Medicate the patient before a medical examination.
   - **d.** Integrating mental and physical health in one setting.
9. A female consumer with severe and recurrent mania argues with outpatient staff about her medication. She does not believe she has a mental illness. Although she takes medication during hospitalizations, she stops taking them after discharge. Which intervention is most helpful in promoting medication adherence?
   - **a.** Assign a new outpatient staff to reduce the conflicts she is experiencing with her current providers.
   - **b.** Explain that the medications will help her and that all medications have side effects, but she can learn to live with these.
   - **c.** Involve her in a medication group that will teach her the types and names of psychotropic medications, their purpose, and possible side effects.
   - **d.** Explore her perceptions and experiences regarding medication and help her to connect taking medications with achieving her goals.

10. Isadora is a middle-aged woman living in a group home after being discharged from a psychiatric institution nearly 20 year ago. Isadora keeps to herself, stays in her room most of the day, and only ventures out for meals. Cassandra, the house manager, encourages Isadora to:
    a. Begin looking for a job
    b. Join a day program clubhouse
    c. Assist in the kitchen washing dishes
    d. Take on a roommate so as not to be alone

Answers

1. **b, c, d, e**; 2. **c**; 3. **c**; 4. **c**; 5. **a, b, c, d, e**; 6. **b**; 7. **b, c**; 8. **d**; 9. **d**; 10. **b**

Visit the Evolve website for a posttest on the content in this chapter: http://evolve.elsevier.com/Varcarolis

Post-Test interactive review

REFERENCES

Benthe, J. (2015). Associations between quality of life and functioning in an assertive community treatment population. *Psychiatric Services, 66*(11), 1249–1252.

Copeland, M., & Jonikas, J. (2014). Wellness recovery action planning: The role of wellness promotion in a new paradigm of community mental health. In G. Nelson, B. B.Kloos, & J. Ornelas (Eds.), *Community psychology and community mental health: Towards transformative change* (pp. 133–151). Oxford, England: Oxford University Press.

De Mooij, L., Kikkert, M., Lommerse, N., et al. (2015). Victimisation in adults with severe mental illness: prevalence and risk factors. *British Journal of Psychiatry, 207*, 515–522.

Funkenstein, A., Hartselle, S., & Boyd, J. (2016). Prior authorization for child and adolescent psychiatric patients deemed to be in need of inpatient admission. *American Journal of Emergency Medicine.* Retrieved from http://www.ajemjournal.com/article/S0735-6757%2816%2900107-8/fulltext.

Göhner, W., Dietsche, C., & Fuchs, R. (2015). Increasing physical activity in patients with mental illness—A randomized controlled trial. *Patient Education and Counseling, 98*, 1385–1392.

Keefe, R., Haig, G., Marder, S., et al. (2016). Report on ISCTM consensus meeting on clinical assessment of response to treatment of cognitive impairment in schizophrenia. *Schizophrenia Bulletin, 42*(1), 19–33.

National Alliance for Caregiving. (2016). *On pins & needles: Caregivers of adults with mental illness.* Retrieved from http://www.caregiving.org/wp-content/uploads/2016/02/NAC_Mental_Illness_Study_2016_FINAL_WEB.pdf.

National Alliance on Mental Illness. (2010). *Grading the states 2009.* Retrieved from http://www.nami.org/gtsTemplate09.cfm?section=Grading_the_States_2009&template=/ContentManagement/ContentDisplay.cfm&ContentID=75459.

National Institute of Mental Health. (2014). *Serious mental illness (SMI) among U.S. adults.* Retrieved from http://www.nimh.nih.gov/health/statistics/prevalence/serious-mental-illness-smi-among-us-adults.shtml.

National Alliance on Mental Illness. (2014). *Road to recovery: Employment and mental illness.* Retrieved from http://www.nami.org/work.

National Alliance on Mental Illness. (2015a). *A long road ahead: Achieving true parity in mental health and substance use care.* Retrieved from https://www.nami.org/about-nami/publications-reports/public-policy-reports/a-long-road -ahead.

National Alliance on Mental Illness. (2015b). *States to use Medicaid money to house homeless people.* Retrieved from http://www.huffingtonpost.com/entry/states-to-use-medicaid-money-to-house-homeless-people_us_565390a8e4b0879a5b0c2d33.

National Alliance on Mental Illness. (2015c). *State mental health legislation 2015: Trends, themes and effective practices.* Retrieved from https://www.nami.org/About-NAMI/Publications-Reports/Public-Policy-Reports/State-Mental-Health-Legislation-2015/NAMI-StateMentalHealthLegislation2015.pdf.

National Alliance on Mental Illness. (2016a). *Family-to-Family Program.* Retrieved from https://www.nami.org/Find-Support/NAMI-Programs/NAMI-Family-to-Family.

National Alliance on Mental Illness. (2016b). *#Iamstigmafree program and pledge.* Retrieved from https://www.nami.org/stigmafree.

Olfson, M., Gerhard, T., Huang, C., et al. (2015). Premature mortality among adults with schizophrenia in the United States. *JAMA Psychiatry, 72* 1172–1181.

President's New Freedom Commission on Mental Health. (2003). *Report of the president's new freedom commission on mental health.* Retrieved from http://govinfo.library.unt.edu/mentalhealthcommission/reports/FinalReport/downloads/FinalReport.pdf.

Substance Abuse and Mental Health Services Administration. (2014). *Substance use and mental health estimates from the 2013 National Survey on Drug Use and Health.* Retrieved from http://www.samhsa.gov/data/sites/default/files/NSDUH-SR200-RecoveryMonth-2014/NSDUH-SR200-RecoveryMonth-2014.htm.

Torrey, E. (2016). A dearth of psychiatric beds. *Psychiatric Times.* Retrieved from http://www.psychiatrictimes.com/psychiatric-emergencies/dearth-psychiatric-beds?GUID=E38AEFDF-01D2-4B63-BCB3-BEC92DC7E284&rememberme=1&ts=27022016.

Weinberger, A. H. (2016). Smoking cessation and adults with serious mental illness. *Nicotine and Tobacco Research, 18*(3), 227–228.

Zagorski, N. (2015). CBT found to be successful in low-functioning patients. *Psychiatric News.* Retrieved from http://psychnews.psychiatryonline.org/doi/full/10.1176/appi.pn.2015.12b14.

33

Forensic Nursing

L. Kathleen Sekula, Alison M. Colbert

ⓔ Visit the Evolve website for a pretest on the content in this chapter: http://evolve.elsevier.com/Varcarolis Pre-Test interactive review

OBJECTIVES

1. Define forensic nursing, forensic psychiatric nursing, and correctional nursing.
2. Describe the educational preparation required for the forensic nurse generalist and the advanced practice forensic nurse.
3. Identify the functions of forensic nurses.
4. Discuss the specialized roles in forensic nursing.
5. Identify three roles of psychiatric nurses in the specialty of forensic nursing.
6. Discuss the roles of the forensic psychiatric nurse within the legal system.

OUTLINE

KEY TERMS AND CONCEPTS

advanced practice forensic nurse
competency evaluator
consultant
correctional nursing
criminal profiler
diminished capacity
expert witness
fact witness
forensic nurse examiner
forensic nurse generalist
forensic nursing
forensic psychiatric nurse
hostage negotiator
legal sanity
nurse coroner/death investigator
sexual assault nurse examiner (SANE)

The rate of violent crimes in the United States increased by nearly 2% in the first half of 2015 (US Department of Justice, 2015). Violent crimes are considered to be murder, rape, robbery, and aggravated assault. Both intentional injuries, which includes self-inflicted injuries, and those caused by acts of violence are among the top 15 killers of Americans of all ages and a leading cause of death for Americans ages 1 to 44. Reducing violence is a goal in *Healthy People 2020* (US Department of Health and Human Services, 2017). Box 33.1 identifies the specific goals for injury and violence prevention.

Violence is often the focus in **forensics**. Forensics is an abbreviation for *forensic science* and refers to the application of a broad spectrum of sciences to answer questions of interest to the legal system. In recent years, nurses formalized a specialty of nursing called forensic nursing, which brings together traditional nursing practice and forensic knowledge to better serve

BOX 33.1 *Healthy People 2020* Goals: Injury and Violence Prevention (IVP) Objectives

IVP-29	Reduce homicides
IVP-30	Reduce firearm-related deaths
IVP-31	Reduce nonfatal firearm-related injuries
IVP-32	Reduce nonfatal physical assault injuries
IVP-33	Reduce physical assaults
IVP-34	Reduce physical fighting among adolescents
IVP-35	Reduce bullying among adolescents
IVP-36	Reduce weapon carrying by adolescents on school property
IVP-37	Reduce child maltreatment deaths
IVP-38	Reduce nonfatal child maltreatment
IVP-39	Reduce violence by current or former intimate partners
IVP-40	Reduce sexual violence
IVP-41	Reduce nonfatal intentional self-harm injuries
IVP-42	Reduce children's exposure to violence
IVP-43	Increase the number of states and the District of Columbia that link data on violent deaths from death certificates, law enforcement, and coroner and medical examiner reports to inform prevention efforts at the state and local levels

From US Department of Health and Human Services. (2017). Injury and violence prevention. Retrieved from https://www.healthypeople.gov/2020/topics-objectives/topic/injury-and-violence-prevention/objectives

victims and perpetrators of violence. In this chapter, we will explore a variety of roles that registered nurses assume within nursing that interface with the legal system.

FORENSIC NURSING

The International Association of Forensic Nurses (IAFN, 2009) defines forensic nursing as:

1. The application of nursing science to public or legal proceedings.
2. The application of the forensic aspects of healthcare combined with the biopsychosocial education of the registered nurse in the scientific investigation and treatment of trauma and/or death of victims and perpetrators of abuse, violence, criminal activity, and traumatic accidents.

Forensic nurses provide direct services to crime victims and perpetrators of crime and consultation services to colleagues in nursing, medicine, social work, rehabilitation, and law. Forensic nurses can offer expert court testimony in cases related to their areas of practice and expertise and provide input on policy changes within forensic settings. They can also offer evaluation services regarding specific medical and psychiatric diagnoses for both victims and perpetrators.

The IAFN was formed in 1992 when 74 nurses—most of whom were sexual assault nurse examiners—came together to create an organization to represent nurses whose practice overlapped with key areas of forensic science and law (Lynch, 1997). A year after its creation, the organization had more than tripled in size, and by 2016, the IAFN's membership had grown to well over 3000 nurses (IAFN, 2016). The group now represents nurses who are forensic nurse generalists, sexual assault nurse examiners, forensic psychiatric nurses, death investigators, risk managers, coroners, and correctional nurse specialists.

The American Nurses Association (ANA) officially recognized forensic nursing as a specialty practice area in 1995. The ANA then combined efforts with the IAFN to develop the first edition of the *Scope and Standards of Forensic Nursing Practice* in 1997 (IAFN and the American Nurses Association, 1997).

The goals of the IAFN (2009) are to:

- Incorporate primary prevention strategies into our work at every level in an attempt to create a world without violence.
- Establish and improve standards of evidence-based forensic nursing practice.
- Promote and encourage the exchange of ideas and transmission of developing knowledge among its members and related disciplines.
- Establish standards of ethical conduct for forensic nurses.
- Create and facilitate educational opportunities for forensic nurses and related disciplines.

Education

Educational programs help prepare nurses for careers in forensic nursing. The IAFN recommends that forensic content be included at all levels of nursing education (Sekula et al., 2012). As nurse graduates became more knowledgeable about forensic issues, additional graduate programs were developed that focused on forensic practice as a specialty area. Forensic education is now offered at all academic levels.

Forensic Nurse Generalist

A registered nurse working in forensics who is prepared at the baccalaureate, associate degree, or diploma level is called a **forensic nurse generalist**. The nurse may acquire additional knowledge and skills by completing a certificate program that comprises continuing education in an area of forensic nursing. Nurses can also gain expertise by taking secondary education electives and/or pursuing a minor in legal topics.

The role of the forensic nurse generalist may vary according to clinical setting but consistent within this role is the need to be proficient in assessment and treatment of victims and perpetrators of violence. The nurse learns evidence collection and preservation, proper documentation, the legal system, and standards of care for both victims and perpetrators.

A forensic nurse generalist may work in a specialty area such as on a trauma team or in an emergency department, corrections, critical care department, outpatient women's health clinic, or may serve as a general resource person for colleagues in the clinical setting. The forensic nurse generalist often provides expertise as a resource for the care provider working with a patient who has been a victim or perpetrator of violence. In addition to addressing patients' physical and psychological needs, forensic nurse generalists are ready to identify and care for victims of violence and know when to collect and preserve evidence.

Advanced Practice Forensic Nursing

Advanced practice certification at the master's level in forensic nursing consists of a portfolio certification process established by the IAFN through the credentialing arm of the ANA—the American Nurses Credentialing Center (ANCC). This credential is called advanced forensic nursing (AFN-BC) and the role is referred to as an **advanced practice forensic nurse**. Nurses in this role have completed graduate education with a comprehensive focus in forensic nursing. Advanced practice forensic nurses may also have obtained credentials as a clinical nurse specialist, certified nurse-midwife, or nurse practitioner. The education provides clinicians with nursing, medical, and legal content and focuses on the collaboration among disciplines in the care of victims and perpetrators. The advance practice registered nurse in forensics also has an educational background in psychiatric assessment and intervention skills, death investigation, forensic wound identification, evidence collection, family violence, sexual assault of all types and in varied populations, introductory law, and principles of criminal justice and forensic science.

Additional advanced training may take place after the completion of a master's degree. Individuals who are prepared with a doctor of nursing practice (DNP) may evaluate and apply evidence-based forensic practice for the improvement of education, clinical practice, systems management, and nursing leadership. A doctor of philosophy (PhD) prepares nurses to initiate and conduct research in an area of forensics to advance nursing science and to ultimately enhance the practice of forensic nursing. Most forensic nursing researchers have completed a doctoral degree or have another advanced degree.

Roles and Functions of Forensic Nurses

In forensic nursing, the nurse-patient relationship occurs based on the possibility that a crime has been committed. However, it is not the role of the forensic nurse to make a decision as to guilt or innocence or whether a victim is being candid in reporting what happened (Sekula, 2016). Basic roles of the forensic nurse include the following:

1. Identification of victims
2. Creation of appropriate treatment plans
3. Collection, documentation, and preservation of potential evidence

The forensic nurse possesses expertise in assessment and treatment related to competency, risk, and danger. Forensic nurses are educated in theories of violence and victimology, legal issues, and nursing science that enable them to objectively assess the circumstances of the case.

An understanding of both the victim and the perpetrator enhances evidence collection. Forensic nurses may apply medical-surgical knowledge to the care of victims and perpetrators or they may function in the legal role primarily as they collect evidence, testify in court, or collaborate with law practitioners regarding victims or perpetrators.

CONSIDERING CULTURE

Historical Trauma in the Dakota Sioux Tribe

In the Dakota Sioux Tribe, an alarming infant mortality rate, chronic obesity, and second-hand drug exposure were identified as primary care issues in children. Adolescents have the highest national per capita rate of suicide. Alcohol and substance use, liver cirrhosis, and kidney failure are too common. Comprehensive health services were seriously underutilized. More than 90% of households met the federal poverty level, and more than 80% of adults were unemployed.

Could historical trauma influence poor health in this population? Settler invasions and religious missions that forced cultural assimilation contributed to the Sioux's historical trauma. Some elders in the tribe experienced abuse after being taken from their families and sent to white boarding schools. These children were forced to cut their hair, were not allowed to speak their native language, and were beaten by their teachers.

In a case report, nurses identified the need for healthcare clinicians to understand the impact of historical trauma on present-day health. They partnered with community members in participatory action, acknowledging the importance of *listening,* and acknowledging pain. Their efforts served to provide a culture where trust, respect, and understanding could develop to begin the process of improving healthcare for this community.

From Heckert, W., & Eisenhauer, C. (2014). A case report of historical trauma among American Indians on a rural Northern Plains reservation. *Journal of Forensic Nursing, 10*(2), 106–109.

Sexual Assault Nurse Examiner

The **sexual assault nurse examiner (SANE)** was the first specialized forensic role for nurses, and it represents the largest subspecialty in forensic nursing. SANEs are forensic nurse generalists who seek training in the care of adult and pediatric victims of sexual assault (SANE-A and SANE-P, respectively). The IAFN has established clear guidelines for the preparation of SANEs and provides certification for nurses, although not all nurses who work in this capacity have achieved certification.

A SANE training course is typically 5 days (40 contact hours) and is available online or in the classroom setting. After course completion, an expert SANE serves as a preceptor for the nurse until the nurse is proficient in conducting the exam. At this point, the nurse can then sit for the national certification exam through the IAFN. Chapter 29 addresses the role of the SANE nurse in more depth.

Nurse Coroner/Death Investigator

The **nurse coroner** or **death investigator** role for nurses was created in the mid-1990s. Traditionally, the coroner is a public official primarily charged with the duty of determining how and why people die. Increasingly, nurses are prepared as death investigators or deputy coroners. Nurses can practice as death investigators in medical examiners' or coroners' offices or independently in private offices. This expanding nursing role involves assessing the deceased through understanding, discovery, preservation, and use of evidence. An entry-level certification, Death Investigator, is available through the American Board of Medicolegal Death Investigation.

Nurses who work as nurse coroners or death investigators possess medical knowledge that allows them to make expert judgments regarding the circumstances of death. These judgments are based on observations of history, symptomatology, autopsy results, toxicology, other diagnostic studies, and evidence revealed in other aspects of the case (Mitchell & Drake, 2016).

Nurses are able to expand the role of the coroner and the death investigator and improve services provided to families, healthcare agencies, and communities by using basic principles of holistic nursing care. Knowledge of anatomy and physiology, pathophysiology, pharmacology, grief and grieving, growth and development, interviewing, outcomes measurement, and other nursing knowledge strengthen the value of nurses in this setting.

FORENSIC PSYCHIATRIC NURSING

A **forensic psychiatric nurse** may be one who is prepared as a generalist or at the advanced practice level. In the generalist role, nurses are prepared at the entry level with a college/university degree, associate or diploma degree, which prepares them to function as direct care providers and patient advocates. At this level, a nurse who practices in a forensic psychiatric setting can gain advanced knowledge through continuing education or certificate programs that provide education in caring for the forensic patient.

At the advanced practice level, graduate education is required, which prepares nurses to function as psychiatric clinical nurse specialists or psychiatric nurse practitioners. Additional graduate work in forensics at the master's and post-master's levels provides the knowledge needed to practice with forensic populations. This specialty requires skills in psychiatric-mental health nursing assessment, evaluation, and treatment of victims or perpetrators. Combining the skills of medical and psychiatric nursing with a thorough understanding of the criminal justice system is pertinent to expert practice (Sekula & Amar, 2016).

Evidence collection is central to the role of the forensic psychiatric nurse. For example, you collect evidence by carefully evaluating the perpetrator's intent or determining if the perpetrator had **diminished capacity** (impaired mental functioning) at the time of the crime. This evaluation aids in determining the degree of crime and may later influence the sentence. Forensic psychiatric nurses who work as competency evaluators collect evidence by spending many hours with a defendant and carefully documenting the dialogue. In this capacity, the role of the forensic psychiatric nurse is not to determine guilt or innocence, but to provide assessment data that can help make a final diagnosis within the multidisciplinary forensic team (Sekula & Burgess, 2006).

The forensic psychiatric nurse should be skilled in interpersonal communications and able to develop collegial relationships with those in other disciplines. A prerequisite is the ability to listen and accept others' values and motivations in a nonjudgmental fashion.

Forensic psychiatric nursing appeals to a particular type of nurse—one who thrives in a stimulating intellectual environment, seeks out opportunities to apply clinical skills to complex legal problems, and enjoys pushing the limits of traditional boundaries. The forensic psychiatric nurse is sometimes viewed with skepticism and with caution in the legal system, often due to lack of knowledge regarding their roles. Responses to skepticism must be met with professionalism in practice, research, and education. Educating colleagues in both forensic science and in the legal system as to the roles of forensic psychiatric nurses is important, keeping in mind the tenets of evidence-based practice.

BOX 33.2 Forensic Psychiatric Nursing Functions

- Psychotherapist
- Forensic nurse examiner
- Competency evaluator
- Fact or expert witness
- Consultant to law enforcement agencies or the criminal justice system
- Hostage negotiator
- Criminal profiler

Roles and Functions of Forensic Psychiatric Nurses

The forensic psychiatric nurse may function as a psychotherapist, forensic nurse examiner, competency evaluator, fact or expert witness, consultant to law enforcement agencies or the criminal justice system, hostage negotiator, or criminal profiler. The roles of the forensic psychiatric nurse depend on the outcomes for which the nurse is contracted to accomplish. The legal system may contract these forensic psychiatric nurses to interface with the perpetrator for a variety of services. Correctional systems or a private organization may also employ forensic nurses to offer direct services to the perpetrator. They can also provide services to the victim in a variety of settings. A list of role functions of forensic psychiatric nurses is provided in Box 33.2.

Nurse Psychotherapist

In addition to the competencies possessed by the generalist, the forensic advanced practice registered nurse in psychiatric-mental health (APRN-PMH) may function as a psychotherapist, providing individual, family, and group therapy. Depending on educational preparation and individual state statutes, an APRN-PMH may have prescriptive privileges and initiate psychopharmacology treatment along with psychotherapy. While this role is seriously limited within the corrections systems due to procedural and economic restrictions, the role is often filled in the private sector for perpetrators with the necessary financial resources.

Forensic Psychiatric Nurse Examiner

Important functions of the forensic psychiatric nurse examiner are to conduct court-ordered evaluations regarding legal sanity or competency to proceed in a court case, to respond to specific medicolegal questions as requested by the court, and to render an expert opinion in a written report or during courtroom testimony. The prosecution, the defense, or the judge may request an evaluation. Evaluations are usually based on the defendant's history along with behavior at the scene of the crime, in jail, or in the courtroom. A comprehensive report is based on clinical data, observations of the defendant's behavior, forensic evidence contained in crime-scene reports or laboratory reports, a summary of psychological testing, and a thorough psychosocial history. The **forensic nurse examiner** interviews the defendant and notes behavior, past diagnoses, personality traits, emotions, cognitive abilities, symptoms of a psychiatric disorder, and the psychodynamics of interpersonal relationships.

The forensic psychiatric nurse examiner must be able to separate personal opinion from professional opinion. Personal opinion is based on one's background, upbringing, education, and value system. Professional opinion is based on scientific principle, advanced education in a specific field of endeavor, and the unbiased standards set by research in that area. Although other members of the treatment staff on a forensic unit strive to be supportive, accepting, and empathetic, the forensic nurse examiner strives to remain neutral, objective, and detached.

Legal sanity is the individual's ability to distinguish right from wrong with reference to the act with which he or she is charged. Legal sanity is also characterized by the capacity to understand the nature and quality of the act and capacity to form the intent to commit the crime. Legal sanity is determined for the specific time of the act.

The forensic nurse examiner must reconstruct the defendant's mental state by reviewing evidence left at the scene, witness statements, the self-report of the defendant's symptoms, and the defendant's motivation. Some of the issues addressed in the forensic nurse examiner's assessment and final report are (1) whether or not the defendant was using drugs, (2) whether a medical condition affected the defendant's reasoning ability, and (3) what the social context of the crime was.

In most states, the presence of a major mental disorder (usually referring to those that cause psychoses—delusions, hallucinations, and disorganized thought—such as schizophrenia) is a prerequisite for a finding of *legal insanity*. However, a defendant who has a mental illness does not have to use this defense. It is the defendant's choice. The forensic nurse specialist must have a clear knowledge of which legal standard is being used and must be able to articulate it to the court and jury. Legal tests of sanity may include use of the McNaughton rules: *irresistible impulse* and *guilty but mentally ill*.

The *McNaughton rules* come from a trial in 1843 in which Daniel McNaughton was tried for the murder of a public official. McNaughton believed there was a conspiracy among the Tories of England to destroy him. In an attempt to assassinate the prime minister who was the Tory leader, McNaughton mistakenly shot and killed the prime minister's secretary. McNaughton was judged to be criminally insane, acquitted of the murder, and institutionalized for life.

There was a public outcry over the leniency of this verdict. The House of Lords convened a special session of the judges to give an advisory opinion regarding the law of England governing the insanity defense. The judges advised that to be considered legally insane, the accused person with a mental disorder either must not know the nature and quality of the act or must not know whether the act is right or wrong. Whether or not the individual is responsible for his action is the underlying issue in the McNaughton rules.

Irresistible impulse was added to the McNaughton rules in 1929. This addition acknowledges that the person may have known the criminal act was wrong. However, it stipulates that if a person could not control behavior because of a psychiatric illness or a mental defect that the defendant is not guilty.

Guilty but mentally ill is another insanity defense. Those who plead guilty but mentally ill are remanded (sent) to the correctional system where they receive treatment for their mental disorder. They are then subject to the correctional system's parole decisions.

Whereas legal insanity is determined by the defendant's thinking at the time of the offense, *competence to proceed* is determined by the defendant's mental condition at the time of the trial. It is the capacity to assist one's attorney and understand the legal proceedings. Because competence to proceed is a determination of mental capacity in the present, the defendant's competency must be determined each time a court hearing is held. A prior finding of incompetence, even if due to a developmental disability or mental illness, does not prevent a finding of competency in a future unrelated case.

Competency Evaluator

Under US federal law, no person may be tried if deemed legally incompetent. If this is the case, the defendant must be sent to a suitable facility, usually a locked unit in a psychiatric facility, for a specified period of treatment to regain competency.

Roles of the **competency evaluator** include assessing mental health or illness, conducting a forensic interview, providing documentation, completing a formal report to the court, and testifying as an expert witness. Competency evaluators work with the defendant in one-to-one and group activities. For competency therapists, the patient is the court, not the defendant, and the products of their work are a competent defendant and a completed report. Becoming an advocate for the defendant, rather than for the process, is a breach of professional boundaries.

Fact and Expert Witnesses

You can use three types of witnesses in the courtroom trial: (1) the principals (plaintiffs and defendants), (2) fact witnesses, and (3) expert witnesses. Each witness has a specific role in the presentation of the case and in establishing the required burden of proof.

The court can subpoena any nurse to testify as a **fact witness**. A fact witness testifies regarding what was *personally* seen or heard, performed, or documented regarding a patient's care and testifies as to first-hand experience only (Sekula & Burgess, 2006).

An expert witness is recognized by the court as having a certain level of skill or expertise in a designated area and possesses superior knowledge because of education or specialized experience. The **expert witness** is used routinely in medical malpractice cases. Nurses functioning in this capacity are capable and qualified to summarize and explain complex and voluminous medical records and terminology to the jury.

A nurse may testify as a fact witness and an expert witness. For example, a SANE may testify regarding the facts of a case in which she examined the victim and collected evidence and may also testify in the case because of her expertise as a certified SANE-A.

Forensic nurses with advanced degrees are more likely to be called upon as expert witnesses. To establish credibility as an expert witness and to have one's opinion given equal weight to that of other professionals in court, the forensic nurse specialist

BOX 33.3 Requirements for Expert Witness Testimony

Establishment of Expertise
- Academic preparation
- Professional training
- Practical working experience in the field
- Involvement in professional organizations
- Research and publications in the area of expertise

Establishment of Trustworthiness and Objectivity
- Comfortable with self
- Good presentation style
- Successful communication to jury
- Dress, manner, and performance that communicate professionalism

must have current and updated clinical expertise, trustworthiness, and a professional presentation style (Box 33.3). Professional credentials indicate clinical expertise. Trustworthiness is indicated by the degree of honesty and strength of opinion that is provided on the witness stand. A professional presentation style is essential. Nurses who are expert witnesses need to be able to communicate in a concise and convincing fashion. In addition, if the expert has conducted research and published in the area, it is an added strength.

Consultant

Over the past five decades, deinstitutionalization has created a need for interagency cooperation between mental health and law enforcement. Although controversial, individuals who previously would have been institutionalized are now commonly homeless and often, intentionally or unintentionally, the focus of law enforcement.

The forensic psychiatric nurse serving in a **consultant** role can provide advice to mental health agencies regarding the care of the individuals with legal issues. Nurses in this role can also consult with law enforcement agencies regarding the status and suggested treatment of individuals with mental illness in the legal system. The nurse may also act as an advocate for families and patients. The focus of the nurse who serves in this capacity is the perpetrator's well-being even if that results in civil detention and admission to a hospital. An entry-level certification is available—Legal Nurse Consultant—through the American Association of Legal Nurse Consultants.

A forensic psychiatric nurse may be used as a resource for education and information about mental illness by either side in a court case. In this consultant role, the nurse may be asked to listen to witness testimony for the purpose of guiding further cross-examination or to assist in the preparation for trial by giving information about mental illness including personality disorders and paraphilic disorders. The nurse may testify about mental health treatment options, medications, and community resources.

Hostage Negotiator

In the late 1970s, the Federal Bureau of Investigation (FBI) began expanding its hostage-negotiation team structure by recommending the use of consultants who could address the mental state of the perpetrator and recommend appropriate negotiation strategies. In the 1980s, local police agencies began to develop specialized teams that included consultants. When the forensic psychiatric-mental nurse functions as a **hostage negotiator**, the role may include the following:

- Being on call around the clock to assist law enforcement officers on the scene
- Providing suggestions regarding negotiation techniques
- Assessing the mental status of the perpetrator
- Providing a link to mental health agencies
- Participating in a critique of the hostage incident
- Assessing released hostages
- Assessing the stress level of the hostage negotiator
- Providing training in communication skills to law enforcement officers

The successful hostage negotiator should be able to think clearly under stress, communicate with persons from all socioeconomic classes, and demonstrate common sense and street smarts. Hostage negotiators need to cope with uncertainty, accept responsibility with no authority, and be committed to the negotiation process.

Criminal Profiler

A **criminal profiler** attempts to provide law enforcement officials with specific information about the type of individual who may have committed a certain crime. This service is usually requested when the crime scene indicates psychopathology or when serial crime is suspected. Historically, criminal profilers came from a variety of backgrounds including law enforcement, psychology, psychiatry, and criminal justice. The criminal profiler collects available data, attempts to reconstruct the crime, formulates a hypothesis, develops a profile, and tests it against the known data.

This is familiar territory for the forensic psychiatric nurse, who is comfortable with the nursing processes of assessment, diagnosis (analysis), planning, implementation, and evaluation. Ann Burgess, one of the founders of the IAFN, was the first identified nurse criminal profiler with the FBI (Burgess et al., 2004). Skilled profilers have the ability to reconstruct the crime using the criminal's reasoning process (Kocsis & Palermo, 2015). Although this requires time and thoughtful consideration, the insights gained are usually critical for diagnosis and treatment. Psychiatric mental health nurses offer special skills as profilers of perpetrators because of their knowledge of psychiatry and human behavior.

CORRECTIONAL NURSING

Correctional nursing is the care of incarcerated patients and presents challenges to the way nurses think about patients. There is debate as to the terminology used when referring to both correctional nurses and psychiatric-mental health nurses within correctional settings. Education is key in determining the level of expertise and whether one merits the title *forensic nurse,* either psychiatric-mental health or correctional. Working in a correctional setting does not qualify one as a forensic nurse. Rather, it is the advanced education and clinical practice that qualifies a person to use the title of forensic nurse (Sekula, 2016).

At the end of 2015, an estimated 2,173,800 persons were either incarcerated in state or federal prisons or in the custody of local jails in the United States (US Department of Justice, 2016). Offenders supervised in the community on either probation (3,789,800) or parole (870,500) account for most of the US correctional population in 2015. The number of incarcerated individuals in the United States had been steadily increasing for both men and women over the past two decades. On a positive note, the numbers have hit their lowest rate since 2002.

Prisoners are the only US population group with a constitutional right to healthcare. Because most of their civil liberties are taken away from them and their movements are severely restricted, prisoners are unable to seek and secure healthcare services on their own. Therefore correctional facilities must provide "adequate" health services to inmates, either directly or through community health services organizations. The issue regarding whether nurses are providing *custody* or *caring* is a major issue when determining the role of the nurse in the corrections setting. This includes treatment for both mental and physical illnesses. The location of the work or the legal status of the patient defines the role of the correctional nurse rather than the role functions being performed.

Incarcerated men and women have higher rates of serious and chronic physical and mental illnesses than the general population, requiring enormous healthcare efforts (Colbert et al., 2013). Treatment and services for inmates with chronic mental health diagnoses are a significant part of the job for correctional staff. According to the US Department of Justice (2015), about one in three state prisoners, one in four federal prisoners, and one in six jail inmates with a mental health problem received treatment during their incarceration, which amounts to hundreds of thousands of incarcerated adults. Additionally, nearly 25% of inmates with a mental health diagnosis have had three or more prior incarcerations.

In addition to those receiving care are the thousands of incarcerated adults known to have a mental health problem who are not receiving treatment. When compared with the rates in the general population (11% of whom have a mental health problem with approximately 55,000 individuals hospitalized at an inpatient psychiatric hospital on any given day), it is clear that correctional facilities carry a disproportionate share of the burden for the provision of mental health services (McKenna et al., 2014).

Correctional nurses provide care for many patients with serious mental illnesses who are caught in a cycle of homelessness, psychiatric hospitals, and jail. Frequently, these individuals become incarcerated as a result of psychiatric emergencies that generally include threats made to others. Because psychiatric facilities for the management of such emergencies are scarce, often these patients end up in jail instead of in a hospital. Once they are in jail, their psychiatric condition often worsens without adequate psychiatric intervention. The fortunate patients end up in a secure treatment unit within the jail where they receive proper medication and psychiatric-mental health nursing care.

Because of the long-term effects on recidivism (repeat offenders) and resource allocation, policy makers and legislators are beginning to recognize the importance of providing treatment for patients who are incarcerated. In a US Department of Justice (2006) survey, the most common mental health symptoms were insomnia and hypersomnia. Commonly reported symptoms were related to major depression. Delusions and hallucinations were the most commonly identified psychotic symptoms with 25% of state inmates, 15% of federal inmates, and 10% of jail inmates reporting at least one of the two symptoms. Especially critical within this population is treatment of those with a history of trauma or posttraumatic stress disorder (PTSD). The correctional setting, however, is not conducive to the intensive therapy required to adequately treat these issues. Therefore the needs of the vast majority of people with PTSD and/or trauma history in the correctional system are not adequately addressed.

Alcohol and substance use is another critical issue associated with incarceration. According to the National Institute on Drug Abuse (NIDA, 2012), about half of all inmates at state and federal prisons meet the criteria for alcohol or substance use disorder, but few receive treatment in jail or prison. There is a great deal of controversy over how to respond to people with substance use problems who commit crimes: Should we incarcerate or provide treatment? Much of the debate revolves around a more basic question of whether incarceration should be punishment or rehabilitation. There is significant evidence to support rehabilitation if the goal is improving safety in communities and reducing crime. Drug courts and alcohol and substance treatment within correctional facilities have all shown to decrease the likelihood of recidivism and increase the likelihood of abstinence from substances and/or alcohol after release.

VIGNETTE: Susan Barnes is a 34-year-old woman recently incarcerated after being arrested for public intoxication and retail theft.

Past History:

- Multiple incarcerations over the past 10 years for drug use and minor property crimes
- Previously diagnosed with bipolar I disorder, she has been on multiple medications
- Past arrests associated with discontinuing medications and self-medicating with crack cocaine and other drugs

She reports being off her medications "for a while." Correctional staff notes that she is acting erratically, pacing the floor, and not sleeping. Her behavior is becoming more aggressive toward others, and the staff has threatened to put her in solitary confinement.

A forensic psychiatric nurse practitioner (NP) interviews Ms. Barnes, who says she "feels great" and "the cops are just out to get me." Her speech is pressured, and she expresses significant hostility. She is diagnosed as being in an acute manic phase. Her plan of care focuses on safety, stabilization, medications, patient education, and sleep hygiene. NP orders her to be housed in the infirmary until stabilization at which time she will be reevaluated for return to the general jail population.

Discharge planning is especially critical since Ms. Barnes' involvement in the criminal justice system coincides with stopping her medications. She will be assessed for Forensic Mental Health Court, which offers specialized services for offenders with severe mental illness. This program provides access to a variety of institutional and community-based services and allows the judge to require participation in treatment and follow-up as terms of release from jail. The treatment plan includes intensive case management upon release to address needs such as housing, healthcare, and food. The NP knows that a key outcome for this patient is preventing a return to jail.

In addition to the needs of people living with mental illness while they are incarcerated, the nurse must also address the needs of those same people when they are released and returning home. The reentry experience is more difficult for persons with mental illness due to factors such as physical health problems and housing and employment difficulties (Colbert et al., 2013). To be effective, services for this population must include comprehensive discharge planning. Nurses working in this setting must try to facilitate ongoing care for people living with chronic mental illness. This may include advocating for alternatives to incarceration because the prison systems are often ill-equipped to deal with the needs of people with severe mental illness, nor is the purpose of incarceration that kind of care. The alarmingly high rates of mental illness in the offender population, often referred to as the "criminalization of mental illness," has encouraged advocates to push for options other than jail or prison, such as treatment programs.

Correctional nurses working in facilities with comprehensive psychiatric services perform psychiatric-mental health nursing role functions rather than forensic nursing role functions. These functions include completing comprehensive mental status examinations and implementing psychiatric care plans. The following vignette illustrates challenging situations facing correctional psychiatric nurses.

VIGNETTE: Suzanne, a 45-year-old woman incarcerated at a state facility, is convicted of assault with a deadly weapon after a confrontation. Psychiatric diagnosis includes major depression and PTSD (severe abuse in childhood and intimate partner violence). She is seen by the facility's psychiatric-mental health nurse practitioner (NP) for medication management.

While watching television in the common area, she attacked a fellow inmate for no apparent reason, screaming and clawing at anyone who approached her. Staff, unable to control her physically, placed her in solitary confinement with mechanical restraints.

The NP reported that Suzanne was having a flashback related to her PTSD and the solitary confinement and restraints were worsening her flashbacks. The staff and the NP were facing a common dilemma in correctional healthcare: custody versus caring. While the NP was focusing on the needs of Suzanne, the correctional staff were focused on the goals of the correctional facility related to violent offenders and protecting the environment. A successful correctional treatment team seeks to balance the two sides of this debate: Creating an environment where possible rehabilitation of offenders is possible without compromising the compulsory "punitive" aspects of incarceration.

EVIDENCE-BASED PRACTICE

How Do Psychiatric Forensic Patients and Nurses View Seclusion?

Problem

Seclusion is widely regarded as a complicated therapeutic intervention with consequences for patients, staff, and the unit. However, for patients and nurses in the psychiatric forensic care setting, seclusion is a reality of care used primarily in situations to protect patient safety and well-being. Clinical staff may use this strategy more effectively if they better understand the experience of seclusion for patients and nurses.

Purpose of Study

The purpose of this study was to describe the lived experience of seclusion in a psychiatric forensic setting from the patient's and nurse's perspectives.

Methods

This qualitative study employed a modified Interpretative Phenomenological Analysis design, which emphasizes the lived experience and perceptions of the world around them. A total of 26 participants, 13 forensic psychiatric inpatients who had experienced seclusion in the previous 6 months and 13 psychiatric nurses who had taken care of a secluded patient in the previous 6 months, were included. Content analysis was used to code and categorize data.

Key Findings

- For the patients, three major themes emerged: experienced seclusion (reaction and impact on mental state), assessing quality of care (specifically while secluded), and space of confinement (the room and physical space).
- The data from nurses also produced three major themes: resorting to seclusion (reasoning and use as last resort), observing and assessing patients, and experiencing seclusion (impact on patient and relationship).
- Both patients and nurses emphasized the importance of maintaining a therapeutic relationship during any period of patient seclusion.
- Patients and nurses found seclusion to be difficult and prefer to see seclusion as a last resort. However, both expressed that it is needed for the safety and well-being of patients.
- Patients requested more information about why they were secluded (after the situation stabilizes) and recommend postseclusion debriefing for patients and others on the unit who may have been affected. Nurses also felt a need for that kind of debriefing themselves.
- The authors stress the importance of recognizing the "bodily" experience of seclusion as part of care.

Implications for Nursing Practice

The use of seclusion with psychiatric forensic patients must be a deliberate clinical choice, and nurses have an obligation to understand the impact of seclusion on patients, the quality of care, and the therapeutic relationship. Specific recommendations from this study about communicating with patients about seclusion in that context can influence care.

From Holmes, D., Murray, S. J., & Knack, N. (2015). Experiencing seclusion in a forensic psychiatric setting: A phenomenological study. *Journal of Forensic Nursing, 11*(4), 200–213.

KEY POINTS TO REMEMBER

- Forensic nursing is an emerging specialty area of practice that combines elements of traditional nursing, forensic science, and criminal justice.
- Psychiatric forensic nursing requires that a nurse gain additional education to serve this unique population.
- The International Association of Forensic Nurses (IAFN) was established in 1992 as the professional association representing this specialty. IAFN offers certification for the sexual assault nurse examiner.

- Forensic psychiatric nurses can fulfill a variety of roles including that of therapist, forensic nurse examiner, competency evaluator, fact witness, expert witness, consultant, hostage negotiator, criminal profiler, and correctional nurse.
- The forensic psychiatric nurse must understand the roles of other forensic nurses to function on teams to provide quality care for all victims and perpetrators of violence.
- Forensic nursing brings together traditional nursing practice with forensic knowledge to better serve all persons within the healthcare system affected by violence in some way.
- The forensic nurse generalist must be proficient in assessment and treatment of victims of violence, evidence collection and preservation, proper documentation, the legal system, and setting standards of care for victims and perpetrators.
- In contrast to other members of the treatment staff on a forensic unit who can be supportive, accepting, and empathetic, the forensic nurse examiner must remain neutral, objective, and detached.
- Correctional nursing is the care of incarcerated patients. Treatment of psychiatric disorders and alcohol and/or substance use is a critical issue that needs to be addressed in the prison population to decrease recidivism and promote a better quality of life.

CRITICAL THINKING

1. Compare and contrast the roles of the forensic psychiatric nurse and the correctional nurse. How do their roles differ regarding their relationship with the patient?
2. Given the varied and complex roles within forensic psychiatric nursing, how does an advanced practice forensic psychiatric nurse prepare for these roles? What educational requirements should be considered?
3. The Institute of Medicine's report on the *Future of Nursing: Leading Change, Advancing Health* (2010) encourages all nurses to be full partners with physicians and other healthcare professionals in redesigning healthcare. How can a forensic psychiatric nurse prepare to be a part of that team?
4. As a forensic psychiatric nurse, describe circumstances under which you might be called to serve as a fact witness versus being called as an expert witness? What types of education and practice requirements are needed for each role?

CHAPTER REVIEW

Questions

1. The forensic nurse examiner is attempting to reconstruct the mental state of an individual accused of a hit and run automobile accident. Which question(s) would help achieve that goal? *Select all that apply.*
   - **a.** "Were you under the influence of illegal substances at the time of the accident?"
   - **b.** "What were you feeling when you realized you had hit someone crossing the street?"
   - **c.** "Have you ever been involved in a hit and run accident before?"
   - **d.** "Can you remember the events leading up to the accident?"
   - **e.** "Had you and your friends been drinking before the accident?"
2. A forensic nurse examiner is interviewing an individual accused of a homicide. Which question should the nurse ask in preparation for a possible legal insanity defense?
   - **a.** "Have you ever been told that you are intellectually deficient?"
   - **b.** "Do you ever hear voices that no one else can hear?"
   - **c.** "What were you doing the day the crime was committed?"
   - **d.** "Did you know the individual who was murdered?"
3. Which nurse would qualify as a fact witness in a case dealing with a physically abused young child?
   - **a.** A psychiatric nurse
   - **b.** A sexual assault nurse examiner nurse
   - **c.** An emergency room nurse
   - **d.** A pediatric intensive care unit nurse
4. Which intervention focused on children supports the *Healthy People 2020* goals related to injury and violence prevention? *Select all that apply.*
   - **a.** Screening middle school-aged children for evidence of bullying.
   - **b.** Identifying risk-taking behaviors among high school students that often result in injury.
   - **c.** Holding a focus group discussion regarding the reasons students bring weapons onto school property.
   - **d.** Holding a community forum to identify the main sources of violence children are exposed to.
   - **e.** Screening to determine the prevalence of unprotected sex.
5. Forensic nursing combines scientific knowledge and inquiry in an effort to serve:
   - **a.** Victims of crime
   - **b.** Perpetrators of violence
   - **c.** Victims and perpetrators of crime
   - **d.** Families of crime victims
6. In understanding the role of victim and perpetrator, the act of evidence collection is enhanced. What knowledge base assists in caring for the injured victim?
   - **a.** Legal aspects
   - **b.** Experience testifying in court
   - **c.** Collaboration with law practitioners
   - **d.** Medical-surgical nursing skills

7. The psychiatric forensic nurse (PFN) has been asked to evaluate an incarcerated patient who has mental health problems for a competency hearing. As the patient is being considered for sentencing, what is the PFN's role? *Select all that apply.*
   a. Assessing the patient for level of competency
   b. Determining whether the patient is guilty or innocent
   c. Assisting in determining the length of the sentence
   d. Completing a formal report to the court
   e. Becoming an advocate for the incarcerated patient
8. To determine a patient's legal sanity or competency, the psychiatric forensic nurse must assess all of the following, *except*:
   a. The patient's ability to distinguish right from wrong regarding the act
   b. The patient's capacity to understand the nature of the act committed
   c. The evidence with respect to the defendant's mental state at the time of the act
   d. The patient's social network
9. You are caring for Naomi who has been arrested and is found to be at risk for alcohol and drug use. Which approach is thought to be most useful in treating Naomi?
   a. Recommending that the patient receive treatment when released from jail
   b. Providing immediate drug/alcohol treatment plan
   c. Immediately withdrawing all medications
   d. Isolating the patient until withdrawal from drugs is complete
10. Which activity does a correctional nurse not fulfill within the corrections setting?
   a. Nursing assessment
   b. Maintain proper safety procedures
   c. Psychotherapy
   d. Document patient progress

Answers

1. **a, b, d, e**; 2. **b**; 3. **d**; 4. **b, c, d**; 5. **c**; 6. **d**; 7. **a, d**; 8. **d**; 9. **b**; 10. **c**

Visit the Evolve website for a posttest on the content in this chapter: http://evolve.elsevier.com/Varcarolis

Post-Test interactive review

REFERENCES

Burgess, A. W., Berger, A. D., & Boersma, R. R. (2004). Forensic nursing: Investigating the career potential in this emerging graduate specialty. *American Journal of Nursing, 104*(3), 58–64.

Colbert, A. M., Sekula, L. K., Zoucha, R., & Cohen, S. M. (2013). Health care needs of women immediately post-incarceration: A mixed methods study. *Public Health Nursing, 30*(5), 409–419.

Institute of Medicine. (2010). *The future of nursing: leading change, advancing health.* Retrieved from http://www.nursingworld.org/MainMenuCategories/ThePracticeofProfessionalNursing/workforce/IOM-Future-of-Nursing-Report-1.

International Association of Forensic Nursing. (2009). *Forensic nursing: Scope and standards of practice* (2nd ed.). Silver Spring, MD: nursesbooks.org.

International Association of Forensic Nursing. (2016). *About forensic nursing.* Retrieved from http://www.forensicnurses.org/?page=WhatisFN.

International Association of Forensic Nurses and American Nurses Association. (1997). *Scope and standards of forensic nursing practice.* Washington, DC: American Nurses Publishing.

Kocsis, R. N., & Palermo, G. B. (2015). Disentangling criminal profiling: Accuracy, homology, and the myth of trait-based profiling. *International Journal of Offender Therapy and Comparative Criminology, 59*(3), 313–332.

Lynch, V. (1997). Forensic nursing. *Virginia Nurses Today, 5*(2), 27.

McKenna, B., Furness, T., Dhital, D., et al. (2014). The transformation from custodial to recovery-oriented care: A paradigm shift that needed to happen. *Journal of Forensic Nursing, 10*(4), 226–233.

Mitchell, S. A., & Drake, S. A. (2016). Murder, assault and battery, stranger danger. In A. F. Amar, & L. K. Sekula (Eds.), *A practice guide to forensic nursing: Incorporating forensic principles into forensic practice* (pp. 243–261). Indianapolis, IN: Sigma Theta Tau International.

National Institute on Drug Abuse. (2012). *Principles of drug addiction treatment: A research based guide.* Washington, DC: Author.

Sekula, L. K. (2016). What is forensic nursing? In A. F. Amar & L. K. Sekula (Eds.), *A practice guide to forensic nursing: Incorporating forensic principles into forensic practice* (pp. 1–15). Indianapolis, IN: Sigma Theta Tau International.

Sekula, K., & Amar, A. F. (2016). Forensic mental health nursing. In A. F. Amar & L. K. Sekula (Eds.), *A practice guide to forensic nursing: Incorporating forensic principles into forensic practice* (pp. 225–242). Indianapolis, IN: Sigma Theta Tau International.

Sekula, L. K., & Burgess, A. W. (2006). Forensic and legal nursing. In C. H. Wecht & J. T. Rago (Eds.), *Forensic science and law: Investigative applications in criminal, civil, and family justice* (pp. 601–627). Boca Raton, FL: CRC Press.

Sekula, L. K., Colbert, A. M., Zoucha, R., et al. (2012). Strengthening the science of forensic nursing through education and research. *Journal of Forensic Nursing, 8*(1), 1–2.

United States Department of Justice. (2006). *United States uniform crime report.* Washington, DC: Author.

United States Department of Justice. (2015). *2015 crime in the United States.* Retrieved from https://www.fbi.gov/about-us/cjis/ucr/crime-in-the-u.s/2015/preliminary-semiannual-uniform-crime-report-januaryjune-2015/home.

United States Department of Justice. (2016). *U.S. correctional population at lowest level since 2002.* Retrieved from https://www.bjs.gov/content/pub/press/cpus15pr.cfm.

34

Therapeutic Groups

Donna Rolin, Sandra Snelson Yaklin

Visit the Evolve website for a pretest on the content in this chapter: http://evolve.elsevier.com/Varcarolis Pre-Test interactive review

OBJECTIVES

1. Identify basic concepts related to group work.
2. Describe the phases of group development.
3. Define task and maintenance roles of group members.
4. Discuss Yalom's therapeutic factors.
5. Discuss seven types of groups commonly led by basic level registered nurses.
6. Describe a group intervention for (a) a member who is silent or (b) a member who is demoralizing.

OUTLINE

KEY TERMS AND CONCEPTS

feedback	group process	maintenance roles
group content	group psychotherapy	task roles
group norms	group work	therapeutic factors
group phases	individual roles	therapeutic group

"It takes people to make people sick, and it takes people to make people well again."

Harry Stack Sullivan (1953)

Humans are fundamentally social and are wired for attachment (Siegel, 2012). We form groups because we are psychologically and physiologically dependent on one another. A **group** is an interconnected and interdependent set of individuals who come together for a shared purpose. These purposes can vary as widely as marriage (a *social group*), inventing cures for cancer, or building a nuclear reactor (*task groups*). Groups can be as large and complex as nations or as intimate as those with whom we share the love, joy, anxiety, fear, sorrow, and doubt that comes with being alive.

FROM GROUP TO THERAPEUTIC GROUP

The first and second World Wars are examples of the fantastic destruction that can arise through human collaboration. These two wars resulted in vast numbers of traumatized veterans and

BOX 34.1 Group Therapy Advantages and Disadvantages

Advantages

- Multiple members can be in treatment at the same time.
- Members of a therapeutic group benefit from the knowledge, insights, and life experiences of both the leader and the participants.
- A therapeutic group can be a safe setting to learn new ways of relating to other people and to practice new communication skills.
- Groups can promote feelings of cohesiveness.

Disadvantages

- Individual members may feel cheated for participation time, particularly in large groups.
- There may be concerns about privacy.
- A member of the group may become disruptive during an emotionally vulnerable point.
- Group identity may discourage dissent.
- Cohesiveness may bind group members together and encourage unacceptable/illegal behaviors.
- Not all patients benefit from group treatment.

People who are acutely psychotic, acutely manic, or intoxicated are not appropriate candidates for group therapy.

civilians. Psychotherapists, in an effort to help the large numbers of psychologically wounded veterans, began to treat individuals in groups. A **therapeutic group** refers to any group of people who meet together for personal development and psychotherapeutic growth.

Group settings provide an efficient method of addressing the needs of multiple individuals. There are drawbacks to this method and group work may not suit every situation. See Box 34.1 for a list of the advantages and disadvantages of group therapy.

Skilled group leaders can usually address and manage problematic group issues. In fact, groups usually provide nurses with excellent opportunities to facilitate growth in patients. This chapter explores concepts central to therapeutic groups, group leadership styles, and various types of group treatment settings.

CONCEPTS COMMON TO ALL GROUPS

Therapeutic Factors

Irvin D. Yalom, an existential psychiatrist, developed an influential approach to **group psychotherapy** (Yalom & Leszcz, 2005). He identified the core principles that make a group therapeutic. These **therapeutic factors** are aspects of the group experience that leaders and members have identified as curative (healing) and crucial for therapeutic change. For example, within a therapeutic group, a member may recognize for the first time that she is not so different from those around her. Yalom calls this factor *universality*—a patient's recognition that other people feel the same way or have had the same experiences. When universality is discovered within a group, it helps create a feeling of belonging and connection.

Group leaders can emphasize certain therapeutic factors that correlate with the desired outcome of the group (DeLucia-Waack et al., 2014). The leader may also role-model some therapeutic behaviors during the initial phase of group development such as *instilling hope* and *imparting information*. Table 34.1 summarizes the curative factors that patients benefit from during group therapy.

Group Content and Process

One of the most fascinating aspects of **group work** is recognizing what is happening on the surface and what is going on underneath. **Group content** is the easiest to describe. If you were to tape record a group's interactions, type up what everyone says, and print it out, you would have a transcript of the content of the group. Minutes from meetings are examples of content.

Group process is the term used to describe everything else that goes on in the group. It refers to the way that group members interact with one another. They may be supportive, interruptive, judgmental, or silent. Their expressions may be concerned, hostile, open, closed, bored, or intense. Speech may be rapid, loud, mumbled, or soft. The group process is the art of doing group work. For groups to be effective and helpful, it is the group process that must be carefully managed and supported.

Groups tend to develop their own identity. Leaders are aware of these identities and may describe them positively with terms such as cohesive and supportive, or negatively with terms such as codependent or disengaged. This shared identity takes the form of group norms. **Group norms** are established expectations or assumptions held by members of a group regarding what kind of behavior is acceptable, good or bad, allowed or not allowed. While group members rarely spontaneously articulate these expectations, they could do so if asked.

Other terms that are central to therapeutic groups are found in Box 34.2.

> *"Everybody is identical in their secret unspoken belief that way deep down they are different from everyone else."*
>
> ***D. F. Wallace (1996)***

PHASES OF GROUP DEVELOPMENT

Group phases represent distinct periods or stages in the process of group development. All groups go through developmental phases similar to those identified for individual therapeutic relationships (refer to Chapter 8). In each phase of the therapeutic group, the group leader has specific roles and challenges to address in support of positive interaction, growth, and change.

Planning Phase

To develop a successful group, planning should include a description of specific characteristics. The following attributes should be identified:

- The name of the group
- Objectives of the group
- Types of individuals (e.g., diagnoses, age, gender) for inclusion
- Group schedule (frequency, times of meetings)
- Physical setting

TABLE 34.1 Curative Factors in Group Therapy

Curative Factor	Description	Example
Interpersonal learning	Members gain insight into themselves based on the feedback from others during later group phases.	"When you speak to me that way, I feel intimidated."
Catharsis	Through experiencing and expressing feelings, therapeutic discharge of emotions is shared.	"This experience allowed me to get in touch with my sadness."
Instillation of hope	The leader shares optimism about successes of group treatment, and members share their improvements.	"You got better, maybe I can too."
Universality	Members realize that they are not alone with their problems, feelings, or thoughts.	"You feel that way too? Wow! I am not alone."
Imparting of information	Participants receive formal teaching by the leader or advice from peers.	"Here is how to take your medication."
Altruism	Members gain or profit from giving support to others, leading to improved self-value.	"I'm sorry that happened to you. I can help you."
Corrective recapitulation of the primary family group	Members repeat patterns of behavior in the group that they learned in their families; with feedback from the leader and peers, they learn about their own behavior.	"Is this the way you speak to your wife at home?"
Socializing techniques	Members learn new social skills based on others' feedback and modeling.	"You took that criticism really well. You didn't appear to become upset. Maybe I can try that."
Imitative behavior	Members may copy behavior from the leader or peers and can adopt healthier habits.	"I like the way you answered that question, maybe I can try that next time."
Group cohesiveness	This powerful factor arises in a mature group when each member feels connected to the other members, the leader, and the group as a whole; members can accept positive feedback and constructive criticism.	"This group has helped me to see that when I complain to my daughter about her father that I am triangulating her by trying to get her on my side. Now I see how unfair this is to her."
Existential resolution	Members examine aspects of life (e.g., loneliness, mortality, responsibility) that affect everyone in constructing meaning.	"I understand that all of us struggle with the inevitable loss."

Data from Yalom, I. D., & Leszcz, M. (2005). *The theory and practice of group psychotherapy* (5th ed.). New York, NY: Basic Books.

BOX 34.2 Terms Central to Therapeutic Groups

Terms Describing Group Work

Group content: All that is said in the group (e.g., the group's topics)

Group process: The dynamics of interaction among the members (e.g., who talks to whom, facial expressions, body language, and progression of group work)

Group norms: Expectations for behavior in the group that develop over time and provide structure (e.g., rules about starting on time, not interrupting)

Group themes: Members' expressed ideas or feelings that recur and share a common thread. The leader may clarify a theme to help members recognize it more fully.

Feedback: Providing group members with awareness about how they affect one another

Conflict: Open disagreement among members. Positive conflict resolution within a group is key to successful outcomes.

- Seating configuration
- Description of leader and member responsibilities
- Methods or means of evaluating outcomes

Other decisions have to do with the type of group being planned. Some groups meet for a specific amount of time to accomplish a certain task while others are open-ended. Additional characteristics of groups are found in Box 34.3.

Planning and structure are especially important when group leaders are likely to change such as in-patient settings where staffing patterns change. When several groups are running simultaneously with a common goal such as in a research study, consistency is crucial.

BOX 34.3 Terms Describing Membership

Heterogeneous group: A group in which a range of differences exists among members

Homogeneous group: A group in which all members share central traits (e.g., men's group, group of patients with bipolar disorder)

Closed group: A group in which membership is restricted; no new members are added when others leave

Open group: A group in which new members are added as others leave (e.g., inpatient group with transient membership)

Subgroup: An individual or a small group that is isolated within a larger group and functions separately. Members of a subgroup may have greater loyalty, more similar goals, or more perceived similarities to one another than they do to the larger group.

Thoughtful consideration of the physical space is important. The size of the room should be functional. A large room for a small group does not encourage intimacy, and an overcrowded room may cause discomfort and anxiety among members. Room temperature, lighting, external noise, and privacy are important comfort measures to consider. Depending on the size of the group, organize the room and its physical boundaries with close nonhierarchical seating. Arranging chairs in a circle conveys equality and allows members to see one another.

Inpatient groups tend to be somewhat different from outpatient groups. In general, inpatient groups require more structure

TABLE 34.2 Comparison of Outpatient and Inpatient Groups

Group Component	Outpatient Groups	Inpatient Groups
Composition	The group has a stable composition.	The group is rarely the same for more than one or two meetings.
Membership selection	Members are carefully selected and prepared.	Patients are admitted to the group with little prior selection or preparation.
Level of functioning	The group is homogeneous with regard to ego function.	The group has a heterogeneous level of ego function.
Motivation	Motivated, self-referred patients make up the group; therapy is growth oriented.	Patients are ambivalent, as therapy is often compulsory; therapy is relief oriented.
Length of group treatment	Treatment proceeds as long as required: may continue for years.	Treatment is limited to the hospital period, with rapid patient turnover.
Boundary	The boundary of the group is well maintained, with few external influences.	Boundary diffuse; events in the milieu affect the group.
Cohesion	Group cohesion develops normally, given sufficient time in treatment.	There may be little time for cohesion to develop spontaneously; group development and work progress may be limited to the initial phases.
Leadership	The leader allows the process to unfold; there is ample time to let group norms evolve.	The group leader structures time and is not passive.
Contact	Members only convene for scheduled group meetings, encouraged to avoid extra group contact.	Patients eat, sleep, and live together outside of the group; extra group contact is endorsed.

Data from Mackenzie, K. R. (1997). *Time-managed group psychotherapy: Effective clinical applications.* Washington, DC: American Psychiatric Press.

due to the acuity level of patients being hospitalized. Table 34.2 compares outpatient to inpatient groups.

Orientation Phase

In the **orientation phase** the group is forming. The group leader's role is active in structuring an atmosphere of respect, confidentiality, and trust. During the first session, the group leader should provide a personal introduction. Members are encouraged to get to know one another through their own introductions. The leader describes the purpose of the group.

Initially, members may be overly polite, quiet, or anxious because they have not yet established trust with one another. Therapeutic interaction is supported when the directive group leader points out similarities between members, encourages them to talk directly to each other rather than to the leader, and reminds members about ground rules for respectful, meaningful interaction.

Participants are urged to treat what happens in the group as confidential. Technology presents several challenges to confidentiality. Mobile phones can be used to record voices and images or to make posts on social media. For this reason and also to reduce disruptive incoming notifications, group members should turn off their phones during group therapy.

Working Phase

During the **working phase,** the leader facilitates communication, the flow of group processes, and group conduct. The group leader's role is to encourage focus on problem solving consistent with the purpose of the group. As group members begin to feel safe within the group, conflicts may be expressed, which should be viewed by the group leader as a positive opportunity for group growth. It is important for the leader to guide and support conflict resolution. Through successful resolution of conflicts, group members develop confidence in their problem-solving abilities and better support one another in their individual efforts to grow and change.

Tuckman (1965) described steps in this working phase, which takes place after the "forming" phase. He called them the classic stages of "storming, norming, and performing" and identified them as natural and necessary in the development of a group.

- Storming refers to the disagreements, attempts at dominance, and personality clashes that must be addressed in order for the work of the group to be done. The authority and legitimacy of the leader may be questioned in this phase.
- Norming occurs when personality clashes and disagreements are resolved and a spirit of cooperation emerges. Team members begin to settle into their respective roles.
- Performing groups have established norms and roles. Group members focus on achieving goals.

The sequence of these phases begins with the generation of group cohesion, followed by completion of group tasks, resulting in insight development. Groups may revert to earlier stages when conflict arises. Leadership activities at different phases of group formation will require different approaches and strategies and ultimately yield team building.

Termination Phase

In the **termination phase,** the leader ensures that each member summarizes personal accomplishments, shares new insights, and identifies future goals. The leader encourages group members to provide both positive and negative feedback regarding the group experience. Feedback refers to information that group members get from other members about how they affect one another. Members may experience feelings of loss or anger about the group ending. At times, the individual can direct these feelings toward other group members or the leader. It is important to openly address such feelings as part of the work toward successful group adjournment.

Post Group Issues: Evaluation and Follow-Up

Evaluation and follow-up are fundamental aspects of a therapeutic group. Objective measures are an important way to demonstrate

TABLE 34.3 Functional Roles of Group Members

Role	Function	Example
Task roles	Coordinator	Tries to connect various ideas and suggestions
	Elaborator	Gives examples and follows up meaning of ideas
	Energizer	Encourages the group to make decisions or take action
	Evaluator	Measures the group's work against objectives
	Information giver	Provides facts or shares experience as an authority figure
	Information seeker	Tries to clarify the group's values
	Initiator-contributor	Offers new ideas or a fresh outlook on an issue
	Opinion giver	Shares opinions, especially to influence group values
	Orienteer	Notes the progress of the group toward goals
	Procedural technician	Supports group activity with physical tasks (e.g., distributing papers, arranging seating)
	Recorder	Keeps notes and acts as the group memory
Maintenance roles	Compromiser	During conflict, yields to preserve group harmony
	Encourager	Praises and seeks input from others
	Follower	Agrees with the flow of the group
	Gatekeeper	Monitors the participation of all members to keep communication open and equal
	Group observer	Notes different aspects of group process and reports to the group
	Harmonizer	Tries to mediate conflicts between members
	Standard setter	Verbalizes standards for the group
Individual roles	Aggressor	Criticizes and attacks others' ideas and feelings
	Blocker	Disagrees with and halts group issues; oppositional
	Dominator	Tries to control other members of the group with flattery or interruptions
	Help seeker	Asks for sympathy of group excessively
	Playboy	Acts disinterested in group process
	Recognition seeker	Seeks attention by boasting and discussing achievements
	Self-confessor	Verbalizes feelings or observations beyond the scope of the group topic
	Special-interest pleader	Advocates for a special group, usually with own prejudice or bias

From Benne, K., & Sheats, P. (1948). Functional roles of group members. *Journal of Social Issues, 4*(2), 41–49.

group effectiveness. Questionnaires can be helpful in refining what patients found helpful. The Therapeutic Factors Inventory-19 (Joyce et al., 2011) is a questionnaire that asks patients to identify which of the therapeutic factors were present in therapy. The Group Questionnaire (Burlingame, 2010) is another tool that evaluates the climate, cohesion, empathy, and alliance of the group. Regardless of the scale or instrument used, group leaders should evaluate all groups to determine if goals set in the planning phase were accomplished and to reevaluate or redesign future groups.

GROUP PARTICIPANT ROLES

We each have a particular style of interacting with others. Some of us tend to sit back and observe, giving an opinion only after careful consideration. Others feel it is important to keep everyone moving in a common direction, or helping maintain order, or actively urging people to continue working. The way we behave in groups is a function of our personalities (e.g., shy or outgoing), socialization (e.g., birth order, prior exposure to groups), and comfort or interest with the context of the group (e.g., topic, members, leader).

Studies of group dynamics have identified functional roles that group members often assume which may either help or hinder the group's development. The classic descriptive categories for these roles are task, maintenance, and individual roles (Benne & Sheats, 1948). **Task roles** keep the group focused on its main purpose and get the work done. **Maintenance roles** keep the group together, help each person feel worthwhile and included, and create a sense of group cohesion. **Individual roles** have nothing to do with helping the group but instead relate to specific personalities, personal agendas, and desires for having personal needs met. For example, a blocker throws up roadblocks to disrupt group progress or to avoid doing his own real work.

Awareness of roles that individual members assume can assist the group leader in identifying behaviors that should be reinforced or confronted. Members' growing self-awareness of their roles may encourage more deliberate and insightful group participation and growth.

Table 34.3 describes the functional roles of group members.

THERAPEUTIC FRAMEWORK FOR GROUPS

Psychiatric-mental health nurses are involved in a variety of therapeutic groups in acute care, long-term, and community treatment settings. For all group leaders, a clear theoretical framework is necessary for analyzing the group dynamics and progress. Table 34.4 describes common theoretical frameworks underlying group work.

NURSE AS A GROUP LEADER

Registered nurses who are trained at the basic level (diploma, associate degree, or baccalaureate degree) have holistic training and educational leadership skills to provide group therapy in a variety

TABLE 34.4 Theoretical Foundations for Group Therapy

Theoretical Base	Focus	Leader Practices
Humanism (patient centered, existential, experiential)	Self-actualization; awareness of subjective experience	Nondirective, active listening, Socratic dialogue
Cognitive-behavioral	Specific maladaptive behaviors and thought patterns	Goal setting, planning, reinforcing, modeling, and monitoring
Psychodynamic (psychoanalytic, Gestalt)	Insight; resolution of intrapsychic conflict	Listening, interpreting, confronting, probing, working through, directing enactments
Psychoeducational	Information on specific topics; coping; emotional and practical support	Teaching, modeling, organizing, leading discussions, assessing
Systems (Adlerian, choice/reality, feminist, family, interpersonal	Positive interaction with social and political milieu; balance between individual and society; social equality	Modeling, analyzing, strategizing lifestyle investigation, activism

From Day, S. X. (2014). A unifying theory for group counseling and psychotherapy. In J. L. DeLucia-Waack, C. R. Kalodner, & M. Riva (Eds.), *Handbook of group counseling and psychotherapy* (2nd ed.) (pp. 24–33). Los Angeles, CA: Sage.

of settings. Registered nurses with basic preparation may lead activity, educational, task, and support groups. Advanced practice registered nurses (APRNs) may lead these groups as well. They are also qualified to facilitate other specialized group treatments including psychotherapy for which more complex skills are necessary. Types of therapeutic groups are discussed in Table 34.5. Support and self-help groups are outlined in Box 34.4.

An important aspect of the group leader's responsibility is modeling sensitivity and respect to both individual and larger cultural differences. The leader initially sets a foundation for open communication by defining the importance of shared respect for group conduct. As group members begin to engage with one another, the leader should be aware of cultural differences that may impact efforts to maintain open respectful communication. Diversity exists in many forms including racial, ethnic, economic, and sexual orientation. Encouraging members to share and explore their cultural assumptions and beliefs promotes genuine rich communication and provides the group with the opportunity to explore similarities and differences in a safe environment.

Styles of Leadership

There are three main styles of group leadership. While we all have preferred methods of interacting that may range from directive to hands-off, in group situations leaders should defer to the group's goals. Ideally, a leader selects the style that is best suited to the therapeutic needs of a particular group.

- **Autocratic leaders** exert control over the group and do not encourage much interaction among members. For example, staff leading a community meeting with a fixed time-limited agenda may tend to be more autocratic.
- **Democratic leaders** support extensive group interaction in the process of problem solving. Psychotherapy groups most often employ this empowering leadership style.
- **Laissez-faire leaders** allow the group members to behave in any way they choose and do not attempt to control the direction of the group. In a creative group such as an art or horticulture group, the leader may choose a flexible laissez-faire style, directing minimally to allow for a variety of responses.

In any group, the leader must be thoughtful about using communication techniques because these can have a tremendous impact on group content and process. Table 34.6 describes communication techniques frequently used by group leaders.

Group Leader Supervision

Clinical supervision is important for registered nurse group leaders. It provides feedback about performance and enhances professional growth. Transference and countertransference issues occur in groups just as they do in therapeutic relationships during one-to-one work (refer to Chapter 8). These issues can be identified and managed effectively with the help of a trusted colleague. Clinical supervision also provides outside input and perspective while supporting a focus on therapeutic goals. Co-leadership of groups is a common practice and has several benefits, which include (1) providing training for less experienced staff, (2) allowing for immediate debriefing between leaders after sessions, and (3) offering two distinctive role models for teaching communication skills to members.

According to the American Nurse Association's *Scope and Standards of Practice* (ANA, 2014), APRNs are able to provide clinical supervision to other clinicians. The purpose of the supervision of other providers is to evaluate their performance and meet the need for peer supervision. With appropriate educational preparation, the APRN may supervise group therapy leaders to help them examine and understand their performances and effectiveness. The APRN clinical supervisor must extend confidentiality to the group leaders under their guidance. APRNs who lead group or individual therapy need to seek their own clinical supervision from a more experienced clinical psychiatric provider.

CONSIDERING CULTURE

Members of the lesbian, gay, bisexual, transsexual, queer (LGBTQ) community are diverse. Group leaders may not know when LGBT patients are in a therapeutic group. Group leaders should be mindful of obtaining supervision and training to ensure that group therapy does not create barriers that would silence or marginalize members of this population (Goodrich & Luke, 2011).

TABLE 34.5 Types of Therapeutic Groups

Type	Purpose
Psychiatric-Mental Health Registered Nurse	
Psychoeducational group	Groups set up to increase knowledge or skills about a specific psychological or somatic subject and allow members to communicate emotional concerns. These groups may be time limited or may be supportive for long-term treatment. Generally, written handouts or audiovisual aids are used to focus on specific teaching points.
Medication education	The psychoeducational group for which the nurse most commonly assumes responsibility is the medication education group. These groups teach patients about their medications, answer their questions, and prepare them for self-management. The group setting facilitates discussion. When patients have concerns about taking medications, it is often the group members themselves who are in the position to most effectively respond to these questions. "Yes, I got a dry mouth when I first started taking that, but it got better. Hang in there."
Health education	Nurses also frequently lead health education groups, including groups on medical conditions and general health topics, such as sex education. The majority of patients with a serious mental illness will have comorbid chronic medical illnesses. Common topics for discussion may include the following: diabetes, hypertension, HIV/AIDS and other sexually transmitted infections, condom use and other forms of safer sex practices for harm reduction, nutrition, and exercise.
Dual diagnosis	Dual-diagnosis groups incorporate learning about coexisting mental illnesses and substance use disorders. Since treatment issues for patients with dual diagnoses can be complex, group leaders must have competency in both mental health and substance use treatment. The goals are to engage patients in treatment decrease their use of substances in a step-by-step, meaningful process and improve psychiatric symptoms.
Symptom management	For patients with common symptoms resulting from a disorder such as anger or anxiety, symptom management groups are ideal. The group focuses on sharing positive and negative experiences so that members learn coping skills from one another. A primary goal is to increase self-control by helping patients develop a plan for action at the first appearance of chronic symptoms to prevent relapse.
Stress management	Stress management groups teach members about various relaxation techniques, including deep breathing, exercise, music, and spirituality. Mindfulness groups focus on developing awareness of the present moment with the intent to induce relaxation and promote insight into thoughts, emotions, and physical symptom responses.
Therapeutic community meetings	With the promotion of patient rights and advocacy, another common group consistently held on inpatient units is the therapeutic community meeting. As every interaction in an inpatient milieu has the potential to be therapeutic, the community meeting is the essential venue at which unit happenings are processed and integrated into treatment. Group members adjust to authority, rules, and tolerance of peers. Patient governance and advocacy matters are ideally managed during these groups and nurses are ideally suited to lead these groups because they model socially appropriate behavior, and are in close daily contact with patients and make frequent individual and unit assessments.
Support and self-help	Support/self-help groups are structured for the purpose of providing patients with the opportunity to maintain or enhance personal and social functioning through cooperation and shared understanding of life's challenges. One of the most important functions of such groups is to demonstrate universality to individuals, as they are not alone in having a particular problem. Group members help one another by telling their stories and providing alternative ways to view and resolve problems.
Advanced Practice Psychiatric-Mental Health Registered Nurse	
Group psychotherapy or group therapy	Group psychotherapy is a specialized treatment intervention led by an advanced practice mental health professional such as an advanced practice psychiatric-mental health registered nurse, psychologist, or social worker. Groups may focus on specific problems such as depression, obesity, chronic pain, or substance use. They may also focus on more general topics such as improving social skills, shyness, anger, or grieving.
Dialectical behavior treatment	Dialectical behavior treatment (DBT) groups were originally developed for the treatment of patients with borderline personality disorder and suicidal behaviors. It has proven to be successful with other illnesses such as eating disorders. DBT groups focus on improving interpersonal, behavioral, cognitive, and emotional skills. At the same time, members learn to reduce self-destructive behaviors by focusing on acceptance and mindfulness. This treatment requires specialized training and advanced education.

ETHICAL ISSUES IN GROUP THERAPY

The *Code of Ethics for Nurses with Interpretive Statements* (ANA, 2015) provides the definition for professional ethical conduct for registered nurses. The nurse group leader has an ethical obligation to inform participants of risks and benefits of group participation (informed consent). They must also discuss both confidentiality and exceptions to confidentiality. Because a group contains individuals who are not bound by a professional code of ethics, there is no way to guarantee confidentiality. Other topics the group leader must address are "Who is free to leave the group?" and "What are the rules about group members socializing outside group?"

A member is only removed from the group as a last resort. One obvious reason is if one member were to become violent or aggressive toward another member. This would necessitate

BOX 34.4 Support and Self-Help Groups

Support Groups
- Bereavement groups for those who have experienced the loss of a loved one
- Suicide survivor groups for those who have lost a loved one to suicide
- NAMI (National Alliance for the Mentally Ill) groups for patient/family support, education, and advocacy
- Cancer support groups for families and patients coping with the ramifications of this terminal illness
- Virtual support groups for a growing number of people, providing online, synchronous interaction and support, which may be perceived as more private or anonymous
- Veterans support groups

Self-Help Groups
- Twelve-step groups that use a common model for recovery: Alcoholics Anonymous (AA)—the prototype for other 12-step groups
  - Gamblers Anonymous (GA)
  - Overeaters Anonymous (OA)
  - Narcotics Anonymous (NA)
  - Co-Dependents Anonymous
  - Adult Children of Alcoholics (ACOA) and Al-Anon (friends and families of alcoholics)
- Recovery International for people who have had a mental illness; groups use prescribed model for managing illness and recovery
- National Mental Health Consumers Self-Help Clearinghouse, an information clearinghouse to guide consumers to the nearly 500 diverse types of self-help groups in operation.

TABLE 34.6 Group Leader Communication Techniques

Technique	Example
Active listening	Eye contact; head nod, "Go on…"
Ask questions	"Could you tell us the last time you did that?"
Giving information	"Antidepressants may take as long as 4 weeks or more to show full therapeutic effects."
Clarification	"What do you mean when you say 'I can't go back to work'?"
Confrontation	"Jane, you're saying 'nothing is wrong,' but you are crying."
Empathizing	"I can see how that experience was very painful."
Reflection	"I noticed you're clenching your fists. What are you feeling right now?" "It sounds like that really upset you."
Summarization	"We've talked about different types of cognitive distortions, and everyone identified at least one irrational thought that has influenced their behavior in a negative way. In the next session, we'll explore some strategies for correcting negative thinking."
Support	"It took a lot of courage to explore those painful feelings. You're really working hard on resolving this problem."

temporary or permanent removal. Other reasons that might require temporary or permanent removal from the group include (1) a member who is consistently unwilling or unable to participate or (2) a member who violates the agreements created for group membership.

Group leaders should obtain appropriate training or credentialing to practice, and must work within the ANA's defined scope of practice. The best way to help patients and at the same time avoid malpractice lawsuits for negligence is for the group leader to consistently follow the ethical guidelines and professional standards of practice.

To protect the integrity of the group therapy process, nurse clinicians should be use evidence-based practice. For instance, brief cognitive-behavioral therapy (CBT) has proven beneficial for depression and anxiety (Bernhardsdottir et al., 2013). Staying current with research helps nurse clinicians to select the best therapeutic modality for the target group audience. Evidence-based practice helps ensure that the therapeutic group maximizes benefit and minimizes harm. See Table 34.7 for some examples of evidence-based groups. Table 34.8 reviews the quality of evidence from the 1990s to the present on group treatment outcomes for different disorders and patient populations.

DEALING WITH CHALLENGING MEMBER BEHAVIORS

Research into group dynamics has identified certain behaviors of individual members that are challenging to manage within a group. Many defensive behaviors used by patients interfere with their ability to function or achieve satisfaction in their lives. Group therapy is about working through problem behaviors and resistance, but some behaviors can be especially disruptive to the group process and difficult for the leader to manage.

In dealing with any problematic behaviors and issues in groups, members may appreciate help disclosing their own feelings and responses. The leader encourages the use of statements that do not focus on what the other one did but the "how" of expression such as "When you speak this way, I feel..." The leader helps by noting that feelings are not right or wrong but simply exist. People tend to feel less defensive when *I feel* statements rather than *you are* statements are used. This approach helps members feel like part of the group, not alienated from it or threatened.

The patient who monopolizes the group, the patient who complains but continues to reject help, the demoralizing patient, and the silent patient are examples (Yalom & Leszcz, 2005), and specific group interventions may be beneficial.

Monopolizing Group Member

One subtle method in dealing with a monopolizing group member is to address the entire group. Provide them with a reminder that, during group work, everyone should have an equal chance to contribute and members should consider whether or not they are dominating the group's time. It may be necessary to speak directly to the monopolizing group member, either privately or in the group setting. In private, you can share your observations and suggest that perhaps nervousness may be a factor causing the talkativeness.

You may then ask the patient to limit contributions to a specific number of times, such as two or three. In the group setting,

TABLE 34.7 Evidence-Based Group Treatment Methods

Theoretical Base	Focus	Leader Practices
Humanist (patient centered, existential, experiential)	Self-actualization; awareness of subjective experience	Nondirective, active listening, Socratic dialogue
Cognitive-behavioral	Specific maladaptive behaviors and thought patterns	Goal setting, planning, reinforcing, modeling, and monitoring
Psychodynamic (psychoanalytic, Gestalt)	Insight; resolution of intrapsychic conflict	Listening, interpreting, confronting, probing, working through, directing enactments
Psychoeducational	Information on specific topics; coping; emotional and practical support	Teaching, modeling, organizing, leading discussions, assessing
Systems (Adlerian, choice/reality, feminist, family, interpersonal	Positive interaction with social and political milieu; balance between individual and society; social equality	Modeling, analyzing, strategizing lifestyle investigation, activism

From Day, S. X. (2014). A unifying theory for group counseling and psychotherapy. In J. L. DeLucia-Waack, C. R. Kalodner, & M. Riva (Eds.), *Handbook of group counseling and psychotherapy* (2nd ed.) (pp. 24 –33). Los Angeles, CA: Sage.

TABLE 34.8 Quality of Evidence from 1990s to Present

Use of Group Treatment	Very Good to Excellent	Promising to Good
Group as primary	Social phobia, panic disorder, obsessive-compulsive disorder, bulimia nervosa, eating disorders	Mood disorders
Group as adjunct	Schizophrenia, personality disorders, trauma-related disorders, medical-cancer, substance use disorders	Medical—HIV, sexual abuse, pain/somatoform

From Burlingame, G. M., Whitcomb, K., & Woodland, S. (2014). Process and outcome in group counseling and psychotherapy: A perspective. In J. L. DeLucia-Waack, C. R. Kalodner, & M. Riva (Eds.), *Handbook of group counseling and psychotherapy* (2nd ed.) (p. 57). Los Angeles, CA: Sage.

the leader may ask the group if they would like to share observations or feedback about other members, thereby offering a chance for redirecting growth. This strategy is probably the most challenging but potentially the most rewarding in that members feel empowered, and the real therapeutic forces of groups are realized.

Demoralizing Group Member

Some people whose behavior is self-centered, angry, or depressed may lack empathy, hope, or concern for other members of the group. They refuse to take any personal responsibility and can challenge the group leader and negatively affect the group process. The group leader should listen to the comments objectively. The leader may choose to speak to the group member in private and ask what is causing the anger. Sometimes this simple exchange can make the patient feel more connected with the nurse and, more importantly, as a member of the group. This intervention will likely decrease hostile behavior and increase the group's benefit. Angry patients may be extremely vulnerable, and devaluing or demoralizing keeps others at a distance and maintains the patient's own precarious sense of safety. Leaders must empathize with the patient in a matter-of-fact manner, such as, "You seem angry that the group wants to support you."

Silent Group Member

Patients who are silent in the group may be observing intently until they decide the group is safe for them. Other silent groups' members may believe they are not as competent as other, more assertive group members. Silence might or might not mean that the member is not engaged or involved, but it should be addressed for several reasons. The person who does not speak cannot benefit from others' feedback on their thoughts, and other group members are deprived of this group member's valuable insights. Furthermore, a silent group member may make others uncomfortable and create a sense of mistrust.

There are several techniques that may help, including allowing the person to have extra time to formulate thoughts before responding. Saying, "I'll give you a moment to think about that," and waiting or coming back to the group member later is often helpful. Another tactic is to make an assignment that every person in the group respond to a certain topic or question. For example, "Let's all write down a positive and assertive response to something that you generally feel helpless about. I'll give you a minute or so to think this over, and then I'm going to ask each of you to share."

EXPECTED OUTCOMES

Expected outcomes of group participation vary depending on the type and purpose of the group. For education groups, such as a medication education group, the expected outcome would be the demonstration of precise knowledge such as the following:

- Patient identifies three significant side effects of prescribed medication.
- Patient recognizes dangerous drug-drug and drug-food interactions for prescribed medications.
- Patient correctly identifies time of day and dose for each prescribed medication.

For therapy groups, the expected outcomes will focus more on insights, behavior changes, and reduction in symptoms. For example, in an alcohol treatment group, an expected outcome might be that the patient develops insight into the connection between drinking and negative consequences. An expected behavioral outcome would be abstinence from alcohol use. In groups that focus primarily on emotional issues such as depression or anxiety, you can use standardized symptom surveys to measure symptom reduction as an outcome of group participation.

KEY POINTS TO REMEMBER

- A group format has advantages over individual therapy including cost savings, increased feedback, an opportunity to practice new skills in a relatively safe environment, mutual learning, and instilling a sense of belonging.
- Yalom's therapeutic factors that operate in groups can lead to therapeutic change for members.
- Groups develop through predictable phases over time: planning phase, orientation phase, working phase, and termination phase. Group leaders need to use specific skills depending upon the phase the group is in.
- For a group to continue and be productive, members must fulfill specific functions known as *task or maintenance roles.* Individual roles are not productive and are based on individual personalities and needs. Nurse leaders should reinforce productive group roles and confront individual roles.
- Clinical supervision is important so that group leaders can analyze group interactions and characteristics, as well as leadership techniques.
- Nurses have many opportunities to lead or co-lead therapeutic groups both in the hospital and community settings.
- Psychoeducational groups, health teaching groups, and support groups are often led by registered nurses.
- Advanced practice registered nurses may lead psychotherapy groups based on various theoretical models.
- Challenging member behaviors such as monopolizing, silence, complaining, or demoralizing can be especially difficult. A variety of interventions are recommended to minimize the disruption to the group and maximize the insight to the patient who is engaging in these behaviors.

CRITICAL THINKING

1. You are automatically a part of several groups during nursing education: your large cohort and smaller course and clinical practicum groups. Review Table 34.3 and think about your position and ways you tend to participate in your current groups at school.
   a. Which task role do you assume in your groups?
   b. Which maintenance role do you assume?
   c. Which individual group role is yours?
   d. In your class groups in general, how would you characterize the norms?
2. While participating in your nursing education groups, you have surely noticed that some groups function better than others. Think about your current or past clinical group and consider the following questions:
   a. How would you describe the dynamics of the group?
   b. Which overall leadership styles have your instructors modeled?
   c. Were group members well prepared to participate in the class/group sessions? If no, how did this affect the dynamic of the group?
   d. How did the group leader handle group monopolization, side conversations, or distraction?

CHAPTER REVIEW

Questions

1. Which outcome would be appropriate for a group session on medication education? *Select all that apply.*
   a. Patient will identify three side effects of prescribed medication.
   b. Patient will verbalize the purpose of taking the medication.
   c. Patient will acknowledge and accept the financial cost of prescribed medications.
   d. Patient will correctly identify time of day and dose for each prescribed medication.
   e. Patient will list two dangerous drug-drug and drug-food interactions for prescribed medications.
2. What question by the nurse leader is helpful in managing a monopolizing member of a group?
   a. "You seem angry. Is there something you want to discuss with the group?"
   b. "Would it be helpful if you had time to think about the question?"
   c. "Would you tell us about experiences that have frightened you?"
   d. "Who else would like to share feelings about this issue?"
3. What advantages does group therapy have over those of individual therapy? *Select all that apply.*
   a. Groups are less expensive than one-to-one therapy.
   b. Groups provide an opportunity to learn from others.
   c. Groups are homogeneous in composition.
   d. Feedback is available from the group leader and group members.
   e. Interpersonal skills can be practiced in a safe environment.
4. What group would benefit most from a laissez-faire leader?
   a. Art group
   b. Grief group
   c. Social skills group
   d. Anger management group
5. The nurse tells group members that they will be working on expressing conflicts during the current group session. Which phase of group development is represented?
   a. Planning (formation) phase
   b. Orientation phase
   c. Working phase
   d. Termination phase
6. Group dynamics can vary widely and at times members are capable of disrupting the group process. Which of

the following participant traits may indicate a need for additional support for a new nurse facilitator? *Select all that apply.*
  a. A member with paranoid delusions
  b. A quietly tearful participant expressing suicidal thoughts
  c. An angry woman who raises her voice
  d. A calm but ineffective communicator

7. The nurse is caring for four patients. Which patients would not be appropriate to consider for inpatient group therapy? *(Select all that apply.)* The patient who:
  a. Has limited financial and social resources
  b. Is experiencing acute mania
  c. Has few friends on the unit
  d. Is preparing for discharge tomorrow
  e. Does not speak up often, yet listens to others

8. Group members are having difficulty deciding what topic to cover in today's session. Which nurse leader response reflects autocratic leadership?
  a. "We are talking about fear of rejection today."
  b. "Let's go around the room and make suggestions for today's topic."
  c. "I will let you come to a conclusion together about what to talk about."
  d. "I'll work with you to find a suitable topic for today."

9. A patient continues to dominate the group conversation despite having been asked to allow others to speak. What is the most appropriate group leader response?
  a. "You are monopolizing the conversation."
  b. "When you talk constantly, it makes everyone feel angry."
  c. "You are supposed to allow others to talk also."
  d. "When you speak out of turn, I am concerned that others cannot participate equally."

10. The nurse is planning care, which includes a dual-diagnosis group. Which patient would be appropriate for this group? The patient with:
  a. Depression and suicidal tendencies
  b. Anxiety and frequent migraine headaches
  c. Bipolar disorder and anorexia nervosa
  d. Schizophrenia and alcohol abuse

Answers

1. **a, b, d, e;** 2. **d;** 3. **a, b, d, e;** 4. **a;** 5. **b;** 6. **a, b;** 7. **b;** 8. **a;** 9. **d;** 10. **d**

ⓔ Visit the Evolve website for a posttest on the content in this chapter: http://evolve.elsevier.com/Varcarolis

Post-Test interactive review

REFERENCES

American Nurses Association. (2015). *Code of ethics with interpretive statements.* Retrieved from http://nursingworld.org/DocumentVault/Ethics-1/Code-of-Ethics-for-Nurses.html.

American Psychiatric Nurses Association, International Society of Psychiatric-Mental Health Nurses, & American Nurses Association. (2014). *Psychiatric-mental health nursing: Scope and standards of practice.* Silver Springs, MD: NurseBooks.org.

Benne, K. D., & Sheats, P. (1948). Functional roles of group members. *Journal of Social Issues, 4*(2), 41–49.

Bernhardsdottir, J., Vilhjalmsson, R., & Champion, J. D. (2013). Evaluation of a brief cognitive behavioral group therapy for psychological distress among female Icelandic university students. *Issues in Mental Health Nursing, 34*(7), 497–504.

Burlingame, G. (2010). Small group treatments: Introduction to special section. *Psychotherapy Research, 20,* 1–7.

DeLucia-Waack, J. L. (2014). In C. R. Kalodner & M. Riva (Eds.), *Handbook of group counseling and psychotherapy* (2nd ed.). Los Angeles, CA: Sage.

Goodrich, K. M., & Luke, M. (2011). The LGBTQ responsive model for supervision of group work. *The Journal for Specialists in Group Work, 36*(1), 22–40.

Joyce, A. S., MacNair-Semands, R., Tasca, G. A., & Ogrodniczuk, J. S. (2011). Factor structure and validity of the Therapeutic Factors Inventory–Short Form. *Group Dynamics: Theory, Research, and Practice, 15*(3), 201.

Siegel, D. J. (2012). *Pocket guide to interpersonal neurobiology: An integrative handbook of the mind.* New York, NY: Norton.

Sullivan, H. S. (1953). *The collected works of Harry Stack Sullivan.* New York, NY: Norton.

Tuckman, B. W. (1965). Developmental sequence in small groups. *Psychological Bulletin, 63,* 384–399.

Wallace, D. F. (1996). *Infinite jest: A novel.* Boston, MA: Little, Brown and Company.

Yalom, I. D., & Leszcz, M. (2005). *The theory and practice of group psychotherapy* (5th ed.). New York, NY: Basic Books.

35

Family Interventions

Laura G. Leahy, Laura Cox Dzurec

Visit the Evolve website for a pretest on the content in this chapter: http://evolve.elsevier.com/Varcarolis Pre-Test interactive review

OBJECTIVES

1. Discuss the characteristics of a healthy family.
2. Identify family structures.
3. Differentiate family patterns of behavior as they relate to five family functions: management, boundaries, communication, emotional support, and socialization.
4. Compare and contrast models of modern family therapy.
5. Construct a genogram using a three-generation approach.
6. Recognize the significance of self-assessment to successful work with families.
7. Formulate outcome criteria for families.
8. Identify strategies for family intervention.
9. Distinguish between the nursing intervention strategies of a psychiatric-mental health registered nurse and those of a psychiatric-mental health advanced practice registered nurse with regard to counseling and psychotherapy.

OUTLINE

KEY TERMS AND CONCEPTS

boundaries
clear boundaries
differentiation
diffuse boundaries
enmeshment
family therapy
family triangle
flexibility
genogram
identified patient
rigid boundaries

In Western culture, the uniqueness of the individual and the search for autonomy are celebrated. Yet we are also defined and sustained by interwoven systems of human relationships including the relationships developed with our family members. Families are the foundation and structure for most societies. Families are defined by reciprocal relationships in which persons are committed to one another.

Healthy family relationships support the well-being of individual family members. When children do not have family support—for instance, in cases of loss due to the ravages of war—they tend to respond with a range of adjustment difficulties and guilt reactions. These reactions can influence their health and well-being for years, if not a lifetime.

In other cases, the family remains physically intact, yet family members do not support one another. Emotional stress or trauma experienced by one family member, as well as complex life challenges faced by the family as a whole, can threaten interactions. For those families and for the members within them, family support and/or therapy are needed.

The family is the primary social system to which a person belongs, and in most cases, it is the most powerful system of which a person will ever be a member. The dynamics of the family subtly and significantly influence the beliefs and actions of individual members across the lifespan. Healthy families tend to deal better with developmental changes than do less healthy families. However, even "normal" changes such as the birth of a child can test the strength of relationships even in the most resilient family.

FAMILY STRUCTURE

When Duvall (1957) described family functioning, she was referring to the nuclear family—mother, father, and children. Today, family structures are more complex. Sutherland (2014) identified the following types of families that exist in the United States:

- Nuclear family: Children living with two parents who are married to each other and are each the biological or adoptive parents to all the children in the family.
- **Single-parent family:** Children living with a single adult of either gender.
- **Unmarried biological or adoptive family:** Children living with two unmarried parents who are the biological/adoptive parents to all the family's children.
- **Blended family:** Children living with one biological/adoptive parent and that parent's spouse.
- **Cohabitating family:** Children living with one biological/adoptive parent and that parent's unmarried cohabitating partner.
- **Extended family:** Children living with at least one biological/adoptive parent and at least one related nonparent adult (age 18 or older) such as a grandparent or adult sibling.
- **"Other" family:** Children living with related or unrelated adults who are not biological or adoptive parents. This includes children living with grandparents and foster families.

As the notion of family has broadened to incorporate nontraditional family structures, it has been a challenge for family therapists to recognize and incorporate similarly broad definitions of family in their work. Fig. 35.1 depicts the family structure of households in the United States by race and Hispanic origin.

FAMILY FUNCTIONS

A healthy family provides its members with tools to guide effective interactions within the family. The family also extends its influence when an individual functions in other intimate relationships, the workplace, culture, and society in general. The tools acquired through activities associated with family life include management activities, boundary delineation, communication patterns, emotional support, and socialization (Nichols, 2013).

Management

Every day in every family, decisions are made regarding issues of power, resource allocation (i.e., who gets what), rule-making, and the provision of financial support. These decisions contribute to adaptive family functioning. In healthy families, it is usually the adults who mutually agree about how to perform these management functions. In families with a single parent, these management functions may often become overwhelming. In chaotic families, an inappropriate member

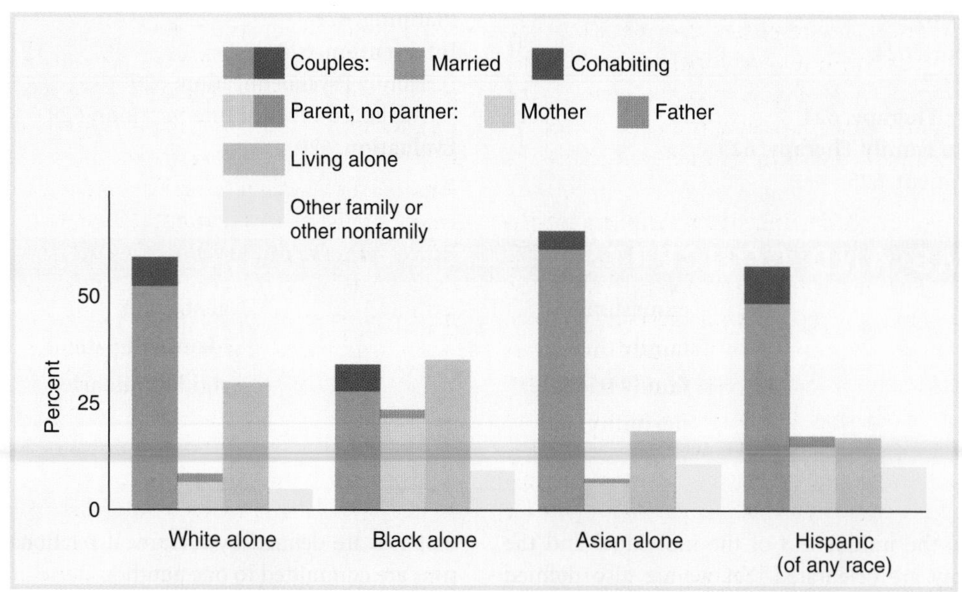

FIG. 35.1 Family structure of households by race and Hispanic origin. US Census Bureau. (2015). *Household by Race and Hispanic Origin. Current population survey, annual social and economic supplement.* Retrieved from https://www.census.gov/hhes/families/files/graphics/HH-7a.pdf

such as a teenager may be the one who makes management decisions.

Although children learn decision-making skills as they mature and increasingly make decisions and choices about their own lives, they should *not* be expected or forced to take on this responsibility for the family. A 12-year-old child, for example, should not be the one to decide whether to pay the gas bill or buy groceries.

Boundaries

Boundaries maintain distinctions between and among individuals in the family. They also distinguish between the family and individuals external to it. Establishment and maintenance of flexible and appropriate boundaries are essential to healthy family functioning.

Minuchin (1974) identified three types of boundaries within families: clear, diffuse, and rigid.

Clear Boundaries

Clear boundaries are adaptive and healthy. All members of the family understand these boundaries and they give family members a sense of self. They are firm, yet flexible, and provide a structure that responds and adapts to change. Clear boundaries allow family members to take on appropriate roles and to function without unnecessary or inappropriate interference from other members. They reflect structure while simultaneously supporting healthy family functioning and encouraging individual growth.

Diffuse Boundaries

Diffuse boundaries result in unclear boundaries and lack of independence. Individuals in families with diffuse boundaries may have problems defining who they are. When boundaries are diffuse, individuals tend to become overly involved with one another. This overinvolvement is referred to as enmeshment.

When boundaries are diffuse, everyone, and thus no one, is in charge. It is not clear who is responsible for decisions and who has permission to act. Diffuse boundaries are particularly problematic when parent/child role enactment becomes blurry, for example, when a parent may be unemployed and one of the children takes responsibility for earning money to meet the family's basic needs.

In families with diffuse boundaries, individual members are discouraged from expressing their own views. Differentiation, or the ability to possess a strong identity and sense of self while maintaining an emotional connection with the family, is also discouraged. To an outsider, it may appear that family members are extremely close, and family members may believe that they are of one mind. They may take comfort that everyone thinks the same way. "No one in our family likes seafood." That sense is typically false, and deeper analysis often results in the discovery of suppressed frustrations, anger, and passive-aggressive behaviors.

Expression of separateness or independence is viewed as being disloyal to the family. Members are prone to psychological or psychosomatic symptoms, probably as a function of the individuals' inability to actually say or even to recognize how they feel. During times of change or crisis, whether the crisis is one of normal development (such as when a baby is born or an elderly grandparent dies) or one that is unanticipated (such as the loss of a pregnancy or serious debilitating injury to a family member), adaptation of both individuals and of the family as a whole is extremely difficult.

Rigid Boundaries

Rigid boundaries are the opposite of diffuse boundaries. Families with this type of boundary demand adherence to rules and roles—some apparent and some less so—regardless of circumstances or outcomes. Boundaries can be so firmly closed that family members are disengaged and avoid one another, resulting in little sense of family loyalty. In families in which rigid boundaries predominate, communication is minimal, and members rarely share thoughts and feelings. Isolation may be marked feature in such family systems.

Disengaged family members lead highly separate and distinct lives. Because they do not learn intimacy in the family setting, individuals from disengaged families do not tend to develop insights into their own feelings and emotions. As a result, they may have a hard time bonding with others and participating in new family structures when they leave their families of origin and begin their lives as adults.

Communication

Communication patterns are extremely important in healthy families. Healthy communication patterns are characterized by clear and comprehensible messages (e.g., "I would like to go now" or "I don't like it when you interrupt what I'm saying"). Healthy communication within the family encourages members to ask for what they want and need and to share their feelings. Thoughts and feelings can be openly, honestly, and assertively expressed in families where communication is encouraged. Alternatively, those in legitimate positions of power within the family, typically the parents, are able to evaluate the appropriateness of family members' requests.

In healthy families, there is a necessary and natural hierarchy for the protection and socialization of younger family members. Parents are the leaders in the family and children are the followers. Despite this arrangement, children can voice their opinions and have influence on family decisions. In dysfunctional families, this seemingly simple hierarchy becomes unbalanced. When communication among family members is not clear and natural hierarchal roles become confused, communication cannot be used as a means to solve problems or to resolve conflict.

The cardinal rule for effective and functional communication in families is "Be clear and direct in stating what you want and need" whether you are in a powerful or a subordinate position. Speak from the "I" position as opposed to deferring to the "you." Clear communication is one of the hardest skills to cultivate in a family system. To be direct, individuals must first have a sense that they are respected and loved and that it is safe to express personal thoughts and feelings. The consequences of being clear and direct may be unpleasant in a family system that does not tolerate openness. Box 35.1 offers examples of unhealthy family patterns of communication.

Emotional Support

All families, regardless of how healthy they are, encounter conflicts. In the most functionally healthy families, feelings of affection generally are paramount, and family members realize that bursts of anger and conflict reflect a short-term response. Anger and conflict do not dominate the family's pattern of interaction.

Healthy families are concerned with one another's needs, and family members' emotional and physical needs are met most of the time. When members' emotional needs are met, they feel support from those around them and are free to grow and explore new roles and facets of their personalities. A family dominated by conflict and anger alienates its members, leaving them isolated, fearful, and impaired emotionally.

Socialization

It is within families that individuals first learn social skills such as how to interact in nonfamily venues, how to negotiate for personal needs, and how to plan. Children learn through parents' role modeling. Children learn through behavioral reinforcement about how to function effectively within the family and, when the system is successful, how to apply those skills in society.

Each developmental phase for family members and for the family as a whole brings new demands and requires new approaches to deal with changes. Parents are socialized into their family roles as they address the growth and developmental needs of each child. Parents' roles change when the children mature and leave home. This may necessitate partners' renegotiation of the patterning of their lives together. As time goes on, the parents may need their adult children's help if they become less able to care for their own needs.

BOX 35.1 Examples of Dysfunctional Communication

Manipulating

Instead of asking directly for what is wanted, family members manipulate others to get what they want. For example, a child starts a fight with a sibling to get attention. Another example is when a request is granted with "strings attached" so that the other person has a difficult time refusing the request: "If you clean my room for me, I won't tell Daddy you are getting bad grades in school."

Distracting

To avoid functional problem solving and resolving conflicts within the family, family members introduce irrelevant details into problematic issues.

Generalizing

Members use global statements such as "always" and "never" instead of dealing with specific problems and areas of conflict. Family members may state, "Harry is always angry" instead of exploring why Harry is upset.

Blaming

Family members blame others for failures, errors, or negative consequences of an action to deflect the focus from them.

Placating

Family members pretend to be well meaning to keep peace in the family. "Don't yell at the children, dear. *I* put the shoes on the stairs."

It is not surprising that families have difficulty negotiating role change. Periods of change increase the overall stress within families. If the family is socialized to manage stress through open, direct communication, the period may be short-lived. However, if the family is not socialized to emotionally support its members or communicate effectively, the stress may linger, deteriorating the family's ability to function.

In response to the demands of change, healthy families demonstrate **flexibility** in adapting to new roles. Through well-organized management activities, firm but flexible boundary delineation, strong and appropriate communication patterns, ongoing provision of emotional support, and adept socialization, healthy families provide tools to their members to facilitate functioning for the present and into the future.

OVERVIEW OF FAMILY THERAPY

As a treatment approach, family therapy began to emerge in the 1920s as social psychologists recognized that behaviors among family members mutually influence the behaviors of individual members (Perreau, 2016). The two major aims of **family therapy** are to:

1. Improve the skills of the individual members
2. Strengthen the functioning of the family as a whole

Family therapists are trained and practice at the advanced level. While you will not be conducting family therapy without an advanced degree, registered nurses often lead family groups for the purpose of education or support. Knowledge of basic family therapy skills will help you with group work. It will also provide you with information you can use for community referrals.

Family therapists use various strategies to assess a family's level of functioning. However, the following areas are almost always explored:

- Cohesiveness—how much time do members spend together as a family unit?
- Communication—do the members respectfully listen to one another's concerns and ideas and allow for open discussion when disagreement arises?
- Appreciation—do the individual members contribute in meaningful ways to the functioning of the family and offer gratitude to one another that supports self-esteem?
- Commitment—do the individual members consider the impact of their actions on the family as a whole and in a manner that promotes unity?
- Coping—do the family members demonstrate the ability to support one another during times of crisis?
- Beliefs and values—does the family identify with or practice within a collective moral, ethical, or spiritual set of standards?

Specific approaches to therapy vary according to the philosophical viewpoint, education, and training of individual therapists. Family therapy's effectiveness is not tied to any particular theoretical approach (Keeney & Keeney, 2012). Table 35.1 lists specific therapies; identifies some of the therapists who contributed to their development and use; and highlights assumptions, concepts, and goals related to each therapy.

Multiple-family group therapy is a useful therapeutic modality for families who are facing similar difficulties. By hearing other families discuss their problems, family members identify and gain insight into their own problems. New skills can be modeled and learned in the context of the group. In the case of multiple-family therapy, several families meet in one group with one or more therapists, usually once a week.

VIGNETTE: Eight-year-old Diego is a Hispanic male who has recently become disruptive at school and at home. He is brought to the community mental health clinic by his mother to be evaluated for attention-deficit/hyperactivity disorder (ADHD). The family includes Diego's married parents, his sister and brother, and a maternal grandmother. Diego's father is unemployed, and his grandmother was recently diagnosed with cancer. Diego's mother plans to file for separation because of constant unresolved arguments with her husband.

The psychiatric-mental health nurse practitioner, Alma, views Diego's problems in the context of his family. His symptoms are influenced by losses and transitions that are stressing the entire family's coping mechanisms. Once the issues within the family are addressed and plans are made to deal with these issues, perhaps Diego's symptoms will subside. Alma refers Diego's parents to a separate couples' therapist. In the meantime, she encourages the couple to focus more on their own issues and less on Diego's behavior. They make an appointment to return to the clinic in 1 month.

CONCEPTS CENTRAL TO FAMILY THERAPY

The Identified Patient

When a family seeks treatment, the first task of the therapist is to address the presenting problem. That problem often belongs to the **identified patient**. The identified patient is an individual in the family typically regarded by family members as "the problem," the family member whose beliefs, perceptions, actions, and responses demand an immediate fix. Sometimes known as the family symptom-bearer, this person is generally the focus of most of the family system's concern.

From a therapeutic point of view, the identified patient may indeed be a problem. Yet this person may also serve to divert attention from other hidden problems of the family. The symptoms of the identified patient may actually serve as a stabilizing mechanism to bring about relatively cohesive behavior in a distressed family, at least in the short term (Goldenberg & Goldenberg, 2008). The identified patient may be aware, even on a remote level, of the role he or she serves in stabilizing the family. For example, adult children may sacrifice their autonomy by staying in the home to hold the parents together. This behavior demonstrates a violation of role boundaries.

The patient may or may not be the one who initially seeks help from inpatient or outpatient services. Some families will enter therapy on the recommendation of a clinician as noted in

TABLE 35.1 Models of Contemporary Family Therapy

Therapy	Theorists	Assumptions	Concepts	Goals
Contextual	Ivan Boszormenyi-Nagy (1987)	Values and ethics transcend generations and drive behaviors and relationships	Family problems arise from conflicts relating to loyalty, entitlement, legacy, and accounting	Gain insight into problematic relationships originating in the past to promote a "balanced ledger"
Family of origin	Murray Bowen (1978) Michael Kerr (1988)	Past issues influence present relationships Anxiety inhibits change Symptoms are indicators of stress and lower differentiation Multigenerational transmission process	Family viewed as a system of emotional relationships Triangulation and cut-off Differentiation of self Multigenerational transmission process Sibling position matters	Foster differentiation and decrease emotional reactivity
Experiential-existential	Carl Whitaker (1978) Virginia Satir (1967)	Battle for structure, initiative, and self-worth Growth occurs through shared experience	Symptoms express family pain Use of nurturing to identify dysfunctional communication patterns	Guide the family to identify and develop their own solutions to dysfunctional behavior patterns
Structural	Salvador Minuchin (1974)	Inflexible structure leads to dysfunction Restructuring leads to improved functioning	Identify patterns of enmeshment and disengagement Clarify boundaries	Improve family relationships through restructuring the family hierarchy and boundaries
Strategic	Jay Haley (1967)	Family members perpetuate problems through their actions People resist change	Symptoms are messages which serve functions in maintaining family homeostasis Family rules are unspoken Incongruous hierarchies	Realign family hierarchy through use of rituals which change repetitive and maladaptive patterns of interaction
Cognitive-behavioral	Aaron Beck (2003)	Family relationships, cognitions, emotions, and behaviors mutually influence one another Cognitive inferences evoke emotion and behavior	Focuses on negative cognitions Uses learning theory to alter patterns leading to destructive behaviors Use of "homework" assignments	Improve patterns of negative behaviors through changing thought patterns, which alleviates symptoms

the previous vignette with Diego's family. In other cases where criminal behavior is involved, a court may mandate family therapy. A family member other than the identified patient may initiate a request for therapy as well.

Family Triangles

Dyads, consisting of two people, are often emotionally unstable. When tension in a dyad builds and communication fails, triangulation may be used. **Triangulation** occurs when one family member will not communicate directly with another family member but will communicate with a third family member. This forces the third family member to be part of the triangle and communication is then routed through the third person.

For example, Lisa is the youngest child of Susan and Bill. Lisa has sensed increasing tension in her parents' marriage since her older siblings left home. When things get especially conflicted between Susan and Bill, Susan vents her frustrations to Lisa and even confided that Bill had an affair. Lisa is afraid that her parents will get a divorce when she goes away to college and is considering going to a local community college rather than her dream university. In this and many other cases, the family triangle (Fig. 35.2) serves to stabilize interpersonal relationships in the short term.

Triangulation can also be a form of splitting within the family system. One person may play a third family member against the one with whom he or she is upset. This splitting is accomplished through exaggeration, telling half-truths, or other manipulation of facts to present an untrue picture of the targeted person.

Although triangles within families tend to be structurally stable, the intensity of the triangulation process varies over time. During stressful times, triangulation may increase. Family triangles are destructive and may create emotional instability over the long-term family lifecycle.

VIGNETTE: Six-year-old Addison is having trouble making friends. Her mother, Megan, has been trying to help Addison connect with other children. Yet Megan uses an overprotective approach that further inhibits Addison. Megan believes that her husband, Shawn, is uncaring and disinterested. He thinks that she should be more relaxed about Addison's social life and let things develop naturally. Because Shawn's job requires that he travel most of the week, he is rarely involved with Megan's daily experiences or in her struggles with Addison.

Megan and Shawn have been avoiding intimacy for almost a year. Megan is angry with Shawn for spending so much time with his parents, which further places him in a peripheral role in their nuclear family. Shawn is angry with Megan due to her rejection of him. Both partners feel isolated and alienated in their marriage. Neither Shawn nor Megan addresses this issue directly. Instead, they play out their anger in the parental arena as they battle over how to handle Addison's social isolation.

Triangulating behavior occurs everywhere, not only in families but also in social situations among friends and in the workplace. You can monitor your own indirect communication and make an effort to communicate directly. Obviously, splitting behaviors are almost always emotionally unhealthy and should definitely be avoided.

Box 35.2 provides an overview of common terms used in discussions of family dynamics.

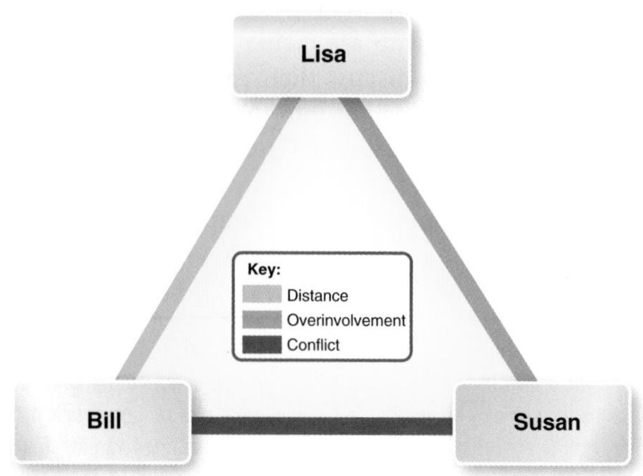

FIG. 35.2 Example of a family triangle.

BOX 35.2 Family Dynamics Terms

Boundaries: Clear boundaries are those that maintain distinctions between individuals within the family and between the family and the outside world. Clear boundaries allow for balanced flow of energy between members. Roles of children and parent or parents are clearly defined. Diffuse or enmeshed boundaries are those in which there is a blending together of the roles, thoughts, and feelings of the individuals so that clear distinctions among family members fail to emerge. Rigid or disengaged boundaries are those in which the rules and roles are adhered to no matter what.

Differentiation: The ability to develop a strong identity and sense of self while at the same time maintaining an emotional connectedness with one's family of origin.

Double bind: A situation in which a positive command (often verbal) is followed by a negative command (often nonverbal), which leaves the recipient confused, trapped, and immobilized because there is no appropriate way to act. A double bind is a "no-win" situation in which you are "darned if you do, darned if you don't."

Family life cycle: The family's developmental process over time; refers to the family's past course, its present tasks, and its future course.

Hierarchy: The function of power and its structures in families, differentiating parental and sibling roles and generational boundaries.

Multigenerational issues: The continuation and persistence from generation to generation of certain emotional interactive family patterns (e.g., reenactment of fairly predictable and almost ritual-like patterns; repetition of themes or toxic issues; and repetition of reciprocal patterns such as those of overfunctioner and underfunctioner).

Scapegoating: A form of displacement in which a family member (usually the least powerful) is blamed for another family member's distress. The purpose is to keep the focus off the painful issues and the problems of the blamers. In a family, the blamers are often the parents and the scapegoat a child.

Sociocultural context: The framework for viewing the family in terms of the influence of gender, race, ethnicity, religion, economic class, and sexual orientation.

Triangulation: The tendency, when two-person relationships are conflicted, to draw in a third person to stabilize the system through formation of a coalition in which the two join the third.

APPLICATION OF THE NURSING PROCESS

Nurses prepared at the basic level meet the needs of patients and families in inpatient and outpatient settings. Their work as part of the healthcare team can contribute significantly to the quality

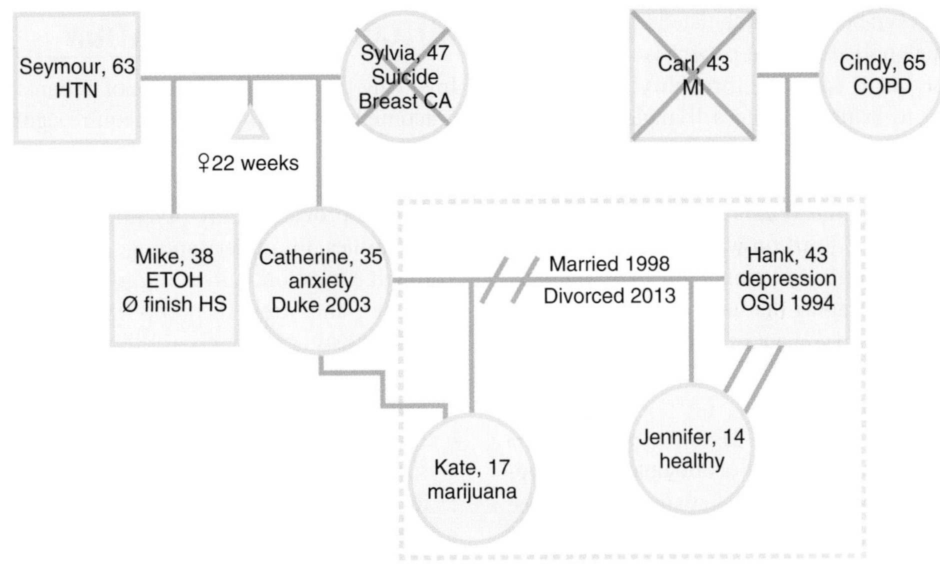

FIG. 35.3 The Smith family genogram.

of intervention and patient outcomes. Psychiatric-mental health advanced practice registered nurses who have graduate or post-graduate training in family therapy may practice as nurse family therapists.

ASSESSMENT

A variety of assessment tools are available to help the nurse and nurse therapist assess how the family functions as a unit. These tools can also help to identify individual members' perceptions of how the family communicates and how they deal with emotional issues such as anger, conflict, and affection. You can even use some tools to show the family how they work together as a unit to plan and solve problems and to demonstrate how they make the important decisions for the family. General assessment tools can show how a family functions.

Genograms

Bowen (1978) provided much of the conceptual framework for the analysis of family relational patterns using genograms. He proposed that the family is organized according to generation, age, sex, roles, functions, and interests. Bowen suggested that where each individual fits into the family structure influences the family functioning, relational patterns, and type of family formed in the next generation. He further contended that sex and birth order shape sibling relationships and characteristics just as some patterns passed from one generation to the next result in persistent, interactive, emotional patterns and triangulation.

The **genogram** is an efficient clinical summary and format for providing information and defining relationships across at least three generations. By creating a genogram, nurses and therapists are able to map the family structure and record family information that reflects both history and current functioning.

The information included on a genogram should include demographic data such as geographic location of family members, their respective occupations, and educational levels. You should also record functional information regarding medical, emotional, and behavioral status. Finally, note any critical events such as important transitions, moves, job changes, separations, illnesses, and deaths. Females are represented in circles and males are represented in squares. Fig. 35.3 provides an example of a genogram based on information from the following vignette.

VIGNETTE: Kate Smith is receiving therapy for depression and substance use. The psychiatric-mental health advanced practice registered nurse develops a genogram of the family based on the following information:

Kate's parents, Hank and Catherine, are both college educated. Catherine, 35, has been treated for generalized anxiety disorder. Her mother, Sylvia, committed suicide at age 47 after a diagnosis of breast cancer. Catherine's family of origin never discusses the suicide. Catherine's brother Mike, 38, "drinks too much" and never finished high school. Her mother miscarried a female fetus before Catherine's birth. From an early age, many expectations were placed on her.

Hank has a history of major depressive disorder. Hank is an only child whose father, Henry, died of a heart attack at age 43, Hank's present age. His mother, Cindy, is 65 years old and has chronic obstructive pulmonary disease.

Hank and Catherine were married for 15 years before divorcing in 2013. Their two daughters, Kate and Jennifer, live with Hank. Kate, the identified patient, is 17 years old. She has been using marijuana. Jennifer is 14 years old and healthy. Kate and her mother have a very conflicted relationship. Jennifer and her father are very close. Kate often finds herself trying to "run interference" between her parents to shelter Jennifer from their parents' arguing.

Self-Assessment

Although nurse generalists do not provide family therapy, they do interact with patients and families. Most nurses come from families, and because no family is perfect, nurses may identify with certain family dynamics, which can trigger uncomfortable feelings. Nurses should be aware that their personal backgrounds, family of origin issues, and styles of interacting might affect their responses to patients and families.

As a nurse, you can even become triangulated into a patient's family system. You may notice that the patient is not speaking directly to his spouse but is speaking through you. A family member may attempt to bring you into a triangle by sharing negative information about the patient, particularly poor treatment by the patient toward this family member. Triangulation makes effective therapeutic intervention difficult. Having an anxiety level greater than the situation warrants is one indication that you are involved in triangulation. Direct communication on your part and encouraging the same in the patient and family members will help keep you out of unhelpful triangles.

NURSING DIAGNOSIS

Families often experience stress in times of anticipated developmental change, as well as in unanticipated change. Severe dysfunctional patterns such as marked relational conflict, sexual misconduct, abuse, violence, and suicide exist within many families. These patterns can lead to physical or mental symptoms, at times requiring professional intervention, among its members. Psychiatric-mental health registered nurses' understanding of family dynamics within a context of broader sociocultural and personal variables assists in the identification of diagnoses.

Numerous nursing diagnoses are useful when working with families. Box 35.3 provides a comprehensive list of nursing diagnoses relevant to families and family functioning.

BOX 35.3 Family-Related Nursing Diagnoses

- *Risk for caregiver role strain*
- *Caregiver role strain*
- *Risk for impaired parenting*
- *Readiness for enhanced parenting*
- *Risk for impaired attachment*
- *Dysfunctional family processes*
- *Interrupted family processes*
- *Readiness for enhanced family processes*
- *Parental role conflict*
- *Sexual dysfunction*
- *Impaired resilience*
- *Readiness for enhanced resilience*
- *Ineffective family health management*
- *Deficient knowledge*
- *Risk for disturbed personal identity*
- *Disturbed personal identity*
- *Risk for ineffective relationship*
- *Ineffective relationship*
- *Readiness for enhanced relationship*
- *Risk for chronic low self-esteem*
- *Chronic low self-esteem*
- *Ineffective role performance*
- *Impaired social interaction*
- *Compromised family coping*
- *Disabled family coping*
- *Readiness for enhanced family coping*

From Herdman, T. H., & Kamitsuru, S. (Eds.). (2014). *NANDA International nursing diagnoses: Definitions and classifications, 2015-2017.* Oxford, UK: Wiley-Blackwell.

OUTCOMES IDENTIFICATION

Involving the family in the care of patients is often an essential outcome for patients who will require significant support. Outcomes should be developed with the input of both patients and families whenever possible.

Nurses provide family psychoeducation to support patients and families in understanding and coping with diagnoses. Through education, nurses reinforce strengths, help to identify resources, and strengthen coping skills. Family teaching may include assisting members as they:

- Learn to accept the mental or physical illness of a family member.
- Learn to deal effectively with an ill member's symptoms, such as hallucinations, delusions, poor hygiene, physical limitations, and disfigurement.
- Develop an understanding of what medications can and cannot do and when the patient or family should seek advice from a professional.
- Learn what community resources are available and how to access them.
- Begin to feel less anxiety and regain or acquire a sense of control and balance in family life.

PLANNING

Nursing care for patients and their families usually occurs within the context of individual care planning. A planning priority is to address the safety needs of the family. For example, a member of the family may be at risk for acting in an aggressive or suicidal manner. A family member may be abusive or may be abused. If so, the nurse will need to determination whether to engage protective services for an abused family member or facilitate hospitalization to protect a suicidal or self-mutilating family member.

Nurses are adept at assisting family members to learn about the physical or mental illness of an afflicted family member; understand the effects, risks, and benefits of medications; and identify support groups and community resources. Planning and education are essential to help the family cope with crisis and improve the quality of life for all of its members. Identification of the extent of the family's knowledge deficit is equally important to organizing appropriate interventions.

INTERVENTION

Nurses prepared at the generalist level may provide counseling to family members utilizing a problem-solving approach. This approach addresses the immediate family conflict or crisis related to health or well-being. Developing and practicing effective listening skills and viewing family members in a nonjudgmental manner are critically important qualities for nurses of all educational and training levels, regardless of the practice setting.

An important function for nurse generalists is to respond to cues from various family members that indicate the degree and amount of stress the family system is experiencing. Some indicators of stress in a family system are the following:

- Inability of the family or a family member to understand and act on treatments
- Somatic complaints among family members
- High degree of anxiety
- Depression or anger
- Problems in the school or work setting
- Substance use

Promoting and monitoring a family's mental health can occur in virtually any setting. Sometimes an informal conversation can have the greatest effect. For example, the question "Do you think you will help your mother taking the medications she's been prescribed?" would likely put the family member on the defensive. An invitation such as, "Tell me your thoughts about the medication your mother has been prescribed" sets a collaborative tone between the nurse, patient, and family.

If extended family members are involved in the conversation, whether on the hospital unit or in a family session, the nurse should consider each member's view. How does the patient's medical regimen impact the way in which the family functions and what the individual members consider a possible solution?

Explain treatment plans in a clear and understandable manner using language common to all family members to help them make informed decisions. This is both a respectful and an empowering way to work with families indicating to them that *they* are the ones who are accountable and responsible for how they choose to use the information.

Elicit and listen to the perspective of each family member. It may seem surprising, but family members often hear the view of another member for the first time in this type of discussion. Personal perspectives may contribute to bewilderment or confusion among family members: "I didn't know you felt that way." The greater the family input, the more options exist for alternative ways of managing problematic situations.

Family Psychoeducation

Often, the most compelling family need is psychoeducation. This is particularly true for families who have a member with a severe mental illness. The primary goal of **family psychoeducation** is the sharing of mental healthcare information. Family education groups help family members better understand their member's illness, prodromal symptoms (symptoms that may appear before a diagnosis is reached or a relapse occurs), and medications needed to help reduce the symptoms.

Educational family meetings or multiple family meetings allow feelings to be shared and strategies for dealing with these feelings to be developed. Families can share painful issues of anger or loss, feelings of stigmatization or sadness, and feelings of helplessness. They can then put these feelings in a perspective that the family and individual members can deal with more satisfactorily.

An area in which family psychoeducation has been applied successfully is in treatment of the patient with schizophrenia. Families are extremely valuable and positive resources for patients, and family work promotes and supports families in coping with a member who has a severe psychiatric disorder. Psychoeducational groups also have proven helpful in parent management training such as teaching a parent to work with a child with a conduct disorder.

Advanced Practice Interventions

Psychiatric-mental health advanced practice registered nurses may conduct family therapy. Care providers have applied family therapy to virtually every type of disorder among children, adolescents, and adults (Abbott, 2012). Treating the whole family appears to be particularly helpful in the treatment of substance abuse disorders, child behavioral problems, marital relationship distress, and as an element of the treatment plan for schizophrenia (Deane et al., 2012).

Although therapists may adhere to different theories and use a wide variety of methods, the psychiatric advanced practice nurse will aim to (Nichols, 2013):

- Reduce dysfunctional behavior of individual family members
- Resolve or reduce intrafamily relationship conflicts
- Mobilize family resources and encourage adaptive family problem-solving behaviors
- Improve family communication skills
- Increase awareness and sensitivity to other family members' emotional needs and help family members meet their needs
- Strengthen the family's ability to cope with major life stressors and traumatic events including chronic physical or psychiatric illness
- Improve integration of the family system into the societal system (e.g., school, medical facilities, workplace, and especially the extended family)
- Promote appropriate individual psychosocial development of each member of the family

Family therapy may not be helpful in some circumstances. For example, when the therapeutic environment is not safe and there is a risk for harm by information, uncontrolled anxiety, or hostility, a shared therapy session should be avoided. If the therapist is fairly sure that family members are not being honest, it is likely that the work being done will not be productive. If parental conflict involves issues of sexuality that are not appropriate for the children, these issues should be discussed in couples' counseling.

In most other situations, however, family therapy is useful. Family therapy is often combined with psychopharmacology in the treatment of families who have a member with a psychiatric disorder such as bipolar disorder, major depressive disorder, or schizophrenia. Other families may choose psychoeducational family therapy and/or self-help groups, which are good options that may be less costly and time consuming. Advanced practice nurses are trained in the provision of these modalities of treatment.

EVALUATION

Both nurse generalists and psychiatric-mental health advanced practice registered nurses should evaluate the effectiveness of interventions. At the basic level, evaluation will address such issues as knowledge of therapeutic regimen, accessing outside support, and improved family coping. At the advanced level, evaluation focuses on the level of family members' individual and group functioning, whether conflicts are reduced or resolved, communication skills improved, coping methods strengthened, and whether family members have been better integrated into the broader societal system.

KEY POINTS TO REMEMBER

- Primary characteristics essential to healthy family functioning are flexibility and clear boundaries.
- The aim of family therapy is to decrease emotional reactivity, enhance awareness, strengthen communication among family members, and encourage personal differentiation.
- The genogram is an efficient clinical summary and format for providing information and defining relationships across at least three generations.
- Registered nurses with basic training can interact and counsel families in most settings. Triangulation with patients and patients' families can be a challenge. Using direct communication and encouraging direct communication within families best address this problem.
- Psychiatric-mental health advanced practice registered nurses who have specialized training may provide family therapy using a variety of theoretical approaches.

CRITICAL THINKING

1. Select a family with whom you have worked. Evaluate this family's status in terms of functionality with reference to the five family functions described in the text (i.e., management, boundary, communication, emotional-supportive, and socialization).
2. Create your own personal genogram including at least three generations. Be sure to include the following:
   a. Location, occupation, and educational level
   b. Critical events such as births, marriages, moves, job changes, separations, divorces, illnesses, and deaths
   c. Relationship patterns such as cutoffs, distancing, overinvolvement, and conflict
3. A family has just learned that their young son has a terminal illness. The parents have been fighting and blaming each other for ignoring the child's ongoing symptom of leg pain, which was diagnosed as advanced cancer. There are two other siblings in the family.
   a. How would you apply family concepts to help this family?
   b. What would be your outcome criterion?

CHAPTER REVIEW

Questions

1. A 24-year-old is leaving the family to start a new job in a city 400 miles away. Which statement made by the patient best demonstrates a healthy sense of family support?
   a. "I've always been independent. That's how I was raised."
   b. "If I get in trouble financially, I know Mom and Dad will help me out."
   c. "I don't need anyone's help. Everyone has their own problems to deal with."
   d. "I'm going to miss everyone terribly, but I know they will support me in this decision."
2. A nurse works with patients whose families are attending family therapy. The nurse should recommend psychoeducational family therapy for which family?
   a. A family whose members have problems establishing and respecting boundaries.
   b. A family whose teenaged children are routinely making major family decisions.
   c. A family whose 18-year-old son has been diagnosed with schizophrenia.
   d. A family who communicates primary using dysfunctional techniques.
3. A 10-year-old shares that he doesn't like spending weekends with his father "now that dad's girlfriend moved in." The nurse will discuss the issues with the child and parents based on an understanding of the stresses present in which type of family structure?
   a. Unmarried biological
   b. Cohabitating
   c. Blended
   d. Other
4. Which statement is an example of a parent demonstrating the dysfunctional communication technique of generalizing?
   a. "I want to be a good mother, but my husband just isn't involved with the kids."
   b. "I keep the peace by seldom asking any of the family to help with chores."
   c. "My wife's priorities are the kids, her parents, and then her job."
   d. "The kids never listen to me even when I threaten them."
5. Just before you escort the Juarez family in for a meeting, their 17-year-old son confides to you that he is gay. He says he has not told any other adult including his parents. What is your best response to him?
   a. "Your parents have a right to know about this."
   b. "How do you think your parents would react if you told them?"
   c. "That's your decision, but you need to be careful about risky sexual behavior."
   d. "Lots of famous people are gay. You don't need to worry."

6. When performing an intake assessment on a family, you wish to map the family's structure and information that reflect both the family's history and current functioning. This assessment tool is called a:
   a. Mini-mental status exam
   b. Beck depression inventory
   c. Genogram
   d. Histogram
7. While you are working with a family whose son was admitted due to a psychotic break, you observe the mother say to her son, "What, no hug for your Mom?" As the son embraces his mother, she stiffens, which results in the young man backing away. She responds, "You only care about yourself." What behavior is this mother engaging in?
   a. Triangulation
   b. Scapegoating
   c. Double binding
   d. Differentiation
8. Which of the following family members should you refer to individual therapy rather than family therapy?
   a. A mother who has anxiety controlled by medication.
   b. A father who is questioning his sexuality.
   c. A son who is verbally abusive toward his parents.
   d. A daughter who has been treated for alcohol use.
9. You are evaluating the family therapy experience. Which behavior would indicate that further family therapy is needed?
   a. Wife talks to husband through the children.
   b. Son's grades have risen from a "D" average to a "C" average.
   c. Daughter's headaches have subsided.
   d. Mother has stopped using illicit substances.
10. Emotional support is an important family dynamic because it allows family members to:
   a. Feel secure enough to explore aspects of their personality.
   b. Feel isolated and fearful even though family members are near.
   c. Grow without boundaries within the family unit.
   d. Have bursts of anger without recourse or shame.

Answers

1. **d**; 2. **c**; 3. **b**; 4. **d**; 5. **b**; 6. **c**; 7. **c**; 8. **b**; 9. **a**; 10. **a**

Visit the Evolve website for a posttest on the content in this chapter: http://evolve.elsevier.com/Varcarolis

Post-Test interactive review

REFERENCES

Abbott, D. A., Springer, P. R., & Hollist, C. S. (2012). Therapy with immigrant Muslim couples: Applying culturally appropriate interventions and strategies. *Journal of Couple and Relationship Therapy*, *11*(3), 254–266.

Beck, A. T. (2003). *Cognitive therapy across the lifespan: Evidence and practice*. Cambridge, UK: Cambridge Press.

Boszormenyi-Nagy, I. (1987). *Foundations of contextual therapy: Collected papers of Ivan Boszormenyi-Nagy*. New York: Brunner/Mazel.

Bowen, M. (1978). *Family therapy in clinical practice*. New York, NY: Jason Aronson.

Deane, F. R., Mercer, J., Talyarkhan, A., et al. (2012). Group cohesion and homework adherence in multi-family group therapy for schizophrenia. *Australian & New Zealand Journal of Family Therapy*, *33*(2), 128–141.

Duall, E. M. (1957). *Family development*. Oxford, UK: Lippincott.

Goldenberg, H., & Goldenberg, I. (2008). *Family therapy: An overview* (7th ed.). Belmont, CA: Thomson.

Keeney, H., & Keeney, B. (2012). What is systemic about systemic therapy? Therapy models muddle embodied systemic practice. *Journal of Systemic Therapies*, *31*(1), 22–37.

Kerr, M. E., & Bowen, M. (1988). *Family evaluation: An approach based on Bowen theory*. New York, NY: Norton.

Minuchin, S. (1974). *Families and family therapy*. Cambridge, MA: Harvard University Press.

Napier, A. Y., & Whitaker, C.A. (1988). *The Family Crucible*. New York, NY: Harper & Row.

Nichols, M. P. (2013). *Family therapy: concepts and methods* (10th ed.). New York, NY: Pearson.

Perreau, F. (2016). *The 4 factors influencing consumer behavior*. Retrieved from http://theconsumerfactor.com/en/4-factors-influencing-consumer-behavior/.

Satir, V. (1967). *Conjoint family therapy*. Palo Alto, CA: Science and Behavior Books.

Sutherland, A. (2014). *Family structure and children's health*. Retrieved from http://family-studies.org/family-structure-and-childrens-health/.

36

Integrative Care

Christina Fratena, Laura Cox Dzurec

Visit the Evolve website for a pretest on the content in this chapter:
http://evolve.elsevier.com/Varcarolis Pre-Test interactive review

OBJECTIVES

1. Define the terms integrative care and complementary and alternative medicine.
2. Identify trends in the use of nonconventional health treatments and practices.
3. Explore the category of alternative medical systems along the domains of integrative care: natural products, mind and body approaches, and other therapies.
4. Discuss the techniques used in major complementary therapies and potential applications to psychiatric-mental health nursing practice.
5. Discuss how to educate the public in the research and safety of integrative modalities.
6. Explore informational resources available through literature and online sources.

OUTLINE

KEY TERMS AND CONCEPTS

acupuncture
aromatherapy
Ayurvedic medicine
chiropractic medicine
complementary and alternative medicine (CAM)
expressive therapies
healing touch
herbal therapy
holism
homeopathy
integrative care
naturopathy
Reiki
therapeutic touch
traditional Chinese medicine

Complementary and alternative medicine (CAM) is the conventional term for medical practices and products that are outside of standard medical care. Standard medical care refers to generally accepted treatments provided by healthcare professionals. CAM includes complementary medicine, alternative medicine, and integrative medicine. The distinctions between the three approaches can be seen in the following statements:

- Complementary medicine uses non-mainstream medicine in conjunction with standard medical care.
- Alternative medicine uses non-mainstream medicine instead of standard medical care.
- Integrative medicine uses non-mainstream medicine in conjunction with standard medical care in a coordinated way.

For the purposes of a psychiatric-mental health nursing textbook, we will discuss these approaches while replacing the word medicine with the word care. Also, we will primarily refer to non-mainstream medicine as integrative care since this approach fits most closely with values in nursing. **Integrative care** places the patient at the center of care, focuses on prevention and wellness, and attends to the patient's holistic needs including the physical, mental, and spiritual (Fontaine, 2015). The emphasis is on the body's ability to heal itself given the right tools and knowledge.

INTEGRATIVE CARE IN THE UNITED STATES

Conventional healthcare is a system of care in which healthcare professionals such as nurses, doctors, pharmacists, and therapists treat symptoms and diseases with drugs, surgery, and radiation. Other terms for mainstream medicine include allopathic medicine, biomedicine, conventional medicine, orthodox medicine, and Western medicine. Conventional healthcare has only been used for around 200 years, whereas CAM has been practiced worldwide for thousands of years (Fontaine, 2015). In the United States, up to 40% of patients use nontraditional approaches to healthcare (Williams et al., 2015). The increased use may be due to a greater availability of CAM-prepared practitioners and practice facilities along with more public exposure to CAM through the media.

One of the essential differences between conventional and integrative healthcare is that conventional medicine focuses on what is done *to* the patient. Integrative practices are patient-centered meaning that the patient participates *with* the provider to heal the body and mind. While Western medicine defines health as the absence of disease, integrative health views health by how well the physical, emotional, mental, environmental, spiritual, and social components interrelate (Fontaine, 2015).

In 1998 the National Institutes of Health (NIH) established the National Center for Complementary and Alternative Medicine. In 2014 this center was renamed the National Center for Complementary and Integrative Health (NCCIH), making it one of 27 institutes and centers of the NIH. The objectives of the NCCIH (2016) are to:

1. Advance fundamental science and methods development
   - Basic biological mechanisms of action of natural products, including prebiotics and probiotics
   - Mechanisms through which mind and body approaches affect health, resiliency, and well-being.
   - New and improved research methods and tools for conducting research studies of these health approaches.
2. Improve care for hard to manage symptoms
   - Developed and improve strategies for managing symptoms such as pain, anxiety, and depression.
   - Conduct studies in "real world" settings to test safety and efficacy of these health approaches.
3. Foster health promotion and disease prevention
   - Investigate mechanisms of action for approaches and practices that improve health and prevent disease across the lifespan.
   - Study safety and efficacy in nonclinical settings such as community and employer-based wellness programs.
4. Enhance the complementary and integrative care workforce
   - Support opportunities to increase the number and qualities of researchers to conduct rigorous, cutting-edge research.
   - Foster interdisciplinary collaborations and partnerships.
5. Disseminate objective, evidence-based information

Trends in use of integrative therapies from 2002 to 2012 were identified in the most recent report from the National Center for Health Statistics (NCHS). This report included nearly 89,000 people with data comparisons from the 2002, 2007, and 2012 *National Health Interview Survey* (Clarke et al., 2015). The use of yoga, tai chi, qigong, homeopathy, acupuncture, and naturopathic approaches increased across all three time points. Fig. 36.1 compares the most common CAM therapies used by adults in the United States.

Consumers and Integrative Care

Consumers are attracted to integrative care for a variety of reasons, including the following:

- A desire to actively participate in their healthcare and engage in holistic practices that can promote health and healing
- A desire to find therapeutic approaches that seem to carry lower risks than traditionally used medications
- Positive experiences with holistic integrative CAM practitioners, whose approach to patients is supportive and inclusive
- Dissatisfaction with the practice style of conventional medicine (e.g., rushed office visits, short hospital stays)

Other reasons individuals might try integrative approaches are listed in Box 36.1.

Integrative Nursing Care

The American Nurses Association (ANA) recognizes holistic nursing as an official specialty within the nursing profession. Along with the American Holistic Nurses Association (AHNA), the ANA publishes guidelines for this specialty in *Holistic Nursing: Scope and Standards of Practice* (ANA & AHNA, 2012). According to the AHNA, holistic nursing is "all nursing that has healing the whole person as its goal" (AHNA, 1998). More specifically, **holism** involves:

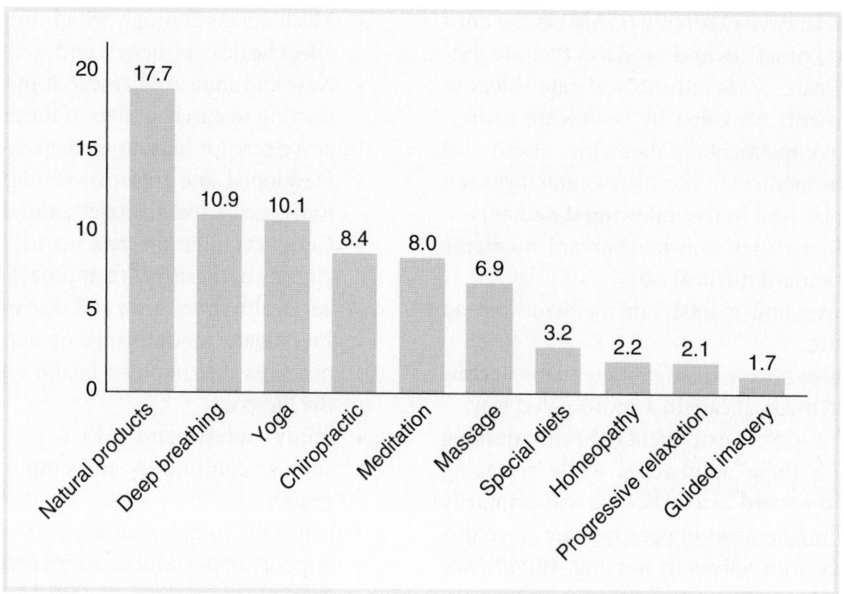

FIG. 36.1 Ten most common CAM therapies used by adults in the United States. From Clarke, T. C., Black, L. I., Stussman, B. J., Barnes, P. M., & Nahin, R. L. (2015). *Trends in the use of complementary health approaches among adults: United States, 2002–2012.* Retrieved from http://www.cdc.gov/nchs/data/nhsr/nhsr079.pdf

BOX 36.1 Factors Influencing Use of CAM

- One or more neuropsychiatric symptoms
- Recommendation by their provider
- Ineffective conventional treatment
- Financial cost of conventional treatment
- Nonsymptomatic, general wellness, and prevention usage
- Recommendation by friends and family
- Use for improvement of energy and immune function

Data from Purohit, M. P., Zafonte, R. D., Sherman, L. M., et al. (2015). Neuropsychiatric symptoms and expenditure on complementary and alternative medicine. *Journal of Clinical Psychiatry, 76*(7), 870–876.

1. The identification of the interrelationships of the bio-psycho-social-spiritual dimensions of the person, recognizing that the whole is greater than the sum of its parts.
2. An understanding of the individual as a unitary whole in a mutual process with the environment.

The traditional psychiatric nursing assessment includes presenting problem, past psychiatric history, substance use, medical illnesses/surgeries, family psychiatric history, and social history. A holistic approach to assessment involves using open-ended questions to identify the patients' view of their experience and concerns. Additional questions concerning nutrition, exercise, relationships, work, cultural and religious/spiritual concerns, and use of herbal supplements should also be part of the assessment. Without prompting, patients are not as likely to disclose to healthcare providers what herbal remedies or supplements they are taking.

Nurses in any setting should have a basic knowledge of treatments used in integrative care. Nursing programs often include basic integrative modalities such as relaxation techniques and guided imagery. Some schools may include energy-based approaches such as therapeutic touch. Inclusion of CAM information in nursing education is important because you will care for patients who use a variety of unconventional modalities. Activities such as assessment and patient education require a basic understanding of integrative approaches.

Consumers typically rely on health information obtained from friends, the internet, and social media. Based on these sources, they may be suspicious about some aspects of conventional healthcare. In fact, up to 80% of those searching the internet are doing so for a health-related purpose (Scarton et al., 2013). Unfortunately, online sources may be inaccurate as often as 50% of the time. Helping consumers actively evaluate the quality of information available to them is an important nursing activity.

Credentials in Integrative Care

Graduate programs in the United States that prepare nurses with a specialty in holistic nursing are increasing. Numerous post-master's certificate programs exist for advanced practice registered nurses. Doctor of nursing practice (DNP) programs with an emphasis in integrative health are available.

The American Holistic Nurses Credentialing Corporation (AHNCC) offers two levels of certification for registered nurses. Both require 2000 hours or 1 year of full-time experience in holistic nursing within the past 5 years. They also require 48 hours of continuing nurse education in holistic care. The holistic nurse–board certified (HN-BC) certification is for diploma or associate degree–prepared nurses. The holistic baccalaureate nurse–board certified (HNB-BC) distinction is for baccalaureate-prepared nurses.

The AHNCC also offers two certificates for advanced practice nurses. In addition to meeting the hours of experience and continuing nurse education previously described for undergraduates, 500 hours of experience in the specialty is required. Registered nurses who have attained graduate status may sit for an examination leading to the credential of advanced holistic nurse–board certified (AHN-BC). The other credential is based on the attainment of an advanced practice nursing degree (e.g., nurse practitioner) and prescriptive authority. This credential is referred to as advanced practice holistic nurse–board certified (APHN-BC).

Credentials are also available for other specific approaches such as acupuncture, chiropractic medicine, naturopathy, and massage therapy. Regulation and licensing of CAM and healthcare providers varies from state to state. Efforts are under way to regulate integrative care through credentialing of integrative physicians and non-physician practitioners including nurses.

HEALTH POLICY

Should Insurance Companies Provide Coverage for Integrative Medicine Treatment?

Some insurers provide coverage for certain modalities, such as chiropractic medicine, nutritional care, massage, mind-body approaches, and acupuncture. The covered benefits are narrowly defined, however. For instance, acupuncture can be used in some plans only as an alternative to anesthesia. This also leaves a wide range of approaches uncovered. In addition, licensed CAM providers are reimbursed less for their services than are conventional providers.

In recent years, a bill was introduced in Vermont that would require insurance companies to reimburse for complementary and alternative medicine (CAM). Proponents say enacting a law that requires third-party payers to provide coverage for CAM services would relieve a financial burden from consumers.

Opponents argue that involving insurance companies could increase restrictions on the CAM. Oversight by the government would require providers to meet strict criteria that currently are not in place. They argue that this would lead to suffering on both the part of the business and the consumer. The amount and type of services could be limited.

Those who use alternative approaches to treatment may not have wanted to pay for commercial insurance because the services they used were not covered. Now that the Affordable Care Act requires every individual to have healthcare insurance, it may make sense for all services, including CAM, to be properly covered.

CLASSIFICATION OF INTEGRATIVE CARE

Integrative care is classified into three domains: (1) natural products, (2) mind and body approaches, and (3) other CAM therapies (NCCIH, 2015).

Natural Products

Natural products include herbal medicine (botanicals) and also vitamins, minerals, and probiotics. With the proliferation of literature on herbal remedies and the accessibility of the products, increasing numbers of consumers are using these products to manage symptoms. A growing number of people in the United States are using herbal therapy for preventive and therapeutic purposes.

The American Association of Poison Control showed that most major classes of pharmaceutical medications have significantly more adverse effects and fatalities than vitamins, dietary supplements, herbs, and homeopathic remedies (Mowry et al., 2015). In 2014 the number one cause of poisoning was pharmaceutical in 1105 (78.5%) of the 1408 fatalities.

Unfortunately, a major drawback to dietary supplements and herbs is that the current regulatory climate is not effective in managing these products. In a recent study, researchers used a test called DNA barcoding that examined 44 bottles of popular supplements sold by 12 different companies. They report that one-third of the samples were contaminated or substituted with plants and fillers that were not listed on the labels (Newmaster et al., 2013). Fig. 36.2 summarizes the findings. Contamination and fillers dilute the effectiveness of otherwise helpful remedies. Using DNA barcoding for authenticating herbal products could improve safety and improve public confidence.

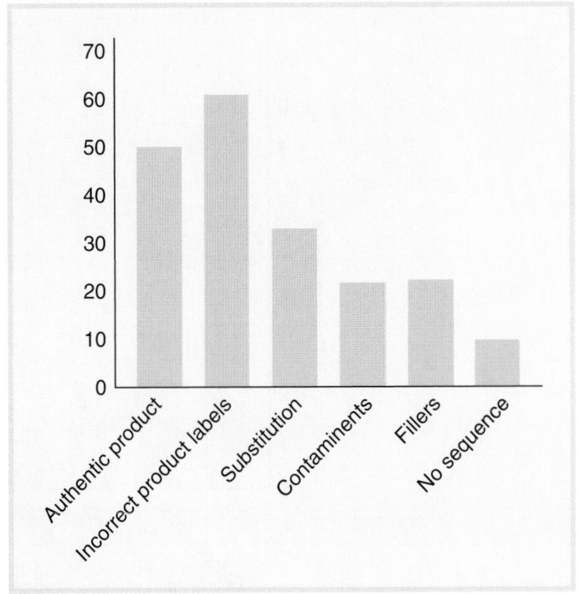

FIG. 36.2 DNA barcode results from 44 herbal products. From Newmaster, S. G., Grguric, M., Shanmughanandhan, D., Ramalingam, S., & Ragupathy, S. (2013). DNA barcoding detects contamination and substitution in North American herbal products. *BMC Medicine, 11*(22:222). Retrieved from https://bmcmedicine.biomedcentral.com/articles/10.1186/1741-7015-11-222.

Some herbs can have negative effects in certain individuals and interactions with other prescription medications. For example, ginseng has anticoagulant effects. Drinking ginseng tea may increase the effects of prescription anticoagulants, and the consequences could seriously affect blood clotting. Although relatively rare, Kava used for anxiety or insomnia can be hepatotoxic. St. John's wort, which is used for depression, can result in serotonin syndrome when combined with pro-serotonergic medications such as antidepressants, triptans, and methadone. It can also induce the metabolism of other medications such as oral contraceptives and some human immunodeficiency virus (HIV), medications.

We use caution with the term "natural" when discussing these products. This term may indicate that the chemicals in these medications are present in nature. The notion of naturalness suggests that alternative medications are harmless. However, just because something is called natural, it may not be safe to use in or on the body.

While there is a wide range of natural products used by consumers, fish oil is the number one product used (Black et al., 2015). Fig. 36.3 outlines the top 10 most commonly used natural products. Table 36.1 identifies commonly used herbal and dietary supplements in psychiatric symptoms and disorders.

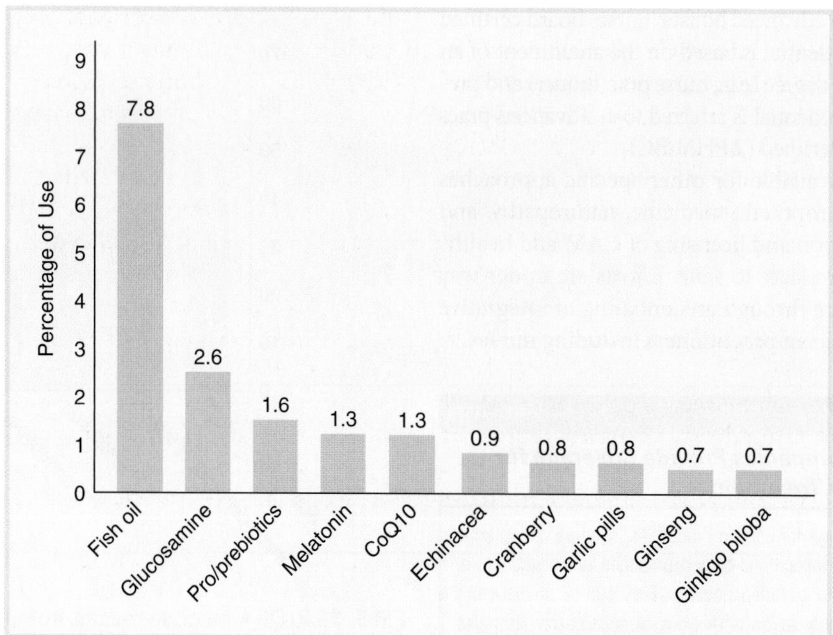

FIG. 36.3 Ten most common natural products used by adults in the United States: 2012. From Clarke, T. C., Black, L. I., Stussman, B. J., Barnes, P. M., & Nahin, R. L. (2015). *Trends in the use of complementary health approaches among adults: United States, 2002–2012.* Retrieved from http://www.cdc.gov/nchs/data/nhsr/nhsr079.pdf

TABLE 36.1 Herbal/Dietary Supplements Used with Psychiatric Symptoms and Disorders

Herbal Supplement	Uses	Cautions
St. John's wort	Depression	• Interaction with other medications • Photosensitivity • Increased risk of serotonin syndrome when combined with pro-serotonergic medications such as antidepressants, triptans, and methadone
Kava (Kava kava)	Insomnia Fatigue Anxiety	• FDA warned against use due to the link to severe liver damage
Golden Root (Rhodiola)	Anxiety Fatigue Depression	• Dizziness, dry mouth, and headaches may occur • Allergic reactions can occur
Valerian Root	Insomnia Anxiety Depression	• Generally considered safe for short time periods • Mild side effects could include morning fatigue, headaches, dizziness, upset stomach
Chamomile	Sleeplessness Anxiety	• Allergic reactions can occur, particularly in those allergic to the daisy family of plants
Lavender	Anxiety Restlessness Insomnia Depression	• Topical use generally considered safe if diluted properly, although breast growth in young boys has been reported • Oil taken by mouth may be poisonous • Teas and extracts may cause side effects including gastrointestinal complaints and headache • Use with medications with sedative properties may cause drowsiness to increase
Melatonin	Insomnia Jet lag Night shift	• May worsen mood in dementia • Side effects uncommon, but possibly drowsiness, dizziness, headache, nausea • Long-term use may affect the body's ability to produce melatonin on its own
SAMe	Depression	• May interact with certain medications • Increased risk of serotonin syndrome when combined with pro-serotonergic medications such as antidepressants, triptans, and methadone • Side effects are uncommon
Fish Oil (Omega-3 Fatty Acids)	Depression Bipolar disorder	• Possible GI effects, like belching, indigestion • Caution with those having fish/shellfish allergies • May increase bleeding time

Source: National Center for Complementary and Integrative Health (NCCIH). Retrieved from https://nccih.nih.gov

Diet and Nutrition

Because psychiatric illness affects the whole person, it is not surprising that patients with psychiatric disorders frequently have nutritional disturbances. Often their diets are deficient in the proper nutrients or they may eat too much or too little. Obesity and diabetes coexist at a greater than average rate in people with psychiatric disorders. Nutritional states may also cause psychiatric disturbances. Anemia, a common deficiency disease, is often accompanied by depression.

The influence of diet and nutrition on general health and mental health has been the subject of much research. The International Society for Nutritional Psychiatry Research (ISNPR, 2013) was established to study nutritional approaches to the prevention and treatment of psychiatric disorders. Topics on their website include:

- The role of vitamin C, vitamin E, and omega-3 fish oil in schizophrenia
- Fermented foods, microbiota, and mental health
- Dietary patterns and suicide in Japanese adults
- Association of diet in women with depression and anxiety

The traditional Western diet tends to consist of highly processed food with little nutritional value. A landmark longitudinal study demonstrated an association between a diet high in saturated fats, refined carbohydrates, and sugar and decreased left hippocampal volume (Jacka et al., 2015). Lower hippocampal volume has been associated with depression.

Another significant study looked at depressive symptoms in relation to diet and followed participants over 10 years (Le Port et al., 2012). This study indicated the following:

- Higher depressive symptoms in men occurred in those who ate a standard Western diet, increased snacking, and ate a large amount of food that was high in fat and sweets.
- Higher probability of depression in women is associated with greater amounts of snacking and larger consumption of foods low in fat.
- Reduced risk of depression was found in those eating regular meals that consisted of more fish, fruit, raw or cooked vegetables, and omega-3 fatty acids.
- Stress may increase unhealthy nutrition and cravings associated with emotional eating.

Megavitamin therapy, also called *orthomolecular therapy*, is a nutritional therapy that involves taking large amounts of vitamins, minerals, and amino acids. The theory is that the inability to absorb nutrients from a proper diet alone may lead to the development of illnesses. This type of therapy should be undertaken with caution because there is the potential for side effects.

Vitamin D. The Vitamin D Council (2012) lists many conditions caused by insufficiency or deficiency in this substance including osteoporosis, cancer, asthma, high blood pressure, diabetes, and autoimmune diseases. The Endocrine Society recommends using the 25(OH)D test to screen for vitamin D levels for at-risk populations, as well as targeting a blood level of, at minimum, 30 ng/ml (Holick et al., 2011).

A randomized-control study found that vitamin D supplementation improved scores on the Beck Depression Inventory (Sepehrmanesh et al., 2015). Another meta-analysis highlighted the risk of vitamin D deficiency even for individuals in sunny climates. They concluded that vitamin D supplementation reduced levels of depression (Spedding, 2014).

Vitamin D is not without side effects. When we convert ultraviolet light to vitamin D in the body, there is no danger of an overdose. Few foods naturally contain vitamin D, although some countries fortify foods with vitamin D. When vitamin D is taken orally as a supplement, people often take too much. Because vitamin D is fat-soluble, it may be stored in the body. Large amounts of this vitamin cause the liver to produce too much 25(OH)D. The 25(OH)D causes high levels of calcium in the blood (hypercalcemia). Symptoms of toxicity include:

- Malaise, fatigue
- Loss of appetite, increased thirst
- Frequent urination, constipation, diarrhea
- Abdominal pain, muscle weakness or pain, bone pain
- Confusion

Omega-3 fatty acids. Researchers continue to study the efficacy of omega-3 fatty acids in the treatment of depression and bipolar disorder. A recent meta-analysis indicated that supplementation of omega-3 was effective for depressed patients along with showing a positive effect for those with bipolar disorder (Grosso et al., 2014). Another systematic review suggested longer-term use (more than several weeks) of folic acid and B vitamins may decrease the onset and severity of depression (Almeida et al., 2015).

Microbiomes. Human beings have up to 100 trillion microbial cells, primarily in the gut. The impact of the human microbiomes and chronic inflammatory states are both becoming more recognized as impacting mental health, particularly depression and anxiety. Healing the gut and body with proper nutrition, probiotics, and fermented foods has shown promise in treating these conditions, as well as others (Selhub et al., 2014).

Mind and Body Approaches

Mind and body approaches are built on theories that focus on the continuous interaction between mind and body (Bartol, 2016). Most of these techniques emphasize the mind's capacity to affect bodily function and symptoms, but the reverse—the effects of bodily illness on mental health—is also part of the equation.

The significance of the mind-body relationship is well accepted in conventional medicine and probably is the domain most familiar to psychiatric-mental health nurses and nurses in general. Many of the mind-body interventions such as cognitive-behavioral therapy, relaxation techniques, guided imagery, and support groups are now considered mainstream and have been the subject of considerable research.

Meditation and Mindfulness

Meditation is an extremely popular method recommended to reduce physical and emotional stress and to promote wellness. It can be most simply accomplished by concentrating on slow deep breathing and focusing on calming thoughts or the breath. Specific types of meditation include Benson's relaxation techniques (refer to Chapter 10) and mindfulness meditation by

Kabat-Zinn, among others. Mindfulness-based interventions have been increasingly useful in conditions such as depression, anxiety, and chronic pain. A recent systematic review indicated that mindfulness interventions were evidenced-based treatments for these conditions, as well as in prevention of illness (Gotink et al., 2015).

Yoga

Yoga is another popular method to both physically strengthen and emotionally relax people. It typically combines a variety of physical postures, meditation, and breathing techniques. Yoga may help, in part, by increasing dopamine and gamma-aminobutyric acid (GABA) levels in the brain, as well as helping to stabilize the hypothalamic-pituitary-adrenal (HPA) axis, thereby decreasing depression (Cramer et al., 2013). In addition to depression, yoga is effective in the treatment of anxiety and pain (McCall et al., 2013).

Exercise

Many patients with psychiatric disorders have low energy and motivation, leading them to become sedentary. This, in turn, can increase symptoms including depression and anxiety. Exercise alters the levels of dopamine, serotonin, and norepinephrine and increases levels of brain-derived neurotrophic factor (BDNF). Exercise also increases cerebral blood flow; reduces oxidative stress levels; increases apoptosis in the brain, which can improve hippocampal function; and can turn on signaling pathways in the brain responsible for cognitive function and behavior (Hamilton & Rhodes, 2015). Extensive research with meta-analysis has been conducted on the positive benefits of exercise in a variety of mental health disorders including the following:

- Exercise was effective in treating substance use disorders including increasing the rate of abstinence, reducing withdrawal symptoms, and reducing symptoms of depression and anxiety (Wang et al., 2014).
- Exercise reduced weight gain and waist circumference, improved positive and negative symptoms, and reduced rates of neurodeterioration in individuals with schizophrenia (Firth et al., 2015).
- Physical exercise resulted in reduced symptoms of attention-deficit/hyperactivity disorder in children (Cerrillo-Urbina, et al., 2015).
- Exercise can cause a decrease in anxiety levels (Ensari et al., 2015).

Acupuncture

Acupuncture is becoming increasingly popular in the United States. A skilled therapist should perform it. Acupuncture involves placing needles into the skin at key points (meridians) to modulate the flow of qi. According to Taoists, qi is a life force that circulates throughout the universe and in our bodies in precise channels called *meridians.*

Sometimes the needles are inserted and removed immediately; sometimes they are twirled and even attached to stimulating electrodes. Another method is to leave them in place for a certain period of time. Following needle placement, patients describe feeling sensations such as rushing, warmth, tingling, or occasionally pain. Acupuncture acts by stimulating and altering patients' physical responses including those affecting cardiac, endocrine, neurological, and immune function. It is commonly used in the treatment of pain and in some blood disorders, as well as for substance withdrawal and certain emotional disturbances.

Guided Imagery

The use of **guided imagery** has been discussed in the nursing literature for decades. Imagery is used as a therapeutic tool for treating anxiety, pain, psychological trauma, and posttraumatic stress disorder (PTSD). Imagery may be combined with cognitive-behavioral therapy to help war veterans and people who have survived natural disasters. Imagery enhances coping before childbirth or surgery, augments treatment, and minimizes side effects of medications. It may help people cope with difficult times if they can imagine themselves as strong, coping, and eventually finding meaning in their experience.

Manipulative Practices

Manipulative, or body-based, practices relate to specific body systems and structures. These include joints and bones, circulation, and soft tissues. Two commonly used therapies—spinal manipulation and massage—fall within this category.

Spinal Manipulation

Spinal manipulation is accomplished through chiropractic medicine, one of the most widely used integrative therapies. The term *chiropractic* comes from the Greek words *cheir and praxix,* meaning "treatment by hand" and "practice," respectively. Chiropractic medicine focuses on the relationship between structure and function and the way that relationship affects the preservation and restoration of health, using manipulative therapy as a treatment tool.

Daniel David Palmer, a grocery store owner, developed the method in the late 1800s in an effort to heal others without drugs. Palmer developed a series of manipulative procedures to bring health to muscles, nerves, and organs that had gotten out of alignment. He referred to these misalignments as *subluxations.* He believed that subluxations were metaphysical and that they interfered with the flow through the body of "innate intelligence" (spirit or life energy).

Contemporary chiropractic medicine continues to be based on the theory that energy flows from the brain to all parts of the body through the spinal cord and spinal nerves. Manipulation of the spinal column, called *adjustment,* returns the vertebrae to their normal positions. Back pain is the most common reason people seek chiropractic treatment. Chiropractic manipulation treats a variety of other conditions including general pain, headaches, allergies, and asthma. Manipulation is also helpful in reducing migraine, tension, or cervicogenic headache pain. Many chiropractors also treat patients with depression, anxiety, and chronic pain. Chiropractic treatment may be done in conjunction with herbs and supplements.

A comprehensive systematic review on the use of chiropractic medicine in disease showed that chiropractic care could improve conditions such as shoulder and neck pain and sports injuries (Salehi et al., 2015). A randomized trial in those with neck pain found spinal manipulation to have greater efficacy than medication (Bronfort et al., 2012).

Massage Therapy

Massage therapy includes a broad group of medically valid therapies that involve rubbing or moving the skin. Massage therapists employ four basic techniques: effleurage (long gliding strokes over the skin), pétrissage (kneading of the muscles to increase circulation), vibration and percussion (a series of fine or brisk movements that stimulate circulation and relaxation), and friction (which is decreased with the use of massage oils). Probably the best-known massage technique in the United States is **Swedish massage**, which provides soothing relaxation and increases circulation. Japanese **Shiatsu massage** was strongly influenced by traditional Chinese medicine and developed from acupressure. It originated as a way to detect and treat problems in the flow of life energy (Japanese *ki*). The shiatsu practitioner uses fingers, thumbs, elbows, knees, or feet to apply pressure by massaging various parts of the body, known as *acupoints*.

Massage therapy has positive benefits in depression and stress. The most recent meta-analysis on this topic found depressive symptoms to be significantly lowered in those using massage therapy (Hou et al., 2010). Another review of the evidence by Deliginnidis and Freeman (2014) found that massage could be an effective tool in perinatal depression.

Other Complementary Therapies

Homeopathy and Naturopathy

Homeopathy is an example of Western alternative medicine. In homeopathy small doses (dilutions) of specially prepared plant extracts, herbs, minerals, and other materials are used to stimulate the body's defense mechanisms and healing processes. Infinitely small doses of diluted preparations that produce symptoms mimicking those of an illness are used to help the body heal itself. Homeopathy is based on the Law of Similars ("like cures like"), and dilutions are prescribed to match the patient's illness/symptom and personality profile. Healing occurs from the inside out, and symptoms disappear in the reverse order they appeared.

Homeopathic remedies are available over the counter. Consumers should have a full evaluation by a homeopathic practitioner before using any treatments. While use of homeopathic remedies may be increasing in the general population, its use in psychiatric conditions is more limited, and homeopathy for psychiatric conditions is mainly used in anxiety disorders (Grolleau et al., 2013).

Naturopathy emphasizes health restoration rather than disease treatment and a naturopathic physician may combine nutrition, homeopathy, herbal medicine, hydrotherapy, light therapy, therapeutic counseling, and other therapies. The underlying belief is that the individual is responsible for recovery.

EVIDENCE-BASED PRACTICE

Does Adding Body-Mind-Spirit Interventions Improve Depressive Symptoms?

Problem

Major depressive disorder is a severe, prevalent, and sometimes fatal illness, which can be difficult to treat and affects the whole person. Body-mind-spirit interventions may be useful adjuncts in the treatment of depression.

Purpose of Study

The purpose of this study was to identify if body-mind-spirit intervention is effective in improving the outcomes of patients with depression.

Methods

Researchers used a sample of 120 adults with depression in a psychiatric outpatient department in India and analyzed data over 6 months. Participants were assigned randomly to either the treatment-as-usual (TAU) group receiving standard treatment only (antidepressants with structured psychoeducation) or the body-mind-spirit (BMS) group receiving BMS intervention plus standard treatment.

Key Findings

- Significant reduction in depression was seen in the BMS group.
- Significant improvement was seen in well-being and quality of life in the BMS group.
- Reduced functional impairment was seen in the BMS group.

Implications for Nursing Practice

This study demonstrated that BMS may significantly improve symptoms of depression. It also highlighted the nurse's role as instrumental in educating and recommending the use of these interventions.

From Rentala, S., Fong, T. C. T., Nattala, P., et al. (2015). Effectiveness of body-mind-spirit intervention on well-being functional impairment, and quality of life among depressive patients—a randomized controlled trial. *Journal of Advanced Nursing, 71*(9), 2153–2163.

Aromatherapy

Aromatherapy, the use of essential oils for enhancing physical and mental well-being and healing, is a popular therapy in the mainstream market. Essential oils, often derived from herbs and plants, may be applied topically, inhaled, or diffused into the atmosphere through a diffuser. You can find many essential oils in a variety of skin-care products, as well as used in baths and compresses. The sense of smell connects with the part of the brain that controls the autonomic (involuntary) nervous system. Depending on the essential oil used, the resulting effects are calming, pain-reducing, stimulating, sedating, or euphoria-producing. Some nurses are trained in this art and have introduced various oils into hospitals, nursing homes, and hospice situations.

There are anecdotal reports that aromatherapy is useful for pain relief, memory improvement, and wound healing. Tang and Tse (2014) found the use of aromatherapy to improve depression, anxiety, and stress in older adults. The National Association for Holistic Aromatherapy (2016) provides guidelines for use and safety. They also list the most common essential oils used for mental health related concerns, which can be found in Table 36.2.

Safety guidelines for use of essential oils include becoming properly trained in their use, not taking oils by mouth,

TABLE 36.2 Essential Oils Used in Mental Health-Related Concerns

Essential Oil	Use
Roman chamomile	Relieving anxiety/stress
Clary sage	Relaxing, relieving anxiety/stress
Ginger	Emotionally and physically warming
Lavender	Calming, decreases anxiety
Mandarin	Calming
Neroli	Relieves and decreases anxiety; antidepressant
Patchouli	Antidepressant
Rose	Relieves and decreases anxiety/stress
Vetiver	Calming
Ylang ylang	Antidepressant

Source: National Association of Holistic Aromatherapy. (2016). *Most commonly used essential oils*. Retrieved from https://www.naha.org/explore-aromatherapy/about-aromatherapy/most-commonly-used-essential-oils/

not using near the eye, keeping oils away from flames, storing in a cool, dark area, keeping oils away from children (use under age 2 is not recommended), knowing which essential oils cause photosensitivity, and using caution with undiluted application and in pregnancy (Buckle, 2016). Some individuals, particularly those with pulmonary disease, may be sensitive or allergic to essential oils when they come into contact with the skin or are inhaled. Before massaging any essential oil into the skin, check for an allergic reaction by diluting the oil, administering a small amount, and performing a 24-hour skin patch test.

Expressive Therapies: Music and Art

Many psychiatric treatment programs including inpatient, partial hospitalization, intensive outpatient, and outpatient programs are incorporating the use of **expressive therapies**. Both music and art therapists are trained in higher education programs and are licensed or certified in their fields. The American Music Therapy Association and the American Art Therapy Association provide guidelines for the care of those with a variety of medical illnesses including mental illnesses. Their respective websites outline numerous research studies that have been conducted on the efficacy of these interventions. One meta-analysis showed music therapy to be one of the essential areas for the recovery process in those with mental illness (Solli et al., 2013).

Energy Therapies

Energy therapy is based on the belief that nonphysical bioenergy forces pervade the universe and people. Explanations vary as to the nature of this energy, the form of the therapies, and the rationale for how healing is believed to occur with its use. Some cultures believe the energy comes from God. Individuals who practice shamanic healing rituals believe the energy comes from various spirits through a priest or shaman. Therapeutic touch, healing touch, and Reiki are the most common energy therapies practiced by nurses.

Therapeutic Touch

Therapeutic touch is a modality developed in the 1970s by Dolores Krieger, a nursing professor at New York University, and Dora Kunz, a Canadian healer. The premise for therapeutic touch is that balancing the body's energies promotes healing. In preparation for a treatment session, practitioners focus completely on the person receiving the treatment without any other distraction. Practitioners then assess the energy field, clear and balance it through hand movements, and/or direct energy in a specific region of the body. The therapist never physically touches the patient. Ideally, after undergoing a session of therapeutic touch, patients report a sense of deep relaxation.

Practitioners of therapeutic touch believe that the therapy is useful for many conditions including pain relief, premenstrual syndrome, depression, complications in premature babies, and secondary infections associated with human immunodeficiency virus (HIV) infection. They believe that therapeutic touch can also lower blood pressure, decrease edema, ease abdominal cramps and nausea, resolve fevers, and accelerate the healing of fractures, wounds, and infections.

Healing Touch

Healing touch is a derivative of therapeutic touch developed by a registered nurse, Janet Mentgen, in the early 1980s. Healing touch combines several energy therapies and is based on the belief that the body is a complex energy system that can be influenced by another through that person's intention for healing and well-being. Healing touch is related to therapeutic touch in the belief that working with people to achieve their highest level of well-being, not necessarily to relieve a specific symptom, is the goal.

Healing touch involves gentle laying on of hands on a clothed body or moving over the body in the energy field. The practitioner may focus on a specific problem area or the full body.

CONSIDERING CULTURE

Amish Use of Natural Treatments

The Amish community relies heavily on what they describe as natural treatments. It is common to consult alternative providers, as well as lay providers/healers, for an array of medical concerns including psychiatric symptoms.

Typical treatments include natural supplements, special diets, chiropractic treatments, reflexology, iridology (diagnosis of illness by examination of the iris), and ridding the body of parasites.

Do these practices occur to reduce costs because most Amish do not have commercial insurance? Maybe in part. Yet members of the Amish community may spend a great deal of money on these treatments. For example, they may make a trip to Mexico to get chelation treatment or spend thousands of dollars on supplements.

The Amish often rely on word of mouth with regard to the treatments. If a close friend or relative quit taking their psychiatric medication in favor of natural pills and did well, an Amish woman with bipolar disorder might do the same. This can result in relapse. At that point, the family is likely to seek out a psychiatric healthcare provider.

From Hurst, C. E., & McConnell, D. L. (2010). *An Amish paradox: Diversity and change in the world's largest Amish community*. Baltimore, MD: Johns Hopkins University Press.

Reiki

The Japanese spiritual practice of Reiki has become an increasingly popular modality for nurses to learn and use. Reiki is an energy-based therapy in which the practitioner's energy is connected to a universal source (many interpret this as God or another sacred being) and is transferred to a recipient for physical or spiritual healing (Thrane & Cohen, 2015). Numerous hospitals, hospices, cancer support groups, and clinics are now offering Reiki in complementary programs. A review of randomized trials suggested Reiki was effective in treating pain and anxiety (Thrane & Cohen, 2015).

Bioelectromagnetic-Based Therapies and Bright-Light Therapy

Bioelectromagnetic-based therapies involve the unconventional use of electromagnetic fields such as pulsed fields, magnetic fields, or alternating-current or direct-current fields. Transcranial magnetic stimulation (TMS) and vagus nerve stimulation (VNS) treatments for depression are in this category and have US Food and Drug Administration approval.

Bright-light therapy has been shown as promising both in the treatment of seasonal affective disorder (SAD) and in non-seasonal depression. One study found bright light treatment to be more effective in non-seasonal major depressive disorder, both in monotherapy and in combination treatment with fluoxetine, than with the use of fluoxetine alone (Lam et al., 2015).

Prayer and Spirituality

Patients with psychiatric disorders often have significant spiritual needs. Some feel angry with God or another higher power for allowing them to suffer with disorders that affect every aspect of their lives. This anger can also be in relation to grief and loss. Some individuals harbor anger, for example, toward friends and family who may have rejected them or been judgmental. Other patients may wish to seek forgiveness because of hurt they have caused others. Many patients rely on a higher power as their source of strength and maintain a deep abiding faith despite the circumstances of their illnesses. Those dealing with substance use issues and attending a 12-step group are directed to identify a higher power.

Table 36.3 identifies CAM uses in psychiatric disorders.

TABLE 36.3 CAM Used for Psychiatric Disorders

Disorder	CAM Used (not all inclusive)
Anxiety	Exercise, yoga, mindfulness-based stress reduction, music, acupuncture, homeopathy, Reiki
Bipolar disorder	Exercise, mindfulness/meditation, yoga
Major depressive disorder	Exercise, nutrition, chiropractic, bright-light therapy, music, Reiki, religious/spiritual, healing touch, qigong, massage
Posttraumatic stress disorder	Guided imagery, yoga, acupuncture
Schizophrenia/psychosis	Exercise, yoga, acupuncture
Substance use disorder	Exercise, mindfulness/meditation, yoga, qigong

Sources: Lake, J. (2009) *Integrative mental health care. A therapist's handbook*. New York, NY: Norton; Wynn, G. H. (2015). Complementary and alternative medicine approaches in the treatment of PTSD. *Current Psychiatry Reports, 17*(8), 600.

Historical Notes Regarding CAM

Traditional Chinese medicine (TCM) provides the basic theoretical framework for many CAM therapies including acupuncture, acupressure, transcendental meditation, tai chi, and qigong. TCM comes from the Eastern tradition, specifically the philosophy of Taoism, and emphasizes the promotion of harmony (health) or to bring order out of chaos (illness).

The main concept in TCM is the movement of life energy or essence, *qi*, which maintains an individual's health and wellness. If this life energy is disrupted, it can seriously impact the mind, body, and spirit (Shields & Wilson, 2016). TCM is a vast medical system based on a constellation of concepts, theories, laws, and principles of energy movement within the body. Therapy addresses the patient's illness in relation to the complex interaction of mind, body, and spirit.

Adherents of TCM say that it addresses not only physiological and psychological symptoms but also cosmologic events that relate to the dynamics of the universe. These meridians become significant in the practice of acupuncture, touch therapy, and the more recent energy-based therapies used to treat emotional symptoms and promote mental health. Forms of movement such as qigong and tai chi may be used, as well as yoga. Viewed as a stressor itself, movement seems to mediate the effects of other stressors.

In TCM, health is the balance between *yin* and *yang*, and illness emanates from imbalances. The TCM practitioner uses the history and physical examination to understand the imbalances of mind, body, and spirit that have caused the patient's illness. Diagnosis involves both questioning and observing body structure, skin color, breath, body odors, nail condition, voice, gestures, mood, and pulse. Eastern goals, perspectives, and stages of healing are useful in treating mental illnesses, many of which are long term. The goals of healing in Eastern medicine include the following:

- Being in harmony with one's environment and with all of creation in mind, body, and spirit
- Reawakening the spirit to its possibilities
- Reconnecting with life's meaning

Ayuvedic Medicine

Ayurvedic (pronounced eye-yur-VEH-dik) medicine originated in India around 5000 BC and is one of the world's oldest medical systems. *Ayurveda* means "the science of life" and is a philosophy that emphasizes individual responsibility for health. Individuals are seen as consisting of the five elements of earth, water, fire, air, and space, which combine to regulate the mind, body, and spirit. Ayurveda views the body as *doshas* (vital energies), *dhatus* (tissues), and *malas* (waste products; Fontaine, 2015). Health is achieved when the doshas are in balance. Imbalance may be treated by nutrition, herbs, exercise, yoga, breathing, meditation, massage, aromatherapy, music, or purification with five procedures, called panchakarma.

KEY POINTS TO REMEMBER

- A philosophy of holism and promotion of therapeutic relationships are at the heart of psychiatric-mental health nursing and are important no matter what modality is used, conventional or integrative.
- Complementary, alternative, and integrative therapies are in demand as consumers seek a broader range of therapies than those offered by traditional medicine.
- Integrative care is classified as (1) natural products, (2) mind and body medicine, (3) other CAM therapies.
- With the availability of information online, consumers are more likely to research their symptoms or condition and identify potential CAM treatments.
- An increasing amount of evidence-based research is available on the efficacy of the majority of CAM treatments used.
- Nurses are ideally positioned to guide patients to reliable resources, such as the NCCIH, that provide up-to-date information for healthcare practitioners and consumers.
- Nurses' knowledge of current research about major CAM therapies will assist in purposeful promotion of holistic integrative care.

CRITICAL THINKING

1. As a nurse, you may have patients who use integrative therapies in conjunction with the conventional therapies prescribed by the healthcare provider. Identify issues that are important to assess and discuss how you would ask about the use of these nonconventional practices.
2. Discuss the role of exercise and nutrition in treating psychiatric illness. Given that many individuals are self-conscious about their weight, how would the nurse present this information to a patient in a nonjudgmental style?
3. How would a nurse educate a patient on the appropriate and safe use of aromatherapy?
4. By visiting their websites, determine how the NCCIH and other informational resources, such as the AHNA, provide information for the consumer and professionals.

CHAPTER REVIEW

Questions

1. Which statement made by the patient demonstrates an understanding of the foundational principle of integrative care?
   - **a.** "My body has the ability to heal itself if we have the knowledge to give it the right tools."
   - **b.** "The integrative care I'm getting is primarily a combination of complementary, alternative, and mainstream medicines."
   - **c.** "Much of the knowledge that integrative care is based on comes from Western cultural traditions."
   - **d.** "The most important focus of my integrative care is the cure of my cardiac illness."
2. When considering the goals of complementary and alternative medicines, which patient would be of particular interest to researchers studying advances in symptom management?
   - **a.** One who experiences chronic pain related to a neck injury
   - **b.** A patient diagnosed with an acute gastrointestinal infection
   - **c.** A pregnant woman diagnosed with gestational diabetes
   - **d.** A child requiring surgery for a clubbed foot
3. Which assessment question regarding a patient's report of pain demonstrates the nurse's attention to the principles of holistic nursing care?
   - **a.** "When did your pain begin?"
   - **b.** "Are you taking any herbal supplements for the pain?"
   - **c.** "Has anyone else in your family ever experienced this kind of pain?"
   - **d.** "How has the pain affected your daily ability to care for yourself?"
4. What medication education should the nurse provide to a patient who has expressed an interest in taking St. John's wort?
   - **a.** Allergic reactions to this herb are common.
   - **b.** Due to liver toxicity, regular liver function test should be conducted while taking it.
   - **c.** St. John's wort should not be taken in combination with antidepressants.
   - **d.** This medication results in gastrointestinal symptoms including bleeding.
5. Which factor is likely to attract a patient to complementary and alternative medicine? *Select all that apply.*
   - **a.** This nonmainstream approach is always less expensive than conventional medical treatment.
   - **b.** A desire to choose personal healthcare practices.
   - **c.** Using these approaches carries a lower risk than many pharmaceuticals.
   - **d.** Traditional medicine has been unsuccessful in providing effective treatment.
   - **e.** Integrative medication practices tend to produce desired results more quickly than conventional practices.
6. In contrast to most Western medicine, integrative care takes into consideration:
   - **a.** The physician's diagnosis and the patient's response
   - **b.** The nurse's ideas about healing in addition to the physician
   - **c.** A whole-person perspective: body, mind, and spirit
   - **d.** The diagnosis before beginning spirit work

7. A nursing student in her last semester has increasing test anxiety. Her professor suggests the student try some integrative therapies. The student reported successful test anxiety reduction with which of the following therapies?
   a. Aromatherapy and breathing exercises
   b. Megavitamin therapy and yoga
   c. Naturopathy
   d. Reiki
8. The nurse is caring for a patient who has a question about the safety of an herbal supplement. Which nursing response is best?
   a. "Herbal supplements are regulated by the FDA."
   b. "Natural ingredients in herbal supplements are harmless."
   c. "Your primary care provider needs to be aware of any supplements you take."
   d. "Marketing for herbal supplements demonstrates that all supplements are safe."
9. A patient asks the nurse if exercise and what she eats can impact her mood. The nurse's best response is which of the following?
   a. "There is no need to be concerned about exercise and nutrition if you take your antidepressant."
   b. "Limited studies are available on exercise and nutrition and mood."
   c. "Exercise is helpful, but you don't need to worry about nutrition."
   d. "Extensive research has shown that exercise and proper nutrition greatly improve mood symptoms."
10. Reviewing prescription medications in the discharge instructions for a patient with a diagnosis of major depression, the nurse would caution the patient about which over-the-counter supplement(s)? *Select all that apply.*
   a. Fish oil
   b. SAMe
   c. St. John's wort
   d. Melatonin

Answers

1. **a**; 2. **a**; 3. **b**; 4. **c**; 5. **b, c, d**; 6. **c**; 7. **a**; 8. **c**; 9. **d**; 10. **b, d**

Visit the Evolve website for a posttest on the content in this chapter: http://evolve.elsevier.com/Varcarolis

Post-Test interactive review

REFERENCES

Almeida, O. P., Ford, A. H., & Flicker, L. (2015). Systematic review and meta-analysis of randomized placebo-controlled trials of folate and vitamin B12 for depression. *International Psychogeriatrics, 27*(5), 727–737.

American Holistic Nurses Association. (1998). *Description of holistic nursing.* Flagstaff, AZ: AHNA.

American Nurses Association & American Holistic Nurses Association. (2012). *Holistic nursing: Scope and standards of practice.* Silver Spring, MD: Author.

Bartol, G. (2016). The psychophysiology of body-mind healing. In B. M. Dossey & L. Keegan (Eds.), *Holistic nursing: A handbook for practice* (7th ed.) (pp. 345–363). Burlington: MA: Jones & Bartlett.

Black, L. I., Clarke, T. C., Barnes, P. M., et al. (2015). *Use of complementary health approaches among children aged 4-17 years in the United States: National Health Interview Survey, 2007–2012.* Retrieved from http://www.cdc.gov/nchs/data/nhsr/nhsr078.pdf.

Bronfort, G., Evans, R., Anderson, A. V., et al. (2012). Spinal manipulation, medication, or home exercise with advice for acute and subacute neck pain. *Annals of Internal Medicine, 156,* 1–10.

Buckle, J. (2016). Aromatherapy. In B. M. Dossey & L. Keegan (Eds.), *Holistic nursing: A handbook for practice* (7th ed.) (pp. 345–363). Burlington, MA: Jones & Bartlett.

Cerrillo-Urbina, A. J., Garcia-Hermoso, A., Sanchez-Lopez, M., et al. (2015). The effects of physical exercise in children with attention deficit hyperactivity disorder: A systematic review and meta-analysis of randomized control trials. *Child: Care Health and Development, 41*(6), 779–788.

Clarke, T. C., Black, L. I., Stussman, B. J., et al. (2015). *Trends in the use of complementary health approaches among adults: United States, 2002-2012.* Retrieved from http://www.cdc.gov/nchs/data/nhsr/nhsr079.pdf.

Cramer, H., Lauche, R., Langhorst, J., & Dobos, G. (2013). Yoga for depression: A systematic review and meta-analysis. *Depression and Anxiety, 30*(11), 1068–1083.

Deligiannidis, K. M., & Freeman, M. P. (2014). Complementary and alternative medicine therapies for perinatal depression. *Best Practice & Research Clinical Obstetrics & Gynaecology, 28*(1), 85–95.

Ensari, I., Greenlee, T. A., Motl., R. W., & Petruzzello, S. J. (2015). Meta-analysis of acute exercise effects on state anxiety: An update of randomized controlled trials over the past 25 years. *Depression and Anxiety, 32*(8), 624–634.

Firth, J., Cotter, J., Elliott, R., et al. (2015). A systematic review and meta-analysis of exercise interventions in schizophrenia patients. *Psychological Medicine, 45*(7), 1343–1361.

Fontaine, K. (2015). *Complementary and alternative therapies for nursing practice* (4th ed.). Upper Saddle River, NJ: Pearson.

Gotink, R. A., Chu, P., Busschbach, J. J. V., et al. (2015). Standardised mindfulness-based interventions in healthcare: An overview of systematic reviews and meta-analysis of RCTs. *PLoS ONE, 10*(4), 1–17.

Grolleau, A., Begaud, B., & Verdoux, H. (2013). Characteristics associated with the use of homeopathic drugs for psychiatric symptoms in the general population. *European Psychiatry, 28*(2), 110–116.

Grosso, G., Pajak, A., Marventano, S., et al. (2014). Role of omega-3 fatty acids in the treatment of depressive disorders: A comprehensive meta-analysis of randomized clinical trials. *PLoS One, 9*(5), 1–18.

Hamilton, G. F., & Rhodes, J. S. (2015). Exercise regulation of cognitive function and neuroplasticity in the healthy and diseased brain. *Progress in Molecular Biology and Translational Science, 135,* 381–406.

Holick, M. F., Binkley, N. C., Bischoff-Ferrari, H. A., et al. (2011). Evaluation, treatment, and prevention of vitamin D deficiency: An Endocrine Society clinical practice guideline. *Journal of Clinical Endocrinology Metabolism, 96*(7), 1911–1930.

Hou, W. H., Chiang, P. T., Hsu, T. Y., et al. (2010). Treatment effects of massage therapy in depressed people: A meta-analysis. *Journal of Clinical Psychiatry, 71*(7), 894–901.

International Society for Nutritional Psychiatry Research. (2013). *About us*. Retrieved from http://www.isnpr.org.

Jacka, F. N., Cherbuin, N., Anstey, K. J., et al. (2015). Western diet is associated with a smaller hippocampus: A longitudinal investigation. *BMC Medicine, 13*(1), 1–8.

Lam, R. W., Levitt, A. J., Levitan, R. D., et al. (2015). Efficacy of bright light treatment, fluoxetine, and the combination in patients with nonseasonal major depressive disorder. *JAMA Psychiatry, 73*(1), 56–63.

Le Port, A., Gueguen, A., Kesse-Guyot, E., et al. (2012). Association between dietary patterns and depressive symptoms over time: A 10-year follow-up study of The GAZEL cohort. *PLoS One, 7*(12), 1–8.

McCall, M. C., Ward, A., Roberts, N. W., & Heneghan, C. (2013). Overview of systematic reviews: Yoga as a therapeutic intervention for adults with acute and chronic health conditions. *Evidenced-Based Complementary and Alternative Medicine, 2013*, 1–18.

Mowry, J. B., Spyker, D. A., Brooks, D. E., et al. (2015). 2014 annual report of the American Association of Poison Control Centers' National Poison Data System (NPDS): 32nd Annual Report. *Clinical Toxicology, 53*(10), 962–1147.

National Association for Holistic Aromatherapy. (2016). *Most commonly used essential oils*. Retrieved from https://www.naha.org/explore-aromatherapy/about-aromatherapy/most-commonly-used-essential-oils/.

National Center for Complementary and Integrative Health. (2015). *Three long-range goals*. Retrieved from https://nccih.nih.gov/about/research/goals.

National Center for Complementary and Integrative Health. (2016). *NCCIH 2016 strategic plan*. Retrieved from https://nccih.nih.gov/about/strategic-plans/2016.

Newmaster, S. G., Grguric, M., Shanmughanandhan, D., et al. (2013). DNA barcoding detects contamination and substitution in North American herbal products. *BMC Medicine, 11*(22).

Salehi, A., Hashemi, N., Imanieh, M. H., & Saber, M. (2015). Chiropractic: Is it efficient in treatment of diseases? Review of systematic reviews. *International Journal of Community Based Nurse Midwifery, 3*(4), 244–254.

Scarton, L. A., Fiol, G. D., & Treitler-Zeng, Q. (2013). Completeness, accuracy, and presentation of information on interactions between prescription drugs and alternative medicines: An internet review. *Studies in Health Technology and Informatics, 192*, 841–845.

Selhub, E. M., Logan, A. C., & Bested, A. C. (2014). Fermented foods, microbiota, and mental health: Ancient practice meets nutritional psychiatry. *Journal of Physiological Anthropology, 33*(1), 1–12.

Sepehrmanesh, Z., Kolahdooz, F., Abedi, F., et al. (2015). Vitamin D supplementation affects the Beck Depression Inventory, insulin resistance, and biomarkers of oxidative stress in patients with major depressive disorder: A randomized, controlled, clinical trial. *The Journal of Nutrition, 146*(2), 243–248.

Shields, D. A., & Wilson, D. R. (2016). Energy healing. In B. M. Dossey & L. Keegan (Eds.), *Holistic nursing: A handbook for practice* (7th ed.) (pp. 345–363). Burlington: MA: Jones & Bartlett.

Solli, H. P., Rolvsjord, R., & Borg, M. (2013). Toward understanding music therapy as a recovery-oriented practice within mental health care: A meta-synthesis of service users' experiences. *Journal of Music Therapy, 50*(4), 244–273.

Spedding, S. (2014). Vitamin D and depression: A systematic review and meta-analysis comparing studies with and without biological flaws. *Nutrients, 6*(4), 1501–1518.

Tang, S. K., & Tse, M. Y. M. (2014). Aromatherapy: Does it help to relieve pain, depression, anxiety, and stress in community-dwelling older people. *Biomedical Research International, 2014*, 1–12.

Thrane, S., & Cohen, S. M. (2015). Effect of Reiki on pain and anxiety in adults: An in-depth literature review of randomized trials with effect size calculations. *Pain Management Nurse, 15*(4), 897–908.

Vitamin D. Council. (2012). *Vitamin D and depression: A patient-friendly summary*. Retrieved from https://www.vitamindcouncil.org.

Wang, D., Wang, Y., Wang, Y., Rena, L., & Zhou, C. (2014). Impact of physical exercise on substance use disorders: A meta-analysis. *PLoS ONE, 9*(10), 1–15.

Williams, H., Simmons, L. A., & Tanabe, P. (2015). Mindfulness-based stress reduction in advanced nursing practice. *Journal of Holistic Nursing, 33*(3), 247–259.

NANDA-Approved Nursing Diagnoses 2015–2017

Indicates new diagnosis for 2015–2017—25 total
Indicates revised diagnosis for 2015–2017—14 total
(Retired Diagnoses at bottom of list—7 total)

1. Activity Intolerance
2. Activity Intolerance, Risk for
3. Activity Planning, Ineffective
4. Activity Planning, Risk for Ineffective
5. Adaptive Capacity, Decreased Intracranial
6. Airway Clearance, Ineffective
7. Allergy Response, Risk for
8. Anxiety
9. Aspiration, Risk for
10. Attachment, Risk for Impaired
11. Autonomic Dysreflexia
12. Autonomic Dysreflexia, Risk for
13. Behavior, Disorganized Infant
14. Behavior, Readiness for Enhanced Organized Infant
15. Behavior, Risk for Disorganized Infant
16. Bleeding, Risk for
17. Blood Glucose Level, Risk for Unstable
18. Body Image, Disturbed
19. Body Temperature, Risk for Imbalanced
20. Breastfeeding, Readiness for Enhanced
21. Breastfeeding, Ineffective
22. Breastfeeding, Interrupted
23. Breast Milk, Insufficient
24. Breathing Pattern, Ineffective
25. Cardiac Output, Decreased
26. Cardiac Output, Risk for Decreased
27. Cardiovascular Function, Risk for Impaired
28. Childbearing Process, Ineffective
29. Childbearing Process, Readiness for Enhanced
30. Childbearing Process, Risk for Ineffective
31. Comfort, Impaired
32. Comfort, Readiness for Enhanced
33. Communication, Readiness for Enhanced
34. Confusion, Acute
35. Confusion, Chronic
36. Confusion, Risk for Acute
37. Constipation
38. Constipation, Perceived
39. Constipation, Risk for
40. Constipation, Chronic Functional
41. Constipation, Risk for Chronic Functional
42. Contamination
43. Contamination, Risk for
44. Coping, Compromised Family
45. Coping, Defensive
46. Coping, Disabled Family
47. Coping, Ineffective
48. Coping, Ineffective Community
49. Coping, Readiness for Enhanced
50. Coping, Readiness for Enhanced Community
51. Coping, Readiness for Enhanced Family
52. Death Anxiety
53. Decision-Making, Readiness for Enhanced
54. Decisional Conflict
55. Denial, Ineffective
56. Dentition, Impaired
57. Development, Risk for Delayed
58. Diarrhea
59. Disuse Syndrome, Risk for
60. Diversional Activity, Deficient
61. Dry Eye, Risk for
62. Electrolyte Imbalance, Risk for
63. Elimination, Impaired Urinary
64. Elimination, Readiness for Enhanced Urinary
65. Emancipated Decision Making, Impaired
66. Emancipated Decision Making, Readiness for Enhanced
67. Emancipated Decision Making, Risk for Impaired
68. Emotional Control, Labile
69. Falls, Risk for
70. Family Processes, Dysfunctional
71. Family Processes, Interrupted
72. Family Processes, Readiness for Enhanced
73. Fatigue
74. Fear
75. Feeding Pattern, Ineffective Infant
76. Fluid Balance, Readiness for Enhanced
77. Fluid Volume, Deficient
78. Fluid Volume, Excess
79. Fluid Volume, Risk for Deficient
80. Fluid Volume, Risk for Imbalanced
81. Frail Elderly Syndrome
82. Frail Elderly Syndrome, Risk for
83. Gas Exchange, Impaired
84. Gastrointestinal Motility, Dysfunctional
85. Gastrointestinal Motility, Risk for Dysfunctional
86. Gastrointestinal Perfusion, Risk for Ineffective
87. Grieving
88. Grieving, Complicated
89. Grieving, Risk for Complicated
90. Growth, Risk for Disproportionate

91. Health, Deficient Community
92. Health Behavior, Risk-Prone
93. Health Maintenance, Ineffective
94. Health Management, Ineffective
95. Health Management, Readiness for Enhanced
96. Health Management, Ineffective Family
97. Home Maintenance, Impaired
98. Hope, Readiness for Enhanced
99. Hopelessness
100. Human Dignity, Risk for Compromised
101. Hyperthermia
102. Hypothermia
103. Hypothermia, Risk for
104. Hypothermia, Risk for Perioperative
105. Impulse Control, Ineffective
106. Incontinence, Functional Urinary
107. Incontinence, Overflow Urinary
108. Incontinence, Reflex Urinary
109. Incontinence, Risk for Urge Urinary
110. Incontinence, Stress Urinary
111. Incontinence, Urge Urinary
112. Incontinence, Bowel
113. Infection, Risk for
114. Injury, Risk for
115. Injury, Risk for Corneal
116. Injury, Risk for Perioperative-Positioning
117. Injury, Risk for Thermal
118. Injury, Risk for Urinary Tract
119. Insomnia
120. Jaundice, Neonatal
121. Jaundice, Risk for Neonatal
122. Knowledge, Deficient
123. Knowledge, Readiness for Enhanced
124. Latex Allergy Response
125. Latex Allergy Response, Risk for
126. Lifestyle, Sedentary
127. Liver Function, Risk for Impaired
128. Loneliness, Risk for
129. Maternal/Fetal Dyad, Risk for Disturbed
130. Memory, Impaired
131. Mobility, Impaired Bed
132. Mobility, Impaired Physical
133. Mobility, Impaired Wheelchair
134. Mood Regulation, Impaired
135. Moral Distress
136. Nausea
137. Noncompliance
138. Nutrition, Imbalanced: Less than Body Requirements
139. Nutrition, Readiness for Enhanced
140. Obesity
141. Oral Mucous Membrane, Impaired
142. Oral Mucous Membrane, Risk for Impaired
143. Other-Directed Violence, Risk for
144. Overweight
145. Overweight, Risk for
146. Pain, Acute
147. Pain, Chronic
148. Pain, Labor
149. Pain Syndrome, Chronic
150. Parenting, Impaired
151. Parenting, Readiness for Enhanced
152. Parenting, Risk for Impaired
153. Peripheral Neurovascular Dysfunction, Risk for
154. Personal Identity, Disturbed
155. Personal Identity, Risk for Disturbed
156. Poisoning, Risk for
157. Post-Trauma Syndrome
158. Post-Trauma Syndrome, Risk for
159. Power, Readiness for Enhanced
160. Powerlessness
161. Powerlessness, Risk for
162. Pressure Ulcer, Risk for
163. Protection, Ineffective
164. Rape-Trauma Syndrome
165. Reaction to Iodinated Contrast Media, Risk for
166. Relationship, Ineffective
167. Relationship, Risk for Ineffective
168. Relationship, Readiness for Enhanced
169. Religiosity, Impaired
170. Religiosity, Readiness for Enhanced
171. Religiosity, Risk for Impaired
172. Relocation Stress Syndrome
173. Relocation Stress Syndrome, Risk for
174. Renal Perfusion, Risk for Ineffective
175. Resilience, Impaired
176. Resilience, Readiness for Enhanced
177. Resilience, Risk for Impaired
178. Role Conflict, Parental
179. Role Performance, Ineffective
180. Role Strain, Caregiver
181. Role Strain, Risk for Caregiver
182. Self-Care, Readiness for Enhanced
183. Self-Care Deficit, Bathing
184. Self-Care Deficit, Dressing
185. Self-Care Deficit, Feeding
186. Self-Care Deficit, Toileting
187. Self-Concept, Readiness for Enhanced
188. Self-Directed Violence, Risk for
189. Self-Esteem, Chronic Low
190. Self-Esteem, Risk for Chronic Low
191. Self-Esteem, Situational Low
192. Self-Esteem, Risk for Situational Low
193. Self-Mutilation
194. Self-Mutilation, Risk for
195. Self-Neglect
196. Sexual Dysfunction
197. Sexuality Pattern, Ineffective
198. Shock, Risk for
199. Sitting, Impaired
200. Skin Integrity, Impaired
201. Skin Integrity, Risk for Impaired
202. Sleep, Readiness for Enhanced
203. Sleep Deprivation
204. Sleep Pattern, Disturbed

205. Social Interaction, Impaired
206. Social Isolation
207. Sorrow, Chronic
208. Spiritual Distress
209. Spiritual Distress, Risk for
210. Spiritual Well-Being, Readiness for Enhanced
211. Spontaneous Ventilation, Impaired
212. Standing, Impaired
213. Stress Overload
214. Sudden Infant Death Syndrome, Risk for
215. Suffocation, Risk for
216. Suicide, Risk for
217. Surgical Recovery, Delayed
218. Surgical Recovery, Risk for Delayed
219. Swallowing, Impaired
220. Thermoregulation, Ineffective
221. Tissue Integrity, Impaired
222. Tissue Integrity, Risk for Impaired
223. Tissue Perfusion, Ineffective Peripheral
224. Tissue Perfusion, Risk for Ineffective Peripheral
225. Tissue Perfusion, Risk for Decreased Cardiac
226. Tissue Perfusion, Risk for Ineffective Cerebral
227. Transfer Ability, Impaired
228. Trauma, Risk for
229. Vascular Trauma, Risk for
230. Unilateral Neglect
231. Urinary Retention
232. Ventilatory Weaning Response, Dysfunctional
233. Verbal Communication, Impaired
234. Walking, Impaired
235. Wandering

From: Herdman, T. H., & Kamitsuru, S. (Eds.). *Nursing diagnoses: Definitions & classifications 2015–2017* (10th ed.). John Wiley & Sons, Ltd. Retrieved from www.wiley.com/go/nursingdiagnoses

INDEX

A

Page numbers followed by *f* indicate figures, *t* indicate tables, and *b* indicate boxes.

D

E

F

J

K

L

O

Q

R

U

V

W

Y

Z